# THE RIVER

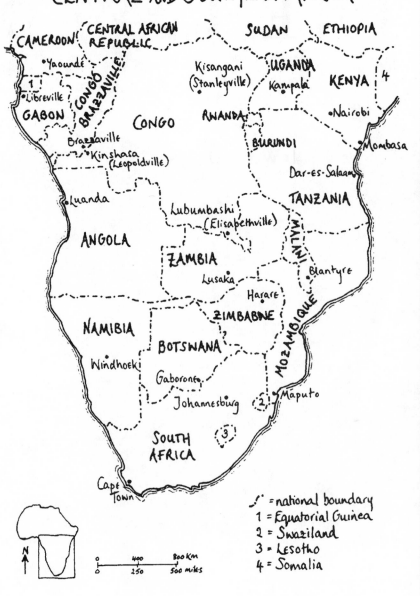

# CENTRAL AND SOUTHERN AFRICA

CAMEROON

CENTRAL AFRICAN REPUBLIC

SUDAN

ETHIOPIA

•Yaoundé

1

•Libreville

GABON

CONGO BRAZZAVILLE

CONGO

Kisangani
(Stanleyville)

Brazzaville•
•Kinshasa
(Leopoldville)

RWANDA

UGANDA

Kampala•

KENYA

4

•Nairobi

BURUNDI

•Mombasa

•Luanda

Lubumbashi
(Elisabethville)

Dar-es-Salaam

TANZANIA

ANGOLA

ZAMBIA

Lusaka•

MALAWI

•Blantyre

Harare•

ZIMBABWE

MOZAMBIQUE

NAMIBIA

BOTSWANA

Windhoek•

Gaborone•

Johannesburg•

2

•Maputo

3

SOUTH
AFRICA

Cape•
Town

N

0       400      800 Km
0     250    500 miles

╭ = national boundary
1 = Equatorial Guinea
2 = Swaziland
3 = Lesotho
4 = Somalia

# THE RIVER

A JOURNEY TO THE SOURCE OF HIV AND AIDS

## EDWARD HOOPER

LITTLE, BROWN AND COMPANY

BOSTON  NEW YORK  LONDON

FIRST EDITION

All maps and charts originally drawn by Sally Griffin
with the exception of those on pp. 744 and 745, by Nigel
Andrews; on p. 832, by Pat Griffin; and
on p. 843 by Brian Foley.

Library of Congress Cataloging-in-Publication Data

Hooper, Edward (Edward Jonathan)
The river: a journey to the source of HIV and AIDS/ by Edward
Hooper; with maps and charts by Sally Griffin.
p.   cm.
Includes bibliographical references and index.
ISBN 0-316-37261-7 (hc)
1. AIDS (Disease) — Epidemiology.   2. AIDS (Disease) — Etiology.
3. Poliomyelitis vaccine — Contamination.   4. Poliomyelitis —
Vaccination — Congo (Democratic Republic) — History.   I. Title.
RA644.A25H663      1999
614.5'99392 — dc21         98-41592

10   9   8   7   6   5   4   3   2   1

MV-NY
Book design by Julia Sedykh
Printed in the United States of America

TO ALL THOSE WHO HAVE BEEN AFFECTED
BY THE AIDS EPIDEMIC, EITHER DIRECTLY OR INDIRECTLY. MANY
HAVE BEEN INSPIRED BY THEIR DIGNITY AND COURAGE — AND
BY THEIR FREQUENTLY REMARKABLE RESPONSES TO ADVERSITY.

*A journey is a person in itself; no two are alike.*
*And all plans, safeguards, policies and coercion*
*are fruitless. We find after years of struggle that*
*we do not take a trip; a trip takes us.*

— JOHN STEINBECK

# Contents

## III

## IV

## V

*List of Maps and Charts*

*Cast of Characters*

ARDOUIN A., Jamaican émigré who died of PCP infection in Brooklyn in 1959.

PETER AABY, Danish physician and researcher into HIV-2 in Guinea-Bassau.

MARGARET AGERHOLM, Oxford-based virologist who wrote to the *BMJ* in 1958, questioning the safety of the CHAT vaccine trials in the Congo.

JAN ALBERT, virologist at the Swedish Institute for Infectious Disease Control.

JENNIFER ALEXANDER, head of microbiology at Witwatersrand University, Johannesburg, and proponent of OPV/AIDS theory.

STEVE ALEXANDER, scientist at Biotech Research Inc., Rockville, Maryland, who developed a version of the Western blot assay.

JONATHAN ALLAN, microbiologist and SIV expert working at the Southwest Foundation for Biomedical Research, San Antonio, Texas.

ARMAND ANDRÉ, former director of blood bank in Liege, Belgium, who tested the bloods of 175 Lindi chimps taken in the fifties.

L. J. ANDRÉ, former captain of the French colonial medical service based at the Institute Pasteur in Brazzaville; vaccinated population around Mitzic in Gabon with Lépine vaccine in 1957.

STEWART ASTON, former head of the virus and rickettsial vaccine production laboratory, Lederle Laboratories.

FRANÇOISE BARRÉ-SINOUSSI, virologist and AIDS specialist based at the Pasteur Institute, Paris.

GEORGES BARSKI, tissue culture expert from Pierre Lépine's virology department at the Pasteur Institute in the early fifties; visited Alexandre Jezierski in the Congo to collect blood samples for polio research.

CLAUDIO BASILICO, microbiologist from the New York University School of Medicine; co-chair of the expert committee convened by the Wistar Institute to examine the OPV/AIDS theory.

ANNE BAYLEY, British doctor and former chief surgeon at the University Teaching Hospital, Lusaka, Zambia.

WILFRID BERVOETS, inspector of hygiene for the Congo at the time of the CHAT trials.

GUNNEL BIBERFELD, virologist from the National Bacteriological Laboratory in Stockholm; specialist in HIV-2 research.

BOB BIGGAR, conducted AIDS research (including some controversial African epidemiological studies) under Robert Gallo in the eighties.

HOWARD BINNS, director of the research institute at Muguga, Kenya, at the time of Koprowski's visits in 1955 and 1957.

DAVID BODIAN, polio researcher from Johns Hopkins University who helped identify the three types of poliovirus; later, conducted poliovirus research in chimpanzees.

MARGERETE BÖTTIGER, Swedish virologist who assisted Sven Gard with polio vaccine research at the Karolinska Institute in the fifties and sixties.

JEAN BRAKEL, sanitary agent for the Laboratoire Médical de Stanleyville in the fifties, who assisted Gaston Ninane with the vaccinations in response to polio epidemics in Province Oriental.

PAUL BRUTSAERT, senior professor from the tropical institute, Antwerp, Belgium, who opened the virus symposium at Stanleyville in September 1957.

LOUIS BUGYAKI, Hungarian vet who worked in Stanleyville between 1956 and 1959 and who helped look after the Lindi chimps.

MARGERETE BUNDSCHUH, German missionary doctor who worked in Tanzania for over 30 years.

FRITZ BUSER, Swiss pediatrician who helped conduct trials of various polio vaccines, including Koprowski's, in Bern in the fifties.

VICTOR CABASSO, Lederle virologist who took over as Herald Cox's deputy after Koprowski left in 1957.

MICHELE CARBONE, Italian scientist who linked SV40 and asbestos exposure to the development of mesothelioma.

DAVID CARR, the "Manchester sailor" who died in 1959 from an AIDS-like illness characterized by PCP and CMV infections.

WILSON CARSWELL, Scottish surgeon who became a leading figure in the fight against AIDS in Uganda.

HUBERT CAUBERGH, sanitary agent who participated in, and documented, the CHAT vaccinations in Ruanda-Urundi between 1958 and 1960.

FRANCIS CHARLTON, Californian physician and father of a brain-damaged child (AAC) who was fed with a Koprowski polio vaccine in 1956 and whose excreted virus was used as the basis for CHAT vaccine.

STEVE CONNOR, science journalist who wrote exposé about the David Carr contamination for *The Independent* in 1995.

ANDRÉ COURTOIS, Belgian physician, son of Ghislain Courtois.

GHISLAIN COURTOIS, Belgian physician who headed the Laboratoire Médical de Stanleyville throughout the fifties and who established Lindi camp in collaboration with Koprowski. Distributed OPV to different parts of the Congo and Ruanda-Urundi, and later helped organize vaccination campaigns with Sabin's OPV in Belgium itself.

HERALD COX, head of viral and rickettsial research at Lederle Laboratories, American Cyanamid, between the forties and sixties.

JOHN CREWDSON, renowned *Chicago Tribune* journalist.

JULIAN CRIBB, Australian scientific journalist and author of *The White Death*, published in 1996, the first book to discuss the OPV/AIDS hypothesis in detail.

JAMES CURRAN, effective head of the CDC's AIDS program from 1981 (when it was known as the Task Force on Kaposi's Sarcoma and Opportunistic Infections) until 1995 (when it was known as the Division of HIV/AIDS); U.S. assistant surgeon-general, 1991–1995.

MICHAEL KENT CURTIS, Tom's brother; a professor of law from Wake Forest University who wrote a lengthy paper about the legal implications of the OPV/AIDS controversy and the suppression of dissent.

TOM CURTIS, American journalist and author of *Rolling Stone* article entitled "The Origin of AIDS."

DANIEL D., Belgian construction worker who worked in central Africa in the seventies, and who died of AIDS-like conditions in 1981.

ROBERT DAENENS, Belgian caretaker at Lindi camp in the late fifties.

DAVID DANE, British virologist who was George Dick's deputy at Queen's University, Belfast, in the fifties and sixties.

WILLIAM DARROW, sociologist and sole nonmedical scientist in the CDC Task Force on KSOI (later, Division of HIV/AIDS).

PAUL DE BRAUWERE, inspector-general of hygiene in Brussels at the time of the CHAT vaccinations in the Congo.

KEVIN DE COCK, Belgian-born physician, epidemiologist, and specialist in HIV-2 research.

EDWARD DE MAEYER, virologist who joined the Rega Institute, Leuven, in 1957.

JEAN DE MEDINA, headed the animal capture station at Epulu, eastern Congo; formerly Camp Putnam.

PIETER DE SOMER, head of virology at Leuven University and Rega Institute, Leuven, from the 1950s onward; cofounder of RIT (Recherche et Industrie Thérapeutif ).

FRIEDRICH ("FRITZ") DEINHARDT, worked under the Henles at the virology department of the Children's Hospital of Philadelphia (CHOP) in the fifties; conducted hepatitis studies at Lindi camp in 1958.

JEAN DEINHARDT, British virologist who joined the Wistar Institute in 1959 and who married Fritz Deinhardt soon afterward.

JEAN DELVILLE, Belgian virologist based at Elisabethville, Congo, in the fifties.

JAN DESMYTER, head of virology, Rega Institute and Univerity of Leuven, Belgium.

RONALD DESROSIERS, Harvard virologist based at the New England Primate Research Center, member of the Wistar's expert committee looking into the OPV/AIDS theory, and a leading proponent of live, attenuated vaccines against AIDS.

PAULETTE DHERTE, nurse and technical assistant at the Laboratoire Médical de Stanleyville and Lindi camp in the fifties.

GEORGE DICK, British virologist who staged trials of Koprowski's OPVs in Belfast, Northern Ireland, in 1956.

PIERRE DOUPAGNE, lab technician who worked at the Laboratoire Médical de Stanleyville in the fifties.

CHARLES DRICOT, chief physician of the Belgian Congo in 1957 when the CHAT field trials began.

PETER DUESBERG, molecular biologist and AIDS researcher who, for more than ten years, championed theory that HIV does not cause AIDS.

GAETAN DUGAS, Canadian air steward who became known as Patient Zero, in allusion to the theory that he was the source (or key disseminator) of HIV in North America.

RENATO DULBECCO, Italian virologist and Nobel Laureate who, in the fifties, developed the techniques of trypsinization and plaque purification.

BLAINE ELSWOOD, San Francisco AIDS activist and one of the developers of the theory that Koprowski's OPVs might have sparked the AIDS epidemic.

JOHN ENDERS, microbiologist who developed tissue culture technique for isolating and growing viruses.

MAX ESSEX, Harvard virologist and AIDS researcher.

MRS. SADAYO F., sixty-year-old Japanese-Canadian who died of AIDS-like infections in Montreal in 1945.

AGNES FLACK, medical director of Clinton Farms, the women's prison in New Jersey; helped with the Ruzizi field trial of CHAT in 1958.

ALAN FLEMING, hematologist and AIDS epidemiologist.

TOM FOLKS, head of retroviral research at the Centers for Disease Control.

DR. MICHEL FORRO, Hungarian doctor who worked for Vicicongo, the construction and haulage parastatal based at Aketi, Congo; officially oversaw the first mass trial of Koprowski's vaccines in 1957.

CECIL FOX, American histologist and tissue culture expert formerly with the National Institutes of Health.

JOHN FOX, virologist from Tulane University, New Orleans, who provided attenuated poliovirus isolates that were used as the basis for several polio vaccine strains, including Fox and P-712.

THOMAS FRANCIS, Jonas Salk's former teacher who helped organize the first IPV trials in the U.S.in 1954.

DR. STIG FRÖLAND, Norwegian physician and AIDS specialist.

PATRICIA FULTZ, American virologist based at Birmingham, Alabama, who reported on altered pathogenicity of SIVs after transfer into new hosts.

DICK G., twenty-eight-year-old engineer and former marine who died of AIDS-like illnesses in Memphis, Tennessee in 1952.

CARLETON GADJUSEK, Nobel Laureate for his work on the prion disease, kuru.

ROBERT GALLO, the first to isolate a human retrovirus, HTLV-I. He also isolated HIV (after Montagnier and Levy) but called it HTLV-III, thereby inaccurately implying that it was from the same family of retroviruses as HTLV-I and HTLV-II.

FENG GAO, virologist and PCR expert with Beatrice Hahn's team in Birmingham, Alabama.

SVEN GARD, Swedish virologist and developer of an improved IPV, used in Sweden since the 1950s.

JOHN GARRETT, virologist at the National Institute for Biologic Standards and Control, Potters Bar, U.K., who conducted experiments suggesting that there was little risk of oral polio vaccines becoming contaminated with SIVs.

LAURIE GARRETT, journalist and author of *The Coming Plague*.

ROBERT GARRY, microbiologist from Tulane University, New Orleans, who found HIV in blood and tissue samples from Robert R.

JAMES GEAR, senior virologist at the South African Institute for Medical Research; developer of South African oral polio vaccine in African green monkey tissues, and long-term associate of Hilary Koprowski.

HENRY GELFAND, virologist from Tulane University, New Orleans, who carried CHAT vaccine from Brussels to Leopoldville for the 1958 vaccination campaign in that city.

PAUL GIGASE, Belgian physician who worked at Katana Hospital, eastern Congo, in the fifties and who, in the eighties, carried out studies of KS and AIDS in the same region.

CHARLES GILKS, parasitologist who proposed theory that the AIDS epidemic originated from malaria research that involved injecting monkey and ape blood into humans.

SERGIO GIUNTA, Italian virologist who proposed that AIDS could have come about through the increased capture of African monkeys for scientific research.

TOM GORDON, associate director of Yerkes primate research center, Atlanta, Georgia.

MICHAEL GOTTLIEB, Los Angeles doctor who, in June 1981, coauthored the first report on AIDS to be published in the medical literature.

SIDNEY GOTTLIEB, CIA scientist who headed a team that developed and tested various experimental drugs and biological weapons in the fifties and sixties.

JAAP GOUDSMIT, Dutch retrovirologist and author of *Viral Sex*, which features a controversial account of the prehistory of AIDS.

VICTOR P. GRACHEV, helped with the mass polio vaccine campaign in the Soviet Union in the 1950s; later worked for the WHO.

SALLY GRIFFIN, research and editorial assistant to the author, 1996/7.

HERBERT H., German concert violinist and bisexual who died from what was almost certainly AIDS in 1979.

BEATRICE HAHN, German-born microbiologist based at Birmingham, Alabama.

BILL HAMILTON, Oxford-based evolutionary biologist and Royal Society research professor, is sometimes considered the originator of sociobiology; perhaps the most eminent supporter of the OPV/AIDS theory.

HERWIG HAMPERL, German microbiologist and specialist in *Pneumocystis carinii* research in the fifties.

JIMMY HARRIES, Kenyan-based physician who, in 1956, discussed possible vaccination schemes in Africa with Hilary Koprowski.

MASANORI HAYAMI, Japanese virologist and head of SIV/HIV research team at Kyoto University.

LEONARD HAYFLICK, biologist who took charge of tissue culture development at the Wistar Institute in 1958; developer of WI-38, a human diploid cell strain.

HÉLÈNE, Congolese woman who died from AIDS-like infections in Kinshasa in 1962.

WERNER AND GERTRUDE HENLE, husband and wife team who ran the virology department at the Children's Hospital of Philadelphia (CHOP) from 1939 until the nineties.

FERGAL HILL, Cambridge-based molecular biologist who collaborated with the author, testing archival tissue and serum samples for presence of HIV.

JOHN HILLABY, British author and scientific journalist who visited Lindi camp in 1957.

MAURICE ("MAX") HILLEMAN, American virologist, codiscoverer of SV40 and developer of Heptavax-B vaccine at Merck Sharpe and Dohme.

VANESSA HIRSCH, American virologist based at the National Institute of Allergy and Infectious Diseases, Bethesda, Maryland.

DAVID HO, director of the Aaron Diamond AIDS Research Center and member of the OPV/AIDS committee convened by the Wistar Institute.

Simon Wain-Hobson, British virologist based at the Pasteur Institute in Paris.

David Huminer, Israeli researcher who identified possible cases of pre-epidemic AIDS from the medical literature.

Klaus Hummeler, German virologist who worked at Children's Hospital of Philadelphia in the fifties and collaborated with Koprowski on polio and rabies research.

Andrew Hunt, visiting physician at Clinton Farms during the fifties, who helped oversee Koprowski vaccine trials at the prison.

Constant ("Stan") Huygelen took over from Pieter De Somer as director of RIT in the early sixties.

Drago Ikic, Zagreb-based virologist who collaborated with Koprowski in Croatian trials of polio vaccines made in monkey kidney and in WI-38.

Duncan Jeremiah, Manchester physician and vaccinator, who wrote to the *British Medical Journal* complaining about Koprowski's approach to vaccine trials.

George Jervis, director of laboratories at Letchworth Village, a center for mentally handicapped children in New York State; helped at the Ruzizi vaccine field trial in 1958.

Alexandre Jezierski, Polish émigré vet who worked in the Belgian Congo in the forties and fifties, and who developed his own sets of live and killed human polio vaccines at the Gabu-Nioka laboratory.

Philip Johnson, American virologist formerly based at the National Institute of Allergy and Infectious Diseases, Bethesda, Maryland.

Yvon K., Belgian man who did voluntary work in the Congo in the seventies, and who later died of AIDS.

Phyllis Kanki, Harvard virologist and colleague of Max Essex.

Moriz Kaposi, Hungarian dermatologist who practiced in Vienna in the nineteenth century; identified several new skin conditions, including the sarcoma named after him.

Anicet Kashamura, Congolese politician, sociologist, and writer; author of *Famille, sexualité et culture*.

Abraham Karpas, Cambridge-based virologist and author of the theory that the AIDS epidemic began with monkey-related sexual practices in central Africa; also proposed an amplification role for reusable needles in the advent of the epidemic.

Olen Kew, polio expert and director of molecular virology at the Division of Virological Diseases, CDC.

Leonhard Kopf, the first patient to be diagnosed with Kaposi's sarcoma, 1867.

Irena Koprowska, married Hilary Koprowski in Poland in 1938, and in 1997 wrote an autobiography entitled *A Woman Wanders through Life and Science*.

HILARY KOPROWSKI, virologist and developer of a set of oral polio vaccines; the first to feed oral polio vaccine to humans in 1950.

ADRIAAN KORTLANDT, Dutch primatologist who visited the Laboratoire Médical de Stanleyville in 1960.

DAVID KRITCHEVSKY, biochemist who worked at Lederle Laboratories and later followed Hilary Koprowski to the Wistar Institute.

KAMIL KUCERA, Czech parasitologist; specialist in *Pneumocystis carinii* research.

WALTER KYLE, New Hampshire attorney, who propounded theory that AIDS epidemic originated from Sabin's OPV, taken topically as an antiherpes treatment.

SENHOR JOSE L., the first known sufferer from HIV-2-related AIDS, believed to have been exposed in Guinea-Bissau by 1965.

GEORGES LAMBELIN, Jezierski's deputy at Gabu-Nioka in the 1950s.

MONIQUE LAMY, virologist at the Rega Institute, Leuven; later put in charge of vaccine production at RIT in the late fifties.

LINDA LAUBENSTEIN, physician and colleague of Alvin Friedman-Kein at New York University Medical Center.

BERNARD LE GUENNO, formerly virologist based at the Pasteur Institute, Dakar, Senegal; now head of research into hemorrhagic fevers at the Pasteur in Paris.

ANDRÉ LEBRUN, in the late fifties, director of the Marcel Wanson Institute of Hygiene, Leopoldville, and effective head of hygiene for the Congo; helped coordinate the polio vaccination campaign in Leo, 1958–1960.

GERASMOS ("MIKE") LECATSAS, chief virologist at the Medical University of Southern Africa (MEDUNSA), Pretoria, and proponent of the OPV/AIDS theory.

JACQUES LEIBOWITCH, French physician, raconteur, and writer on AIDS.

EDWIN LENNETTE, virologist who worked with Koprowski at the Yellow Fever Research Service in Rio during the Second World War; later tested various biological agents for the U.S. Army Chemical Corps.

JOHN LEONARD, senior registrar at the Manchester Royal Infirmary when David Carr was a patient in 1959.

PIERRE LÉPINE, head of virology at the Pasteur Institute in Paris from 1941 for several decades; developer of an inactivated polio vaccine administered in many Francophone countries.

JAY LEVY, San Francisco virologist who identified retrovirus ARV (later called HIV) shortly after Luc Montaigner.

GILBERT M., Belgian mine official who worked in the Congo, and who died of AIDS-like diseases in 1977.

EDNA MAHAN, governor of the women's prison at Clinton Farms for forty years, including the period of the Koprowski vaccine trials.

BRIAN MAHY, British virologist, director of the CDC's division of viral and rickettsial diseases.

JONATHAN MANN, American physician; head of *Projêt SIDA* in Kinshasa in the early eighties and head of the WHO's Global Program on AIDS from 1986 to 1990. Killed in plane crash in 1998.

MARIA, Rwanda-born HIV-infected wife of Daniel D.

BRIAN MARTIN, sociologist of science who heads Science and Technology Studies at the University of Wollongong, Australia; proponent of the OPV/AIDS theory, and publisher of Louis Pascal's paper: "What Happens When Science Goes Bad?"

PRESTON MARX, American primatologist and expert in HIV/SIV research; frequent visitor to West Africa; representative of the Aaron Diamond AIDS Research Center at LEMSIP (the Laboratory for Experimental Medicine and Surgery in Primates).

JOSEPH MELNICK, dean emeritus of Baylor College, Houston; respected commentator on polio vaccines for several decades.

KARL MEYER, Swiss-born doctor who headed the George Williams Hooper Foundation, a San Francisco–based research institute, from the forties onward; helped set up vaccine trials for Koprowski in California.

HECTOR MEYUS, director of the hygiene service of Ruanda-Urundi at the time of the Ruzizi vaccinations in 1958.

JEAN-LOUIS MICHAUX, Jean Sonnet's assistant at Lovanium University Hospital, Leopoldville, in the fifties and sixties.

PHILIP MINOR, principal virologist at the National Institute for Biologic Standards and Control, Potters Bar, U.K., in the nineties.

LUC MONTAGNIER, head of virology at the Pasteur Institute, Paris; generally considered to be the first person to identify HIV (which he called LAV) as the cause of AIDS.

JAMES MOORE, member of the National Institute for Drug Abuse, Lexington, Kentucky, who arranged for retrospective HIV testing of stored sera from drug addicts taken in 1971 and 1972.

JOSEPH MORTELMANS, primatologist and chimpanzee expert; worked in Stanleyville as a vet in 1956.

JACQUES MORVAN, researcher from the laboratory of clinical biology at the army medical school in Bordeaux, France.

ARNO MOTULSKY, American geneticist from the University of Washington, Seattle, who collected blood samples in the Belgian Congo and Ruanda-Urundi in 1959.

KARY MULLIS, inventor of the polymerase chain reaction (PCR) technique for molecular analysis.

GERRY MYERS, director of the HIV Sequence Database, Los Alamos, New Mexico, which produces HIV/SIV sequences and phylogenetic trees.

ANDRÉ NAHMIAS, professor from Emory University, Atlanta, who retrospectively tested African blood samples and found L70, the HIV-positive
  sample from Leopoldville, taken in 1959.

ANDERS NAUCLER, Swedish doctor based in Guinea-Bassau, who wrote
  Ph.D. thesis on HIV-2.

TOM NELSON, superintendent of Sonoma, a Californian center for handicapped children, in the fifties; collaborated with Koprowski in testing
  OPVs in child patients.

GASTON NINANE, Belgian virologist who worked under Ghislain Courtois at
  Stanleyville in the fifties; helped vaccinate in the Ruzizi Valley and Province
  Oriental.

ARVID NOE, Norwegian sailor (between 1961 and 1965) and one of the
  world's earliest confirmed AIDS fatalities, in 1976.

THOMAS NORTON, chief laboratory technician under Koprowski at Lederle
  Laboratories until 1957; later on, assistant director at the Wistar Institute,
  Philadelphia.

LOUIS O., Belgian cartographer who worked in the Congo until 1968 and
  who died of AIDS in 1988.

BASIL O'CONNOR, lawyer and friend of Franklin D. Roosevelt, headed the
  National Fund for Infantile Paralysis and launched the "March of Dimes,"
  which raised public funds for polio research.

JAMES OLESKE, Newark-based pediatrician who cared for some of the first
  children with AIDS in North America, including a girl who may have been
  infected in 1973 or 1974.

PAUL OSTERRIETH, Belgian physician and virologist who worked at the
  Laboratoire Médical de Stanleyville between 1957 and 1960.

JOSEPH PAGANO, trained at the CDC Epidemiology Intelligence Service (EIS)
  and followed Stanley Plotkin to the Wistar Institute, where he organized
  several polio vaccine trials.

LOUIS PASCAL, philosopher and armchair researcher; founding father of
  OPV/AIDS theory.

LOUIS PASTEUR, French veterinary scientist, developer of first vaccine against
  rabies; the Pasteur Institutes found in Francophone countries around the
  world are named after him.

STÉPHANE PATTYN, worked at Laboratoire Médical d'Elisabethville under
  Jean Delville in the fifties and staged polio antibody studies around the
  Belgian Congo; now an eminent virologist at the tropical institute in
  Antwerp.

JULIAN PEETERMANS, joined the Belgian vaccine house, RIT, at its inception in 1956 and effectively headed vaccine production there until the
  nineties.

MARTINE PEETERS, virologist at the Institute of Tropical Medicine in Antwerp, Belgium; has published several papers on SIV-positive chimpanzees.

ROBERT AND JOAN PHILLIPS, husband-and-wife photographer and journalist team who reported on the Ruzizi vaccinations in March 1958.

TONY PINCHING, London-based immunologist and AIDS researcher.

PETER PIOT, Belgian AIDS researcher and latterly head of UNAIDS, the United Nations AIDS program.

STANLEY PLOTKIN, Koprowski's former associate at the Wistar Institute and, in the nineties, managing director of Pasteur Merieux, the vaccine and pharmaceutical giant.

DR. ANNE-GRETHE POULSEN, Danish specialist in HIV-2 research who worked with Peter Aaby in Guinea-Bissau.

DR. EDMUND PRESTON, Quaker physician from Moorestown, New Jersey, who helped organize the first small-scale U.S. trial of Koprowski vaccines in the open community.

ABEL PRINZIE, Belgian virologist who worked at the Rega Institute, Leuven, from 1954 onward, and later, in the sixties, at RIT.

F. ("SMITHY") PRZESMYCKI, head of virology at the state institute of hygiene, Warsaw, who collaborated on the Polish trials of CHAT and Fox.

ROBERT R., St. Louis teenager who died from an AIDS-like condition in 1969.

GRETHE RASK, Danish surgeon who worked in the Congo and who died of AIDS in 1977.

HERBERT RATNER, Chicago physician who proposed theory that Salk's IPV, contaminated with SV40, was the source of the human AIDS epidemic.

ROBERT REDFIELD, AIDS researcher based at the Walter Reed Army Medical Center.

TOM RIVERS, Rockefeller Institute virologist, and arbiter of polio vaccination policy in the forties and fifties.

GILBERT ROLLAIS, French hunter who captured chimpanzees for Lindi camp.

ROBERT ROOT-BERNSTEIN, author of *Rethinking AIDS,* which proposes a multifactorial theory of origin.

GIOVANNI ROVERA, director of the Wistar Institute after Koprowski's departure in 1991.

RUTH RUPRECHT, Harvard virologist who has challenged the safety of the live AIDS vaccine proposed by Ronald Desrosiers.

ALICE S., twenty-two-year-old secretary who died of *Pneumocystis carinii* in 1964 in Pullman, Washington.

ALBERT SABIN, virologist who developed a set of oral polio vaccines that, since 1961, have been adopted around the world.

CARL-RUNE SALENSTEDT, director of vaccine production at the National Bacteriological Laboratories, Stockholm, Sweden, since the fifties.

JONAS SALK, virologist who developed an inactivated polio vaccine that was administered to millions in Britain and America, before being superseded by Sabin's oral vaccine.

KINGSLEY SANDERS, British tissue culture specialist who worked for the Medical Research Council in the fifties and sixties, and who investigated the suitability of African monkey kidneys for preparing polio vaccine.

CARL SAXINGER, conducted AIDS research under Robert Gallo at the National Cancer Institute, Bethesda, in the eighties.

MEINRAD SCHAR, chief of sera and vaccines at the Swiss Public Health Department; helped organize trials of several OPVs and IPVs in the fifties and sixties.

BARRY SCHOUB, senior virologist at National Institute of Virology, South Africa.

GORDON SCOTT, British vet, formerly based at Muguga, Kenya, who visited Alexandre Jezierski at Gabu Nioka in 1954.

JOHN SEALE, British venereologist who proposed theories that AIDS epidemic might have originated through Cold War biological weapons research, or through increased availability of reusable needles and syringes in central Africa.

JACOB AND LILLI SEGAL, East German husband-and-wife team who proposed theory that American biological weapons research sparked AIDS epidemic.

PAUL SHARP, British molecular biologist who has written extensively on the phylogeny of HIV and SIV.

RANDY SHILTS, San Francisco–based journalist and author of *And the Band Played On*. Died of AIDS in the early nineties.

JOSEPH SMADEL, chief of viral and rickettsial research at the Walter Reed Army Medical Center in the fifties; later the associate director of the U.S. Public Health Service.

A. SMORODINTSEV, Soviet virologist who participated in the testing of the Sabin vaccine strains in the USSR.

EVA LEE SNEAD, San Antonio physician and health activist who lost her license, and then wrote *Some Call It "AIDS" — I Call It Murder!*, which proposes that AIDS came from SV40-contaminated IPV.

JEAN SONNET, Belgian physician based at Lovanium University Hospital, Leopoldville/Kinshasa, in fifties and sixties; pioneering AIDS researcher until his death in 1992.

FRED STARE, nutrition expert from Harvard University who received chimpanzees from Lindi camp.

Tom Starzl, controversial scientist from University of Pittsburgh and leading proponent of xenotransplantation — in this case, transplanting
baboon livers into humans.

Ernest Sternglass, American physicist who proposed theory that low-
level radiation exposure was the principal causative factor behind the AIDS
epidemic.

Jan Stijns, director of the medical laboratory at the tropical institute in
Leopoldville who *may* have been responsible for collecting L70, the first
HIV-positive blood sample, in 1959.

Joseph Stokes Jr., Quaker who headed pediatric department of Children's
Hospital of Philadelphia in the fifties; collaborated on Koprowski's polio
vaccine trials. Later appointed director of CHOP.

Robert and Theodore Strecker, fraternal American right-wing AIDS
activists who proposed that the Soviets and the WHO had produced the
AIDS virus as a biological weapon.

Trevor Stretton, senior house officer at the Manchester Royal Infirmary
in the fifties; tended to David Carr.

Raphael Stricker, San Francisco immunologist who cowrote articles on
OPV/AIDS with Blaine Elswood.

Wolf Szmuness, Polish émigré virologist who pioneered studies of the
hepatitis B vaccine, Heptavax-B, in the United States and elsewhere in the
late seventies and early eighties.

Max Theiler, Rockefeller Institute virologist and developer of live vaccine
against yellow fever.

Lise Thiry (formerly Quersin-Thiry), head of virology at the Pasteur
Institute satellite in Brussels; also taught at the Université Libre de
Bruxelles. Later a socialist politician.

Geoffrey Timms, physician in charge of vaccine procurement in Kenya at
the time of Koprowski's visit in 1957.

Mike Tristem, British molecular biologist, former student of Fergal Hill;
now head of the virology labs at Imperial College, Ascot.

Philipe Van De Perre, Belgian AIDS specialist based in Kigali, Rwanda.

Rachel Van Der Meeren (née Yeld), British researcher who monitored
Rwandan Tutsi refugees in Tanzania in the early sixties.

Jean Vandepitte, chair of microbiology at the University of Lovanium
in the Belgian Congo in 1959, when he helped Arno Motulsky collect
blood samples. Temporarily headed the Laboratoire Médical de
Stanleyville in 1958.

Michel Vandeputte, established the first virology laboratory in
Leopoldville in 1956 and moved to the Rega Institute, Leuven, in
1960.

BERNARD VANDERCAM, Belgian AIDS physician who took over from
Dr. Jean Sonnet at St. Luc Hospital, Brussels, in 1992.

BORIS VELIMIROVIC, former WHO official who worked in the Congo in the
early sixties.

JACK ("BLACK MAMBA") WALDEN, former brigadier of the Tanzanian
People's Defence Forces who played a major role in the invasion of Uganda
in 1978/9.

KARL F. WEFRING, Norwegian pediatrician who helped care for Arvid Noe's
youngest daughter.

ROBIN WEISS, British virologist and AIDS researcher.

HANS WIGZELL, former head of the National Bacteriological Laboratory,
Stockholm, and, latterly, Rektor of the Karolinska Institute. Cochair of
consultative group on live AIDS vaccines for the WHO.

TADEUSZ J. WIKTOR, Polish-born vet who served in the Congo in the fifties
and met Hilary Koprowski in Kenya in 1955. Joined the Wistar Institute in
the sixties, to work on rabies research.

GEORGE WILLIAMS, pathologist who conducted autopsy on David Carr and
who provided tissue samples from that autopsy that tested HIV-positive
by PCR.

JOHN ROWAN WILSON, author of *Margin of Safety*, a history of polio vaccines published in 1963.

ZOFIA WROBLEWSKA, Polish researcher at the Wistar Institute.

JOHN WYATT, St. Louis pathologist who identified CMV in tissues of Dick G.

GEORGE Y., Japanese-Canadian who died of PCP at Toronto General
Hospital in 1959.

VERONIQUE Y., Congolese woman, wife of Louis O., who left the Congo in
1968 and died of AIDS in 1987.

DANIEL ZAGURY, French doctor based in Kinshasa, Congo, who injected
himself and other volunteers with an experimental AIDS vaccine in the
mid-eighties.

*Foreword*

W. D. HAMILTON

Every time two people put their heads together, Truth suffers; when many put their heads together, she suffers more. A major point of this book is that when the heads are great ones and have owners with much to lose (employed perhaps in giant companies or government departments), Truth can be made so ill that we should all shiver.

Evasion and untruth have long been known to be beneficial at many levels and useful to people in many ways. They can be presented as virtues — the little bads that add to a greater good, with a proviso, of course, that the good is of a kind that the colluders believe only they know how to attain. "Don't we have faith in ourselves? — let's keep it simple for their — for all our sakes." Even for God's sake: this version has been abundantly illustrated by religious leaders ever since Christianity became official in the Roman Empire, with disastrous effects upon other faiths — and a fiery impact upon a myriad of free-thinking "witches," as well as the occasional literary loner like Giordano Bruno. Once there is acceptance by an "establishment," there is often no need to whisper about it anymore: in those who have jointly suffered to win, say, the Queen's Commission in the British armed forces, or the privilege of saying the Hippocratic Oath, a solidarity springs up automatically, and with it a deep conviction that the purpose of the discipline, whatever it be, must be good. And yet, knowing the untruths that emotions arouse, especially in groups, Plato amazingly denied roles even for poetry and music in his ideal Republic.

Most of the daily untruths communicated need not be taken too seriously: we have become accustomed to them and in a sense self-vaccinate. However, when eminent rivals in an ancient profession are seen to be uniting to crush an outside critique, and when the best-funded branch of science, to which the rivals belong, draws almost all its practitioners into line behind them (as Louis Pascal and then Tom Curtis in the case treated in this book had already experienced, even before Hooper), and when an expectant and immensely wealthy international industry is also seen marching in step with the profession in question, it is time for the rest of us to wake up.

The thesis of *The River* is that the closing of ranks against inquiry may, in this case, be preventing proper discussion of an accident that is bidding to prove itself more expensive in lives than all the human attritions put in motion by Hitler, Stalin, and Pol Pot. Furthermore, essentially unwarned by what we have recently done, we may be moving rapidly toward further and perhaps even worse disasters of the same kind. Some aspects of genetic engineering may indeed be dangerous, but a situation in which the general public has greater concerns about mystical subversion of the chemicals in soy sauce than about the risk of viruses in live animal products that are already administered, almost compulsorily, to our bodies, is near to absurd. In parallel to this, our doctors' Hippocratic Oath warns them of various temptations and dangers, but it says nothing of how they need to guard themselves, and their profession, against the effects of the millions of profit that dangle before the nascent industry proposing to transplant organs into humans from other species.

These are the foreground dangers emphasized by Hooper in this book. Its background has another danger, which is still more insidious. Litigation has been used to suppress the publication of discussions about a hypothesis; litigation is again being used as a threat to Hooper. In the same vein and equally unsettling, we have seen the best known and seemingly most independent science and medical journals join forces on the side of the countercritique, while generally avoiding publishing details of the original issue. Again it is time for us to wake up and consider what is happening to freedom of discussion and to the spirit of science.

It is the foreground, the potential repercussions in the next thirty or so years, which will probably most arouse the reader of this book. Perhaps something is being tardily seen by the establishment. A few months ago the British Medical Association announced revisions to the Hippocratic Oath British doctors must take; then just a week ago, as I write, the Association's organ, the *British Medical Journal,* published for the first time an admission of a likelihood that Simian Virus 40, established as an infection in millions of humans by the Salk polio vaccine, is causing human cancers. "Salk," it may be remembered, is the "dead" and therefore safer polio vaccine — safe supposedly not only from reversions to virulence but from the possibility of "extraneous agents." It is quite different from the type focused upon in this book — the type we now all receive. On another front, committees in recent months have enjoined slowness and caution with xenotransplants, but not before the first baboon liver transplant into a human was attempted — an operation that perhaps fortunately failed. Meanwhile heart valve implants from pigs, a species known to harbor retroviruses that can live in human tissue cultures, are in trial and application.

All this is why the world still very much needs lone researchers like Edward Hooper. They reach truth faster than committees. Shortly after I first knew him I introduced him to someone as a journalist, knowing he had formerly been one in Africa. Later he asked me, pained, "Why journalist? Couldn't you call me a *writer?*" I did so from then on but stayed puzzled. Weren't journalists supposed to be the guardians of our free world, the para-predators ranging our savannah and making even the most lordly lions take care of their actions? Weren't they (the best at least) even cousins to us scientists, ferrets setting themselves to bolt the most willfully concealed and elusive truths of history where we scientists deign only to chase the immobile targets, such as atoms and missing links? Why should one not want to be a journalist? After reflection and listening to the talk of "paparazzi" and the like that came after Princess Diana's death, I think I see better now the perspectives that journalists dread — but just as hyenas do less scavenging and far more primary predation than was once thought, so also do the best journalists.

Whatever, this book, with its almost 2,500 footnotes, demonstrates how Hooper has finished up. Not only is he the kind of predator that all in Big Science should fear, but he is a writer and historian as well. Even that is not all. He has self-taught his way to "honorary" status in several branches of science — to be almost virologist, almost geneticist, almost evolutionist. To most of us, however, these achievements just provide the reassurance that he is writing sense in his diverse fields; in contrast it is the writing itself and the history — dare I say even the first-class journalism? — that will keep us bent over the pages that follow. What scoops, what personalities, what landscapes, what far places! Above all what enigmas, what awful inexorable tragedy (tragedy at its deepest, gnawing within millions of homes — a scale perhaps grander than any ever before described) stand there behind!

In 1995, in Africa for another purpose, I tried to help Ed by looking for some of the Ugandan friends who had helped, nearly a decade earlier, with the research for his first book, which described the AIDS disaster in that focal area close to the shores of Lake Victoria. There were two men in particular whom he wished to contact and to thank. As I discovered after some questioning, both had died. I was led to the father of one, and he in turn took me to a neat private graveyard in his *matoke* plantation and showed me the newly heaped mounds, six in all. They were for his wife and all his children. One mound, with a stone slab, was for the son Hooper knew, a local government official (who had been, perhaps, a little more important locally than the others). The old man sat on a corner of the slab and read the letter Ed had sent, while two grandchildren, come into his care after the last death, watched from nearby. The children were lively and healthy but very quiet, and I hoped the infection was going to miss them. Such graveyards, I found, were everywhere in the district, though they are not much seen from the roads. Orphans, too, were everywhere: a generation had been scythed out from between those who were too young and too old to be readily infected. I saw children in groups ranging from teens to tots seemingly loose and self-foraging in the countryside, which included as it happened trying to forage from me, the passing foreigner. Presumably these were the children not lucky enough to have grandfathers and grandmothers who were still alive. Both in the robust elderly and in these youthful gangs I felt I was seeing how Africa would survive, if only after a period of great suffering. Yet it may end up less changed, it seemed to me, than will the continents of the First World, in spite of our lower expected mortalities.

After that brief experience in southern Uganda — a few days only — I understood better what had been driving Hooper to follow up on the lighter and more emotional book he had already written about the epidemic in Africa. I suspect he had no idea, at the start, of the magnitude of what he was undertaking, nor of the nine-year odyssey of research and travel it would require. Even before he read Louis Pascal's extraordinary paper "What Happens When Science Goes Bad . . ." and had realized the full tragic possibility about the origin that it raised, he had been aroused by personal indignation to far more energy over the epidemic than had most of the rest of us. In the late eighties in Nairobi and Kampala, he had seen friends sicken and die around him. Despite this, in the nineties he was still finding Westerners who claimed it was all untrue, and that there was no epidemic. Instead, false trails and absurdities were glibly promoted; hypotheses were floated that seemed aimed, even from the first, to lead into impenetrable bush. At the same time, as he found later, much better hypotheses about the epidemic were studiously ignored and had needed tortuous paths to achieve any public notice at all. The ideas and research of New York–based Louis Pascal, for example, had to be published in Australia, and the investigations of science journalist Tom Curtis went perforce to an outlet in a popular magazine, *Rolling Stone*. Neither piece was much followed up.

Without question it is science that will shape the human world of the Third Millennium. Even if science can only direct us back to a dark age it will still be our cause and our guide. But it could be made to do better or worse. There is a risk that science is going to lose its fertility and change radically away from that spirit of free inquiry and exchange that first inspired the Greek and then later the Renaissance experimenters and philosophers. Indeed, this process seems to be starting already; patenting and secrecy about gene sequences are perhaps one symptom. Science may bring on us not so much a dark age in the old sense, via some spectacular collapse, but rather a super-technological state whose monstrous futures — if they could be shown to us clearly through the present smoke of excitement about more and ever more technology — would only arouse our dread. While still working its miracles on the outskirts, science may already, at its center, like a great city, be slowly dying of its very success. Dictators and businessmen everywhere want to use all the technical products of science and, if possible, to control the rights and the how-tos for creating more. They would also like to be free to hide the results of their unsuccessful or disastrous experiments.

After reading Pascal's paper, it was a great shock to me that when I passed out copies to others whom I thought would be interested, including a journalist who had written on AIDS for a major popular science magazine, I met with exactly the wall of silence Pascal had described. From being at first impressed mainly by his theme about the origin of AIDS, I thus began to believe his arguments about scientific integrity as well — arguments that at initial reading had seemed to me just overreactions generated in a sensitive, frustrated man. Only one person (from the medical fraternity, surprisingly) replied to my mailing with any sign of taking the paper seriously. Even my old mother, a doctor, told me, "You are going to be very unpopular if you pursue that one — polio of all things, that one is sacred! Anyway, if it's true, it's all happened and what could you do?" Well, personally I didn't pursue anything very far; after several tries with the editors of both *Science* and *Nature,* I lapsed back again into the general silence. Overall I have left it to Pascal, Curtis, Julian Cribb, and now Hooper. I have simply watched from the sidelines as each in turn has held aloft his blazing but strangely unregarded torch. However, I have become, with each new revelation, and particularly with the discoveries of Hooper, which you can now read about for the first time, more and more a convert to the underlying theme. The new facts in the case still tend to be widely separated and none by itself amounts to a proof; however, taken together the steady trend and accumulation has become very impressive. At the very least the OPV theory of the origin of AIDS now merits our acute attention.

I have pondered very much about what sorts of people should be encouraged to try which sorts of tests: Hooper also in the book gives his list. There are some that could be decisive. However, the factual case was already quite strong after Pascal, and the present situation adds up to reiterating that Pascal was also right in his other theme, and that very major questions need to be asked about why supposedly "free" science has been so slow to listen to what should have been taken very seriously from the first. If the topic had somehow been far from Big Science and had lacked any implications touching on issues like politics and professional pride, I have little doubt that its questions would have been much more discussed and investigated by now. I very much hope this book will cause the questions to be asked and the tests to be undertaken, and that it will also stimulate a lot more of the kind of sociology and science critique which Brian Martin in Australia promoted during (and supportative to) the building of the present story. How much more useful his effort is than so much that is done under the name of the sociology of science!

Forensic high-tech analysis has been enthusiastically applied to the hair of a historic corpse, Napoleon, in order to try to separate the natural events, accidents, and malfeasance that might have played a part in his death. He was a great man by any standard and also, looked at a bit more sourly, was instrumental in causing hundreds of thousands of deaths. Most would agree that these attributes of Napoleon justify the considerable interest historians have in how he died. But this level of interest makes it all the more remarkable that another historical issue with already far more deaths to its tally, and its Waterloo not even in sight, receives currently only a single historian's effort. Vaccine vials, which are surely much more accessible than samples of Napoleon's hair, stay untested in the Wistar Institute freezers. Through turning a blind eye to the OPV/AIDS hypothesis, our establishment actively avoids testing and hearing about the plentiful though scattered evidence that the AIDS epidemic may have had a medical accident at its origin — an accident possibly compounded, more recently, by a desire by certain protagonists to conceal the evidence.

In getting together the materials for his book, Hooper has worked harder and for much longer than any of his forerunners. Several times he has countered my plea for a start on the writing by saying there just had to be this further trip to Belgium or that one to the United States. His work has amounted to more than six hundred interviews in all, he tells me, and this says nothing of the library research. I believe no one, not even a person "speaking as a scientist," is going to call this book "the wildest of lay speculation" — the criticism that was leveled, even then unfairly, at Tom Curtis's much briefer accounts in *Rolling Stone*. If the OPV theory of AIDS origin comes to be proved, I think the new standards of *evolutionary* caution in medicine that their publications will eventually engender (especially regarding all treatments that use live products from other animals on humans) should merit for Hooper and Pascal jointly a Nobel Prize. As a species we ought to have known somehow in our culture, or even genes, that intimate invasions of live animal products, especially those coming from closely related species, are inherently dangerous. I have conjectured elsewhere that these dangers may be the main reason why separate species exist generally. That notion and what happens next in the present case are all in the lap of the gods. There are as stated, however, tests which can prove convincingly whether or not AIDS was our medical mistake. Meanwhile, Hooper deserves great praise for having so tenaciously carried through his investigation and for bringing to light so many more facts affecting the main question — facts that are almost all further challenges to the null hypothesis of "coincidence only." Even if the OPV theory is eventually rejected or remains permanently in limbo, he has done a great service in putting so many details of the early spread of AIDS on record. He has in fact given us the best history of the epidemic.

I have seen the cost the task has had for him manifested in many stages of tiredness, illness, and despair, which however he has always managed to overcome. Truly it has been like watching an explorer — Burton or Living-stone — making his halting progress toward some center of mystery that is far inland from the obvious coastal hills which we have all been seeing. Most strangely, as it may seem at first, his story wends toward exactly the same center of Africa as those Victorian explorers sought. This comes to seem a little less strange, however, once we reflect on our evolutionary origins. What dramas on all scales have been played out in the human population in the same geographic region, around the spine of Africa and in those places where the savannah and the forest meet. Almost all of these things were happening long, long before there was anyone who could write or even speak about them. Upright we became . . . trying for new social structures, for tools, for speech, for fire . . . Finally out of Africa, our home, there came this new disease and on its heels, in this case, a *written* drama of *how* it came. Both themes are gravid with our future, and the written one is like Sherlock Holmes, Professor Challenger, Augustus Caesar, and Mark Antony all rolled into one.

Everyone should read this book, both for its story and in order to think hard on all that it implies — all this before Truth, more white and sick even than with AIDS, quietly rejoins us through another door.

# THE RIVER

What is a source? Where does a river begin? In this valley is a spring, but higher up the hillside lies a dripping rock. Between the two points, a trickle of water bubbles among stones and disappears underground. (In another sense, in time, the source may be different again: a nudging of continents, a crumpling of uplifted land, a new mountain emerging to draw rain from passing clouds.)

That ultimate source on the ground is almost never easy to identify, and some would say the search is meaningless. But the resulting geography — the nick in the hillside, the steep-edged valley, the mature river, the floodplain, the estuary — although it never ceases to evolve, remains firm enough to allow description, and depiction on maps. These features are the visible consequences of that tiny source, and it is these that make their immense impact on humanity.

It is a strange place this, with its fish eagles and parched, but distinctively British gardens. Known as the Ripon Falls, this is where the waters of Lake Victoria, extending more than thirty thousand square miles but draining an area of nearly a million, breach the shallow surrounding walls and tumble northward on their four-thousand-mile descent to the Mediterranean. The young river Nile is narrow here, and the proximity of the opposite shore gives a vivid sense of the volume of water that is spewing forth.

A hundred and fifty years ago, a great and bearded controversy raged in Britain about this very place. John Speke claimed that here, at the point where the waters erupted from Lake Victoria, he had found the source of the river Nile. Richard Burton, his erstwhile companion, proposed a different map, and eventually taunted the troubled Speke to shoot himself — though whether by accident or design is uncertain.

Afterward, the colonial British — decent, earnest chaps, builders of railways and hospitals, spreaders of the gospel — decided that Speke was right, and that this place represented the origin of all that water which descended through the pink-hued territories of Uganda, Sudan, and Egypt, and which made them viable entities as British protectorate and condominium. Control the Nile, they said, and you control Africa. They erected a small plinth to indicate the significance of the place.

The plinth still stands today, but its presumptions are incorrect on two counts. First, in terms of discovery. This place had clearly been discovered, and its significance realized, long before the arrival of Victorian explorers (though it was they who made the connections between the broken blue lines on the map). Second, and more significantly, in terms of geography. For this is not the source of the Nile at all.

There is a slight, but distinct, current that flows across Lake Victoria toward the Ripon Falls from the southwest. The source of that current is the Kagera, the main feeder to the lake. And if one traces the Kagera back from its mouth, near Lukunyu on the border between Uganda and Tanzania, one ends up at a small spring near the village of Kyriama, in southern Burundi. It is this spring, in reality, that is the fabled "source of the Nile."

And so, although the official version of truth was recorded on the colonial plinth, and in the great contemporary textbooks and atlases published in London, Paris, and New York, we now know better. The real truths, of course, are not always those enshrined on brass, stone, and vellum.

The controversy surrounding the source of the Nile — its passions, false hopes, misconceptions, the assumptions and lies that misled explorers — is strangely echoed by another controversy of a century and a half later, the long-running debate about the origins of AIDS. For a while, many commentators were pointing to the shores of Lake Victoria and saying: This is where it begins. But, like the Victorian explorers, they were wrong. They needed to trace the evidence a little further back in place and time.

*Introduction*

JOHN SNOW AND THE WATER PUMP

It is now nearly twenty years since it began. Or, to be more accurate, since anyone knew that it had begun. The story is by now so well known that its rhythms and cadences have begun to settle deeply — if not comfortably — in the communal psyche, like folktales and scriptures. It rings forth, this great, sad anthem, though there is something here too with qualities of insinuation, of infiltration, like the more irritating of advertising jingles. The song has been sung so often that it is all too easy to pick up the tune and mouth the words in time. It is altogether hard to contemplate a different version.

So much has happened in these two decades, so much has changed. But already most of us have forgotten what we were like (the overt, but also the more subtle differences in outlook and behavior) before it started. And yet the epidemic has brought good things as well as bad. We have had to grow up fast. Nowadays in our schools we teach about gays and straights, about high-risk and low-risk sex, about the use and abuse of narcotics. In newspapers and on TV, we read about techniques which allow HIV-positive couples to have babies with minimal risk, we compare condoms, we mull over the joys of mutual masturbation. The other side, of course, is that AIDS has scarred the spirit and emotional fitness of an entire generation, has inhibited not only sex for fun, but also sex as an integral step in the process of forming relationships, of finding a partner or mate. Many have been wounded — not just those who have gotten the virus.

Perhaps, as further years go by, the syndrome will work its way even further into our communal consciousness, and the tale of its arrival in our midst will be taught at mother's knee. In the meantime, it will perhaps be useful to replay those first few, memorable bars — to help any who need help to lock on to the great, sad anthem which thrums away softly in the background.

It is April 1981. Over the last seven months, five young men have appeared at different hospitals around Los Angeles district, all gravely ill with a variety of unusual symptoms. In each case the symptoms have included PCP, a rare pneumonia caused by *Pneumocystis carinii*, a microorganism to which most people have been exposed, but which causes disease in very few. These few include those with congenital immunodeficiency, and those whose immune systems have been devastated by cancers and leukemias, or deliberately inhibited by the administration of radiotherapy or immunosuppressive drugs during, for instance, cancer treatment or transplant operations. Yet such factors do not apply in any of these cases. There is, however, a common denominator among the five patients, for all are homosexual.

Four of the five have candidiasis, or thrush, of the mouth or esophagus, caused by *Candida albicans*, a relatively harmless fungus better known for colonizing the vagina. In addition, laboratory tests reveal that all the patients have high titers (levels) of cytomegalovirus (CMV), with four of them having specific CMV infections of the lungs, eyes, or windpipe. Most significantly, all of the three men so tested have very low quantities of T-cells (white blood cells), indicating an immune dysfunction.

By May, two of the five are dead, and the coincidence of time, place, and sexuality has convinced some of the Los Angeles doctors that something new and serious is afoot. Two of them, Michael Gottlieb and Wayne Shandera, decide to approach the Centers for Disease Control (CDC) in Atlanta, and to submit a brief report to the CDC's *Morbidity and Mortality Weekly Report (MMWR)*, a booklet that is mailed out at the end of every week to physicians around America, keeping them up-to-date with the latest disease outbreaks across the nation. The *MMWR* allows for fast-track publication, instead of the lengthy process of submission, peer review, revision, and acceptance, which obtains for more mainstream medical journals.

A report extending over a page and a half, entitled simply "Pneumocystis Pneumonia — Los Angeles,"[1] appears some few days later and features conjecture about the cause of the disease, its etiology. Is this a condition sparked by environmental factors, such as drugs, or is it an infectious disease, perhaps a new disease entirely? Gottlieb and his coauthors observe that none of the five men knew each other or had mutual partners, though two of the five reported having had sex with multiple partners. All five had apparently used nitrite inhalants, and one had injected hard drugs. The final editorial comment includes the following rather laborious observation: "The fact that these patients were all homosexuals suggests an association between some aspect of a homosexual lifestyle or disease acquired by sexual contact and Pneumocystis pneumonia in this population."

The date is June 5, 1981; the AIDS epidemic — or pandemic — has officially begun.[2] In reality, of course, the AIDS epidemic started some years earlier, but June 5, 1981, is when information about the newly recognized condition was first released to the medical profession and the general public. How long it might have taken for such a diffuse condition to be recognized, had its presence not manifested itself among such a clearly defined group as homosexual men, is a debatable subject.

June 5, 1981, thus provides a convenient watershed, a Year Zero, a medical equivalent of Anno Domini 1. All that follows that date can be viewed as part of the recognized spread of AIDS across the globe. All events prior to that date can be said to have occurred before the epidemic.

In fact, the Los Angeles team is not the first to recognize the new condition, but rather the first to announce its existence in print. Four weeks later another piece appears in *MMWR*, this time cowritten by several doctors from New York and California, headed by Alvin Friedman-Kien and Linda Laubenstein of the New York University Medical Center.[3] It transpires that for the past thirty months, these doctors have been seeing another rare disease in homosexual men — this time a malignant condition known as Kaposi's sarcoma. KS is normally confined to people from equatorial Africa and elderly men of Jewish or Mediterranean origin, but since the start of 1979 it has been seen in twenty-six young or middle-aged gays: twenty from New York and six from California. Several of these men have subsequently experienced other serious infections, including PCP, chronic candidiasis, toxoplasmosis of the central nervous system, and cryptococcal meningitis. These are called "opportunistic infections" because they are caused by pathogens that are normally harmless, but that have a propensity for exploiting bodies in a state of lowered immunity. The report ends with the information that a further ten gay men with PCP have appeared in California, bringing the total in that state to fifteen, and that in New York there have been four cases of gay men with severe and progressive herpes simplex infections of the anus, three of whom have already died. The editors conclude: "Physicians should be alert for Kaposi's sarcoma, PC pneumonia and other opportunistic infections in homosexual men."

Thus, as the second half of 1981 begins, forty-five gay American males, mostly in their thirties and forties, are known to have died or become gravely ill as a result of diseases rarely seen in young and healthy people. Immunological assessments of these patients reveal that their bodily defenses are universally compromised, and that they all have some unexplained defect in their white blood cells, especially their T-cells. A new, or newly recognized, condition of immune deficiency has entered the male homosexual population, and already the doctors involved with these patients are wondering what the new factor might be, what has changed.

In these early days, it is called GRID, or Gay-Related Immune Deficiency, but before the end of 1981, clusters of similar cases begin coming to light in nonhomosexual groups. The first such group to be recognized is that of intra-venous drug users, IVDUs, suggesting that the unknown causative agent can also be acquired parenterally (via the bloodstream) and by either sex.[4] The the-ory of spread outside the gay community gains currency when it is realized that several Haitians — both men and women — are apparently suffering from the same condition.[5] Before long, parenteral transmission is confirmed in the worst possible manner, as cases are retrospectively recognized among hemophiliacs who have been treated with the clotting agent Factor VIII,[6] and recipients of blood transfusions.[7] Soon afterward, children born to IVDUs join the list, sug-gesting that the agent can also be transferred perinatally, from mother to child.[8] People start referring to the "Four Hs"— homosexuals, heroin-users, hemo-philiacs, and Haitians. It takes rather longer for them to realize that the fourth H should perhaps stand for heterosexuals rather than Haitians, and that the four Hs are in fact one: *Homo sapiens.*

Everyone who has ever had sex, who has ever received a blood product or a jab with an unsterilized needle, is potentially at risk — and for those who pre-fer to live their lives in the harsh glow of divine judgment and retribution, then the sins of the fathers can indeed be said to have been visited on the sons (hav-ing called on the mothers first). Indeed, one of the greatest tragedies of this new and horrible condition is that it all too swiftly brings out the stentorian lan-guage of blame and accusation, especially among those who, by their own lights, should know better.

As it becomes clear that "GRID" is not just a gay disease, and that gay men were merely the unfortunate group among whom the agent first became widely disseminated in the West, the title is replaced by a broader one: Acquired Immune Deficiency Syndrome, or AIDS. "Acquired" indicates that the unknown causative agent is transmitted to human beings exogenously, from external sources in the course of their natural life span (rather than passed endogenously, in the germ line); "immune deficiency" indicates that symptoms result from a fault in the immune system, the very bodily mechanism that has evolved to combat disease; and "syndrome" indicates that there is a range of symptoms associated with the infection, rather than a single disease presentation.

As it happens, the causative agent will not remain unknown for very much longer. By late 1983, Professor Luc Montagnier and his team from the Pasteur Institute in Paris have identified a retrovirus* in the blood of people with AIDS and with the lymphadenopathy (a swelling and inflammation of the glands) that seems to precede full-blown AIDS. The French christen their agent "LAV,"

---

* Retrovirus: Only discovered in the 1970s, retroviruses are comprised of RNA (rather than the more usual genetic material, DNA) and use an enzyme, reverse transcriptase, to convert the RNA to DNA so that it can be incorporated into the host cells.

for Lymphadenopathy-Associated Virus. Soon afterward, Jay Levy and his team in San Francisco isolate a virus from AIDS patients, which they call ARV, or AIDS-Related Virus. And nearly a year after the French, Professor Robert Gallo and his team from the National Institutes of Health announce that they have located the AIDS agent — and christen their virus HTLV-III, thus bracketing it with the two other Human T-Cell Lymphotropic Viruses that Gallo has already discovered.

As it turns out, they have all isolated the same retrovirus — but Montagnier and Levy are right and Gallo wrong, for LAV/ARV/HTLV-III is not an oncovirus* (like HTLV-1 and HTLV-2), but rather a lentivirus,† so named for its slow pathogenic course within the body. Gallo and Montagnier spend several years tussling for primacy, but in March 1987 at a press conference in Washington, President Reagan and French prime minister Jacques Chirac announce an agreement whereby the two men will henceforth be credited with codiscovery of the virus, which has by now been rechristened HIV, the Human Immunodeficiency Virus. Amidst the handshakes and backslappings, few notice that Jay Levy and his group have not been included in the cosy compromise.

In fact, as John Crewdson ably demonstrates in a remarkable article that appears two years later in the *Chicago Tribune*,[10] Gallo's HTLV-III isolates almost certainly originated from LAV samples sent him by Montagnier. At the very least, cross contamination had occurred, and although an NIH investigation launched to determine whether or not such contamination was accidental eventually clears Gallo of misconduct, it leaves a number of key questions unanswered. A report issued soon afterward by the Office of Research Integrity (part of the Department of Health and Human Services) is more forthright, finding that Gallo's claim that he had been unable to grow a sample of LAV provided by the French was "knowingly false when written," accusing him of "irresponsible laboratory management," and concluding that the episode represents "a tragedy for science."[11]

Throughout these years, scientific and public perceptions of AIDS and its causative virus, HIV, have steadily broadened. So has an understanding of their history and prehistory. Gaetan Dugas, a Canadian air steward who has had sex with some 250 men a year for the better part of a decade, comes posthumously to be known as Patient Zero, after Randy Shilts popularizes the theory that he was the key disseminator of the virus in North America and, indeed, might even have been the first to introduce the virus from elsewhere.[12] As to the identity of that "elsewhere," opinions are divided, but people begin to hypothesize that

---

\* Oncovirus: A subfamily of retrovirus that causes cancer (as well as other diseases).

† Lentivirus: A subfamily of slow-acting retroviruses; includes the immunodeficiency viruses (HIV, SIV).

American gays might have become infected in the Caribbean, or in Europe. And by the middle of the eighties Western scientists begin to hypothesize publicly — albeit cautiously — that the origin of HIV, like so many other life-forms including *Homo sapiens,* might lie in Africa.

---

All this we know. We also know that many of those medics and scientists who have spent long years working with HIV and AIDS are now deeply tired in body and spirit, and that these people tend to have a stock reply to questions about how the epidemic began. "I haven't got time to worry about that," they say. "I'm too busy worrying about where this thing's going. I'm too busy trying to save lives to bother about archaeology."

This is a strange response, even if the caring and commitment of these doctors is not in question. It is strange because an appreciation of how diseases started — of the where and the when — is usually a key step toward understanding how to stop them dead in their tracks.

Take one classic example — that of John Snow, whose pioneering investigation of the terrible cholera outbreak in south London in the middle of the nineteenth century, which caused some five hundred deaths in ten days, led to his removal of the handle of the water pump in Broad Street, and hence to the prompt termination of the epidemic.[13] That memorable event took place on September 7, 1854 — and one wonders whether a similar date, denoting a "Eureka moment" for AIDS, will ever be written into the medical textbooks. Few scientists, of course, believe that the AIDS epidemic is susceptible to such a straightforward solution, but there again few of his fellows were impressed by the epidemiological approach favored by John Snow when he arrived in Broad Street a century and a half ago. Perhaps even today the simple epidemiological approach is underrated as a scientific tool.

Snow's investigations may seem staggeringly obvious today, but then it is partly his clear and original thinking that have rendered them so. He began by mapping out the residences where people had died, and then added the locations of the various pumps in the area, thus demonstrating dramatically the role of one public pump. He collected additional anecdotal evidence, too — the workhouse in Poland Street that was surrounded by fatalities, but where only five of 535 inmates had died (it had its own private well); the woman victim from Hampstead, north London, who used to live in the Broad Street area, and who so loved the taste of its water that she paid a carter to bring her a fresh bottle every day.

The initial questions that John Snow asked about cholera in 1854 were: "When did it first appear?" and "Where did it first appear?" Next he asked: "How does it spread?" and his research produced the only logical answer — through the water supply. Finally, he inquired about the specific source. Once that had been identified, it was time to ask around for monkey wrenches.

With respect to AIDS, we already know the answer to the transmission question (sexually, perinatally, and parenterally), and although the HIVs are mutating faster than any other viruses known to man, most scientists believe it unlikely that any new routes of spread (via water, for instance, or air) will be added to the list. Of course, God help us if ever they are.

This leaves us to resolve the when and the where of that first appearance in humans. And to these questions — as we shall see — might be added a third, involving just two words: "Why now?"

Let us take a brief look at some of the possibilities. In 1990, when this book began, the world was still in a panic about AIDS, and both the popular press and the scientific journals were awash with different theories of origin. These ranged from the worthy and plausible, through gently wacky conspiracy theories, to the exploitative, the paranoid, and the products of serious madness.

According to these versions, AIDS came from God, and it punished homosexuals, junkies, and other perverts and reprobates. Or it came from man, who was aiming at roughly the same groups that God was after. It came from outer space, on the tail of a comet. It came from Africa, through people eating monkeys. It came from Africa, through kinky stuff with monkeys. It came from Haiti, and had something to do with swine fever and voodoo rites. It came from scientists, from a hepatitis B, or smallpox, or polio vaccine gone wrong. It had always been around, but had escaped only recently from the confines of an isolated tribe. It had always been with us, and was merely syphilis, malnutrition, TB, the effects of hard drugs — or combinations of the above — lumped together and given a new name. There were other theories about the source, but these embrace the broad categories. These are enough to be getting on with.

The diversity — and frequent weirdness — of these explanations was entirely understandable. The sudden arrival in our midst of an insidious, frightening, and fatal disease, which appeared to be spread by the very activities that some would say make life worthwhile or, indeed, enable life to exist, was bound to engender speculation about its origin. Perhaps, given the emotional stakes, it was inevitable that much of the speculation would be wild, and would tend to confirm preconceived fears and prejudices.

However, in the second half of the nineties, as I write these words, some — at least — of the panic engendered by AIDS is over. People all over the world have learned to confront this condition full in the face, to acknowledge the price it levies, to respond intelligently to its demands — to the things it allows and those it does not. We know, for instance, that unlike pathogens endemic in the tropics, such as those that cause malaria and the diarrheal diseases, the onward transmission of HIV can be halted (albeit by what some would consider a radical change of behavior). And at long last, as we begin properly to understand the way the human immunodeficiency virus works, AIDS is starting to lose that air of mystery, that odd sense that somehow it falls outside the range of normal human experience. At long last, we can begin to see it for what it is — a condition caused by a not especially infectious virus, but one which, when contracted, bears a dreadful inevitability.[14]

That said, it must swiftly be added that nowadays, as the millennium approaches, there is great and justified optimism because of the emergence of drug treatments such as "triple therapy."[15] But despite this, HIV infection still has dreadful consequences. The new treatments represent a wonderful breakthrough, but they do not provide an answer for the 90 percent of infectees around the world who cannot afford them. Furthermore, they represent a palliative, rather than a cure, for AIDS.

Nonetheless, even if those early, hasty predictions about a vaccine or magic bullet turned out to be wildly premature, we are now able to claim at least one truly significant against "this diabolical virus." And we are entitled to hope that perhaps one day it will prove possible to immunize against HIV, or that a drug will be developed that will not merely keep HIV in check, but will enable existing infectees to rid themselves entirely of the virus. Of course, those days — the days when AIDS becomes a preventable or a curable condition — probably still lie far in the future.

In the meantime, nearly two decades have passed since Year Zero. Perhaps now, for the first time, we are ready to return once more to that vital question about origin, and to see where the answers lead us. And perhaps this time we can examine the arguments without prejudice, without self-interest, and without fear.

---

Insomuch as a *book* can be said to have a source, this book probably began at one of those pavement cafés with wobbly tables that lie scattered across the cobblestones of Covent Garden in central London. It was June 1990, and I had arranged a final meeting with Professor Alan Fleming, a hematologist, who was just about to return to southern Africa to take up his new posting at the Baragwanath, the huge hospital serving Soweto. We ordered coffee and some expensive, sugary pastries; I had my notebook open on the table, so I could jot down any final words of wisdom he might have to impart. To this day, the relevant pages have a tendency to stick together.

I originally became interested in Fleming's work in 1988, after coming across a long, detailed article of his entitled "AIDS in Africa," which contained a superb review of early epidemiological studies of HIV in Africa.[16] It was exhaustively referenced and scrupulously detailed — listing, in every instance, the geographical location, the year of testing, the size of the cohort (or group) tested, the number and percentage of HIV-positives, and the precise assay (test), or combination of assays, that had been used to establish HIV-positivity.

The data supported the hypothesis that HIV might have been present, sporadically, earlier in Africa that elsewhere, but it also suggested to Fleming that HIV was a relatively new virus in *Homo sapiens*. He reminded me that in 1985, two years after the French discovery of "LAV" in the blood of AIDS patients, American and French researchers had announced the discovery of a second human immunodeficiency virus in the blood of persons from West Africa.[17] (Shortly afterward, this virus was named HIV-2, with the original HIV being renamed HIV-1.) This in itself was remarkable enough — that two HIVs, causing two AIDS epidemics, should have been discovered in so short a space of time.[18]

But this still offered no information about how long the HIVs might have been present in man — and the best way to find out more about that was clearly to search out ancient stored specimens of human blood or tissue. And yet such samples are few and far between. There is simply not enough room in the freezers, or on the dusty shelves of pathology departments, and such materials tend to get cleared out every few years, or else be destroyed by fire, flood, or other natural disaster.

However, a different kind of historical evidence *was* still available, Fleming pointed out, as a result of events that had taken place more than a century earlier, and that are still described, albeit perhaps nowadays euphemistically, as "the slave trade." The rape of west Africa and west central Africa by the British, French, Dutch, Portuguese, and, latterly, Americans, in the three centuries preceding 1866, resulted in more than ten million Africans being kidnapped and transported to the New World — in particular to the Caribbean, Brazil, and the southeastern seaboard of the United States. Leaving aside the incomprehensible scale of the human violation, this mass exodus also constituted a mass experiment in terms of human biology and virology.

Fleming explained that there was no serological evidence to suggest that either HIV-1 or HIV-2 had been brought to the Americas with the slaves, prior to 1866. By contrast, Robert Gallo's human retrovirus, HTLV-1, was now widely disseminated within black populations in the United States and on most of the islands in the Caribbean, showing that it had been exported from Africa to various destinations across the Atlantic.[19] HTLV-1 and the HIVs are transmitted by similar methods, and this radically different epidemiology therefore offered strong support to the hypothesis that the two HIVs have emerged as human viruses much more recently than the HTLVs, and are probably both less than 130 years old.

We talked about a lot of other issues as well, that June afternoon, but the discussion kept returning to those two words: "Why now?" Why have immunodeficiency viruses only begun to appear in humans within the last century or so?

And why have two geographically distinct epidemics of AIDS, related to HIV-1 and HIV-2, emerged in the space of just five years? What is the new factor in the equation? Answer that one, we agreed, and then start looking around for the pump handle.

Before he left, Alan Fleming had one final piece of advice to offer. "If you're serious about finding out more, you should get yourself to a decent medical library, and spend a few weeks doing some research. There's a lot to be found out, if someone takes the trouble." We shook hands, a sticky handshake, and the tall, fair-haired figure strode off purposefully, cutting a swathe through the crowds of tourists.

Later that afternoon, I walked beneath the white tower of Senate House, the centerpiece of the University of London, and entered a smaller, less imposing building in its lee. Here, in Keppel Street, is the home of the London School of Hygiene and Tropical Diseases, and upstairs on the first floor is housed one of the finest medical libraries in the world.

A few minutes later, I pushed open the door into the great oak-paneled hall of the Barnard Room, and began my search for the source of the epidemic. I started by looking into different theories about the origin of AIDS. Then I set about searching through the literature for early cases of AIDS, both those reported in the first years of the eighties, and those identified retrospectively, from the late seventies. And after that, I began to look for other possible archival cases, for instances of unexplained immunodeficiency and opportunistic infections from even further back in the past.

And quite soon I began to understand the lure of this sort of research. It becomes a bug. It creates its own passions, its own gratifications and rewards. And all too easily, it grows exponentially, with each article producing its own batch of footnotes to follow up, its own sources to check, its own ideas to pursue. Back at home, the reading begins, the papers get read and annotated and filed. New shelves go up on walls; folders of different colors spread slowly around the room. Only slowly does one learn to discriminate, to sort the wheat from the chaff.

I had no way of knowing it then, but that June afternoon was to be the first of many spent searching out articles in the upstairs stacks, twisting and turning the great heavy volumes over a hot photocopy machine, or stretched out comfortably in one of the great leather armchairs by the windows, with a pile of books on the sill, and the plane trees swaying to and fro across the street. Over the next eight years, the Keppel Street library was to become a home from home, as I set about trying to work out what might have happened.

# I

## THE RIVER IN CROSS SECTION:

## FROZEN MOMENTS OF FLOW

*We shall not cease from exploration*
*And the end of all our exploring*
*Will be to arrive where we started*
*And know the place for the first time.*

— T. S. ELIOT, "Little Gidding"

# 1

FROZEN IN TIME: 1959

Let us take a moment in time. Let us freeze it. Let us watch as the crystals form, as it becomes translucent. Let us mount it on a slide and lift it carefully to the microscope stand. Using strong light and mirrors, adjusting the focus, let us see what can be seen.

Truth, like beauty, resides in the eye in the beholder. Whatever the material on that glass slide — be it a moment in history or a cluster of cells — it is inevitable that what you see and what I see will be different. I may see colors, a myriad of dots, a divine impressionistic sweep of light and shade. You, the historian, may see a pattern, a grand design, the beginning of a chain of cause and effect. Now let us change the eyepiece, increase the magnification. This time I may see a meaningless smudge with specks of darkness within, while you, the biologist, may see a nucleus and mitochondria, the beauty of simplicity, the pulsating potential of a cell ready to divide.

How will we describe our truths, you and I, for the blind man, for the child without a microscope? And whose description will be more accurate? While I pack away the lenses, and you put the glass rectangle into its slot in the velvet-upholstered case, remember this. Empirically, the image that you see and that which I see are the same. What differs is our relative clarity of vision, level of understanding, power of analysis — and the language we choose to describe what lies beneath the lens.

---

It is the February of 1959. It is a particular moment in the history of the world. The old order is breaking up; the barriers of time and space are tumbling. The first jet planes are taking off, heading for destinations — Hong Kong, Nairobi, Sydney — that once were days away, but are now just hours. There is a new type of global language too, as people talk of atom bombs, the cold war, of international power blocs, and the arms race.

It is also a particular time in the history of Africa. The wind of change is blowing hard: in the last two years Ghana and Guinea have attained independence, and across the continent the clamor is rising. The old colonial powers — the British, the French, the Belgians — are, each in their own time, recognizing the inevitability of the process, acknowledging that these are the final days of the Raj; only the Portuguese are still defiantly opposed. Here, in the Belgian Congo, amidst the wide, gracious, tree-lined avenues of the capital, Leopoldville, the first round of riots has just ended, with more than fifteen hundred Africans arrested. The Belgians are bewildered. People returning to Brussels tell the man from the London *Times* that "something untoward is brewing at Stanleyville," the town a thousand miles upstream at the great bend in the river.[1]

Meanwhile two doctors, one American and one Belgian, are traveling around the capital immersed in their own world, which is one of scientific inquiry. The American, funded by grants from the U.S. Public Health Service and the Rockefeller Foundation, arrived in Leopoldville just after the end of the unrest, and neither saw evidence of its impact nor, one suspects, would have had much appreciation of its significance had he done so. The Belgian, for his part, has just been appointed chair of microbiology at the newly built university of Lovanium, eight miles from the city center on the banks of the Congo River — but for all that, he is happy for the chance to collaborate with such a rising star in the firmament of human genetics. These are impassioned men operating in an era that reveres their activities, in an era when science is the new religion, and the men in white coats its prophets and priests.

Over the next few weeks the American, Arno Motulsky, and the Belgian, Jean Vandepitte, with the help of other local doctors, start collecting blood samples from medical staff, hospital patients, and police recruits in Leopoldville, and from a large group of villagers living to the south, near the Angolan border. Motulsky is keen to investigate the relative incidence of two genetic traits in different ethnic groups in sub-Saharan Africa, and their possible relationship to malaria. Later, he visits several other regions of the Belgian Congo and the neighboring territory of Ruanda-Urundi, administered by the Belgians as a trusteeship since Germany was dispossessed of its African colonies after the First World War. At the end of three months, he and his Belgian colleagues have collected nearly eighteen hundred blood samples from eight different population groups, including pygmies from the Ituri Forest, hospital patients from Stanleyville, and schoolchildren from the two principal ethnic groups in Ruanda-Urundi, the Tutsi and the Hutu. Most of these samples are finger-prick specimens mounted on glass slides and examined in local laboratories the same day, but more than seven hundred are samples of whole blood, which are then refrigerated and flown back to Motulsky's department at the University of Washington in Seattle.

As Jean Vandepitte bids farewell to Arno Motulsky at the airport, neither man has any inkling of the additional significance which one of these 5-milliliter blood samples will assume just over a quarter of a century later.

————

Independence arrives, and the countries where Motulsky obtained his specimens subsequently become known as the Republic of the Congo,[2] Rwanda, and Burundi. Over the next few years, all three experience tragic events, as ethnic tensions and the meddling of foreign powers combine to promote upheavals, violence, and bloodshed. Meanwhile, back at the University of Washington, various tests are conducted on the blood samples, and a series of papers published in journals of genetics.[3]

Several years later, Moses Schanfield, a professor from Emory University, contacts Motulsky to ask if he can undertake further genetic studies on the Congo cohort, and the remaining 672 frozen plasmas are flown to Atlanta. Finally, in 1985, they change hands once more, and are given to another Emory professor, André Nahmias, who has an entirely different interest. He wants to test them for the presence of antibodies to a virus that has suddenly entered the medical limelight — the virus that causes AIDS. He examines not only the Motulsky samples, but a further 500 plasmas originating from South Africa, Mozambique, and Congo-Brazzaville, and collected at various times between 1959 and 1982.

Over the next few months, the specimens are examined exhaustively, first at Emory and then at Harvard; the results are then confirmed at two other laboratories, by a total of four different testing procedures.[4] Of all the plasma samples, just one comes out strongly positive on all the tests. Its code number is L70, and it comes from a group of ninety-nine specimens taken in 1959, somewhere in or around Leopoldville.

In the mid-eighties, scientists are just awakening to the possibility that HIV (as it will soon become known) may have been present in sub-Saharan Africa for some years before the recognized start of the AIDS epidemic in North America and Europe in 1981, and the Nahmias investigation provides the first really dramatic evidence in support of this hypothesis. No further details appear to be available, however, about the source of the L70 sample. In the 1986 letter to *The Lancet* in which he reports the results of his investigations, Nahmias comments simply: "The identity of the donor is no longer known."[5]

Nearly four decades have passed since his trip to Africa, but Arno Motulsky, now professor emeritus, still lives in Seattle and is still a man of spiky brilliance. And his papers do reveal a little more about the identity of the L70 donor. They record that the blood was taken from a Bantu male, one of seventy-eight men in the group of ninety-nine designated as "Leo."[6] Unfortunately, of all the twelve groups tested by Motulsky,[7] there is less documentation about the "Leo" series than any of the others. Motulsky says that most of them were normal members of the population, and that around 20 percent were hospital patients.[8] The identity of the hospital is not recorded, although Jean Vandepitte, now professor emeritus at the University of Leuven and the Institute of Tropical Medicine in Antwerp, believes that it was probably that at Lovanium, the great campus the Belgians constructed on the outskirts of Leopoldville, and which many consider to have been their parting gift to the country they ruled for seventy-five years.[9]

Whatever, it appears that this tiny amount of blood, taken in 1959 from an unknown man living in the city now known as Kinshasa, the bustling capital of the Congo, represents the oldest specimen of the human immunodeficiency virus in existence. We shall return to it later in the story.

———

As with the early course of a river, where water may seep unnoticed through sphagnum bogs, or plunge underground through limestone, so with the early course of a new disease. It is, of course, entirely possible that the first traces of an unusual and hitherto unseen condition (especially a disease syndrome with a diverse range of presentations and a long latency period, like AIDS) will pass by unremarked. There again, perhaps because of serendipity, or an especially conscientious team of doctors, it can also happen that the crucial clues are noticed and recorded for posterity.

On January 31, 1959, just as Arno Motulsky was leaving for Africa, a twenty-five-year-old man from Reddish, a working-class suburb adjoining Manchester, was getting engaged. At the same time (though he could not have known it) he was becoming involved in a chain of events that would end up with his becoming public property, part of global folklore. For this man, David Carr, was about to become inextricably entwined with the early history of the AIDS epidemic.

By that year, Reddish was a place in decline. Cotton manufacturing was moving overseas to new nations where wages were lower, and the town's huge mill finally closed its doors at the end of 1958. Many were reemployed at the breweries and railway repair yards, but the soul of Reddish seemed to have departed, together with much of its disposable income. There was only a light scattering of TV aerials on the long terraced roofs around the mill. For the fortunate few in the black-and-white flicker below, Harold Macmillan was meeting with General Eisenhower, issuing joint communiqués from Chequers, reminding Britons that — with a nuclear deterrent of their own — they were one of "The Big Three," telling them they had never had it so good.[10] Not all believed him.

The country that had, until recently, viewed itself as lying at the fulcrum of global activity was now in reality a leviathan, grown loose-eyed and sleepy, still touched by memories of wartime sacrifice and ration books. Its grandiose dreams were fading, as one by one the countries of Africa and Asia were granted freedom; the sun was setting on an empire over which, it was once boasted, the sun never set.

———————

Dave Carr was a former seaman, a local Reddish lad with crinkly eyes and wavy brown hair. "Elsie," his fiancée, was from northern Manchester; she had a strikingly trim figure and bright red hair, worn in a perm. They worked within yards of each other in the city center — he as a printer on the *Manchester Evening Chronicle;* she as a mantle machinist, making ladies' gowns and raincoats. Each had a good sense of humor, but whereas Dave was easygoing, Elsie was strong-willed and known for speaking her mind. Their friends thought them a perfect match. To save money, they had bought the engagement ring from a pawnbrokers' shop — a pledge made but broken, never redeemed.

Whether or not Dave and Elsie were planning an early wedding is a moot point, for since the end of the previous year, Dave's health had suddenly collapsed. Throughout 1958 he had suffered from small but persistent ailments — chronic gingivitis, and a funny measles-like rash on his back and shoulders, for which he attended a local skin clinic on a monthly basis, receiving steroid creams and two courses of radiotherapy. In November, he had to have part of his lower gum removed in a gingivectomy, but for some reason, the wounds never healed properly. Then, toward Christmas, he developed a nagging cough and began having serious problems with his breathing. He had only to walk a few hundred yards or climb a flight of steps to end up gasping, panting, propped up against wall or lamppost. He was losing weight as well — a lot of it.[11]

In the weeks that followed the engagement, Dave Carr got substantially worse. In February the hemorrhoids and *pruritis ani* from which he had suffered intermittently for years suddenly became more inflamed, and he developed a painful sore around the anus. The weight loss, night sweats, and fevers also became more pronounced, and now his chronic cough began bringing up mucus which was flecked with blood. He began to take more and more time off work at the *Chronicle,* and after work, over a pint, his mates would talk in undertones about leukemia, or about his picking up some strange bug while swimming in the local canal or during his National Service in the navy.

In March, Dave began seeing a private consultant, Dr. Charles Don. On the morning of his second appointment, in early April, a telegram was delivered, requesting a postponement, but Dave's parents told him to turn up anyway. It was as well that he did. Dr. Don took one look at his patient's anal fissure, now three inches long, and arranged for him to be admitted to the Manchester Royal Infirmary. Ward M4 (male) at the MRI was to become Dave's home for the next five months.

The physicians in charge of the ward, notably the senior registrar, John Leonard, and the senior house officer, Trevor Stretton, were baffled by David Carr's various maladies — the weight loss, persistent cough, breathing difficulties, the sore on his bottom, and the small "blind boil" that had appeared at the tip of his left nostril. All they knew was that here was a man just a few years younger than themselves, who until recently had appeared quite healthy, and who was now wasting away before their eyes, strafed by a series of apparently untreatable infections.

Their first response was to suspect miliary TB, an unusual form of tuberculosis, but when Dave failed to respond to the appropriate drugs, they wondered about sarcoidosis,[12] and the collagen diseases (nowadays known as autoimmune disorders). They had already checked all the known cancers and lymphomas, but now they began to wonder about the possibility of an unknown malignancy.

Of course, they asked him questions about his past, about his time in the navy — and noted that he did not recall having any tropical diseases. They tested for syphilis and found him negative, but they did not question him about his sexuality, for such matters were less frequently and openly discussed in 1959 and, in any case, did not seem relevant to the case. They tried further radiotherapy, together with chemotherapy, steroids, and an even wider range of drugs. Once or twice he picked up briefly, for a week or two, but the remission never lasted.

By June, Dave's fevers were becoming more frequent, and his breathing steadily worse. The spot in his nostril became an ulcer, which started eating away at his nasal cartilage and upper lip; shaving became impossible, so he grew a mustache, but it did little to hide the spreading open wound from view. The anal lesion also grew, until it became an excavated sore the size of a small football, covering most of his buttocks. A cradle was placed over him to keep the weight of the blankets from his body. But most dramatic of all was the emaciation. One year before, David Carr had been a strapping lad of 185 pounds, broad-shouldered and somewhat overweight for his five foot seven inch frame. Now, however, his face was drawn and his bones clearly visible through the skin. Elsie and his parents called at the hospital every day, but Dave began to discourage visits from friends.

Just a few days before Dave and Elsie's engagement, an unusual death occurred in Canada, at Toronto General Hospital. The deceased was a thirty-six-year-old Japanese-Canadian man, who had been admitted six weeks earlier with severe breathing difficulties. Eventually he suffocated to death. At autopsy, Dr. John Barrie, a British émigré pathologist, found a honeycomb of cyst-like cavities throughout the man's lungs, which he ascribed to *Pneumocystis carinii,* a rare pathogen that takes advantage of a state of lowered resistance in the human host.

However, in the case of this patient, George Y., there were no clear indications as to what might have caused his resistance to be diminished, and for this reason Dr. Barrie wrote a paper about the case, which was published the following year.[13] "We are not aware of any reports of deaths in adults which have been caused primarily by infection with *Pneumocystis,*" wrote Barrie, in the introduction. He reported that the patient had been well until March 1958, when he had experienced a five-day fever with chills, headache, and nonproductive cough, an episode that was repeated several times in the following months. In late October, he began to experience sharp pains in his chest, drenching night sweats, and pronounced weight loss. By December 1958, when he was admitted to hospital, he was losing weight dramatically, had chest pains, and would become breathless after the slightest exertion. The physicians administered a range of drugs in a bid to save his life — culminating in 100 milligrams (a very heavy dose) of a steroid, prednisone, every day for the final fortnight. At the autopsy, the only contributory factor noted was a mild cirrhosis of the liver, presumably from drinking.

In 1991, I located Dr. Barrie, by then in his late eighties, and he managed to procure a copy of his original autopsy report. This revealed that George had worked as a sawmill operator during the forties and then, for ten years from 1948, as a carpenter in Edmonton, Alberta. In 1958, however, he abandoned his steady job and migrated north to work in the Northwest Territories. It was when he arrived there in March that he suffered his first illness, followed by another in May, when "he developed . . . a virus infection common in the camp in which he was working at that time." Something, it seems, had caused George Y. to become immunocompromised at some point during the final year or so of his life, leading to his demise from PCP in January 1959.

———

A few months later, in June of that year, *Pneumocystis carinii* pneumonia was responsible for another most unusual adult death at the Kings County Hospital in Brooklyn, New York. The patient, Ardouin A., had been born in Jamaica of Jamaican parents, but the family had moved to Haiti when he was seven, and he emigrated from there to the United States ten years later, marrying a Haitian émigré soon afterward. Ardouin was an attractive man, with slicked-back hair, a thin mustache, and sharp dress sense — and he apparently had several girl-friends on the side. He also had several jobs, but after the Second World War began working as a shipping clerk for a dress manufacturer on Seventh Avenue in Manhattan — a post he was to keep for the rest of his life.

Ardouin had never been seriously ill in his forty-nine years, but in March 1959 his smoker's cough became more severe and productive of large amounts of sputum, and he began losing weight. By June, his chest pains and wheezing had gotten so serious that he was admitted to hospital, where he was quickly placed on a respirator and treated with steroids. His doctors asked many questions and wanted to know whether he had ever been to Nevada, which suggests they thought he might have been present at an atom bomb test; he had not. They also tested his blood, bone marrow, and urine (including a check for beryllium content, since he had apparently broken a fluorescent lamp some while earlier), but found nothing untoward. Ardouin, meanwhile, became weaker, and told his family that he wanted to be buried in his blue suit. His prognosis was correct, for on June 28 he had to have a hole cut in his windpipe to assist his breathing, and he died later the same day.[14]

His widow was terrified, fearing that voodoo was involved — while the pathologist, Gordon Hennigar, was mystified as to why he could find no underlying disease that might explain why the *Pneumocystis* infection had taken hold and proved so remorseless. The case was sufficiently unusual to be written up in two medical journals,[15] and although one of the papers pointed out that the white blood cell count had sometimes been high (which might suggest a leukemoid reaction), its conclusion was that Ardouin represented "the first reported instance of unassociated [*Pneumocystis carinii*] disease in an adult." Dr. Hennigar, meanwhile, decided to pickle Ardouin's lungs for posterity.

---

While Gordon Hennigar filled his bell jar with formalin, back in the Manchester Royal Infirmary, David Carr's symptoms were progressing inexorably. By July, the latest theory of his doctors was that he was suffering from Wegener's granulomatosis, a fatal disorder of the connective tissue that often involves the respiratory tract. Altogether, just fifty-six cases of Wegener's had been recorded in the medical literature.[16]

Dave kept cheerful to the end, but by August he and Elsie and his parents all knew that he was dying. At this stage, pustular ulcers were appearing on his stomach, inner thighs, and fingers, over both his lips, and inside his mouth. He developed spiking fevers and found it more and more difficult to breathe. He had what appeared to be an untreatable pneumonia, and sometimes he became cyanotic, with his extremities turning blue from lack of oxygen and his fingers swelling at the tips. In the final week of his life, he was put in a separate room and treated with Euphoricus, a sedative cocktail of morphine, cocaine, and gin. At three o'clock on the afternoon of August 31, as he was being lifted on to the commode, he died.

It was only when the tissues taken at autopsy were examined microscopically by pathologist George Williams that two unexpected conditions were identified. One was disseminated "cytomegalic inclusion disease," a condition caused by a virus that, the following year, would be renamed cytomegalovirus, or CMV. The other was *Pneumocystis carinii* pneumonia, PCP.

Thus, in the first eight months of 1959, three apparently healthy men from different parts of the world died primarily as a result of PCP, a disease previously unrecognized in healthy adults. During the next twenty-five years, the doctors who had been involved with these three patients, either alive or dead, continued to be intrigued by their illnesses, and by the continuing mystery of underlying cause. At times they would review their papers, and wonder about this possibility or that — exposure to some toxic agent, an undiagnosed cancer or leukemia, a congenital immunodeficiency that they had failed to spot. But none of these tentative explanations was entirely convincing. It was only in the eighties, after the recognition of the AIDS epidemic, that a solution to the mystery seemed to have emerged — for between 1983 and 1987, several researchers proposed that these three deaths might represent pre-epidemic cases of AIDS.[17]

Were they right? Was David Carr in Reddish an antecedent of the coming epidemic? Were George in Toronto and Ardouin in New York? Were these men the harbingers of a new disease beginning its global spread, the earliest, unfortunate infectees with some new pathogen that was already — in 1959 — becoming widely dispersed, albeit extremely thinly? This is one of the hypotheses that we will be investigating in some detail in the course of this book.

---

As the condition of David in Manchester deteriorated ever faster, and as Ardouin in Brooklyn entered the final week of his life, a very different event was taking place in Washington, D.C. Whereas the savage disease processes affecting these two men were graphic reminders of how, even in the best-equipped medical systems in the world, nature could still get the better of doctors, this latter event was essentially a celebration of the triumph of modern medicine over disease.

Poliomyelitis, until then the most dreaded of illnesses, the one that caused authorities to close down schools and swimming pools, and that persuaded people across America to donate their small change to the March of Dimes, was about to be vanquished, and the world's pre-eminent virologists and physicians had gathered in the national capital to witness the coup de grâce.

The event was called the First International Conference on Live Poliovirus Vaccines, and among the seventy attendees from the ranks of the great and the good were two doctors — Albert Sabin and Hilary Koprowski — who had probably done more than any others to bring about this hugely popular scientific achievement, this metaphorical lunar landing of the fifties. Both of them had developed their own sets of oral polio vaccines (OPVs), and all the indications were that the United States was about to adopt either Sabin's or Koprowski's strains. In fact the stakes were even higher, for it was apparent that whichever vaccine set was approved in America would — in all probability — be adopted by the rest of the world also.

The principle of vaccination is that a tiny amount of a virus (either a weakened live virus, or else a virus that has been killed by chemicals like formalin) is introduced to the vaccinee, whose immune system responds by producing the appropriate antibodies. The subject will then be protected against exposure to the "wild" form of the virus found in nature, which might otherwise cause serious disease. In the case of poliomyelitis, the first vaccine to be adopted for general use in America — in 1955 — was the killed vaccine developed by Jonas Salk. Referred to by scientists as an inactivated polio vaccine, or IPV, this preparation had already, by 1959, been given to millions of children around the world. It was, however, gradually falling out of favor by the end of the decade — and not just because sugar lumps are more popular with kids than shots in the arm. More crucially, there were demonstrable problems with its safety and effectiveness. In one infamous episode, the "Cutter incident," hundreds of vaccinees and their close contacts contracted polio because a batch of vaccine had been improperly inactivated.[18] Furthermore, by the end of the decade, an increasing number of vaccinees were becoming paralyzed even after receiving the full course of three shots, showing that not all batches of the vaccine were protective.

By 1959, many virologists were persuaded that the more easily administered oral vaccines of Sabin and Koprowski were also capable of giving longer-lasting protection. On the question of safety, opinions were more divided. The live poliovirus in OPVs has first been weakened, or attenuated, by a series of passages* through animals (such as rodents and monkeys) or through tissue cultures (layers of cells — typically from chicken embryos or the kidneys of monkeys — that are kept alive under laboratory conditions). However, the theoretical side of attenuation (relating to what causes the poliovirus to become

---

\* Passage: With regard to a virus, passage involves inoculating the virus into a foreign host (a different animal species from its natural host) or foreign tissue culture, allowing it to multiply, and then harvesting it again. This often causes genetic modifications to the virus, including a reduction in its ability to cause disease.

innocuous for humans, and what keeps it that way) was still shrouded in mystery.[19] For this reason there was considerable interest when, in a discussion session on the fourth day of the conference, Professor Albert Sabin made a dramatic accusation.[20]

He repeated a claim that he had first made three months earlier, in an article in the *British Medical Journal*,[21] that at least one batch of his rival Koprowski's CHAT vaccine, which had been fed to hundreds of thousands of vaccinees in the Belgian Congo, had been contaminated with an unidentified simian virus, one that had nothing to do with polio — but which, like polio, was cytopathic (it killed cells when introduced into monkey kidney tissue culture). The unspoken inference was clear — that such a virus might also do damage when introduced into human beings.

A renowned Swedish virologist, Dr. Sven Gard, who had been on several months' sabbatical at Koprowski's research center, the Wistar Institute, spoke up in his defense. Gard said that he had tested the same lot of vaccine for the presence of extraneous virus, both in Sweden and the United States, and had found nothing.[22]

And there, apparently, the matter rested. Certainly there is no further reference to the affair in the published record of the conference. But by voicing his concern, Albert Sabin had invoked a specter that was hovering over the proceedings — the fear that OPVs, even while they were bringing the most feared viral disease of the era under control, might also be introducing new and perhaps more sinister viral agents into mankind, ones that proliferated during the process of vaccine manufacture.

This was a fear that was to become very much more substantial over the years that followed, as virologists began to learn a lot more about tissue cultures, especially monkey kidney tissue cultures, and the many ways in which they could become contaminated. Naturally, new procedures were introduced to ensure the safety of vaccines. But many of these men, when they looked back years later with the benefit of hindsight, would shiver at the risks which they had inadvertently taken in those days of blissful ignorance, those days of hope and courage, in the fifties.

---

Put the slide back in the case. Pick another. Here, try this one, from the nineties. Let us see whether it provides a different perspective — one that benefits from the accumulation of scientific wisdom. Perhaps try another lens, too. Some, of course, may have the corrective properties of hindsight.

It is March of 1993. The intervening years have seen further great victories for vaccination programs and the public health system, with the conquest of smallpox, and the suppression of malaria, measles, and cholera. But they have also witnessed significant reverses, such as the emergence of AIDS and the re-emergence of tuberculosis.

And now, almost thirty-four years after that first international conference on live poliovirus vaccines, Albert Bruce Sabin has died peacefully at his home in Washington, D.C., at the age of eighty-six. Despite his many achievements during more than six decades of scientific toil,[23] he was always best known for his development of the OPVs, which would later be adopted in almost every country in the world. Now, in 1993, the World Health Organization is promoting a campaign of global poliomyelitis eradication by the year 2000.[24] Even if this may be optimistic, polio is likely to become only the second viral disease to be conquered by human intervention, a state of affairs that owes much to the success of Albert Sabin's slightly dirty-looking sugar lumps.[25]

One of Sabin's many other achievements was to identify a herpes virus of monkeys (B virus, or herpes B), which is harmless to its natural host but almost invariably fatal when transferred into humans, as evidenced by the deaths of some two-dozen monkey handlers and laboratory workers since the thirties.[26] Sabin's discovery of herpes B virus identified what then seemed the most formidable danger inherent in handling monkeys and their organs, and facilitated the adoption of minced monkey kidneys as a tissue culture for *in vitro* research and for the cultivation of viruses. This in turn paved the way for the golden age of virology in the fifties, and the production of polio vaccines on a commercial scale.

During his final years, Albert Sabin became increasingly concerned by the problem of AIDS, and wrote articles and letters about the problems inherent in developing an effective vaccine against the syndrome. The last of these was published in *Nature* a fortnight after his death.[27] Like its predecessors, it predicted that attempts to vaccinate against HIV would prove unsuccessful, and ended with the words "In my judgment, it would be disastrous to continue the current inadequate methods of study of HIV and SIV* vaccines, and to carry out large scale tests in humans of vaccines without adequate evidence that such vaccines can protect against natural infection." From such an *eminence grise,* these were powerful final words of warning.

Five weeks after Sabin's death, an obituary was published in *Nature.*[28] It opened with a reference to "the heroic age of poliomyelitis research" and an acknowledgment that Sabin had been "one of the heroes," before moving on to review Sabin's life and works. By this stage of the obituary, the observant reader might have begun to suspect that writer and subject had not always been in agreement.

---

\* SIV: Simian immunodeficiency virus, the monkey equivalent of HIV.

This was frankly admitted in the final paragraph, which read:

At one time, Sabin and I became adversaries over the selection of polio virus strains to be used as oral vaccines. This did not affect our long-lasting friendship and mutual respect. In a letter to me written just a year ago, reviewing a paper speculating that AIDS started with polio vaccination in the Belgian Congo,[29] Sabin expressed his opinion that this was "a most irresponsible and uncritical communication." Courageous and wise. This is how I see him. I will miss him sorely.

The obituary was signed Hilary Koprowski, from the Wistar Institute in Philadelphia.

Several of the scientists who knew the two men from the time of their great rivalry in the fifties and early sixties were intrigued by the obituary. They too had vivid recollections of the period, though their memories were rather different from Koprowski's. They spoke of two Jewish émigrés from Eastern Europe, both possessed of keen intellects and quick tempers — coupled, however, with great powers of persuasion (and, in Koprowski's case, of charm). They spoke of two men cast from the same mold, men who shared many of the same tendencies and personality traits — but who had somehow evolved into polar opposites.

Few of them recalled any tangible friendship (let alone one that was long-lasting) between Sabin and Koprowski, or remembered demonstrations of mutual respect. Instead, they spoke of a bitter enmity that had been barely — if at all — concealed in their respective articles in the medical literature and papers delivered at the great virology conferences of the day. They remembered the occasions when the great men had posed together, smiling, for the photographers, and then each had swiftly turned on his heel the moment the cameras were packed away.[30] This rivalry, some of them hinted, had perhaps stemmed from the fact that Koprowski had been the first to feed an oral polio vaccine to humans in 1950, fully three years before Sabin had entered the field — and yet it was Sabin's vaccines that had been licensed, Sabin who had won the lasting acclaim. "Koprowski and Sabin hated each other," one contemporary told me.[31] "Salk, Sabin, Koprowski, Cox — I would have loved to see them tag-team wrestling," said another, referring to the four great polio vaccine-makers.[32] "They were fighting like dogs over a bone — about who would make the vaccine of choice," said a third.[33]

Given this history, many scientists were dubious about Koprowski's motivation for praising Sabin's wisdom — particularly as, in the same breath, he noted Sabin's rejection of a theory that suggested that one of his (Koprowski's) vaccines had given birth to AIDS. Perhaps in 1993 few scientists would have recalled that, back in 1959, it was Sabin who had introduced the first slither of doubt about the safety of this very vaccine.

All in all, there was much that the obituary left unsaid, some of which has great relevance for the story that follows. We shall return to the tale of the obituary writer, and his uneasy relationship with his subject — a relationship that helped define the characters of both men — later in this book.

# 2

FROZEN IN SPACE:

A RURAL EPICENTER IN AFRICA

Sometimes a statement or a version of events gets repeated so often that it becomes accepted by a large part of humanity as fact, even when the supporting evidence has been disproved long before. This is one of the ways in which myth can take over from reality. An example of a commonly accepted myth in the public mind would be that HIV came from the African green monkey — a claim that began with an erroneous report based on a lab contamination in the mid-eighties, but which is still believed by many people to this day. Like many myths, if taken literally this version of events is incorrect, but if regarded as a broad representation of the truth that the human viruses causing AIDS originated from viruses found in various African monkeys, then it has some merit.

This chapter introduces several different aspects of the origins investigation by focusing on another popular AIDS myth — that the disease emerged from the area bordering Lake Victoria in eastern Africa, and specifically from Rakai district in Uganda and Kagera region in Tanzania. This scenario began with the observation that a particular area was heavily stricken with AIDS, and continued through local mythology (attempts to explain the calamity) to another sort of mythology, peddled by Western reporters: that here, perhaps, lay the source of the global pandemic. Such versions of events met the needs of specific groups of people at particular moments in time — and although they contained a kernel of truth, a figurative integrity, the reality, as we shall see, was rather different.

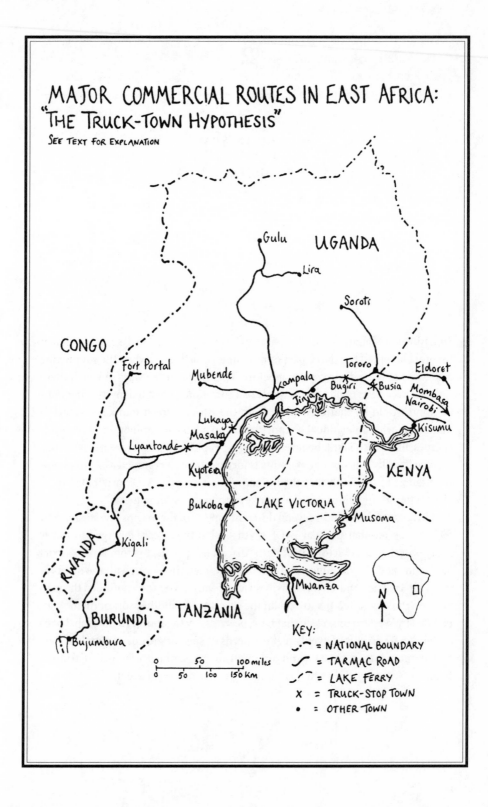

MAJOR COMMERCIAL ROUTES IN EAST AFRICA:
"THE TRUCK-TOWN HYPOTHESIS"
SEE TEXT FOR EXPLANATION

UGANDA

Gulu

Lira

Soroti

CONGO

Fort Portal

Mubende

Tororo

Eldoret

Kampala

Bugiri

Busia

Mombasa
Nairobi

Jinja

Lukaya

Masaka

Kisumu

Lyantonde

Kyotera

KENYA

Bukoba

LAKE VICTORIA

Musoma

RWANDA

Kigali

Mwanza

N

BURUNDI

TANZANIA

Bujumbura

KEY:
= NATIONAL BOUNDARY
= TARMAC ROAD
= LAKE FERRY
X = TRUCK-STOP TOWN
• = OTHER TOWN

0      50     100 miles
0    50   100   150 KM

(Kasensero, southwestern Uganda, August 1986)[1]

Down at the lakeshore, the water fell in tiny waves on the beach. The waves made light, careless slaps as they fell on the shallow sands, and the rhythm was uncertain, varying as it did with the vagaries of the onshore wind. The waves pressed forward one after the other, not quite reaching as far as the long, narrow fishing boats, which had been dragged up on the beach, among the rubbery lacustrine shrubs that grew there. A few cattle grazed lazily on these shrubs, their great lyre-shaped horns rising and falling, sometimes knocking against wooden gunwales, as one or other tried to flick away the flies that swarmed in the noonday heat. Fifty yards away, back in the village, smoke curled up as the first of the day's catch was committed to the fire.

Half an hour later the French photographer Roland Neveu and I took our places on a couple of wooden crates in the strip of shade beneath a corrugated iron roof, and began eating chunks of oily Nile perch from enamel bowls swirled with garish color. The fish would have tasted sweet even without the long, bumpy drive that had occupied much of the morning — from the village of Kyebe, up on the hill, over the rutted tracks of the smugglers' road as it wound across the swamp toward Kasensero.

Babies played in the dirt near the drainage channel that ran between the huts, and every few minutes a woman would emerge, stooping, adjusting her *khanga* around waist or breasts as she did so, to scoop up an infant who had strayed too far, or to hang out washing. Sometimes she would smile across at the strangers who sat on the crates. Most of the people of the village seemed to be young: in their teens or early twenties.

Lunch over, I wandered off to locate one of the few men in the village who spoke English. John had arrived in Kasensero from Masaka, the regional capital, a few months before: there were hints of trouble at home and a forced departure. Since his arrival, he had become relatively wealthy — from fishing, he claimed, though most of the local youths were also involved in smuggling sacks of coffee, car tires, batteries, and blankets across a small arc of Lake Victoria from Tanzania, a few miles to the south. Whatever, John was rich enough to have a girlfriend, and to see her two or three times a week. The rest of the time she worked as a bar-girl at one of the mud-walled hostelries in the main street; on these evenings she usually spent the night with other men.

John looked fit and healthy. He felt so, too. He was not, he explained, one of those affected by this strange sickness that had recently appeared in the region, causing so much death and misery.

In the late afternoon, as the shadows lengthened beneath Kasensero's single tall tree, one of the elders called a meeting, so that the villagers could tell us about the disease, which had first arrived there some four years earlier. Since that year of 1982, over a hundred people — both Kasensero residents and those who came down to the lake to fish, or smuggle, or sell their bodies — had succumbed to the new disease. These persons had died in a variety of nasty ways. The mouths and throats of some had filled with a strange, creamy paste that would not go away; others had been racked with coughs and fevers, had developed sores on face and body, or had been plagued with constant diarrhea.

The one common factor seemed to be that nearly all had become thin and shrunken, like the wraiths and ghouls and nightwalkers that are a constant theme in Kiganda folklore. It was perhaps for this reason that the Baganda peoples of Kasensero and the surrounding district of Rakai (and, later on, the central part of Uganda around the capital, Kampala) readily identified the sickness as something unprecedented in their area — and as a single entity, rather than a syndrome of many different conditions.[2] And since this was clearly a new disease, they chose a new name for it: a descriptive name, but also one that was sweet and rather sad. The Baganda love playing with words and, given the violence of their recent past, have developed an affinity for hidden meaning and double entendre. What is more, as a nation of shopkeepers, they have taken brand names and the other paraphernalia of capitalism to their hearts. And so, with a playful nod to the cut then popular in Western shirts and to the elfin figures then fashionable among Western women, they called this new disease "Slim."

The shadows moved on the ground, and the people beneath the great tree spoke out. They said that Slim had come from over the border, from Tanzania. Some said it had started because of witchcraft, after Ugandan traders had cheated their Tanzanian counterparts. Others denied this, saying it had come with the soldiers who had invaded the country and overthrown its tyrannical ruler, Idi Amin Dada, seven years earlier. Some remembered a morning of bombardment by rocket, *saba saba* in the local slang, which caused Amin's soldiers to flee the area — and they said Slim started then, on that day of madness and crescendo. Another, older man said that it was a punishment from God — divine retribution for too much greed and loose living. Yet another speaker had heard about this sickness on the radio — about the fact that it was rife in America among men who loved men, and among those who took drugs. This was not an African disease, he explained, this was something brought by the whites, by the *bazungu*. There were murmurs of agreement, and a sudden shriek of nervous laughter from one of the men at the back.

Several of the speakers identified the first case of Slim as being a woman called Regina, who had died in 1982. She had been a trader and part-time prostitute who had conducted regular trips to Lukunyu, the small port some six miles south of Kasensero, just past where the great Kagera River unloads into Lake Victoria, but still a mile or two from the border with Tanzania.

Presently, somebody asked us what we knew about Slim: what could be done about it; what medicines were available to fight the disease? Embarrassed, we looked at each other; eventually it was I who spoke. There were no effective drugs at present, I told them — though, Roland added, some of the best scientists and doctors in the West were searching hard for a cure. The only way to fight this thing, I went on, was to avoid having injections with needles that had been used on other people and that had not first been sterilized in a flame, or in boiling water — and, above all, to avoid having sex unless one was protected by a condom. Earlier, we had seen a few condoms on sale at a store in the trading center of Kyebe, up on the hill, but there seemed to be none in Kasensero. A while later the meeting broke up — and some of the villagers were visibly and audibly disgruntled as they moved away.

Down on the shoreline, the waves slapped away lightly — slip, slap, slip, slip, slap. These were love-slaps, tenderly given, like those which some Ugandan women bestow on their men when they have finished making love.

---

I still look back on that day with a mixture of sadness and horror. I replay the scene over again, and hear the villagers' question: what can you tell us to help us save our lives? And I recall how we answered: go and buy a small package from a store which is three hours' walk away, something that most of you cannot afford and that many of you do not know how to use and that, even when you do know, you will hate with an angry, stubborn passion. You men, unaccustomed as you are to public speaking about sex, will make boyish jokes about it being like sucking a sweet with the wrapper still on. While you women, less inhibited perhaps — at least among yourselves — will throw up hands and shriek and laugh, and then claim, indignantly, that such a tiny, sticky thing would become lodged in the vagina, and prove impossible to extricate. I hear your voices now; I hear your mirth, your indignation, your embarrassment. "Skin on skin," I hear you say; "it is the only way."

Some years later, I phoned Roland at his new home in Los Angeles, and we talked about Kasensero. God, he said, I wonder how it is today. I wonder how many are still alive. We talked about the people who had helped us for those few days in the August of 1986 — about the grave, dignified council chairman Joseph Ssebyoto-Lutaya, about Jimmy Ssemambo, the health assistant who was always smiling, always eager to help, and Perpetua, the woman who did the injections with a few blunt needles in the front room of her house, and who insisted, in a whisper, how she boiled them after every use. We recalled those bumpy drives around Kyebe subcounty when, bearing cameras and notebooks, we joined the great throngs at the funerals among the banana trees. We remembered how Joseph and Jimmy led us to trading centers to talk with knots of worried youths, to smallholdings where grandparents had only grandchildren left to care for, and to houses where young men and women were dying dreadful, fetid deaths, laid out on pallets of straw in their own front rooms.

When I first wrote this passage, in 1995, I was thinking of Joseph and Jimmy and others like them, in the hope that despite the desperate unfairness of being born in that time and that place, with a fatal virus lying in wait in bloodstreams all around, threatening such awful consequence for such small and innocent transgression . . . in the hope that, despite all this, they were not too stubborn. And that somehow, miraculously, they had managed to survive.

Just a few months later, a friend of mine visited Kasensero, and returned with sad news. Joseph, he told me, had died of Slim in November 1992, and his wife two months later. Jimmy had also succumbed, in the June of 1995. Like so many others in Rakai district, and in Uganda, and elsewhere around the world, they too had ended up paying an inappropriate price for those few brief moments of pleasure and intimacy.

---

They were successful — the articles, the photographs, the video.[3] They struck a chord. And in the months that followed a new profession — journalists — joined the fishermen, smugglers, and bar-girls bouncing along the long, rutted track down to Kasensero. By that stage, it was certain that Slim disease was a form of AIDS, albeit a more enteropathic presentation than that usually witnessed in Europe and America (largely because the pathogens in a tropical African environment are different from those present in San Franciscan bathhouses or shooting galleries in Edinburgh). By then, doctors in Kampala had taken blood from hundreds of patients with Slim, including some from the lakeside port, and determined that the great majority contained antibodies to HIV.[4]

The patient histories strongly suggested that here was an AIDS epidemic driven by straight sex, rather than by gay sex or by junkies sharing needles, and the Western press was awestruck by the implications. Here was something else to have come "Out of Africa," they informed their readers: here was the dark, sinister counterpoint to the mellow vision that had swept the 1985 Oscars. Many could not resist this apocalyptic vision of a new virus, incurable and fatal for humans, which had somehow escaped from the lakes and forests to begin its slow, inexorable sweep around the globe.

The newspaper and magazine reports that followed varied from the carefully researched to the sensational, but they all bore the underlying sense that what was happening in Kasensero, in Rakai district — indeed, in Uganda and in sub-Saharan Africa as a whole — might be happening before long in a neighborhood closer to home.[5]

The questions which most fascinated the reporters were the obvious ones: how had HIV arrived here, and what had caused such a cataclysmic explosion of AIDS in the general population of such a remote place? Clearly something extraordinary had happened, for in 1987 there was no other rural zone in the world that had seen devastation like that in Rakai district and the neighboring Tanzanian region of Kagera. Such was the impact on visiting reporters that some even went so far as to claim that these lakeside villages represented the source, the "core of infection," of the global pandemic.[6]

The first question that needs to be asked about these small fishing villages alongside Lake Victoria is therefore a simple one. Were the reporters right — is this where AIDS began?

---

The official version of the arrival of AIDS in Uganda was given by the chairman of the Ugandan AIDS Control Program, Dr. Samuel Ikwaras Okware, in his address to a national seminar about the syndrome held in August 1987.[7] At that time, suggestions that AIDS might have been present in Africa earlier than elsewhere still had explosive potential, especially for the careers of African doctors involved in AIDS control. Sam Okware, therefore, did not beat about the bush. "AIDS," he began, "is a new disease in Uganda.

"Towards the end of 1982," he went on, "several local traders engaged in illicit trade and smuggling across the border died at Kasensero fishing village on Lake Victoria. This was almost two years after the disease had been reported in the USA and elsewhere in Africa. When they died the population took it lightly, because it was believed that such misfortune was a result of natural justice against cheats and smugglers. Decent businessmen smiled, but smiles stopped when spouses of the AIDS victims started dying. Everyone got concerned; the survivors fled inland to the towns, taking with them the infection. Many spent sleepless nights, especially those who had had affairs with prostitutes."

This account, which by and large concurs with the one that Roland and I were given in Kasensero in 1986, is not, however, the last word on the matter. Several of the Western journalists who followed us to "the AIDS villages of Uganda" asked the same questions that we had asked, but came up with rather earlier dates. Badru Rashid, the local political leader of Rakai district, told several reporters that the first cases had appeared in 1979;[8] others reported the key year as 1980,[9] but all sources agreed that the first deaths had occurred shortly after the liberation war of 1978/9 that had resulted in the overthrow of Idi Amin.

Perhaps the most convincing interviewee was Dr. Folgensius Mwebe, head of Kalisizo Health Center, at that time the only large medical facility in Rakai district, who told the writer Alex Shoumatoff that he thought AIDS had made its appearance by 1980.[10] In that year, one of Dr. Mwebe's uncles died of Kaposi's sarcoma, seven years after which the man's widow and one of his girlfriends succumbed to "classic AIDS immunosuppression."

Such dates are lent further substance by Dr. Wilson Carswell, a Scottish surgeon who became a leading figure in the early fight against AIDS in Uganda. He believes that in 1979 or 1980 some of Amin's ex-soldiers may have died of AIDS in Luzira Prison, just outside Kampala. He recalls seeing some of their corpses, which apparently weighed only about half of the normal body weight of an African male, and he believes that certain of these men had suffered from fever, diarrhea, and tuberculosis (the classic presentations of African AIDS).[11]

Also significant is the evidence of Dr. Teasdale Corti, a Canadian missionary who worked as a surgeon at Lacor Hospital, Gulu, in northern Uganda, from 1961 until her death from AIDS in August 1996. During those years she conducted more than three thousand war surgery operations, many of them on soldiers and civilians wounded in the liberation war in 1979; she had to remove many of the shards of bone by hand, and often cut herself in the process. She learned that she was HIV-positive in 1985, but according to her biographer, Michel Arseneault, was already showing many of the symptoms of AIDS (including weight loss, pneumonia, candidiasis, and coughing) as early as 1982. He believes that Dr. Corti was most likely to have been infected during one of the many 1979 operations, which would be consistent with HIV having already infected either Ugandan or Tanzanian soldiers by that year.[12]

These dates are supported by evidence from the other side of the border. As in Uganda, there is an official version, which has it that AIDS first appeared in Tanzania in 1983, in the form of three cases from the south of Kagera region, which adjoins Rakai district in Uganda.[13] Laurie Garrett's excellent 1988 reports for *Newsday* also mention 1983, but move the location fifty miles northward, up to the border; she records the first case as involving a Tanzanian woman from Lukunyu.[14]

All sources agree, however, that Kagera region, at least in the early days, was the worst-affected part of Tanzania. In 1987, for instance, more than 60 percent of all Tanzania's reported AIDS cases came from there.[15] Garrett, in 1988, reports that "nearly one in five" of the one thousand inhabitants of Kanyigo, a village near the border, had died of AIDS, and quotes local doctors as saying that over half the young adults and over 80 percent of the bar-girls in the regional capital of Bukoba were now HIV-positive.[16] Even if a serological survey conducted in 1987 revealed rather lower HIV prevalence (for instance 24 percent for adults in Bukoba, and 10 percent for adults in the surrounding rural districts), these were still very high figures for so early in the epidemic.[17]

But to get a more accurate idea of the first appearances of AIDS in Tanzania, personal testimony is once again important. Dr. Margerete Bundschuh is a German missionary doctor in her seventies, who worked in the country for thirty-one years. Until 1980, she was based at Kagondo hospital, to the south of Bukoba in the middle of Kagera district, and during this period she saw no cases that — even in retrospect — were suggestive of AIDS.[18]

But at the start of 1981 she moved to the hospital at Mugana, situated fifteen miles northwest of Bukoba and a similar distance south of Lukunyu. She recalls that in June 1981 five women from one of the border villages "in the free-trade zone beside Lake Victoria" attended the hospital. All were suffering from anaer-obic ulcers, which had destroyed the anal sphincter and the whole perianal region. A man from the same area also visited at around this time; his penis was apparently "half rotted off." After quite lengthy treatment, but without any clin-ical improvement, the patients returned home and were never seen again. Dr. Bundschuh thought that the cause was the virus *Molluscum contagiosum,* com-plicated by "serious immune-deficiency." It seems very possible that the disease cluster may have represented a geographically localized group who had been dually exposed to both HIV and *M. contagiosum* (or some other sexually trans-mitted pathogen).

Dr. Bundschuh continues: "About one year later, we observed patients with the full picture of AIDS — [wasting], candidiasis in mouth, serious diarrhea, pneumonia — death. We had the impressions — sex infection, three to six months of slow deterioration, then acute serious disease and death. At that time there was no long stage of undetectable AIDS."[19]

This valuable personal testimony, which appears to put back the arrival of AIDS in Tanzania by one or two years, also serves to confirm some of the phe-nomena observed in Uganda — that the arrival of the "new disease" seems to correlate in place and time with the smuggling trade and the liberation war — and that some of the earliest cases may have been extremely rapid compared to the slow progression to AIDS that is familiar today.[20]

This hypothesis is strengthened by one other case history: that of Craig H., a forty-seven-year-old Scottish economist who worked in Tanzania between November 1979 and 1981. He first reported to a Tanzanian hospital with fever and weight loss in March 1981, but when his illness worsened he flew to Stockholm, where he was treated for what would now be termed AIDS-Related Complex, or ARC.[21] He eventually died of AIDS-like symptoms (CMV, toxo-plasmosis, *Klebsiella* pneumonia, and a cerebral lymphoma) in Glasgow in December 1982,[22] and the diagnosis was confirmed when his stored blood later tested HIV-positive.[23] A friend of the deceased has revealed that he had sexual relationships with hundreds of women in the course of various postings, but that his steady Tanzanian girlfriend in Dar es Salaam — a former prostitute — had been showing signs of weight loss and unexplained fever from as early as June 1980, and that she subsequently died in her early thirties.[24] If indeed this woman was the source of Craig's infection, then it took only a year or so for him to develop his first symptoms, and three years for him to die of AIDS. We shall return to the subject of the speed of progression to AIDS at a later point.

———

It would seem, therefore, that the first East African cases of Slim were appear-ing in the Rakai/Kagera region in about 1980, and that occasional cases may have been cropping up in the main Ugandan and Tanzanian cities, Kampala and Dar, at around the same time. Although this is relatively early in the epidemic — before the syndrome was recognized and named in the United States — it certainly does not represent the first appearance of AIDS in *Homo sapiens,* for (as we shall presently see) AIDS cases were cropping up in North America, Europe, and elsewhere in Africa back in the seventies. It is therefore highly unlikely that this region represents the source of AIDS.

However, the rural zone of Rakai and Kagera does appear to have been the first area in the world to have witnessed a raging epidemic among the general population. Why should this be? To examine this further, we need to look at how the virus might have arrived here, and why — once it entered the community — it spread so rapidly, and to such disastrous effect.

First it is worth examining the views of those living in Rakai and Kagera, in the apparent epicenter. As already explained, the local explanations for the arrival of this calamity included "fallout" from the *saba saba*[25] rockets used by the Tanzanians in the liberation war of 1978/9, divine retribution for worldly sins, and revenge wrought by Tanzanian witch doctors on Ugandan traders who had welshed on their debts.[26] Another explanation involved *buwuka* — tiny insects, which were said to pass between partners during sex.[27]

There are variations on these themes. Amid the glut of articles about the AIDS villages that followed those first reports from Rakai district in 1986,[28] undoubtedly the best was by Alex Shoumatoff, whose journey "In Search of the Source of AIDS" ended down at Kasensero with the following passage: "The sick ones here say the people of Ukerewe and Kome [islands in the Tanzanian part of Lake Victoria] did it to them. . . . It came from there. I wonder if it is worth taking a boat to Ukerewe and Kome, and decide against it. . . . Some more enterprising quester can chase the elusive source over the next rise."[29] In fact, Ukerewe and Kome are both large, quite populous islands situated over a hundred miles away on the far shores of the lake — and a study published in 1995 found that HIV prevalence on Ukerewe was very low compared to the rest of Tanzania.[30]

However, there is another possible interpretation. In 1986 I had been told that AIDS came from the "Bakerebwe," a group of Tanzanian witch doctors whose exact location was never specified, but who were said by some to come from small islands in Lake Victoria.[31] Shoumatoff's people from Ukerewe island (or "Bakerewe") may therefore represent another version of the witch-doctor myth. This is supported by the fact that the traditional name for the lake in Luganda, the tongue of the Baganda people who live in these parts, is also Ukerewe.[32] On this level, therefore, the Bakerewe could be simply "people of the lake."

Across the border in Tanzania, where AIDS has been christened "Juliana," a slightly different explanation obtains. According to Laurie Garrett, the tale involves a Ugandan trader who, at the beginning of the eighties, used to sell a beautiful, patterned cloth called Juliana on both sides of the border. A young Tanzanian woman from Lukunyu coveted this cloth to make a *khanga*, but lacked the necessary money — so the trader had sex with her in lieu of payment. Other women also were attracted to the unusual pattern and some of them, also, paid for it with sex — and these were the women, some time later, who were the first to fall sick, starting with the woman from Lukunyu.[33] The locals concluded that the Ugandan trader must have been a witch.

The story of the merchant and his cloth has the same irresistible appeal and moral imperative as tales from the Old Testament. However, it is not the only explanation, for others who have lived and worked in Kagera region claim that Juliana is also the local name for a prostitute.[34]

Again, the ninety-six-year-old chief of Gwanda parish in Kyebe told a visiting epidemiologist about a woman from Busungwe island (which lies a mile outside Lukunyu) who "had a black seed."[35] The chief said that the woman was "very, very beautiful," and implied that she had had sex with many of the men from Lukunyu and Kasensero.[36] This would seem to represent a composite version of the tale of Regina, the prostitute, and the mysterious people from the islands in the lake.

There are thus several versions of origin, from both sides of the border, that point to Lukunyu as the place where the epidemic "began" — and these do, of course, contain a kernel of historical truth. Due to those straight lines drawn on maps in Berlin in 1885, Lukunyu is administratively part of Uganda, even though its only natural connections by land are to villages lying farther south in Tanzania. The fact that it is cut off from the rest of Uganda by the Kagera River means that, even more than Kasensero, it has become a de facto duty-free port and a center for contraband and prostitution. Beginning in the mid-seventies, as the Ugandan economy collapsed in the wake of Amin's expulsion of the Asians, the two lakeside villages became key venues for smuggling, especially of coffee. They attracted young and energetic entrepreneurs who were willing to run the gauntlet of Amin's infamous Anti-Smuggling Unit, whose officers were not renowned for taking prisoners.[37] Not only Ugandans and Tanzanians were involved: according to various sources, Kenyans and Congolese also paid regular visits to the border region, and it is certainly possible that Burundians and Rwandans did also.[38] Later, as the black market economy prospered, an increasing number of young women from the region were drawn here to share in the wealth. Some of them ran lodges and eating-houses for the smugglers and fishermen; others worked as bar-girls and prostitutes.

The border village of Lukunyu is therefore the place where reality and myth coalesce. Part of the reason why both Ugandans and Tanzanians from this area identify Lukunyu as the source of Slim is that its ambivalent nationality allows both peoples to blame the other for its introduction. In much the same way, the English, French, Italians, and Spanish sought to blame each other for the sudden emergence of syphilis ("the Italian disease"; "the Spanish pox"; *"morbus gallicus"*) in western Europe at the end of the fifteenth century.

---

Apart from lakeside smuggling, one of the other phenomena that local people recognized as having played a key role in the emergence of AIDS was the liberation war at the end of the seventies, which resulted in the overthrow of the Ugandan dictator Idi Amin — even if some suspected that the barrage by *saba saba* had somehow been involved. Once again, historical evidence lends substance to the legend. In order to illustrate this, it is necessary to review, albeit briefly, the history of that war.

In May 1978, in a bid to divert attention from the parlous domestic situation, Idi Amin[39] accused Tanzania of having staged military incursions into Rakai district. In October, in response to these phantom incursions, thousands of Ugandan soldiers invaded the "Kagera Salient," a 500-square-mile expanse of floodplain lying between the straight colonial border and the most easterly section of the Kagera River, where it debouches into Lake Victoria. During the three weeks that followed, fifteen hundred Tanzanian civilians were killed, movable items were looted, and many of the women and girls in the area were raped. According to one report, a thousand or so civilians of both sexes were abducted to Uganda, and there put to work at a labor camp near Kalisizo, in the north of Rakai district, with many of the women presumably forced to act as soldiers' concubines.[40] Amin subsequently visited the Salient to be photographed, heroically, with a pile of captured Tanzanian weapons, and Radio Uganda announced that the border now lay along the Kagera River.

By November, as the Tanzanian military machine began to mobilize, Amin realized that he had blundered badly. His first response was a typical piece of public relations buffoonery: to avoid unnecessary casualties on the battlefield, he would meet Tanzanian president Julius Nyerere in the boxing ring, in a bout to be refereed by Muhammad Ali. Later, he ordered the Ugandan army to retreat to the north of the internationally accepted border, but it was too late. President Nyerere, infuriated by his counterpart's several years of bullying and provocation, had already ordered the conscription of forty thousand members of the People's Militia (who had received basic training at village level), thus doubling the strength of the national army, the Tanzanian People's Defence Force (TPDF). Some forty-five thousand soldiers, two-thirds of them new conscripts, moved up to Kagera region,[41] and Kyaka bridge, the only crossing-point over the Kagera, was quickly retaken and the central span rebuilt.

Between November 1978 and January 1979, the TPDF brigades set up camp in different villages to the south of the Salient, while the militia were given a crash course in fighting techniques; some village populations swelled from a few hundred to six thousand or more.[42] On January 20, three brigades crossed over Kyaka bridge and reoccupied the Salient, to be greeted by the devastation wrought by Amin's troops. Two brigades, the 206th and the 208th, moved along the main road to the border post of Mutukula, which they retook without difficulty. Meanwhile the 207th, under Brigadier Jack Walden, advanced farther east to the village of Minziro, where they found that most of the population had been massacred. At the end of January, Nyerere and his military commanders took a major policy decision, and launched a punitive counterattack on Uganda.

To begin with, the invasion met with problems. The two brigades on the main road were held up by Amin's artillery in the Simba Hills, while to the east, the 207th had to take Katera, a hill just across the border which overlooks the trading center at Kyebe and the road to Kasensero. Katera was occupied by five hundred Amin soldiers with armored vehicles, but Walden decided to march his entire brigade, artillery and all, through a swamp — a fifteen-mile journey that took three days, but that afforded the element of surprise. Following a bombardment by *saba saba,* the brigade took the hill with ease. The 207th — now jokingly referred to as "The Amphibious Brigade"— rested up briefly, before marching westward to help resolve the impasse at the Simba Hills. A contingent was left behind at Katera camp, and remained there for the better part of a year.[43]

After that, progress was much smoother. The TPDF front line moved northward to Kyotera and Masaka with minimal opposition, and took Kampala, the main city, in April. Amin was secretly flown to Libya a few days later, and on April 13 a civilian government was sworn in and the eight-year reign of terror was officially over. Some of Amin's troops continued to resist, but the TPDF completed the occupation of the country on June 3, 1979. There was rejoicing throughout Uganda, although in reality the celebrations had now been going on for five months, especially along those routes taken by the victorious armies.

When they had freed Uganda, most of the Tanzanian soldiers went back home, although several thousand remained until June 1981, helping to police the peace before and after the Ugandan elections. The large number of Ugandan children with Tanzanian fathers testifies to the debt of gratitude felt toward the liberators.

---

As a recent report on AIDS in the armed forces expressed it: "Military personnel are among the most susceptible populations to HIV. They are generally young and sexually active, are often away from home and governed more by peer pressure than accustomed social taboo. They are imbued with feelings of invincibility and an inclination towards risk-taking, and are always surrounded by ready opportunities for casual sex."[44] It is therefore not surprising that the events described above had enormous reverberations in terms of HIV and

AIDS, particularly on those places where the TPDF, and the various Ugandan forces, stopped and rested.

By the time the last Tanzanians were returning, the first cases of the new disease were cropping up on both sides of the border, in the districts adjoining Lake Victoria. Slim went on to take a dreadful toll. By the end of the 1980s, more than half of the women in their twenties living in trading centers in Rakai, and a quarter of those living in rural areas, were HIV-positive,[45] while one in eight of the children in the district as a whole were believed to have lost at least one parent to AIDS, rising to very nearly one in five in Kyebe subcounty.[46]

Elsewhere in Uganda, things were little better. Reliable HIV antibody tests (including the national HIV serosurvey conducted in 1987/8, only the second such survey in the world) revealed a dreadful and vivid picture of a virus apparently percolating outward from a core of infection in Rakai. Furthermore, the movements through Uganda of the TPDF brigades in 1978/9 appeared to be correlated — on three of the four military axes — with subsequent areas of high HIV-positivity.

The 207th brigade had entered Uganda at Katera, in Kyebe subcounty, and proceeded via Masaka to occupy Kampala; by 1987, a quarter of the women in each of the latter towns were HIV-positive, and Kyebe was famous as an epicenter of AIDS. The so-called Task Force, consisting of the 206th and the Minziro brigades, marched through western Uganda, from Mbarara and Kasese through Fort Portal, Hoima, and Masindi, and up to West Nile; in 1987, 29 percent of all urban adults in Western province were found to be HIV-positive.[47] The 205th had taken another route from Masaka through central Uganda (Mubende and Hoima) up to the town of Gulu. Unrest in 1987 prevented the HIV survey being carried out in Gulu, but by that year it was well known as a major secondary epicenter of the Ugandan AIDS epidemic. By contrast, HIV prevalence in eastern Uganda, where the other two TPDF brigades, the 201st and 208th, spent several months in mid-1979, was far lower, with the 12 percent prevalence recorded at Tororo apparently representing a peak.[48]

TPDF troop movements also seem to correlate well with the sequence in which AIDS was first recognized in these areas. Save for the unconfirmed reports about Amin soldiers in Luzira Prison, the first reports of AIDS in Uganda come from Kyebe subcounty and Kyotera, starting around 1980. In 1984 and 1985, the new disease began to be noticed in Kampala itself, and in cities like Masaka and Gulu, where the 207th and 205th brigades had spent some weeks or months during early 1979.[49] As for western Uganda, the troops never stopped in one place long enough for many local women to become infected in any one place, so the dissemination of the virus in local communities perhaps took a little longer. Nonetheless, by 1986 and 1987, AIDS cases were beginning to appear at urban and rural hospitals throughout the region, suggesting that the long march of the

"Task Force" may have played a role in the initial seeding. By contrast, AIDS was virtually absent from the towns of eastern Uganda, which were visited only by the 201st and the 208th brigades, until well into the nineties.[50]

Meanwhile, across the border, the seeding of infection in Tanzania started as the TPDF soldiers began returning to their home areas in June 1979. Many would have gone to the main city, Dar es Salaam, which is where the Scottish economist was probably infected at the end of 1979. Since the start of the nineties, despite its epidemic being far less publicized than that of Uganda, Tanzania's AIDS case total has kept pace almost exactly with that of its northern neighbor.[51] What is more, HIV would appear to have spread to even the most remote of Tanzania's districts — exactly as one might expect, given the stress which Julius Nyerere and the TPDF high command always placed on having a regionally and ethnically balanced army.[52] If this theory has merit, then the events of the liberation war would not only have caused the seeding of HIV in Kampala and the towns of southern and western Uganda, but also in the home districts of the Tanzanian fighters.

---

Further evidence supporting the role of these two factors — lakeside smuggling and the liberation war — in the emergence of AIDS in Rakai district is provided by some fascinating research conducted by Susan Hunter and Andrew Dunn for the British arm of the Save the Children Fund (SCF). They made a study of orphans based on a census of all parents who had died from 1971 onward in nine of Rakai's thirteen subcounties.[53] From this they compiled cumulative death charts, which provide a remarkable microcosmic view of the impact of AIDS.[54]

Four of the nine subcounties witnessed a dramatic rise in parental deaths in the early eighties. The most notable examples were Kyebe and Kakuuto, the two subcounties along the Tanzanian border, where a steep upward curve began in 1982. Deaths in Mabiyasu subcounty, which occupies the lakeside area immediately to the north of Kyebe and east of Kyotera, rose steeply from 1983 onward. The fourth badly affected subcounty was Kalisizo, which lies along the main road in the northeast of the district; here the steep rise in deaths began in 1984, and quickly outstripped that in Mabiyasu.

By 1988, each of these four subcounties had witnessed more than a thousand parental deaths (eighteen hundred in the case of Kyebe). By contrast, two subcounties lying to the west of the Kyotera-Masaka road (one of which contained the administrative center of the district, Rakai town) presented normal increases in cumulative deaths — still under a hundred by 1988. One must conclude that the massive differential in death rates was largely due to AIDS, and that HIV was not introduced until much later to these inland areas where smuggling activities

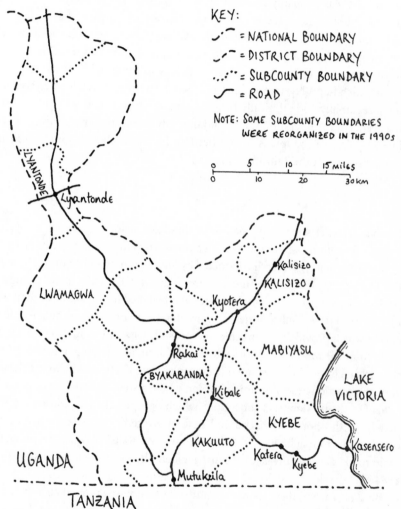

# SUBCOUNTIES OF RAKAI DISTRICT

KEY:
- ⌇ = NATIONAL BOUNDARY
- ⌇ = DISTRICT BOUNDARY
- ⋯ = SUBCOUNTY BOUNDARY
- ⌇ = ROAD

NOTE: SOME SUBCOUNTY BOUNDARIES
WERE REORGANIZED IN THE 1990s

```
0        5       10      15 MILES
|___|___|___|___|___|___|___|
0       10      20      30 KM
```

LYANTONDE

Lyantonde

LWAMAGWA

Kalisizo
KALISIZO

Kyotera

MABIYASU

LAKE
VICTORIA

Rakai
BYAKABANDA

Kibale

KYEBE

Kasensero

KAKUUTO

Katera
Kyebe

UGANDA

Mutukula

TANZANIA

SOURCE: BARNETT & BLAIKIE, "AIDS IN AFRICA" (LONDON: BELHAVEN PRESS, 1992), p. 30

# Cumulative Numbers of Deaths of Parents by Subcounty, Rakai District, Uganda, 1972-1988

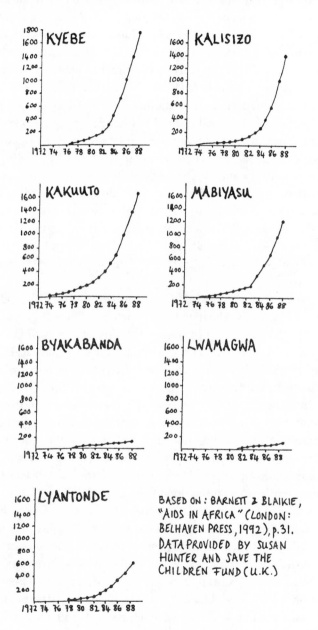

Based on: Barnett & Blaikie, "AIDS in Africa" (London: Belhaven Press, 1992), p.31. Data provided by Susan Hunter and Save the Children Fund (U.K.)

are minimal and through which the TPDF did not pass in the course of its long liberation march. The SCF data thus offers strong support to the hypothesis that both smuggling and the TPDF movements in 1979 played important roles in HIV transmission in Rakai.

A third pattern can be detected in Lyantonde subcounty, in the northwest of the district, where the report shows parental deaths increasing more gradually, to reach a total of five hundred by 1988. Although this suggests that HIV arrived here later than in eastern and southern Rakai, other data indicate that by 1989 HIV prevalence in this village had overtaken that in all other centers in the district, almost certainly because of its role as a truck stop.[55]

This in turn offers support to another theory of HIV spread, the "truck-town" hypothesis.[56] The small town of Lyantonde lies astride one of the main arterial roads in East Africa, and features perhaps the most infamous truck stop in the whole of Uganda. The TPDF did not pass through here in 1979, but it did spend time in Masaka and Mbarara, some fifty miles to east and west. It seems that the absence of the soldiers may have delayed the seeding of HIV in Lyantonde, but thereafter the truck stop appears to have served as a reservoir of infection from which HIV was channeled to and fro along the highway. To the southwest, the highway extends to Rwanda, Burundi, and eastern Congo; to the east, it passes through Kampala, and then on to Tororo, Nairobi, and the Kenyan coast.[57]

This theory was first investigated in 1986/7 by a team of Ugandan doctors under Warren Namaara who found that 67 percent of the bar-girls of Lyantonde were HIV-positive, as were 17 percent of all pregnant women in the village.[58] Farther east along the road, in the regional capital of Masaka, 26 percent of adults were reportedly infected, as were 24 percent of pregnant women in the capital, Kampala, and 12 percent in the eastern town of Tororo.[59] Across the border in Nyanza district, the first in Kenya, HIV prevalence was apparently around 6 percent, and nearer 2 percent in Nairobi, the Kenyan capital, a further two hundred miles along the road. Infection levels in Mombasa, the port city at the end of the highway, were somewhat higher at 4 percent, but this was not surprising, given the large prostitute population in the city, and the fact that truck crews spent more time here on "turnaround."[60]

The validity of the truck-town hypothesis was reinforced when, in late 1986, a team led by Wilson Carswell carried out tests in Kampala's main truck park, and found that 40 percent of drivers and 26 percent of the "turnboys" who serviced the vehicles were HIV-positive. During the previous three years, most of the truckers had traveled frequently between Mombasa, Kenya, and five countries of the immediate hinterland: Uganda, Rwanda, Burundi, Tanzania, and Congo.[61] When the adults of Lyantonde were carefully retested in 1989, a horrific 52.8 percent were found to be infected, which must be one of the highest levels of HIV infection ever recorded in the general population of any town in the world.[62]

All this suggests that it was the arrival of the warring armies in the vicinity of the smuggling zone of Rakai and Kagera in 1978 that either planted the seeds of HIV in a fertile soil, or that provided essential fertilizer, which allowed existing seeds to germinate. It seems that thereafter it was the movement of those armies, especially certain TPDF brigades, during and after the liberation war that facilitated further dissemination of the virus in Uganda and Tanzania. At a somewhat later date, an important tertiary role in HIV spread was played by prostitutes and truck crews plying the main commercial routes of eastern Africa.[63]

---

But if this three-stage hypothesis is correct, the primary question still remains: how did HIV-1 arrive in Rakai and Kagera in the first place? At its simplest level, there are three possible solutions: that the virus was introduced to the border region by Amin's armies; that it was introduced by the TPDF; or that it was already present in the free-trade zone, and that the epidemic began when the virus was transferred into a new, sexually active and mobile population as the soldiers passed through.

There are three pieces of evidence that suggest that the third scenario is the most plausible. First, almost all the earliest cases of AIDS were seen in the lakeside smuggling villages on both sides of the border, rather than in the villages farther inland where the Ugandan army and the TPDF were based. Second, in both countries it was prostitutes, traders, and smugglers who were the first to fall ill, although the soldiers of the two armies were also having sex with local village women who were not prostitutes.

The third piece of supporting evidence comes, once again, from the SCF charts for the various subcounties of Rakai. Although the steep rises in cumulative death rates began between 1982 and 1984 for the four subcounties situated along the lakeshore and the Kyotera road, all of them (unlike the five other subcounties assessed) had already experienced a slight, but perceptible, upward tilt in the graphs during the seventies. This was most pronounced in the two border subcounties where the smuggling ethos was strongest. It therefore seems that something was causing a gradual increase in mortality among young to middle-aged adults in these areas even prior to the liberation war. This suggests that HIV was perhaps already present in the black market community, causing occasional deaths that went unremarked in the late seventies — but that it was the arrival of the TPDF that sparked the explosive epidemic.[64]

It may therefore be that the true significance of the rural AIDS epicenter in the border region of Rakai and Kagera is that it was the site for an important transfer of HIV — from a small smuggling community to an invading army. It seems, in short, that the Tanzanians who fought so heroically in 1979 may actually have won a Pyrrhic victory. From the perspective of AIDS, they too were among the losers, having had the great misfortune to liberate the wrong place at the wrong time.

_____

Why the Rakai/Kagera epidemic should have been so explosive is to some extent explained by our latest understanding of the way that HIV works within the body. It is now widely accepted that the two times when a person is most infectious (the times of peak viremia) are during the first few weeks of infection (until the subject seroconverts, and produces the first wave of antibodies against HIV), and during the eventual decline into ARC and full-blown AIDS, when the sheer number and variety of viral strains within the body finally overwhelm the immune system.[65] Few people have sex when they are feeling really ill, but the same does not apply to the first few fateful weeks after infection, when the worst an infectee is likely to experience is a transient "seroconversion illness," which is usually little more than fever and general malaise. Just prior to that illness, the host is probably shedding virus, and there is a much greater chance that he or she might infect others.

One can therefore imagine the damage that could be done in the space of a few days or weeks when HIV is introduced into an unknowing, highly sexed population that, unlike the more conservative segments of society, is not inhibited about sharing partners. Or that, to be more precise, is having sex with as many partners as possible. Examples of persons in this category that come readily to mind include military gangs enjoying an officially sanctioned spree of looting, rape, and murder; victorious soldiers and relieved civilians celebrating the toppling of a repressive dictator; wealthy smugglers and the prostitutes who are willing — for a consideration — to share their unhealthy lakeside habitats; gay men, armed only with a can of Crisco and a bottle of poppers, lying naked and facedown in bathhouse cubicles.[66] It is for this reason that the border regions of East Africa and the gay metropoles of North America both appear to have served as seedbeds for the virus.

There have been various hints in the course of this chapter that in certain cases, individuals living in Rakai and Kagera may have developed AIDS very soon after infection, perhaps even within a year or two. This provides an important insight into the way in which viruses may behave when they enter a new community, or a new host.

Studies conducted in Uganda and Kenya indicate that the average time of progression from initial infection to full-blown AIDS tends to be much briefer in Africa than in the United States (less than four years, as compared to just under ten), as does the time between the first development of AIDS symptoms and death.[67] This is perhaps because the overall burden of pathogens in tropical Africa is greater than in temperate climes. Nonetheless, studies conducted on the San Francisco City Clinic cohort conclude that a small percentage (roughly 1 percent) of HIV-positive Americans go on to develop AIDS quickly, within two years of infection (presumably either because of poor host resistance, or because these particular individuals have encountered unusually virulent strains of HIV).[68] It would therefore not be surprising if a rather larger proportion of those Ugandans and Tanzanians who were exposed to HIV during the time of the 1978/9 war went on to develop ARC or full-blown AIDS in the year or two that followed.

"Fast-track AIDS" is also entirely credible from an evolutionary viewpoint. When a virus enters a new host population, there is likely to be a wide range of responses to the pathogen, from rapid progression to disease to very slow progression (or no disease at all). It is only after some time that the host and pathogen establish a more stable relationship.[69] It may therefore be that the Rakai/Kagera region, like other early epicenters of AIDS (including New York, and Port-au-Prince in Haiti), experienced an especially rapid burst of deaths shortly after HIV entered those communities.

---

Whether it be witch doctors, tiny insects, the people from the lake, the Juliana salesman, or deadly germs from *saba saba* — these various stories of how Slim came into being are all part of the communal need to explain the inexplicable, an attempt to come to terms with the arrival of calamity. However, within some of these explanations lie seeds of truth, and certainly they are no more ridiculous, or strange, than the attempts made elsewhere in the world to rationalize and cope with the disaster of AIDS by implicating God, the CIA, the KGB, voodoo rituals, or comets from outer space.

Next, we need to gather some more hard evidence by attempting to trace the early footprints of the epidemic — the directions in which HIV-1 was moving in those first years of AIDS, the years immediately preceding Year Zero.

# II

FROM TRICKLE TO FLOOD:

THE EARLY SPREAD OF AIDS

*Stop it at the start; it's late for medicine to be prepared when disease has grown strong through long delays.*

— OVID, Remedia Amoris

# 3

## "A MYSTERIOUS MICROBE":

## EARLY EVIDENCE OF AIDS IN NORTH AMERICA

There have been several accounts, many of them superb in their color and detail, about the early days of the epidemic in North America, the foremost of which is the Randy Shilts book *And the Band Played On.*[1] This chapter, and the following three, will begin with some of the early events described by Shilts, but will then take the story in the opposite direction, backward in both time and space. What follows is a survey of the early epidemiology of HIV and AIDS, as based on noncontroversial sources, both published and unpublished. Later, we shall look at certain more controversial cases, many based solely on clinical diagnosis, from even further back in time.

They play it down now, many of them, with Reaganesque diffidence. They shrug and say it's all in the past. They explain that — in any case — they've been ordered to destroy their notes. (Some have; some haven't.) But these were the men and women who were standing on the levee when the cracks appeared and the first waters trickled through, and who valiantly attempted to staunch the flow as AIDS, in all its many manifestations, burst the banks — and began its awful roll across America.

During the sixties and seventies, some of their predecessors, both in America and elsewhere, had predicted that scientific and technological advances would soon enable humanity to curb the pathogenic power of Nature, to tame that great river and force it through channels of concrete. But during the seventies the river rose and kept on rising until, on June 5, 1981,[2] it broke through, knocking aside human arrogance and artifice like rotten timber.

The CDC Task Force on Kaposi's Sarcoma and Opportunistic Infections (KSOI) was set up in July 1981, shortly after the second published report in the *MMWR* had linked both Kaposi's sarcoma and *Pneumocystis carinii* pneumonia (PCP) to the new — and as yet unnamed — syndrome.[3] From the beginning, it was run by Jim Curran, who somehow combines the chumminess of a favorite uncle with the evasiveness of a seasoned politician. Although he shared the chair with Denis Jurannek, from the CDC's division of parasitic diseases, it was Curran who ran the show, and who recruited the first members of the team: the hardworking Mary Guinan and the intense but rather witty Harold Jaffe — both veterans of previous campaigns, such as that against hepatitis B.

Other members of the KSOI Task Force included Selma Dritz, the seasoned expert on sexually transmitted diseases (STDs); Alex Kelter from toxicology; and Harry Haverkos from parasitology. And there were representatives from the CDC's very own fire brigade, the Epidemiology Intelligence Service (EIS): Pauline Thomas from New York and Dave Auerbach from Los Angeles. In addition, there was one member of the task force who was not a medical scientist at all, but a sociologist: Professor William Darrow.

---

From the point of view of reconstructing the early history of the AIDS epidemic in America, it is perhaps unfortunate that the understandable concerns about patient confidentiality have led to an excessive degree of caution, and the loss of much relevant material from the public domain. One suspects that much more medical and epidemiological information about the earliest cases could have been released through the simple expedient of anonymization. As for the rather dry statistics that do appear in the published literature, they provide some general background, but not a lot more.

The key paper, which retrospectively summarizes the early course of the epidemic, is entitled "AIDS Trends in the United States, 1978–1982,"[4] and was written by Curran, Haverkos, and a CDC colleague, Richard Selik. Published in March 1984, it details the number of AIDS cases diagnosed in America, by quarter year, from the start of 1978 until the first quarter of 1983 (the earlier cases having been diagnosed retrospectively). Of the four so-called risk groups specified in this paper, the first case of AIDS in homosexual or bisexual men is documented as having occurred in the first quarter of 1978, the first cases in intravenous drug users (IVDUs) and Haitians both feature in the first quarter of 1980, and the first case in hemophiliacs in the last quarter of 1981. Apparently four AIDS cases were diagnosed in the United States in 1978, and eight in 1979. Eleven of these twelve cases involved gay men, eight of whom lived in New York, two in California, one in Illinois, and one in an unspecified state. The twelfth case involved someone "without apparent risk factors" —

possibly a woman, a child, or a heterosexual man. Nine of the twelve patients presented with Kaposi's sarcoma (KS), one with *Pneumocystis carinii* pneumonia (PCP), and two with other opportunistic infections (OIs).

Other papers reveal that just one of these cases resulted in death before 1980. The patient in question was a twenty-seven-year-old gay, black hospital guard from New York City, who died in December 1979 after an eight-month history of PCP, latterly complicated by amebiasis and candidiasis of mouth and throat.[5] This case still represents the first generally accepted death from AIDS in an American gay male.

Not all of the mooted early cases are reliable, and this applies especially to those in which KS was the main presenting symptom. At this stage in the epidemic, the appearance of just a single lesion of Kaposi's sarcoma in a person under the age of sixty was sufficient for a presumptive GRID, or AIDS, diagnosis. In retrospect, some of these patients appear to have had the relatively benign "classical" type of Kaposi's sarcoma that traditionally infects certain older men of Jewish and Mediterranean origin, a type that is normally confined to arms and legs, and is not part of the spectrum of AIDS.[6]

Reports elsewhere in the medical literature about the 1979 cases in the "AIDS Trends" paper provide enough additional detail about patient histories to suggest that at least five of the eight were almost certainly genuine cases of AIDS, resulting in death in 1979 or 1980. The four cases from 1978, however, appear far more problematical, and the two that can be tentatively identified both look very much like cases of classical KS. But even if some of the earlier AIDS diagnoses may have been questionable, the underlying message contained in these papers is absolutely accurate. Whatever the exact date of the first case, an epidemic of immune deficiency, evinced by a variety of different symptoms, had indeed begun attacking the gay community of North America by the end of the 1970s.

------

In the twelve short years that followed the Stonewall riots of 1969, as the various American states ceased to define homosexuality as a psychiatric disorder or criminal offense, homosexual life was transformed. After centuries of repression and prejudice, there was suddenly a new self-belief and pride. As more and more came out, the trend became a movement, and the movement assumed the sassy, unashamed title of "gay." During the seventies, especially in the main urban centers of America, many gay men came to view impersonal bathhouse sex as the easiest and most affordable way of achieving gratification,[7] and the getting of sexually transmitted diseases as both an occupational hazard and a badge of political commitment.[8] As the pendulum swung, and as gays made up for lost time, there was an intensive cultivation of hedonism, sexual athleticism, and physical excess. And it was into this fertile soil, at some stage as yet unknown, that the seed of HIV was planted.

One of the early infectees, in all likelihood, was "Donald Lombardo," a twenty-nine-year-old gay man from Staten Island, New York. On April 7, 1992, ten months after the appearance of Gottlieb's paper in the *MMWR*, and five days before the CDC announcement that 248 gay American males had now been diagnosed with Gay-Related Immune Deficiency, Donald was interviewed in the course of one of the CDC's AIDS studies. His history is of interest, in that he was a fairly typical member of the New York gay community of the early eighties, as members of that community were beginning to fall sick, but before they became fully aware of the cause, or the seriousness, of the situation.

Donald had been displaying signs of immunosuppression (and, in all probability, what would later come to be called prodromal AIDS or ARC — AIDS-Related Complex) since September 1981. In addition, he was a sexual contact of two men who had themselves contracted AIDS.

At the time of interview, Donald — who originated from mixed European stock — had been a practicing homosexual for some twelve years. During this time, he had had sex with approximately 200 men and four women, a total of male partners which is not atypical for the New York gay community of that era.[9] Since 1977, he had averaged some thirty partners *per annum*, though during the year before interview he had limited his sexual activity because of a general feeling of listlessness, combined with frequent skin infections and mouth ulcers. During that last twelve-month period he had had sex with fifteen different men, of whom ten were one-night stands, three were occasional partners, and two regular partners (the latter defined as partners on at least ten occasions). In each of these fifteen instances, the two men had had mutual oral sex, and in most cases anal sex, with both parties taking active roles. On rarer occasions he and his partners had practiced mutual rimming (analingus, or oral-anal sex) and on one occasion fisting — the insertion of hand or fist into the partner's rectum.

Donald had had hepatitis B ten years earlier, but in retrospect it was clear that his general level of health had begun a sharp deterioration in 1978. In the years since then, he had experienced a wide range of sexually transmitted infections and diseases, including gonorrhea (three times), syphilis, rectal warts, pubic lice, and chronic scabies. He had also suffered a variety of enteropathic conditions, including hepatitis A and, on four occasions, severe diarrhea caused by either amebiasis or giardiasis — all of which were probably sexually transmitted.

Since the start of his sexual life, Donald had always lived within the five boroughs of New York, save for brief sojourns in New Jersey and on Fire Island, the thirty-mile strip of beaches and pine trees to the east of New York which had long ago been adopted by the gay community as a summer resort. His only overseas trip had been a holiday in Puerto Rico. For most of the seventies he had worked as a clerk for banks and shipping lines, but in 1979 he began working for specifically gay enterprises: as a cook in a Fire Island restaurant, as a cashier at the Club Baths, and doorman at the Mineshaft bar, both in Manhattan. The latter was probably the most infamous of the anything-goes establishments where, in the so-called wild back room, consenting adults could fist-fuck, defecate on each other, play water sports, or insert small mammals up each other's rectums.

Donald had a limited disposable income, much of which was spent on drugs. He had taken a wide range of street drugs, including marijuana (on a daily basis) and, less frequently, cocaine, amphetamines, barbiturates, and LSD, but, significantly, he had never taken any drug by injection. Since the late sixties, he had used amyl nitrate "poppers" (a sexual stimulant that also relaxes the muscles of the anal sphincter) a couple of times a month, and had occasionally sniffed ethyl chloride.

Although Donald's subsequent medical history is not available, it seems highly probable that he was indeed infected with HIV — and via the sexual route. It is not, of course, known when he first became infected, but his increased number of sexual partners from 1977 onward, and his deterioration in health which began in 1978, afford some clues.

Donald Lombardo's sad history has been recounted here because there were soon to be hundreds — and later still hundreds of thousands — of men like him, in the United States and in other countries around the globe.

––––––––

Within a day or two of Gottlieb's report in the *MMWR* of June 1981, calls came in from several doctors who believed that they had seen similar cases. Jim Curran and Denis Jurannek flew up to New York City to see Alvin Friedman-Kien and Linda Laubenstein, both to interview some of the thirty-one men with KS and PCP whom they had on their books, and to get details on others who had already died. They also spoke further with Fred Siegal, an immunologist at Mount Sinai Medical Center, who had seen four gay men with chronic perianal ulcers caused by *Herpes simplex,* only one of whom was still alive.[10] When they returned to Atlanta, Curran got together with Haverkos to draw up a working case definition — one that was subsequently to be greatly enlarged, but that still forms the basis of the AIDS clinical case definition of today.[11]

Essentially, they defined GRID as a state of underlying cellular immunodeficiency in otherwise healthy persons who had no other known cause for, or predisposition to, disease (like, for instance, a genetic susceptibility, cancerous involvement, or a medical history that featured the administration of radiotherapy or steroids), and they listed the various opportunistic infections that signaled the syndrome. The most notable of these, then as now, were the fungal diseases such as PCP, disseminated candidiasis, and cryptococcosis, the protozoal disease toxoplasmosis, the viral infections associated with cytomegalovirus

(CMV) and *Herpes simplex,* and the atypical bacterial infections caused by *Mycobacterium tuberculosis, M. avium-intracellulare,* and *Klebsiella pneumoniae.* In addition, the case definition included two specific cancers: Kaposi's sarcoma and B-cell lymphoma.[12] Of these conditions, KS alone had an age limit: only those aged sixty or below were to be included in the case definition for GRID.

Next, the task force members set about reviewing pathology logs from eighteen major cities. They found that GRID cases were not spread throughout the United States, but seemed to be cropping up almost exclusively in the four centers of New York, Los Angeles, San Francisco, and Atlanta. At this stage, all the cases were in gay men, and it was clearly of paramount importance to discover why this group was — apparently uniquely — vulnerable to the syndrome. It was thus that a few weeks later, sociologist Bill Darrow was requisitioned to join the team.

As soon as he arrived, he drew up the interview form for a case-control study, a twenty-one-page questionnaire designed to establish the main risk factors for GRID. Fortunately, one of the subjects that most intrigues "sex-positive" people[13] is their own sexual activity, and the eight physicians whom Darrow trained in Atlanta during August and September apparently had little difficulty persuading their interviewees to answer the sixty-two subdivided questions. From September to November 1981, his team interviewed fifty GRID patients, and 120 controls (gay men without symptoms of GRID), from the four key cities. They concluded that the main differences between cases and controls were the number of sexual partners per year and the proportion of those partners met in bathhouses. Also associated with illness were such factors as having a history of sexually transmitted diseases, and exposure to feces — notably during rimming and fisting.[14] The typical GRID patient was an openly gay man in his thirties, who had enjoyed an energetic sex life based around bars and bathhouses for some years, and who used amyl nitrate "poppers" as a sexual stimulant and relaxant.

None of these conclusions was unexpected. Indeed, by this stage, most of the task force members were "willing to bet their salaries" that GRID was caused by a new — or hitherto unrecognized — infectious agent. Alvin Friedman-Kien and colleagues at the New York University Medical Center were beginning to identify sexual connections between some of their GRID patients, but nobody thus far had documented or proved such links. And until such proof did exist, there were other possibilities to be considered, such as a genetic predisposition to disease (for it had been discovered that 26 percent of the KS cases, as against 9 percent of controls without KS, were of Italian ancestry), exposure to a toxic agent (such as poppers), exposure to an immunosuppressive agent (sperm, or the steroid creams increasingly used to treat venereal diseases),[15] or immunological overload — as a result of the many chronic diseases to which sexually active gay men had become especially susceptible in the seventies.

On March 3, 1982, Bill Darrow sent Jim Curran a memorandum about time-space clustering of cases of Kaposi's sarcoma,[16] in which he mapped out all the cases of KS reported from Manhattan up to the start of 1982, and illustrated that, with four exceptions, they all came from either the Greenwich Village area or the Upper West Side. In the same memorandum, Darrow analyzed the first fifteen cases of KS in New York males, all of which had a date of onset before 1980. Most of these men identified the same places as favorite pickup spots: bathhouses such as the St. Mark's, Everard, the Club, and Dakota, bars such as the Mineshaft, "action stores" such as the Christopher Street Book Shop,[17] and parks — most notably that in Washington Square. Among the fifteen men were four who would later feature under different identifying codes (Patient O, NY1, NY2, and NY3) in Darrow's case-cluster study.[18]

One particular cautious sentence in the memo indicates the lines along which Darrow was now thinking. "One might even speculate," he wrote, "that a mysterious microbe might have passed among certain homosexual men who congregated at certain places for sociosexual interactions at various times during the late 1970's." But there was still no absolute proof.

Shortly after this, Dave Auerbach phoned from Los Angeles with a fascinating story to tell. Darrow immediately flew out to join him, and during the next few days they conducted the study that would effectively confirm the theory of causation that most of the task force scientists, and several of the men suffering from GRID, had long intuited.

Darrow and Auerbach's elegant case-cluster study has a fascinating background, which, were it not so tragic, would have all the makings of a Mensa brainteaser. In October 1979, three long-established gay couples shared the same table at a fund-raising dinner in Los Angeles. The following summer, two of the couples attended a small party beside the backyard pool at one of their houses; they also invited a male prostitute, described as "a $50 trick off Santa Monica Boulevard."[19] During the evening, each of the five men had sex with each of the others. Soon afterward, some of the men started feeling lethargic and losing weight, and by March 1982, one of the partners from each of the original three couples had died of AIDS. One of the surviving partners was so concerned by the fact that each of the three men had died on the sixth day of the month, resulting in the ominous figure "666," that he called up Dave Auerbach at the CDC.

Darrow and Auerbach visited this man a few days later. Unimpressed by the Beelzebub theory, they decided that the fact that only two of the deceased had attended the backyard party confirmed that the cause of their deaths was unlikely to be either environmental (like contaminated water in the swimming

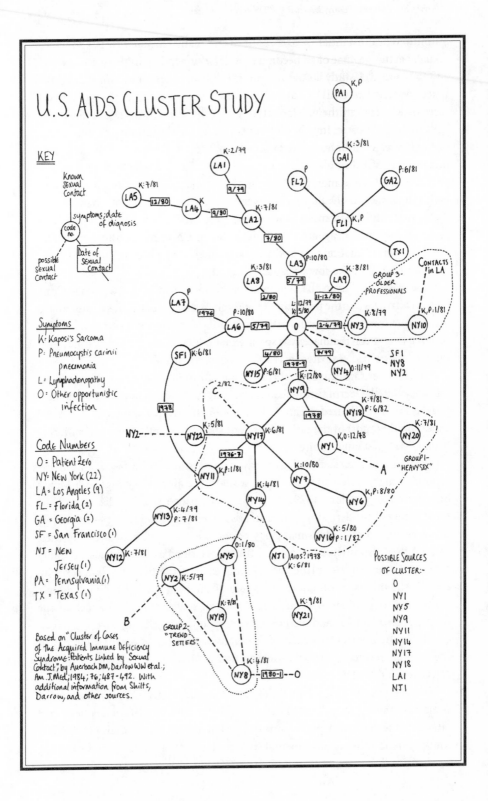

pool) or circumstantial (a bad lot of drugs). But then the real connections began to emerge. One of the dead men from the pool party (who would later be given the cluster study code LA2), turned out to have had sex with two other men who also had GRID, one of whom was an air steward (LA1), who had traveled widely around the world in the previous six years: in 1976 to Kenya and Tanzania, in 1977 to Italy and Greece, and in 1978 to France and England.[20] Soon afterward it became apparent that one of the other dead men from the pool party, LA3, had also had sex with an air steward who was suffering from KS, and that this man, a Canadian, had himself had sex with three other Los Angelinos with GRID. At long last, there was hard evidence to support the oft-suspected theory of causation. GRID appeared to be caused by an infectious, sexually transmitted agent, most probably a virus.

As in a reversed loop of film, the whole tumbling cascade of cards suddenly — and surprisingly — re-formed into a neat deck. The Canadian air steward, Gaetan Dugas,* who was given the code "Patient O" (since, as regards the Los Angeles cluster study, he was the patient from "Out of California"), turned out to have also had sex with a further four GRID patients from New York. This placed Dugas at the hub of a wheel that had eight gay men with AIDS around its rim, with each of whom he had had sex between 1978 and December 1980.[21] These eight were, in turn, connected by sexual contact to another thirty-one, thus placing Patient O at the center of a group of forty AIDS cases, representing almost one-sixth of the 248 U.S. cases then reported. Given Dugas's apparently central role in the cluster, it was not long before everyone involved in the research, including the CDC people, abandoned "Patient O" for the rather more graphic sobriquet of "Patient Zero."

Apart from Dugas, the cluster of forty included nine men from Los Angeles, twenty-two from New York,[22] and one each from New Jersey and San Francisco.[23] Also included was a small subcluster of six men (two each from Florida and Georgia, and one each from Texas and Pennsylvania). As the links were tracked down and corroborated in just a few days of intensive interviewing, Darrow and his colleagues realized that they were tracing their way through a spider's web of sexual connections within the gay community, a network that included many who had multiple sexual partners, as well as a few who were in long-standing (albeit not exclusive) loving relationships.

CDC memoranda and reports from 1982,[24] combined with historical details gleaned from the texts of Randy Shilts and other documenters of the period, permit some further unraveling of the cluster of forty, including some dates of sexual contact, onset of disease, and dates of death. The first thing that becomes

---

* Dugas, and a few other persons with AIDS (or AIDS-like symptoms) who feature in this book, have already been identified in books and television documentaries, and for this reason their real names have been retained. Otherwise, aliases or first names have been used.

## ADDITIONAL INFORMATION ABOUT THE CLUSTER

| Code No. | Identity | Date of Death | Possible Place of Exposure in U.S. | Notes |
|---|---|---|---|---|
| 0 | Patient Zero, Gaetan Dugas, French–Canadian | 3/84 | St. Mark's Baths, Mineshaft Bar | Flight attendant: Europe (incl. France, UK), Florida Keys, Caribbean, Haiti |
| NY1 | Black | 7/82 | Everard's Baths | Flight attendant: Haiti and Caribbean |
| NY2 | Rick W., schoolteacher | 12/80 | — | — |
| NY3 | — | 12/80 | St. Mark's Baths | — |
| NY4 | — | 8/80 | — | — |
| NY5 | Nick R., cruise ship staffer | 12/80 | — | Visited Haiti and Caribbean |
| NY6 | — | 8/82 | Everard's Baths | — |
| NY7 | — | — | St. Mark's and Everard's Baths | — |
| NY8 | Jack N., window dresser | 9/81 | Flamingo Disco | — |
| NY9 | French ballet teacher | — | Everard's Baths, Mineshaft Bar | Fister |
| NY10 | — | 11/81 | St. Mark's Baths | — |
| NY11 | "Cosmic Energy" | 2/82 | St. Mark's Baths, Mineshaft Bar | — |
| NY12 | — | — | — | — |
| NY13 | — | 1/82 | — | — |
| NY14 | — | — | Everard's Baths, Mineshaft Bar | — |
| NY15 | — | 8/81 | — | — |
| NY16 | — | 6/82 | Everard's Baths, Mineshaft Bar | — |
| NY17 | Leather shop employee | — | St. Mark's and Everard's Baths | — |
| NY18 | Italian | — | — | Fister |

| Code No. | Identity | Date of Death | Possible Place of Exposure in U.S. | Notes |
|---|---|---|---|---|
| NY19 | Enno P., German graphic designer | — | — | — |
| NY20 | — | — | — | Fister |
| NY21 | — | — | — | — |
| NY22 | — | — | — | — |
| LA1 | — | — | — | Flight attendant: Kenya, Tanzania, Italy, Greece, France, UK |
| LA2 | — | 3/82 | Pleasure Chest Leather Shop | Fister |
| LA3 | — | 2/82 | — | — |
| LA4 | — | — | — | — |
| LA5 | — | — | — | — |
| LA6 | Fashion photographer | 6/81 | 8709 Club | — |
| LA7 | — | — | — | — |
| LA8 | — | — | — | — |
| LA9 | Hairdresser | — | 8709 Club | — |
| FL1 | — | — | — | — |
| FL2 | — | — | — | — |
| GA1 | — | — | — | Fister |
| GA2 | — | — | — | — |
| SF1 | Michael M., Italian–American hairdresser | 7/82 | — | — |
| NJ1 | — | — | — | — |
| PA1 | — | — | — | — |
| TX1 | — | — | — | — |
| A | Black | — | — | Visited Haiti, 1980/81 |
| B | — | — | — | — |
| C | — | — | Pleasure Chest Leather Shop | — |

clear on the basis of this information is that there cannot have been a single source for the entire cluster.

Though it was the Los Angeles cases that established the infective agent principle, it is the New York side of the cluster that (with the exception of LA1) contains most of the really early cases, and that provides the most illumination about the early spread of HIV in America. Bill Darrow managed to identify three main groups of New Yorkers with whom Gaetan Dugas had had sexual contact.

The first of these he described as the "heavy sex group," which was centered around NY9 (a French ballet instructor who hosted private parties in his loft, and with whom Dugas had sex at the Mineshaft in 1978 or 1979) and NY17 (an employee of the Pleasure Chest, a leather and sex toys shop in Lower Manhattan). Members of the heavy sex group tended to frequent the New Everard Baths (or "Everhards," as it was affectionately known) and the Mineshaft bar.

Others from this group, like NY18 and NY20, were members of sadomasochistic clubs, most notably the "Fist Fuckers of America" (FFA). This elite club had chapters in New York, Philadelphia, Los Angeles (where LA1 was a member), and other major gay centers, and its 300-strong membership list featured international globetrotters and a wide variety of VIPs — including, for instance, certain members of the New York Philharmonic Orchestra. FFA parties often lasted the entire weekend, and featured not only fisting, but also activities like scat, rimming, and water sports, which involved playing with — or ingesting — feces or urine. The sex was generally perked up, or washed down, with a catholic cocktail of street drugs.

In retrospect, it seems likely that fisting and other sadomasochistic practices involving the rectum were ill-advised from a medical perspective even before HIV came on the scene, in that they tended to traumatize the anal mucosa, allowing a portal of entry for any pathogens that might later come into contact with the wounds. This is borne out by the fact that, whether or not they contracted AIDS, fisters proved to be susceptible to a wide range of viral and intestinal infections. Darrow's research identified at least nine men who attended FFA meetings in New York who had developed AIDS by early 1982. Not all, however, could be connected with certainty to the cluster — and it is worth noting that even those who could be connected were not — save for LA1 — among the earliest cases.

One noteworthy member of the heavy sex group was NY1, the only black man in the cluster. NY1 was yet another flight attendant, the third in the group of forty and, as his code number indicates, the first New Yorker in the cluster to display the symptoms of AIDS (in December 1978). He had one sexual encounter with NY9 at the New Everard in 1978. Through his job he was a frequent visitor, from 1974 onward, to Haiti and the Caribbean.

The second discernible group in the cluster is described by Darrow as "the trend setters." Many members of this group had steady professional jobs and had been together since 1976 or 1977, sharing apartments and a rented seafront summer house on Ocean Walk, Fire Island. Including schoolteacher Rick Wellikoff; Nick Rock, a bartender on gay Caribbean cruises; window dresser Jack Nau; and Enno Poersch, a graphic designer, they were connected to the main cluster via NY14, who was part of the "heavy sex" group. Jack, Rick, and Nick were among the first people to die of AIDS in New York City, and their stories are told in some detail in *And the Band Played On*. It was their friends, most notably the writer Larry Kramer and the businessman Paul Popham, who later set up the first AIDS support organization, Gay Men's Health Crisis.

The third group consisted mainly of fairly active, older professional men who were more discreet about their homosexuality — at least while at work. They would generally take alcohol in preference to drugs, they visited the New St. Mark's Baths (which were less heavy-duty than some others), and they traveled a lot, often having anonymous encounters while on the road. Only two members of this group could be linked with certainty to the cluster study.

At this point, it clearly becomes important to discover more about the history and lifestyle of Gaetan Dugas, "Patient Zero." He was born in February 1953, was adopted soon afterward, and spent his early life in Quebec City, in Francophone Canada. Witnesses recall his arrival in Toronto's gay scene as being in 1971 or 1972, and it seems that he averaged roughly 250 partners a year over the next decade. His first job was as a hairdresser, but in 1975 or 1976 he moved to Vancouver to improve his English in preparation for a job with Air Canada, the national airline. By 1977, Shilts records him as being based in Halifax, Nova Scotia, and it is known that he flew to Paris, London, and to "many cities in Europe" — perhaps including Copenhagen and Amsterdam. Significantly, Darrow records in one of his many memoranda that Dugas visited Haiti in 1977, and that the Canadian remembered having had sex with "black men who spoke French."

Over the next three years, Dugas flew regularly between Toronto, Vancouver, New York, Los Angeles, and San Francisco. When in Manhattan, he picked up most of his partners at bars like the Mineshaft and Twelve West, or at the New St. Mark's or Club Baths. He was a well-known figure in gay society, being noted for his blond, boyish good looks, and was apparently sometimes paid to appear at parties. Toward the end of these three years, Dugas spent more time in San Francisco, which Darrow sees as being potentially connected to the fact that the epidemic in that city lagged a year or so behind those in New York and L.A.

Dugas developed lymphadenopathy in December 1979, and KS the following year; by mid-1981, he was attending Alvin Friedman-Kien's clinic for treatment. Later, he was transferred to Montreal and then Vancouver, but because there was still no proof that his illness was infectious, he stubbornly continued to attend the baths. He eventually died back in the town of his childhood, Quebec City, in March 1984. Shilts points out that it was finally kidney failure — rather than a recognized opportunistic infection of AIDS — that killed him,[25] which in turn suggests that many AIDS deaths may be overlooked in the course of retrospective reviews of pathology records. The case-cluster study, in which Dugas played such a key role, was published that same month.

Since then, it has been widely assumed that "Patient Zero" must have been the source of the other thirty-nine HIV infections in the cluster, or even the source of all infections in North America — but neither assumption is sound. Dugas has the highest number of direct confirmed contacts within the cluster — eight, including three, or even four, of the ten earliest cases. However, there are several men who have multiple links — including two with five known connections. Indeed, the central position of Dugas may well be an artifact of the inquiry, since it was his cooperation, and his address book, that provided many of the crucial leads, and because other key figures may already have died by the time the inquiry began. Furthermore, one of the crucial observations of the cluster study is that Patient Zero's partners developed AIDS between four and thirty months (and on average 10.5 months) after having had sex with him. This raised far fewer eyebrows in 1984, when the concept of a long latency period was only just being grasped, than it would today, when it is estimated that — in the West, at least — the average time between HIV infection and the onset of full-blown AIDS is approximately a decade.[26]

There are two possible readings of this. One is that Darrow and Auerbach were right about the central role played by Dugas, and that the clinical course of many of the early HIV infectees in America was far swifter than it is today — perhaps because (as in Rakai and Kagera) the virus was making its first inroads in a new population.[27] The other interpretation is that Darrow was wrong, and that many of these men were infected with HIV prior to any sexual contact with Gaetan Dugas. One thing is certain. Had the CDC Task Force realized in 1982 that it would be confronting an asymptomatic period of ten years rather than ten months, there would have been even greater alarm — for, of course, the longer the asymptomatic period, the greater the potential for infectees to unknowingly infect others.

In fact, an analysis of the known dates of sexual encounters between couples and the dates of onset of AIDS suggests that there are nine other men, apart from Patient Zero, who could quite plausibly have introduced HIV to the central part of the cluster, any of whom could have directly or indirectly infected Dugas himself.[28] It is noteworthy that of these ten possible "sources," four (O, LA1, NY9, and NY18) had links with Europe, one (LA1) had visited Africa, and three (O, NY1, and NY5) are known to have visited the Caribbean and, in particular, Haiti, prior to onset of symptoms.

Alternatively, of course, the initial seeding of HIV in North America might have involved a sexual conservative who, perhaps, infected just one other person, neither of whom would necessarily appear in the group of forty. Besides, there were almost certainly other important sexual contacts within the cluster that were never tied down — some of which are alluded to in passing in the various unpublished CDC reports and memoranda.[29]

It is clear that, if indeed there was a "Patient Zero" for North America, then there are several plausible candidates for the role. It is equally clear, however, that even if the role played by Dugas may have been exaggerated, many of the key events of the early dissemination of HIV and AIDS in North American gays are contained within the borders of Darrow and Auerbach's cluster study diagram.

---

All this while, the CDC Task Force was also on the lookout for even earlier cases of AIDS. Two possibilities are described in the Selik/Haverkos/Curran paper: a forty-nine-year-old heterosexual Haitian who had died of PCP in Brooklyn, New York, in 1959, and a fifty-seven-year-old white woman from Shreveport, Louisiana, who had been diagnosed as having PCP in 1975 and again in 1979. Neither, they conceded, appeared from lymphocyte and blood cell counts to be typical cases of AIDS. The authors added that apart from the man's Haitian ancestry,[30] the two had no known risk factors, and concluded that "we are skeptical that [they] are part of the current AIDS epidemic."

Other possible archival cases that were investigated by the CDC's Task Force on AIDS, or its subsequent incarnation, the Division of HIV/AIDS, were later mentioned in interview by Jim Curran's deputy, Peter Drotman. They included a woman from Hawaii who died in 1978 of disseminated toxoplasmosis and cryptosporidiosis — an enteropathic condition more commonly found in sheep than humans;[31] a man from Philadelphia who succumbed to disseminated actinomycosis — another unusual fungal disease — in the mid-seventies;[32] and a teenager from St. Louis, Missouri, who died in 1969 of disseminated, aggressive KS, lymphedema, and chlamydia.[33]

In addition to these, I came across certain other possible cases among existing reports in the medical literature. One involved a forty-eight-year-old gay man from Boston who fell ill in March 1979 with diarrhea and massive weight loss caused by cryptosporidiosis. By the time he died in April 1980, he also had disseminated CMV infection and evidence of *Klebsiella pneumoniae*.[34] Although this case had already been published in September 1981, and although nowadays such an array of symptoms in a gay man would readily be diagnosed as AIDS, it apparently was not included in any of these early AIDS reviews.[35]

---

There is of course another, more accurate technique for tracking AIDS within a specific environment — and that is to look not for clinical presentations typical of the disease, but for antibodies against the causative virus, HIV. This virus was first identified (as LAV) in 1983, and the original antibody tests (developed by Robert Gallo's lab) became available in 1984. Many of the early assays were notorious for having a high ratio of false positives — and the first truly reliable tests appeared only in 1985 and 1986. Since then, seroepidemiological studies of archival North American sera have been relatively few and far between. Certain collections of frozen sera have, however, been thawed and retested, and these retrospective studies have been most illuminating.

The earliest archival evidence of HIV being present as a contaminant of blood products in the U.S. comes from 1978. Retrospective screening by Bruce Evatt and his CDC colleagues showed that a two-year-old hemophiliac child from the Children's Hospital of Los Angeles seroconverted (developed antibodies) in that year, after receiving both Factor VIII concentrate and blood transfusions, either of which may have been responsible.[36] The earliest instance on record of an American getting AIDS after a blood transfusion involved a nineteen-year-old man who had a car crash in December 1979. He developed the opportunistic infection *Herpes zoster* in September 1981 and died in March 1983. Investigations revealed that one of the two donors was a gay man with multiple partners who had had unexplained lymphadenopathy since 1979.[37]

A much larger collection of frozen blood samples derives from a cohort, or group, of gay and bisexual men in San Francisco who enrolled for a trial of a vaccine against hepatitis B in the late seventies. Stored blood samples from 320 of the participants in the San Francisco vaccine trial show that in 1978, the earliest year for which information is available, just one participant was HIV-positive. The vaccine trial cohort consisted, however, of "hepatitis B virgins," specially selected because, although sexually active, they had apparently not been exposed to that virus. Because the two viruses are transmitted in similar ways, the trial group therefore consisted of gay men who were also at relatively low risk of HIV infection. A far better gauge of early HIV prevalence among the sexually active in the city is derived from a cohort of 6,875 gays and bisexuals who were screened between 1978 and 1980 by Nancy Hessol, Paul O'Malley, and coworkers at the San Francisco City Clinic, a treatment center for sexually transmitted diseases. When, in 1984, approximately a tenth of the sera taken in 1978 were retrospectively tested by the earliest available HIV assay,[38] a surprisingly high 4.5 percent were found to be HIV-positive. This rose to 12.6 percent of those taken in 1979, 24.1 percent for 1980, and a horrifying 67.4 percent for 1984.[39] Paul O'Malley has revealed that when the samples were retested by more accurate methods[40] in 1985/6, there was little appreciable difference in the results, and says he suspects that the first seroconversions may have occurred in 1977.[41]

For comparison, 378 homosexually active men were assessed for HIV by Cladd Stevens's group, who were in charge of the hepatitis B vaccine trials in New York City. Of the sera taken in 1978 or 1979, 6.6 percent were HIV-positive — a prevalence very similar to that in San Francisco.[42] Stevens has been testing even earlier banked sera from New York, and so far the earliest confirmed HIV-positive specimen comes from a gay man bled on September 6, 1977.[43]

———

In 1985, Dr. James Moore of the National Institute for Drug Abuse arranged for the HIV testing of more than eleven hundred stored sera originating from addicts held in 1971 and 1972 at the National Institute for Mental Health research center in Lexington, Kentucky. (In those days, convicted drug addicts were sent to Lexington, rather than to prison.) He sent the samples to Steve Alexander of Biotech Research, Inc. — a company that, according to Dr. Moore, was closely associated with Robert Gallo's laboratory. Three of these sera appeared to be repeatedly positive on two different ELISA assays and a Western blot test, though the title of the letter that the researchers wrote to the *New England Journal of Medicine* testifies to their wariness: "HTLV-III Seropositivity in 1971–1972 Parenteral Drug Abusers — a Case of False Positives or Viral Exposure?"[44]

Several years later, their doubts were confirmed, when a team led by Robert Lange managed to trace eight of the ten addicts whose blood from the early seventies had given positive Western blot readings: seven were alive and healthy, the eighth had died in a car crash in 1985.[45] Further blood samples were also taken from the two ex-addicts who had provided the most reactive 1971 sera, and these latest samples were found to be HIV-negative. Lange concluded that the original findings were false positives — adding that it was "conceivable" that this was caused by the sensitivity-enhancing technique used by Biotech for the Western blot assays. Lange further concluded that, given the size and geographic spread of the addict cohort tested, it was unlikely that HIV had been present in the American IVDU community in 1972.[46]

The earliest evidence of HIV in North America comes from another route entirely. In 1982, it was realized that women also could get AIDS, as could their children. Retrospective analysis of children with AIDS in New York City by Pauline Thomas and colleagues in the city's Department of Public Health has identified six who were born in 1977. Since they were presumably infected perinatally, we may assume that their mothers were also HIV-positive by that year. All six mothers were intravenous drug users: two came from the Bronx, two from Manhattan, and one each from Brooklyn and Staten Island. Five of the six children were born in the last four months of 1977, but one (who later died) was born in February, and this child's birth provides the earliest presumptive evidence of HIV transmission in North America.[47] Additional evidence comes from San Francisco, where an HIV-positive child was born in 1977 to "Mrs. Profit,"[48] a drug-injecting Caucasian prostitute who had not traveled outside California, but who is known to have had a wide range of clients of all races. Mrs. Profit gave birth to two further HIV-positive children in 1979 and 1981, before dying of AIDS in 1986.[49]

Thus seven children born in different parts of the United States in 1977 — all of them to mothers who used intravenous drugs — later proved to be HIV-positive, with no known risk factors other than their parentage. (The possibility of exposure of these children to HIV through sexual abuse, transfusion, or contaminated injection was, in each case, investigated and rejected.) The HIV status of only three of the mothers is known, and all three were HIV-positive.[50]

There is thus retrospective evidence that strongly suggests that HIV was already present in two North American groups — male homosexuals and drug injectors — by the year 1977. There is considerable disagreement about the extent to which the two groups overlap, but certainly a small percentage of male homosexuals inject drugs.[51] The difference in timing — a mere seven months — between the earliest mooted perinatal infection and the first proven homosexual infection is far too small to permit a confident determination of which came first. Besides this, it must be borne in mind that babies can be infected postnatally through breast milk[52] and thus, theoretically at least, the baby born in February 1977 could have been infected by a mother who herself only seroconverted in late 1977 or even 1978.

A further forty-four children who later proved to be HIV-positive were born to drug-injecting mothers in New York by the end of 1978.[53] This sudden increase in children with HIV reflects the even more dramatic increase in HIV prevalence in gay cohorts at around the same point in time, and is suggestive of a virus newly introduced to the two communities, probably at some time during 1977 or 1976.

We are still left, however, with several hypotheses as to how HIV might have arrived in the United States. One classic theory, as espoused by Randy Shilts, is that the virus arrived on board one of the ships or planes carrying visitors to the Bicentennial celebrations in July 1976. The fact that seven drug-injecting mothers from two port cities — some of whom financed their habit through prostitution — appear to have been infected by 1977 is consistent with the theory. So is the fact that a decade after the publication of *And the Band Played On* there is still no incontrovertible evidence (such as a proven instance of HIV infection in the United States in 1975) to confound the Shilts hypothesis.[54]

There are, however, several alternative theories, each of which has its merits and demerits. One, to which we shall return later, proposes that HIV and AIDS were present in North America for years before 1977, but at such a low level that the virus has never been detected among the few archival sera screened, and the disease was not remarked upon by doctors at the time. After all, it took a sudden and ferocious outbreak in a clearly-defined risk group in 1981 before the syndrome was recognized by the best-equipped medical surveillance system in the world.

Another theory is that HIV was introduced in the mid-seventies by contaminated blood imported from Africa or the Caribbean.[55] Yet another is that HIV was brought to North America by Americans who were international travelers, and here the voyages of flight attendants, including Patient 0, NY1, and LA1, and cruise ship attendants, like NY5, may be of relevance. All four men are believed to have visited cities either in the Caribbean, western Europe, or eastern Africa between 1974 and 1977 and, as we shall see in future chapters, there is evidence to suggest that HIV may already have been present in each of these places by these years.

The most frequent of all the common denominators appears to be the mooted link between North America and Haiti. Since Haiti was becoming an increasingly popular winter vacation spot for gay men during the seventies, there is some historical evidence to support such a scenario. As well as gay cruise ships, Haiti has voodoo, men in dark glasses, and African swine fever — all of which have, at different times, been proposed in connection with the onset of the AIDS epidemic. It is time to find out whether any of these exotic rumors have substance.

# 4

## HIGH DAYS AND HOLIDAYS:

## THE HAITIAN INTERCHANGE

The entry for Haiti in the eleventh edition of the *Spartacus International Gay Guide,* published in February 1981, four months before the official advent of AIDS, starts as follows:

> Haitians are cheerful, honest and have a very easy-going attitude towards sex in general. Extreme poverty and extreme happiness abound everywhere.... Haitian men are very beautiful and very well-endowed, and have a great ability to satisfy, whatever it is you are looking for.... They are lovely people, and as they are often treated as "meat," your affection and tenderness will be greatly appreciated and warmly returned.... If you are turned on by beautiful black guys, and can adjust to Haiti's extreme poverty and lack of creature comforts, you may indeed find Haiti a paradise.[1]

This is one of the warmest recommendations in the *Spartacus* guide, which covers the entire world with the exception of the United States. A warning, however, is also included. "Early in 1980, several boys, aged 14 to 16, were hospitalized as a result of sodomy injuries caused by sadistic Caucasian tourists. The result of this was an outbreak of police attacks on the former free-and-easy gay scene and several places have subsequently been closed down. It is advisable for the time being to stay away from Haiti, as it is no longer the paradise it used to be." Despite this inconvenient interruption to normal service, the guide lists several gay hotels, bars, and "houses with boys" — in Cap Haitien on the north coast, Jacmel on the south coast, and the capital, Port-au-Prince, where many of the establishments were located in the Carrefour district down by the quay, Haiti's main center of both male and female prostitution.

---

Haitian tourism almost died out in 1957 when François Duvalier came to power, but picked up again in the late sixties, when he began courting American tourists, inviting them to visit a country that he described as "close, beautiful and politically stable."[2] By 1970, 100,000 were taking up this invitation from Papa Doc, one of the world's great despots, and by the end of the decade, with Club Mediteranée about to open a resort, the annual figure had risen to 150,000.

Precisely when Haiti became known as a holiday hot spot for gay men is harder to determine, but its reputation appears to have been growing throughout the seventies, with Port-au-Prince becoming an increasingly focal stopover on gay cruises, like those on which Nick Rock was employed.[3] The black air steward known as NY1 used to travel there from 1974 onward, and Gaetan Dugas apparently visited the country in 1977, before it became part of the Air Canada network, which suggests that Haiti's attractions were already well known.[4] By 1980, because of the growing poverty, Haiti had become very much a buyer's market, and the fairly discreet gay scene of the sixties and early seventies had been transformed into something much more overt and geared toward foreign tastes.[5]

In late 1981, the CDC began getting reports of AIDS-like conditions occurring in Haitians living in the United States.[6] By mid-1982, a total of thirty-four Haitian AIDS patients had been recorded in Miami, Brooklyn (New York), and elsewhere in the United States.[7] All but four of the thirty-four were men, yet none of them reported any homosexual activity, and only one admitted to a history of intravenous drug use. Some of the CDC interviewers realized, however, that Haitians viewed them with suspicion, as members of the establishment, even of the CIA. Many of the patients were refugees and many had entered the United States illegally. None would wish to admit to anything that might lead to imprisonment or deportation.[8]

A report on the Haitian cases was published in the *MMWR* on July 9, 1982. That same day, Alvin Friedman-Kien wrote to Jim Curran, saying that he too had seen "a number of patients who have had direct exposure to individuals in Haiti itself, or Haitians here in the United States" at his Manhattan clinic, thus providing further evidence for the infectious-agent hypothesis.[9]

Almost immediately, alarmist newspaper articles started appearing, some of which suggested that AIDS had originated in Haiti. The impact on Haitian tourism was instantaneous. Visitors fell away from 75,000 in the winter season of 1981/2 to a mere 10,000 the following winter.[10] In June 1983, the CDC announced that 5 percent of the 1,641 AIDS cases in the United States had involved persons born in Haiti, and took the extraordinary step of formally identifying those of Haitian nationality — alongside homosexuals, intravenous drug users, and patients with hemophilia — as a specific risk group for AIDS.[11] Journalists substituted "heroin-users" for IVDUs, and began making facile references to the "4H Club." By the mid-nineties, Haitian tourism had still not recovered from the bad publicity: there was only one cruise line (running both gay and straight vacations) still calling at Haiti, and then only at Labadie, a 260-acre "private tropical paradise" on the northwest coast.[12] Disembarking passengers were not told that they were entering Haiti, nor was this fact mentioned in the glossy brochures.[13]

By 1983, American and Haitian doctors were writing to medical journals, suggesting that the origin of AIDS might somehow be linked to the recent outbreak of African swine fever in Haitian pigs and the eating of undercooked pork, to bloodletting as a medical practice in rural areas of Haiti, or to voodoo rituals, which allegedly involved the drinking of animal or human blood.[14] One such letter appeared under the facetious title "Night of the Living Dead II: Slow Virus Encephalopathies and AIDS: Do Necromantic Zombiists Transmit HTLV-III/LAV During Voodoo Rituals?"[15] Meanwhile, back in Haiti, several hotels went bankrupt, and a group of Port-au-Prince hoteliers threatened to sue the CDC.

Haitian complaints that most of the Haitian-American cases should have been placed in the homosexual or bisexual category, because it was considered "extremely shameful to acknowledge homosexuality in their culture," were largely ignored.[16] Two years later the CDC reversed its decision, reclassifying most of the Haitian cases as "homosexuals" and the rest in the "other/unknown" risk category, but by then the damage had been done.[17] Haiti's most prominent AIDS researcher, Jean Pape, subsequently claimed that American researchers had "made a serious error in the interpretation of epidemiological data. The CDC never wondered why 88% of the early Haitian AIDS cases in the U.S. occurred in males. In 1983, our group had identified risk factors [such as] bisexuality and blood transfusion in 79% of Haitian AIDS patients."[18] Dr. Pape also commented that "The disparity in the data from the United States and Haiti may be attributable, in part, to a greater willingness of Haitians to provide reliable responses to personal questions in their native country and language."[19]

Among that first group of Haitians with AIDS questioned by Pape's group, by far the most important risk factor turned out to be bisexuality, being cited by exactly half of Haitian AIDS patients in 1983. Significantly, the proportion fell to just 1 percent by 1987, which gives some idea of the impact of the Haitian AIDS scare of 1982/3, and of the key role played by gay tourism in the years preceding. Other key factors were the Haitian government's announcement, in 1983, that homosexual men would henceforth be jailed for six months and then spend an additional six months in "rehabilitation" and its request that foreigners who owned gay establishments should leave the country forthwith.[20] It would seem that many Haitian men were willing to swing both ways when paid to do so, but reverted to more traditional sexual habits when homosexuality became dangerous and the stream of rich, gay foreigners dried up.

---

What this does not tell us, however, is whether in the first instance HIV was brought to America by Haitian immigrants, or by American gays returning from the Caribbean, or whether the movement was in the other direction, with U.S. gays introducing the virus to the island of Hispaniola (which contains Haiti and the Dominican Republic). It is here that the early footprints of HIV and AIDS in the Caribbean offer some intriguing clues.

Jean Pape's first paper about AIDS in Haiti, published in October 1983, depicts the course of a rapidly escalating epidemic.[21] He and his colleagues recorded seven retrospective cases of AIDS in 1980, sixteen cases in 1981, and thirty-seven in the first ten months of 1982. Pape also launched a determined search for pre-1980 cases. A review of hospital records at three private hospitals in Port-au-Prince revealed no plausible cases of AIDS, but a review of work performed between 1978 and 1982 at the Albert Schweitzer hospital, which serves 115,000 people in the rural area around Deschapelles, did reveal a plausible case: a previously healthy twenty-year-old man who had generalized seizures in July of 1978, who died a fortnight later, and who was revealed at autopsy to have toxoplasmosis of the central nervous system. Three further suggestive cases were seen in Haiti in 1979, and a further four cases of AIDS occurred in 1978/9 in Haitian émigrés (three living in Montreal and one in Miami).[22]

It is interesting that the earliest AIDS cases among Haitians and Americans apparently occurred in the same year — 1978. However, calculating cases-per-population gives a very different picture. Haiti's total of eight pre-1980 cases out of approximately 5.5 million people (allowing for 500,000 living overseas) is over twenty-seven times greater than the twelve AIDS cases recorded in 1978 and 1979 among the population of the United States.

Furthermore, seroepidemiological studies indicate that HIV was far more prevalent in the general population in Haiti than it was in the United States in the early eighties. For example, research by Pape and coworkers in 1986/7 detected an HIV prevalence of 9 percent among adults tested in Port-au-Prince, and 3 percent among rural adults.[23] The seroprevalence among Haitian immigrants to the United States was 4.6 percent.[24] HIV infection among American adults in the first half of the eighties appears to have been roughly a hundred times lower.[25]

It may be that, in addition to sexual networking, factors such as the popularity of medical injections, both self-administered and given by local folk healers or *piquristes*, facilitated a rapid early spread of HIV in Haiti.[26] However, this data also suggests that HIV may have arrived earlier in Haiti than in the United States.

In fact, four separate incidents provide circumstantial evidence that HIV was already present in urban areas of Haiti between 1976 and 1978. All involved foreign nationals, and three of the four certainly occurred outside the homosexual/bisexual milieu. In September 1978, while on honeymoon in Port-au-Prince, a French geologist had a car crash, which required his being transfused with eight units of blood; he developed AIDS in 1981, and died the following year.[27] And a Swiss woman developed AIDS in 1982, five years after holidaying in Haiti. During her 1977 vacation she also contracted hepatitis B infection, and her lack of other risk factors suggests that she may have acquired both viruses heterosexually. Another Swiss citizen, a man of unknown sexual orientation, developed AIDS in 1980 after vacationing in Haiti in 1978.[28] And in 1981, a fifty-two-year-old Canadian woman died of AIDS in Montreal. For twenty years, up to 1972, this woman had worked in Haiti as a nun, but from then until 1979 she concentrated on more earthly work, helping to rehabilitate prostitutes in Port-au-Prince. At some point in those seven years she apparently had a single sexual encounter — and according to Jacques Leibowitch, this occurred in or before 1976.[29]

Leibowitch also has some interesting observations to offer about the purchase of blood from Haiti. From the beginning of the seventies, he writes, the use of Factor VIII blood-clotting concentrates became widespread among American hemophiliacs. Each batch of concentrate was prepared from the pooled plasma of several thousand donors, and in the early part of the decade much of that blood was purchased from the Caribbean and Latin America, most notably from Port-au-Prince. There the lucrative business was monopolized by the Hemo-Caribbean Company of Haiti, owned by Joseph Gorinstein, a New York stockbroker, whose links to the Haitian government involved Luckner Cambronne — the minister of defense and Papa Doc's brother-in-law. Leibowitch claims that most of the blood used in North America prior to 1975 came from Haiti, but that after a series of scandals about the methods of procurement, the U.S. Food and Drug Administration would no longer license Haitian blood after that year.[30] He believes that this shows that HIV was not present in Haiti before 1976.

Piet Hagen's book, *Blood: Gift or Merchandise,* has a slightly different sequence of events.[31] According to him, Jean-Claude Duvalier, the Baby who succeeded Papa in 1971, was angered by the bad press[32] and closed down Hemo-Caribbean in November 1972, prompting Cambronne to flee the country. But Hagen adds that Gorinstein later tried to reopen the Port-au-Prince facility, and he cites reports from 1975, 1979, and 1981 that suggest that the commercial collection of blood had resumed in Haiti. Although there is no evidence as to where such blood was sold or utilized, it is worth noting that the first recorded hemophiliac seroconversion in the United States was not until 1978,[33] by which time the source of contamination could well have been an American gay or IVDU blood donor.

---

In fact, there is further circumstantial evidence that suggests HIV may have been present in Haiti as early as 1973 or 1974. The greatest influxes of Haitians to North America have taken place since 1972, when boat people started setting off from the north coast of Haiti, bound for Florida. That flow became a torrent when a lengthy drought caused famine in 1975–1977, and by 1980 there were 40,000 official Haitian refugees in the United States, and a further 100,000 to 300,000 illegal immigrants.[34]

The three greatest expatriate concentrations of Haitians are found in Miami, New York City (and, in particular, Brooklyn), and Montreal, and in 1983, doctors from these three cities published papers on AIDS cases among Haitian immigrants. Twenty patients seen between April 1980 and December 1981 were reported from Miami, three of whom had entered the United States in 1976, 1975, and 1974.[35] Another ten Haitian patients were seen between January 1981 and July 1982 at the Kings County Hospital in Brooklyn, some of whom arrived in the United States as early as 1973/74.[36] The same pattern, only more pronounced, is revealed from Montreal. Of the first eight Haitian patients with AIDS, three had arrived in Canada in 1976 and one in 1974.[37] In all three cities, the patients questioned claimed to have had no sexual contact with people back in Haiti or with other Haitian immigrants since moving to North America, and admitted to no other risk factors. If correct, this would mean that they could only have been exposed to HIV infection in Haiti before emigrating in the mid-seventies.

There is one further report that offers supporting serological evidence. In November 1984, soon after the advent of the HIV antibody test, researchers from the Pasteur Institute of Cayenne, the capital of French Guiana, tested the sera of 211 apparently healthy Haitians living in the area,[38] and found six to be HIV-positive. At least one of the six had arrived in Guiana from Haiti in 1974.

When examined in toto, this substantial circumstantial evidence — involving nine early émigrés — suggests that HIV may well have been present in Haiti as early as 1973 or 1974, though at a very low prevalence. This in turn suggests that the Hemo-Caribbean episode might well represent a close shave, in that the first outbreak of AIDS in the United States could so easily have occurred among hemophiliacs in the mid-seventies, three or four years before the actual outbreak in gay men.

---

Let us assume for a moment that HIV really was present in Haitians in 1974. This still leaves open the question of who infected whom. In essence, there are two possible scenarios: that "international gays" infected Haitians (presumably prior to 1974), or that Haitians infected gay visitors (between 1974 and 1977).

What limited evidence there is lends some support to the scenario of an initial straight-to-gay interchange, for 40 percent of the earliest cases of AIDS in Haiti, seen in 1980 and before, occurred in women.[39] This dropped dramatically to 9 percent in the series reported by Jean Pape for 1981 and 1982, before rising again to 27 percent for 1983–1985, and 31 percent for 1986–1988. This data, although too limited to attain statistical significance, could be interpreted as suggesting that HIV was initially present in Haitian heterosexuals, that it transferred to the gay community in Port-au-Prince in the second half of the seventies (causing an increase in AIDS in bisexuals and homosexuals at the start of the eighties), but that it began to reassume a more evenly balanced sex distribution after the AIDS scare of 1982.[40]

What *can* be proposed with some confidence is that Port-au-Prince in the seventies may have represented a key interchange for HIV on its world tour, that a pivotal role may have been played by Haitian bisexuals in the latter half of the seventies, and that this is possibly where HIV first entered the gay community. By 1980, the flow of the virus was almost certainly bidirectional: northward from Haiti by plane, and on board those overcrowded boats as they lumbered across the Great Bahama Bank toward the Florida coastline — and southward by plane and cruise ship from Miami, Montreal, and the "pink triangle" cities of New York, Los Angeles, and San Francisco.

---

All this returns us once more to the question of source. As we shall see later, the early theories of origin, which saw AIDS emerging from pigs, bloodletting, and necromantic rituals in Haiti, appear to have been based more closely on Hollywood depictions of voodoo and zombiism than on a real appreciation of *vodun* as a complex religion with its roots in Africa.[41] Allegations that voodoo rituals include practices such as cannibalism and the drinking of human blood appear to be without substance and are, in any case, irrelevant to the story of the origin of AIDS — unless one proposes that HIV could have arrived in Haiti with slaves originating from central Africa, two centuries or more ago. The same goes for the untrained "injectionists" with their syringes and needles — they may conceivably have played a role in the early transmission of HIV in Haiti (although this is disputed),[42] but cannot be relevant to the origin of the virus. So, let us instead examine two rather more plausible hypotheses as to how HIV might have arrived in Haiti.

The first proposes that HIV came to the country with Haitians returning from the central African country of Congo in the sixties and seventies. The history of this rather unexpected connection is as follows. After the mass exodus of the Belgians at the time of the Congo's independence in 1960, and again after the upheavals of 1964, the Congolese government sought replacements for the professional and technical positions previously filled by their former colonial masters, who had themselves signally failed to train adequate African replacements. They turned to Haiti, a black, independent, French-speaking nation, many of whose better-educated inhabitants were more than ready to depart the land of Papa Doc and his feared militia, the Tontons Macoutes. From the early sixties through the seventies, several thousand Haitians left to work in the Congo.[43] At least a thousand of these were employed by the United Nations, and got home leave every two or three years. However, many of them, fearing that they might have problems leaving Haiti if they ever returned, preferred to spend their vacations in places like Belgium, the United States, and Canada.[44] Again, although many thousands of these technocrats eventually returned to Haiti during the seventies and eighties, some of them (after tasting freedom and privilege overseas) later reemigrated to North America or Europe.

In 1984, a fascinating study of risk factors for AIDS was initiated among Haitians living in Miami and New York, using Creole-speaking interviewers. The report, published in early 1987,[45] found no significant correlations with a history of injections or tattoos, past homosexual experience, or past travel to central Africa. And yet the tables of results revealed a fascinating fact — of the fifty-five Haitian-Americans with AIDS involved in the study, one had indeed visited central Africa — which almost certainly meant the Congo.[46]

As will be explained later, there is increasing evidence from the virologists and phylogeneticists (who have analyzed a wide range of HIV isolates* and have drawn up detailed viral family trees documenting ancestry) that there is a single source for the various HIV-1 strains found in North America, Europe, and the Caribbean — nearly all of which belong to a clade, or group, called "subtype B." One can therefore postulate that a single Haitian who became infected in the Congo (where, as we shall see, HIV has been present for some time) and who later returned to Haiti before reemigrating to the United States, might theoretically have been the source of the epidemic of HIV-1 subtype B, the so-called Euro-American strain.

However, there is a second scenario, equally plausible, which posits that the initial introduction of HIV to Haiti might have occurred within the gay community, rather than the straight. Haiti's growing popularity in the seventies as a gay holiday venue, as a place for affordable sex, drugs, and *reggae,* meant that

---

* Isolate: a microorganism found in an infectee and cultivated on tissue culture.

it also attracted many men from Europe, and one group made its presence felt in a number of ways. That caustic editorial comment in the 1981 edition of the *Spartacus* guide makes it clear that the sadistic tourists who had put local teenagers in the hospital with rectal injuries were "predominantly German and Swiss."

The possibility of a German connection is reinforced by the fact that one of the first AIDS patients in the United States was a thirty-three-year-old German homosexual who died in Manhattan in December 1980.[47] What is not recorded in the literature, however, is that this man had not come to the United States direct from Germany. Between 1977 and the summer of 1980, he had been living in Haiti, working as a chef, and throughout this period he had suffered from inflammatory bowel disease. One of his New York doctors, Donna Mildvan, says that in retrospect this may have represented a prodrome — or early symptom — of AIDS (in which case it is possible that he was already HIV-positive prior to settling in Haiti). Indeed, the patient's chart also records that "he did travel to the Caribbean often," suggesting that this man may have visited Haiti some years before moving there in 1977.[48] Given the circumstantial evidence that Haitians may have been HIV-positive as early as 1973 or 1974, this could be significant.

This second possibility — that HIV might have been introduced to Haiti by gay visitors from Europe — would clearly become a lot more plausible if it could be demonstrated that there were even earlier traces of AIDS on that continent. It is time to take a look at the first traces of HIV in the Old World.

# 5

## EARLY TRACES IN EUROPE

The bare bones of the story so far — concerning the emergence of AIDS in North America and Haiti — are probably familiar to those with a basic knowledge of the history of the epidemic. By contrast, the history of the emergence of AIDS in Europe is less well known, although it is one that almost certainly extends even further back in time.

All over Europe, in the early eighties, gay men who had previously vacationed and had sex in North America were themselves contracting AIDS. If we leave aside David Carr, the first known fatality from AIDS in Britain was a forty-nine-year-old gay man who died in the fall of 1981 from PCP and CMV infections; he had visited gay friends in Miami on an annual basis up to the year of his death.[1] One of the next to die, in March 1982, was a personnel director with a blue chip company, whose work required him to travel widely throughout Europe, and who vacationed at least twice in the late seventies in America, with most of his time being spent in San Francisco.[2]

However, the links with America were not always so clear-cut. One of the first countries in Europe to experience the new syndrome was Denmark. In retrospect, it would appear that the first man to present with symptoms was a thirty-seven-year-old agricultural engineer who died of PCP and arthralgia in September 1980. He is believed to have been bisexual, and during 1979 he studied in New York. However, his first symptoms — a chronic cough, poor appetite, and persistent weight loss — had occurred in October 1978, and he apparently had not visited the United States before that date.[3] It may be, therefore, that if he had lovers during his time in New York, then far from getting infected by them, he transmitted his infection to them. This is the first suggestion that the passage of HIV across the Atlantic may — even in these early days — have been in both directions.

Much mention is made of contact with America in the first published paper on AIDS in Denmark which appeared in July 1982,[4] but of the four patients described, only one had himself visited the United States (and he only in the year preceding onset of symptoms), though one of the others lived with a man who made regular transatlantic visits. Once again, it is unclear whether the virus was on board the outward or return flights. However, a subsequent paper reported that there was a significantly higher risk (more than sevenfold) of having a low T-cell count among Danish gay men who had visited the United States (versus those who had not), and that this increase first became apparent in persons who had visited in 1980 and after.[5] This shows that even if contacts between local and American gay men were crucial to the early dynamics of the Danish epidemic, they were not necessarily pertinent to its source.

However, the European country that provides the earliest evidence of AIDS among gay men is Germany. There are two intriguing cases, both of which precede any of those thus far described as regards both date of onset and date of death.

The first case involves a twenty-one-year-old soldier who came from one of the Rheinland towns to the south of Bonn. He fell ill in October 1977 with ill-defined pains in his abdomen and unexplained weight loss. During 1978, he developed further symptoms, and spent several months at the large military hospital at Koblenz, before being transferred to the university hospital at Ulm. There his doctors, under the director of internal medicine, Hermann Heimpel, ran a battery of tests and discovered that his lymph nodes were full of macrophages (white blood cells), which were themselves full of an unusual mycobacterium, *M. fortuitum*. They realized that they were dealing with an unexplained T-cell deficiency that was probably not congenital, but were at a loss as to how to treat him. Finally, in January 1979, the young soldier died.

Unfortunately, samples relevant to the case were destroyed in a fire in 1986, so it is unlikely that it will ever be known with certainty whether HIV was responsible. When questioned sixteen years later, however, Professor Heimpel said that he was "sure that this was a case of AIDS." The soldier had neither had a transfusion, nor had he traveled away from home, apart from the eight months spent at a single German army base, and there were no physical indications that he had been sexually abused or raped. Nobody ever thought to question him about his sexual preferences, but Dr. Heimpel believes that the patient once volunteered that he was homosexual.[6]

In the same month, January 1979, another German man also died from what was almost certainly AIDS, but his was an entirely different personality from that of the young soldier. Herbert H., a fifty-two-year-old concert violinist who had played with one of Cologne's symphony orchestras, was completely open about his homosexuality, although this fact was not mentioned in the original 1979 paper that reported his death from multiple-site Kaposi's sarcoma, meningitis, and a battery of infections including *Molluscum contagiosum,* oral thrush, and perianal warts.[7] In April 1983, however, his doctors, under Wolfram Sterry, a dermatologist at the University of Cologne, wrote to the *Lancet,* declaring that their patient had been gay, and proposing that his mysterious immunosuppression and death might have been caused by AIDS.[8]

There were certain additional features about their patient that they did not, however, reveal. The first was that Herbert was not simply homosexual, but actively bisexual. He clearly had a large appetite for life, which included a penchant for orgies. For these, it was not essential that women be present, but when they were, he apparently preferred them to be big-breasted — "the bigger the better," according to Sterry's recollection.

Dr. Sterry also remembers that Herbert spent several months of each year traveling around Europe, where he had several lovers in different countries. He spoke of visits to France, Italy, and Austria (particularly Vienna) — though he apparently never visited America or the Caribbean. And although nobody has tested stored sera or tissues, Sterry is now certain about the diagnosis: "It was AIDS — I'm quite confident of that," he says.[9] It is noteworthy that Herbert's first symptoms began in December 1976, more than a year before symptoms began appearing in American gays.

These two cases — and that of Herbert in particular — suggest that HIV may have arrived earlier among German gays and bisexuals than among their American and Haitian counterparts.[10] However, given the variability of the asymptomatic period, this is far from proven; the Germans may, for instance, have been infected with a more virulent strain.

There are further clues also. The family of the German chef who worked in Haiti and died of AIDS in New York at the end of 1980 come from Gelsenkirchen in the Ruhr,[11] which lies some fifty miles from Cologne, where Herbert lived, and roughly a hundred miles from the hometown of the soldier. Cologne is the main urban center of this part of Germany, and the possibility that HIV may have been circulating in the vibrant gay clubs and leather bars of the city during the seventies has to be admitted, as does the possibility that the Gelsenkirchen chef was already infected by the time he first visited Haiti.

Running against this hypothesis is the fact that no other German AIDS cases were reported until 1982, and that six of the seven patients recorded in that year were believed to have been infected by American homosexuals, and the seventh by Factor VIII.[12] It would appear, therefore, that if HIV did enter the German gay scene at an early stage, it may have burned itself out without sparking a local epidemic (even if the sparks may have traveled rather farther afield).

---

By September 1983, 243 AIDS cases had been diagnosed in Europe, of which 221 were evaluable for probable source of infection. A detailed report on these cases documents that 33 percent involved gays who had probably been infected in the United States; 10 percent gays who had probably been infected in Haiti; and 21 percent gays who had not had sexual exposures in either the United States or Haiti, but who had had contacts with other European men. Just a handful of cases had occurred in IVDUs, or persons exposed to blood products. However, fully 29 percent of the 221 cases involved Africans. The report emphasizes, in italics, that *"A new group at risk of developing AIDS has emerged in Europe . . . namely patients originating from central Africa."*[13] It soon became clear that not only Africans, but persons who had visited equatorial Africa, or who had had sex with people from that region, were at risk.

France is the country that best exemplifies the different groups that were demonstrating susceptibility to AIDS at the end of the seventies. It is also the European country that identified the most pre-epidemic cases, with seven recorded from Parisian hospitals alone up to the end of 1979.[14] However, four of these involved middle-aged gay men who were diagnosed with KS in 1974, 1975, 1978, and 1979, but who were all still alive in 1983. These men are no longer mentioned in reviews of early AIDS in Europe, which strongly suggests that they had the more indolent, "classical" form of KS, which is uncomplicated by HIV infection.[15]

The fifth pre-1980 patient seen in France was an African with opportunistic infections; specific details of this case were never published. The sixth and seventh cases involved Europeans with African connections. One was a thirty-two-year-old French woman who had been living in the Congo between 1971 and 1976 with an apparently healthy Congolese husband. The other was a thirty-five-year-old Portuguese man who, from 1968 to 1974, had been driving trucks from one coast of Africa to the other, between the then colonies of Angola and Mozambique. He was heterosexual, and had occasionally had sex with prostitutes. Both of these patients presented with PCP at the Tenon hospital in Paris — the woman in October 1976 and the man in June 1978[16] — and both died soon afterward. (However, as was later revealed, the man was actually infected with "the second AIDS virus," HIV-2.)[17]

Jacques Leibowitch and Jean Baptiste Brunet, the two leading figures in the Study Group on the Epidemiology of AIDS in France, were increasingly persuaded that the AIDS epidemic was linked to Africa. By 1982, they were encouraging fellow doctors to look out for unusual diseases in their African patients, and by early 1983 they were traveling up and down the east coast of America, delivering papers about their "African hypothesis."[18]

In March 1983, this group had an important letter published in the *Lancet* concerning the first twenty-nine AIDS cases seen in France. Even if, in retrospect, most of the eleven "KS only" cases look dubious as instances of AIDS, the eighteen cases of opportunistic infections are clearly significant, as the French doctors ably demonstrated in their analysis. Eight of these OI cases involved homosexuals, six of whom had traveled to the United States in the previous five years. The other ten involved heterosexuals, only one of whom had ever been to the United States, but five of whom had visited Haiti. Of the remainder, four had lived in Equatorial Africa — the two Europeans mentioned above, plus two Congolese men. "We suggest that Equatorial Africa is an endemic zone for the supposed infectious agent(s) of this illness," the French doctors wrote.

They were not, however, the first to air this hypothesis in print. In the previous week's edition of the *Lancet*, a group of Belgian doctors under Nathan Clumeck had reported five Africans with AIDS, three of whom were women and four of whom came from the Congo.[19] The letter concluded: "This preliminary report suggests that black Africans, whether immigrants or not, may be another group predisposed to AIDS."

A month later, in response to these letters from France and Belgium, two further letters from European doctors appeared in the *Lancet*, both reporting early cases of clinical AIDS with an African connection. A Danish woman surgeon who had worked for much of the seventies in rural Congo fell sick with wasting and PCP in 1976, and died in Copenhagen in 1977.[20] That same year, a Congolese airline secretary from Kinshasa reported to a hospital in Brussels with a wide range of typical AIDS infections. She returned to the Congo, where she died early in 1978.[21] A subsequent article about African AIDS patients in Belgium noted that the husband of a Congolese woman with prodromal AIDS had himself died in Brussels in 1976 from infections which, the authors observed, represented "a picture consistent with AIDS."[22] Suddenly, therefore, a number of much earlier AIDS cases were being recognized, all of which had links with equatorial Africa.

The distribution within Europe of these African-linked cases was extremely significant, for most of the patients were appearing in Belgian hospitals, and were Congolese. By August 1983, Belgium's total number of AIDS patients was thirty-eight, of whom thirty-four were African, and two were Europeans who had had sexual relationships with Africans.[23] These were remarkable statistics, given that just six thousand to eight thousand persons from central Africa were living in Belgium at the time, and that most of the African cases had apparently emerged from within this immigrant community. "The [African] cases seen in Belgium are probably only the tip of an iceberg," wrote Nathan Clumeck,[24] adopting what would quickly become the most overemployed metaphor of the epidemic.

By contrast Britain and France, both of which had once enjoyed far larger colonial holdings on the continent, had seen far fewer cases of AIDS. By late 1983 France had seen twenty-two cases in persons presumed to have been infected in central Africa (many of whom came from former Belgian colonies).[25] Britain had seen none.[26] These figures clearly suggested that certain specific areas of Africa (most notably the former central African colonies of Belgium and, to a lesser extent, France) might be high-risk areas for AIDS.

If plausible archival cases were being retrospectively diagnosed in the central African population living in Europe, and among Europeans who had recently lived or had sex in central Africa, then it seemed reasonable to hypothesize that AIDS might have been present for some time in this region, but had gone unrecognized as a new disease syndrome amidst the welter of infections already present. Not all European doctors agreed, however. Some who had themselves worked in Africa insisted that they would certainly have recognized a condition as striking as AIDS — especially its more uncommon presentations, like candidiasis of the esophagus — had it been common in the sixties or seventies. Others, mindful of the political sensitivity of such claims, maintained a cautious silence.

During the rest of the eighties, only one further substantial European case study emerged to bolster this hypothesis of an earlier AIDS epidemic in Africa, and this took the form of yet another letter to the *Lancet*, written in 1988, which came from an unexpected quarter.[27] In 1976, three Norwegian family members — a father, mother, and nine-year-old daughter — all died in southern Norway with symptoms typical of AIDS, and now sera from all three, drawn in the early seventies, had tested HIV-positive. The father had presented with his first symptoms as early as 1966, and it seemed likely that he had infected his wife, who had in turn infected the daughter perinatally. The Norwegian doctors noted: "The father had been a sailor and had visited foreign countries, including African ports, several times before 1966. In this period he had contracted sexually transmitted diseases at least twice." This raised the possibility that on one of those occasions he could also have become infected with HIV.

In the light of this overwhelming evidence, Africa also becomes our next port of call.

# 6

## HIV and AIDS in central africa

First, we need to take a further brief look at AIDS in the former British colonies of eastern Africa. We have already seen that the border region between Uganda and Tanzania was a significant staging post for HIV-1, even if this region was probably not the place where the first AIDS cases emerged. But a thousand miles to the south of Kagera lies the Zambian capital of Lusaka, where another very significant episode in the history of AIDS occurred. For it was here, in early 1983, that an African form of AIDS was first recognized by an Africa-based physician — Dr. Anne Bayley.

During the seventies and eighties, Dr. Bayley was professor of surgery at the University Teaching Hospital (UTH), the only public hospital in Lusaka. She clearly recalls the "Eureka moment"— the day when she realized that something different was happening with the KS cases in her ward. "I had been seeing about eight to twelve cases every year since 1978 — a very steady level," she explains. "And then one day — it was in the January of 1983 — I went into my ward to do a round, and I realized that there were nine cases of KS in there at once." Many of these were of a very different, more aggressive type of KS, accompanied by swollen lymph nodes. "I realized that I was seeing a new manifestation of the disease. And I remember being frightened. I'd never seen this range of presentations before, and I knew this disease well. These people responded to chemotherapy, but then the disease recurred within two, three or four months." Dr. Bayley also began to realize that the socioeconomic background of the patients was changing, and that a different, wealthier, more educated group appeared to be more susceptible to this new form of the disease.

During the first five months of 1983, she gradually became persuaded that this new form was the same as the aggressive KS being seen in American gays.

By the end of the year, she had seen ten of the old-style KS patients, all ten of whom were still alive and well, together with thirteen of the new-style KS patients — eight of whom had died.[1] Absolute confirmation of causation came in 1985, when one of her 1983 patients returned to the hospital, and his blood was found to be HIV-positive.

Later, Dr. Bayley realized that she had almost certainly seen three of the atypical KS cases before 1983: one in each of the three previous years. The first of these patients came to UTH in January 1980: a woman of fifty-five from Chipata, in eastern Zambia, who presented with aggressive KS, a blue swelling under her tongue, an enlarged spleen, and lymphadenopathy (both of the neck and deep within the abdomen). With her considerable experience of African KS and African AIDS, Dr. Bayley feels that this clinical picture was probably indicative of the latter.[2]

And this was not the only presentation of AIDS she was witnessing. Dr. Bayley also recalls, retrospectively, other patients from the early eighties who exhibited a range of AIDS-like opportunistic infections. The first of these was a young Zambian-based Englishman who developed full-blown AIDS in 1983, but who had been unwell since August 1980 with weight loss, lack of energy, and "vague aches and pains."

If correct, this pushes the advent of the Zambian epidemic back by three years from its *official* beginning in 1983 — a proposal that is supported by three clinical histories from a small hospital at the mining center of Kalalushi, near the town of Kitwe in northern Zambia. The patients were two female secretaries (who had shared the same male lover) and a young male worker. All three died from typical presentations of AIDS in 1985, and the one patient whose blood was tested for HIV proved to be positive. The medical charts reveal that symptoms of immune-suppression began in 1979 in one case, and in 1980 in the others.[3]

One other pertinent case of AIDS from Zambia involved a fifty-eight-year-old Englishman who presented with typical AIDS symptoms in 1983. He had lived in Africa for a total of twenty-five years, but between 1978 and 1980 he had been based in Rwanda, which, according to Dr. Bayley, is very possibly the place where he became infected.

In all likelihood, therefore, AIDS was occurring in three distinct areas of Zambia — the Copper Belt in the north, Chipata in the east, and Lusaka in the center — by 1980, or even 1979. The geographical diversity of the sightings suggests that the well-developed road and rail network in Zambia may have played a significant role in early spread. Although there was no explosion of AIDS in Zambia, as occurred in Uganda as a result of the liberation war, there was a steady rise in HIV prevalence, so that by the start of the nineties over 30 percent of adults in Lusaka were infected.[4]

In Kenya, the other major English-speaking country in East Africa, retrospective serosurveys of blood taken from female prostitutes and attendees at STD clinics suggest that HIV was not present until 1981,[5] while the first known case of AIDS did not occur until 1983, in a Nairobi-based Ugandan journalist.[6] The fact that Kenya is situated on the coast to the east of Uganda offers further support to the hypothesis of a virus percolating outward from a central African source.

All this suggests three important conclusions. First, the personal testimonies and records of experienced African-based physicians are revealed, once again, to be as useful as the published literature in terms of identifying the first appearances of AIDS. This may be partly because poorer resources in Africa, and the greater overall disease burden, mean that fewer unusual cases are thought noteworthy enough to be written up for journals. Second, it seems unlikely that the former British colonies of East Africa represent the source of AIDS, in that North America, the Caribbean, and Europe all witnessed probable cases before the earliest plausible reports from Uganda, Tanzania, Zambia, and Kenya. Third, there are clues from Zambia and Uganda[7] (and further evidence from Belgium and France) that suggest that some of the early cases in those countries may have been infected in Belgium's former central African colonies of Rwanda, Burundi, and the Congo.

In early 1985 Belgian doctors based in Kigali, the capital of Rwanda, wrote to the *Lancet* about finding a cluster of HIV infections in a Rwandese family comprising a mother, father, and three sons, aged six years, five years, and eighteen months.[8] The history went back a long way. Within three months of the birth of the first boy in 1977, the mother had experienced a range of unexplained symptoms, including chronic diarrhea, dramatic weight loss, lymphadenopathy, disseminated dermatitis, and oral candidiasis. She was still alive in 1984, but had a depressed T-cell count, as did her husband, who was otherwise healthy. All three of the children had experienced inflammation of the salivary glands, and the youngest also had a swollen spleen and persistent oral thrush. In retrospect, it seems likely that the mother was presenting with early symptoms of AIDS in either 1977 or early 1978, thus predating the first official case of AIDS in Rwanda by at least five years.

The likelihood that HIV was already spreading in this immediate region by the mid to late seventies is further supported by the case of a thirty-one-year-old Dane who died of PCP and CMV infections in August 1983, after a year of ill health. The man had lived in Rwanda between 1974 and 1976, and in Bujumbura, the capital of neighboring Burundi, between 1976 and 1981. In the latter country he had been "frequenting Tutsi bar-girls" and had been treated for syphilis and, on several occasions, gonorrhea.[9]

Evidently HIV infection was spreading rapidly in Rwanda by the early eighties, for in July 1984, a group of thirty-three female prostitutes in the second city,

Butare (home of a large army camp and the national university), were tested, and an astonishing twenty-nine — or 88 percent — were found to have HIV antibodies. Even today, this represents one of the highest prevalences ever recorded for prostitutes, or for any other risk group apart from prospective AIDS patients. These women had an average of forty-four partners a month, and their reported sexual activity was strikingly conservative, with over 95 percent involving straightforward penile-vaginal sex, and with oral and anal sex making up the remaining 5 percent in equal measure. (This helped give the lie to those Western "experts" who claimed that the AIDS epidemic in Africa stemmed from a predilection for anal intercourse, or its use as a contraceptive method.[10]) That HIV was not restricted to those who sold sex was demonstrated by the fact that 12 percent of a control group of nonprostitute women from Butare also tested positive.[11]

1984 was the year when HIV antibody testing began, and many of the early ELISA tests were subsequently found to register high levels of false positives. Nonetheless, the overall validity of the 1984 Butare survey would seem to be corroborated by follow-up studies conducted eight years later, which found that fourteen of the twenty-nine HIV-positive prostitutes had died with symptoms suggestive of AIDS, while of the others one had been murdered, two lost to follow-up, and twelve were still alive. The survivors were generally those who were younger, or who had had higher T-cell counts in 1984.[12]

In December 1986, Rwanda became the first country in the world to stage a national serosurvey of HIV-1 prevalence which embraced all age groups from infants to the elderly. The results were staggering, for they revealed that 17.8 percent of urban dwellers and 1.3 percent of rural dwellers were HIV-positive.[13] The specific results for individual prefectures were published in 1988 in an article in Rwanda's own medical journal, the *Revue Médicale Rwandaise*.[14] Butare was not the town with the highest HIV prevalence; in fact, it was only the fourth, at 16 percent. Ahead of it came the capital, Kigali, with 21 percent prevalence, but the list was dramatically headed by two small towns in the Hutu heartland of western Rwanda: Ruhengeri (22 percent) and Gisenyi (31 percent). The latter statistic is quite startling, and the article further reveals that more than half of all persons aged twenty-six to forty in that lakeside town on the Congolese border were already HIV-positive by the end of 1986.

One small crumb of encouragement was that rural prevalence was comparatively low, which was clearly significant in a country in which about 95 percent of the population live in rural areas. However, Rwanda also has the highest population density in Africa, meaning that very few people live far from a town. Even in 1986, few doctors doubted that significant urban-to-rural HIV diffusion would occur within a fairly short period of time.[15]

In October 1983, prompted by the evidence of AIDS among Africans in Europe (as reported in the letters to the *Lancet* in March 1983 from doctors in Brussels and Paris),[16] two teams of European and American doctors set off for Rwanda and the Congo to investigate the pattern of AIDS in central Africa. By this stage, certain doctors in Kinshasa and Kigali, as well as Anne Bayley in Lusaka, were beginning to report increases in diseases like cryptococcus, tuberculosis, esophageal candidiasis, KS, and enteropathic conditions such as Slim — and it was important to determine whether these were genuine cases of AIDS and, if so, just how they compared to the spectrum of diseases that was associated with AIDS in the West.[17]

A joint team of Belgian, Dutch, and Rwandan doctors spent four weeks in Kigali, and readily identified twenty-six cases of AIDS and prodromal AIDS, equally divided between the sexes. Nearly all cases involved employed urban middle-class people: only one came from a strictly rural area (Bugarama, in the extreme southwest).[18] The paper concluded that "Urban activity, a reasonable standard of living, heterosexual promiscuity and contact with prostitutes could be risk factors for African AIDS."[19]

Meanwhile, a team of American, Belgian, and Congolese doctors spent three weeks in the Congolese capital, Kinshasa, and identified thirty-eight AIDS patients. Once again, those affected were relatively affluent, more than half of them having attended hospitals that catered mainly for private patients.[20] The findings of the Rwandese and Congolese teams were published side by side in the *Lancet* in July 1984.

The Congo paper, the lead author of which was Peter Piot (later head of the United Nations joint program on AIDS, UNAIDS), was especially interesting. It demonstrated an equal sex ratio (even though the mean age of female AIDS patients was twenty-eight years, versus forty-one years for men, probably as a result of patterns of sexual behavior). It showed that the immunological characteristics of AIDS patients in Africa and the United States were the same, and it discounted homosexuality, transfusion, or intravenous drug use as risk factors. It concluded powerfully: "The findings of this study strongly argue that the situation in central Africa represents a new epidemiological setting for this worldwide disease — that of significant transmission in a large heterosexual population."

In addition to the thirty-eight AIDS patients, there was commentary about several further anecdotal cases, which included two clusters, each involving five people who had had heterosexual contact with at least one of the others. All ten persons had died, the earliest death occurring in 1980, and the chronologies suggested that both male-to-female and female-to-male heterosexual transmission had taken place. At that stage, only a handful of potential male-to-female transmissions had been described in the United States, and no transmissions had been reported from women to men.

Mention was also made of thirty-five cases of cryptococcal meningitis that had occurred in Kinshasa since 1981. A key paper had already been published on this subject in 1982,[21] in which fifteen cases of this unusual disease were described (fourteen of them fatal, and five involving coincidental TB infection). All fifteen cases had occurred in two Kinshasa hospitals in the space of eighteen months, and it was pointed out that, in contrast, only one case per year had been reported from the same hospitals during the previous two decades, most of which had responded to treatment with a powerful antifungal drug.[22] In addition, cases of aggressive KS had apparently increased eightfold in Kinshasa in 1981 alone.

The Piot paper was also the first to postulate a possible AIDS link between the Congo and Haiti, pointing out that between the early sixties and the mid-seventies, "several thousand professional people" from Haiti came to the Congo to fill posts that had formerly been held by Belgians. The authors stressed, however, that "only one case of AIDS has been recorded in a Haitian in the Congo, and that was in 1983 in an unmarried woman. We are unaware, therefore, of any facts implicating either central Africa or Haitian immigrants from central Africa as the origin of the disease, and such speculation must be viewed with scepticism unless substantive data appear."

Some, of course, might take the view that even one Haitian with AIDS out of a grand total of forty-nine cases reported from Kinshasa demonstrated that Haitian immigrants, just like Congolese citizens, were getting exposed to HIV, and that this supported the Congo-Haiti transmission hypothesis. It will be recalled that, in an uncanny echo, one of the fifty-five Haitians with AIDS who participated in the risk-factor study conducted in the United States in 1984 had a history of previous travel to central Africa. In all probability, this meant that this man, also, had lived and worked in the Congo.[23]

---

In their landmark paper, Peter Piot and colleagues interpreted the AIDS epidemic in the Congo in similar terms to that among American gays and drug injectors, as involving a sudden explosion of cases occurring at or around the start of the 1980s.[24] Indeed, several contemporary papers propose this scenario — partly, one suspects, out of a desire for political correctness. There is, however, a snag to the theory, for in the case of the Congo, there is substantial evidence that people had been dying of AIDS for several years prior to 1980.

There are numerous such cases relating to the years 1979 and 1978, some of which will be referred to later. At this point, however, it seems more appropriate to take a look at some of the significant cases that occurred before 1978 — before, that is, AIDS became apparent in North America, the Caribbean, or East Africa.

The first involves the thirty-four-year-old airline secretary mentioned previously. She flew to Brussels in August 1977 in order to bring her three-month-old daughter, who had been suffering oral candidiasis from birth, to a Belgian hospital. As it turned out, the daughter was readily cured — and turned out later to be HIV-negative[25] — but within a week the mother herself fell sick with fever, fatigue, headache, and sinusitis. During the next five months, she baffled her Belgian doctors by developing a staggering range of opportunistic infections, including polyarthralgia, weight loss, oral candidiasis, genital and peri-anal herpes, generalized cryptococcosis, severe diarrhea, plus four different bacterial infections. Eventually, at her own request, she flew back to Kinshasa, where she died in February 1978.[26]

Further clinically defined cases originating from the Congo related to 1976 or earlier, two of which have been referred to in the previous chapter.[27] A third such case involved a twenty-nine-year-old Belgian man who had lived in Kinshasa from 1971 to 1976, when he returned to Brussels to seek treatment for persistent lymphadenopathy, dermatitis, and *Herpes zoster*. He later returned to Africa, this time to Burundi, where he married a young Tutsi refugee from Rwanda. He died of clinically defined AIDS in 1981, and although his blood was never tested for HIV, his Rwandese widow was found to be HIV-positive in 1985 and later developed ARC.[28]

But not all these early Congolese AIDS patients came out of Kinshasa. One of the most famous was the surgeon from Denmark, Grethe Rask, who after feeling exhausted and weak throughout 1975, then fell sick with drug-resistant diarrhea, chronic fatigue, wasting, and universal lymphadenopathy the following year. She died in Denmark in December 1977, after suffering a range of typical AIDS diseases, including PCP.[29] At the time she first fell ill, Dr. Rask was working in Kinshasa, but prior to that, between 1972 and 1975, she had been based at a small up-country mission hospital in the village of Abumonbazi, in the Equateur province of northern Congo. Frequently this hospital ran short of vital supplies, and it is believed that Dr. Rask may have performed operations without wearing surgical gloves. A great friend and colleague of hers in the Congo was Dr. Ib Bygbjerg, who has since gone on to become one of the leading lights in the fight against AIDS in Denmark. He says that Grethe Rask was a very serious person: "She wasn't drinking, or going out with Congolese men, or anything like that."[30] Bygbjerg clearly believes that the most likely explanation for Dr. Rask's infection was her up-country surgery. Grethe Rask's stored blood was assayed in Copenhagen in 1984, on a very early version of ELISA, which had poor sensitivity; it tested negative.[31] However, the Rask sample has since apparently tested positive on two antibody assays conducted in America — results that were never formally reported in the literature.[32]

The probability that Grethe Rask was HIV-positive was considerably strengthened by a subsequent report, which concluded that as early as 1976 there was a low but detectable level of HIV infection around Yambuku, a mission hospital situated just sixty miles to the south of Abumonbazi by road. In the same year there was an outbreak of Ebola hemorrhagic fever in that area, and teams of experts from the WHO and CDC flew in to perform heroic work isolating and treating infectees. When they flew out again, they took with them a number of blood samples from local villagers, and it was these that were retested nine years later for the presence of HIV. To the amazement of many, five out of 659 proved to be positive.[33]

Another CDC group returned to the region in November 1985, and its members attempted to trace the five HIV-positives. They found that three had died with symptoms typical of AIDS: a twenty-seven-year-old woman in 1977 or 1978, a forty-eight-year-old woman in 1981, and a sixteen-year-old boy in 1984. Two subjects, however, were still alive, and still tested positive for HIV-1: a fifty-nine-year-old woman (who had a normal T-cell count), and a fifty-seven-year-old man with an abnormally low T-cell count, who was the widower of the woman who died in 1981.

Two of these people are of particular significance. The first woman to die, in 1977 or 1978, had worked as a *femme libre* (a "free woman," or casual prostitute) in Kinshasa between 1971 and 1975. The virus itself was isolated and sequenced from the blood sample that she gave in 1976 — and it was this isolate (Z321) that, twenty years later, still represented the earliest sample in the HIV Sequence Database at Los Alamos.[34] And if (as seems possible) the boy who died in 1984 was indeed a perinatal case, he would have been born in 1967 or 1968 to an HIV-positive woman — thus taking the history of HIV even further back in time.

These findings were so interesting that the following year, 1986, the American team returned to take further blood samples from the area. They tested the blood of fifty-five prostitutes from Yandongi (the village nearest to Yambuku hospital) and others from the two nearest towns of Bumba and Lisala, and found that 11 percent were infected.[35] (This compares with 27 percent in a prostitute group in Kinshasa, and 88 percent in the group tested in Butare, Rwanda, at around the same time.) Then they tested patients from the hospitals in Yambuku, Lisala, and Bumba, some of whom had symptoms of AIDS, and five were found to be HIV-positive. Finally, they took blood from another cross section of villagers from the zone around Yambuku, and found that three samples out of 388 were positive — a prevalence of 0.8 percent, almost identical to that detected ten years earlier. This apparently stable seroprevalence over a ten-year time span in a rural area, which contrasted with a steadily rising seroprevalence in Kinshasa during the seventies, led them to hypothesize that "HIV infection and AIDS could have existed and remained stable in [this] rural area of Africa for a long period," and that "the disruption of traditional lifestyles and the social and behavioral changes that accompany urbanization may be important factors in the spread of AIDS in central Africa." This was an early expression of the "isolated tribe hypothesis," which, as we shall see later, is rather more controversial than it may at first glance seem.

In a future chapter, there will be further discussion of this theory that HIV and AIDS may have existed unnoticed in a remote part of Africa for many years — and that only recently have they "escaped" to large cities like Kinshasa and thence to the outside world. Suffice it for now to point out that both the very presence of fifty-five prostitutes in a rural area like that around Yandongi, and their significant level of HIV infection, suggest that there may have been a substantial level of traffic on the north-south road through the village, which would make it unlikely that HIV would have been contained in such an area for very long.

By a remarkable and tragic twist of fate, there was another freak event that also took place in 1976 and that demonstrated the presence of the virus in yet another part of the Congo. In November 1976, a Canadian transport plane carrying mining equipment from Belgium to Lubumbashi was due to make a final stopover at Kisangani on the river Congo, but adverse conditions forced it to put down in a forest clearing near Opala, some 150 miles to the southwest. The sole survivor of the crash landing, flight engineer Ron M., sustained a compound fracture of the right leg and a serious neck injury, but was transported by truck to Kisangani, where he spent several days at the University Hospital.[36] Here he was transfused with two units of blood donated by Congolese volunteers (the only blood he received while in Africa).

Later, he was transferred back to Edmonton, Alberta, and though he was discharged from hospital in time for Christmas, he never fully recovered from the accident. By 1977, Ron began to suffer oral candidiasis, and he eventually died, in June 1980, from respiratory distress syndrome, disseminated *Herpes simplex* infections, and septicemia. Years later, stored blood samples were tested and found to be HIV-positive.[37] He therefore represents the earliest serologically proven and generally accepted case of AIDS on the North American continent.[38] Ron's history also provides strong circumstantial evidence that HIV was present in the Kisangani region in 1976.

The possibility that further cases of AIDS, unreported in the medical literature, were already occurring in the Congo by the mid-seventies is supported by Arnold Voth, the same Canadian doctor who accompanied the injured flight engineer on the plane from Kinshasa to London. Dr. Voth was based at Mama Yemo Hospital in Kinshasa between 1974 and 1978, and he recalls that during these four years he and his colleagues "saw a lot of cases which in retrospect probably were HIV [related]. Patients presenting with uncontrollable diarrhea and weight loss and going on to die were well-known to clinicians at that time.

They became even more well-known in the following ten years." Dr. Voth writes that it was not until he returned to Canada in 1983 and read reports about the new syndrome that he realized what he had been seeing in the Congo almost ten years earlier.[39]

Voth's view is reinforced by that original *Lancet* paper on AIDS in the Congo by Piot and coauthors. The conclusion reads: "It was impossible to date the onset of AIDS in Kinshasa. A chart review revealed syndromes including weight loss, lymphadenopathy and invasive KS in young adults as far back as 1975, but information was inadequate to diagnose AIDS definitely."

In fact, there are certain even earlier cases of AIDS in people from the Congo — some clinically likely, and others serologically confirmed — all of which involve children. One such was the son of a Congolese government official. The boy, born in August 1974, began presenting with typical symptoms of AIDS five months later in Kinshasa. In 1978, the whole family (mother, father, and three children) moved to Stockholm, where the boy eventually died in September 1982, at the age of eight. Stored blood samples taken between 1978 and 1982 later tested HIV-positive,[40] and other information subsequently released by one of his doctors makes it clear that this was almost certainly a case of perinatal infection. His two siblings, born in 1970 and 1972, both tested HIV-negative.

The earliest persuasive evidence of clinical AIDS in Kinshasa, however, comes from one of the children of the Congolese airline secretary mentioned earlier. Before she flew home to die, she told her Belgian doctors that though all the children of her first marriage were healthy, the first and second children of her second marriage had each died aged less than a year, the first from a respiratory infection, the second from septicemia. Both had also had oral thrush. Dr. Jean Vandepitte, one of the doctors who reported this case to the *Lancet*, subsequently revealed that these two children were born in 1973 and 1976. If, as seems likely, the two children and the mother all died of AIDS, then the mother is likely to have been infected at some point between 1970 (the year of birth of her last healthy child, by the first marriage) and 1973.[41] Quite possibly the source was the second husband. No HIV serology was ever done, however, on the mother's blood — and apparently no information was recorded about the health of her second husband.

---

Not all the cases above were confirmed by HIV serology. There is, however, independent proof that HIV was present throughout the seventies in Kinshasa — proof that is not available for any other place in the world. Doctors from the Rega Institute in Belgium, under Jan Desmyter, have tested 498 deep-frozen blood samples from apparently healthy Kinshasa mothers from 1980, and a further 805 samples from a similar cohort, taken in 1970. Those found positive on the ELAVIA assay were then subjected to three further confirmatory tests,[42] each of which gave identical results, yielding fifteen confirmed HIV-positives from 1980 (a seroprevalence of 3 percent) and two positives from 1970 (a prevalence of 0.25 percent). The authors of this communication concluded: "An increase of true positivity of about ten-fold[43] in ten years is compatible with slow, predominantly heterosexual spread [of a virus] possibly introduced in about 1940 in central African cities."[44]

There is one even earlier HIV-positive serum from Kinshasa — the most famous positive serum of all — that takes us at least part of the way back to Desmyter's mooted "introduction date" of 1940. This, of course, is the serum investigated by André Nahmias, which suggests that a man from Leopoldville was infected with HIV back in 1959.[45] We shall return to this serum later.

So, to sum up, we see AIDS in the United States, Haiti, and Europe in the late seventies; but in the Congo the syndrome is present in the early seventies. Furthermore, we have evidence that HIV-1 was already present in the Congo in the late fifties. A pattern is beginning to emerge.

---

More than ten years have passed, and our perspective on the early AIDS epidemic in the Congo is now that much clearer, but it only reinforces the impression that physicians such as Nathan Clumeck, Peter Piot, and Arnold Voth got it just about right back in 1983 and 1984. They were indeed observing the tip of an iceberg.

Is this the end of the trail leading back toward the source of HIV and AIDS? Does the Congo represent the natural hearth for the HIV-1 virus? We shall return to this question later, but suffice it for now to say that we appear to be getting close. In the past, it has been suggested that HIV might have been imported to the Congo by American Peace Corps workers, or by a colonial official with a salty past. However, the many examples of AIDS and HIV infection witnessed in the Congo during the seventies and their apparent absence in other continents, combined with the much greater genetic variability of HIV isolates from the Congo (indicating that they have been evolving for a longer time), begin to suggest that the virus must have originated somewhere in this part of central Africa and spread outward, rather than vice versa.

If indeed the Congo was an early center of HIV prevalence, then we should contemplate for a moment the many ways in which the virus might have spread thereafter. In addition to noting such groups as European ex-patriates (Belgians and Greeks in particular), Congolese émigrés, and Haitian technocrats who came and then left again, armchair theorists have postulated roles for groups as disparate as European mercenaries,[46] Cuban soldiers, early overland travelers, development agency workers, and the many thousands who attended the Ali–Foreman fight in Kinshasa in October 1974.[47] The Rumble in the Jungle. Yet another overworked metaphor with a peculiar resonance for the world of AIDS.

———————

There is an interesting footnote to these early reports of AIDS in the Congo — one that is directly relevant to the development of an AIDS vaccine, a subject that assumes greater importance toward the end of this book. Western research teams were, of course, not slow to realize the significance of the AIDS epidemic in central Africa, and in 1984 a major U.S.-funded AIDS research program, Projet SIDA, was set up in Kinshasa, initially under Robin Ryder and Jonathan Mann — who was to become better known later in the eighties as head of the WHO's Global Program on AIDS. For the next seven years, until its closure following the riots in Kinshasa in 1991, Projet SIDA was a major player in HIV research in Africa.[48]

Other important AIDS research was conducted at the French-funded Institut National de Recherches Biomedicales (INRB), also in Kinshasa, and this included some controversial work by the French doctor Daniel Zagury. In 1986, to the surprise and shock of many of his colleagues, Zagury announced that he had already injected himself, some of his colleagues, and an unspecified number of Congolese "volunteers" with a genetically engineered AIDS vaccine. (This vaccine comprised the vaccinia virus that is used as a vehicle for smallpox vaccine, plus a portion of the envelope, or outer coat, of HIV-1.) This constituted the first human trial, anywhere in the world, of a vaccine against AIDS. Although Zagury was loath to answer questions about the trial,[49] it was reported elsewhere that the volunteers had included about a thousand Congolese soldiers, and a French colleague who had previously accidentally pricked himself with an HIV-infected needle.[50] Zagury issued brief reports on part of this work in a letter and a paper published in 1987 and 1988;[51] in these, he claimed that the trial had been sanctioned by the Zairean Ministry of Health. One of his collaborators, and the final author on the 1988 paper, was Robert Gallo.

Many years later the concept and conduct of the trial were investigated, and severely criticized, in a report issued by the Office for Protection from Research Risks (OPRR) at the National Institutes of Health.[52] Among other things, it was revealed that the vaccine virus had originally been supplied by an NIH scientist, and that a French version of the vaccine had also been used in the trials. It was further revealed that the "volunteers" had actually included eighteen HIV-negative Congolese children aged between two and eighteen. The volunteering, Zagury alleged, had been done by their mothers, all of whom had AIDS and who had urgently requested that their children be included in the experiment.

No independent verification of the children's subsequent health status was available. The report also documented a further vaccine trial involving "approximately 30 HIV-seronegative adults, including military volunteers." The results of this trial were never published, although, once again, Zagury informed the investigators that the subjects remained healthy. The OPRR subsequently placed restrictions on Robert Gallo's research activities involving human subjects, and forbade Zagury from pursuing any further research involving U.S.-provided materials or technology.

Writing about the children's vaccine trial in 1991, Carol Levine observed: "This example indicates how easily ethical considerations can be swept aside under the rubric of 'humanitarianism' or 'compassion.' The children had escaped perinatal transmission; they were not at risk through casual contact with their mothers. There could be no possible benefit to them and there was potentially serious harm."[53]

In fact, there was another, perhaps even more important question: whether others in the community might not also have been put at risk through the introduction of a new — and potentially transmissible — viral agent. For Zagury's was a live vaccine, containing a viable portion of HIV's envelope. The full implications of this well-intentioned, but potentially very dangerous, experiment would become apparent only in the nineties, when molecular biologists began to reveal the uncanny ability of lentiviruses to recombine, and to pass slabs of genetic information from one to another. For instance, writing in 1995, Paul Sharp and colleagues concluded their paper on "cross-species transmission and recombination of 'AIDS' viruses" with the following comment: "Recombination provides the opportunity for an 'evolutionary leap' in so far as the genetic consequence is far more drastic than the steady accumulation of individual mutations, and so a future hybrid virus may have significantly altered biological (and pathogenic) properties."[54]

Some observers, at least, believe that Zagury and Gallo had been drumming their fingers on the lid of Pandora's box.

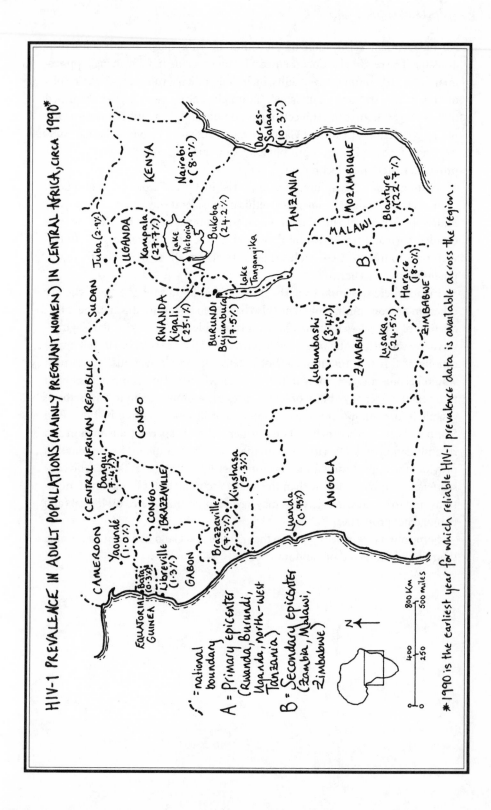

HIV-1 PREVALENCE IN ADULT POPULATIONS (MAINLY PREGNANT WOMEN) IN CENTRAL AFRICA, CIRCA 1990*

Yaoundé (1.0%)
Bangui (7.4%)
Libreville (1.3%)
Bata (0.3%)
Brazzaville (7.3%)
Kinshasa (5.3%)
Luanda (0.95%)
Juba (2.9%)
Kampala (27.7%)
Bukoba (24.2%)
Kigali (25.1%)
Bujumbura (17.5%)
Nairobi (8.9%)
Dar-es-Salaam (10.3%)
Lubumbashi (3.4%)
Lusaka (24.5%)
Harare (18.0%)
Blantyre (22.7%)

CAMEROON
CENTRAL AFRICAN REPUBLIC
SUDAN
UGANDA
KENYA
CONGO
CONGO-BRAZZAVILLE
GABON
EQUATORIAL GUINEA
RWANDA
BURUNDI
Lake Victoria
Lake Tanganyika
TANZANIA
MOZAMBIQUE
MALAWI
ANGOLA
ZAMBIA
ZIMBABWE

N

400  800 Km
250  500 miles

⌐⌐ = national boundary

A = Primary epicenter (Rwanda, Burundi, Uganda, north-west Tanzania)

B = Secondary epicenter (Zambia, Malawi, Zimbabwe)

*1990 is the earliest year for which reliable HIV-1 prevalence data is available across the region.

# 7

## FALSE POSITIVES,

## AND THE SPECTER OF CONTAMINATION

Of course, just as important as knowing where HIV and AIDS were in the years before the recognized epidemic[1] is knowing where they were not.

Unfortunately, the picture has become muddied, because some of the clinically plausible cases of pre-epidemic AIDS that appear in the medical literature (especially those lacking the confirmation of a positive HIV antibody test) may in fact not be AIDS at all.[2] Many presentations *resembling* AIDS can be caused (and presumably have always been caused) by other factors such as cancers or leukemias, congenital immunodeficiency, combined immunodeficiency diseases (like Nezelof's syndrome), or the presence of other viruses that, exceptionally, can have an immunosuppressive effect.[3] What is more, the lack of specificity in the early case definition allowed several "classical KS" cases to be wrongly diagnosed as AIDS. Caution is therefore warranted.

Another factor is that the early assays used to evaluate whether or not someone was infected with HIV (most of which actually tested for antibodies to the virus) were of variable quality. In 1984 and 1985 in particular, a lot of strange results — many of which would now be termed "false positives" — were encountered, because the techniques then in use had poor sensitivity or specificity. (Sensitivity relates to the ability to detect small amounts of antiviral antibodies; specificity, the ability to identify accurately the virus that is causing them to appear.) At the time, the standard explanation for such false positives was that old sera, especially those which had been thawed and refrozen on a number of occasions, tended to become "sticky." In addition, sera from places like Africa, where most people have been exposed to a large number of different viruses and bacteria, are more difficult to interpret than Western sera, because antibodies of pathogens other than HIV can, on occasions, also adhere to the assays.

Furthermore, the assays themselves were of variable accuracy. Some (such as ELISA — the enzyme-linked immunosorbent assay, and EIA — the enzyme immunoassay) involve the addition of a reagent; if it changes color, the serum is judged to be HIV-positive. Similarly, IFA — the immunofluorescence assay — relies on a subjective assessment of a fluorescent reaction. Other assays like the Western blot (WB) are based on the antibodies to various proteins producing discernible bands on a testing strip[4] — or, in the case of RIPA, the radioim-munoprecipitation assay, an autoradiograph. Once again, the problem is one of interpretation, especially with "weakly reactive" readings.[5] Even when the p24 antigen test (which measured the presence of the major core protein of HIV-1) became available later in the eighties, there were still problems with reliability and interpretation.

---

Several of the most notorious early papers, which reported what are now known to be false positive results, were those dealing with old, stored African sera. These misleading reports often went on to infer that HIV and AIDS had been present in parts of Africa for many years or, indeed, that the virus was endemic (regularly found) in those regions, as distinct from epidemic (occurring in sporadic outbreaks). Because they caused so much scientific and political confusion, it is necessary to analyze such researches in a little more detail.

Some of the earliest claims relate to the Republic of South Africa. In 1986 Professor Hans-Dieter Brede, a German microbiologist based at the Tygerberg Hospital near Cape Town, apparently reported at an AIDS conference in Istan-bul that he had found several archival South African sera to be HIV-positive, the oldest of which dated from 1963. Dr. Brede also claimed that he had knowledge of several cases of rapidly fatal AIDS-like illnesses, such as aggressive KS, pneu-monia, and meningitis, which had occurred between 1959 and 1974 among migrant workers originating from central Africa.[6]

The reality, however, is rather different. When I interviewed him by phone and letter several years later, Dr. Brede denied having said anything about an HIV-positive serum from 1963, and later agreed that he was probably thinking of the 1959 serum from the Belgian Congo investigated by Nahmias. Regard-ing the potential archival AIDS cases, he said that during the sixties his col-leagues in internal medicine and dermatology had acquainted him with many cases of strange illnesses in migrant workers from Uganda and Malawi. He told me that between three and six such patients had presented every year with aggressive forms of KS, PCP, and an atypical form of tuberculosis, and that there was some literature about these cases in the *South African Medical*

*Journal.* "Retrospectively," he added, "it is quite sure these were cases of HIV [infection]."[7]

However, a careful review of the said journal for these years reveals just a single brief reference to a case of KS and TB, and two other case reports of disseminated KS (without additional opportunistic infections).[8] Although any of these three fatal cases might conceivably have been AIDS, the reports feature far too little supporting evidence for such a diagnosis to be made with any confidence. Neither are there any cases featuring pneumonia, meningitis, or atypical mycobacteria that are suggestive of AIDS. In short, there is nothing to support Professor Brede's certainty that South Africa was host to dozens of cases of AIDS in the fifties and sixties.

Neither do early seroepidemiological studies support the professor's hypothesis. In a 1987 study of more than 2,500 sera collected between 1970 and 1974 from mineworkers originating mainly from Mozambique and Malawi, but also from Lesotho, Botswana, Angola, Swaziland, and South Africa itself, just two sera tested HIV-positive on two (notoriously nonspecific) assays — and negative on two others. The authors conclude: "In testing serum from Africans that has been stored frozen, false positive results and lack of uniformity in the results of various methods can be expected. The results of the present study fail to provide conclusive evidence of HIV infection in southern Africa in the early 1970s."[9]

Several other claims of early HIV-positivity relate to West Africa. The best-known report involves sera that were originally taken from 144 children from the West African country of Upper Volta (now Burkina Faso), during a measles and smallpox vaccination trial conducted by Harry Meyer in 1963.[10] In 1985, scientists from the U.S. Food and Drug Administration (FDA), including Meyer, reported that two of these sera had been retested and found positive for HIV antibodies,[11] and concluded that "these results support the hypothesis that a virus antigenically related to [HIV] may have been present in West Africa prior to the AIDS epidemic," a claim that has been frequently repeated in subsequent books and articles.[12]

In fact, one serum tested positive only for a single protein (p28) on Western blot; the other demonstrated the presence of four proteins which are far more typical of HTLV-1 than of HIV.[13] The evidence therefore suggests that the FDA team identified the wrong retrovirus.[14]

Another anomalous report was made in 1989 by a group headed by Tatjana Frenkl. This team found that over 5 percent (21 of 404) of blood samples taken from three Ghanaian tribes from various years during the sixties, starting in 1960, were positive for HIV-1 envelope proteins on EIA. Dr. Frenkl claims that "this assay has been shown to have high specificity and sensitivity." However, the apparent failure to confirm the unexpected results using other assays, and the lack of correlation with more recent data from Ghana, which shows that none of 896 stored sera from 1977 were HIV-positive, does not encourage confidence in Dr. Frenkl's findings.[15]

---

Arguably, these dubious results did little real damage except, perhaps, in the countries so identified as early hosts to HIV and AIDS. Similar papers relating to eastern Africa, however, had serious and lengthy repercussions with respect to governmental and popular attitudes toward AIDS and AIDS researchers. Probably the most notorious study was one published in 1985 by Carl Saxinger and his boss, Robert Gallo, from the Laboratory of Tumor Cell Biology at the National Cancer Institute in Bethesda.[16] This retrospectively found that two-thirds of a small group of children bled between 1972 and 1973 in the Ugandan district of West Nile had been positive for HIV. This cohort had a mean age of 6.4 years, and had been clinically healthy at the time of bleeding. But in Saxinger's hands, fifty-five of the seventy-five children tested positive for HIV antibodies on ELISA, and fifty of these positives were then confirmed by a "newly developed . . . enhanced sensitivity . . . immunoblot," which detected several typical HIV proteins. Unfortunately, it now appears certain that the sensitivity was so enhanced that it came up with false positive results for negative sera.

The authors postulated that perhaps the reason why high levels of HIV infection had gone unnoticed for so long was that African populations had been exposed to the virus for a lengthy period, and that present-day infectees exhibited only subclinical infections (those that do not cause disease). However, in another paper, which appeared five months later, there was a degree of back-tracking.[17] The serum reactivity was now described as representing "a unique pattern"; and it was added that "the antibody status of this group was unlike any normal or acquired immunodeficiency syndrome-risk group previously tested." There was also, for the first time, mention of "relatively low titers" — or weak reactivity. Nonetheless, Saxinger and Gallo continued to propose that they had detected "a relative or predecessor of [HIV]" or "[HIV] itself but in a population acclimatized to its presence." They added, moreover, that their research "suggest[ed] a likely African origin of [HIV]."

A similar 1984 letter from Gallo's lab, this time with Bob Biggar as lead author, reported that 12.4 percent of sera from apparently healthy outpatients at a remote rural hospital in the Kivu region of eastern Congo had tested positive for HIV on ELISA,[18] with "excellent" confirmation by the same enhanced-sensitivity Western blot.[19] A later paper by Biggar and Gallo reported very high levels of HIV exposure among Kenyans, including more than 50 percent of ninety-nine Turkana people tested between 1980 and 1984 in the remote north-western region.[20] Again these results were based on ELISA tests, with the results being "supported by Western blot analysis of a subset of sera."

The inclusion of Steve Alexander of Biotech Ltd. of Rockville, Maryland, as a coauthor, suggests that this (and the previously mentioned papers) may have employed his avidin-biotin sensitivity-enhanced Western blot, which was later responsible for the false positives found in James Moore's study of Lexington addicts in 1971/2.[21]

Shortly after this, Bob Biggar and colleagues wrote another article for the *Lancet,* reporting that the HIV antibodies detected by ELISA assays used in his Kivu studies "correlated strongly with levels of antibodies against *Plasmodium falciparum,*" the malaria parasite.[22] He offered a variety of hypotheses to explain the unusual reactivity, including the possibility that HIV might be transmitted by mosquitoes, or that other, hitherto undiscovered retroviruses might be involved. One year later, he had discarded most of these explanations, as shown by a letter he wrote to the *New England Journal of Medicine* in which he conceded that patients with recurrent malaria could show false positive reactions in HIV tests "prepared in a manner that enhances sensitivity at the expense of specificity."[23]

This cautious retraction was to Biggar's credit, but it took other researchers to show that Saxinger and Gallo's 1972/3 results from West Nile were highly improbable. First, a group under Jay Levy in San Francisco published a 1986 paper that demonstrated that not a single serum from 199 children and adults bled in 1968 in West Nile was positive for HIV.[24] Also in 1986, Wilson Carswell bled seventy-six apparently healthy adults who were resident in West Nile. Using a competitive ELISA technique, which is much more specific than the direct ELISA that had been used in Gallo's laboratory, he found just one serum to be HIV-positive. By contrast, he found that 15.4 percent of healthy adults from West Nile who were resident in Uganda's main city, Kampala, were HIV-positive, a percentage that was typical of healthy adults resident in the city.[25] In other words, HIV was most unlikely to be endemic in West Nile, and citizens of West Nile were not innately prone to HIV infection although, like others, they became highly infected when they moved to a high-risk urban center.

Despite Biggar's communications about malarial antibodies causing false positives, and the potential implications for the Kivu results, neither he nor Saxinger nor Gallo ever formally accepted that the Kenyan and West Nile data must also have consisted of false-positive results, or specifically retracted these papers. Nor did any of them ever attempt to explain how they could have been detecting antibodies to the malarial parasite, rather than HIV, not just on one assay but on two very different ones.

---

Of course, the finding of false positives is not the only type of laboratory error that can occur. Potentially far more serious is the specter of contamination of one sample with material from another. It is ironic that the so-called African green monkey theory, which is probably the theory of origin best known to the nonspecialist, happens to be based on a laboratory mix-up that was uncannily reminiscent of Robert Gallo's earlier experiences with "HTLV-III."

The story, unfortunately, is rather complicated. In 1985, Max Essex and Phyllis Kanki of Harvard University identified a retrovirus in the sera of the African green monkey, *Cercopithecus aethiops,* and, in accordance with the Gallo HTLV-III nomenclature, decided to call their virus STLV-IIIagm. Essex and Kanki proposed that STLV-IIIagm might have been transmitted to humans in central Africa, giving rise — perhaps after a series of mutations — to HTLV-III (or HIV-1, as it was later known).[26]

Later in 1985, the discovery of a second human immunodeficiency virus among persons from West Africa (LAV-II, later to be renamed HIV-2) was announced by French and American doctors, and early in 1986 another group, from Luc Montagnier's laboratory at the Pasteur Institute, announced that it had found LAV-II in the sera of West African AIDS patients.[27] By this time, however, Essex and Kanki had announced that they, too, had discovered another human retrovirus, probably nonpathogenic, among asymptomatic prostitutes from Senegal in West Africa, and this they named HTLV-IV. Furthermore, they claimed that this HTLV-IV was almost identical to STLV-IIIagm.[28]

Doubts arose, however, when others were unable to isolate viruses from AGMs using Essex and Kanki's techniques. In a 1988 letter to *Nature,* Harry Kestler and Ronald Desrosiers from the New England Regional Primate Research Center resolved the mystery by pointing out that both HTLV-IV and STLV-IIIagm were virtually identical to an isolate of another virus, SIVmac, which had been obtained from an immunosuppressed rhesus macaque at their facility. Essex and Kanki had been working with this very isolate, SIVmac251, in their laboratory during 1985,[29] and cross contamination had apparently occurred, meaning that, in reality, all three viruses were one and the same. In an accompanying letter, Essex and Kanki acknowledged their mistake,[30] and a commentary by Carol Mulder observed: "This episode should serve as a strong warning for all virologists working with multiple isolates to check any new isolates against viruses present in the laboratory. I am aware, or have been told, of at least five instances in other laboratories in the United States and Europe where noninfected cell cultures became infected with HIV-1 in the same containment hood."[31] One of these instances may well have been the alleged contamination of the HTLV-III isolate in Gallo's lab by Montagnier's LAV.

Yet again the desire for primacy seemed to have prompted a team of virologists to make rushed and mistaken claims, which ended up simply retarding the course of AIDS research. Such errors only reinforced African perceptions that the West was determined, at all costs, to blame Africa for AIDS, and to "attribute everything that is bad and negative to the so-called dark continent."[32]

Later in 1988, when the sequence of a genuine isolate of SIV from the African green monkey (SIVagm) was announced by a Japanese team under Masanori Hayami,[33] it became apparent that the African green monkey SIV was actually only distantly related to HIV-1 and HIV-2, which meant that although SIVagm might be an ancient ancestor of the HIVs, it could not have been the immediate source.[34] Nonetheless, the African green monkey myth persists to this day.

<hr />

My one meeting with Robert Gallo (or "Bob," as he likes to be known) took place entirely by accident in the fall of 1990. Toward the end of a trip round the States, I arranged to interview Carl Blattner, an acknowledged *éminence grise* on HTLV-I and HTLV-II, at the National Cancer Institute in Bethesda.

Perhaps an hour into the interview, a rather debonair-looking man swung into the lab where we were talking, and strode across toward us, his hand already extended in greeting. "Now why do I get the feeling," he inquired with an easy smile, "that you and I are going to get along?" During the previous months, Gallo had been getting a roasting from John Crewdson of the *Chicago Tribune* about the LAV/HTLV-III affair, and it seemed possible that he saw in me an opportunity to tell his side of the story.[35]

Gallo told me that, having heard of my visit, he had taken leave of a seminar for a few minutes in order to arrange a time when he could talk with me. In the end, we met over breakfast, arranged by him at the swankiest hotel in Bethesda.

It was a fascinating meal, which lasted some two hours, with all manner of appetizing items jostling for space with my tape recorder on the table. At the start, I said I assumed he would want to talk with me about the LAV controversy, and I would be glad to hear what he had to say — but that I would first like to ask him some questions of my own. He readily agreed, and I found him to be a sympathetic listener and a good talker, with a decent sense of humor to boot. Only occasionally, when I probed a little deeper, did he show that he could also be prickly.

Gallo suspected that HIV was not a new virus, but one that had been in humans in rural Africa for some generations and had only attained epidemic status because of social changes in the last forty or so years. All right, I said, but why did two epidemics emerge at the same time? "They didn't," he answered quickly. "The epidemic we see is just HIV-1. Without it, we wouldn't even know HIV-2 existed." It was an interesting point, though considering the sheer number of HIV-2-related AIDS cases that were then appearing in hospitals around West Africa, I felt that it might be fairer to say that without the HIV-1 epidemic, the sister epidemic might have gone unrecognized for another few years after 1986. Gallo went on to suggest that HIV-2 might have come into man from a West African monkey a few hundred years ago, while HIV-1 perhaps crossed from a chimpanzee about a hundred years ago. On the other hand, he added, those epidemics could have been going on for millennia, with small pockets of infection, and people dying off before they had had a chance to spread the virus. Then the same thing might have happened again a few centuries later. "I can't really think of anything to refute that explanation," he added.

When we turned to vaccines and therapies, he gave me a rundown of his latest investigations, including his collaboration with Daniel Zagury in Kinshasa. He told me about their immunotherapy work, using killed, whole virus, but made no mention of the previous trials of a live AIDS vaccine. Gallo said that he was supplying Zagury with some purified proteins, and "some intellectual input."

All this was fascinating, but his manner changed noticeably when the conversation turned to LAV/HTLV-III. He became indignant and, at times, quite garbled in his attempts to explain and justify what had happened, and how he had been victimized and ill served by others. He said that, unlike the Pasteur Institute, he had no lawyers and no public relations people working for him. He went on to claim that "material" had been sent to several newspapers and magazines, especially *New Scientist,* and so "a lot of things were said which were untrue"— things that he had never had a chance to clarify. He and his team had, he said, been "partly framed." Someone, he said, had altered certain key documents, and he was "99 percent sure of who did it; he's a key source of Crewdson's information," but he feared being sued if he named the person. When I asked if the Pasteur LAV isolate had been in any way incorporated in his own HTLV-III isolate, he said that "the short answer is 'no,' but there's lots of innuendoes." Montagnier, he said, had published on just one detection of the virus whereas he, Gallo, had published on forty-eight. "The worst interpretation is that one of the forty-eight, and the one used in the blood test, was an accidental contamination with LAV," he said. "Every active lab has contaminations every year or two," he added, by way of explanation.

When we got onto the subject of Crewdson, Gallo said that he had never in his life "heard or seen the style of investigative journalism of this man. Let's just say that about 20 percent seems to me to be totally false, and I'm surprised that he doesn't know the truth." What of the other 80 percent, I asked. "Eighty percent of the article is true, but in a vicious, detailed way that in my view misleads the reader," he responded.

I asked him about the name of the virus — did he now accede to the common nomenclature of HIV-1, which had been in use for the last three years, or did he still think of it as "his" virus, HTLV-III? "It's still HTLV-III, just a different name," he responded. I pointed out that HTLV-1 and HIV were from different families of retroviruses. "So what if it's a different family? You call it hepatitis A, B, and C; they don't even belong to the same category; they're completely different viruses of different families. HIV and HTLV are retroviruses, human T-lymphotropic retroviruses," he retorted. He added that in 1983 he and the British virologist Robin Weiss had signed an agreement to the effect that all future human retroviruses that primarily targeted T-lymphocytes would be called HTLV-III, IV, V, and so on. I wondered what legality or force he and Weiss had felt that such a document might have; did they feel that others would feel constrained by it too? But it was getting toward the time for my first scheduled interview of the day, so I let it go at that.

Later that afternoon, as I was leaving the main NCI building after a long series of meetings, I ran into Bob Gallo once again, and he offered me a lift. He wanted to know how I had got on and whom I had seen. I told him about my meeting with Bob Biggar, and confessed that when Biggar had started to justify himself about the African false positives I had lost my temper with him.

I asked Gallo why Biggar and Saxinger had never written letters to the journals concerned to withdraw their erroneous HIV-prevalence results, and in response he said two very interesting things. First, he laughingly questioned the competence of one of the two scientists in question — I will not say which — saying that he had always been a bit of a bungler, or words to that effect.[36] And second, he said that his own input to the various erroneous papers had been minimal, if any. He explained that, as head of the laboratory, his name simply went on the paper automatically.

However, it was not until years later that I realized the full story. For although Robert Gallo's name appears on four of the five publications that wrongly claimed that there were remarkable levels of HTLV-III-positivity in Africa, it is absent from both of the articles and the letter in which Bob Biggar admitted that there might have been some mistake. It was then that I began to suspect that when I had shouted at Biggar, I had actually been shouting at the wrong man.

———————

Contaminations and false readings are bad enough from a scientific perspective, but with a topic as sensitive as AIDS, they necessarily have far wider repercussions. Between 1985 and 1988, this being the period immediately following the publication of these erroneous results by Biggar, Saxinger, Gallo, and others, the response of African scientists and politicians and of their Western sympathizers was understandably incandescent. There was much talk of the deliberate slanting of results in order to further the racist agenda that HIV and AIDS had come out of Africa. A typical accusation was the following, from a book entitled *AIDS, Africa and Racism* published privately in 1987 by a Zimbabwean social scientist and an Australian doctor, Richard and Rosalind Chirimuuta:

"Much of the confused, contradictory and simply nonsensical conclusions reached by the scientists about AIDS in Africa can be attributed to their attempts to square their research findings with their racist preconceptions, rather than objective scientific reality."[37]

This book, and others like it, accused Western scientists of resorting to the politics of blame, and falling back on old, safe, traditional targets. Many of them quoted the reported AIDS totals from each country in a bid to "prove" that the AIDS epidemic must be an American export. This was somewhat disingenuous, for by mid-1987 it was widely known and acknowledged that although the 4,500-odd cases reported from the whole of Africa were considerably fewer than the 37,000 reported from the United States,[38] the former certainly represented a profound underreporting of the real situation on the ground — if only because, in Africa, many of the sick never resorted to the official health system. Other commentators attempted to pour oil on troubled waters, by adopting the line that HIV and AIDS must have arrived at around the same time in America, the Caribbean, Europe, and Africa.[39] But as has already been demonstrated, this claim was more politically than epidemiologically correct.

Having rightly pointed out the inconsistencies in the reports of men like Saxinger and Biggar, the Chirimuutas then emphasized the several studies that had failed to indicate any evidence of HIV in Africa before 1980. The largest such study was that conducted by Alan Fleming and his German colleagues, which showed that, of some six thousand blood samples taken between 1976 and 1984 — mainly from West Africa, but including nearly six hundred collected from areas close to the capitals of Kenya and Uganda[40] — the earliest HIV-1-positive sample dated from 1981.[41] Another such study had reported zero HIV-prevalence among 340 Aka pygmies who had been bled between 1975 and 1978 in Congo-Brazzaville and the Central African Republic;[42] the result was interesting, in that pygmies are hunter-gatherers, and have direct contact with a wide variety of forest monkeys.[43]

Unfortunately, the Chirimuutas then moved on to the serosurvey by Nahmias, which had detected the HIV-positive sample from Leopoldville/ Kinshasa in 1959,[44] and suggested that a solitary HIV-positive result like this might also be caused by human error or contamination.

Of course, it is relatively easy to find areas of Africa where HIV was not present in the fifties, sixties, seventies, and early eighties. But in their determination to prove that AIDS did not come from Africa, the Chirimuutas — and others like them — entirely overlooked the substantial number of genuine HIV-positive results that had emerged from sera taken throughout the seventies in places like Kinshasa and the Equateur province of the Congo. By ignoring the fact that HIV was beginning to spread in very specific areas of Africa during the seventies, they ended up biasing their findings in the very same way as, according to them, the "racist" scientists had done before them.

Sadly, conclusions similar to the Chirimuutas' were reached by certain African politicians, some of whom clearly felt it beneficial to represent the African AIDS epidemic as either a Western import or a Western fabrication. And so it was that in 1986 and 1987, when the true HIV-prevalence figures for sub-Saharan Africa were already spectacularly bad, exceeding 15 percent of the adult population in several urban centers,[45] the false-positive reports allowed certain African governments to conceal the true situation behind a smoke screen of accusations about racist propaganda. During those two years, the Kenyan government, for instance, often seemed more concerned about preserving its lucrative tourist industry than with informing its own people about the gravity of the situation.[46]

And yet, at that very moment, there was a desperate need for the correct message about AIDS to be broadcast, for in the late eighties many Africans retained a cavalier attitude about the risks of having unprotected sex. In Tanzania at around this time, AIDS became extrapolated as *"Acha Inwe Dogedoge Siachi,"* which is Kiswahili for "Let it kill me; I shall never abandon the young ladies." And in the Congo, SIDA (the French acronym for AIDS) was translated as *"Syndrome Imaginaire pour Decourager les Amoureux"* — an even more blatant demonstration of the popular belief that AIDS was little more than a Western propaganda ploy designed to dampen the sexual ardor and reproductive capacity of the African.[47]

---

Before leaving the question of lab contaminations and false positives, it is important to point out that nowadays, in the nineties, there is a far more sensitive technique for identifying not antibodies to the virus, but the presence of the virus itself in a tissue or serum sample. This technique is known as PCR, or the polymerase chain reaction. The PCR, which was first developed in the mid-eighties by Kary Mullis (who won a Nobel Prize for his efforts), represents a real breakthrough for laboratory analysis, one which permits the detection of even tiny quantities of DNA from any organism, including viruses.[48]

At its most basic level, this is how PCR works. The following ingredients are combined in a test tube: a sample of DNA extracted from the tissue being examined, "primers" (short stretches of DNA which, it is hoped, will latch on to complementary sequences of DNA in the tissue), together with a quantity of the four nucleotides (adenine, cytosine, guanine, and thymine — A, C, G, and T, the basic building blocks of DNA), an enzyme, and a buffer solution. The tube is then subjected to a series of temperature changes. First it is heated to 95°C, to separate the double-stranded DNA in the target tissue into single strands; then cooled to about 55°, to allow the primers to stick themselves to the single strands; and then raised again to about 70°, to allow the enzyme to synthesize new double-stranded DNA, using the nucleotides provided.[49] Thus the stretch of DNA between the primers is doubled in each cycle — an exponential increase. This process is repeated through several cycles, at the end of which the target DNA has hopefully been amplified a million times or more. (In the early days of PCR this was a complicated and lengthy procedure, but in the nineties it became possible to carry out the entire process on a single machine.)

After a specific fragment of DNA (for instance, from a virus in the target tissue) has been amplified, it can be characterized genetically, or "sequenced." (As might be expected, the DNA sequence — the order in which the building blocks of DNA appear — varies from one organism to another.) The first PCR amplification and sequencing of an HIV isolate was reported in 1987.[50]

Being far more sensitive than any of the assays that preceded it, PCR gives researchers by far the best chance of detecting a virus in an archival sample that contains HIV. There are two caveats, however. One is that a *negative* result on PCR is not, by itself, conclusive. In a stored serum sample or wax-embedded tissue block, the viral DNA may be very degraded, or the desired fragments may not be detected by the primers.

The second caveat is that considerable precautions have to be taken to avoid contamination, because even a minute quantity of HIV DNA introduced to the sample from another source can be amplified instead of the target DNA. This rogue DNA could be from a contaminated pipette, an aerosol spray, or equipment originating from another laboratory where other HIV isolates have been tested in the past.

A positive PCR result represents very powerful evidence that a specific virus is present in a sample. However, the potential for PCR contamination remains a real and constant danger, one that was subsequently to play an important role in one of the most celebrated and controversial archival cases of AIDS — that of the so-called Manchester sailor, David Carr.

# 8

## THE MANCHESTER SAILOR

Glance again through the photographs: the toddler in the back garden; the eager young teenager in football gear; the twenty-year-old on holiday — confident, surely, but a bit cocky too; the burly young man holding up the blackboard inscribed with "D. Carr" and his service number — harder now, less open, more difficult to read. Then look at these of the best man at the wedding in his smart suit; and then, finally, the photo from the hospital, the one of his nose and mustachioed mouth and the ugly, spreading ulcer that is eating through them. Take one last look, search in the eyes for any message, any communication from across the years.

Now clear the desk. Let the mind run free. Allow it to focus on the detail that sticks out, which seems important — or strange. What is the truth here? What really happened? We have a beginning and an ending. What went on between?

———

Another small scene frozen precisely in memory, fixed in time. The voice on the tape still retains the distinctive rhythm and lilt of Manchester. For the past few minutes it has been reliving the blind hope that something, somehow, will turn the tide. But now, for the first time, the voice grows thin and starts to waver, as Elsie, Dave's one-time fiancée, talks about the day of his death.

"That day I'd taken time off work to go to the hospital earlier. Usually I used just to go after work, but this particular day, I decided for some reason I would go early, and I went in my lunch break. And I went in to the room with him, and he said, 'Oh, hi kid,' just like he always did. And we sat there talking for a while.

"And then his mum came, and we all talked. And then, all of a sudden, his mind just started to wander, and he was saying: 'Aren't those flowers beautiful? And the fields — they're so lovely.' Now his mum looked at me and I looked at her. We were in a hospital room in Manchester — where were the fields and the flowers? And then he came right back to the present — no mention of it, as if he didn't realize that we'd been there, or that he'd been talking about fields and flowers. It put a bit of a scare in me, that did . . . and for good reason.

"He suddenly said that he needed to use the toilet. He called the nurse and she came in, and she asked if we would mind just leaving the room for a little while. So we did. And while we were waiting outside, Dave's dad came. And the next minute there were bells ringing — aah, mad bells ringing through the hospital, and doctors went running into his room. And they were in there for such a long time. And then a doctor came out and said that he was very sorry, but that Dave had just died."[1]

There is a long pause, and the sound of somebody composing herself, someone who — even after all these years — still mourns the husband she never had. Then a click, as Elsie switches off the recorder.

———

Dr. Leonard signed David Carr's death certificate, and as cause of death entered what he and his colleagues still considered the most likely of the working diagnoses: Wegener's granulomatosis. Nobody, however, was very surprised when George Williams's autopsy report — and its findings of a CMV infection[2] and PCP — proved them all wrong.[3] However, there was still the unresolved mystery of underlying cause.

During the postmortem, George Williams had taken several small chunks from the body and preserved them in blocks of paraffin wax, themselves affixed to pieces of wood to facilitate handling and the cutting of sections. He decided to store these blocks for possible reappraisal in the future, for a time when medical advances might allow a fuller diagnosis.

Some weeks after the death, two of the doctors involved made significant observations. Dr. Stretton wrote to Jack Nowlan, Dave's GP, to inform him that his patient had died of something "extremely rare . . . it seems possible that the condition is on the increase, and one may learn more of the disease in the future." The president of the Royal College of Physicians, Sir Robert Platt, had also been consulted about the case, and he now wrote to Stretton: "I have often wondered, in the last year or two, if we are in for some new wave of virus disease now that the bacterial illnesses are so nearly conquered." The latter comment was typical of the overconfidence of the times: the medical world had yet to confront the problems of antibiotic-resistant bacteria. On the other hand, Dr. Platt's thoughts about viral diseases were to prove remarkably prescient.

A year later, in October 1960, doctors Williams, Leonard, and Stretton wrote up their case of adult PCP and CMV infection in a four-page report for the *Lancet,* illustrated with striking photos of the oral and anal ulcers.[4] The article ends with the key observation: "very rarely both infections described have been found together in adults in association with serious underlying diseases; no underlying disease was identified in this patient."

On many occasions during the next two decades, when the three doctors bumped into each other in the MRI, the talk would turn to the death of David Carr. Then, in 1981, came the reports of the new disease affecting gay men. Dr. Leonard started clipping articles on GRID and AIDS, and when he next met Trevor Stretton, they both agreed that there were strong similarities between David's case and those of the American homosexuals. Eventually, the two doctors got together with George Williams to write a letter to the *Lancet,* entitled "AIDS in 1959?"[5] which was published in November 1983. This letter ended with the following: "Could he have had AIDS? He had previously been well. While in the navy (1955–57) he had traveled abroad. He was not married and we know nothing of his sexual orientation. . . . Perhaps AIDS is not a new disease; rare examples may in the past have masqueraded under various diagnoses."

No blood or sera from the patient had been preserved, so even when the first HTLV-III/LAV antibody assays became available in 1984, it was not possible to test for the presence of the causative virus. But the tissue blocks were still in storage, and so after the invention of PCR in the late eighties,[6] George Williams persuaded Gerald Corbitt, chief virologist at the University of Manchester Medical School, and head of the Virology Unit at Booth Hall Children's Hospital, the main center for virological research in Manchester, to test them for HIV by the new method. Four of the six samples tested positive.

The results were published in July 1990,[7] and they prompted a wave of media interest, much of it focused on where David Carr had traveled during his time in the navy. Several British newspapers said that he was believed to have contracted the infection in Africa,[8] and one stated that he had probably been to the Congo.[9] Later articles were more cautious, quoting Stretton as saying that he was not sure whether the unnamed patient had served in the Royal Navy or the Merchant Navy, and that the only clue to the places he visited was that he had been asked whether he had experienced any tropical diseases, which implied "that he had travelled through tropical climates."[10]

But it was an article a few weeks later in the mass-market paper, the *Sunday Express,* which really blew the case open. Graham Bell's exposé, which ran under the headline "Revealed: David Carr, the West's First Aids Victim,"[11] was the first to name David, and also the first to feature a photo of him — albeit as a young teenager, in the colors of his local football club, Central Rovers. Bell claimed that David had chosen to serve three years in the Merchant Navy in lieu of National Service, and that for these three years "he was a crewman based at Gibraltar. His ship regularly traversed the Straits, loading and unloading cargoes around the North African ports. . . . This suggests he caught AIDS in the early part of his National Service, during his frequent African visits."

---

In November 1990, I arranged to meet the two doctors who had tended to David more than thirty years before. Back then, they had been almost at the beginning of their medical careers, but now they were eminent physicians on the point of retirement. John Leonard, who had been the senior medical registrar for various wards including David's, proved to be friendly, avuncular, and eager to discuss the case. He was at pains to explain just how many tests had been conducted in a bid to arrive at the correct diagnosis and save the man's life. However, even after they received George Williams's autopsy report, the case had remained a mystery. "The question was why had this man died from infections which were usually of low virulence. You or I would have shaken off these organisms, but they proved lethal to this young man. In other words, there was something wrong with his immune mechanism."

Dr. Leonard also vouchsafed that he had recently had contact with David's former fiancée. He was unable to name her or tell me where she was living, but he did say that, brokenhearted by David's death, she had left England many years before, and had now settled abroad and married. An account of the "Manchester sailor" case had appeared in her local newspaper, and she had written to the MRI doctors to inquire whether it was David — and, if so, whether she too might be at risk. John Leonard had written back to reassure her that it was most unlikely that she herself was infected, but he also seized the opportunity to ask what she recalled about David's travels in the navy. He was still awaiting her reply.

Trevor Stretton, who, as senior house officer, had probably had closer contact with David than any of the other doctors, was more reserved than John Leonard and far more cautious. But over the months and years that followed I grew to appreciate his integrity and his thoughtful, carefully worded responses to questioning. He had recently been telephoned by the New York Times medical writer Lawrence K. Altman, who had asked him whether, had the patient died of another opportunistic infection, like tuberculosis, they would have thought any more of it — and Stretton had had to acknowledge that they would not. Altman's point was well made: cases of AIDS with less striking presentations could well have occurred — unremarked and unrecognized — even further back in time.

Dr. Stretton pointed out that it was only during the 1960s, when doctors began deliberately suppressing the immune systems of transplant patients to ensure that they did not reject donated organs, that conditions like PCP and CMV disease became widely recognized medical problems. It struck me as remarkable that in less than ten years two new factors had come into play that could cause a distinct and novel form of immunosuppression — one of which, HIV, had apparently emerged naturally, while the other, transplant therapy, resulted from human intervention.

I also wanted to see the men who had been responsible for the recent PCR revelations, beginning with the chief virologist at Booth Hall, Gerald Corbitt. I found him energetic and brisk, sporting a pair of broad-lensed glasses the size of lab goggles, and looking a lot younger than his forty-nine years. He also proved to be an impressively precise and fluent speaker, who was prepared to give a meticulously detailed account of how he (and his chief technician, Andrew Bailey, who had conducted the PCR work) had investigated the case.

Apparently George Williams had been encouraging the virology department to investigate the case for some years, and had first supplied them with wax-embedded blocks from the autopsy some three or four years earlier, in the hope that they could be analyzed by a version of the p24 antigen test. None of the samples proved positive — although, given the relative lack of sensitivity of this assay when applied to tissue samples rather than sera, this was perhaps hardly surprising.

But then came the invention of PCR. Corbitt arranged for a special PCR laboratory to be set up, and Bailey spent several months improving his facility with the process. Finally, at the end of 1989, he began work on four of the tissue samples that Williams had already provided from the "sailor" — and he discovered evidence of HIV in all four.

Early in 1990, it was decided, before going any further, to restart the investigation in the form of a double-blind study, which, if it also came up positive, would provide acceptable scientific proof of their work. Williams told Corbitt that, as a control, he could supply tissues from a road accident victim, matched for age and sex, who had died in the same year. Corbitt apparently advised him to take special precautions to avoid any cross contamination in his laboratory, counseling him either to use different knives while cutting the sections or, if that was not feasible, to clean the knife carefully with alcohol before sectioning from a new block. Soon afterward, twelve coded samples from case and control arrived at Booth Hall.

Bailey carried out the PCR investigation, taking even more stringent measures to avoid contamination, and once again he got positive results. Then, just to be certain, he repeated the work from scratch. Eventually, one day at the end of May 1990, he drove up from the university to Booth Hall, and told Corbitt that four of the twelve samples had tested repeatedly positive. There and then, Corbitt called Williams, who cracked the codes down the phone: as Corbitt read out a code number, Williams would say "case" or "control," as appropriate. Corbitt came out of his office and told Bailey that all six of the samples from the road accident case were negative, and that the four positives had come from the kidney, bone marrow, spleen, and pharynx of their index case.[12] "Well, thank God for that" was Bailey's response. Virologists, as they themselves like to say, are a pretty phlegmatic bunch.

Corbitt told me that they had just started on the really exciting work — that of sequencing the virus (determining the order of its nucleotides, in order to establish its precise genetic composition). At that stage, the oldest sample of HIV to have been sequenced was that from the Yambuku *femme libre,* from 1976.[13] The 1959 sample was therefore potentially of enormous importance. Perhaps its sequence would be radically different from current HIVs; it might even be similar to one of the SIVs found in certain species of African monkeys. I asked Corbitt what he anticipated finding, and he told me: "I rather suspect that we won't find a great deal of difference somehow. Don't ask me why. It's just a feeling." Given the rapid rate of mutation of HIV, and the fact that the 1976 sample had been quite highly divergent from modern strains, this answer surprised me somewhat.

The final meeting I had in Manchester was with Dr. George Williams, the Scottish pathologist whose foresight in storing tissue sections from the body had allowed the case to be reinvestigated thirty years later, with such remarkable results. We met at his laboratory in the MRI, shortly before his formal retirement from the pathology department. He was smartly dressed, urbane, quietly self-confident, and rather charming, with a habit of producing knowing smiles at key moments. He also proved to be surprisingly adept at giving a quotable sound bite.

We started off by discussing his postmortem report, and I asked Williams to go through the findings with me. At one point, when he described the lesions on the patient's shoulders, thighs, and pelvis as "raised reddish papules" between one and two centimeters across, I casually inquired whether they could possibly have been examples of Kaposi's sarcoma. He answered straightaway: "Oh, I think so. That would be a rational explanation." I was rather surprised at the apparent success of my amateur diagnosis, especially since KS had never been previously mentioned in this case.

Williams went on to say that the patient's lymph nodes had been large, fleshy, and prominent, especially those in the center of the body. But the really interesting thing was that under microscopic investigation, instead of being packed with lymphocytes in response to the various infections, these nodes turned out to be markedly depleted in lymphocytes. Furthermore, Williams found a tiny swelling in the cerebral cortex, suggesting that infection had also reached David's brain.

He told me that the autopsy had taken about an hour and that the fifty tissue samples he had extracted had included those from heart and arteries, brain and spinal cord, the bone marrow, and the viscera (including spleen, liver, kidneys, and pancreas). Apparently he had also sampled many of the skin lesions.

He admitted that later, when the HIV antibody test became available, he regretted the fact that he had not taken any serum. Clearly by this stage he strongly suspected that the patient might have had AIDS. Even after Corbitt and Bailey failed to find any trace of HIV using the antigen assay, he was still determined to carry on. "The important thing was that we weren't prepared to leave it at that. We weren't prepared to take a negative answer. The question was — was there another test, or would one evolve which might give us a more definitive answer? So in the end it was the combination of chance that this [PCR] test came along, the availability of tissues, and persistence on the part of those involved."

I returned to the subject of the fifty paraffin blocks, and asked if they were still in existence. At this he started laughing, and went on doing so for some little time. "The answer is numerically yes," he began, "but they're a lot slimmer than they were to begin with, because they've been done [sliced] once or twice. And the blocks to begin with were relatively thin."

This seemed to me to be of little relevance, since it was clear that only a small number of the fifty blocks (perhaps half a dozen or, at most, ten) should now be "slimmer." I asked whether it would be possible for me to see them, and he told me not these specific ones. I explained that I merely wanted to take a photo of him with the blocks, but he told me they were "essentially private property." Amazed, I asked to whom they belonged. Dr. Williams took a long time to reply, and then said: "They're officially the property of the institute that holds them."

I asked whether Corbitt and Bailey would have enough to complete their PCR sequencing, and he replied: "They would have to decide that. That's their problem. My supply is perforce limited, and when they're finished, they're finished."

Although Dr. Williams said that he would have another think about whether or not I could see and photograph the blocks, and although I gently reminded him of this in months to come, he never did allow it. Neither did he ever agree to show me the full autopsy report, to which he had referred at several stages in the course of the interview. I was left feeling taken aback at his thinking of autopsy samples in terms of "private property," and wondered what David Carr's next of kin would have felt about all this.

---

The doctors had helped elucidate the medical history, but it was David's surviving family, friends, and workmates who provided a growing sense of him as a personality. Slowly, a picture of the man and of the times began to emerge. He was born to Dave and Agnes Carr in November 1933, an only child, and he lived most of his life at a rented semidetached house in Naseby Road, built just before the war. Reddish was then a close-knit working-class community surrounded by cotton mills, breweries, railway sidings, and canals. Dave, as the young boy was known, lived just three doors away from his aunt Jessie and cousins Val and Keith.

His upbringing was unremarkable. He went to two local primary schools, where he was known as being bright and enthusiastic, albeit something of a prankster. After the war he moved to Stockport Junior Technical School, and became an enthusiastic member of the Boy Scouts and the local football team. The goalie, the ebullient Clary Mills, recalls that Dave dated one or two of the girls who, according to Val, used to "fight to hand out the lemons at half-time." Both informants stressed, however, that in that era such teenage liaisons were still innocent affairs, involving little more than kissing and hand-holding down by the river, in a milk bar, or in the back row of one of the local fleapits.

In 1950, at the age of sixteen, Dave Carr started work as an apprentice compositor at Kemsley House in the center of Manchester. Until its closure in 1988, this was the largest print shop in Europe, and possibly the world. For the next five years, he learned his trade in different departments, but spent most of his time working the morning shift, which produced the *Manchester Evening Chronicle*. Like the other apprentices, he had a day release each week to study at the local technical college. Printers were then among the best paid of British workers, but because of the unsocial hours they tended to stick together and organize their own activities. They had their own football and cricket leagues, motor clubs, and golf clubs, and during the fifties, these tended to be all-male preserves. At lunchtimes, when the shift ended, Dave would often join the others for a few beers.

In the summer of 1953 or 1954, Dave and two of his friends spent a fortnight in Douglas, on the Isle of Man. In those days, before foreign holidays became commonplace, a sizable percentage of the teenage population of northern England went to the island in the summer. A dog-eared photo still exists of the three lads, accompanied by an older man and a buxom woman, apparently Scottish, with whom they spent much of the holiday. They are seated outside a boardinghouse, with Dave at the rear, leaning back in his chair and looking wryly at the camera. He is wearing a casual jacket and open-necked shirt; his curly hair is pushed up high with brilliantine. He feels confident with these people, that is clear, and is not embarrassed to show it. Apparently the photo was taken by another Scottish woman who was Dave's girlfriend for much of the fortnight.

Dave was long overdue for National Service, which had been deferred until he could complete his five-year apprenticeship. He was finally called up in November 1955, shortly before his twenty-second birthday. He had already joined the Royal Navy Volunteer Reserve the year before, a maneuver that now allowed him to join the navy, instead of square-bashing in the army with the other "national heroes." The only certain memory about Dave's naval travels came from his elderly aunt Jessie, who recalled that he was stationed at Gibraltar for a while, although Val thought that she remembered discussions about "dry desert heat." The only other clues are the mementos that he brought back. Once he gave Val and Jessie a set of "black japanned" trays, each bearing the design of a Japanese flower garden burned into the wood. Another time he returned with an elongated gazelle carved from a soft pale wood, and a dark wooden bust of a long-necked woman wearing a headdress and jewelry, which his father apparently used to say Dave had bought in Africa.

Dave was released from the navy in November 1957, and returned to his job at Kemsley House. Some of his friends, however, thought he had changed. One, in particular, said he was more serious, as if something had happened to him that he didn't want to talk about. We now know that Dave was already having problems with his gums and visiting the skin hospital every month for X-ray treatment to his back and shoulders, but none of his family or friends appear to have known about this. However, early in 1958 he met Elsie and they started walking out together. Elsie was widely admired, and so there was general approval when, a year or so later, she and Dave announced that they were to get married.

By this stage, however, his friends had begun to notice that Dave was seriously unwell. He began taking days, then weeks, off work, and of course this sparked a lot of rumors. One of his Kemsley House friends, who had served in the army and knew about the British nuclear tests on Christmas Island, believed that Dave might have attended these tests, and was keeping quiet about it because he had signed the Official Secrets Act. His parents, meanwhile, began telling people that he was sick with fever, that it was something he had caught while abroad.

Nonetheless, nobody could really believe it when, in the late summer of 1959, David Carr died. Val recalls finding Elsie at Naseby Road the night after his death, and the two of them crying in each other's arms on the sofa. Elsie told her over and over that it was because of the ring, that everyone knew it was bad luck to buy an engagement ring at a pawnshop.

Some days after the funeral, Dave's ashes were scattered, and a rosebush planted in the Gardens of Remembrance, with a small plaque beside it. In 1965, when Agnes died (from a broken heart, according to Val), her name was added to the inscription. Soon afterward Elsie emigrated, in a bid to leave the sad memories behind her, and in 1974 Dave senior also passed away. In the days before his death, he moved in with one of his sisters, and apparently spent long periods talking about his son and weeping for him.

---

How did such a pleasant and unexceptional young man as David Carr become the world's first recorded case of AIDS? How had this virus — at that time an extremely rare virus — come to intrude upon his life? Just where had he been exposed? Some observers thought, given the ten years of latency that is typical of HIV, that he must have been infected in the late forties — but, given his history and the fact that he was then still at school, this seemed highly improbable.

So what were the potential risk periods of his life? There was that first holiday away from home, on the Isle of Man, when he was nineteen or twenty — and then there were his two years in the navy, which clearly constituted the likeliest period of exposure. Unfortunately, nobody recalled very much about these years, such as where he had traveled.

Then there was the question of Dave's sexuality. Some I had spoken with felt that the anal lesions, which had possibly been caused by a herpes virus,[14] were significant. Could these be an indication of the portal of entry for both herpes and HIV? Could Dave have been bisexual — or had he, perhaps, been raped by one of his fellow sailors? This was possible, of course, but if so, where were the other sailors who should also have died of AIDS at around the same time? Besides, Dr. Stretton, his physician in 1959, said he had since seen similar lesions in AIDS patients who were not homosexual and who claimed never to have had anal intercourse.

Dave's friends and family were all convinced that he was exclusively heterosexual. Val, who recalled his fondness for Jane Russell and other hourglass-figured pin-ups of the day, hypothesized that "he must have gone along with some shipmates to a brothel somewhere." But if a prostitute in a foreign port had been infected with HIV in the second half of the fifties, then why had the global pandemic not begun until 1981?

The gap in the information about Dave's time in the navy began to be filled when two officials from his print union came up with an old, inky filing card, which confirmed that Dave had definitely been in the Royal Navy (not the Merchant Navy) and provided the exact date of his induction into the "senior service." Val, as next of kin, agreed to help further by writing to the navy to request details of where he had served.

---

The response, a week or so later, gave David Carr's service number, the dates of his joining (November 7, 1955) and discharge (November 6, 1957), and the information that he had served as a stores accountant in the victualling section. It went on to state that he had joined the Royal Navy at H.M.S. *Victory,* and had served on board H.M.S. *Drake,* H.M.S. *Ceres,* H.M.S. *Warrior,* and H.M.S. *Whitby,* before being released from H.M.S. *Drake.* The letter contained neither the dates when he had been on the various ships, nor the order in which he had served on them.[15]

The next week, I went up to the Maritime Museum at Greenwich, where a few minutes of research in the 1950s editions of *The Navy List* revealed a number of interesting things. I found that three of the "ships" on which Dave Carr had served were actually "stone frigates"— meaning bases and training schools on land. But it was when I started looking through other books, in a bid to find out more about the two oceangoing vessels, *Warrior* and *Whitby,* that I discovered there might be rather more to this story than met the eye. For H.M.S. *Warrior,* I learned, had served as the headquarters ship for Britain's nuclear test program in the Pacific during 1957, code-named Operation Grapple.

I spent the next week examining the appropriate ships' logs at the Public Record Office at Kew, unraveling where the ships had sailed, and when. The itinerary of the *Whitby* had been relatively mundane. Save for a fortnight spent in Gibraltar in February 1957, and a week in Malmo, Sweden, at the start of June 1957, the *Whitby* spent the rest of 1956 and 1957 based in London- derry, Northern Ireland, or hunting submarines in exercises along the Ulster coastline.[16]

The *Warrior,* by contrast, had traveled rather farther afield. In 1955 and 1956 she underwent a series of refits that converted her into one of the best-equipped aircraft carriers in the British fleet.[17] She sailed from Portsmouth at the start of February 1957, and squeezed through the Panama Canal, arriving at Christmas Island in March 1957.[18] Apart from a brief recreational trip to Hawaii, she spent the next two months shuttling to and fro across the five hundred miles of ocean between the two islands where the British military was to detonate its H- bombs — Christmas and Malden. She was then used as the headquarters ship for the first three detonations of Operation Grapple; it was from her flight deck that the visiting scientists and journalists viewed the blasts.

Officially, three H-bombs "in the megaton range" were detonated a few thousand feet over Malden Island, on May 15, May 31, and June 19, 1957 — one of which, the second, was supposed to have had an especially large yield.[19]

After the third explosion, the five Avenger aircraft that had been loaned for the tests by the Americans were dumped overboard into the Pacific. Soon after- ward, the *Warrior* sailed north to Pearl Harbor, so that the crew could enjoy some R and R, after which she returned to Britain by the long route, via Cape Horn, stopping off at seven ports on what was billed as a mission to "show the flag" to the South Americans. She made one other stop, at Gibraltar, on the way back to Portsmouth. Despite several cases of VD in the sick bay, and a pitched battle in an Argentinian dance hall, the public relations trip was such a success that the *Warrior* was sold to the Argentinian navy a few months later. The thousand- strong crew of the aircraft carrier, the men who — without being asked — had formed the front line for the Grapple tests, finally went on leave on October 14, just three weeks before Dave Carr's discharge from National Service.

Other details featured in the logbooks were rather more embarrassing to the British military, which has always insisted that the *Warrior* was moored some twenty-seven miles away from Ground Zero at the time of the H-bomb blasts, this being a safe distance that ensured that none of the men could have been exposed to significant levels of radiation. For the logs revealed that within ninety minutes of each of the detonations, the aircraft carrier steamed down to Malden Island, and then spent the afternoon and night drifting offshore, often just a mile or two from Ground Zero. On the last occasion, a boat was launched for what was described as a "fishing party to Malden," and returned two hours later. It looked very much as if the crew of the *Warrior*, a vessel that — after the blasts — was kept away from British ports for four months and then swiftly sold, had actually served as nuclear guinea pigs, just like their American and Soviet colleagues during the same mad, bad, Cold War period.[20]

One thing that all this revealed for certain was that — contrary to several newspaper reports about David Carr's travels — he had never visited Africa with the navy. However, this still left open the question of whether he had traveled to the Pacific tests with the *Warrior*, or stayed in Europe with the *Whitby*. The fact that the *Warrior* had returned to England just a few weeks before Dave's release from the navy, combined with the hunch of one of Dave's friends that he might have been constrained by the Official Secrets Act, suggested that he had probably been aboard the nuclear vessel.

I decided to place some "Calling Old Shipmates" adverts in naval magazines, and the results were not long in coming. Over the next six months or so, I interviewed over twenty men from the *Warrior*, including her commodore, Robin Hicks, various officers, the chaplain, and a number of enlisted men and national servicemen.[21] I learned that since 1957, many of the ship's crew had contracted unusual diseases, including leukemias and cancers. The first fatality had been a radar officer, David Franklin, who died of aplastic anemia and leukemia in August 1958, at the age of twenty-nine, amid a security crackdown by the navy.[22] Many others had died at an unusually early age, including at least two storekeepers. Of course, it was not possible, in any one individual instance, to prove that radiation was the cause of death, but the sheer number of such unusual deaths among a group that had shared a unique experience was highly suggestive.

Many of the men who were present at the 1957/8 tests at Malden Island and Christmas Island, and the atomic trials staged in Australia in 1952–1957 have joined the British Nuclear Test Veterans Association (BNTVA). A very large proportion of BNTVA members — perhaps as many as half — are now suffering from leukemias, cancers, autoimmune conditions, and hypothyroidism (low performance by, or atrophy of, the thyroid gland, often caused by radiation exposure). In addition, many of their children and grandchildren have been born with deformities.

I was given a copy of a paper that one of the BNTVA researchers had un-covered at the Public Records Office, proving that in 1953, the military had wanted to see how atomic blasts would affect "ships, stores and men"— in that order.[23] There was much more evidence along similar lines. One particularly sinister aspect was that dosimeter badges, even when issued, seemed generally to have gone missing in the intervening years, or else to have readings indicat-ing zero radiation exposure. None of this inspired confidence, and yet most of the BNTVA members still vigorously defended the concept of Queen and Country, and were loath to blame the British military for what had befallen them since.

I became increasingly alarmed as I read through the BNTVA records. One man, an artillery officer on H.M.S. *Diana* who had twice sailed through an atomic cloud off western Australia in 1955, had died thirty years later with *Pneumocystis carinii* pneumonia (PCP), non-Hodgkin's lymphoma, multiple skin infections, and weight loss, which sounded like a typical diagnosis of AIDS. By this stage, I had come across two other cases in which people had developed symptoms typical of AIDS after having apparently been exposed to radiation from a nearby nuclear facility, or while working in a uranium mine. And I had unearthed possible associations between outbreaks of PCP and uranium min-ing in Czechoslovakia and the former Belgian Congo.

It was then that I began to investigate that other human retrovirus, HTLV-1. Was it merely coincidence that the place where this virus was first found to be pathogenic, as adult T-cell leukemia (ATL), was the area around Nagasaki?[24] I began to wonder whether HIV and HTLV-1 might in fact be old, nonpatho-genic viruses, which only caused AIDS and ATL among those who had become immunocompromised through prior radiation exposure.

It was during this research that I first heard about Ernest Sternglass's theo-ries, which included the proposition that the French atomic blasts in the Sahara in the late fifties and sixties had released radiation that later "rained out" in the tropics, and in particular around the Great Lakes of Africa, in the very area where the AIDS epidemic emerged in the general population two decades later. His idea was that low-level radiation exposure had immunosuppressed an entire generation, and had perhaps also caused a crucial mutation to the retro-viral ancestor of HIV.[25] By this stage, I was beginning to get serious about this idea, and began following up other possible radiation links such as nuclear acci-dents, areas of high natural radiation, and even levels of fish consumption among different African lakeside tribes.

But amid all the excitement, I had forgotten one rather important thing. I had still not managed to confirm that David Carr had actually been on board the *Warrior* for the Malden Island tests. It was when I located the third (and then the fourth and fifth) persons who had served in the *Warrior*'s naval and victualling stores in 1957, and still nobody recognized his photograph or recalled him, that I realized something must be wrong.

Finally, in 1992, this growing suspicion was confirmed. By a considerable stroke of luck, I managed to find out where Elsie, Dave Carr's former fiancée, lived. I decided to write her an all-or-nothing letter, one that made it clear that if she did not reply, I would not bother her again.

Ten days later, I received a lengthy and very courteous reply, containing all the information about Dave that Elsie could remember. It also contained two photos of him. The fuzzier of the two featured Dave and two other "pussers" (wearing the matelot's gear of the supply branch) standing in front of a statue of a fat man astride a horse. The top of the photo was faded, as if it had been poorly fixed or shot into the sun, but one could just make out that the roof of the building behind was crenellated.

The architecture looked northern European, but could also possibly have been from one of the older sections of a South American port. To resolve this, I paid a visit to the local library. I started by looking through several tourist guidebooks, and within a few minutes I had the answer. For there, in a book about Sweden, was a large photo of a rather plump King Karl X, sitting on top of an equally burly horse. The base of the plinth, and the shape of the buildings behind, were indisputably the same as in the snapshot from Elsie. The picture had been taken in the Stortorget, the main square of Malmo.

The letdown was instantaneous. There was only one time that David could have been in Malmo, and that was in June 1957. This meant that he must have been serving on board the *Whitby* at that time, rather than on the *Warrior* at the bomb tests in the Pacific.

This had two immediate implications. First, it meant that the cornerstone of the theory on which I had been working on and off for the previous year had been split asunder. Second, it meant that if David had served on board the *Warrior* at all, it could only have been during her tour of British ports, before she left for Christmas Island. In other words, the only places he had visited out-side the British Isles would have been Malmo and Gibraltar, while he was aboard H.M.S. *Whitby*.

Just where, I thought once again, had this unfortunate man contracted HIV?

# 9

## AIDS in the pre-AIDS era?

However Dave Carr might have contracted HIV, one conclusion was strongly indicated. It was unlikely that he was the solitary archival case of AIDS.

One of my earliest interviews for this book was with the first scientist to claim he had unearthed a positive sample of HIV from 1959: André Nahmias, professor of epidemiology and immunology from Emory University, Atlanta.[1] The professor's schedule did not allow a meeting during working hours before I was due to leave Atlanta, so he called at my hotel room at around eleven one evening, and we talked for the next two and a half hours. Born in Egypt, Nahmias has a *basso profundo* voice, a large body, and an imposingly forthright presence.

Sadly, he was unable to provide any further details about the donor of the L70 sample, save that he was an unidentified Bantu male from Leopoldville in the Congo. But he did give me a detailed account of the testing procedures. It was 1985 when he acquired the several hundred Congo samples from his Emory colleague, Moses Schanfield, and having tried without success to involve the CDC in the testing, Nahmias decided to take on the job in his own labs. He and his technicians started by using the ELISA test from Abbott Laboratories, which proved to be far from specific: according to the first round of results, over 90 percent of the 1959 sera were antibody-positive for HIV! Later, the sera were sent to Harvard, where Max Essex and Phyllis Kanki brought the number down to just three positives by using IFA, the fluorescent antibody technique, and then Western blot. One of these three positive samples, L70, also tested positive by RIPA, and these positive readings were later confirmed by two other labs. Significantly, L70 tested positive for HIV, but negative for the SIVs, which were just then being found in Asian macaques in American primate centers; in retrospect, this made it look very much like a sample of HIV-1, rather than HIV-2. Given the number of assays, and the amount of cross checking in different laboratories, this seemed to be a very good bet as a genuine HIV-positive sample — and Nahmias was understandably indignant that some researchers still doubted the veracity of his findings.

L70 might, of course, have represented a contamination with a modern HIV-1 isolate — but it was difficult to see how this could have affected just one of the several hundred archival samples he tested unless it had happened deliberately, at source, before the sample was subjected to the various different assays.

There was one other interesting point. It was popularly believed by other researchers that Nahmias had used up all of the L70 sample in the course of the copious testing.[2] But when I commented that it would be marvelous if L70 could be confirmed and sequenced by PCR, Professor Nahmias made it clear that a small amount of the serum still remained. However, he warned, PCR was well known for giving you false positives. But there was still a possibility of looking into this at some time in the future, when PCR technology was more advanced.

André Nahmias was convinced that HIV was a new virus, and pointed out that any virus that caused violent disease and death was not yet well adapted to its host, and had probably crossed over recently from another species. The reason why HIV was so "diabolical," he added, was that it had the persistence of DNA viruses (which stay permanently in the body, facilitating onward transmission), but the mutability of an RNA virus, which lent it great variation due to replication errors, and allowed it to escape the attentions of the immune system. Furthermore, it was well adapted to sexual transmission, and without sex, there was clearly no future for the human species.

Nahmias felt that getting a fix on HIV's beginnings, on how old the virus was in humans, could only improve scientific understanding of whether HIV would eventually become attenuated — and how long it would take before people could develop resistance to it. His guess was that without medical intervention it would take forty generations, eight hundred to a thousand years, before humans were able to coexist happily with HIV.

---

I was greatly impressed by Professor Nahmias, and his testimony only fired my determination to search for other early traces of HIV and AIDS. That search had in fact already begun two months earlier, in June 1990, when the first article I photocopied at the Keppel Street library was one which had been quoted in several of the epidemiological papers by Alan Fleming. Entitled "AIDS in the Pre-AIDS Era" and written by David Huminer and two colleagues from an Israeli hospital,[3] it presented the results of a literature search for pre-epidemic cases of AIDS, based on the CDC's surveillance definition of the syndrome.[4]

The authors had excluded children under five and persons aged over sixty, and all those patients for whom there was evidence of predisposing illnesses like congenital immunodeficiencies or cancers, or past treatment with steroids or radiotherapy. They also excluded suggestive cases in which the reports featured insufficient information to merit an AIDS diagnosis. Despite this, Huminer's team came up with nineteen "probable" cases of AIDS, based on clinical criteria, between 1950 and the end of the seventies. Their list included ten from North America, eight from Europe, and just one from Africa (though this was possibly because so few African case studies get written up in medical journals). The earliest mooted case was from 1952.

I was intrigued, and began my own research into the literature, using Huminer's cases as a starting point. I became even more intrigued when, a month after beginning the research, the *Lancet* letter about the 1959 case from Manchester demonstrated that in this instance, at least, the presence of HIV had been confirmed by PCR analysis.[5] Another plausible case, dating from 1968/9, had also been confirmed by positive HIV serology,[6] and these corroborating reports, combined with the serological evidence that HIV had been detected in Leopoldville/Kinshasa in 1959 and 1970,[7] further reinforced the feeling that this was a worthwhile approach.

It seemed increasingly plausible that sporadic early cases of AIDS might have been occurring over the years, some of them recorded in the medical literature, but "masquerad[ing] under various diagnoses."[8] It was, it appeared, just a question of searching. In August 1990, four weeks after the confirmation of HIV in the tissues of the "Manchester sailor," another *Lancet* letter entitled "Tracking AIDS Epidemic in Libraries," by a Dutch epidemiologist, proposed this very approach, with the comment: "Astute physicians have always felt the urge to write down and publish the unusual. My preliminary hunt makes it likely that early reports of isolated AIDS patients are hidden in medical journals."[9]

Over the first few weeks of my research, some burrowing through the literature and a few phone interviews persuaded me that seven of Huminer's cases should be disqualified, since they were probably not true AIDS cases. Three of these seemed unsafe because they were based on a disease (progressive multifocal leukoencephalopathy, or PML) that appeared to be capable of killing people with or without the presence of HIV. I discarded four other cases on the basis of advice from the doctors who had been directly involved — for example, if it was clear that congenital immunodeficiency, not HIV, had been the cause of illness.[10]

This left twelve cases of clinically plausible AIDS, which seemed to divide fairly naturally into six cases from the seventies, and six more debatable cases from the sixties and fifties. Five of the former six cases came from the latter half of the seventies, and have already been described in previous chapters (the gay American from Boston; the two Germans — the gay violinist and the soldier; and two women — the Danish doctor and the Congolese secretary — who appeared to have been infected in the Congo). All — with the possible exception of the young German soldier[11] — seemed to be plausible cases of AIDS, linked either to the gay scene in the West or to sexual or parenteral exposure in Africa during the late seventies, this being a period when HIV was certainly already present in both milieux. The sixth case, involving a disseminated bacterial infection (strongyloidiasis) in a Ugandan man who died in 1973, was less certain, in that only scant clinical details were supplied.[12] It may or may not have been a genuine case of AIDS.

The six cases from before 1970 were more controversial, although they were certainly not far-fetched, for the visible beginning of any epidemic is usually preceded by a few sporadic, isolated cases. In any case, Huminer was not alone in his suspicions, for by 1984 three of the six had been proposed elsewhere in the literature as possible cases of AIDS.[13]

The six were as follows: a teenager from St. Louis, Missouri, who died in 1969;[14] a young woman from Washington state (1964);[15] Ardouin A. from New York (1959);[16] David Carr, the Manchester sailor (1959); George Y. (Toronto, 1959);[17] and a young man from Memphis, Tennessee (1952).[18]

Since five of these cases came from North America I decided, in August 1990, to fly to the United States in order to do some follow-up on the ground. By then, I had also identified another possible case of AIDS from before the beginning of Huminer's survey (a Japanese-Canadian woman who had died in Montreal in 1945),[19] and I decided to include her in the investigation also.

Before leaving England, however, I received two important pieces of advice from the London-based immunologist Dr. Tony Pinching. First he warned me that some opportunistic infections, like lymphomas, can be misleading. If, for instance, a patient had presented at a hospital twenty years ago with an extensive lymphoma and PCP, it would nowadays be difficult to determine if the PCP had been the result of immunosuppression caused by the lymphoma (and/or its treatment, which would often include radiotherapy and steroids), or if HIV had caused both conditions. One way of knowing, of course, would be to test any available tissues or sera for the presence of virus. However, he also warned once more about the vagaries of the various HIV assays, and stressed that several different tests that indicated the presence of both core and envelope proteins of the virus were needed if one was to be absolutely confident that HIV really was present. The warnings were timely.

I spent several weeks of that summer in North America, traveling slowly but comfortably to and fro by Amtrak, and interviewing en route. I returned in the summer of 1991, this time buying an old car and selling it again after five weeks. I found that the attempt to unravel the human stories underlying the case histories was invariably fascinating, and usually worthwhile to boot, for it turned out that most of these patients had been involved in certain unusual events or experiences — very few of which had emerged in the published papers or medical chart. These episodes might or might not have had bearing on the unusual nature of their deaths, but clearly it was legitimate to consider the possibility that there was some connection.

In the end I found I was able, in each case, to propose a plausible hypothesis to explain the mysterious collapse of the immune system.

Three of the scenarios of causation that follow (relating to Robert R., Alice S., and George Y.) are advanced tentatively, and three (relating to Ardouin A., Dick G., and Sadayo F.) with rather more confidence. These six cases are detailed here partly because they are interesting investigations in their own right. Mainly, however, it is because they provide some valuable perspective on the true nature of AIDS.

In the descriptions of these cases, details sometimes differ from those already presented in published papers. This is because examinations of the medical notes, interviews with the protagonists, and further research have provided more accurate information.[20]

———————

Robert R., a black youth from St. Louis, Missouri, was just sixteen when he died in May 1969. He had first begun experiencing swellings in his legs some two and a half years earlier, and as time passed the abnormal buildup of fluid in his tissues (known as edema) progressed remorselessly until it included his genitalia, lower abdomen, and, finally, his chest. For some unknown reason, his lymphatic system seemed to be blocked. Beginning in mid-1967, he was admitted "a few times" to the City Hospital in St. Louis, but by November 1968, when his condition started to cause breathing difficulties, he was moved to the Deaconess Hospital, where he spent the final six months of his life. By this stage he was in a miserable state, with what seemed like "a big continuous bag" of fluid underneath his skin, which moved to and fro like a wave in a water bed.

The doctors at Deaconess found Robert surly and unresponsive to questioning — an attitude that apparently became more pronounced as he grew more ill. In later notes, Robert is described as having a "mild psychotic reaction" and "moderate mental retardation." Apparently the only time he relaxed during those final months was when he was undergoing physiotherapy, and the picture that emerges is of a shy, awkward adolescent who was terrified by what was happening to him.

The doctors did what they could for Robert, and successfully drained the lymphatic fluid from his legs and chest, removing up to five liters at a time. Eventually the patient became so debilitated from the lymphatic disorder, and the pressure on his lungs so great, that he contracted pneumonia, and died a few days later.

At autopsy, the pathologist William Drake noted that with the fluid drained, the corpse was that of an emaciated boy, weighing "probably 75 pounds." As he was examining the skin of his legs and scrotum, which had become woody and elephantine in texture, he noticed a small nodule on the boy's left thigh. After the microscopic examination, he realized that the nodule was of Kaposi's sarcoma, and that this condition was aggressive and widespread, involving not just the lower body beneath the skin, but also the bone marrow, lymph nodes, and the pleural cavity. Some KS lesions were also present, together with some hemorrhoids, near the anal sphincter. Previously, the patient had always vigorously refused a rectal examination. Robert had also been infected with the bacteria *Chlamydia* (which is often sexually acquired).

In 1973, a paper was published in *Lymphology* on the case, written by Memory Elvin-Lewis (a *Chlamydia* specialist) and Marlys Witte, who had treated Robert at the City Hospital at the start of his illness.[21] The paper made only passing reference to the KS, but emphasized the finding of *Chlamydia* throughout the body, pointing out that it was conjectural whether this had played a primary or secondary role in the patient's illness. The authors stated that Robert had "admitted to frequent sexual intercourse," and hypothesized that the *Chlamydia* might have been acquired venereally.

Eleven years later, in 1984, Marlys Witte and her husband wrote a letter to the *Journal of the American Medical Association,* this time with Dr. Drake as coauthor, in which they proposed that the widespread chlamydial infection and disseminated KS "makes AIDS a compelling diagnosis in retrospect." The letter included the claim that "While he admitted to heterosexual relations for several years, a homosexual history was not specifically elicited."[22] However, the hemorrhoids and anorectal KS might, it suggested, indicate an anal portal of entry for a venereal infection.

In their freezers, Witte and Elvin-Lewis still had samples of serum, together with samples of spleen, brain, lymph node, and liver taken at autopsy. In June 1987, Witte sent some of these samples to Professor Robert Garry, a young microbiologist from Tulane University, New Orleans, for further analysis. Garry tested the serum by Western blot, and detected antibodies to all the major proteins of HIV-1. Later, he apparently detected HIV-1 virus in all four tissue samples, using the p24 antigen test.[23]

However, as I discovered when I started looking into the case, there were still a considerable number of loose ends. The first concerned Robert's sexual history, knowledge of which was not helped by the fact that the patient had been so uncommunicative. The two women doctors who were responsible for arranging the testing both claimed retrospectively that the autopsy had shown that Robert R. had probably had regular passive anal intercourse; one stated that he could have been a male prostitute.[24] But both Drake and William Cole, the physician who had spent most time with Robert, were much more cautious. They suspected that Robert *might* have been gay, on the basis that the KS had been found around the anus but not elsewhere in the gastrointestinal tract, yet they pointed out that there were several other possible explanations.

I was unable to find out much about the gay scene in St. Louis, which was described by one informant as being "one giant closet" in the nineties, let alone the sixties. However, it seemed far more productive to investigate Robert's heterosexual activity, which was not in dispute — even if the extent of that activity was. The only evidence about this subject in Robert's medical records featured in the autopsy notes, where it was recorded that "The patient dated his physical disability from an instance of sexual relations with a neighborhood girl." With the help of some local journalists[25] I located the mother, who stoutly insisted that her son had not been gay, and who told me she only knew of his having had sex with one girl, whom she named and described. She added that the woman was still alive, and that she "moved from house to house" as a vagrant. Later, her account was apparently confirmed by a group of men whom I found drinking beside a barrier in the same street where Robert had gone to grade school, and where he and his family had been living in the late sixties. One man knew of a woman of the right name, age, and description who, he said, he had last seen some six months before. If indeed she was the same woman, this meant that the main suspect for infecting Robert was still alive more than twenty years after his death, making her an unlikely source for his apparent HIV infection.

The more I looked into the case, the more doubts I had about whether Robert R. had really died of AIDS. There was no proof that he had been promiscuous, gay, or an IVDU, so it was hard to imagine what his risk factor could have been. And although he had had disseminated KS, the rest of his symptoms did not represent a typical presentation of the syndrome. It was hard to imagine a case of AIDS cropping up this early and so far from Africa — the apparent source of the HIV-1 epidemic. And furthermore, there appeared to be some uncertainty surrounding the fate of some of the tissue samples. When, at my request, William Drake tried to relocate some of the wax-embedded blocks from the autopsy at Deaconess in 1990, he found that they had disappeared.[26]

Then there was the question of the HIV testing. First, it seems that the Western blot test used may have been the sensitivity-enhanced Biotech assay, which had produced false-positive results in the case of James Moore's 1971/2 Lexington drug injectors.[27] And in the late summer of 1990 there was further mystery, when somebody apparently broke into Garry's office, taking the notes on the Robert R. Western blot tests and a couple of the Western blots themselves.[28]

Soon after Garry's paper on Robert R. was published in October 1988, there was talk about sequencing the virus by PCR. The job was eventually entrusted to John Sninsky, an acknowledged PCR expert from the Cetus Corporation in

California. But as the years went by, and no sequence was published, virologists became more and more nervous about the veracity of the original HIV-positive results.[29]

All this, of course, leaves unanswered the question of what might have caused Robert's illness. Robert had told his doctors that his grandfather had suffered "the same symptoms." Could he have had some sort of congenital immunodeficiency, perhaps exacerbated by a venereal infection with *Chlamydia* and KS? It is certainly possible, but it seems an inadequate explanation.

There is, however, another possibility — one which involves one of the more shameful episodes in American history. In June 1980, research conducted by the Church of Scientology revealed that during the early summer of 1953 the Army Chemical Corps conducted secret open-air chemical warfare tests in St. Louis — involving thirty-five aerosol releases at various places in and around the city, including the Monsanto plant.[30] The army provided a cover story to city officials and the local press, claiming that the experiments were intended to see whether smoke screens could protect the city from attacks by Soviet bombers.[31] These experiments were part of a much larger chemical and biological testing program operated by the army (sometimes in conjunction with the CIA), which involved hundreds of similar releases staged in cities across the United States between 1949 and 1968.[32]

Information released by the army in July 1994 revealed that the house where Robert was living in 1953 was sited less than half a block from the "How" test site, one of the two 25-square-block areas where most of the releases took place.[33] This area was described as a "slum district," with a population density that was "possibly one of the highest of any residential district in the country." Apparently the choice of socioeconomic group was "to minimize public questions about the tests."[34]

The St. Louis tests all involved zinc cadmium sulfide, a yellow crystalline substance that appears to be a mixture of zinc sulfide and cadmium sulfide. It is sometimes referred to as "FP" for fluorescent particle, because it glows in ultraviolet light, making it easy to trace in diffusion experiments. According to an army spokesman talking in 1980, these FP tests "were completely safe and no one's health was endangered."[35] Others, however, have disputed this claim. Cadmium, in particular, is a highly toxic metal; because of its "extraordinary facility for accumulation in the kidney it is associated with kidney damage, but it also leads to cirrhosis of the liver, and severe damage to the lungs." Apparently digestive absorption of cadmium is low, but "absorption of cadmium from the air is very much faster."[36] FPs can cause lung damage similar to that from bronchopneumonia, while acute cadmium poisoning can cause pulmonary edema, pneumonitis, and death.[37]

One of the prominent findings at Robert R.'s autopsy was bronchopneumonia, and another (not mentioned in any of the published papers) was "acute passive congestion" in the kidney. It is certainly possible that the cause of Robert's edema (for so long his principal symptom), pneumonia, and kidney problems could have been cadmium poisoning, with the KS and chlamydial infections only playing a secondary role.

This may be less implausible than it seems. Between May and June 1953, when the zinc cadmium sulfide tests were staged so close to his home in St. Louis, Robert would have been aged between three and five months. Infants are immunologically vulnerable, especially during the first three months of life, when they are highly susceptible to invasion by foreign antigens.[38] It may be that Robert was also congenitally immunodeficient, and therefore more at risk from the diffusion experiments than other infants living in the same area. Furthermore, several of the FP tests staged in the United States involved simultaneous releases of allegedly harmless biological substances like *Serratia marcescens* bacteria and *Lycopodium* spores, and there is no guarantee that the St. Louis tests were not of this type.[39]

This is but a tentative scenario. I am not stating that there is necessarily a link between these tests by the Army Chemical Corps in 1953 and Robert R.'s death sixteen years later, but the coincidence of geography and timing seems remarkable, and worthy of further follow-up.

---

As it happens, it is possible that the second of these pre-AIDS-era patients, Alice S., may also have been an accidental victim of Cold War experimentation. In September 1964, a young married couple from Pullman, in the east of Washington State, died within ten days of each other from *Pneumocystis carinii* pneumonia, PCP. At the time, Larry S. was a twenty-six-year-old store manager, while his wife, Alice, was a twenty-two-year-old secretary at the local university. In both cases, the course of the illness was rapid; they suffered their first symptom (a cough) just a few weeks before their deaths, and both partners sought medical advice only when they had less than two weeks to live. The reason that Alice alone has been mooted as a possible case of AIDS is that her husband had been suffering from leukemia for the previous five months, even though it was supposedly "in good remission" by the time of his death.[40] She, by contrast, apparently had no underlying condition to explain her sudden demise.

The 1965 paper that reported these tragic deaths was entitled "*Pneumocystis carinii* Pneumonia in a Family," because it also described a respiratory-tract infection suffered by the seven-year-old daughter during June and July 1964. It claimed that there was "strong presumptive evidence" that PCP was involved here too, although in her case the microorganism was never isolated.[41]

The background to the case was intriguing. Larry's family (he, his parents, and two siblings) were natives of Moscow, Idaho, just ten miles from Pullman across the state line, but during the forties they lived in several places in eastern Washington and western Idaho. Members of the family had experienced repeated health problems since 1945. Three of the five (including Larry) suffered from hypothyroidism or thyroid dysfunction; both the parents developed diabetes and arthritis in later life; the mother was admitted to hospital with bleeding stomach ulcers on three occasions (one of which was considered life threatening), while Larry eventually developed leukemia.[42] The family's collective medical history, with its autoimmune diseases and leukemia, is strongly suggestive of exposure to radiation or other toxic materials.

Alice grew up in Port Angeles on the west coast of Washington, moving to Pullman to begin a college course at Washington State University in September 1960. A woman with whom she lived during this period recalls her "being ill more than once with respiratory ailments." At some point in 1962 she began going out with Larry, who already had a five-year-old daughter by a previous marriage.

In May 1963, however, Alice and her flatmate decided to leave Pullman, and headed south to the bright lights of the Bay Area of California. They moved into an apartment in Mountain View, and Alice soon found a job in nearby Palo Alto, but then Larry turned up, asking her to marry him. She accepted, and followed him back up north at the end of June.

They were married in September 1963, after which they moved into a basement apartment in Pullman. By that winter, Larry was frequently getting tired, and his body began to take on bruises. In March 1964, he was admitted to hospital with pains in his arms and chest, and a second hospital visit in April revealed that he was suffering from acute lymphatic leukemia. He began a course of steroids and, despite experiencing a remission, continued to feel unwell throughout the summer.

By June 1964, Alice was looking after both Larry and his daughter, who had developed a cold and a persistent cough, though her condition cleared up after a course of antibiotics. Later that summer, Larry and Alice spent a week alone together on the Snake River and did some waterskiing. When they returned in early August, Alice had a rash, as if she had been in the sun too long, and soon afterward she developed a cold and a dry, hacking cough, which caused her to consult a doctor at the end of the month. She was admitted to the hospital with severe breathing problems on September 4, and despite being put in a tent, the lack of oxygen in her brain caused her to ramble and hallucinate. During her more lucid moments, she told the nurses she was worried about her family. She died six days later.

Larry, who had also started coughing at the end of August, was readmitted to hospital in Spokane the day after Alice's death, with similar symptoms. Like her, he deteriorated steadily, and died on September 20. In addition to the PCP, his discharge summary cites acute lymphoblastic leukemia (in remission) together with hyperplasia of the prostate and an unspecified blood disease.

Samples from Larry's lung and spleen were apparently sent to the virology lab of the state department of health, but no virus was isolated. A member of that laboratory says that there are no remaining records about these tissues, and that they would have been discarded after the negative findings. Neither, it seems, were any of Alice's autopsy tissues retained.

Larry was clearly profoundly unwell with leukemia and was on steroid therapy, and it is therefore not surprising that having been exposed to the *Pneumocystis carinii* organism (and devastated by the death of his young wife) he succumbed quickly. It is now thought that most of the adult population has been exposed to *Pneumocystis*,[43] and there have been several reports of PCP being transmitted nosocomially (within a hospital environment), from carriers to persons whose resistance has been lowered by leukemia or lymphoma.[44] One of the explanations advanced for the occasional susceptibility of otherwise healthy elderly people and infants is that they may have encountered an unusually virulent strain.[45] Perhaps Larry, suffering from leukemia, was exposed to such a variant of the pathogen.

Despite concerns in the local community that Larry's daughter might have caught something contagious from her parents, she was found to be in good health when reexamined by doctors shortly after their deaths.[46] Indeed, thirty years later she was still eminently alive and healthy, and in the mid-nineties gave birth to her first child.

However, the question of what caused Alice to die of PCP remains unresolved. It certainly seems that she was immunocompromised by September 1964, but did she die of AIDS, as Huminer has hypothesized? There are reasons for being skeptical. First, the course of her illness was unusually rapid, and it has been reported that the progress of PCP is usually much slower in AIDS patients than in other immunocompromised hosts.[47] Second, she showed no sign of any of the other typical opportunistic infections of AIDS. Third, as a woman who apparently had only had two sexual partners (one of whom was still alive and well in 1992) and was not injecting drugs, she was not at high risk of HIV exposure (presuming that HIV was even present in America in 1964).

So what did cause Alice to succumb so rapidly to PCP, when she was an apparently healthy twenty-two-year-old? Already we know that there are many factors, including infancy, old age, cancer, cancer therapy, or exposure to radiation, that can cause suppression of the immune system and can make one vulnerable to an opportunistic pathogen such as PCP. Alice does not appear to have had an undiagnosed cancer, and she is excluded from the other categories — save the last. For like hundreds of thousands of others in eastern Washington State between the forties and the sixties, Alice was a "Downwinder." She may, in other words, have been exposed to radiation or radionuclides, simply as a result of where she was living.

In the east of Washington State lie the reactors of Hanford where, in 1945, the Nagasaki A-bomb was made. Between 1944 and the mid-sixties, radioactive particles were, on many occasions, vented into the air from the Hanford stacks, whence they were carried mainly eastward, toward the Idaho border. In addition, large amounts of radioactive waste were dumped into underground pits or the Columbia River.[48] The medical histories of Larry and his family suggest that they may all have been exposed to radiation in the forties or fifties. And although Alice only arrived in the "downwind" area in 1960, she too may have been one of the unlucky ones.

In such an irradiated environment, she may have ingested or inhaled a harmful amount of radioactive material in any number of ways, most of which can no longer be identified. However, there were also three specific episodes in which she would seem to have been in the wrong place at the wrong time.

On September 3, 1963, there was an accident at the PUREX (Plutonium Uranium Extraction) plant at Hanford, when sixty curies of radioactive Iodine-131 were released into the atmosphere — four times the quantity that escaped during the Three Mile Island accident of 1979.[49] No announcement was made at the time of the accident. Three days later, on September 6, 1963, Alice, Larry, and his daughter drove westward to Port Angeles, on the day before their wedding. It is believed that they took the direct route via Othello, which lies immediately north of Ringold and the Hanford reservation. The main way in which I-131 is absorbed into human bodies is by being deposited on grass, eaten by cows, and then drunk as milk. Is it possible that they bought some milk en route or breathed in dust through an open car window? Alternatively, could they have been among the human volunteers who, it was later revealed, were deliberately exposed by inhaling I-131 from the air or by drinking milk from cows that had grazed on contaminated pastures at the time of a deliberate 1963 release from Hanford?[50]

Another way in which radioactive particles may be absorbed is through eating irradiated fish. The Columbia River has special fish ladders that allow salmon to return upstream to spawn; one salmon hatchery is even situated at Ringold, opposite where Hanford used to vent much of its waste.[51] In July 1964, just two months before their deaths, Larry caught a thirty-pound salmon in the Strait of Juan De Fuca, near Port Angeles. It is believed to have been a Coho salmon, which is one that migrates hundreds of miles up the Columbia River, to Hanford and beyond, to spawn; some, at least, probably nibble on the odd piece of radioactive moss en route. It is conceivable that this particular fish was heavily contaminated, and that its consumption triggered a rapid disease process in the young couple. However, the facts that Alice and Larry suffered fatal diseases of the lungs (not the digestive system), and that other family members also ate the fish and emerged unscathed, both argue strongly against this hypothesis.

The final scenario is even more fantastic, at least in prospect. Fred Allingham, who heads an organization called the National Association of Radiation Survivors,[52] told me about a man who had been in the army, based at Fort Louis, near Tacoma, Washington, in 1958, and who claimed to have participated in a radiation experiment conducted along the Snake River that summer. It had apparently involved the detonation of a small, tactical nuclear weapon, and the monitoring of responses among army "volunteers." As part of this test, he had to drive along the Snake River at night, through what he believed was the detonation area, to collect water from a small town across the Idaho border.[53]

There are no official records of any such small nuclear weapons being detonated in eastern Washington in 1958. However, in 1993 the U.S. Department of Energy admitted that hundreds of secret, unannounced nuclear tests had been staged on American soil.[54]

The only place where there is a road running alongside the Snake River for more than a few miles is Wawawai River Road, which begins some twenty miles southwest of Pullman, and continues for about thirty miles as far as Lewiston, the first town in Idaho.[55] This is apparently the same stretch of river where Alice and Larry used to go swimming and waterskiing, and is very likely to have been where they spent their week's vacation in the summer of 1964. Their decline into serious ill health began days later.[56]

It is not essential, of course, to invoke a nuclear incident or an exposure to radiation to explain Alice's sudden decline and death.[57] There are also other, rather more mundane explanations that may be more realistic. Perhaps, for instance, the young couple had been exposed to *Pneumocystis* some time before, and were then further exposed to a serious bacterial pathogen which compromised their immune systems — such as *Legionella* — during the waterskiing trip.[58]

One thing, though, can be stated with some confidence. Alice S. is most unlikely to have died as a result of HIV infection. Quite simply, she lacked risk factors, and her clinical course was one of a patient with a suppressed immune system who had previously been exposed to a possibly virulent form of *Pneumocystis,* rather than that of somebody declining slowly into AIDS.[59]

---

Before Alice in 1964, there were three patients (George Y., Ardouin A., and David Carr) who all died with AIDS-like symptoms in 1959. The background histories of these cases have already been described, as have the reports that HIV was apparently present in the tissues of David Carr and in the L70 serum sample from Leopoldville. By the early nineties, 1959 did appear to be the watershed year, the earliest for which there was persuasive evidence of the existence of HIV.

However, further investigation into the two North American cases also began to unearth other possible factors, apart from HIV, that could have caused their illnesses. The clue to what probably happened to Ardouin A., the Jamaican man who died of PCP in Brooklyn in June 1959, comes in the reference to "a fluorescent lamp [which] had broken near him some time before his admission to the hospital."[60] In reality, the episode was rather more serious. According to Isolde, his daughter-in-law,[61] a friend who used to work with Ardouin in the garment factory on Seventh Avenue talked about his having "to break up a lot of fluorescent light bulbs in the factory. Perhaps they were accumulated in a box somewhere, and they had to go."

In a review of chronic beryllium disease published at the end of the sixties, thirty-seven of the sixty cases studied were found to have been working in the fluorescent lamp manufacturing industry.[62] This report states that the industry voluntarily chose to eliminate the use of beryllium compounds in 1949, but it is not known whether all manufacturers complied with this decision immediately. Neither is it known whether fluorescent lamps containing beryllium were imported from overseas after that date. Apparently, the incident described by Ardouin's friend had taken place "not too long before he got sick" (which was in March 1959, three months before his death). Of course, if the lamps had been stored for a long time, it could well have been that some had been made in the forties, before the ban.

Ardouin's urine was analyzed for beryllium content, and found to be positive, but "within the normal range";[63] however, a handbook on clinical testing reports that "urinary excretion is variable in exposed workers and does not correlate well with beryllium disease."[64]

It seems, therefore, that the death of Ardouin A., which in the past has often been claimed as the first adult case of PCP to be unassociated with any other disease, may well have been caused by beryllium exposure. In this case, *Pneumocystis*, the supreme opportunist, may have invaded only at a later stage, perhaps during the patient's three weeks in hospital, when he would anyway have become immunosuppressed as a result of the heavy steroid therapy.

So Ardouin does not seem to have been suffering from AIDS. This conclusion was apparently confirmed in 1992, when a lung tissue sample from his autopsy was analyzed by PCR by Fergal Hill, a molecular biologist based at Cambridge University, and found to contain no trace of HIV.[65]

---

What about George Y., the Japanese-Canadian carpenter — did *he* die of AIDS? Is it possible that he was infected with HIV sexually, perhaps in Edmonton

(where he lived for ten years), or in 1958 in the camp in Northwest Territories (NWT)? Once again, the clinical history offers little support to this scenario.

It is noticeable that it was almost immediately after his move to NWT in March 1958 that he fell sick with a fever, chills, headache, and a chronic cough; others in the camp were also suffering from what was thought to be the same "viral infection." Was there really some viral epidemic taking place up there — or could it be that the men were all affected by something quite different: by an environmental factor, for instance?

This brings us back to the question of what might have persuaded George to abandon his steady job in Edmonton and travel up to the far north. The most plausible answer, of course, is money. It turns out that the late fifties was a boom period for uranium production in Canada, particularly NWT, and in 1958 it became the leading producer of uranium ore in the Western world. In the previous year, a new uranium mine and mill had opened on the Marian River, northwest of Yellowknife, and there was increased exploitation of the famous old mine at Port Radium on Great Bear Lake, near the Arctic Circle, which had supplied ore for the Manhattan Project.[66] At the latter mine, the grade of ore was at least three times higher than anywhere else in Canada, making it profitable for half of the production to come from old surface tailings.[67]

If indeed this was the reason for George's sudden departure from Edmonton, it is conceivable that the apparent "virus infection" that affected him and his fellow workers was linked to the inhaling of radon gas and high-grade radioactive dust from the mine or the tailings dump.[68] Residual racism against those of Japanese stock might have resulted in George being given more than his fair share of dangerous tasks.[69]

This seemed a reasonable hypothetical scenario — but at this point I found that the trail ran cold. Neither the pathologist, Dr. Barrie, nor I was able to find any further information about George Y. from the mining companies, the town clerks of various communities in NWT, or from the Workers' Compensation Board.[70] However, Dr. Barrie agreed that exposure to radiation, or to the effects of uranium dust, was a plausible explanation for the immunosuppression and lung problems[71] — and that this, when combined with the massive steroid treatment over the final fortnight in Toronto, might have caused George's sudden demise from PCP. Alternatively, the steroids alone might have been enough. They would have suppressed George's immune system, and "brought the *Pneumocystis* sprouting out," admitted Dr. Barrie, laconically.

Either of these scenarios seemed a far likelier explanation for George's death than HIV infection. There was, however, one other possibility, which related to his Japanese ancestry. It is not known from which part of Japan he originated, but Gallo's retrovirus, HTLV-1, is endemic on parts of the Japanese islands of Kyushu and Shikoku[72] — and this virus can, on occasion, cause immunosuppression

that resembles that of AIDS.[73] Unfortunately, none of George's autopsy tissues remain, so this hypothesis cannot be tested.

---

The case that chronologically precedes these involves an engineer called Dick G., who died in Memphis, Tennessee, in 1952. The life and death of this man is of particular interest, partly because he features as Patient No. 1 in Huminer's "AIDS in the Pre-AIDS Era" article, and partly because his wide range of opportunistic infections apparently represents such a classic picture of AIDS.

Dick fell ill with a fever, malaise, and persistent cough in February 1952, while working on a road project in Louisiana. He returned to Memphis and was admitted to the Baptist Memorial Hospital, where he developed a rash all over his body, and his respiratory embarrassment developed into pneumonia. In May, it became clear that his illness was serious and he had exploratory lung surgery, during which the lower left lobe was removed and sectioned.

Soon afterward, Dick's employer decided that it was worth seeking a second opinion from the renowned Mayo Clinic. Dick was flown to Minnesota carrying lung and skin biopsy samples, but the Mayo physicians apparently concluded that nothing could be done for him, and recommended that he return to Memphis to die. Over the next few weeks, increased cortisone therapy brought some respite, but then he was readmitted to hospital, where he had a bone marrow biopsy. He died quite suddenly of septicemia two days later, at the end of July, leaving his young widow to look after their seven-month-old son.

Sections of Dick's lung were reviewed by three other pathologists, one of whom, John Wyatt of St. Louis, identified the giant cells typical of "salivary gland virus," which usually limited its pathogenic appearances to infants and small children. Wyatt proposed that the term "cytomegalic" be coined to describe the cellular condition[74] and later, in 1960, the virus was renamed cytomegalovirus — or CMV.

Wyatt's paper about Dick G., published in 1953, reported that although there had been no visible signs of cancer or lymphoma either in life or at gross autopsy, the microscopic autopsy had revealed some lymphoma-like cells in the lungs. But he concluded that these might have been the result of the salivary gland virus (which, he said, can "simulate certain morphological features of cancer"), and that even if they were genuine, they were not the primary cause of the illness.

In 1955, the description and microphotographs of Dick's lungs from Wyatt's article were reviewed by the German pathologist Herwig Hamperl, who stated that it was "highly probable" that he had also been suffering from PCP,[75] a conclusion that was further supported by a Los Angeles physician in 1982.[76] This death of an otherwise apparently healthy man of twenty-eight from CMV and

PCP (together with multiple skin infections and "difficulty in swallowing," which may have been caused by candidiasis) began to sound uncannily similar to the demise of David Carr seven years later. Was it possible that Dick G. had been suffering from AIDS?

Despite Dick's wide range of opportunistic infections, I began having doubts about this case as well.[77] Among Dick's copious medical records is a five-line letter from Dr. John McDonald of the Mayo Clinic, who, after reviewing slides from the skin and lung lesions in May 1952, concluded that both conditions were a result of "reticulum cell sarcoma," perhaps complicated by his steroid treatment. I corresponded with Lester Wold, the current chair of the department of laboratory medicine and pathology at the Mayo Clinic, who told me that "reticulum cell sarcoma" would nowadays be designated as non-Hodgkin's lymphoma (NHL) of large cell type. He also concluded that the patient had most certainly been immunosuppressed, but that it was "improbable" that he had been suffering from HIV infection or AIDS.

So what if the Mayo Clinic was right and John Wyatt wrong, and there had been a tumor? Apart from Kaposi's sarcoma, non-Hodgkin's lymphoma (or B-cell lymphoma) is the only tumor that is recognized as being a "serious manifestation of AIDS."[78] But, as Anthony Pinching had warned me at the start of the investigation, general immunosuppression can be caused either by HIV or by the tumor and its treatment. Given the fact that it was 1952, it seems much more likely that the tumor began independently, without any HIV involvement, and that it was this (plus the steroid treatment) that was responsible for Dick's syndrome of illnesses.

This conclusion is supported by the patient history. It seems that the only time Dick traveled outside America was during his sixteen months of war service in the Pacific islands and Australia (where the first cases of AIDS were detected only in 1987 and 1982, respectively).[79] He certainly never visited Africa, and all in all the likelihood of his having been infected with HIV in the forties or fifties seems extremely remote.

Sebastian Lucas, a physician who specializes in AIDS, has since confirmed that back in the early fifties, it would not have been possible to distinguish between B-cell and T-cell lymphomas: Dick could have had either. Unlike the B-cell lymphoma, the T-cell variant is caused by a retrovirus, HTLV-1 — and one of the few areas of the world where HTLV-1 infection is endemic is the South Pacific.

Dick's widow made further inquiries about his military service, and discovered that in late 1943, Dick joined a marine bombing squadron at its base on Green Island in the Solomon Islands, a thousand miles northeast of Australia. During the next year and a half, he shuttled to and fro across the South Pacific and Melanesia, calling at Hawaii, Tuvalu, Guadalcanal, and other islands.

It is here that Dick's photo album comes into play. For there, among the standard war-time photos of VJ-Day celebrations, and grinning GIs holding armfuls of Japanese skulls, are pictures of various women who appear to have been girlfriends, including one Chinese woman and one South Sea islander.[80] Dick's widow says she cannot be certain, but she thinks he probably did have some "local" girlfriends during the war.

The whole of Melanesia (which includes New Guinea, the Solomon Islands, and Vanuatu) has very high rates of HTLV-1 infection.[81] It seems likely that many of the marines who had sex in the South Pacific during World War II may have become infected with the virus. However, it is only rarely pathogenic, so only a small proportion of the men would have developed adult T-cell leukemia-lymphoma (ATL) or tropical spastic paraparesis/HTLV-1-associated myelopathy, its two major disease presentations. A far smaller number would be expected to develop an even more serious disease presentation in which HTLV-1 infection leads not only to ATL, but to an almost total immune breakdown, very similar to AIDS.

An example of such a clinical course was reported by two New York doctors in 1987. It involved a case of ATL of the entire intestinal tract and "an acquired immune deficiency" in a thirty-seven-year-old Hispanic man who was infected with HTLV-1, but not with HIV. Their patient suffered from lymphadenopathy, profuse diarrhea, weight loss, night sweats, and a wide range of opportunistic infections.[82] He eventually died from septic shock, in an uncanny echo of Dick G.'s death three decades earlier.

In conclusion, it seems highly unlikely that when Dick G. died of an acquired immune deficiency in 1952, HIV was responsible. A far more likely hypothesis is that HTLV-1 (and treatment for a related tumor) was the cause.[83]

---

The last of the six archival cases concerned a sixty-year-old Japanese-Canadian woman, Mrs. Sadayo F., who died in Montreal in 1945 from "inclusion-disease pneumonitis." This was again a reference to cytomegalic inclusion disease (caused by CMV), and the presence of *Pneumocystis* was once again detected retrospectively by Herwig Hamperl.[84] Sadayo first fell ill in June 1945 with breathing difficulties, sleeplessness, diarrhea, and weight loss. During the next six weeks she developed penicillin-resistant pneumonia, which progressed steadily, and she died at the end of July. At autopsy, she was diagnosed with a wide range of ailments, including bronchopneumonia, pleurisy, vitamin A deficiency, a thrombosis of the femoral vein, and adenomata (a benign tumor) of the thyroid.

The patient history and autopsy report revealed that during the final month of her life she had suffered from oral candidiasis — yet another opportunistic infection typical of AIDS patients and the otherwise immunocompromised. Her sole surviving daughter, now in her seventies, told me a great deal more about Sadayo's background.

She had been born in Nagoya, central Japan, in 1885, and emigrated to Canada in 1913, where she began working as a nurse near Vancouver. In 1931, she returned to Japan, where she trained in chiropractic. By the time she returned to Canada in 1937, she was the proud possessor of a bulky electromagnetic bed, "a wonderful piece of machinery" designed to help back sufferers. Apparently she had been well all her life until the summer of 1945.

On the phone, her daughter told me that she had always thought that her mother had died of stomach cancer, but that she would like to know if the diagnosis had been incorrect. I explained that the medical records revealed there had been infections with CMV and *Pneumocystis carinii* — two conditions which are nowadays typically found among persons infected with HIV. The daughter told me that she knew of no blood transfusions and that her mother had been "a very religious individual. . . . I don't think she had other relationships; she was too straitlaced." On the face of it, Mrs F. seemed an unlikely candidate for HIV infection.

The daughter's belief that her mother had died of cancer is supported by the second differential diagnosis at the end of her mother's case history, which was "G.I. neoplasm" — cancer of the gastrointestinal tract — a type to which those of Japanese ancestry are especially prone. The pathologist who reported the case in the literature was Dr. Gardner McMillan and, in a letter to me, he acknowledged that many of Mrs. F.'s symptoms had been nonspecific and that the diarrhea and weight loss might suggest bowel cancer.

In his article about the case, he had concentrated on the interesting finding of "inclusion-disease pneumonitis" (which was only the second such adult case to be reported in the literature), rather than speculating about the possible etiology. In answer to my question about whether he felt that an autopsy conducted today might have come up with different findings, Dr. McMillan wrote: "Today one would document a list of tests and circumstances known to influence the immune system (but many not operative in 1945). These would include leukemias, radiation, antineoplastic [anticancer] drugs, chemicals that injure the bone marrow, steroids, drugs used in transplantation surgery and of course tests and cell counts related to HIV infection. One or more of these might yield relevant information."

As it turned out, it was possible to conduct tests for HIV infection in this case. Dr. Serge Jothy from McGill University in Montreal managed to unearth some glass-mounted slides from the autopsy, including one from the spleen and one from the bone marrow. At my prompting, he sent these two slides to Fergal Hill at Cambridge, who tested them using PCR, but was unable to find any evidence of HIV-1.[85] As far as can be determined, therefore, Mrs. Sadayo F. did not die of AIDS.

Because she was born in Japan, one can only speculate whether HTLV-1 infection might have played a role in the etiology of Mrs. F.'s disease. From the perspective of this narrative, it is enough to state that she may well have had a cancerous process, which was not detected by the relatively unsophisticated diagnostic tests of the forties — and that it was very probably the immunosuppression caused by this (and perhaps its treatment) that led to the PCP and CMV infections.

Most, though not all, of the aforementioned research had been conducted by the spring of 1992, by which time I was beginning to feel skeptical about several of these potential early cases of AIDS. Although the involvement of HIV had apparently been confirmed in the cases of David Carr and Robert R., and though the case of Dick G. was intriguing, the other cases struck me as being less than convincing.[86]

But despite the wrong turnings (including the apparent link between radiation exposure and the earliest cases of AIDS, which had appeared, and then disappeared just as suddenly, when Elsie's letter proved that Dave Carr could not have been at the Pacific nuclear tests), I did not feel that the time had been wasted. What I had gained was considerable perspective on the true nature of AIDS. I concluded that in early, sporadic, geographically dispersed "cases" such as these, it was unsafe to make an archival diagnosis of AIDS on clinical grounds alone.

I was now persuaded that since the dawn of *Homo sapiens,* there had been a low but fairly constant background level of cases in which humans died, not as a result of HIV infection, but because their immune systems had been destroyed by other factors. These included congenital immunodeficiency (which might possibly have played a role in Robert R.'s case), exposure to ionizing radiation or radionuclides (as might have happened to Alice and George), exposure to toxic substances (Ardouin and possibly Robert R.), undiagnosed cancer and cancer treatments (Sadayo and Dick), and HTLV-1 infection (another possible factor in the latter two cases).[87]

The research also engendered two other valuable side products. First, it provided some invaluable perspective on the extent to which dangerous field tests of atomic, biological, and chemical substances were carried out on unknowing civilians and military "volunteers" by arms of the U.S. and British governments during the Cold War period of the fifties and sixties.[88] Second, the fact that, despite my continued efforts, I had been unable to come up with any evidence that either HIV or AIDS had existed before 1959 only reinforced the possibility that hypotheses placing the first arrival of the virus in humans in the fifties might have merit.

---

Shortly after this, to my surprise and pleasure, there was some independent confirmation of the concept of general immunosuppression without HIV involvement, and it came from the heart of the AIDS research community. In July 1992, at the Eighth International Conference on AIDS in Amsterdam, several pillars of the scientific establishment suddenly announced the existence of "AIDS without HIV," as it was swiftly christened by reporters. This development came about after a scientist from California, Sudhir Gupta, told the press that he had found an AIDS-like disease in an HIV-negative sixty-six-year-old woman. In an attempt to quell the growing media hubbub, an emergency press conference was called at which it was announced that doctors were already following up on some thirty similar cases involving unexplained opportunistic infections, which were typical of AIDS, but which had occurred in the absence of HIV.

At this press conference, Dr. Jeffrey Laurence gave details of five individuals (including two gay men, one promiscuous heterosexual man, and one female transfusion recipient) who were negative for HIV-1 and HIV-2 on PCR, but who had very low CD4 counts, and a variety of opportunistic infections. The most dramatic case involved a patient without any recognized risk factors — a heterosexual of Italian origin who developed inflammatory bowel disease followed by candidiasis, PCP, *Herpes simplex* infections, and a profound wasting syndrome, and who died after ten months of illness. Like two of the other patients, he was also tested for HTLV-1 and HTLV-2, with negative results.[89]

Since the scientists reporting this apparently new phenomenon (who included Luc Montagnier and David Ho) clearly had mixed opinions as to the cause, it was hardly surprising that reporters were unsure what to make of HIV-free AIDS.[90] In the popular press, it was widely reported as a major new development, one that might indicate either that HIV did not cause AIDS (as proposed by molecular biologist Peter Duesberg), or that there was yet another unknown virus that produced symptoms similar to AIDS. Amid the clamor, the only skeptical voices belonged to some of the older and more experienced immunologists, who were already familiar with rare instances of late onset adult congenital immunodeficiency, and who were therefore little surprised by such reports.

For the rest, however, the picture only became clearer six months later, when four related articles on "HIV-free AIDS" (now officially titled Idiopathic CD4+ Lymphocytopenia, or ICL) were published by the *New England Journal of Medicine*.[91]

Before long, Peter Duesberg claimed ICL as a vindication of his hypothesis, but in fact the recognition of ICL by the AIDS establishment, far from weakening the case against HIV as the cause of AIDS, had actually strengthened it, by making the description of true AIDS more specific. Essentially, the CD4+ lymphocyte counts of ICL patients are often over 300, whereas those of AIDS patients are usually below 200. The causes of the former syndrome (which is not always fatal) are still unclear, whereas for AIDS there is only one known and proven cause.[92]

A short time after this, there was a significant moment in the history of the AIDS epidemic. By this time David Ho, director of the Aaron Diamond AIDS Research Center, was becoming widely acknowledged as perhaps the leading figure at the cutting edge of AIDS research. When Dr. Ho, like so many before him, finally lost patience with the selective reasoning of Peter Duesberg and his followers, and their intransigent refusal to take on board the increasingly clear-cut evidence about the causation of AIDS, he resorted to the cry of the exasperated parent who has just been asked the same question for the umpteenth time, and who no longer has the patience to explain, gently and sensibly, just what is going on.

"It's the virus, stupid" was how Ho expressed it.[93]

# 10

One of the lovely things about starting a new area of research is that one wakes, throws back the curtains, and looks out over a pristine field of snow. No tracks, no footprints; no preconceptions, no arrogant certainties. In those first few weeks at the Keppel Street library, and during interviews with some of the proponents of the various hypotheses of origin, I retained the wonderfully liberating sense that anything was possible. Admittedly, several theories seemed crazy from the outset — their well-meaning proponents (some bearing the sympathetic stigmata of the zealot; others rendered huge and bombastic by their burden of absolute certainty) having either misinterpreted information, or else rushed to judgment on the basis of some seemingly crucial — but actually worthless — nugget of "evidence." But even these, I came to realize, sometimes contained some item of value, which could usefully be winkled out and put to one side.

After several months of investigation, I felt better equipped to sort wheat from chaff, and so this chapter outlines a wide range of hypotheses, together with a summary of the reasons why most can be refuted.[1] This is interesting historically, but is also vitally important in that it helps establish the criteria that need to be met if we are to explain how the immunodeficiency viruses arrived in humans, and how AIDS began.

Broadly speaking, the different hypotheses concerning the origin of AIDS can be split into five categories. Three of them — the heavenly, the malevolent human, and the unwitting human — interpret AIDS as a syndrome that has appeared only recently in the human race. The fourth category treats AIDS and HIV infections as older conditions that have existed (probably unrecognized) for centuries, millennia, or longer, and the fifth proposes AIDS as a chimera, a creation of semantics — one that describes assorted diseases that have always existed, but which have only recently been lumped together and given a new name.

The first group of hypotheses — which embrace the idea that AIDS somehow came *ex caelo,* from the skies — is, because of its innate fundamentalism, both the easiest and the most difficult to confront logically.

Many religious groups in different parts of the world have ascribed AIDS to an angry, interventionist god: one who has grown unhappy about recent developments on earth, such as the spread of drug addiction, homosexuality, and promiscuity, and who is teaching miscreants a well-needed lesson.[2] Such hypotheses become still harder to sustain when applied to other groups such as newborn children, hemophiliacs, recipients of blood transfusions, and the monogamous wives of men with multiple partners — persons whom even the disciples of blame and retribution would presumably find it hard to view as deserving victims. Whatever, since such explanations of AIDS are based on faith rather than scientific argument, I shall not discuss them further in this book.

Another oft-quoted theory of celestial origin is rather more scientific in tone, and is commonly ascribed to the former British astronomer-royal, Sir Fred Hoyle. He and his colleague Chandra Wickramasinghe have written three books on the subject of the galactic origin of microorganisms,[3] and are said to have argued that HIV could have arrived on earth in the form of viral debris, as part of the tail of a comet. However, when I asked Sir Fred about this, his testy fax reply read: "This is irresponsible journalism. I have *never* said Aids is a space-incident and do not hold that view." I later discovered that this hypothesis apparently began with a 1986 *Nature* article that opened — snappily enough — with the words "Sir Fred Hoyle may hold the view that the AIDS . . . virus is of extra-terrestrial origin."[4] Three years later, a feature in the *British Medical Journal* went one stage further, claiming: "Sir Fred Hoyle believes HIV to be of extra-terrestrial origin."[5] The game is called Chinese Whispers, and gathers its own natural momentum.

––––––––

From the celestial to the unremittingly worldly. The next group of theories treats AIDS as evidence of Man's evil, as the result of manipulations by scientists and generals in their laboratories of biological warfare.

One of the most beguiling examples appeared in 1989 in an American newspaper, and proposed that the AIDS epidemic was in fact caused by "Virus Q," a secret weapon developed by German scientists during the last world war.[6]

According to "Rudolph Kessler, an 80-year-old former German staff officer now living in Brazil," Virus Q was considered worthless by the scientists who developed it, since it took years to kill, and was spread only by blood or sexual contact, but Adolf Hitler, who considered the Americans "a bunch of sex-crazed degenerates" whose armies were "riddled with homosexuals," thought otherwise. A bomber laden with the virus was dispatched on a secret route toward America but, unfortunately, was shot down over central Africa; we learn that "Hitler was outraged, and doubly so when the Virus Q biological lab was destroyed in a bombing raid the next day." Nothing more was heard of Virus Q until many years later, when the first reports of a new disease gradually emerged from the African jungles.

Not all the conspiracy theories are quite so pleasingly transparent. The most notorious of them proposed that American scientists (with, it was inferred, the involvement of the U.S. Army, and perhaps the CIA) had developed HIV at Fort Detrick, Maryland, as a weapon of germ warfare. This theory has received extensive coverage since the mid-eighties and, for this reason, its convoluted history deserves some attention.[7]

The story first appeared in October 1985 in a Soviet literary weekly,[8] and was then picked up by the wire services. Much of the theory appeared to be based on the ideas of John Seale, a British venereologist who, for more than a year, had been arguing that AIDS was artificially created, and that it might be linked to biowarfare programs.

An expanded version of the hypothesis appeared in September 1986, at a conference of the Non-Aligned Movement held in Harare, Zimbabwe, where copies of a fifty-four-page report entitled "AIDS, Its Nature and Origin," by two retired East German scientists, Jakob and Lilli Segal, were circulated among the delegates.[9] The Segals proposed that HIV was in reality a genetically engineered recombinant of the visna virus of sheep and the HTLV-1 discovered by Robert Gallo, and that it had been developed as a germ warfare agent at Fort Detrick in 1977. They proposed that this "new germ" was tried out later that year on male prisoners who had become practicing homosexuals during their incarceration and that, upon their release, it spread to the gay community in New York.[10] The story was widely publicized around the world throughout 1987, causing serious damage to America's reputation, particularly among Third World nations.

While all this was going on, right-wing American groups were simultaneously broadcasting the claim that the Soviets were responsible for the AIDS epidemic. The first example of the genre, entitled "AIDS and the Security of the Western World," comprised an interview with John Seale that appeared in the magazine *Executive Intelligence Review* in October 1985. At one point in the interview, Seale says: "Employing the AIDS virus, transmitted on a drug addict's needle, is an infinitely more cost-effective strategic weapon and far less destructive for the USSR than using nuclear warheads or conventional forms of military might."[11]

The "Soviet AIDS" conspiracy theory gained further ground in 1986 and 1987, largely as a result of the activities of two brothers from Los Angeles, Theodore and Robert Strecker, a lawyer and a doctor, respectively. In March 1986 they composed an eleven-page paper entitled "This Is a Bio-Attack Alert," which claimed that they had "stumbled across a written order for the AIDS virus and a written plan to inject disease during preventive vaccinations for experimental purposes."[12] They further alleged that HIV had been deliberately created from the combination of two animal retroviruses — visna virus and bovine leukemia virus (BLV) — grown in human tissue culture.[13] Like the Segals, the Streckers believed that HIV was created at Fort Detrick, but they claimed it was Soviet scientists who were responsible.[14]

The following year an article by a Strecker disciple, William Campbell Douglass, enlarged upon the theory by claiming that HIV was genetically engineered in 1974. Douglass asserted that the WHO and "Communist conspirators" had first spread their new virus in Africa through the smallpox vaccination program, and then done the same in America via contaminated oral polio vaccine and the hepatitis B vaccine given to homosexual men.[15]

Many might feel that the claims of the Segals, the Streckers, and their supporters are so patently absurd that they themselves smack of disinformation campaigns. Others would simply argue that they do not merit serious attention. Perhaps the best way to respond, however, is to cite examples of watertight archival samples from before 1977 or 1974, when HIV was apparently "created": for example, the 1959 sample from Leopoldville or any of the three Norwegians whose blood from 1971 and 1973 later tested HIV-positive.[16] Furthermore, we now know that visna, HTLV-1, and BLV are only distantly related to HIV, far too distantly to have played a role in its origin (see chapter 11). The credibility of such theories was dealt a further blow in 1992 when Yevgeni Primakov, the former head of the Soviet Union's foreign intelligence service, publicly admitted that "the KGB planted stories in the late 1980s which alleged that the HIV virus was the result of a Pentagon experiment."[17] Sadly, supporters of the Streckers have continued to peddle their ill-informed and outdated versions of the myth, blaming variously the Soviets, the CIA, the Germans, and the World Health Organization well into the nineties.[18]

Even if we can therefore dismiss the Strecker/Segal theories of origin, we cannot yet leave such conspiracy theories about the origin of AIDS altogether. Although the term *retrovirus* did not come into use until 1970, tissue culture techniques developed in the early fifties allowed countless simian viruses — including foamy viruses and oncoviruses (both types of retrovirus) — to be grown and studied in the laboratory. During the fifties and sixties, one of the standard techniques used by military researchers to manipulate viruses was to attempt to alter their pathogenicity and host range by passaging them through different tissue cultures, different animals, or both. Is it possible that in the course of such research SIVs from African primates (unrecognized as such, of course, at the time) were among the viruses manipulated, and that a new version was discovered that was found to be an effective killer of humans? SIVs were certainly present in U.S. primate labs by the early sixties, and perhaps even earlier than that.[19]

Also during the fifties and sixties, the CIA and the Chemical Corps of the U.S. Army were secretly testing a variety of drugs and chemical and biological agents in many different American cities under the aegis of the MKULTRA program.[20] If they were prepared to take such risks on home soil, is it not possible that they mounted overseas trials as well?

There are certain historical facts (and a related rumor) that lend some substance to such a scenario. In September 1960 Dr. Sidney Gottlieb, the CIA scientist who had headed MKULTRA since the early fifties, arrived in Leopoldville, capital of the newly independent Democratic Republic of Congo, carrying a biological weapon intended for the assassination of the country's first head of state, Patrice Lumumba. This weapon, variously described as a toxin, a poison, and a lethal virus, "was supposed to produce a disease that was . . . indigenous to that area [of Africa] and that could be fatal." It seems most unlikely, however, that the biological weapon could have been HIV, for even if the virus had been accidentally discovered by 1960, it would have made a poor "lethal agent" in comparison to virulent forms of smallpox, yellow fever, anthrax, or tularemia. In any case, whatever the agent was, it was reportedly never used — for Gottlieb and the CIA station chief in the Congo, Larry Devlin, each testified that they personally dumped it into the river Congo.[21]

Nonetheless, there are rumors that a "secret military installation . . . involved in CBW [chemical and biological warfare] research . . . was installed in Zaire [Congo] in the wake of [Gottlieb's] visit."[22] This is not an absurd notion, for the U.S. Army displayed an intense interest in agents of biological warfare that continued through the rest of the sixties. And intriguingly, in 1969 a U.S. Department of Defense spokesman claimed that "Within the next 5 to 10 years, it would probably be possible to make a new infective microorganism which could differ in certain important respects from any known disease-causing organism. Most important of these is that it might be refractory to the immunological and therapeutic processes upon which we depend to maintain our relative freedom from infectious disease."[23] Superficially at least, this sounds like a description of HIV. Is it conceivable that this was one of the agents which the military scientists were working to develop — or even one that they had already developed — by accident or design?

The biological weapon hypothesis is so vague, and so unsupported by historical evidence about the nature of the rumored lethal agents (or even the location of the alleged base in the Congo), that it is difficult to counter. Unless, that is, one wishes to cite the HIV-positive 1959 blood sample from

Leopoldville, which predates Gottlieb's Congo visit. If that is proven genuine, then the theory is swiftly blown from the water.

---

Many of the theories of origin that attempt to address the perceived newness of AIDS have seen the hand of Man as being involved, but not all believe that the disease is a deliberate creation. Another whole group of theories propose AIDS as a product of unfortunate human happenstance or — more often — Man's blundering. Such theories have tended to move in and out of fashion just as the perceived place of origin of the epidemic has shifted from one region to another.

At the start of the eighties, when AIDS was called Gay-Related Immune Deficiency (GRID) and was believed to be restricted to the homosexual community, one of the most widely circulated explanations for the epidemic, especially in gay circles, related to a vaccine against hepatitis B ("Heptavax-B"), which had undergone trials among male homosexual cohorts in six U.S. cities (New York, San Francisco, Los Angeles, Chicago, St. Louis, and Denver) in the late seventies and early eighties.[24] The vaccine had been prepared from the sera of chronic hepatitis B carriers, including gay men, many of whom by corollary would also have been at risk of HIV infection, so there was some real basis for the fear that certain vaccine batches might have been contaminated with HIV, which had somehow survived the inactivation process.[25]

However, once again, the timing is all wrong. The existence of HIV-positive blood samples from different parts of the Congo dating from 1976, 1970, and 1959 clearly demonstrates that the Heptavax-B vaccine cannot have been involved with the *origins* of HIV and AIDS. But is it possible that these early trials could be connected to the start of the North American epidemic?

The first full-scale American trial of Heptavax-B involved over a thousand gay New Yorkers (half of whom got the vaccine, and half a placebo), and ran from November 1978 to October 1979. Clearly this cannot have infected the gay New Yorker who was HIV-positive in September 1977. Similarly, the trial in San Francisco began in April 1980, but gay men were testing positive in that city from 1978 onward.

However, there is a small fly in the ointment, for the aforementioned were all Phase 3 trials, designed to assess the efficacy of the vaccine. Prior to these there were, between 1975 and 1977, Phase 1 trials (to assess safety) and Phase 2 trials (to measure antigenicity and the ability to produce antibodies) of early versions of the vaccine. Some sixty-six of these first vaccinees were mentally handicapped children from Willowbrook State School, but a further sixty-six were defined merely as "antibody-positive subjects" — who may, of course, have been gay men.[26]

On the basis of timing alone, we therefore cannot completely dismiss the possibility that one of these Phase 1 or Phase 2 vaccine lots was contaminated with HIV.[27] But what clues there are do not support the hypothesis. In New York, only two of 826 gay vaccinees, and none of more than 1,100 "low-risk" vaccinees (660 dialysis patients and 442 medical staff) had developed AIDS by early 1983.[28] Furthermore, in the mid-eighties an experimental lot of Heptavax-B was apparently prepared from HIV-positive sera, and then subjected to inactivation procedures identical to those for the original vaccine. The end product was found to be free of viable HIV.[29]

Nonetheless, it is regrettable that nobody — to my knowledge — has gone back to test early samples of the vaccine (such as lots 559, 723, and 751, which were used for the Phase 1 and 2 trials) to establish whether or not they were contaminated with HIV-1. Given the controversy surrounding these trials, especially in the U.S. gay community, such an initiative could have helped dispel lingering fears that the vaccine might have played a role in the beginnings of the U.S. AIDS epidemic.

Heptavax-B was not the only vaccine to fall under suspicion. In 1987 Herbert Ratner, a family practitioner from Chicago, proposed that Jonas Salk's inactivated polio vaccine (IPV) had started the AIDS epidemic.[30] Between 1954 and 1960, several million doses of IPV were injected in the United States and elsewhere, before it was discovered that a simian virus known as SV40, originating from the macaque kidneys in which the vaccine had been prepared, had survived the inactivation process.[31] Dr. Ratner, who had always had profound reservations about the Salk vaccine, came to believe that, with its oncogenic nature and known ability to hybridize with other viruses, SV40 could well have spawned HIV. In the same year, 1987, an alternative physician called Eva Lee Snead made a similar allegation about Sabin's oral polio vaccine, which was also known to have contained SV40.[32] Later, other polio vaccines would also fall under the spotlight. These are very different theories, and will be dealt with in more detail later.

Another set of theories linked to a perceived place of origin of AIDS came into vogue in 1983, when the CDC officially defined Haitians as a risk group for AIDS. One hypothesis was advanced by Jane Teas and John Beldekas, who for several years pursued the idea that AIDS might be a vaccine-modified form of African swine fever (ASF) that had become transmissible to humans, probably in Haiti, where it was then transmitted to visiting American gays.[33] They based their ideas on the observation that ASF caused symptoms similar to AIDS (fever, lymphadenopathy, appetite loss, and immunosuppression), and that the two conditions seemed to have emerged more or less simultaneously in the case of Haiti and certain other developing countries.[34]

Other Haitian practices to fall under suspicion were the ritual drinking of animal blood and bloodletting "cures" administered by voodoo priests called *houngans*.[35] In addition, there was apparently an "underground theory," never

published or in any way substantiated, that male and female prostitutes working in Carrefour had been deliberately infected by the CIA with "viruses"
(including, one must infer, HIV) in the course of antibiotic injections given at
local STD clinics.[36] (This latter scenario is best dismissed in the same breath as
the "germ warfare theory," discussed elsewhere in this chapter.)

Later the spotlight moved from Haiti to Europe, and before long a theory of
origin emerged to explain the posited emergence of AIDS on that continent.
Noting that fellow scientists had proposed that there might be close links
between the AIDS virus and visna, an infectious lentivirus that is endemic in
many European flocks of sheep, a Canadian pediatrician put forward his own
hypothesis. "Cases of AIDS," he wrote to the journal of his national medical
association, "have been reported from certain urban areas in north-western
Europe noted for their varied and lax sexual mores. One could speculate that a
homosexual community in such an area may have become infected by one
member's having had sexual contact with a diseased sheep." The writer advocated "further epidemiologic and viral studies," but provided no further clues as
to the location of the morally lax homosexual community — or of the diseased
sheep.[37] In 1988, Harold Katner, a leading proponent of a Euro-American origin for AIDS, pointed out that men from those two continents were known to
have had sex with horses, goats, and cows, all of which are host to their own
lentiviruses — and posited that perhaps here lay the origin of HIV.[38]

Now, in the nineties, we are able to sequence these viruses, and it is apparent
that the differences between HIV and SV40, ASF virus, visna virus — and other
lentiviruses found in farmyard animals (such as equine infectious anemia virus,
caprine arthritis encephalitis virus, and bovine immunodeficiency virus) — are
far too great for HIV to have recently derived from any of them.[39] The theories
involving SV40 contamination of polio vaccines, altered forms of ASF vaccine,
and bestiality can therefore be dismissed.

By the mid-eighties, the AIDS focus had shifted again, this time toward
Africa. Sure enough, an African theory of origin, involving both African monkeys and esoteric sexual practices, soon emerged. The author this time was
Abraham Karpas, who wrote two letters to scientific journals[40] about an anthropological work published in 1973, *Famille, sexualité et culture,* by one Anicet
Kashamura.[41] A large part of the book is taken up with an analysis of the sexual
practices of peoples from the Rift Valley region. One section, entitled "Magies
d'Amour," describes the following technique: "In order to stimulate a man or
woman and induce them to intense sexual activity, one inoculates them in the
thighs, the pubic region and the back with blood from a male monkey (for a
man) or a female monkey (for a woman)." Read fifteen years later, this sounded
like an ideal method for transferring a monkey virus to humans.

Kashamura's book begins with the preamble: "In the countries of the Great
Lakes, and in particular on Idjwi, one encounters a great variety of magic rites

involving love." Anicet Kashamura himself comes from Idjwi island in Lake Kivu on the Congo/Rwanda border, which makes it all the more likely that he is describing a practice of his own tribe. And yet there is no evidence of early AIDS cases emanating from Idjwi island — and there can be little doubt that had the disease occurred in such a naturally segregated community, it would have been swiftly noticed, since there is a major hospital at Katana, just ten miles from Idjwi on the Congolese shore, and another at Bukavu, the terminus of the lake ferry that serves the island. An exhaustive survey of the mammals of Idjwi, published by the Swiss primatologist Urs Rahm in 1966, found that there was only one monkey species present, *Cercopithecus mitis schoutedeni* (a variety of blue monkey).[42] No SIV has ever been found in *C. m. schoutedeni,* nor in any members of the Congolese subgroup of *Cercopithecus mitis.*[43]

A further African theory involved yet another vaccination campaign, this time against smallpox. In May 1987, the science editor of the London *Times,* Pearce Wright, wrote a front-page article postulating that the WHO's smallpox eradication program, conducted between 1967 and 1980, might have triggered the AIDS epidemic.[44] Wright wrote that the most heavily vaccinated part of Africa, where 97 million smallpox inoculations had been given, consisted of the very countries (Congo, Rwanda, Burundi, Uganda, Tanzania, Zambia, and Malawi) that now constituted the "AIDS epicenter." What is more, by 1987, Brazil (the only South American country to have been included in the eradication program) had the highest incidence of AIDS in that continent, as did Haiti within the Caribbean (and Wright claimed that fourteen thousand Haitian nationals had received the smallpox vaccine while working for the U.N. in central Africa).

The article referred to a recent case of smallpox vaccination in an HIV-positive, but asymptomatic, nineteen-year-old U.S. Army recruit, which had prompted a rapid decline to AIDS and death.[45] It also pointed out that the vaccination needles used in Africa had each been employed an average of forty to sixty times, being waved across a naked flame between inoculations, a "perhaps not totally satisfactory method of sterilisation."

Contrary to the claims of many subsequent commentators, Wright was not proposing that the smallpox vaccine was itself contaminated with HIV. He was rather suggesting that the smallpox vaccine might have prompted subclinical HIV infections to become more pathogenic and progress to AIDS in certain HIV-positive vaccinees, or that the campaign might have accelerated person-to-person transmission of HIV as a result of inadequately sterilized needles.[46] Strictly speaking, therefore, this should be described as a theory of dissemination rather than a theory of origin.

Wright's article had, however, been partly based on an internal WHO discussion paper commissioned from a consultant immunologist, which went considerably further, by suggesting that the vaccine itself was probably contaminated with HIV.[47] It pointed out that all the countries in the AIDS epicenter had their peak year of smallpox vaccine delivery prior to 1972, whereas those African countries where AIDS was not (in 1987) viewed as a major public health problem — such as Ethiopia and Nigeria — had had peak delivery after 1972. Observing that "particular campaigns using certain virus stocks [of smallpox vaccine] correlate with the appearance of AIDS," the consultant concluded that this suggested a fifteen-year latency period for HIV. The discussion paper went on to note that the smallpox vaccine had been produced in sixty-four different laboratories, of which nine were in Africa, and that in 1968 alone, fifteen different strains of *vaccinia* virus had been used. Between 1967 and 1978, the WHO had tested the vaccine and "concluded that more than 80% of the test batches were satisfactory, [but] this level of quality control would not now be acceptable in a commercial vaccine."[48]

This theory of a contaminated smallpox vaccine would appear to be scientifically unsound, for there is no reason for either HIV or SIV to be accidentally present in a vaccine that was prepared in the skin of cows, sheep, or water buffaloes, or in tissue cultures of chick embryo or rabbit kidney.[49] HIV and SIV could simply not survive in such preparations, unless human or monkey cells were also present.

Another misadventure theory, one that sought to explain the early emergence of AIDS in central Africa, the Caribbean, and the east and west coasts of North America, was proposed in 1986 by the American physicist Ernest Sternglass, whose background included an honorable whistle-blowing book about the dangers of low-level radiation exposure, following events like the Three Mile Island disaster.[50] He maintained that atmospheric nuclear testing conducted in the fifties (and rising to a crescendo in 1962 and 1963, before the atmospheric test ban treaty)[51] could have had a dual impact. First, it might have caused the mutation of "an AIDS-related indigenous human or animal retrovirus"; second, it might have damaged the immune defenses of an entire generation, irradiated during the crucial first trimester in the womb.[52]

Sternglass assembled some persuasive evidence in support of his claims. He pointed out that 90 percent of fallout is brought to earth in the form of precipitation, and that areas of low rainfall (such as North Africa, or the American Midwest) had witnessed relatively few cases of AIDS, in marked contrast to apparent early epicenters of the syndrome — such as the Congo and the two North American seaboards. He demonstrated that levels of strontium-90 in the diets of residents of different American cities had risen threefold between 1961 and 1963, following the major tests, adding that the greatest explosive increase in AIDS in America had occurred some nineteen years later, between 1980 and 1982, when the infants of the early sixties were reaching sexual maturity. And he pointed out that the earliest available global data for strontium-90 in human bone found these levels to be highest in the Belgian Congo and Liberia — two countries that were already, in 1986, suspected to be close to the epicenters of the HIV-1 and HIV-2 epidemics.

Sternglass's epidemiological data was intriguing, and his research into the impact of low-level radiation exposure, though controversial, was extremely well documented and supported. By contrast, his proposal of retroviral mutation was far more hypothetical and sketchy. It failed, for instance, to address the similarity between the HIVs and the SIVs, or to explain why a species jump from monkeys to humans might have occurred.

Some of the aforementioned scenarios may seem incredible from the perspective of the nineties, but that does not mean that the concept of the "unwitting human" causing AIDS is to be dismissed. There are, of course, countless examples of human intervention in the global ecosystem having disastrous consequences, and it could be that one of these was the factor that initiated the epidemic.

---

Another set of theories portrays AIDS as an older condition, one that has been in humans for some while, but that has only recently been recognized.

PCR technology has allowed virologists to sequence the DNA in the genes of viruses, and has allowed some remarkable breakthroughs in terms of determining the ancestry of HIV. In 1989 and 1990, the simian immunodeficiency viruses (SIVs) from two African primates — the sooty mangabey and the chimpanzee — were sequenced, and these viruses (SIVsm and SIVcpz) were found to be very similar to HIV-2 and HIV-1, respectively.[53] The SIV of the African green monkey, by contrast, was found to be only distantly related to both of the HIVs.[54]

When two viruses are similar genetically, it is apparent that either they share a common ancestor, or that one is derived from the other via a chain of infection. When the similar viruses are found in two different hosts, then it is clear that the chain of infection may have involved a cross-species transfer in the not-too-distant past. The discovery that SIVcpz and SIVsm were so closely related to HIV-1 and HIV-2, respectively, therefore provided the clinching evidence about the lineage of the HIVs. The "AIDS viruses" had, as was widely suspected, emerged out of Africa.

The genetic evidence led, in turn, to what is now the most widely accepted hypothesis of how AIDS came into being. It has gone under various titles, but "natural transfer" seems the most appropriate to use here. It proposes that the HIVs originated from chance transfers to humans of the SIVs that are found naturally in certain species of African primate.

In African monkeys, these viruses do not cause visible signs of disease, but they can and do cause disease when transferred from one species to another —

an event referred to as "crossing the species barrier." The first recognized instance of this happening was in American primate research laboratories where, in the late sixties and seventies, Asian monkeys — various species of macaque — began falling sick with diseases that are nowadays called "simian AIDS."[55] Retrospective sequencing of the viruses revealed that the Asian monkeys had become infected with SIVsm — the SIV found naturally in an African monkey, the sooty mangabey. In its new hosts, the virus was pathogenic, and eventually fatal — which clearly presented a model for how the human AIDS epidemic might have started.

But if this theory had merit, how might the transfer of an SIV from monkey to human have occurred? Some non-Africans of a lurid bent proposed that perhaps Africans were in the habit of having sex with monkeys.[56] More sensibly, others suggested that local people might have become infected after eating monkey meat,[57] which constitutes a regular or occasional part of the diet of several million Africans.[58] Perhaps, they proposed, in exceptional circumstances a monkey had been eaten raw, or so rarely cooked that a simian virus might have survived to infect the human consumer. Others again suggested that the likeliest origin for the crucial transfer was for an African hunter to have been infected through a bite or scratch from a wounded monkey.[59]

Nowadays, however, most adherents of natural transfer believe that the riskiest activity might well be preparing the monkey for pot or fire. If the cook (usually the hunter or his wife, depending on which ethnic group is involved) has small cuts or wounds on the hands (from working in the fields, from clearing bush, or from subduing a wounded monkey), there is clearly a potential for exposure to fresh monkey blood during the process of skinning and butchery.

This hypothesis of natural transfer is in many ways the most straightforward explanation for the appearance of AIDS. All the necessary ingredients seem to be present — there are two plausible primate candidates for the ancestral host species of HIV-1 and HIV-2 (the chimp and the sooty mangabey), which seem to live in more or less the right parts of Africa, and both species are known to have been hunted and eaten by man.

There is, however, a worm in the apple, an intrinsic flaw. The fact that the African monkeys live comfortably with their SIVs suggests that the simian viruses have been present in these species for a considerable period of time, and that the two have adapted to each other. By contrast, the fact that both HIV-1 and HIV-2 cause AIDS in humans suggests that virus and host are not in equilibrium, and that the HIVs are comparatively recent introductions to *Homo sapiens*. And yet African monkeys and apes, we can safely presume, have been hunted and skinned since the dawn of our species. So, why have the HIVs not emerged before now — and not once, but twice, in the space of a few years in the latter half of the twentieth century?

Some have pointed out that there might have been an increase in the consumption of monkey meat over the last four or five decades — either because population growth has prompted a corresponding rise in the number of poor people prepared to eat protein from any source, or because of the growing availability of firearms. If one accepts monkey butchery and eating as a risk, then this might affect the scale of the risk, but not its existence.

However, over the years most adherents of natural transfer have maintained that AIDS is an "old" disease, which has only recently become widespread, and been recognized. They have sought to explain this belated recognition through secondary theories, such as the post-colonial emigration of isolated rural groups to towns, or the sudden availability of needles and syringes. These, and other theories, will be discussed more fully below.

According to the "isolated tribe" hypothesis, the virus could have first been transferred to humans living in a remote rural area. Proponents of this theory, which include both of the official "codiscoverers" of HIV-1, Luc Montagnier and Robert Gallo,[60] argue that the traditional sexual mores in such an area would have meant that the virus was seldom transmitted between humans, and that even when it was, its pathogenic impact would perhaps have gone unrecognized in an area with few diagnostic facilities,[61] and against a normal background of high morbidity and mortality.[62]

The recent recognition of AIDS as a phenomenon could then be explained through the opening up of the African interior by roads, railways, and riverboats in the course of this century and, in particular, by the mass migration to urban areas, which followed decolonization in the late fifties and early sixties. According to this scenario, one or more of the members of this isolated tribe, encouraged by the freedom of movement afforded by new transport routes, and by the social freedoms that accompanied independence, made their first visits to towns and cities, where the mixing of different ethnic groups and sexual contacts between them allowed the virus to break free from its previously restricted range of infectees.[63]

However, where are these isolated tribes? One of the prime candidates, the pygmies, a people who hunt and live in close proximity to various monkeys, appear not to have come into contact with HIV until well after the beginning of the present epidemic.[64]

Furthermore, would ancient AIDS really have gone unrecognized and unremarked? Although typical AIDS symptoms such as fever, TB, wasting, and pneumonia would not be expected to cause ripples of concern in a rural hospital in the first half of the twentieth century, the same could surely not be said of rarer presentations, such as cryptococcal meningitis or esophageal candidiasis.[65] Experienced doctors of the caliber of Jack Davies in Uganda and Jean Sonnet in the Belgian Congo insist that such conditions were simply not seen prior to the 1960s.

Other adherents of natural transfer favor a different explanation. They point out that viruses such as those that cause Lassa fever and measles often fail to cause disease until they are released into new, susceptible populations (in towns, for instance) and then become more virulent as they are passed rapidly from one infectee to another.[66] Could this also have applied to the first rural infections with HIV? Could they have been of low pathogenicity for humans — or indeed nonpathogenic, producing no clinical symptoms?[67]

This seems unlikely, for the following reasons. One of the few documented examples we have of early HIV infection in a rural area came about as a result of the blood samples taken at the time of the Ebola epidemic of 1976 from Yambuku/Yandongi in northern Congo. Some 0.8 percent of blood samples subsequently tested positive for HIV-1 — and when a cross section of the population was again tested in 1985, exactly the same percentage was infected.

This, therefore, would appear to be a good example of a stable rural epidemic of HIV-1. And yet these were certainly not invisible, or subclinical, infections.[68] Three of the five HIV-positive people detected in Yandongi in 1976 had already died of AIDS-like disease by 1986, and one of the other two was clearly immunocompromised and in decline. Yet only one of these four (the *femme libre*), had ever lived outside rural Equateur province — in Kinshasa — and it is hard to imagine that the other three were all infected as a result of contact (indirect or direct) with her.[69] In other words, these three appear to have been living a typical rural lifestyle, and yet they too were vulnerable to AIDS. HIV was, it seems, already pathogenic in this rural setting in the mid-seventies, even if it failed to spread as dramatically as it was about to do in the more hedonistic urban environment.

When one considers that steamers were traveling up and down the Congo River between Leopoldville/Kinshasa and Stanleyville/Kisangani from the 1880s onward,[70] and that river ferries — carrying blacks as well as whites — were plying the great, brown thoroughfare through the heart of the rain forest from the early decades of the twentieth century, one finds it harder to consider any Congolese community that was connected even remotely to the main river (for instance by a series of tracks and footpaths) as being truly "isolated."[71] In other words, once HIV arrived in a rural community, it would presumably have required only one trip to the capital by a young, sex-positive man or woman for the AIDS epidemic to begin in earnest.

All this suggests that the steadily rising graph of HIV infection seen in Leopoldville/Kinshasa from 1959 through 1970 and 1980 was not merely indicating the sudden arrival of an old rural virus in the national capital, but rather the arrival of a new virus that had not previously been seen in *Homo sapiens*.

However, there are other subsidary theories that seek to explain why AIDS has only recently become recognized. Commentators like Abraham Karpas and

John Seale emphasize the importance of the arrival in African marketplaces of needles and syringes, which quickly became the preferred means of administering medicines such as antibiotics. Both men believe that it was person-to-person needle-borne spread of HIV that allowed the virus to break free from an isolated group of human infectees and enter its epidemic phase (in which sexual and perinatal spread took over as the main modes of onward transmission). Karpas proposes that syringes first arrived in Africa at the same time as antibiotics, shortly after the Second World War; Seale believes that it happened some time in the fifties.[72] On the face of it, this seems a plausible hypothesis — and it is one to which we shall return later in the book.

Another intriguing theory was proposed by two Italian virologists, Sergio Giunta and Giuseppi Groppa. They maintained that the massive use of African primates for virological work and for the testing and manufacture of polio vaccines led to an enormous increase in demand from the 1950s onward. This in turn led to an unprecedented exposure of humans (especially Africans) to these simians in the course of capture, caging, and shipping to primate laboratories and vaccine plants in the Western world. Live capture clearly could involve more potential risk for the hunter than slaughtering for the pot.[73] This theory seems rather less plausible, if only because relatively few chimps and sooty mangabeys were used in research and vaccine manufacture.

There are two other theories that need to be mentioned. Both, by rights, should be categorized with the "unwitting human" group, but they are described here for convenience, because they relate to viral transfers from African monkeys. The first featured in a 1987 report published in Britain by the National Anti-Vivisection Society.[74] This proposed that it was the transmission experiments initiated in 1966 in American primate research laboratories and at facilities run by the National Institutes of Health that inadvertently produced both simian and human AIDS. The carefully documented report related how at primate research facilities such as that at Davis, California, scientists had attempted to passage unknown monkey viruses "from monkey to monkey, species to species," and pointed out that "a virus may be forced to mutate and may become more dangerous in the process, simply by being transferred across the species barrier." The viruses being tested included those suspected of causing cancers, and what were then termed "slow viruses"; perhaps they had also included an SIV. Accidental transfer of SIV to a lab worker might, they proposed, have given birth to HIV and the human epidemic. Of course, although this hypothesis appears to describe a way in which AIDS could have arrived in America, it fails to provide an explanation for its epidemic emergence in Africa.

In 1991, another theory of origin was published, one that attempted to link the origin of HIV-1 and HIV-2 to specific cross-species transfers from the chimp and the sooty mangabey. It was put forward by a young professor of parasitology, Charles Gilks, who had unearthed articles about malaria research conducted in the United States and Europe since the beginning of the twentieth century.[75] Some of the experimentation had included the inoculation of "volunteers" (sometimes the scientists themselves, but often prisoners) with malarial blood originating from different primates — a perfect method, he posited, for the simultaneous transfer of simian retroviruses. Gilks cited thirty-four instances of people receiving inoculations of fresh chimpanzee blood, and a further thirty-three of persons being injected with blood from these primary human inoculees. Gilks also referred to "far fewer, perhaps two" instances of people being inoculated with mangabey blood, but did not specify the species of mangabey. The theory was covered in detail by the *New York Times*, in an article that featured enthusiastic comments by Robert Gallo, who called it "astounding and fascinating . . . it deserves to be followed up and all leads on it pursued."[76]

Gilks's theory proposes a plausible means for the transfer of a chimpanzee SIV to man — but it is epidemiologically unconvincing, because the experiments mainly occurred in the first four decades of the century, and almost exclusively in the United States, Belgium, and Germany, where, as we have seen, AIDS was not recognized until the late seventies.[77] As for the two experiments in which mangabey blood was injected directly into man, these occurred nearly a century ago, and seem likely to have involved the wrong type of mangabey.[78]

Speaking some years later, Gilks insisted that he had proposed a testable hypothesis for the origin of AIDS, which, to his horror, had resulted in his being "vilified." However, he then added, with commendable candor, "I have to say I *don't* think my theory was right."[79]

————

Let us return for a moment to those who believe that AIDS is an ancient disease. Certain investigators pointed to specific disease outbreaks of the past, and proposed that these might have been early presentations of the syndrome. Some (like Robert Root-Bernstein and Harold Katner) trawled back through the medical literature to unearth pre-1980 cases of some of the relatively rare AIDS indicator diseases — such as PCP, cryptococcal meningitis, and Kaposi's sarcoma.[80] The problem with this approach — as I had discovered — was that without serological support, none of these could be proved as cases of HIV infection, and there were many other causes for generalized immunosuppression.

Others searched through even older historical records and medical archives and proposed mystery diseases of the past as AIDS. Three American doctors wrote to the *New York State Journal of Medicine* about AAA disease, "a scourge of the first magnitude," which is apparently mentioned fifty times in four papyri from ancient Egypt.[81] They pointed out that AAA translates as "semen" or "poison," and postulated that the disease might have prompted or reinforced a taboo against anal intercourse, which perhaps then remained in place (keeping AIDS at negligible levels) until modern times.

In 1987 a French military doctor proposed that the European epidemic of syphilis at the end of the fifteenth century might in reality have been an early outbreak of AIDS.[82] A not dissimilar theory was floated by Belgian doctors, who wondered if the widely traveled Dutch humanist Erasmus, who apparently had many lovers and who may have been bisexual, was actually the first recorded AIDS patient.[83] Erasmus died in 1536, having suffered fevers, diarrhea, skin swellings, arthritis, carbuncles on the buttocks, and general lymph node enlargement in his final years (diseases that, at the time, had been ascribed to syphilis).

Such mooted "ancient cases" are hard to disprove, but it should be stressed once again that no persuasive instances of AIDS or archival samples of HIV have been discovered from before 1959. Furthermore, none of the ancient scourges cited above closely resembles the AIDS that we know today. AAA could be almost any viral or bacterial illness, whereas in the cases of Erasmus, and the soldiers who died at Naples, it sounds very much as if the original diagnoses — of syphilis — were correct.

———————

Such historical conjecture leads naturally to the final batch of theories, which can best be summarized as questioning the causative role of HIV in AIDS. The fact that syphilis and AIDS have similar modes of transmission and (some maintain) similar pathogenic courses, that syphilis has many manifestations, which vary according to climatic area and which appear to have changed over the centuries, and that many of the traditional diagnostic tests for syphilis are fallible, encouraged some commentators, like Joan McKenna and Harris Coulter, to take the hypothesis one step further, and to propose that the two conditions were one and the same.[84] Again, this theory has been disproved by genetic sequencing.

Others, like Joseph Sonnabend and Robert Root-Bernstein,[85] suggested that AIDS is a multifactorial disease, which has been occurring sporadically for centuries and is caused by a variety of different agents and factors, exposure to many of which has become more common in recent times. The multifactorialists questioned the importance of the role that HIV plays in AIDS, believing it to be merely one of several elements that contribute to a condition of immunological overload. At an early stage of the epidemic, Sonnabend suggested that AIDS could also be caused by exposure to hard drugs like heroin or cocaine (in the case of IVDUs and crack smokers), to sperm (in the case of gay men), blood products (in the case of hemophiliacs and transfusion recipients), or malnutrition (among the peoples of the Third World and the inner-city poor of the

West).[86] Other commentators have added exposure to carcinogens like dioxin[87] to the list of multifactors that, they maintain, may cause AIDS.

Others again have suggested that infectious microbiological cofactors, such as CMV (cytomegalovirus), HTLV-1, or *Mycoplasma incognitus,* are also involved in the etiology of the disease.[88] But nowadays the chief proponent of multifactorialism, Root-Bernstein, is less sure of his position, being willing to say only that he is "not certain that HIV is the cause of AIDS," either alone or as a cofactor.[89] For this reason, there seems little point in discussing this theory further.

The logical end point of arguments that question the role played by HIV is provided by Peter Duesberg and his followers, who maintain that what they term "the HIV-AIDS hypothesis" is entirely invalid.[90] The Duesberg school maintains that HIV is itself harmless and that, far from causing AIDS, it is actually a passenger virus, which commonly appears after a subject has already become immunosuppressed by other factors. They claim that those who contract AIDS in North America and Europe have taken drugs (not only the injectable variety, but also hallucinogens, amphetamines, and poppers), and that those who get AIDS in Africa have actually fallen ill with other diseases, which have recently been lumped together and given a new name. Some would say that Duesberg and his supporters do not really have a theory of the origin of AIDS, since their central argument depends upon what AIDS is not (the result of HIV), rather than what AIDS is.

I spent an afternoon with Peter Duesberg at his Berkeley lab in the summer of 1990, and during the course of a four-hour interview, he explained the basis for his position. For most of that time he appeared confident and persuasive. But on two or three occasions, when I asked a question about the African epidemic, for instance, he got up and left the room, and returned five minutes later already talking about Koch's postulates, or some other unrelated argument.[91]

Back in the late eighties, Duesberg asked the scientific community some very valid questions about HIV. Yet almost all of the central questions that he legitimately raised have now been answered. In several experimental cohorts, those with HIV have progressed to AIDS, while those without HIV have not.[92] The basic mechanism of HIV infection within the body (which he questioned) has now been explained — and turns out to be a remarkable revelation.[93] AIDS has different presentations among different risk groups and in different continents simply because (naturally enough) different ecological niches are populated by different pathogens. Meanwhile, Duesberg's claims that there is no AIDS epidemic in Africa,[94] that there would be no AIDS epidemic in Thailand,[95] and that drugs are the cause of AIDS in America and Europe[96] have all been demonstrated to be false.

Duesberg's increasingly selective use of data, and his repeated tendency to misrepresent the content of other papers, raises serious questions about his approach and methodology. This became most obvious when he claimed, wrongly, that the authors of an article in *Nature,* which showed that only HIV-positive drug-injectors progressed to AIDS, had fabricated data.[97] And yet Duesberg continues to be an anti-establishment hero, especially among HIV-positive people who are in denial, or those conspiracy theorists who believe that we are being kept in the dark about the "true nature" of AIDS.

Since the 1996 publication of his *magnum opus,* entitled *Inventing the AIDS Virus,*[98] to widespread critical opprobrium, Peter Duesberg has been less vocal about his theories. One likes to think that perhaps he has finally had to confront some of the shortcomings of his arguments. It would be even more heartening were he to acknowledge some of those logical errors publicly. In particular, many would wish him to retract his oft-repeated offer to inject himself with "pure" HIV in order to prove its innocuous nature. He has never delivered on this promise, claiming that he cannot be certain that any viral sample is not contaminated with some other pathogen. Many find this unpersuasive, and feel that a doctor who has persuaded so many others that HIV is not to be feared should either admit he is wrong, or else put his theory to the ultimate test.[99]

---

I may have missed some, but as far as I know the foregoing includes all the major theories of origin of AIDS — from the carefully reasoned to the seriously wacky — which had been formally published up to December 1991. But what was intriguing was that although by that date, ten years into the recognized epidemic, most of the early theories could be disproven, there were still obvious intrinsic flaws even in the theory that, by then, had emerged as the most plausible and widely accepted — that of natural transfer.

For although by the end of 1991 it was increasingly clear that AIDS was caused by HIV — and that HIV had originated from the cross-species transfer of a closely related simian virus, SIV, from monkeys to humans — the mechanisms of that transfer (and the reasons why two such transfers should have taken place in the space of a few years) were anything but apparent.

To my mind, it seemed more and more likely that some new factor must have been involved — that something must have happened in the 1950s or thereabouts to cause the emergence of AIDS. But what could it have been?

As time passed, I began to realize that the best answers I had heard to this question had featured in an interview I had conducted many months earlier, back in the fall of 1990, in the high desert plateau of New Mexico.

# 11

GERRY MYERS AND

THE MONKEY PUZZLE TREE

Sometimes, nowadays, I have a sort of vision. I cannot remember how it started. Perhaps it was a daydream; perhaps a real dream from a fitful sleep after a day of hard research.

There is a bearded man in a white galabia, standing in an arid landscape and holding a large bunch of keys. He is not a jailer or a janitor, but the keeper of the keys for a garden with high walls and a single large door. In the center of that garden, improbably, stands a single tree, a monkey puzzle, with branches heading off in many directions. The branches are thick with needles, and they are difficult to disentangle, or even to discern. Outside the walls, the bearded man looks on, sometimes fingering this key or that. Over the years, he has found several that fit the keyhole. But he has not yet found the one to turn the lock.

---

It was late in the September of 1990, a few weeks into my first research trip to the United States, and the place was Lamy, New Mexico, a small halt in a dry valley a few miles south of Santa Fe. The long, slow diesel train wound its way into the station, just as older models had done in countless movies; looking out, I half expected horses and a stagecoach lined up beside the track. Instead, there were half a dozen four-wheel-drive vehicles, beside one of which stood a man with a beard, surveying the disembarking passengers.

After my bags were loaded in his car, we stood and watched as the Jeeps and pickups swung away up the road, and then the train rolled out again toward

Kansas City, leaving behind an impressive silence. I found myself wondering if this was how the physicists bound for the Manhattan Project had felt as they arrived in Lamy inconspicuously, in twos and threes, almost half a century before.

The bearded man, Dr. Gerry Myers, director of the HIV Sequence Database, was based at the same site — Los Alamos — as the men who made the bomb, but his mission in life was rather different. Robert Oppenheimer, after witnessing that first predawn blast at Alamogordo, that light of a thousand suns, had been moved to quote from the *Bhagavad-Gita*: "Now I am become Death, the destroyer of worlds."[1] Myers's job in life was to monitor and counteract cataclysm, rather than create it — and the cataclysm he was confronting, though silent and slow, was potentially every bit as damaging as the tumultuous product of milliseconds of fission.

As befitted a man with such a weighty mission, Myers was thoughtful and soft-spoken. Since he rarely leaves New Mexico and is visited only infrequently by inquiring reporters and scientists, Myers has taken on certain of the attributes of the visionary, whose ideas about simian and human immunodeficiency viruses, honed in contemplation and isolation from the mainstream scientific community, are surprisingly original. But it is only when one meets him in person that one realizes the full extent of that originality, for this gentle man is actually a revolutionary, a Sufi in the desert. Myers, of course, does not see it like that. As far as he is concerned, he is merely a logical thinker.

Over the next twenty-four hours, until the next day's eastbound train rolled in, we talked about the origin and history of AIDS, and of the family tree of primate immunodeficiency viruses (PIVs) that places the late-twentieth-century human epidemics in context.

A little background. Although every organism has its own unique genetic structure, it is made up of just four DNA nucleotides (adenine, thymine, cytosine and guanine — A, T, C, and G), which are the basic building blocks of life. (The only exceptions are RNA viruses, in which uracil replaces thymine.) The structure of the organism is determined by the order in which those nucleotides are joined together — its DNA sequence. Given a sample of that organism, the molecular biologist should be able to determine its sequence by methods such as PCR. The phylogenetic analysis of such sequences is the most precise method of determining how closely different organisms are related. In the broadest terms, however, if the sequences of two organisms are very similar, then we can be confident that they are closely related — that one has evolved from the other, or that both have evolved from a common ancestor. The relationships between different organisms — humans, for instance, or pigs, or viruses — can be readily depicted on phylogenetic trees, which look very much like family trees.

The HIV Sequence Database and Analysis Project was set up at Los Alamos by the NIH in 1985, shortly after the first DNA sequence of the HIV genome* — which revealed it to be a single molecule, 9,700 nucleotides in length — had been prepared. Gerry Myers's primary task, with the assistance of Kersti MacInnes, and later Bette Korber, was to launch an "investigation of the molecular facts pertinent to the origin of AIDS."[2]

The Database team began with a computer search of all known genetic sequences stored in international databases, to compare these with the known sequences of HIV, and they repeated the search in 1986 and 1988. Their conclusion was that HIV had not arisen through the recombination of any viruses, either known or unknown, "either naturally or through human agency." What this established was that HIV was almost certainly not the result of a genetic engineering experiment.

The only rational interpretation of their sequence analysis was that HIV must have arisen from a closely related monkey virus, an SIV, which had recently "crossed the species barrier" and infected a human. The fact that this is now taken as given by every serious AIDS researcher is largely because of the solid, incontrovertible proof provided by the Database.[3]

We sat down in the front room of Dr. Myers's adobe-style house, looking out over Santa Fe, and I started in with that prickly question posed by the monkey puzzle tree: Why now? Why had the HIV-1 and HIV-2 branches suddenly produced their dreadful blooms now, rather than in previous seasons? Myers started by confirming the importance of what Alan Fleming had pointed out in Covent Garden, a few months earlier — the newness of the HIVs. He explained that other human retroviruses like HTLV-1 and HTLV-2 had been around for a long time, at least centuries, perhaps much longer. He said that the former virus had certainly been exported, via the slave trade, from Africa to the Caribbean and the Americas — and in all likelihood also to Kyushu and Shikoku, the two southwesterly islands of Japan, where Portuguese mariners, with sailing ships crewed by Africans, traded and evangelized for three decades in the mid-sixteenth century.[4] Since the incidence of disease is so low among HTLV-1-infected individuals, he added, its presence could easily have gone unnoticed in those places for generations.

HIV, however, was another matter. The fact that neither HIV nor AIDS seemed to have arrived in the Caribbean or the southeastern United States before the 1970s (even though the slave trade had transported some ten million Africans across the Atlantic between the early sixteenth and mid-nineteenth centuries) lent support to the hypothesis of a recent HIV crossover.

---

* Genome: The total complement of genetic material contained in an organism.

"I think it's simply a case of a virus moving out of a simian population," he said. "Why did it happen now, rather than fifty years from now or fifty years before? I don't know." But he did have some ideas. "It would appear to be independent events in two different parts of Africa, with two very different simian/human viruses. The only sense I can make out of that is either increased handling of animals for whatever reason, or an increase in health-care procedures, namely vaccinations, that might allow entry of these viruses into the human population at that particular time."

Myers reminded me that from the 1950s onward, African monkeys had been exported by the tens of thousands to Western medical laboratories and zoos, and this had inevitably led to increased handling. He added that Third World vaccination programs, including some that involved live vaccines, had also been very big in the late fifties and sixties. For a moment I thought he was talking about the smallpox eradication campaign in Africa,[5] but it turned out that he had a better candidate for SIV contamination. "Since polio's grown on monkey kidney tissues to prepare the vaccine, that could be a possible route," he said.

I suggested that surely such a theory could be checked by looking back through the old stocks of vaccine, but he said that it was not as easy as that, since it might be difficult to design the right PCR primers to detect the simian precursor to HIV. Furthermore, he said, many of the polio vaccines had been prepared not in the United States, but in other places (such as Poland and Czechoslovakia),[6] and it might prove difficult to check the latter stocks.

I countered that if children were vaccinated with an SIV-contaminated vaccine in around 1960, we would have seen AIDS cropping up in lots of slightly older children in the mid-sixties. Not at all, he responded quickly — for two reasons. First, because the chance of a simian virus crossing into humans was very small, and it might be that only certain lots of vaccine were contaminated with a variant of SIV that could infect humans. Second, the SIVs are lentiviruses, slow viruses, so that even if people vaccinated in 1960 became infected with such a virus, they might have to carry it for a while — until they were adults, even — before it became pathogenic and showed up as a disease, or before they could pass it on to a second person. He clearly took this hypothesis very seriously. "I admit that it's a rare possibility," he continued, "but when you think about your original question, why did the virus come forward when it did, any other hypothesis becomes more difficult. . . . Are you going to say that it was because of a hole in the ozone, or the greenhouse effect?"

He went on to give examples of adventitious viruses that had accidentally contaminated vaccines. First, he said, hundreds of thousands of Americans had been infected with a simian virus, SV40, through the Salk and Sabin polio vaccines.[7] This was actually the fortieth contaminating monkey virus to be discovered in monkey kidneys, but fortunately it appeared that neither SV40, nor any of the others, had increased people's susceptibility to diseases such as cancer.[8] Similarly, a yellow fever vaccine prepared in eggs, made at around the same time, had been contaminated with avian leukosis virus, a retrovirus that causes leukemia in chickens but that seems, fortunately, to have been harmless to humans. He also cited the "Marburg incident," in which monkeys brought into a German vaccine facility were infected with a highly virulent simian virus related to Ebola, which killed many of the people working there — the only positive side being that tissues from these monkeys were never used to make vaccine. However, this did highlight the fact that, especially in these early days, animals used for experimental purposes, or in the manufacturing of biomedical materials, were quite often carriers of unidentified viruses. Myers stressed that since the SV40 episode, new procedures had been put into place that made such contamination far less likely than it was back during "the heavy program of Third World vaccinations."

Having heard countless theories of origin over the previous few months, I felt less than convinced by this latest one. And it seemed to me that despite what Myers said, it would not be too difficult to put the theory to the test. If some of these polio vaccines had been produced in America, then surely they, at least, could be examined for the presence of a contaminating retrovirus. As it turned out, however, his caution was amply justified. I still had a lot to learn.

Later, Myers mentioned two other possible explanations for the recency of AIDS. One was that recent deforestation might have forced monkey populations closer to towns, causing unprecedented contact between monkeys and humans. He said a colleague had recently visited Sierra Leone, and had returned with photos showing kids holding monkeys, apparently as pets.[9] Was this, he wondered, a modern development? The second was that poor sterilization of needles used in a vaccination program might have had an amplification effect on a virus that was already present among one or more of the vaccinees, transmitting it mechanically, from arm to arm.

What was striking about all this was Gerry Myers's willingness to consider the controversial possibility that *Homo sapiens* might have played a part in the beginnings of the AIDS epidemic.

---

In due course, I told Myers about my search for early cases of AIDS, and he listened with interest. He agreed that the best way to trace the history of a disease was to try to locate the earliest cases, but he also seemed to have reservations. He had just been sent a draft copy of a book by the medical historian Mirko Grmek, called *History of AIDS*,[10] and he told me that whereas Grmek and I had "looked for anecdotes," he himself was more interested in the rise in cases, the first little visible blip on the graph. The reason for his skepticism became apparent when he said: "The one 1959 case that Nahmias reported, that's questionable.[11] Apparently the Manchester case is not so questionable. It doesn't surprise me if there are rare and fascinating cases out there prior to the seventies. But what I'd like to emphasize is that clinical chart review . . . doesn't show any evidence for a significant rise of cases prior to the early seventies." He also expressed doubts about the Robert R. case from 1969, since the virus had proved impossible to sequence by PCR, even after two years of effort.

At that stage, I did not share his doubts about the authenticity of some of these earliest samples of HIV. But as it turned out, he was more right than I was, for of these first three samples of HIV from the fifties and sixties, two subsequently turned out to be probable contaminations. The third, however, did not, and it was this positive proof of HIV's existence that, in the end, was the most important.

---

Later, Myers told me about the latest findings from the HIV Sequence Database, which at that stage contained one hundred HIV and fifty SIV isolates, and about a thousand different sequences from different parts of those isolates. What these various sequences showed was that there was a very wide spectrum of SIVs and HIVs (or primate immunodeficiency viruses — PIVs — which is how he collectively referred to them). He was especially excited about two new viruses, which had just been isolated by Beatrice Hahn and her team from rubber workers at the Firestone plantation in Liberia, West Africa. These people were asymptomatic, showing no signs of AIDS, and it was not known when they had been infected, but their viruses were more like SIV than HIV-2. In fact, they were so similar to the SIV of the sooty mangabey that "for all the world they look like simian viruses simply being carried by humans."

Myers had used his Database to construct a PIV "phylogenetic tree," a family tree of the various HIVs and SIVs, which demonstrated how — and potentially when — they had evolved one from another. By introducing a base substitution rate (an estimate of how quickly genetic changes were occurring in these notoriously unstable viruses), it was possible to estimate the approximate date at which two viruses had evolved in different directions, depicted on the phylogenetic tree as the divergence of two branches. Even ten years earlier, few scientists would have dreamed that such insights into the evolutionary history of AIDS would become possible.

But in 1990 the construction of the PIV phylogenetic tree was still in its early stages. What was clear was that SIVsm (the sooty mangabey SIV), SIVmac (the macaque SIV, which was presumably derived from SIVsm), and HIV-2 all clustered together on a single branch. The range of the sooty mangabey, he added, overlapped the area of West Africa where HIV-2 disease was mostly found.

SIMPLE PHYLOGENETIC TREE REPRESENTING
RELATIONSHIPS BETWEEN THE FIVE MAJOR GROUPS
OF PRIMATE IMMUNODEFICIENCY VIRUSES (PIVs)

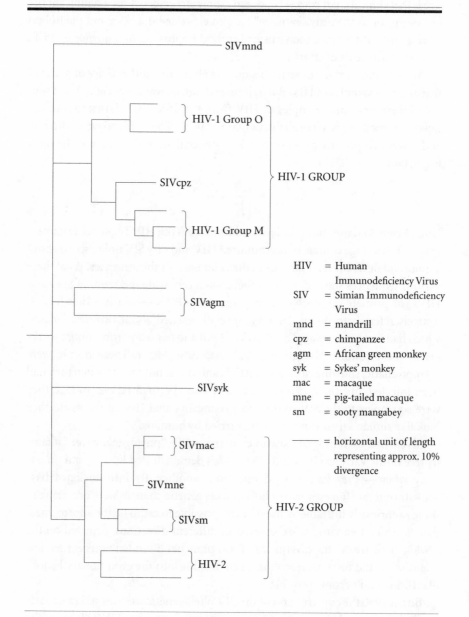

SOURCES: A. J. Leigh Brown and E. C. Holmes, "Evolutionary Biology of Human Immunodeficiency Viruses," *Ann. Rev. Ecol. Syst.*, 1994, 25, 127–165. G. Myers, K. MacInnes, and L. Myers, "Phylogenetic Moments in the AIDS Epidemic," in S. S. Morse (editor), *Emerging Viruses* (Oxford University Press, 1993), pp. 120–137.

Intriguingly, he proposed that similar viruses would also turn up in other primates, such as the baboon.[12]

Similarly, he said, it was quite clear that the chimpanzee virus, SIVcpz, was from the same branch as the HIV-1 isolates — even if there was more difference between them than between SIVsm and HIV-2. So far, only one chimp SIV isolate had been sequenced, and some observers were pointing out that since the animal had been recaptured from poachers, humans could have inadvertently infected the chimp with HIV, rather than vice versa. But Myers added that other chimp isolates were awaiting sequencing, and if they proved similar to the first sequence, this would resolve the problem. Although it was less certain that chimps provided the reservoir from which HIV-1 emerged than it was for mangabeys and HIV-2, there once again seemed to be some geographical correlation, for chimps are found in the parts of central Africa where HIV-1 disease was first seen. Furthermore, it was clearly possible that further research would reveal further SIVcpz isolates which were even closer to the human virus.

Myers told me that Belgian researchers had recently announced the discovery of a new human lentivirus from Cameroon,[13] which some scientists were beginning to call "HIV-3," but added that the isolate would probably be more accurately classified as a highly divergent HIV-1. (Eventually this divergent virus would be redefined as the first member of "HIV-1 Group O," while the main group of HIV-1 isolates would be renamed HIV-1 Group M, to highlight the fact that the two groups, though similar, represented separate introductions of SIVs from primate to man.)[14] But even leaving aside this Cameroonian variant, it was gradually being realized that there were several subtypes within the main HIV-1 branch. It had long been known that one could distinguish between "Euro-American" and "African" variants of HIV-1, but intrinsic differences between HIV-1 isolates from different parts of Africa had recently been identified — indicating that these too represented different subtypes, or clades, of the virus.

Altogether, he told me, there were at least five major branches on the PIV phylogenetic tree. Apart from the HIV-1 branch and the HIV-2 branch, there was an SIVmnd branch, represented by two isolates from mandrills from Gabon,[15] and an SIVagm branch, representing the African green monkey (AGM) isolates,[16] which, Myers explained, subdivided into a bough representing viruses from the West African subspecies of AGM,[17] and another bearing the East African subspecies viruses.[18] The fifth branch, only just discovered, was represented by viruses found in an East African relative of the AGM called the Sykes' monkey.[19]

Of all these viruses, only those found in the Asian macaques housed in primate research centers, and HIV-1 and HIV-2 in humans, were associated with disease, which clearly suggested that these viruses represented recent cross-species introductions, in which virus and host had not yet adapted to each other. As far as anyone knew, none of the African SIVs were pathogenic in the wild, suggesting that these viruses had become adapted to their simian hosts over a much longer period. However, Myers added, nobody could be certain about this, for so far nobody had spent much time actually studying wild African monkeys to determine if the SIV-positive animals experienced any different diseases from their SIV-negative counterparts. In all likelihood, he said, African monkeys with SIV were asymptomatic, but it could be, for instance, that a small proportion did develop mild symptoms.[20]

Proof positive of the pathogenic potential of these viruses once they crossed the species barrier had been provided by Patricia Fultz, who had passed a sooty mangabey SIV through a pig-tailed macaque, and discovered that the resultant virus killed other macaques and SIV-negative sooty mangabeys within one to two weeks.[21] This "killer virus" did not cause anything resembling simian AIDS, but instead destroyed animals by breaking down the walls of their guts. "So here just a small number of genetic changes was sufficient to take an essentially non-pathogenic virus, and turn it into a killer," commented Myers.[22]

Apparently the latest research was revealing that a large proportion (30 percent to 50 percent) of African green monkeys living in the world were naturally infected with SIV.[23] Myers pointed out that these SIVagm isolates represented a "highly diverse reservoir of viruses," and he conceded that this might indicate that they were older than the other PIVs. He added that there was "a very rich pool out there, from which all you needed was one or two events" (by which he meant cross-species transmissions) to lead to the two epidemics of human AIDS. In saying this, he was not suggesting that human AIDS had come directly from the African green monkey. He was rather proposing that over a long period of time, a couple of species jumps could, for instance, have taken SIV from the AGM to the chimpanzee and then to man (to produce HIV-1), while another two jumps could have transferred an SIV from an AGM to a sooty mangabey and thence to man (to produce HIV-2).

Later, Myers came up with further evidence to support the hypothesis that the HIV-1-related pandemic, the main epidemic of AIDS, had started in Africa. He explained that there was considerably more variation between different African isolates of HIV than different American isolates. The latter were delineated by a dense bushy outcrop on the phylogenetic tree, suggesting that they were all descended from a single virus, which had first infected someone in North America around the mid-seventies. The similarity of these isolates from a common source was a phenomenon known as "founder effect." The greatest range of variation between American viruses was 7 percent, this denoting the difference between "Time Zero" (which Myers estimated at 1977 for the United States) and a sample from 1986; the rate of divergence therefore appeared to be just under 1 percent a year. By contrast, the variation among different African viruses was approximately 20 percent, suggesting that divergence had been going on almost three times as long, since around 1959 or 1960.[24] I noted that once again we were back at the "watershed year"— 1959.

---

I was gratified that Gerry Myers saw the study of the origins of the HIVs as considerably more than a mere intellectual pursuit. He went on to explain that an appreciation of the past history of the HIVs would facilitate an understanding of their likely future evolution, and that an ability to forecast how the epidemic was likely to progress was vital in terms of the search for antiviral agents, and in devising vaccine trials.

He said that approved, small-scale Phase 1 and Phase 2 trials of AIDS vaccines — dealing with toxicity and potential side effects — were already under way in the United States, but that Phase 3 trials, which would seek to determine efficacy, were a different matter. Only those who are likely to be exposed to the virus can usefully participate in Phase 3 trials — those involved had to be "at high risk, and suitable for a trial." In North America and Europe, he said, this effectively limited the field to "a few thousand people," which I took to mean gay men who continued to be sexually active, since he was clearly intimating that intravenous drug users made unreliable research subjects. For this reason, "everyone thinks about vaccine trials in Third World countries. That's a sticky matter. Maybe those people shouldn't have that . . . you know vaccine trials are risky."

He told me that Jonathan Mann, the head of the Global Program on AIDS at the WHO, was trying to counsel African ministers who wished their countries to be included in HIV vaccine trials, about what to ask for, and about the pros and cons of allowing their territories to be used for such research. He also made some comments about a recent trial of a live AIDS vaccine in Africa, saying that he and several of his colleagues had profound misgivings about whether the participants had actually been volunteers, and about the apparently secret manner in which the trials had been staged. He asked that further particulars should be off-the-record.

Myers pointed out that if one intended to stage Phase 3 trials in a particular area, it was vital to know which HIV subtypes were present there, so that a vaccine effective against those variants could be prepared. Similarly, to develop an AIDS vaccine that would be effective on a global scale, one had first to know which subtypes were most common around the world. These were further practical reasons why sequence analysis of HIV isolates from different regions was of pressing importance.

---

Gerry Myers told me that he was just completing an article entitled "Phylo-genetic Moments,"[25] in which he would identify the two key moments depicted on the primate immunodeficiency virus tree. The first moment was when the five major PIV branches had diverged from each other, an event that he would later refer to as a "Big Bang," because he felt that all the branches had split at roughly the same time.[26] The second was when the human AIDS pandemic began. One of the key questions, of course, was how to date these two events.

In 1988, he and some colleagues had come up with a minimum estimate for the divergence of HIV-1 and HIV-2 of thirty-seven years, which meant that the two viruses could have evolved from a common ancestor (probably a monkey virus) as recently as 1951.[27] However, this estimate was largely based on a com-parison of HIV-1 samples dated between 1976 and 1985, and was heavily dependent on the earliest sample (Z321, the isolate from Yambuku) not being atypical in any way.[28] But he added that the estimate that appealed most to him had been proposed by a group of French researchers who had calibrated their molecular clocks using the year of 1933, when a sheep lentivirus (visna) was known to have arrived in Iceland. Applying the same rate of lentiviral diver-gence to other branches on the tree, the French concluded that the divergence of HIV-1, HIV-2, and SIVagm (the Big Bang, in Myers's parlance) had occurred about two centuries before.[29] Other geneticists had proposed that this event had occurred between 150 and 280 years ago.[30]

Yet Myers was acutely aware that the basic assumption might be wrong, and the estimates far too short. This was because most of them were calculated on the mutation rates of the last two decades, when viral evolution might well have been "epidemic driven," with the greater number of infected people encourag-ing a higher rate of mutation.

However, there was another significant clue, which suggested that the arrival of immunodeficiency viruses in primates might have occurred within the last three centuries. African green monkeys had been brought with the slave ships to Caribbean islands such as St. Kitts during the seventeenth century,[31] but the Caribbean AGMs showed no signs of SIV.[32]

Even if the dating of the first phylogenetic moment was problematical, Myers felt that there was strong epidemiological evidence placing the second phylogenetic moment, the onset of the global pandemic of AIDS, in the mid to late 1970s. (He was less certain about the HIV-2-related epidemic, but felt that its onset was only a matter of years removed.) He pointed out that even the minimum estimate of 1951 for HIV-1/HIV-2 divergence was "really too long ago to account for the second moment, [which] seems to have occurred in the seventies. So what happened between the fifties and the seventies, that's your job. That's what you're trying to reconstruct," he said, encouragingly. It was an elegant way of putting it, and it took me some time to work out what he meant.

Then I realized that the main event that had occurred between his first moment and his second was the transfer of at least two simian viruses to humans.

This struck me as a sensible approach for a government official to take. Myers was willing to look at the beginnings of the PIVs, and the beginnings of AIDS, but he would leave that intervening phylogenetic moment — the one when the monkey viruses got transferred into man — for somebody else to investigate. For this, of course, was the one that might prove too controversial for comfort.

However, he had already provided several indicators about his own line of thinking. From the very start of our conversation, he had made it clear that he did not favor the "lost tribe" hypothesis — that HIV-1 and HIV-2 diseases had been around for a long time in isolated pockets of people, and that they only emerged on to the broader stage when those groups began to move into the cities in the late fifties or sixties.

Instead, he clearly believed that the sort of events that would have allowed the two AIDS epidemics to emerge almost simultaneously in Africa were likely to involve human interventions, possibly even human blunders. These would include things like vaccination campaigns, the increased handling and exportation of monkeys for medical research, the destruction of monkey habitats, or the increased use of needles — through either inoculation programs, or the sudden availability of reusable needles in the African marketplace.

The following afternoon, Gerry Myers drove me back to the station in Lamy. Just before we arrived, I asked him once again for his ideas about the middle "phylogenetic moment" — the one when the first PIVs arrived in humans. And this time he ventured an answer. "I think that [probably] has to be some time between 1940 and 1960," he said. "I can't pin it down any better than that. But again . . . that could be a pseudoquestion if simian viruses can infect humans and be passed on. I don't think it makes sense to talk about the day it became a human virus."

I took his point — that to begin with there would be an SIV infecting a human (as might have happened with the Liberian rubber workers), and one had to decide at what point the virus could be redefined as an HIV. Perhaps that would be the moment when there was onward transmission to another human. Whatever, I was glad, at last, to have heard his best guess for the date.

As I shook Gerry Myers's hand and walked toward the tracks, I felt invigorated with his theories and ideas, but at the same time almost overwhelmed, weighed down, with what felt like the excess baggage of new information. On this particular occasion, I was not able to take it all on board. For the time being, some quite important pieces were to be left behind on the platform. This was because of the revelation, some weeks later, that Dave Carr might have served on board Britain's nuclear testing ship, H.M.S. *Warrior*. This led me up the blind alley of radiation research, and much of the import of the conversation with Gerry Myers got lost in the excitement. Nonetheless, I believe that many of his ideas remained lodged deep in memory, like a motif playing in the distant background. Sometimes, over the next few months and years, the theme would re-emerge, unbeckoned. *The hand of man*, it was playing, *the hand of man*.

———————

A few days after my meeting with Gerry Myers, and at his suggestion, I went to interview two of his collaborators in phylogenetic analysis, Philip Johnson and Vanessa Hirsch, at their laboratory in the National Institute of Allergy and Infectious Diseases (NIAID), part of the NIH complex at Bethesda and Rockville. Although the meeting was only an hour long, they told me a lot about their characterization and phylogenetic analysis of SIVs from different AGM subspecies and from the Sykes' monkey, and they lent perspective to a number of other issues.

They emphasized that the problem with phylogenetic analysis was not the branching order — on this the trees could offer very useful information — but the timing. "We don't know where to put the root on Gerry Myers's trees" was how Philip Johnson expressed it. In other words, the estimates of the rates of divergence for the various PIVs could be out by an order of magnitude, or even more.

Their own research supported the idea of a far more ancient PIV divergence than the one that Myers favored. They felt that the wide range of SIVs among African green monkeys living in different parts of Africa suggested that the various SIVagm subgroups might have diverged at the time of speciation — when the various monkey subspecies evolved one from another, an event thought to have occurred around ten thousand years ago.[33]

Like Myers, Johnson and Hirsch thought that the evidence of the SIV-negative Caribbean AGMs was significant, but added that these monkeys had also tested negative for STLV-1 — the simian ancestor of HTLV-1. Since this virus is ubiquitous in African monkeys, and since the human descendant, HTLV-1, had clearly been in existence since the time of the slave trade, this suggested that the monkeys exported across the Atlantic might have been "particularly clean" ones.[34]

They also reemphasized a crucial point. None of the SIVs, they reminded me, appear to cause disease to their *natural* hosts — namely, African monkeys. At Yerkes Primate Center, they said, there were two hundred SIV-positive sooty mangabeys running around, all apparently fit and healthy. This only further emphasized how unusual the terrible disease presentations in humans and Asian monkeys were. "So what AIDS says to us is that HIV-1 isn't a human virus — that it came from a monkey and is in an unnatural host. You'd hope that over a period of time it would adapt, but it could take a very long time," said Johnson.

When I asked about the likely mechanism of cross-species transfer to humans, Vanessa Hirsch gave an answer that had some relevance to the two Liberian rubber workers with their SIV-like viruses. "Probably [through] bites," she said. "Also when cutting up meat. We obviously can't test SIVsm by injecting it into humans and seeing if it would infect, though it infects human cells in culture . . . so all it would take would probably be a sufficient dose of the virus getting into a human to establish a transient infection. Then the question is: Can the virus change sufficiently rapidly to allow itself to . . . reproduce in the human, and then be transmitted?" She could not, however, explain why such transient infections, if they occurred fairly frequently, were usually not transmitted to further partners — until recently, when the HIV-2-related AIDS epidemic began.

––––––––––

As it happened, a natural experiment had just begun that would help answer this very question: whether or not SIVsm could infect humans and then adapt inside their bodies to become a transmissible virus, an "HIV-2." For at the Delta Regional Primate Center in Tulane, Louisiana, there had been a needlestick accident in which a technician had self-injected a tiny amount of blood from a macaque that had previously been infected with sooty mangabey SIV.[35]

Virologists knew that during the next few years, this unfortunate technician would provide important information about whether or not an SIV would "take" in humans — and, if it did, how damaging it would be. The technician would be bled, and although the scientists could not inject his blood into another human, they would inoculate it into human cells in culture, to gauge whether the simian virus became more readily transmissible, or more pathogenic. At long last, these scientists would be able to monitor a live experiment into the origin of AIDS.

# III

A NEW HYPOTHESIS OF SOURCE

*Out of this nettle, danger, we pluck this flower, safety.*

— WILLIAM SHAKESPEARE,
Henry IV, Part I

*You do not know what the full implications of*
*discoveries are, until you have made them. Epidemic*
*poliomyelitis is an example of this. It was, in effect,*
*created by hygienic measures designed to deal with*
*other diseases. The measures designed to protect the*
*world from polio may, in their turn, for all we know,*
*lead to some other quite unexpected consequence*
*which may be to man's disadvantage.*

— JOHN ROWAN WILSON,
Margin of Safety *(published 1963)*

# 12

## AIDS AND POLIO VACCINES

In the space of a few days in the early spring of 1992, two theories were published that linked the origin of AIDS to the contamination of oral polio vaccines (OPVs).[1] Both theories came from unexpected sources, and between them, they caused a considerable commotion.

This was a year and a half and two hundred interviews after my long conversation with Gerry Myers in the summer of 1990, when — in very general terms — we had discussed a similar theory. However, since I had taken few notes during that meeting, and had not yet reviewed the tapes, I had largely forgotten his comments. In the meantime a British virologist had also told me of a theory of polio vaccine origin, and had promised to send me some papers on the subject, which had never arrived. I phoned her a few times, and she said she had mislaid the documents, and there the matter rested. Years later, I learned that the papers had been written by Herbert Ratner, who believed that a different type of vaccine, Salk's inactivated polio vaccine (IPV), had introduced HIV to humans.[2]

The first of the OPV articles appeared in the *Lancet* in March 1992, in the form of a "Viewpoint" piece written by a New Hampshire attorney, Walter Kyle.[3] In the course of medico-legal research into a case of paralysis in a contact of a polio vaccinee, Kyle discovered that one particular lot of Albert Sabin's OPV, made by Lederle in 1976, had contained small amounts of a simian Type C retrovirus which, however, was "unlike any of the known type-C viruses." After being held back for further testing by the U.S. Bureau of Biologics (BOB) for an unprecedented twenty months, this lot, 3-444, was released for human use in 1977, on the grounds that it "contained fewer than 100 organisms per dose and did not contain viruses 'known to be harmful to man.'"

Kyle went on to point out two additional pertinent facts. The first was that lot 3-444 had been grown in a tissue culture made from the kidneys of the African green monkey (AGM), a species that is naturally infected by an SIV related to the HIVs of humans. He added that SIV infections cause no visible disease in their natural hosts, and thus nobody would have attempted to exclude apparently healthy, but nevertheless SIV-infected, AGMs from vaccine production prior to 1985, when the virus was first identified.

Second, Kyle cited documents that showed that, from the early seventies onward, certain doctors in Israel and America had been advocating a treatment regime for herpes sufferers that involved taking multiple oral doses of Sabin's OPV.[4] Such patients, he extrapolated, would have been exposed to more of the unknown retroviral agent in the vaccine than the single dose allowance stipulated and permitted by BOB. His hypothesis, therefore, was that multiple doses of contaminated OPV given in the 1970s to American gay men suffering from herpetic lesions may have represented the source of the human AIDS epidemic. He further argued that the relevant polio vaccine lots should be reexamined, to determine whether or not any did indeed contain SIV contaminants.

Kyle's theory is intriguing, but a number of objections present themselves. The first, and most telling, is that Type C retroviruses are not from the same retroviral group as the SIV and HIV lentiviruses — and there was no evidence that lentiviruses had been responsible for the contamination. Second, sequence analysis shows that HIV-1 and HIV-2 are only distantly related to the SIVs found in African green monkeys, so that even if the unknown retroviral contaminant found in the Lederle vaccine was in fact an SIV, it seems unlikely to have represented the origin of the AIDS epidemic in America. The third problem is that the herpes treatment advised (four drops of OPV given monthly, for three to six months) is hardly an exponential increase on the standard dose, given to millions as a polio preventative. Fourth, the herpes treatment was presumably given to persons of both sexes and sexual persuasions, whereas (at least to begin with) only gay men and intravenous drug users developed the new disease. Last, Kyle's records reveal that lot 3-444 was finally released for use on September 30, 1977,[5] but we now know that by that date, at least one New Yorker — the gay man whose blood taken on September 6, 1977, later tested positive — was infected with HIV.[6] This, of course, is in addition to the evidence of HIV infections prior to September 1977 elsewhere in the world, including Europe and Africa.

Kyle claimed that at least two other polio vaccine lots from the same period showed signs of retroviral contamination, but a position paper prepared by the FDA and CDC in November 1994 specifically denied this. The paper instead stated that the original electron micrographs had been reexamined by three different experts, who concluded that the particles seen "were not retroviruses and were likely to be byproducts of cellular debris."[7] Given the importance of the findings, it is surprising that a more detailed version of this paper has not been formally published in the medical literature.

Even though the weight of counterevidence against Walter Kyle's theory is substantial, he still made an important contribution to the origins debate. Above all, he highlighted the possibility that, prior to 1985, polio vaccines prepared in monkey kidney tissue culture might have been contaminated with simian viruses. As he aptly puts it: "What you do not know exists, you cannot check for!"

———————

The second article also pointed the finger of suspicion at an OPV, but not one of Albert Sabin's. It was written by Tom Curtis, a freelance journalist from Texas, and was published in a magazine that was almost guaranteed to elicit thinly disguised hauteur from the medical and scientific communities. The rock magazine *Rolling Stone,* bane of the establishment back in the sixties, has managed to survive the end of the hippie era by broadening its beam and allowing itself to drift discreetly into the mainstream. Despite this hint of middle-aged tubbiness, it is still eminently capable of sudden brave forays against the current, including the publication of high-quality investigative journalism. Curtis's article "The Origin of AIDS," which appeared in the issue dated March 19, 1992, is a good example.[8] However, the article is essentially one that proposes a hypothesis, rather than reports proven facts, and this key element was highlighted by the subtitle, which reads: "A Startling New Theory Attempts to Answer the Question 'Was It an Act of God or an Act of Man?'"

It is a beautifully crafted piece of sustained narrative writing, and is illustrated with some stunning photos, including one of a long queue of black people waiting to be vaccinated, while a white woman in a pith helmet squirts vaccine into the mouth of a baby. The article itself opens with an account of Curtis and his family lining up in the local high school, in 1962, to receive their sugar lumps speckled with drops of Albert Sabin's vaccine. After a brief résumé of the development of inactivated and oral polio vaccines, ending with the discovery that many of the lots injected and fed during the fifties had been inadvertently contaminated with simian viruses, it proposes that another OPV from that era "may have inadvertently infected its recipients with an even more fearsome and insidious virus — the one that causes acquired immune deficiency syndrome — AIDS."

Curtis explains that the vaccine in question, called CHAT, was developed by Hilary Koprowski and his colleagues at the Wistar Institute in Philadelphia, and that between 1957 and 1960 it was fed to more than three hundred thousand Africans in the countries now known as the Congo, Rwanda, and Burundi —

the very area now thought by many scientists to be the hearth, or source, of the epidemic of HIV-1-related AIDS.

Curtis points out that in those early days of tissue culture technique, virologists were loath to cultivate vaccines in human cells, for fear of spreading cancer-causing agents, but were nevertheless slow to realize the potential dangers of introducing to humans a vaccine grown in monkey kidneys. Some of the more obviously dangerous simian viruses (like the herpes B virus discovered by Sabin) were successfully excluded from these vaccines, but others were not, most notably SV40 in the fifties. There was, Curtis reports, widespread alarm among virologists and vaccine makers when it was announced, at the start of the sixties, that SV40 could cause tumors in hamsters and could "immortalize" (render cancerous) human cells in a test tube. For a while, virologists feared that they might have introduced a cancer-causing agent to millions of humans, and although as the decades passed these fears eased, Curtis notes that certain epidemiological studies had detected a higher frequency of childhood cancers, or brain tumors, in persons given either IPV or OPV during the fifties.

Curtis goes on to describe the 1967 outbreak of Marburg disease, caused by a simian virus that was harmless to its natural host (African green monkeys from Uganda), but highly pathogenic in humans. The virus was transferred to technicians working in polio vaccine labs who had handled the animals, their organs, or tissue cultures made from those organs. The condition spread from these initial cases to infect hospital personnel and the wife of one of the index patients; altogether thirty-one people fell sick and eight died before the outbreak was brought under control. Fortunately, the human impact of Marburg virus was so dramatic that its presence was discovered long before it contaminated any polio vaccines — and thus the general public. Nonetheless, it served as a stunning object lesson in the potential dangers of making vaccines from monkey tissues.

After this preamble about the dangers of unknown simian viruses in human vaccines, Curtis examines the possibility that some vaccine lots might have been contaminated with simian immunodeficiency viruses, including the precursors of HIV-1 and HIV-2. Since the SIVs were only discovered in the 1980s, there would have been no way in the fifties of establishing whether or not such a virus might have been present in a polio vaccine, but Curtis notes the claim made in 1959 by Albert Sabin that he had found a cell-killing virus in the CHAT vaccine that Koprowski had used in his Belgian Congo trials. He also notes the response that Koprowski made later that year: that other scientists had also tested CHAT and found no such contaminant. This is placed in perspective by veteran virologist Joseph Melnick, who comments that contaminating viruses may infect some batches of vaccine and not others.

Most tellingly, Curtis reveals that there is real uncertainty about which species of monkey provided the kidneys in which CHAT was manufactured. He interviews Hilary Koprowski, who initially insists that it must have been the African green monkey, but later says: "I have a suspicion the virus was grown in the rhesus monkey at the original beginning. . . . Now when we switched to green monkeys, I have no idea." Koprowski explains that the relevant records no longer exist, and that all the people who helped make the vaccine, such as his long-term associate Thomas Norton, have since died. He goes on to say that the Wistar Institute used to purchase kidneys that were already excised, which, Curtis observes, means that they could have come from any species. Curtis also comments that it may not be that crucial which type of monkey was used, for in those days monkeys of different species were often caged together, and viruses could therefore have passed from one species to another before they were sacrificed to provide kidneys for tissue culture work.

Curtis goes on to investigate which Africans might have received the vaccine. Medical articles reveal that in 1957 and 1958 nearly 30,000 people were given CHAT in the city of Stanleyville (now Kisangani) and in other towns in northeastern Congo; that in 1958 another 215,000 received the vaccine in the Ruzizi Valley, along the borders of what are now eastern Congo, Rwanda, and Burundi; and that between 1958 and 1960 some 75,000 children were fed CHAT in Leopoldville (now Kinshasa, Congo's capital city).[9] But Koprowski tells him that, over and above these 320,000, a further 200,000 or so could have been vaccinated before the pre-independence upheavals disrupted the program. Apparently these civil disturbances also prevented any long-term follow-up of vaccinees.

When Curtis puts it to Koprowski that his field trials with CHAT might have unwittingly introduced the AIDS virus to Africa, Koprowski "dismisses the idea with a deep laugh: 'Ho, ho, ho, ho, ho.'" Curtis presses him, and Koprowski responds that the latency period (the period of time between initial HIV infection and falling ill with AIDS) is nine years — so if CHAT was to blame, why did cases of AIDS not emerge earlier? Curtis comments that early cases did occur in this very region, and that perhaps even earlier cases occurred but were not recognized; alternatively, the virus may have taken longer to become established in the rural regions where CHAT was mainly fed, and where people tend to have fewer sexual partners.

In the course of his interviews with the other two leading polio vaccine manufacturers of the fifties and sixties, and with some of the current luminaries of AIDS research, Curtis comes up with a range of opinions both supporting and decrying the hypothesis. Jonas Salk refuses to discuss the theory, asking: "What value is it to anyone to try to imply such a cause and effect relationship?" Albert Sabin is equally skeptical, and insists that the AIDS virus won't survive swallowing (thus exonerating both Koprowski's OPV and his own).

Tom Folks, the head of the retrovirus laboratory at the CDC, provides some cautious support — all tissue cultures, he maintains, also contain small

amounts of lymphocytes, the white blood cells that are one of the primary targets of SIVs and HIVs, so the theory is at least technically viable. Others, like
William Haseltine of Harvard University, and David Heymann of the WHO's
Global Program on AIDS, flatly reject the theory, on the grounds that it is "of
no importance," or "distracting . . . non-productive . . . [and] confusing to the
public."

Robert Gallo, described by Curtis as "the federal government's preeminent
AIDS researcher" to whom "all roads lead," is more willing to discuss the theory,
but finds little to commend it: he doubts that a lentivirus like SIV could be
absorbed into the body orally, through the mucous membranes of the mouth and
throat, and he points out that, even if the kidneys of SIV-infected African green
monkeys *had* inadvertently been used to make the vaccine, it could hardly have
led to the genesis of HIV-1, since the two viruses, though related, are only distantly related. Nonetheless he backs Curtis's suggestion that someone should put
the theory to the test by examining the seed stocks of CHAT virus. When Curtis
puts the same suggestion to Koprowski, the Wistar director says "yes," but uncer-
tainly, and goes on to argue that HIV or SIV could not survive in kidney cells.

Curtis ends his article by stressing that all three of the polio vaccine pioneers
had clearly acted with the best of intentions, but that their vaccines had all been
inadvertently contaminated with monkey viruses. "If the Congo vaccine turns
out not to be the way that AIDS got started in people, it will be because medicine was lucky, not because it was infallible," he concludes.

When I first read Tom Curtis's article, in June 1992, I was riveted. I checked a few
points in my files, and then went out for a long walk on the South Downs. When
I got back, I read the piece through again, from start to finish. In several respects,
the theory seemed more plausible than any of the fifteen or so others that I had
examined. What is more, my own research of the previous two years lent some
considerable support to the hypothesis. Curtis had merely observed that the map
of CHAT vaccinations, which had been published in an article in the *British
Medical Journal* in 1958,[10] "corresponds roughly . . . to the regions of highest
HIV infection in equatorial Africa." I knew, however, that there were much closer
correlations than that, and that several of the oldest archival cases of AIDS and
HIV infection on record emanated from the very places (such as Kinshasa and
Kisangani in the Congo, and Bujumbura in Burundi) where CHAT vaccine had
apparently been used. And this, it seemed to me, was the very best litmus test for
the CHAT hypothesis. It was important to compare those areas where the vaccine had been fed, not so much with the current prevalence of HIV and incidence of AIDS, but with the earliest available evidence of virus and disease.

I also had some reservations, however. Despite the cogent way in which Tom
Curtis had presented his arguments, there were some weak points. One was the
fact that he had quoted from the 1985 article by Bob Biggar, which claimed to

demonstrate a high prevalence of HIV (especially in children) in parts of Kivu province in eastern Congo where CHAT had been fed.[11] Biggar's team had found little evidence of AIDS in the area, but Curtis remarks that excess child mortality might have gone unremarked in an area where childhood deaths from infectious diseases were common. However, Curtis was apparently unaware that the Biggar study had been effectively retracted by its author in 1986, when he discovered that his assays had been measuring exposure to the malaria parasite, rather than HIV.[12]

Another apparent weakness in the article stemmed from its apparent vagueness about the monkey species that provided the tissue cultures that might have introduced an SIV contaminant into CHAT. Curtis had ably demonstrated the confusion surrounding the donor monkeys, and the fact that Koprowski himself was unable to say which species had been used — but his article gave the impression that the SIV from the African green monkey was the most likely source of contamination. However, he had also mentioned, in passing, that Koprowski had tested the CHAT vaccine at a colony of chimpanzees at Camp Lindi, near Stanleyville. Here, surely, was a realistic opportunity for contamination from a species that was known to be host to the closest simian relative to HIV-1 — yet Curtis surprisingly let this fact go unremarked.

There was one particular allusion in the article that intrigued me. Curtis had made a passing reference to an early field trial of Koprowski's vaccines, which had been planned for Belfast, Northern Ireland, in 1956, but which had been scrapped because of reports that some of his attenuated (weakened) OPVs had reverted to their original wild and virulent form. With the help of a friend from Belfast I did a little preliminary research, and discovered that in fact small-scale trials of two of Koprowski's vaccines had gone ahead.[13] It was only later, after completion of these trials, that the British doctors in charge had expressed fears about the safety of the vaccines.

This was especially fascinating, because the letter from Elsie, received a few weeks earlier, had proved beyond doubt that David Carr must have been based in Londonderry, Northern Ireland, at the end of 1956 and through most of 1957. This was immediately after Koprowski's polio vaccines — including the immediate precursor to CHAT — had undergone their field trials in Belfast, just eighty-five miles away. Was it possible that there could have been a link between the Royal Navy rating and the Belfast vaccinations?

Clearly I needed to try to track down some of those who had been involved with these early trials. However, my initial forays into the medical literature on poliomyelitis had convinced me that this was not a subject that was easily assimilated by the layman. First, therefore, I visited some libraries and began to read all I could about the history of poliomyelitis and of polio vaccination.

# 13

THE RACE TO CONQUER POLIO:

EARLY RESEARCH AND INACTIVATED POLIO VACCINES

The story of the battle against poliomyelitis, and the development of inactivated polio vaccine (IPV) and oral polio vaccine (OPV), is a glorious mélange. It features some great and inspired thinking, a lot of hard work, certain crucial lucky breaks, examples of good and bad judgment, of both informed and irresponsible risk-taking. It also, on occasions, features some substantial economies with the truth.

Nowadays it is sometimes forgotten that it was not until after the Second World War that poliomyelitis became, quite suddenly, the most feared of all Western diseases, occupying much the same position in the public consciousness that AIDS was to occupy in the final two decades of the century.

There were, perhaps, two main reasons for this. The first involved its victims — the young, but also the hitherto fit and healthy among the adult population. Indeed, for a time during the first half of this century, it began to look as if polio worked against all the recognized maxims of public health policy and disease prevention.

Only a very small proportion of persons exposed to polioviruses develop anything worse than a mild flu-like illness, but in a few instances the virus migrates to the spinal cord, where it causes paralysis. As a society becomes cleaner and more hygienic, as more foodstuffs are produced under sterile conditions, as sewage is treated more efficiently and there is wider access to running water so that more hands get washed, fewer of that society's members are exposed to naturally occurring polioviruses during infancy (when individuals are still passively protected by antibodies passed on from the mother) and early childhood. In such a society, fewer youngsters develop protective antibodies against the disease, so that when wild (and virulent) polioviruses begin to circulate among the population during an epidemic year, a higher percentage of older children and adults are struck down with paralysis than in years gone by.

The second reason for polio's sudden assumption of bête noire status involved its public image. It was not only the graphic news photos of children wearing metal braces, of stricken adults in iron lungs. Poliomyelitis acquired special notoriety in America because it was responsible for the crippling of Franklin D. Roosevelt. Although FDR made great efforts to conceal his affliction from the public gaze, the fact that he died at the very moment of triumph, after leading his people through the trauma of the Second World War, virtually guaranteed that — once the war ended — the United States would be at the forefront of the fight against the disease.

It was partly due to America's admirably gung-ho approach to problem-solving, and partly to its aggressive marketing of medicine (a process that accelerated rapidly in the postwar years), that this magnificent scientific enterprise, of controlling polio, began on occasions to resemble a scramble, a desperate race. It was, of course, a race with well-merited and glittering prizes, but it was also one from which many of the runners — had they known at the outset what it would involve — might well have withdrawn, in that it caused some frightening and unexpected injuries to participants and bystanders alike.

----

The story of the first vaccination — by Edward Jenner in 1796 — is well known the world over.[1] Having observed that milkmaids suffering from a cattle disease, cowpox, did not seem to experience the much more severe human disease, smallpox, Jenner inoculated an eight-year-old boy with the contents of a cowpox pustule from a milkmaid's arm. The boy suffered a headache and fever, and a pustule developed on his own arm, but the pustule fell off after a few days. Six weeks later, in an experiment to test the efficacy of his technique — one bold enough to make twentieth-century doctors blanch — Jenner inoculated the boy again, this time with material taken from a smallpox pustule. The boy survived the challenge unscathed; he was apparently protected from smallpox. We now know that exposure to the cowpox virus had provided Jenner's young human guinea pig with immunity to the closely related smallpox virus, but in those days the mechanisms of protection were not fully understood. What was clearly seen was that here was a technique that worked. It came to be known as vaccination, in commemoration of the fact that the original inoculum had derived from a bovine disease.[2]

It was late in the nineteenth century before the next major advance in vaccination occurred, when the great French veterinary scientist, Louis Pasteur, developed vaccines against two animal diseases, chicken cholera and rabies. He was experimenting with cultures of a material lethal to chickens — one that, when inoculated even in small doses, caused them to develop chicken cholera. By serendipity, he tested an old culture of this material, and found that it no longer caused chickens to develop the illness. Just as Jenner had done, he then challenged the birds with a fresh, lethal dose of the chicken cholera material, and found that they were protected from the disease — they were immune. Pasteur intuited that under certain conditions, disease-causing organisms stored in cultures in test tubes could become weakened, or attenuated. He then investigated which factors (such as varying temperatures, the passage of time, exposure to oxygen) might cause this attenuation, and realized that a key factor was transplantation of the disease-causing organism from one experimental animal (or culture) to another.

Next, Pasteur managed to attenuate the rabies virus by passaging it through rabbit brain and spinal cord. (Passaging involves inoculating a viral or bacterial sample into a foreign host — a different animal species — or a foreign tissue, leaving it for a while, and then harvesting the end product. The passage through the "alternative host" often produces subtle changes in the microorganism, including a lessening of its ability to cause disease.) Pasteur used this weakened virus to protect dogs against rabies and then, in an historic experiment in 1885, he successfully immunized a young French boy, Joseph Meister, who had been bitten by a rabid dog a few days earlier. For the first time, humans now possessed a degree of understanding of the mechanisms of disease (the germ theory) and of conferring immunity against disease. Effectively, this was the moment when the disciplines of microbiology and immunology were born.

As the years went by, understanding of the underlying processes improved. It was found that all infectious organisms have chemical substances called antigens, which, when introduced into the body of a foreign host, be it human or animal, cause the production of protective antibodies specific to that organism. And in time, three effective approaches to immunization were discovered.

The first involves injecting the subject with serum containing antibodies from animals or people who have already been exposed to the appropriate infection. This is called passive immunization, and provides only a short-term solution. The other two approaches (which will be examined in greater detail) are both examples of active immunization. One involves inoculating a subject with bacteria or viruses that have first been killed. This is still the favored method for immunizing against diseases like typhoid and cholera, and it confers immunity for a limited period, so that revaccination is required at regular intervals. The other involves introducing a live but attenuated (or weakened) form of a disease agent, a technique that is effective against diseases like rabies, smallpox, and yellow fever.

Both approaches involve a modicum of potential risk. The killed technique can prove dangerous if the virus or bacterium has not been properly treated, and is not completely dead at the time of its inclusion in a vaccine; the live approach becomes unsafe if the infectious agent proves to be insufficiently attenuated or else — after being introduced to the host by swallowing or injection — begins to change its character and "revert to virulence." However, it should be stressed that when modern vaccines are properly administered, the benefits by far outweigh the risks.[3]

Poliomyelitis was first identified as a separate disease in 1840, and though cases certainly occurred before that, it would seem that they were relatively rare. The first small polio outbreak to be described occurred in Stockholm in 1887, but it was not until 1916 that a major epidemic broke out, resulting in twenty thousand polio cases and six thousand deaths across the United States, most notably in New York. At this point, poliomyelitis was still generally thought of as a new disease (or, by some, as an ancient, harmless disease that had suddenly grown savage), and one that particularly affected Americans. It was not yet understood that this was a disease of the modern, sanitized era.

In 1908, it was proved that poliomyelitis was caused by a virus, and that it could be transmitted to monkeys by injecting material from a human patient's spinal cord directly into their brains. But there was no dramatic progress in the research laboratory until 1934, when two vaccines against polio were announced almost simultaneously, and both by press conference, still a rare event in the medical world of the day. The first, an IPV developed by Maurice Brodie and his boss, William Park, from the New York City Health Department, consisted of the pulverized spinal cords of polio-infected monkeys, which had been inactivated — or killed — with formalin. Dr. Park reassured reporters that it was not dangerous, adding that it had already been tried out on six volunteers, including the two doctors themselves. Two days later, Dr. John Kolmer, director of a private establishment in Philadelphia, the Research Institute of Cutaneous Medicine, announced that he too had developed a polio vaccine, this time a live one. Kolmer's preparation, which was also administered by injection, again consisted of polio-infected simian spinal cords, which he had apparently "attenuated" by further monkey passages; as a final safety measure, he had treated his vaccine with a cocktail of chemicals. Like Brodie's, Kolmer's vaccine had been tested on a few humans, but neither vaccine had been subjected to careful clinical trials. Despite this, the two teams were allowed to embark on vigorous vaccination campaigns, each inoculating some ten thousand children in the course of 1935.

The first real indication that something was dramatically wrong came toward the end of that year, when polio struck several of the children who had received each of the vaccines. Other laboratories began checking the safety of the preparations, and finally Dr. Tom Rivers announced that monkey safety tests conducted at the Rockefeller Institute indicated that neither vaccine provided any effective immunity against poliovirus and, furthermore, that Kolmer's live vaccine actually caused polio by reverting to the virulent form of the virus. By the end of the year, it was revealed that twelve children (nine of Kolmer's vaccinees and three of Brodie's) had contracted polio shortly after being vaccinated. Six of them had died, including five of Kolmer's charges. Dr. James Leake, medical director of the U.S. Public Health Service, was eventually moved to make a formal plea to Kolmer at a conference in St. Louis, saying: "I beg you to desist from the public use of this vaccine."[4] Kolmer, to his credit, showed some real, if belated, remorse and humility, confessing: "Gentlemen, this is one time that I wish the floor would open up and swallow me." However, it was not Kolmer whom the earth devoured, but his rivals Brodie and Park, each of whom died in 1939, very possibly of poliomyelitis, contracted from their own inadequately refined vaccine.[5]

These, then, were the highly inauspicious beginnings of killed and live vaccination against polio. Sadly, far from echoing down the years as a plangent warning to those who followed, these dissonant chords were to be struck on many more occasions during the next few decades, as — all too often — the very same errors were made. Partly this is testimony to the highly dangerous nature of poliovirus, once it attacks the brain and spinal cord. Partly, however, it is an indication of the highly experimental nature of some of the procedures. Even by the fifties, and the first pink glimmerings at the dawn of virology, there was still a substantial amount of whistling in the dark by the high priests of the new science.

---

At the very end of the 1940s came two discoveries that had tremendous significance for the development of polio vaccines. First, the gentleman scientist John Enders, based at Harvard, discovered by chance (so often, it seems, the catalyst of great scientific breakthrough) that it was possible to grow poliovirus in cultures of nonnervous tissue — in this instance derived from human embryos.[6]

Such tissue cultures are pieces of living tissue, which are broken down by fine mincing or enzyme activity and then combined with a chemically balanced fluid and a nutrient-packed growth medium such as beef broth, and maintained in laboratory glassware under sterile, controlled conditions. Prepared in this fashion, it is possible to grow living tissue in the test tube and, indeed, to manufacture it in vast quantities. The tissue culture technique was originally developed in 1907, but it was only in the forties, with the advent of antibiotics, that scientists were able to keep the cultures alive for lengthy periods, whereupon tissue culture work swiftly became the basic tool of microbiological research.

Enders's serendipitous discovery, followed up by painstaking confirmatory experiment, proved that the given wisdom (that poliovirus could survive only in the tissues of the central nervous system) was incorrect — and that it could quite easily be grown in cells from the embryo, the skin, the lung, or the kidney. After this breakthrough (which earned Enders and his colleagues Weller and Robbins a Nobel Prize in 1954), other microbiologists began to realize that the natural habitat of the poliovirus was the alimentary canal, and that its migration to the brain and spinal cord (the sites where it caused disease) was but a rare occurrence. Furthermore, now that poliovirus could be mass-produced in tissue culture, and then inactivated or attenuated, there was no longer any obstacle to commercial vaccine manufacture.

In that same year, 1949, a team under David Bodian of Johns Hopkins University discovered that there was not simply one type of poliovirus, but three. This finding was subsequently confirmed in a huge operation in which viral samples from large numbers of polio sufferers were tested, and only the same three polioviruses identified. This laborious work, which involved the use of some thirty thousand monkeys as test animals, was completed in 1951. The most dangerous poliovirus, Type 1, was found to be responsible for 80 percent or more of all paralytic cases, and the great majority of the world's polio epidemics. At long last the nature of the beast was known, and the time was ripe for a courtly knight to gallop onto the scene.

As it happened, there was already a suitable candidate for the shining armor, in Jonas Salk, a good-looking, confident, and yet pleasingly self-effacing microbiologist from a working-class background in the Bronx. In 1951, Salk was the newly appointed director of the virus research laboratory at the University of Pittsburgh. Already known as a tough-minded, hardworking scientist, he had spent much of the previous two years participating in the polio typing investigation, and was one of the principal proponents of an inactivated polio vaccine, IPV.

By the early fifties, polio epidemics were an annual occurrence, and high summer was known, fatalistically, as "the polio season." People had grown so afraid that many would no longer visit swimming pools, or would drive past a city where an outbreak was occurring with car windows wound up tight. There was great pressure on the scientists to come up with a prompt solution, and in this respect IPVs held an inbuilt advantage over OPVs, for it was clearly far easier to kill the three poliovirus types in one fell swoop (for instance, by adding formaldehyde) than gradually, by trial and error, to attenuate them. This was the main reason why Salk and his killed-vaccine research received the immediate backing of that powerful private charity, the National Foundation for Infantile Paralysis.

The NFIP had been inaugurated in honor of Roosevelt in 1938 and, since the early forties, had been headed in ineffably self-confident style by FDR's longtime friend Basil O'Connor. Despite being a lawyer by profession, O'Connor turned out to be an inspired salesman and public relations man. He was largely responsible for the fund-raising effort known as "The March of Dimes," which was so successful in tapping into the hopes, fears, and sympathies of the general public that it managed to raise over $25 million a year for the next two decades. Throughout that period, the NFIP was to wield huge power within the United States, including the organization of the first truly mass trial of polio vaccines in the world.

The NFIP gave Salk free rein to proceed as quickly and effectively as possible, with money no object. His first priority was to choose which particular strains of poliovirus he wished to incorporate in his vaccine, and he decided to employ three of the most virulent — Mahoney for Type 1; MEF for Type 2; and Saukett for Type 3. These, he felt, would also produce the best antibody response, the best immunity. Of course, in order to adopt this approach he had to be absolutely confident that his method of inactivation would comprehensively destroy any traces of poliovirus in the vaccine. He first grew the polioviruses in tissue cultures made from the kidneys of the rhesus macaque monkey, and then killed them with formaldehyde. Already Albert Sabin, a vocal member of the OPV lobby, was decrying Salk's approach and insisting that the inactivation procedures were inadequate and that the resulting immunity would be short-lived. Much later, when it became known that some of the vaccine manufacturers had experienced difficulties in inactivating the vaccine according to the Salk recipe, some would think back to Sabin's prognoses of doom. But at this early stage, such skeptics were very much in the minority.

In 1952, Salk staged his first small trial of a killed vaccine against Type 1 virus on a group of Pennsylvania children who were protected by naturally acquired Type 1 antibodies (they had already been infected by relatively harmless Type 1 polioviruses circulating in the community). When this experiment went without a hitch, he proceeded the following year to vaccinate a group who lacked antibodies. Again he was successful and, as public acclamation and excitement grew, it was decided that a mass trial of a Salk vaccine containing all three poliovirus types should be staged in the first half of 1954. Surprisingly, however, it was decided that the NFIP, rather than the government, would organize the trial. Thomas Francis, Salk's former teacher from the University of Michigan, was brought in to introduce some scientific order and method — and only just in time, for by this stage O'Connor had begun promising certain towns and states that they would be included in the trial. Francis agreed that these promises had to be honored, but insisted that the rest of the trial should comprise a double-blind study, with half of the children receiving the vaccine, and the other half (matched for sex, age, and demography) comprising a control group. He got his way, and between April and June 1954, more than 1.8 million American children received a shot — either of Salk's polio vaccine or a placebo. Then Francis and his team retired to Michigan to analyze the results.

There were no sudden outbreaks of illness among the vaccinees, so it was clear that the vaccine was essentially safe, but it remained to be seen whether or not it was effective. During the next twelve months, the country waited for Francis to complete the data analysis, and the mood grew more and more expectant. O'Connor, never a patient man, and with millions of dollars of funds burning a hole in his bank account, tried unsuccessfully to persuade Francis to speed up his research. Eventually the NFIP boss decided that he could wait no longer, and placed an advance order for 27 million doses of the Salk vaccine with the six pharmaceutical houses that had been approved as manufacturers. His reasoning was that if, as he anticipated, the Francis report was favorable, enough vaccine would be available to ensure that a large proportion of America's children could be vaccinated in 1955, before the start of the summer polio season. It was a massive gamble on his part, and something of a pre-emptive move with regard to Francis.

It was finally decided by Francis and O'Connor that the results would be announced publicly on April 12, 1955, the tenth anniversary of Roosevelt's death, rather than by the time-honored method of publication in one of the nation's medical journals. The announcement was to be made at Francis's alma mater in Ann Arbor, with leaders of science and medicine invited to attend, and movie theaters across the country hired to screen the event live on closed-circuit television, for the benefit of local doctors. The highly detailed results were essentially positive, though less so than some had hoped. Between 62 and 70 percent of the vaccinations were effective, though unfortunately the Type 1 component afforded the least complete protection. None of the vaccine was dangerous, but not every batch provided effective immunity. It had already been decided that, following the Francis address, a committee of experts would sit for a couple of hours to discuss the issues raised, after which the vaccine would receive its official license (again before the TV cameras) that same afternoon — thus telescoping a process that would normally take months into the space of a few hours. Vaccination of American children began almost immediately, but many of those involved would subsequently have cause to regret the unseemly haste shown on that spring day in 1955, a day that ended with the ringing of church bells and the wailing of sirens across the land.

The reason for this was the so-called Cutter incident, which began a fortnight later. On April 26, five California children were reported to have contracted polio just a few days after immunization and, in an uneasy echo of the Brodie episode twenty years before, the first symptoms appeared — in every case — in the same limb that had received the injection. Many other cases of post-vaccination paralysis were reported in the days that followed, and it was quickly realized that all the affected children had received one of a small group of vaccine batches made by Cutter Laboratories, based in California. Clearly, in at least one vaccine house, something had gone dramatically wrong with the manufacturing process. Much later it was learned that, at Cutter, some of the cell debris created when poliovirus is grown in monkey kidney tissue culture had formed into clumps, and that small amounts of virulent Mahoney virus had remained alive in the center of these clumps — even after the nine-day treatment with formaldehyde, which Salk had deemed adequate to ensure total inactivation. This live virus featured, to deadly effect, in some of the production batches of the vaccine.

One of the most worrying aspects of the crisis was the indecisiveness of the official response. At the request of Surgeon General Leonard Scheele, Cutter immediately withdrew all batches of its vaccine, but in an attempt to minimize panic, Scheele announced publicly that this was a "safety precaution" and that there was "no cause for alarm." A few days later, he cryptically announced that the Salk vaccine "can be safe." This did little to calm the nerves of worried parents as dozens of further cases were reported from states as far apart as Georgia and Idaho. Worse still, cases began to be reported among contacts of the vaccinees, indicating that the inadequately inactivated virus had the capacity to spread. For a while, there was very real concern that the mass vaccination might itself spark a major epidemic of a highly virulent polio strain.

It was not until May 6, ten days after the start of the incident, that Scheele banned the release of any further lots of Salk vaccine from any source, a move that he rescinded later in May, only to reimpose a few days afterward. Much later, when the final reckoning was done, it was found that 94 of the vaccinees and 166 of their contacts had been paralyzed, and that eleven of them were dead. What is more, the public attitude to polio vaccination had shifted, within the space of a month, from bell-clanging euphoria to stunned disbelief.

Clearly the safety margins had been underestimated. In the orgy of recrimination and finger-pointing that followed, it emerged that almost everyone involved bore a degree of responsibility — from O'Connor for bulldozing through the results of the field trial and the licensing process, to Salk for his miscalculation about inactivation times, to members of the Laboratory of Biologics Control for failing to impose adequate safety tests in the vaccine houses, to those at the Cutter Laboratories who had made the vaccine.

That the Cutter incident did not totally destroy the future of IPV was largely because of the huge efforts exerted by O'Connor to calm the situation. He stressed that the episode had resulted from an unforeseeable combination of circumstances, and that once the specific causes had been eliminated, many thousands of lives would be saved by Salk's vaccine. Within weeks, two key changes had been ordered to the manufacturing and testing procedures: a mandatory filtration stage was introduced, to eliminate the possibility of cell clumping, and it was decided that the monkeys used in safety tests should first be given cortisone, to render them more susceptible to infection, and more likely to be affected by any residual trace of active poliovirus that might still be present in the preparation. Following this, in July, the vaccination program was allowed to resume, and by the end of 1955 seven million children had been vaccinated without further incident, though very few had received the full course of three injections that was now felt to be necessary to ensure full immunity. As it turned out, O'Connor and the NFIP had already ridden out the worst of the storm, and during 1956 tens of millions of young Americans began lining up in school halls to be inoculated. There were no reprises of the Cutter episode, and the incidence of paralytic poliomyelitis in the United States fell from slightly more than 15,000 in 1955 to 8,000 and 2,500 in the two following years. Between 1955 and 1962, Salk's IPV was the accepted poliovaccine in America and in most other countries around the world, and hundreds of millions of people — mainly children — received his "magic shots."

In Britain, however, reaction to Cutter was more severe (partly, perhaps, because the United Kingdom had just received delivery of a large consignment of Salk vaccine at the time that the news first broke). Eventually it was decided to reject Salk's IPV (on the grounds that it contained the virulent Mahoney Type 1 poliovirus) in favor of an inactivated vaccine containing the milder, and consequently less immunogenic, strain known as Brunenders, which was first field-tested in Britain in 1956.[7]

However, IPV was not the only vaccine in the field, and there was already a large body of opinion that favored immunizing by mouth with live, attenuated polio vaccine. There were many reasons for backing this view, but the principal ones were that oral polio vaccine (OPV) was cheaper and easier to administer (without the need for syringes, clinics, or queues of petrified children), that it mimicked the natural route of infection, the alimentary canal, and that it was able to confer lifelong immunity in a single dose for each poliovirus type. By contrast, IPV required three shots to establish effective immunity, and further booster shots to prevent the diminishing of immunity as time passed.

It was, however, more difficult to manufacture and prepare an OPV. The process involved isolating a sample of poliovirus and subjecting it to repeated passage — making it reproduce in a succession of live animals and culture media, continually removing the viral progeny and transferring them to a new animal or culture until, by a process of trial and error, a modified, attenuated virus was produced. The trick was to attenuate to a point where the virus was safe for humans, but not so far that its power to infect and immunize humans was lost.

In the words of a later commentator, John Rowan Wilson, the difference between preparing IPV and OPV "is the difference between slaughtering an ox and breeding from it, between wringing a parrot's neck and teaching it to talk."[8] By 1955, the animal husbandry work and avian elocution lessons were already well under way.

# 14

## THE RACE TO CONQUER POLIO:

## ORAL POLIO VACCINES

In fact, an attenuated oral polio vaccine had already been developed and tested in humans even earlier than Jonas Salk's first human inoculations. On February 27, 1950, Hilary Koprowski became the first scientist in the world to administer OPV to a human being.[1]

Koprowski was Polish-born, and had emigrated to America nearly six years earlier, swiftly progressing to the post of assistant director of viral research at Lederle Laboratories, the pharmaceutical arm of the chemical giant American Cyanamid. By 1950, he was already being viewed as the star of the show at Lederle — and in more ways than one, for not only was he an inspired and frequently brilliant scientist, but he also played piano to concert standard, spoke several languages, and was apparently a connoisseur of beauty, the arts, good food, and fine wines.

His immediate boss at Lederle, Herald Cox, could hardly have been a more contrasting character. During the forties, Cox had earned a solid reputation through his use of developing chick embryos to prepare numerous vaccines against animal viruses and rickettsial diseases, but his successes apparently came as a result of long hours and dogged determination. Furthermore, he was uneasy with the human demands of leadership, and would sometimes express this unease through bouts of overwork, followed by fits of profound depression. The contrast between these two men, the cosmopolitan peacock and the self-proclaimed "Hoosier,"[2] was to become increasingly pronounced as the fifties progressed. It developed into mutual distrust and, eventually, a deeply felt and lasting enmity that was to play a significant part in the unfolding of the OPV story.

Koprowski's first polio vaccine was developed over the last four years of the forties, and was therefore not based on the tissue culture techniques of Enders. It consisted of a suspension of polio-infected mouse brain, which was then attenuated by several passages through cotton rats. Apart from humans, the only animal susceptible to poliovirus by the oral route is the chimpanzee, and Koprowski duly fed this attenuated Type 2 virus to nine chimpanzees, without apparent ill effect. When he later challenged the chimps with virulent Type 2 virus, they showed no signs of illness, suggesting that they had been successfully immunized. He also attempted to establish whether the vaccine virus could cause paralysis — whether it was neurovirulent — by injecting it directly into the brains and spinal cords of monkeys. (Although this was a crude safety test, it was a logical one, since monkey species — like humans — were known to have central nervous systems that are susceptible to poliovirus.) Again, the lack of paralysis indicated real attenuation.

Having satisfied himself as to the efficacy and safety of his vaccine, Koprowski named it TN, in honor of his chief laboratory technician and close colleague, Tom Norton. Norton had come to Lederle from Max Theiler's laboratory at the Rockefeller Institute, where they had just developed the 17D vaccine against yellow fever, for which Theiler would subsequently win a Nobel Prize. In later years, Theiler would comment wryly to scientific colleagues that Koprowski's TN bore a close resemblance to a Type 2 poliovirus that he had been adapting to mouse brain while Norton was still working for him.[3] Even this first OPV, therefore, was not entirely free from controversy.

In March 1951, Koprowski publicly announced the first human vaccination with TN at a conference in Hershey, Pennsylvania, and many of his peers were taken by surprise.[4] By this stage, a year after the first feeding of the vaccine, Koprowski and Norton had fed TN to twenty children, all of whom went on to develop Type 2 antibodies. Furthermore, no ill effects had been detected during several months of follow-up: a significant development after the dreadful Kolmer episode of fifteen years earlier. Many in the audience were impressed by the meticulously careful research; Koprowski had clearly gone to great trouble to ensure that this was not another public relations disaster for OPV. Others were impressed by his courage in proceeding with human trials — for however many the safety tests, this first artificial feeding in humans was still essentially a leap of faith, which, had it gone wrong, would probably have destroyed his reputation and career.

There was, however, widespread disquiet about the secret manner in which the work had been undertaken. According to Koprowski's own account of the Hershey conference, given some years after the event, Tom Francis, sleepy after the exertions of lunch, had to be convinced by Jonas Salk that children, rather than monkeys, were the subject of the trial, while Albert Sabin apparently "got all perturbed and said to me later, 'Why have you done it? Why? Why?'"[5] Another who was alarmed by Koprowski's initiative was Tom Rivers, by now head of the virus research committee of the NFIP, whose views on such issues tended to be treated as if written on tablets of stone. When approached in advance by the New York state authorities about Koprowski's proposal to con- duct the human experiment, he had apparently advised against it on the grounds that it was both unethical and dangerous. He was appalled to learn that the trial had nonetheless gone ahead.[6]

When Koprowski's seminal paper on this first feeding of OPV was published in 1952,[7] several observers were intrigued about the test subjects. Throughout the article, they were referred to merely as "volunteers," and the only clue to their identity was that some, including the very first volunteer, had had to be fed vac- cine through stomach tubes. In fact, the participants were — to use the argot of the times — "feeble-minded children," and the volunteering had been done by others (their parents). Soon afterward, an editorial note in the *Lancet* com- mented wryly on the research, as follows: "One of the reasons for the richness of the English language is that the meaning of some words is continually chang- ing. Such a word is 'volunteer.' We may yet read in a scientific journal that an experiment was carried out with twenty volunteer mice, and that twenty other mice volunteered as controls."[8] The issue of volunteer status in vaccine trials would continue to bedevil polio vaccine development throughout the fifties.

Koprowski, meanwhile, was attempting to develop a Type 1 vaccine. Herald Cox, after all his successes in producing vaccines in chick embryo, was con- vinced that this was both the safest and most efficacious substrate (or culture medium) for polio work. Indeed, another member of his laboratory, Manuel Roca-Garcia, had already managed to attenuate another strain of Type 2 poliovirus, named MEF1,[9] in chick embryo material — essentially a fertilized hen's egg, kept naturally sterile by its shell. Accordingly, Koprowski mixed two Type 1 strains (a relatively mild isolate known as Sickle, and the more virulent Mahoney), transferred them into mouse brains, and then passaged them several times through chick embryo tissue culture (produced in a test tube, instead of inside an eggshell), to produce an attenuated Type 1 vaccine, which he called SM. Because of the dangers of Type 1, his first experimental feeding of SM was to just three children.[10]

This took place in 1953, at a time when the initiative was moving very firmly across to Salk's IPV, backed by O'Connor and the NFIP millions. In October of that year, Koprowski attended a conference on viral and rickettsial infections in Detroit, where he gave a talk on the practical application of live vaccines.[11] He was not yet ready to report his SM work, but he did bring the audience up to date on his original TN vaccinees, who were still showing good antibody pro- tection up to three years after having ingested the vaccine. However, during the discussion at the end of his address, Albert Sabin got up to speak.[12]

Born in 1906 at Bialystok, at that time part of Imperial Russia, Sabin had emigrated to America in 1921. He was a brilliant student at New York University, and worked briefly under William Park, witnessing the Brodie debacle at first hand, before moving on to the Rockefeller Institute, where he was the first person to grow poliovirus in the nervous tissue of monkeys. In 1939, he transferred to a position in the pediatrics department of the University of Cincinnati, an institution with which he would retain close links until the end of his days. By the early fifties, Sabin was widely acknowledged as a deep thinker and a scrupulously careful scientist. He was also a fine tactician, for although firmly opposing the IPV lobby on grounds of efficacy, he was shrewd enough to acknowledge that it possessed the only polio vaccine then available. However, in the wake of the Enders discovery, he began quietly working away, attempting to attenuate the three types of poliovirus.

At the time of the Detroit symposium, Sabin's hair was already beginning to turn snowy white, and with his uncompromising manner and his fierce, eagle-eyed gaze, he gave the impression of being considerably older than Koprowski, even though the age gap was only ten years. When he rose to speak, he began with a respectful reference to his younger colleague, but a sentence or two later he dropped his bombshell. He announced his belief that the best way to attenuate polioviruses was not to pass them through unnatural hosts (like rodents or chick embryos), but rather to pass them rapidly through their natural hosts — the same hosts in which one would assess their neurovirulence. Indeed, he said, he had already managed to attenuate poliovirus strains representing Types 1, 2, and 3, as evidenced by their lack of neurovirulence for the cynomolgus macaque (an Asian monkey), and he had done this by rapid passages in a tissue culture made of cynomolgus kidneys. Although he had not yet tested his vaccines in humans, it seemed that he was not far from doing so.

Not only had Sabin already managed to attenuate one more poliovirus type than Koprowski, but he was working in a medium that seemed far more suitable for manipulating polioviruses. Koprowski might still be a year or so ahead in terms of clinical trials, but Sabin's five-minute speech must have revealed to Koprowski (if he did not know it before) that he had a serious rival in terms of OPV development.

During the next three years, the rivalry intensified — though it was only after the Cutter incident in April 1955, when it became apparent that OPVs might after all be able to challenge IPVs, that the race really began in earnest. Koprowski was having some difficulty with his Type 1 vaccine, SM, which he found difficult to maintain in chick embryo tissue culture (CETC), forcing him to alternate the chick embryo passages with passages in monkey kidney tissue culture (MKTC) in order to keep the attenuated virus alive.[13] (He did this in spite of the fact that Herald Cox disapproved of MKTC as a substrate, considering it potentially unsafe, on the grounds that it might contain simian viruses that could all too easily adapt to man.)[14] By 1955, Koprowski had still not developed a Type 3 vaccine, but he was gradually refining SM and TN, his Type 1 and Type 2 strains, and feeding them to slowly increasing numbers of mentally handicapped children in homes in New Jersey and California.

But despite his late start, Albert Sabin was by now ahead of Koprowski. Sabin was a notoriously hard taskmaster, and the amount of work he and his assistants managed to get through in these years is little short of breathtaking. Between 1953 and 1956, he tested his candidate strains on a total of 9,000 monkeys and 150 chimpanzees, and finally embarked on human trials in 1955, when he tested his strains on 163 volunteers at Chillicothe, a men's prison in Ohio.[15]

He was not easily satisfied, however. Two years into the work, finding that two of his three original vaccine strains still retained a very slight degree of neurovirulence for monkeys, he decided to abandon them and start again from scratch. He arranged to test eight other "naturally attenuated strains" of poliovirus (from people with no visible symptoms, who had had no known contact with paralytic polio cases), which he then further attenuated in the laboratory using methods that, by this stage, were considerably more sophisticated than those of his rivals. He was still employing rapid passages in monkey kidney tissue culture, which, it was becoming clear, was a far better substrate than chick embryo. (In fact, according to Sabin's own experiments, CETC was incapable of growing poliovirus at all — and his occasional asides on this topic tacitly questioned the whole basis of allegedly "egg-adapted strains" like Cox's MEF1 and Koprowski's SM.) Furthermore, he was now also incorporating the plaque purification technique pioneered by the highly respected Italian virologist Renato Dulbecco.[16]

This involved growing a small amount of poliovirus in a single layer of monkey kidney cells cultured on a gel, so that the area of cell death around each individual viral particle could be identified, and a sample removed to seed a new culture. When repeated three times (triple plaque purified), this was considered to effectively guarantee the purity of a viral strain. Using this method, Sabin eventually developed three strains that he considered to be truly attenuated and safe (LSc, P712, and Leon, representing Types 1, 2, and 3, respectively), and he reported this work in an impressively detailed paper published in the *Journal of the American Medical Association* at the end of 1956.[17]

Sabin also produced some significant work on the theory of attenuation, including the important observation that there was a gradient of intestinal susceptibility to poliovirus, with man at the top, descending through the chimpanzee to the cynomolgus macaque, the monkey he used for his safety testing and vaccine production. By contrast, he observed, the gradient of central nervous system susceptibility featured the same animals — monkey, ape, and man — in reverse order.[18] This had a number of significant implications. It showed that humans could readily be infected, and immunized, by the alimentary route, whereas monkeys could not. In the middle were the chimps, which could be infected orally, but which (unlike humans) did not excrete the virus. There was therefore no test animal that could really substitute for *Homo sapiens* in efficacy trials. Furthermore, the best types of human guinea pigs were clearly children, who had lower levels of naturally acquired antibodies than adults.

However, there were very effective substitutes for assessing safety, since both chimps and — in particular — monkeys were clearly more sensitive than humans to the presence of poliovirus in the brain. If injections of a polio vaccine into monkeys' brains, or of large amounts of that vaccine into chimps' brains, failed to produce paralysis or damage to the spinal cord, then that vaccine seemed likely to be safe for human use.

During 1955, another important issue came to a head — that of the best substrate — or species of tissue culture — in which to manufacture polio vaccines. This became important in the spring of that year, when the Indian government temporarily banned the export of rhesus macaques, at the very moment that this monkey had become the most popular for IPV production and testing, and was being increasingly accepted for OPV work.[19] The ban was later rescinded, but not until there had been real panic in several laboratories and vaccine houses. During that panic, several researchers investigated the possibility of obtaining monkey supplies from elsewhere, for instance from the Philippines or Africa.[20]

By the middle of 1955, Koprowski needed to speed up the pace of his research in order to catch up with Sabin, and he found just the man to help him do it. The British virologist George Dick offered to stage small, carefully controlled trials of SM and TN in the British province of Northern Ireland — a significant step forward from trials in closed communities like mental homes and prisons. The Belfast trials were staged in the first six months of 1956 and, to begin with, all looked rosy. However, Dick began to notice discrepancies between his results and those which featured in Koprowski's prior reports on the strains — most notably a tendency of SM to spread from vaccinee to nonvaccinee, and of TN to become far more virulent after passing through the human gut. These were not the characteristics of safe, stable polio vaccines, and when Dick announced his results in January 1957, he suggested that neither vaccine was suitable for large-scale human trials or, indeed, for further clinical trials.[21] Dick's announcement dealt a serious blow to Koprowski's credibility, and matters finally came to a head between Cox and himself. Koprowski left Lederle shortly afterward, to take over the directorship of the Wistar Institute in Philadelphia, taking Tom Norton and a number of other scientists with him.

Once installed at the Wistar, however, Koprowski and Norton began to turn things around with remarkable speed. They swiftly announced the development of a new Type 1 strain, CHAT, derived from the fourth human passage of the old SM strain, and a Type 3 strain known as Fox — both of which they were producing in monkey kidney, employing Dulbecco's triple plaque purification technique.[22] By the end of 1957, they were also experimenting with a version of Sabin's P712 for Type 2. The Lederle team, meanwhile, regrouped under Cox and a new deputy, Victor Cabasso, and produced a series of vaccine lots using their own candidate strains: an improved version of SM for Type 1, plus MEF1 and Fox. They too had changed course and were now using triple plaque purified MKTC instead of chick embryo. So it was that by the start of 1958, Sabin, Cox, and Koprowski were effectively neck and neck, each possessing three new, purified oral polio vaccine strains.

The intensity of the competition among them can be gauged by their respective addresses to the increasingly frequent polio conferences of the day. Sabin's were precise and sometimes obsessively technical, making no concessions to the listener. Koprowski's were usually less detailed, and full of classical quotation and sideswipes (sometimes witty, sometimes scornful) at his rivals. Cox was not a great conference man, but he delegated to Cabasso, who promptly produced one of the most detailed, clear, and informative addresses on the production and safety testing of a polio vaccine ever to be delivered.[23]

Suddenly, this was a very good time to be involved in OPV research. The Salk vaccine was still being injected into millions of arms, but there were increasing doubts about its long-term efficacy, for it was becoming evident that, as with many killed vaccines, immunity dwindled as time passed. As opinion shifted, so did the cash. Sabin was by now receiving significant research funding from the NFIP and from industry, Cox was still backed by the huge resources of American Cyanamid, while Koprowski was now getting grants from the National Institutes of Health, which he augmented through successful fundraising initiatives.

If 1957 was the year for perfecting sets of attenuated vaccine strains, then 1958 was the year for testing them out in mass trials. The starting flag had been dropped by an expert committee convened by the World Health Organization in July 1957, which had advised that — under certain specific circumstances — large-scale field trials could be mounted of plaque-purified live polio vaccines that had already been proven safe in monkey tests and small-scale clinical trials. These circumstances included situations where a polio epidemic was impending or already under way ("in the face of an epidemic"), or where the administration of inactivated vaccines was deemed to be impractical.[24]

Both situations obtained most frequently in the poorer, less sanitized countries of the developing world, where the majority of the population was naturally immunized by circulating polioviruses within the first few years of life, but where occasional epidemics were still liable to occur among the small percentage of persons who lacked antibodies. And it was here that Koprowski enjoyed a real advantage over his rivals. In 1956, in collaboration with expatriate doctors in the Belgian Congo, he had set up a chimpanzee colony just outside Stanleyville where he could test his polio vaccines. The caretakers of this colony were themselves vaccinated with live vaccine, in order to protect them from the virulent viruses that would be used in some of the vaccination and challenge experiments. When these vaccinations proceeded smoothly, Koprowski managed to persuade the medical director of the colony to approve larger-scale vaccine trials as, for instance, in the face of epidemics. Early in 1958, he fed his CHAT vaccine to the populations of four Congolese villages that had experienced epidemic outbreaks of polio, and then staged the large field trials in the Ruzizi Valley, mentioned previously.

Koprowski's claim that the vaccinations he conducted in the Congo and Ruanda-Urundi in early 1958 had been recommended by the WHO's expert committee was later undermined by the secretary of that committee, who wrote to the *British Medical Journal* to explain that "contrary to some reports, the 'test' in the Belgian Congo was not supported by WHO."[25] By August, however, Koprowski had embarked on a much more carefully monitored trial in Leopoldville, the Congolese capital, which was aimed at all children below the age of five.[26] Furthermore, in October 1958, he managed to arrange a small-scale trial of CHAT in his native Poland, with a view to initiating a mass-vaccination program there if all went well.[27] Not for the first time, his great energy and self-confidence had apparently enabled him to steal a significant march on his rivals.

They, however, were not far behind. Cox and his Lederle associates staged a small trial of SM among infants in Minnesota in 1957,[28] and then began to embark on mass trials in Latin America. Roughly half a million people were vaccinated with all three of the Lederle strains in Nicaragua, Uruguay, and Colombia, including a campaign in response to a Type 1 epidemic in the latter.[29] Sabin, meanwhile, revealed the most ambitious plans of all, for he had managed to negotiate a remarkable deal with the authorities of *his* native land for the feeding of the Sabin strains in the U.S.S.R. After a gradually increasing series of small-scale trials in 1957, larger trials began in 1958, but no details were published. By mid-1959, several million people had been vaccinated with the Sabin strains in the various Soviet republics — an achievement that undoubtedly owed much to the fact that the only volunteering was performed by the state, rather than by individuals. In addition, more than a million doses of his OPVs had been fed in Singapore (in the face of an epidemic), Holland, Mexico, and Czechoslovakia, and Albert Sabin was ready to stir from his naturally taciturn state to announce his achievements to the world.

The First International Conference on Live Poliovirus Vaccines, staged in Washington, D.C., in June 1959, was attended by all the leading figures in the field, and was seen by many as representing the crucial showdown, which would determine who — Sabin, Koprowski, or Cox — would eventually win the race to have their OPV strains approved and licensed.[30] The opening address at the conference was made by George Dick, who set the tone for what followed by issuing a grave warning about allowing open trials of live vaccines that had not been properly tested, whose potential for spread had not been determined, and that were then inadequately monitored. He made particular reference to Koprowski's 1958 mass vaccination in the eastern Congo and Ruanda-Urundi, and to the latter's claim that no illnesses had been observed among the 244,596 CHAT vaccinees. Dick pointed out that — even under normal circumstances — 150 of these persons would have died of natural causes in the space of a month, and many more would have fallen sick.[31] Koprowski, for his part, made no attempt to provide further information about the original vaccinations, but instead gave an impressively detailed account of the CHAT vaccination of 45,000 under-fives in Leopoldville.[32] His reports were, however, completely overshadowed by those concerning four and a half million vaccinations with the three Sabin vaccines.

This was the moment where, if anyone ever doubted it, Albert Sabin — so often the victim of Koprowski's sidelong flicks and jabs[33] — showed that he was capable of throwing some good, clean punches of his own. Virtually no advance information had been released about the Soviet vaccinations, which had mainly been staged in Kazakhstan, Lithuania, and Estonia, so the fact that there had apparently been no untoward complications made a dramatic impact. Of particular importance was the fact that the Sabin strains appeared to suffer no significant reversion to virulence, so that spread to nonvaccinees (which, he conceded, did occur) was actually a desirable quality, since it only added to the "herd immunity" of the population.

This was also the moment when Sabin confirmed that he had found a contaminating virus in a sample of the CHAT vaccine fed in the Congo.[34] In an article published shortly before this, he had made an additional claim: that Koprowski's CHAT and Fox both showed a tendency to revert to virulence.[35] All these allegations were vigorously denied by Koprowski,[36] but they carried considerable weight, because by now most independent scientists were deferring to Sabin as the leading expert in the OPV field. The press took the same view, as was illustrated a few months later, when *Time* magazine reported baldly that Sabin had attacked Kropowski's vaccine, "charging that it contains viruses that cause disease in monkeys and might be dangerous for man."[37]

Sabin's observations received some support from Roderick Murray, director of the Division of Biologics Standards at the NIH — who reported his own independent assessments of the relative neurovirulence of the different sets of vaccine strains. Murray's findings for all three types suggested that the Lederle strains were the most virulent, and Sabin's the least, with Koprowski's falling somewhere in between.[38] The trend was confirmed by another expert virologist, Joseph Melnick from Baylor College in Houston, but his analysis was limited to just two vaccine sets — those of Sabin and Cox — because none were submitted by Koprowski. Despite his clear preference for Sabin's vaccines, Melnick nonetheless pointed out that all the strains tested had been more neurovirulent than their makers had claimed, and emphasized that, as in 1954 and 1955, when the large-scale trials of Salk's IPV began, it was still important to proceed with caution.[39]

The wisdom of this view was reinforced in early 1960, when hurriedly organized trials of Cox's Type 1 strain, SM, in West Berlin and in Dade County, Florida, appeared to run into problems with reversion to virulence, as a number of vaccinees became paralyzed.[40] Effectively, this put the Lederle vaccines out of the running. For his part, Koprowski had been working hard throughout the previous year, and had organized the vaccination of more than seven million Poles with CHAT Type 1 and Fox Type 3.[41] All had gone smoothly, but he was still handicapped by his lack of an effective Type 2 strain. He had done some work with P712 in Philadelphia and New Jersey, and found it worked well, but this was little comfort, in that it was widely regarded as Sabin's strain. Koprowski had also tried, unsuccessfully, to produce an effective Type 2 vaccine by passing MEF1 in MKTC, and was even beginning to work once more with the old, discredited TN strain, this time adapted to MKTC by a series of passages at different temperatures. But it was a case of too little too late. By the time of the Second International Conference on Live Poliovirus Vaccines, in June 1960, Sabin was once again far ahead of him, this time announcing a total of 55 million vaccinations.[42]

---

With the wisdom of hindsight, it is perhaps surprising that while so much effort was being expended on mass trials, and on guaranteeing the attenuation of poliovirus strains, relatively little research had been done on guaranteeing the purity of the substrate in which the polioviruses were grown. Since live vaccines clearly cannot be inactivated, any latent viruses that might be present in the monkey kidney will necessarily be grown along with the weakened polioviruses. Identifying and eliminating such "adventitious agents" is far from easy, since one can test only for those contaminating viruses of which one is aware.

Herald Cox wrote a powerful article warning about the potential dangers of adventitious agents in MKTC in 1953,[43] and the first evidence of contaminating viruses in this substrate was announced by Rustigian in 1955.[44] Far more comprehensive reports of simian viruses in MKTC were published by Hull early in 1956,[45] and by two South Africans, Malherbe and Harwin, who reported on viruses in African monkeys in 1957.[46] However, it was really only at Washington in June 1960 that this became an issue of burning importance. By then, thirty-nine simian viruses had been recognized in the course of six years, most of which were relatively easy to identify and exclude from the final vaccine. But now Maurice Hilleman, of the vaccine house Merck, Sharp and Dohme (the same virologist who helped organize the hepatitis B vaccine trials in the seventies), announced the discovery of a new and far more dangerous monkey virus in the tissues of rhesus and cynomolgus macaques from Asia — the same monkeys that had been used to make most of the IPV and OPV administered to humans during the fifties.[47] This virus, SV40, was found to have the ability to immortalize cells, suggesting that it might promote cancer. Sure enough, shortly after this it was discovered that the fortieth simian virus could also cause tumors in the cheek pouches of hamsters — an area that is often used in biomedical testing, since it falls outside the range of the animal's immune system.[48] Was it conceivable that SV40 could also cause cancer in humans? The scientists were thrown into panic at the possibility that in their honest attempt to save lives and reduce suffering by eliminating one viral threat, they might have paved the way for another, potentially far more serious.

Meanwhile, however, the great momentum that was building up behind the Sabin strains of OPV could no longer be denied. In June 1960, during the second OPV conference in Washington, the WHO Expert Committee on Poliomyelitis made their deliberations, and shortly afterward produced a report that favored the Sabin strains above those of Koprowski and Cox, on grounds of both efficacy and safety.[49] Finally, in August 1960, the surgeon general, Leroy Burney, bowed to the inevitable and gave the official nod of approval to Sabin's three vaccines.[50] However, despite pressure from a now bullishly self-confident Sabin, he refused to be rushed into issuing licenses, and advised Americans to continue using the Salk vaccine until the problems of reversion to virulence had been completely eradicated from OPVs. Lederle, which had invested some $13 million in OPV research over the previous fourteen years, swiftly abandoned the Cox strains, instead applying to become one of the manufacturers of the Sabin vaccines. Koprowski, for his part, dispatched a flurry of letters to the surgeon general, the *British Medical Journal,* and the WHO, disputing some of the adverse findings, and trying to argue a case for at least using his Type 3 strain, Fox.[51] But he was already pursuing a lost cause, for it was clearly far easier for one complete set of vaccines to be adopted.

At the same time, Koprowski turned his attention to the contentious issue of the substrate, and was soon presenting a dramatically new set of opinions. In the wake of the SV40 revelations, the WHO had convened a Study Group on Requirements for Poliomyelitis Vaccine, to meet in November 1960, and had invited all the major vaccine-makers to submit their suggestions on the subject of vaccine safety. The documents submitted by Sabin, Cox, and James Gear from South Africa were all strongly worded, but none more so than that submitted by Koprowski and a young and trusted Wistar associate, Stanley Plotkin, which included a quite remarkable passage about the risks of contamination. It reads:

> Any tissue obtained from a normal animal may be parasitized by viruses probably harmless to the host most of the time. When such an organ is removed from the host and the cells allowed to multiply outside the control of the whole organism, as, for instance, in tissue culture, the virus "infected" cells seem to multiply (perhaps even at an advantage over the "non-infected" cells) and the virus which parasitized them is released. The number of viruses to be recovered from tissue culture explants of freshly removed animal organs is directly proportional to the number of biological assay systems employed for determining their presence. . . . [In] all probability, all vaccine lots fed to millions of people around the world contained at least one of these agents in addition to the attenuated strains of poliovirus. . . . [E]limination of these viruses from each lot of vaccine prepared from monkey kidney may present insurmountable obstacles for successful launching of the manufacture of the vaccine.[52]

The two virologists went on to suggest that, as a stopgap measure, a small quantity of such latent viruses could be permitted in a vaccine, adding that since each polio vaccine pool is diluted 100 to 500 times before use, this would mean that only very small amounts of extraneous viruses would be ingested by vaccinees. As a more permanent solution, they proposed that human cells could be employed as a substrate, instead of freshly removed monkey kidney. Controversially, they proposed that vaccines made from HeLa* cultures might, in fact, be safer than those made from MKTC "even though [HeLa] originated from a malignant tumour of man." As an alternative, they wrote, tissue cultures based on semistable human cells could be used. It so happened that at that very moment, Leonard Hayflick from the Wistar Institute was perfecting just such a substrate, WI-38, a human diploid cell strain that — in years to come — would be accepted by many virologists as perhaps the safest substrate for vaccine production.[53]

It took more than a year before the U.S. Public Health Service was finally persuaded that OPV was definitely a better and safer option than IPV, but licenses for Sabin's three oral polio vaccine strains were finally issued between August

---

\* HeLa: A vigorous *cell line* originating from the cervical tumor of Henrietta Lacks, who died in Baltimore in 1951. HeLa is one of the classic tumor cultures used for virus research in laboratories the world over, but as far as is known, it has never been used for vaccine production.

1961 and March 1962 — some months after OPV had been officially adopted in other countries, such as Great Britain. Surgeon General Burney praised the "great contributions" made by Cox and Koprowski, saying that large-scale field trials of their vaccines had shown "the hazards to man to be very, very slight." Their vaccines were not approved for commercial production.[54]

Not all the bouquets went Sabin's way, however. After small-scale trials of Koprowski's polio vaccines made in Hayflick's WI-38 human diploid cell strain (HDCS) in Switzerland and Sweden in 1962,[55] nearly 200,000 children were successfully fed his HDCS-prepared polio vaccines in Croatia (then part of Yugoslavia) beginning in 1963.[56] And although WI-38 has never been widely adopted as a polio vaccine substrate, it has been extensively used for other vaccines such as rabies and rubella.[57]

Lederle, meanwhile, perfected a trivalent vaccine called Orimune[58] — a single-dose cocktail of the three poliovirus types, which overcame the problems of interference between different types that had bedeviled other manufacturers, and which eventually went into large-scale production using the full set of Sabin strains. And in the seventies, Lederle became the sole OPV manufacturer in the United States, so the company's fifteen-year involvement with polio vaccine development in the forties and fifties did not, in the end, go unrewarded.

As the years passed, Sabin alone had to contend with the continuing problems of OPVs, such as the occasional reversions to virulence, which caused certain vaccinees (especially Type 3 vaccinees) to develop paralysis,[59] and the constant threat of further unknown simian viruses cropping up in the monkey kidney tissue cultures, which even today continue — largely for economic reasons — to be employed as the principal polio vaccine substrate.[60] As for SV40, epidemiological studies conducted in the sixties and seventies did not provide any hard proof that the simian virus could cause cancer in humans,[61] and it was only after Sabin's death in 1993 that the first really alarming data linking the simian virus to human cancer was published. A young Italian, Michele Carbone, found SV40 in the lungs of people with mesothelioma (a rapidly fatal tumor affecting the membranes lining lungs, heart, and viscera), and proposed that SV40 and asbestos had acted as cofactors in the neoplastic process. In 1996, Carbone also found SV40 in bone cancers called osteosarcomas.[62]

The original infections with SV40 must have taken place some four decades earlier, for by the middle of 1961 SV40 was being eliminated from vaccines, as manufacturers shifted from using the kidneys of Asian monkeys, to using those of the SV40-free African green monkey. Unfortunately, African greens were later found to have their own contaminating viruses — including, of course, an SIV, which was only discovered in the eighties.[63]

To Sabin, therefore, the victory. But what of Hilary Koprowski, the first man to develop and test an OPV in humans — what did he feel after spending fifteen years of his life on OPV research? In interviews he tended toward magnanimity, to say that he was glad not to have become a hero figure, to point out that when Albert Sabin had gone to Brazil, the children had sung beneath his hotel window — and that he, Hilary Koprowski, could not have borne such adulation.[64]

However, it would be surprising if, on sleepless nights, he never felt the merest twinge of envy. Be that as it may, Dr. Koprowski has not had to swallow the bitterest pill of all, for none of the four great rivals in the field of polio vaccination was ever awarded the ultimate prize. Perhaps because of the controversies, setbacks, and errors that had littered the history of IPV and OPV development, Jonas Salk, Albert Sabin, Hilary Koprowski, and Herald Cox were never to receive that gilded invitation to visit Stockholm in tie and tails, like John Enders and Renato Dulbecco.

# 15

## DR. DICK AND DR. DANE

Having learned something of the background to poliomyelitis vaccination, I felt it was important to gain some perspective on Hilary Koprowski, by talking with some of those who had worked with him or with his vaccine strains. The obvious place to begin was with the doctors who had been involved in the first major controversy of Koprowski's polio research — the Belfast trials of 1956. In the back of my mind, of course, was the fact that the apparent "first case of AIDS," David Carr, had spent nine months of his National Service just a two-hour train ride away from the trial site.

When I first interviewed him in 1992, George Dick was seventy-seven and had been officially retired for many years, although he retained a lively interest in medicine and was busily writing his memoirs. He and his wife were living in comfortable rural isolation in Sussex, in a Tudor house that boasted an unbroken view over rolling parkland. Tall, white-haired, and patrician in appearance, Professor Dick was nonetheless approachable and eager, with an almost boyish sense of humor. Now something of an *éminence grise*, he vividly recalled his involvement in one of the great medical controversies of the fifties.[1]

Feelings of injury usually diminish with the passing of time — unless, of course, they are bottled up. In that case they tend to concentrate, through steeping in their own juices. George Dick had not told his side of the story for some time but, thirty-six years after the events in question, was still in no doubt that he and his colleague David Dane had been sorely misled. Nonetheless, I was surprised by the faint hissing sound as the cork was unstoppered and he started recalling his experiences with Dr. Koprowski. "He told us the vaccine virus was completely safe, that there were no problems. Old Hilary was living in fairyland . . . he was just trying to promote his vaccine," he explained in a calm tone, which did little to conceal his indignation. "I think we were very, very badly let down, because we were presented with background information which I don't think was honest. I didn't know Hilary well then," he added.[2]

Fascinated, I asked Professor Dick to start the tale at the beginning. He had made his name, he told me, in the forties, working first in Mauritius, where he undertook a detailed epidemiological study of a wartime polio epidemic,[3] and then in Uganda, where he not only discovered a new pathogen called Mengo virus, but — in one of the less trumpeted traditions of virology — became accidentally infected with it. At the end of the decade he moved to the United States, and took a degree course at Johns Hopkins, where he worked on poliovirus inactivation, and studied under such luminaries of polio research as David Bodian. In 1955, after a spell with the Medical Research Council in London, he was invited to take over the new chair of microbiology at Queen's University, Belfast, and managed to recruit David Dane, a young and diligent researcher freshly returned from Australia. In retrospect, Dick regards Dane as "equal best brain with David Bodian in the whole field of poliomyelitis research."

One of the big attractions of working in Northern Ireland was the autonomy it offered, for in those days the province had its own parliament, and thus enjoyed a degree of independence from the political and medical grandees in London. It also offered a discrete and stable population, and one that had a reputation of cooperating with medical researchers. In the spring of 1955, the Cutter incident had introduced the first major doubts about the safety of Salk vaccine and, bearing in mind the successful live vaccines against smallpox and yellow fever, Dick and Dane were eager to investigate the viability of a live vaccine against polio. Their initial research involved testing the local population's antibody status against the three polio viruses.[4]

Dick had met Koprowski on several occasions during his years in America, and when they bumped into each other again in London in early 1955, Koprowski briefed him on his OPV strains, SM and TN. By this stage, Koprowski had already staged small clinical trials in homes for mentally handicapped children on the east and west coasts of America,[5] and was keen to mount larger trials in the general community, but knew that he would never receive U.S. government approval as long as IPV — the leading candidate vaccine — was undergoing efficacy trials in many different parts of North America.[6] After reflection, Dick told Koprowski that he might be able to organize a carefully controlled trial of SM and TN in Belfast. At this time, IPV was still in relatively short supply, and had still not undergone full-scale field trials in Britain, so Dick's proposal of step-by-step trials in an unvaccinated population, which would progress from the investigators themselves, through university volunteers and their children, to the children of volunteers from the general public, was both a valid test regime from the British perspective, and one that could be of real benefit to Koprowski's vaccine program.

It is clear that Dick and Koprowski — both iconoclasts — quickly fired each other's enthusiasm for the project. Dick sought approval from the powers-that-be in both London and Belfast (and was duly told that he personally would have to bear responsibility if anything went wrong). But by the time that final approval was granted, in the fall of 1955, Dick was also proposing the Koprowski strains for trial in other areas that fell under British protection.[7] One plan involved the immunization of small groups of children in Kenya. He also supported a proposal by Koprowski and the South African virologist James Gear to immunize the entire population of Tristan da Cunha, the volcanic outcrop in the South Atlantic, in a single day. These plans had already been approved by the Medical Research Council (MRC) before they were vetoed, apparently on ethical grounds, by "higher authorities" in the Colonial Office.[8]

The Belfast trials, however, went ahead as planned.[9] To begin with, Dick and Dane repeated the safety tests, and here Koprowski made a contribution by providing the services of one of his Lederle technicians, Doris Nelsen, who spent some weeks helping Dane inoculate different concentrations of the vaccines into the brains of mice. They also tested the Type 1 vaccine, SM, in the brains and spines of rhesus monkeys. All these tests produced results consistent with Koprowski's own, and so, in February 1956, the human trials began, to a small fanfare of publicity in the provincial press.[10] The first three volunteers, including George Dick, swallowed capsules containing a very small amount of SM, but only one of them was immunized.

Early in March, Koprowski flew to Belfast to address a meeting at Queen's University. Here he assured faculty members of the safety of his vaccines, and was apparently successful in persuading many to volunteer themselves and their children for the test program. Two days later he was in London, addressing an MRC clinical trials committee, with Dick and Dane once again present. Koprowski reassured the meeting that his research in America revealed that the SM strain was "not contagious" and that it did not increase in virulence after human passage.[11]

In April, a total of ten university staff members took a much larger dose of SM, and this time all developed antibodies. Then two infants were fed the vaccine in milk, and they too were successfully immunized. The minister of health and local government, Dame Dehra Parker, announced that the Northern Ireland government approved of the trials, and hoped that a larger test, involving children of different ages, could be staged by year's end.[12]

As the next element in the trials, Dick vaccinated his own four-year-old daughter. (This was consistent with one of the great democratic traditions of medical research, that innovators should first be prepared to implement their ideas at home.) Since his wife and their two other children all lacked Type 1 antibodies, this was a good test of whether the vaccine virus could spread in a normal family setting. To Dick's great surprise, it did. Five days after the girl's vaccination, her two-year-old brother also began to excrete virus and to develop

Type 1 antibodies, and then Mrs. Dick also demonstrated a low-level antibody response. More worryingly, when tested in monkey brains some days after passing through the human gut, the excreted vaccine virus showed evidence of an increase in neurovirulence (a small, but nonetheless ominous, "reversion to virulence"). In both these respects, SM was performing differently in the hands of Dick and Dane to its reported performance in the hands of Dr. Koprowski.

Here a little background is needed. Early in the summer of 1955, Koprowski had conducted his first full-scale trials of SM at Sonoma, an establishment for mentally handicapped children in California. In the course of these he and Tom Norton, assisted by a phalanx of nurses, had conducted two contact experiments, in one of which a group of six children who had been fed SM and who were excreting virus in their stools were kept "in very intimate contact" with another eight children who lacked Type 1 antibodies. In practice, this meant that for the next twenty days the children (all of whom were incontinent) were allowed to play together for three hours a day on a plastic mat, which, although it was washed down to prevent its becoming grossly soiled, was deliberately not disinfected. In the course of the experiment, three of the unvaccinated children became infected with Type 1 virus. By contrast, none of the nine nurses involved in the experiment (all of whom took careful precautions against infection, wearing caps and gowns and washing their hands after every contact with a child) developed Type 1 antibodies — and on this basis, somewhat surprisingly, Koprowski concluded that SM vaccine was not contagious. "It is quite clear," he wrote, "that when principles of simple personal hygiene are practiced, the attenuated SM virus . . . may be completely prevented from passing from one subject to another."[13] One year later in Belfast, the Dick family was finding differently.

If the Belfast findings on SM were surprising, those resulting from the trial of the TN Type 2 vaccine were little short of astonishing. Type 2 poliovirus is much less dangerous than Type 1 (accounting for less than 5 percent of all naturally occurring polio cases), and Koprowski had already fed TN to 150 children over a period of six years without apparent mishap. On these grounds (and after repeating the safety tests), Dick and Dane felt justified in feeding a sizable dose of TN to a larger group, comprising 21 adults and 169 children and infants.[14] David Dane and his children were among the TN volunteers.

In terms of immunization, the results were startlingly poor: only 22 percent of adults tested, and 77 percent of children, developed immunity. Those who were successfully immunized excreted TN virus in their stools for three weeks or longer after vaccination, and it was this excreted virus that produced the really disturbing finding. For whereas TN *vaccine* virus was found to be nonpathogenic, the virus was radically transformed by passage through the human gut. The *excreted* TN virus proved to be highly pathogenic, causing severe paralysis to half of the twenty-two monkeys injected in intracerebral safety tests. Dick and Dane concluded that TN vaccine was both unstable and potentially unsafe.

When I asked him about this, George Dick commented: "If we'd taken Koprowski's word and organized a large-scale trial, I have no doubt at all that we could have paralyzed a number of children and, if this had happened, this would have set back the introduction of oral polio vaccine for quite a long time."[15]

The 1956 annual report of the MRC referred to Dick and Dane's studies as "the first trial of live poliomyelitis vaccines in a normal community,"[16] and the investigators were obviously shaken to the core by having staged open trials of what they now considered a potentially dangerous vaccine — one that they had also fed to family members and recommended to friends and colleagues.

Some time in October or November 1956, Koprowski heard of the preliminary results and immediately flew to London, where he met with Dick, Dane, and a dozen other British scientists at the Savoy.[17] He attempted to argue that the Belfast results were equivocal. Eventually, he made it clear that he was prepared to jettison TN, although he proposed that the SM strain could be retained in a modified form. He was listened to politely, but his visit had no effect on the Belfast men's resolve, for their three papers on SM and TN were published in the *British Medical Journal* in January 1957.[18]

The first two papers, detailing the course of the Belfast experiments, are couched in typically restrained scientific language. But the gloves are removed for the final paper, entitled "The Evaluation of TN and SM Virus Vaccines." After pointing out the many differences between their test results and Koprowski's, Dick and Dane examine the key issue of safety. First, they describe how SM was readily transmitted in a normal household. Then they turn to TN. Koprowski had reported that TN virus was only rarely excreted, and then only at very low concentrations; and that, because of the character of the virus, there were "formidable odds" against the contagiousness of the vaccine strain.[19] By contrast, Dick and Dane found that TN virus was excreted by all but one of the vaccinees they tested, that it was excreted for lengthy periods, and that, after multiplication in the alimentary tract, the excreted virus was "as virulent as many naturally occurring polio strains." Furthermore, although they had not set up their trials to examine this possibility, they observed that "there is no reason to assume that it may not spread." If a polio vaccine possessed the capacities to revert and to spread, then it also had the potential to spark a full-scale epidemic.

Dick and Dane concluded as follows: "it does not seem that SM and TN fecal viruses differ in any measurable way from naturally occurring strains, and therefore we do not consider that SM and TN vaccines should be used at the moment on a large scale." They were recommending that SM and TN should never again be used in human trials. Nor were they.[20] Indeed, six months later, in an unusually forthright statement, the WHO Expert Committee formally declared TN vaccine to be unfit for human use.[21]

Nowadays, David Dane has retired, and lives in a house on the edge of a wood near the Hog's Back, to the southwest of London. He has not stopped working, however, and has played a significant role in some of the more celebrated medico-legal cases of the last few years, such as that brought by British hemophiliacs who were given HIV-contaminated Factor VIII, and by the parents of children who, in the seventies, were fed growth hormone made from the pituitary glands of human corpses. The hormone, it was later learned, was contaminated with a tiny protein particle, a prion, which causes Creutzfeldt-Jakob disease or CJD — a usually fatal brain condition similar to scrapie in sheep and BSE (mad cow disease) in cattle.

When reviewing his work on polio vaccines, David Dane is quiet and cautious, sometimes almost painfully careful in phrasing his replies to questions, and in the course of several lengthy interviews spread over six years, I came to value greatly his considered judgments. During this time, we attempted to unravel the enigma of the Belfast episode: the true sequence of events, the question of who had known what — and when they had known it.

In retrospect, David Dane concedes that their findings on SM — the small indications of a reversion to virulence and the evidence of spread within George Dick's family were "of arguable importance."[22] But his natural caution vanishes when it comes to discussing the Type 2 vaccine. "The situation was quite different with TN. This was a striking kind of reversion. . . . To other virologists, this must have looked like a major boob by Koprowski." He added that the virulence of the excreted TN virus was roughly a hundred times greater than for any Type 2 vaccine that has been tested before or since.

One of the main reasons for Dick and Dane's initial indignation back in the fifties was their belief that Koprowski must have known about the less promising qualities of TN and SM from his own trials, but that he had nevertheless allowed them to proceed blind. However, after reviewing several of the relevant papers that I had brought with me, David Dane began to change his mind. He began to ponder whether it was possible that Koprowski and Norton had been so confident about TN that they had never actually tested the viruses excreted by vaccinees in MKTC. If so, it was a dramatic error.

Later, David Dane started recalling details about a polio conference held in New York in early 1957, at around the same time that their articles had appeared in the *British Medical Journal.* At this meeting, George Dick had apparently told the audience that TN had "gone in like a lamb, but come out like a lion," and Koprowski made an interesting response. By this time, he had presumably had the opportunity to check the preliminary Belfast results against stored fecal samples from his own TN vaccinees, and he now performed a complete volte-face, acting as if he had known about this tendency all along. "I remember him saying at Belfast and at the MRC meeting that TN was noncytopathogenic, and that very little virus was recovered [from the stools] after feeding. But then in New York he said — with exactly the same aplomb — that excreted TN *was* cytopathogenic. It amused George and me. He talked very persuasively — you could very easily be sold a pup," Dane explained. Later, he added: "All my generation of virologists know that Koprowski is a good virologist [and that he is] charming, amusing, and something of an intellectual, but we wouldn't actually trust him all that much."

The conference in question was on "Cellular Biology, Nucleic Acids and Viruses," convened by the New York Academy of Sciences, and staged at the Waldorf Astoria between January 7 and 9, 1957.[23] Intriguingly, the published record of this conference, which appeared in December 1957, entirely omitted Dick's metaphor about lambs and lions, and contained a dramatically rewritten version of Koprowski's address, one that made no reference to TN, and that dealt only briefly with SM.[24] Instead, this published version of the speech concentrated almost entirely on Koprowski's work on his two brand-new polio vaccines, CHAT Type 1 and Fox Type 3.

Various references appended to the published version of Koprowski's speech make it clear that it must have been written at least five months after the conference was held, and probably at the latter end of 1957, shortly before the volume's publication in December. At that time, the vice president and president-elect of the New York Academy of Sciences, and chairman of its section of biology (effectively responsible for the conference), was Dr. Hilary Koprowski.[25]

---

The Belfast episode encapsulates an important ethical dilemma for scientists. When the stakes get high, and when there is the realistic possibility of achieving an important scientific or medical breakthrough that may be of real benefit to humanity, can the potential rewards ever justify being so bold and fearless that the health and safety of human guinea pigs, of "volunteers," is placed in jeopardy? Alternatively, let us put the question in reverse. Is the scientist morally bound to protect volunteers from harm at all costs, even when this will quite possibly result in the loss of data and information that might, in the future, save many more lives?

Dick and Dane's *BMJ* articles, and Dick's forthright dismissal of TN and SM as vaccine strains at the New York conference,[26] prompted many of Koprowski's peers to the thought that the fecal samples had well and truly hit the fan. The published accounts reveal only the most basic details of what happened next — but the events of January 1957 apparently brought matters between Koprowski and his boss, Herald Cox, to a head,[27] and Koprowski and Norton left Lederle Laboratories shortly afterward, to re-emerge at the Wistar Institute.

We also know that, despite the Belfast debacle, Koprowski — now, at long last, his own boss in name as well as deed — was still eager to carry out vaccine field trials in the open community. And even though he had been frustrated a year earlier with Tristan da Cunha and Kenya, his gaze seems to have fallen, once again, on the continent of Africa.

———————

My first interview with George Dick took place in the morning, and with David Dane in the afternoon of a particularly balmy day in the August of 1992. Late that evening, as the temperatures began to drop, I drove home slowly, turning over in my mind what had been said, and trying to work out just how — if at all — the Belfast vaccinations might have impacted on the story of David Carr and his fatal illness. My initial instinct was that there was only a remote possibility of a genuine link between the two events. Since SM had been prepared by alternate passages through monkey kidney tissue culture and chick embryo tissue culture, there was a theoretical possibility of contamination with a simian virus. However, it had been fed only to eleven adults, all members of staff from Queen's University in Belfast. TN had been fed to nearly two hundred subjects in Belfast and Oxford — and possibly in other unspecified towns in Northern Ireland. But since it had been manufactured in a suspension of rodent brains and spinal cord, there seemed to be no possibility that contamination with a monkey virus could have occurred.

However, in the days and months that followed, I did some further research. This revealed that in 1956 the War Office (concerned by the possible exposure to polioviruses of persons serving in epidemic areas, like West Africa) had given polio vaccine — IPV, presumably — to most of the children of its personnel serving in overseas commands.[28] No details were provided about vaccinations of the servicemen themselves, though it seemed entirely possible that at least some would also have been immunized. Later, I noticed that the MRC polio meeting of March 7, 1956, the one that had been addressed by Hilary Koprowski, had been attended by Brigadier G.T.L. Archer, who was at the time consulting pathologist to the army and therefore directly responsible for polio vaccination.[29] The minutes of another committee meeting from this period reveal a proposal to stage a trial of the Sabin strains on troops going to Kenya, which highlights the fact that the military personnel of the period were viewed as providing a reliable and amenable source of "volunteers" for vaccine experiments.[30]

It was clear that the military was interested in the potential of OPV, and it seemed entirely plausible that, while using IPV for most of the early vaccinations, the service chiefs might also have decided to test the oral version on certain of their troops during 1956 and 1957. It occurred to me that perhaps, on the advice of Brigadier Archer, they elected to assess Koprowski's strains, and perhaps, like George Dick, they decided to use the province of Northern Ireland as an accessible, but pristine, testing ground. If so, then might they not have included men serving in Londonderry, such as the crew of H.M.S. *Whitby*?

A few months later, I went to Northern Ireland to investigate this hypothesis. In Derry, now peaceful again after the Troubles of the seventies and eighties, I got a sense of what it must have been like when David Carr was based there. In those days the British sailors used to wander freely around the town, laughing and drinking with the locals in the pubs and dance halls, the main disruptions coming not from snipers and bombers, but from the B Specials, the notorious military police. I questioned a local doctor who had had some experience of H.M.S. *Sea Eagle*, the "stone frigate," which was the local base for H.M.S. *Whitby*, but he knew of no evidence to suggest that Koprowski's polio vaccines had ever been fed to the military there. Later, a kind local librarian did some research among her friends and among various elderly doctors, and reported back about a series of vaccinations conducted on women working in the local shirt factories in the fifties and sixties. However, without exact dates, or certainty about which vaccines had been given, the information was simply not usable.[31]

Soon after this, however, I discovered another extraordinary coincidence. There was one European country where Koprowski's CHAT vaccine had been fed during 1957, the same year as the first experimental CHAT trials in the Belgian Congo, and this was Sweden. A total of eighty-five people from Stockholm had been vaccinated with CHAT in the course of a household study conducted by Professor Sven Gard and colleagues from the Karolinska Institute.[32] The first feedings (of the infants in each family) had begun in November 1957, and vaccinations had continued through to February 1958. Since I now knew that David Carr had visited Malmo, Sweden's third city, in the June of 1957, I wondered if it was possible that CHAT (or SM) could have been fed informally by private doctors to Swedish adults in the months preceding November 1957. If so, was it conceivable that a young adult vaccinee could have become infected with an SIV contaminant in that vaccine, and then onwardly transmitted this virus, perhaps sexually, to a visiting British sailor such as David?

I had to admit that, even more than the Londonderry scenario, this seemed absurdly far-fetched. There were some correlations of place and time, to be sure, but when examined more closely, they really didn't hold up. Vaccinations with Koprowski's strains had apparently occurred in the same countries where David had been, but in different towns, and at slightly different times. Although it was tempting to claim synchronicity, the links were probably spurious, mere artifacts of the inquiry — unless, of course, some new information emerged.

# 16

"WHAT HAPPENS WHEN SCIENCE GOES BAD"

A couple of months after reading the *Rolling Stone* article,[1] I decided to write a letter to Blaine Elswood, the AIDS activist based at the University of California whom Tom Curtis had credited as being the original author of the OPV/AIDS hypothesis.[2] By this time Elswood, together with an immunologist from San Francisco, Dr. Raphael Stricker, had written a brief letter to the *Lancet* in support of Curtis's article, in which they proposed that the origin of AIDS was a vitally important subject to research for three reasons. "The sociological reason," they wrote, "is that victims of the disease should not be blamed for starting it; the scientific reason is that new therapies for AIDS could be developed from an understanding of its origin; and the ethical reason is that the sequence of events culminating in AIDS should never be allowed to happen again."[3] The two researchers also cited a more detailed paper on the hypothesis, which they had submitted to *Research in Virology,* a French journal edited by Luc Montagnier, but which was still "in press" several months later. In my letter to Elswood, I asked a number of questions, and requested the address of Tom Curtis, together with a draft copy of their latest manuscript.

A few days later Curtis phoned me from his home in Houston; he had received a copy of my letter, and was answering direct. He was friendly and helpful, and wanted to know my thoughts about the *Rolling Stone* piece. I told him that I found much of it persuasive, but also outlined my principal reservations. We talked about the vagueness concerning the species used for the tissue culture work on CHAT. I said I thought that an SIV from chimpanzees was a much likelier bet for an HIV-1 precursor than one from African green monkeys; Curtis responded, quite correctly, that Koprowski's uncertainty on this issue only emphasized that almost any species of kidney could have been used. I also told Curtis that opponents of the theory would doubtless argue that if CHAT were the cause of HIV-1, then why had HIV-2 emerged at roughly the same moment in time? Surely the theory would be more persuasive if there were evidence to suggest that a second and similar vaccination campaign had occurred around the same time period in West Africa, the hearth of HIV-2. Curtis was less convinced.

He added that he had written several follow-up articles, including one for the *Washington Post*,[4] and that a sequel was planned in *Rolling Stone*. Koprowski, he told me, was now refusing to answer further questions, and the Wistar Institute had apparently set up a scientific committee to respond to his article, and to decide whether or not to release samples of the original vaccines for testing — as he had advocated at the end of his piece. He asked if I knew of a laboratory that was experienced in PCR work, and I told him I was in contact with one that would be pleased to collaborate.

A week or so later Tom Curtis phoned again, and in the course of the conversation he told me about a mysterious man called Louis Pascal from New York City, who communicated only by letter. Pascal had apparently been working on the OPV/AIDS hypothesis for several years, but had never managed to get anything published on the subject in a medical journal — until, that is, December 1991, when the University of Wollongong, near Sydney, Australia, had published a lengthy working paper by him, entitled "What Happens When Science Goes Bad."[5] This paper had contained essentially the same hypothesis as that proposed by Elswood, Stricker, and Curtis (which Pascal had apparently arrived at before any of them) — and a lot more besides. The first Curtis had learned about Pascal's existence was when he received a letter from him, shortly after the publication of his feature in *Rolling Stone*. Curtis now gave me Pascal's address, as well as details of the Wollongong paper.

The next morning a letter and a package of papers arrived from Raphael Stricker, including a draft of the article that he and Elswood had submitted to *Research in Virology*.[6] It was immediately apparent that their research had been the source for many of the ideas in the Curtis article, but their article was most effective in those places where it augmented what Curtis had written. It included an illuminating passage on early vaccine accidents, such as the experimental plague vaccine from 1902 that had killed nineteen Punjabi villagers, due to a tetanus contaminant, and the cholera vaccine that had become contaminated with plague bacilli, and that had caused the death of thirteen American prisoners in the Philippines in 1906. The draft article also detailed the infamous 1942 hepatitis B epidemic, which eventually affected a third of a million people, after some fifty thousand U.S. servicemen had been given a yellow fever vaccine stabilized with human serum that was contaminated with hepatitis B virus.[7] This highlighted the potential for exponential disaster that new and inadequately tested vaccines represented, and helped place the alleged African episode with CHAT in proper context.

Also included in the package were several of Curtis's newspaper articles, which detailed a number of important developments to the OPV/AIDS story and showed that he had managed to keep that story on the boil for the better part of six months.[8] This in turn had prompted further coverage in eminent science journals like *Science*[9] and the *Lancet*.[10]

The thing that most intrigued me about Stricker's letter was his response to my comment that evidence of an early vaccine trial having been staged in West Africa would make the OPV/AIDS theory even more persuasive. He wrote back: "I can only say that (as you surmised) the Congo vaccine trial was *not* the only trial performed in Africa at that time. Further information on this issue, however, will require some tough investigative work, perhaps by an inquisitive journalist." This was more tantalizing than revealing, but a fortnight later I got a follow-up letter from Blaine Elswood, who wrote: "I have just noticed your comment about the 'geographical synchronicity' of the HIV-2 epidemic and [SIVsm] infections in West Africa. It is very probable that vaccines used in that region were manufactured there using local species. The French scientists in Gabon and Cameroons were racing the Americans with their own vaccines. Dr. Leonard Hayflick claims that they were using all sorts of primate species, including baboons."[11]

---

By this stage I had received my copy of Louis Pascal's "Working Paper No. 9," from Brian Martin, head of the Science and Technology Analysis Research Program at the University of Wollongong. It bore the promising title "What Happens When Science Goes Bad. The Corruption of Science and the Origin of AIDS: A Study in Spontaneous Generation," and it turned out to be an absolutely remarkable document. After reading just a few pages, I knew that this paper was more than just the product of hard work and enterprising research. Louis Pascal (a striking name, evoking thoughts of Louis Pasteur and the great seventeenth-century writer and thinker Blaise Pascal) was clearly a very unusual man indeed.

In the course of his 19,000-word treatise, Pascal reveals nothing about himself other than the fact that he had once contributed a chapter to a fairly eminent anthology on ethics.[12] In terms of science, he appears to be no more than an enthusiastic amateur. And yet such is his clarity of thinking and intellectual rigor, that most of his observations are stunning in their perspicacity. In certain passages it is hard to escape the conclusion that here one is in the presence of genius. And yet, as with so many of the works of geniuses, there is a worm in the apple. There is a sense in which Pascal's masterful creation leaves one with a strange, sour sensation on the tongue, one that is hard to place, but that seems to bear the tang of obsession and a stubborn refusal to conciliate. One can understand how some might not find this strong, uncompromising flavor to their liking, and how editors of scientific journals, in particular, might react negatively.

Pascal traces his interest in the origin of AIDS to a radio broadcast in May 1987. On the last day of that month, he was listening to a WABC show entitled *Natural Living with Gary Null* — a medley of alternative medicine, New Age therapies, and inspired and wacky ideas.[13] An extraordinary woman from San Antonio, Eva Lee Snead, was being interviewed by Null; she described herself as a physician, although her license to practice medicine had been revoked. Ms. Snead believed she had discovered the origin of AIDS. She told Null that oral polio vaccines had been made from the kidneys of African green monkeys, that these monkeys were frequently infected with simian viruses, including SV40 and SIV, and that SV40 was the cause of the AIDS epidemic. Pascal listened spellbound to Snead's presentation, and immediately realized that if there were any truth at all in these claims, then they ought to be seriously pursued. A modicum of research proved to him that the first two claims were absolutely correct — even though Snead's third proposal, blaming AIDS on SV40, was so implausible that it led to the suspicion that she was not an altogether discriminating researcher.[14]

Pascal began researching at the local library, and soon located articles about the SV40 contamination of polio vaccines. Then he found the source of Snead's central assertion — an article by Phyllis Kanki and Max Essex of Harvard, describing the isolation of an SIV from the African green monkey.[15] Toward the end of this article, he found the following observation: "Much of the oral polio vaccine (OPV) used throughout the world is produced on primary cultures of kidney cells from this species." This piece had been published in November 1985, but by May 1987, it seems, only Eva Lee Snead had thought to ask the obvious follow-up question.

Pascal did some more searching, and he came across the key article in the *British Medical Journal*, which described the 1957/8 CHAT trials in the Belgian Congo and Ruanda-Urundi.[16] Suddenly he realized that these, the earliest mass feedings of OPV in the world, had been staged in three of the countries (Congo, Rwanda, and Burundi) that now had some of the highest HIV-prevalence figures in the world, in the very part of Africa where many suspected the AIDS epidemic to have begun. He also found Sabin's articles about the contamination of this very same OPV batch with an unknown simian virus, and Koprowski's articles about the follow-up trials in Leopoldville, starting in August 1958, just a few months before the world's first-ever HIV-positive blood sample was taken from a man in the same city.

In his working paper, Pascal points out that in 1958 the population of the capital of the Belgian Congo had been just over one-ten-thousandth of the world population, thus highlighting what he calls "the extraordinary . . . coincidence in time and place." He also quotes Koprowski's response to the problem of simian contamination, delivered at the Second International Conference on Live Poliovirus Vaccines, in June 1960: "If, indeed, somebody were to poke his nose into the live virus vaccine, he might find a non-polio virus in all the preparations currently available," and his conclusion that this mattered little, since every day people were exposed orally to many viruses in their food.[17] Pascal rejects Koprowski's response as inadequate, for three reasons. The first is that it was impossible that polio vaccine, as then manufactured, could have been rendered free of contaminating simian viruses, and that Koprowski therefore had an obligation to pronounce these contaminants harmless — or to abandon his polio vaccine altogether. (Attenuated poliovirus was grown on monkey kidney tissue culture and the vaccine prepared by filtering the culture fluid, thereby removing bacteria but retaining the polioviruses — and any other viruses that might be present in the kidney.) The second reason is that humans are not, in the normal run of things, exposed to monkey viruses, and that even those who eat monkey meat would presumably not eat it raw. (Here he adds that the best way to introduce a virus to a new species is to give it to infants, whose immature immune systems are less likely to reject it, and that newborns were indeed among those fed the vaccine in Africa.) His third reason is that viruses introduced to virgin populations for the first time often become especially virulent and contagious (like flu viruses among Eskimos, and smallpox virus to Incas and Aztecs).

Pascal then launches into Koprowski, opining that he failed to take into account the potential consequences if his assumption (that simian viruses in vaccines were harmless) was wrong. "On arguments that a mere schoolchild could see were no more than wishful thinking he risked hundreds of millions of lives, and was never even aware of it," he writes, before continuing: "But his arguments were wrong. It was completely predictable that monkey viruses would get started in a new species never exposed to them before. And it was almost completely predictable that not all of them would be harmless. And now this almost completely predictable disaster has occurred. In fact it occurred right off the bat. This very first batch of vaccine gave us AIDS."

It was ironic, of course, that five months after giving that reassuring speech at the second Washington conference, Koprowski completely changed his stance about MKTC. In November 1960, he began urging people to abandon this substrate in favor of WI-38, the Wistar's very own human diploid cell strain. By that time, however, he had already given millions of people his vaccine made in monkey kidneys — most of whom came not from Africa, but from Poland, where over seven million were fed his strains.

Pascal goes on to deride the standard theory of AIDS origin, which developed soon after the 1985 discovery of SIVs in monkeys. He refers to this mockingly as the "monkey bite theory," although it actually embraces a much wider spectrum of contacts between humans and simians, extending from hunting, catching, skinning, and eating monkeys, to keeping them as pets. (This is the theory that I have characterized as "natural transfer.") Pascal proposes that even if scientists had known about SIV at the time of the first mass feedings of OPV in 1957, and had possessed a test enabling them to identify and exclude SIV from lots of the vaccine, that as time passed and the number of vaccinees rose from thousands to millions and to hundreds of millions, it was almost inevitable that someone in a vaccine lab would get careless and make a mistake, and that a contaminated batch of vaccine would get through. As it was, of course, the SIVs were discovered only after the advent of AIDS, and before then no test for their presence existed. Up to 1985, the only effective precaution against SIV was the exclusion of sick-looking monkeys from tissue culture work — and yet, of course, SIV does not cause green monkeys to fall sick. In any case, concludes Pascal, "[r]egardless of the precautions scientists might have been taking, it simply goes without saying that when, two decades after embarking on such a procedure, the monkey disease *is* found to have crossed over into our species, the first place one should look is to the procedure, and not to a monkey bite."

He goes even further, pointing out that many different monkey species have been found to carry SIV infections and, furthermore, that each individual species may be infected with more than just one SIV. Humans, for instance, can be infected with a total of three polioviruses, and at least two HIVs. He notes that two molecular biologists, Sharp and Li, estimate that both HIV-1 and HIV-2 entered the human race shortly before the year 1960,[18] adding that these two viruses were discovered only in 1983 and 1985, respectively. Using these as models, Pascal calculates that vaccines made in monkey kidney (such as those against poliovirus and adenovirus)[19] may have caused other SIVs to transfer into humans, and that this might have been occurring every one to three years since the late fifties, with each new arrival being recognized only when it had spread to a large number of people — perhaps a million or more.

This was a highly controversial proposition, but it did not take long for events to provide empirical support for the hypothesis. Just months after Pascal's paper was published, in 1992, the first formal reports appeared of a third strain of human immunodeficiency virus in AIDS patients and asymptomatic persons from Cameroon and Gabon. (This is the virus that Gerry Myers had told me about, and that would later come to be called HIV-1 Group O — to distinguish it from the "classic" HIV-1, now officially known as HIV-1 Group M.)[20] The closest simian relative of both these HIV-1s seems to be SIVcpz, the SIV found in the common chimpanzee, *Pan troglodytes,* though both of the human viruses seem to represent a separate transfer of SIVcpz from chimp to man.

The original thinking in Pascal's paper testifies to the fact that he approaches AIDS from the perspective of an interested amateur and armchair theorist, rather than a scientific specialist in this or that small field (one who is unable, or unwilling, to look out over the hedge to gain the larger view). In this spirit, he digresses a little from his main theme, in order to calculate that "several hundred millions" of the world's present population are likely to become infected with HIV in the course of their lifetimes.[21] He concedes that this estimate does not allow for behavior change in the face of AIDS, or for the possible development of a vaccine or cure in years to come. But he adds, ominously, that no vaccine or treatment has ever been developed against a lentivirus,[22] and indeed, in his opinion, AIDS is likely to become more infectious and transmissible as time passes, and as it becomes better adapted to its new host, *Homo sapiens.*

The foregoing subjects take up perhaps half of Pascal's working paper. In the second half of the treatise, he shifts his focus to concentrate on the story of his own frustrated attempts to alert the world. Until 1991, when Brian Martin of Wollongong University agreed to publish "What Happens. . . ," he had labored for four and a half years, without managing to get any of his research made available to a wider audience. As those years passed, and as his letters and papers continued to be ignored, Pascal became more and more obsessed by the thought of the further millions who would die as a result of the failures of those in positions of influence and authority to take heed of his warnings, and to make sensible responses.

He describes and dates his odyssey of disillusionment in some detail. After hearing the Eva Lee Snead radio broadcast in May 1987 and doing his initial research, he produced his first paper on the subject, laying out his central evidence, in November 1987.[23] The following month he sent out copies to seven biologists, six AIDS researchers, and several others, receiving only one brief acknowledgment in reply. He also submitted the paper to three scientific journals, all of which rejected it (the *Lancet* without reason, *New Scientist* without reply, and *Nature* on the strangely inaccurate grounds that whereas the theory "cannot be ruled out, it does not seem to fit the epidemiology of AIDS"). He also posted it to two multidisciplinary publications, which responded that it belonged in a scientific journal. When he sent copies to some of the philosophers whose work had been published together with his in the book *Applied Ethics,* he did receive some responses, and in August 1988 R. M. Hare forwarded the paper to the *Journal of Medical Ethics.* The editor, Raanan Gillon, wrote to inform Pascal that the article, as it stood, was inappropriate for his journal, but requested another much shorter version, which would outline the OPV/AIDS theory but concentrate on the ethics of the various editors' rejections. Apparently Pascal received the letter containing this offer only in the spring of 1990, by which time he felt himself unable to write the article requested. Instead he wrote his 19,000-word treatise, which was completed in April 1991. It was rejected by the *Journal of Medical Ethics*,[24] but accepted by Brian Martin.

Pascal makes much of Gillon's rejection letter, which featured the sentence: "There is just no way that I can publish a 19,000 word paper, even if I thought it was going to save *millions* of lives as you suggest (and I have to say that I remain unconvinced by this speculation)." He claims that Gillon has "withheld extraordinarily vital information from the world for three years now, waiting for a version more to his liking."[25]

Nowhere, however, in his attack does he acknowledge his own failure to submit an article of a length that the journal's editor felt to be appropriate. Pascal's attitude seems to be that the information he has to impart is so vitally important that normal rules do not apply. Even if there is a 10 percent chance, or a 1 percent chance, of its being correct, he says, then the editors are duty bound to publish, when failure to do so might have such catastrophic consequences.

One sees his point, and one can sense his anguish. But one worries about the attitude, the style — which seems almost to guarantee the project's failure. And it is this same stubborn, perhaps heroic refusal to compromise (some might say egocentricity) that permeates the rest of his paper. As far as Pascal is concerned, his hypothesis is so clearly correct that any who don't see it as such must be either foolish or corrupt. If he is aware that his confrontational stance tends to alienate, he shows no inclination to adapt.

And herein lies the tragedy of Pascal's work. The more frustrated he grows, the more uncompromising and virulent he becomes in his denunciations of those who, he feels, have reneged on their responsibilities. A vicious circle develops, with those who are best placed to respond sensibly becoming ever more defensive. Furthermore, he makes no allowances for the exceptional integrity and courage it would take for a leading scientist of the nineties to address, publicly, his momentous allegations about the safety of vaccines — allegations that affect millions. Instead, he seems intent on rubbing noses in the mess.

He ends by listing the groups that have neglected their responsibilities by failing to follow up on Essex and Kanki's article of November 1985, when SIV was effectively "discovered." These include vaccine researchers and AIDS researchers, people involved in the life sciences, science reporters who should have been following up such suggestive clues, and journal editors whose job it should be to broadcast vital new developments (but whose actual purpose, he says, seems to be the preservation of the status quo). Why had none of these "gatekeepers of knowledge," these supposedly informed sources and inquiring minds, asked the obvious question about whether oral polio vaccines (and, in particular, Koprowski's CHAT as used in central Africa) might have sparked the AIDS epidemic?

In a passage that typifies this section of the paper, Louis Pascal delivers the following stinging rebuke:

> I spent weeks carefully sifting through hundreds of articles and distilling them down to a picture so clear no one could have failed to understand it. . . . The research that the scientists should have done themselves a long time ago, I did for them. . . . They had nothing to do but check it out, using the references supplied, references from their own medical journals. Even this was beyond them. And it is not a matter of a single editor or scientist being particularly stupid or particularly irresponsible. It happened over and over. Unless one is prepared to argue that those journals and researchers I sent my work to were a few rotten apples entirely unrepresentative of science as a whole, one must reach the conclusion that people of this caliber typify science.

Toward the end of the paper, he issues a challenge.

> Much that I have said in this piece is of an extreme nature, and extremely uncomplimentary to scientists, editors, and indeed the whole human race. But again, these conclusions follow so immediately from the extremity of the facts, if they are as I allege, that the best if not only way around them is to disprove the allegations. You are quite welcome to try. I think you will find there is a good deal more evidence for my position than I have given here. . . . I think that in fact I have understated things, in places quite considerably.

It was a fine gauntlet he had thrown — one which I, for one, felt to be a legitimate challenge.

# 17

LOUIS PASCAL

I had written to Louis Pascal immediately after getting his address from Tom Curtis, and in mid-September 1992, a fortnight or so after his working paper arrived from Australia, I received an extraordinary package from the man who has quite rightly become known as the founding father of the OPV/AIDS hypothesis. This marked the beginning of a lengthy and sometimes volatile correspondence that would last for some years.

The sheer quantity and detail of the material Pascal sent was quite remarkable. Together with a long and amicable letter was a "documentation packet," as he called it, containing nine batches of supporting articles, or sets of correspondence, on different subjects. It took me several days to read — and more to digest — the contents.

Pascal cleared up one mystery at the start of his letter. It was not he, he explained, who had sent a selection of articles about polio vaccines and AIDS to the British virologist Myra McClure, but rather Herbert Ratner, a physician who had been the public health director for Oak Park, a suburb of Chicago, at the time of the first vaccinations with Salk's inactivated vaccine in the spring of 1955. Because he had reservations about the safety of that vaccine, Ratner, alone among his peers, postponed the immunization in his area. A fortnight later, the Cutter incident proved that his skepticism was justified, but even after changes were ordered to the manufacturing process, Ratner continued to insist that it was Salk's inactivation recipe, rather than Cutter's implementation of that recipe, that was inadequate, and that, in reality, many IPV lots released after mid-1955 contained residual amounts of live Mahoney poliovirus. This stance earned him huge opprobrium among fellow public health officials, and eventually cost him his job. Nonetheless, various of his articles prove that several

famous virologists, including Herald Cox of Lederle and Sven Gard from Sweden, offered Ratner support.

In July 1987, Ratner proposed a far more contentious theory when he wrote a letter to the *Lancet* in which he sought to link Salk's IPV to the AIDS epidemic. (This came shortly after Eva Lee Snead's similar broadcast warning about OPVs, but before the first of Pascal's articles.) In his letter, Ratner pointed out that SV40 was known to have survived the inactivation process and to have been present in the IPV doses given to millions of people between 1954 and 1961. Like Snead, Ratner proposed that, once inside human cells, SV40 had hybridized with other viruses to produce HIV, and to spark the AIDS pandemic. The letter was rejected by the *Lancet,* but he published it the following year in *Child & Family* (a small medical journal which he himself edited).[1]

Pascal included a set of Ratner's articles from *Child & Family,*[2] and I later received further information in a letter from the man himself. It seemed to me that the first part of Ratner's premise was reasonable, in that a vaccine injected directly into the bloodstream is an even more likely vehicle than an oral vaccine for unintentionally transferring a viral contaminant. There were major problems with the rest of his hypothesis, however. The first was that whereas traces of SV40 usually survived the inactivation procedures, SIV (a far more labile virus) is readily destroyed by exposure to formalin. The second centered on the epidemiology. IPV had been used across America, but only minimally in Africa. The areas where HIV and AIDS first appeared simply didn't match the areas where the vaccine had been injected. The third problem, however, was the clincher, for by the early nineties, it was quite apparent that SIV, rather than any hybrid of SV40, was the cause of AIDS.

Though finally misguided, Ratner's work did highlight one important detail. Just as Pascal had done, Ratner concluded that if the AIDS virus came from monkeys, then we should not look to a monkey bite as the means of transfer, but rather to the millions of vaccinations that were known to have been transferring monkey viruses wholesale into our species since the start of the fifties. Just like Pascal, he had sought to publicize the dangers of vaccines made in monkey kidneys and his warnings, like those of Pascal, were being ignored.

Ratner's ideas were thought-provoking but, to my mind, it was Pascal's that were really exciting. He continued his letter to me by addressing the "monkey bite theory," which, he said, suffered from an intrinsic problem. If (as seemed increasingly likely) the SIVs had been present in African monkeys for many thousands of years, why was it only now that any of these viruses had been transferred into humans? He also rated the "lost tribe" refinement to the theory as highly implausible — first because sexual behavior in African cultures had always been diverse (and had always included promiscuous cultures), and second because there had never been any tribes so isolated that they could not have spread such a newly acquired virus to their neighbors, and they to theirs. In any case, with HIV-2, there was now a need for two lost tribes. "Why is it," inquired Pascal, whimsically, "that lentiviruses are so good at infecting lost tribes, having managed to do it twice, yet have never ever managed to infect any of the vastly more common non-lost tribes?" The point was excellently made, even if the titles he gave to the theories were inherently pejorative.[3]

Pascal was now warming to his theme. Although he had no hard evidence to support the contention, he reckoned that a vaccine (perhaps made from the kidneys of the sooty mangabey) was by far the most likely explanation for the birth of HIV-2 as well. He conceded that if it could ever be proved that HIV-2 had resulted through transfer from a monkey bite, then "that would slightly increase the chances that HIV-1 did too." But such a hypothesis was incapable of hard proof. By contrast, if, as he maintained, he had already produced weighty evidence to suggest that HIV-1 had arisen through a vaccine, "then this would significantly increase the chances that HIV-2 did too." The only real evidence for the natural transfer of HIV-2 from a monkey was the geographical coincidence, but on the other hand, the transfer "could have arisen from an experimental vaccine made and used in that part of Africa, or from the Portuguese [using] monkeys easily obtained from their African colonies as a substitute for difficult-to-get rhesus and cynomolgus monkeys, and testing the vaccine so produced on their subject peoples rather than on their own citizens."

"In any case," Pascal continued, "wherever the HIVs came from, it is crystal clear that they *could* have come from monkey kidney vaccines, and this should lead everyone, regardless of their position on where in fact they did come from, to want to ban such vaccines and other sources of exposure to unsterilized primate material (and unsterilized material from other animals, also). This has not occurred, and does not seem close to occurring."

He pointed out the "virtual certainty" that monkeys had other lentiviruses, which were yet to be discovered, and juxtaposed this against the recent transplant, in Pittsburgh, of a "great mass of simian material" (a baboon liver) into a human.[4] The patient's immune system had of course been suppressed to prevent organ rejection, and Pascal added that the doctors clearly hoped that the patient could be kept alive for many years — which would inevitably allow any foreign microbes in the baboon liver the time to adapt to human physiology (and perhaps the opportunity to be transmitted onward, to other humans).

---

In my letter, I had addressed him as "Dr. Pascal," but he now vouchsafed the information that he was neither a doctor nor a biologist. He did, he confided, have a degree in the physical sciences, and he had "a long-term interest in certain aspects of evolution." This information, plus his chapter in the anthology on ethics, made it apparent that, far from being a dilettante, here was a self-educated man who possessed a remarkable degree of both insight and determination.

He went on to explain how he had become involved in AIDS research.

> This whole odyssey began because elementary evolutionary consider-
> ations were being so utterly ignored with this disease. When I failed to
> interest evolutionary biologists in writing on this topic, I resolved to do
> it myself, since however unqualified I might be, I could at least take the
> discussion far beyond the junior high school understanding of AIDS
> researchers. But my AIDS research turned up one thing after another that
> these people were doing wrong, the final straw coming when I learned
> they had started the whole thing themselves, an eventuality that had not
> even occurred to me when I started out. One of the many reasons I am so
> angry derives from my very lack of qualifications: it does seem to me that
> if a self-taught person can do all this on his own, then those who are pro-
> fessionals, if not competent enough to do it for themselves, ought at least
> to be competent enough to understand when someone else shows them
> how to do it.

He continued:

> Medicine has wholly abandoned . . . common sense in an attempt to
> avoid blame for its earlier misbehavior, blame they could have placed on a
> few foolish members of their profession but which they have now thor-
> oughly and indelibly smeared all over themselves. A few people trans-
> ferred AIDS. Then the whole medical and scientific establishment
> covered it up for years.

This, certainly, was science with the gloves off, armchair theorizing without the antimacassar. It was thrillingly uncompromising and uninhibited, and was driven by a real inner fury.

---

The documents that accompanied Louis Pascal's letter, nearly two hundred sides of paper in all, told their own painful and powerful story. Here were cop-ies of all his earlier pieces, from his first 10,000-word article on the subject, completed in November 1987 and entitled, unblushingly, "Modern Medicine Started AIDS," to a far simpler version, completed in October 1990, called "How AIDS Began." They were more than just early versions of his Wollongong paper. They were part of a body of work that needed to be read in its entirety.

Also included were many of the source papers for his different articles, including several collages of clippings, notes, and extracts. Here were lists of additional reading. Here too were copies of correspondences with various scientists and editors, many of whom, it seemed, had eventually fallen short of his expectations. Featured among these was correspondence between Pascal and David Sharp, deputy editor of the *Lancet*. Sharp had written to inform Pascal that the journal was just about to publish Walter Kyle's "Viewpoint" article and, having acknowledged that Pascal had written them with a different theory about the origin of AIDS several years earlier, invited him to review Kyle's paper and to submit a letter to the editor "which could be published very quickly." Pascal failed to respond for more than two months, and then, when he did, sent an angry letter that criticized Kyle's article, and then inquired: "One wonders why, on a matter of historic importance, you print a paper you know contains serious errors in preference to one you can find no errors in" (his own). He declined to submit the suggested letter to the editor, and instead offered the journal the 19,000-word Wollongong paper, on the basis that it be reprinted in its entirety. Now it was the *Lancet* that failed to respond, either to this letter or to Pascal's two follow-up letters requesting a decision.

The same story was repeated over and over, and it was not difficult to see why Pascal had experienced so much difficulty getting published. Whether because of the length, or his intransigence, or occasionally through sheer bad luck (one journal, *African Commentary*, closed down just when it was about to publish his piece), none of Pascal's articles had ever appeared in print, other than the Wollongong working paper,[5] and Pascal's own photocopied versions. These failures, which were partly a result of his immense rage, also added to it. I found myself thinking of a canister of liquid nitrogen, which, with lid removed, would simply start to fizz and boil away.

---

One of Pascal's most important discoveries concerned the precautions that were taken to try to ensure the safety of OPV preparations during the fifties. The vaccine actually consisted of the supernatant, the fluid that remained after attenuated polio virus had been introduced to the monkey kidney cells, and allowed to grow inside them (eventually killing them). The supernatant was later filtered to remove bacteria, fungi, and dead kidney cells, and diluted in saline solution. Since this was a live vaccine, no antiviral agents could be introduced, so this was essentially the material that was fed to vaccinees. As regards the monkeys that provided the kidneys for the culture, they were observed for visible signs of sickness and tested for various known infections (such as herpes B virus). Once they had been sacrificed, the tissue cultures made from their kidneys were also kept under observation (typically for three weeks), which was felt to be long enough to pick up traces of the more obvious "adventitious agents."[6]

However, many viruses do not cause visible disease in their natural hosts. Examples are SV40 (which does not cause illness in Asian monkeys) and the SIVs (which cause no detectable illness in the various species of African monkey). Only when these viruses are transferred into foreign hosts — when, for instance, SV40 is put into African green monkeys, or SIV into Asian macaques — do they cause disease. Indeed, this is how SV40 was first discovered in 1960. Equally, many viruses do not cause any visible damage (or "cytopathic effect") in cell culture during the twenty-one-day observation period. Although forty simian viruses had been detected by 1960, and some seventy-five by the mid-eighties, many others were not picked up by the screening procedures of the day. This is dramatically demonstrated by the fact that African green monkey tissue cultures were used to make OPV between 1961 and 1985, and approximately half of all African green monkeys in the wild are infected with SIV; yet no evidence of SIV contamination of OPV was discovered during those twenty-four years. It is fortunate, Pascal notes, that SIVagm does not appear to be transmissible to man — in contrast to other SIVs, like that from the sooty mangabey.[7]

Pascal sums up in his customary forthright style, as follows: "Thus was a system set up for the selective transfer of slow and difficult-to-detect diseases from other species into the human race."

Having proposed that Koprowski's 1957/8 trials in Ruanda-Urundi and the Belgian Congo were the most likely moment for the transfer of an HIV-1 precursor to the human race, Pascal makes another important observation. He notes that the Ruzizi trial, the first mass OPV trial in the world, was conducted on a quarter of a million people, several years before the first licensing of an OPV (Sabin's) in the United States, and adds that another OPV made by the South Africans (and prepared in the kidneys of local African green monkeys) was fed to roughly a million Kenyans in 1959/60, some time before the first use of this vaccine in South Africa. "There is a well-grounded suspicion," comments Pascal, "that poor black Africans were used as guinea pigs to test a vaccine made by rich Americans and South Africans who were not sufficiently convinced of its safety to want to test it in their own countries."

Pascal uses the story of the moon rock brought back to earth aboard *Apollo 11* in 1969 as a metaphor for the dangers of introducing living agents into an entirely new environment. He points out that before anyone on earth was allowed to handle these lunar samples, elaborate precautions were taken to avoid the potential risk of terrestrial contamination by germs from outer space.[8] The scientists of the late sixties saw clearly that the potential impact of a mistake in their calculations about "space germs" was so great (the end of mankind, or even of life on earth), that if they were to err at all, it had to be on the side of caution.

Pascal then gives examples of the disastrous impact of "virgin soil epidemics" that *have* occurred after a pathogen has been introduced from one species to another, or even from one geographical subgroup of a species to another. The classic example is the experimental introduction, in 1950, of myxoma virus (a South American virus that causes warts in the local species of rabbit) to a small group of wild European rabbits living along the Murray River in Australia. This created the biological equivalent of a nuclear explosion, killing a billion or more rabbits (90 percent of the continental population) in the space of three months. Similarly, after the crew of a British ship brought measles to the Fiji Islands in 1875, the virus killed a quarter of the local people, again in some three months. As for cross-species transfers, relatively harmless simian viruses like herpes B, Marburg virus, and (in all probability) the closely related Ebola virus cause devastation when transferred to human populations.

Pascal argues that because of the genetic proximity of the hosts, monkey viruses are much more likely to be transferable to human beings than, say, cat viruses or pig viruses. There is, he goes on, a very real risk (which should have been realized even back in the fifties) that untreated monkey kidney tissue cultures might effect the transfer of an unknown, unidentified monkey virus to humans, and that such a transfer could be disastrous in its impact.[9] Furthermore, he writes, such a transfer clearly had the potential not only to establish a new disease in *Homo sapiens,* but to spark a worldwide epidemic of that disease, for once a foreign virus becomes established in and begins to adapt to a new host, natural selection (the survival of the fittest) demands that the virus will become more transmissible. This is because variants of the virus that transmit easily will prosper and their progeny will spread quickly, while those that transmit poorly will spread slowly, and eventually tend to die out. Why, he asks, did the scientists of the fifties not treat their live polio vaccines grown in monkey cells with the same elaborate precautions that they subsequently took to protect against the remote possibility of "space germs"?

"A fire alarm," he writes, "must be built to go off *every* time there is a fire, and at the earliest possible moment. This means there will be cases where it goes off and there is no fire. But such false alarms are the price we pay for the assurance that when a fire does break out, we will be warned in time."

---

When he wrote like this, with such candor and common sense, it was impossible not to empathize with him. How could it be, one felt, that the words of this man of clear vision were not heeded, were not treated with the respect they deserved?

Jennifer Alexander (who was clearly greatly impressed by Pascal's work) has tried to provide an explanation for this in a letter to Brian Martin, in which she wrote:

> Pascal's style is accusatory — [his argument is] presented as a *fait accompli* without giving all the facts, figures, irrefutable results and analyzing these in a dispassionate, third person, and detached manner. . . . Most "scientists" these days are not men [and] women of vision. Their world and work is driven by technology and tunnel vision. They have ink in their veins and shrug off ideas or concepts which do not appear in the text-books. . . . Editors of scientific journals are not independent. They rely on editorial panelists who probably largely fall into the above category. . . . Should Pascal's claims have any validity this would so seriously impact on the medical profession that the status they have assumed to themselves would be destroyed.

The discrediting of the medical profession — this was exactly the sort of repercussion that Pascal himself claimed to be a necessary and unavoidable corollary of his work. The stakes, undoubtedly, were getting higher.

# 18

THE COUNTERATTACK BEGINS

During August and September 1992, I began collecting everything I could get my hands on about the OPV/AIDS theory. Much of the most recent material, sent me by Blaine Elswood and others, related to Tom Curtis's articles. What was immediately apparent was that the hypothesis had caused rather more than a "minor blip on the horizon," as Curtis had modestly described it to me. Indeed, Anthony Fauci, director both of the National Institute of Allergy and Infectious Diseases (NIAID) and of the Office of AIDS Research of the National Institutes of Health (NIH), had stated that the articles by Curtis and Kyle had unleashed a "major firestorm" of controversy.[1]

Although it was dated March 19, 1992, Curtis's article[2] had actually been on the streets since the end of February,[3] and throughout March the article prompted extensive coverage, for instance on the wire services and on CNN's *Larry King Live*. The first feedback in a scientific journal, however, was a "News and Comment" piece, which appeared in *Science* on March 20. Written by Jon Cohen, it bore the sardonic headline "Debate on AIDS Origin: *Rolling Stone* Weighs In," which established the tone for the entire piece.[4]

Cohen's line was that "the rock-and-roll magazine's hypothesis" was but the latest of a long line of "wild speculations" and, furthermore, that many of those quoted in the story felt that their viewpoints had been distorted, or that Curtis had used their discussions selectively. Koprowski, for instance, tells Cohen in a statement that "immunization of children in Africa against polio could be used as a model for the approach to the mass immunization against AIDS once a vaccine becomes available. It is a pity in a sense that instead of using his journalistic skills to show this, Curtis chose to misconstrue the information . . . to propagate a hypothesis without basis in fact." Koprowski then tells Cohen that he used "macaques from the Philippines and India" in making his polio vaccine, and adds that no wild monkeys from Asia have ever been found to be infected with SIV.

Cohen goes on to cite Gerald Quinnan, deputy director of the Food and Drug Administration, who says that he deliberately tried to infect monkey kidney cells with SIV and failed. "It is not possible for SIV to be present in polio vaccines in any substantial amount," Quinnan concludes. At the end of his piece, Cohen reveals that "if the Wistar can find frozen samples of Koprowski's vaccine — or, more likely, the initial 'seed stock' used to make it — researchers will test for HIV and SIV."

Curtis responded to many of these points in an article that he wrote for the *Washington Post* in early April. First he highlights the growing confusion about which monkeys Koprowski used for his OPVs, pointing out that at different times Koprowski had claimed that he was using African green monkeys, rhesus macaques, monkeys "from the Philippines" (which would seem to indicate cynomolgus macaques), and ready-to-use kidneys from a supplier. Curtis then reveals that a spokesman for Lederle Laboratories, which since the mid-seventies has been the sole U.S. manufacturer of OPVs, informed him that since 1985 Lederle had "sometimes found SIV in the early stages of its vaccine production process," but that the virus had of course been eliminated when found. "What about vaccine produced and administered before 1985?" Curtis had inquired, to which the spokesman replied that "if you don't know something's there, you can't test for it."

At the end of May, three further letters about the controversy appeared in *Science*.[5] The first contribution, by Cecil Fox, starts by characterizing Cohen's article as "lightweight," before ably summarizing the likelihood of AIDS emerging through two very different processes — the preparation of monkey meat, and the administration of polio vaccines. Both hypotheses are viable, Fox concludes, but only the latter can be tested.

In the course of this letter, Fox makes two especially pertinent contributions to the debate on polio vaccine manufacture. The first is that foamy viruses, or spumaviruses (which, like the SIVs and HIVs, constitute a subfamily of retroviruses), "are sometimes referred to as the 'crabgrass' of polio-vaccine manufacture." He stresses that while such vaccines "have been free of cultivable foamy viruses for many years," it is not known what retroviruses were present in early vaccine preparations. (The point is well made, for a perusal of the literature reveals that the ubiquitous foamy viruses are constantly being mentioned — as presumably harmless contaminants of tissue cultures — throughout the fifties and early sixties.)[6] His second point is even more compelling. He says that there is no good evidence to suggest that lentiviruses like the SIVs will infect kidney cell cultures, but that "there is abundant evidence that either HIV or SIV can grow in cultured lymphocytes or macrophages." (These are white blood cells and scavenger cells, which are likely to have been present in some of the early vaccine tissue cultures.) Fox adds that many lots of these early polio vaccines, especially those used in the Third World, were not produced under FDA control, but rather produced at minimal cost by manufacturers who were unlikely to have screened extensively for other viruses, or to have adopted "good laboratory practice for their monkey kidney cell cultures." He suggests that, in order to test the Curtis hypothesis, and if samples of polio vaccines produced between 1952 and 1982 still exist, such samples could be screened for the presence of various retroviruses by PCR.

In the second of these letters, Tom Curtis takes Jon Cohen to task for maintaining that there is not "a picogram of evidence" to support the theory; instead, he writes, "there is a strong, if circumstantial, case." He also denies Cohen's allegations of misquotation.

In a brief rejoinder printed at the end of this letter, Jon Cohen once again states that the theory is "highly improbable," and that there is no proof that any single polio vaccine lot has ever been infected with SIV or HIV. He admits that nobody has yet tested Hilary Koprowski's Congo vaccine, but reminds the reader that this vaccine "was made at Philadelphia's Wistar Institute, not some backwater lab run by a low-bid contractor in a loosely regulated country." Cohen closes his letter by making a significant admission about the sources for his previous statement about the types of monkey Koprowski used, claiming "I based what I wrote both on what he told me and on what he published at the time."

However, the 1961 article by Koprowski, which Cohen quotes as a reference,[7] makes no allusion to the species that Koprowski himself used. It merely states that "The material used for growing polioviruses in tissue cultures consists of living cells obtained from the freshly harvested kidneys from monkeys brought to the United States either from India or from the Philippines" (meaning the rhesus macaque and cynomolgus macaque, respectively). The context makes it clear that this refers to the species of kidneys that are *generally* used to make polio vaccines, rather than to the species Koprowski's own laboratory had been using. This section of the article is entitled "The Host Cell," and is concerned specifically with the question of the latent presence of contaminating viruses in the tissues of specific monkey species. Koprowski's lack of specificity about his own laboratory's practice is therefore a striking and puzzling omission.

In their published papers of the fifties, other polio vaccine workers furnished full details about the monkey species they used — both for safety testing, and for growing their vaccines. Sabin, for instance, used the cynomolgus macaque;[8] Gear, the African green monkey;[9] and Cox, both cynomolgus and rhesus macaques[10] for making their OPVs. As for IPVs, Lépine employed the Guinea baboon,[11] and although Jonas Salk never himself specified in print the species used, it was frequently reported by others as the rhesus macaque.[12] Koprowski stands alone among the major polio vaccine developers in that details about the species of monkey he used as vaccine substrate are never revealed in the fifties literature. In fact, it is not until 1964 that his Croatian collaborators publish details about the species in which he grows his polioviruses (and by this time, like everyone else, he had switched to using AGM kidneys).[13] This omission is all the more remarkable, given the fact that Koprowski published over sixty articles about polio, and that he frequently acknowledged the use of rhesus monkeys for safety testing.

Tom Curtis's letter to *Science* appears to have served as the last straw for Hilary Koprowski. In August 1992, almost six months after the *Rolling Stone* article had first appeared in the bookstores, he issued a written response to the OPV/AIDS hypothesis in the form of a letter to *Science*.[14]

"As a scientist, I did not intend to debate Tom Curtis when he presented his hypothesis about the origin of AIDS in *Rolling Stone*," Koprowski begins. "The publication of his letter in *Science*, however, transferred the debate from the lay press to a highly respected scientific journal. I would therefore like to state my views, based on facts, in order to counter and thereby repudiate Curtis' hypothesis about the origin of AIDS."

In fact, Hilary Koprowski's attempt to repudiate Curtis is a quite remarkable document, for many of the claims in his letter are either contentious or demonstrably wrong. Koprowski does legitimately correct Curtis for the one major error in his article: that of quoting Biggar's discredited HIV-prevalence figures for Kivu province, which (as we have seen) had been acknowledged by Biggar as likely false positives.[15] Thereafter, however, his submission is littered with errors.

The following are among the mistakes and contentious statements that feature in Koprowski's letter to *Science*:

1. Koprowski claims that he and Tom Norton succeeded in attenuating the three types of poliovirus between 1949 and 1952, but papers published by himself and others in the fifties show that his first successful attenuation of a Type 3 poliovirus (Fox) did not occur until 1956.[16]

2. Koprowski claims that the Ruzizi Valley, where the bulk of the 1958 vaccinations occurred, lies in the northwest of Burundi, and not in the Kivu province of the Congo. In fact, it forms the border between the two countries and the Ruzizi vaccinations were divided almost equally between the two, with a small area of southwest Rwanda also included. This is an extraordinary error, first because he seems not to know the location of this, the first mass trial of OPV in the world, and one which involved his own vaccine — and second, because it is a fact that is so easy to check.

3. He quotes HIV-prevalence figures of 0.7 percent for rural Burundi and 1.3 percent for rural Rwanda. These figures are correctly quoted, but they are hardly representative. HIV prevalences in the early eighties for certain of the rural districts of Burundi that had been involved in the 1958 CHAT trials were more than twelve times higher, as I was later to discover.[17]

4. Koprowski concedes that the urban areas of Rwanda and Burundi are heavily infected with HIV, with prevalences rising as high as 25 percent to 30 percent, but says that the vaccine fed in the Ruzizi Valley cannot be responsible, since that area is rural and HIV appears to have spread from urban to rural parts of Africa, rather than vice versa. This ignores the fact that the spring 1958 campaign involved the feeding of CHAT in a major town (Bujumbura) as well as in rural areas. If indeed there was SIV contamination of some batches of CHAT, then one would expect to find individuals and occasional small clusters with HIV infection and AIDS in the more sexually conservative countryside but, much more strikingly, the early emergence of heavy HIV infection and large numbers of AIDS cases in local towns. This is exactly what one finds. By 1986, five towns in Rwanda had adult HIV-prevalence figures of between 16 percent and 31 percent,[18] as did one (Bujumbura) in Burundi.[19]

5. He claims that the same pool of vaccine was used in Leopoldville and in Poland. Strictly speaking this is true, but the information is far from complete. Seventy-six thousand children from newborns to age five were fed pool 13 of CHAT in Leopoldville (now Kinshasa), whereas fewer than three thousand children were fed this same pool in Poland.[20] The vast majority of vaccinations of CHAT in Poland (more than seven million) were with a different pool — 18.[21]

6. He writes, "Inasmuch as the prevalence of AIDS in Kinshasa today is 25 to 30% and Poland had the lowest incidence of AIDS in Europe, one would have to undertake super-speculative acrobatics to incriminate the vaccine as the source of the AIDS in Africa." Koprowski means the prevalence of HIV, not AIDS. Furthermore, most reports from 1992 indicated that HIV prevalence among Kinshasa adults was below 10 percent[22] not "25 to 30%."

7. "Even the supposedly early cases of AIDS in Africa were clinically diagnosed several thousand kilometers away from the Kivu region." In fact, the putative early cases to which he refers in the referenced article are from Kinshasa, Bujumbura, and from towns in Shaba.[23] His vaccines were used in the first two cities, and the towns in Shaba are actually less than a thousand (not several thousand) kilometers from Kivu and the Ruzizi Valley. In fact, as I was later to discover, the correlations between the early putative AIDS cases mentioned and vaccinations with CHAT were far closer than this suggests.

8. In a key passage, Koprowski unequivocally states that after his original Type 2 vaccine, TN, which was made in cotton rat brain, "all other batches were produced in kidney tissue obtained from rhesus monkeys (*Macaca mulatta*) captured either in India or the Philippines." Not only does this certainty conflict

with his earlier uncertainty when speaking to Curtis, but even this statement is erroneous. *Macaca mulatta* (the rhesus macaque) does indeed come from India, but the species from the Philippines used for vaccine production is the cynomolgus macaque, *Macaca cynomolgus.*[24]

9. Koprowski now claims that the "Congo preparation" in which Albert Sabin found "an unidentified cell-killing virus" was not a vaccine, but rather a seed-lot of virus. Certainly if anyone knows the facts, it should be Koprowski, but all the evidence from 1959 suggests that this new claim is incorrect. When discussing this issue at the First International Conference on Live Poliovirus Vaccines in 1959, both Albert Sabin and Sven Gard (who was then working at the Wistar Institute) referred to the fluid that they had tested as CHAT *vaccine,* as did Joseph Melnick, another very precise scientist, when introducing the subject.[25] Koprowski himself, in a letter rebutting Sabin's claims, which was published in the *British Medical Journal* in May 1959, merely refers to the CHAT pool tested by Sabin, without specifying whether this was a vaccine pool or the parent seed-lot of attenuated poliovirus.[26] The significance of this debate is that if indeed there was an SIV contaminant, it would be much more plausibly found in a sample of the final vaccine (made up in kidney tissue culture from an unknown monkey species) than in the plaque-purified seed-lot of poliovirus, from which further batches of vaccine would be made.

10. With respect to his sudden switch, in the fall of 1960, to advocating human diploid cell strains like WI-38 as a suitable substrate for growing polio vaccines, rather than monkey kidney tissue culture, Koprowski now writes that "the desire to replace the monkey kidney vaccine did not arise from concern about its safety." This is a remarkable statement, and is at odds with statements made by himself and other virologists in 1960 and 1961, when the announcement of the presence of the apparently tumorigenic SV40 in polio vaccines made in rhesus and cynomolgus kidneys (as he now claims his were) was causing genuine alarm. In the "Host Cell" section of his own 1961 article from the *Journal of the American Medical Association,* which he cites, Koprowski does indeed *begin* by arguing that there is no cause for alarm, in that hundreds of millions of the world's population have already been exposed to SV40 in IPV and OPV "without any known harmful consequence." However, in the next two sentences he strikes an entirely different tone, stating: "it would be more difficult to justify scientifically a stand that nothing should be done in the immediate future about the host cells in which polioviruses are grown. Not only has the existence in monkey tissue of the dreaded B virus (which is definitely pathogenic for man) been known for some time, but it is clear that tissues obtained from the next batch of killed monkeys may contain more 'virus surprises.' "[27]

11. Finally, more than half of the twenty-four numbered footnotes in the text of the letter fail to correlate with the references at the end.[28] If this does little

to reassure about the thoroughness and reliability of the author, it also says very little for the subediting process at *Science.*

————————

Toward the end of his letter to *Science,* Koprowski reveals that "there is no vaccine stored at the Wistar Institute," but that "there are a few vials of tissue culture supernatants available that may represent seed lots used for vaccine production between 1957 and 1959." He says that any competent research laboratory could test these seed-lots of attenuated poliovirus if it also used the appropriate positive and negative controls. But then he adds a rider. "If the seed lot is found free of exogenous retroviruses (which is highly probable), contentious individuals could still argue that this does not represent what might have been present in the large lot of vaccine." He begins, in other words, by appearing to encourage independent scientists to test the samples, but ends by arguing against it.

Koprowski closes the letter as follows: "The current anxiety among parents of children who have been or are going to be vaccinated against polio followed dissemination by the lay press of unproved theories about the origin of AIDS. This was unnecessary and harmful, particularly because the vaccine was tested thoroughly before any vaccination was done; the vaccine was and continues to be safe."

Although this sounds conciliatory, it actually confuses the issue. Koprowski seems to be implying that any criticism of CHAT (as made in the fifties) also impugns the safety of the current Sabin OPV. In fact, Curtis had made it very clear that he had no wish to initiate a panic about the safety of current polio vaccines.

Furthermore, Koprowski's claim about the safety of CHAT is not backed up by any factual evidence in the article. It would have been far more reassuring had his letter itemized the specific safety tests that were conducted on CHAT before it was used on humans (which are only rather vaguely described in the literature), and if — in a spirit of scientific openness — he had advocated the release of stored samples of the CHAT seed-lots and vaccine samples for retrospective testing.

It would also have been more reassuring if this — his response to Curtis's questioning of the safety of CHAT, submitted after he had had nearly six months to marshal his thoughts — had not been so riddled with inaccuracy and error.[29] In the end, it was this very letter — his sole published attempt to defend himself against the questions raised by Curtis's article — which convinced me that the OPV/AIDS theory, in contrast to so many of the others, merited some further serious investigation.

————————

His remarkable *Rolling Stone* piece notwithstanding, perhaps the greatest contribution made by Tom Curtis to the debate on the origin of AIDS was the series of follow-up articles he produced for his "local paper," the *Houston Post,* throughout 1992. Written either alone or in conjunction with staff writer Patricia Manson, they represent a remarkably well-focused summary of Wistar-related events, and of scientific developments relevant to the hypothesis. Significantly, he was able to elicit the support of famous figures such as Anthony Fauci, Joseph Melnick, and Frederick Robbins (the latter a Nobel winner with John Enders for pioneering work on tissue cultures) for the proposition that batches of suspect polio vaccine from the fifties should be examined for HIV and other retroviruses by PCR analysis.[30]

These articles give the impression that Curtis had scented blood, and was now swaying in the air like a hungry mosquito. He kept buzzing members of the expert committee that the Wistar had set up to examine the theory, to inquire about the progress of their deliberations, and about the number of polio vaccine samples that had been located during the search of the Wistar's freezers. His most frequent source of nourishment was the cochair, Claudio Basilico, who was also chairman of the microbiology department at the New York University School of Medicine. Eventually Basilico vouchsafed that "no more than 100" samples had been found, some of which "were very likely to have been used" in Africa, but that "it may not be all that easy to find people to do this testing because it's a lot of work." Curtis promptly announced that Dr. Robert Bohannon, a PCR specialist, was prepared to test all hundred samples for HIV, SIV, HTLV-1, HTLV-2, spumaviruses, and Type D retroviruses.[31]

Basilico responded that this offer was premature, and that Bohannon should wait until his committee had issued its report. Meanwhile, Dr. Warren Cheston, a Wistar vice president (who was not himself a member of the blue ribbon panel of experts) announced that although some of the samples dated from the fifties, only those that could be directly linked to the Congo trials should be tested. The committee, he said, would recommend at least three laboratories to test any such samples identified.[32] Curtis, meanwhile, was circling around David Ho, director of the Aaron Diamond AIDS Research Center, who was also a committee member. When, in August, Curtis asked him why he thought no scientists had yet tested any of the stored polio vaccines, Ho replied: "If you really think about it, what do you have to gain and what do you have to lose?" He declined to be more specific. He did, however, acknowledge that monkey viruses were a worry — and not just those in vaccines. With reference to the recent transplantation of a baboon liver to a human, Ho acknowledged: "The baboon thing gave many of us a lot of concerns because you don't know what's in there, what could possibly be transmitted. . . . If the person lives, are we at risk of starting an epidemic from some primate virus or agent? . . .

[The transplant] was done in a hurry, and it's clear many things were not thought out."[33]

_____

Finally, on October 22, 1992, Claudio Basilico delivered the eight-page report of the Wistar-convened committee at a press conference in New York.[34] Although not all the committee members were present, he spoke on behalf of the five other members, including his cochair, Frank Lilly, professor of molecular genetics at the Albert Einstein College of Medicine; the aforesaid David Ho; Eckard Wimmer, chair of microbiology at SUNY at Stony Brook; Ronald Desrosiers, director of the New England Regional Primate Research Center and professor of microbiology at Harvard Medical School; and Clayton Buck, director of scientific development at the Wistar Institute, and its only representative on the committee. Also attending were a number of reporters, including Tom Curtis.

The report summed up the committee's findings as follows: "[W]e consider the probability of the AIDS epidemic having been started by the inadvertent inoculation of an unknown HIV precursor into African children during the 1957[35] poliovirus vaccine trials to be extremely low. Almost every step in this hypothetical mode of transmission is problematic. The contamination of the poliovirus vaccine lots with SIV/HIV particles, if any, is likely to have been extremely small. Transmission by the oral route is extremely rare for HIV or SIV. Finally, the evolutionary distance between known monkey immunodeficiency viruses and HIV-1, the prevalent virus in the AIDS epidemic, probably took decades or even centuries to be bridged and not a few years. The most telling evidence is the case of the Manchester sailor who appears to have been infected with HIV-1 even before the poliovirus trials began in Congo." The latter point is contentious, for the first vaccinations in the Congo occurred in February 1957, whereas David Carr's first AIDS-like symptoms did not begin until December 1958. Theoretically, twenty-two months is easily enough time for him to have been infected (either directly or indirectly), and to have progressed to AIDS.[36]

Despite this fairly comprehensive dousing of the "firestorm" of controversy sparked by Curtis's article, the report did feature some significant statements that were supportive of the hypothesis. One was the admission that: "Unfortunately, the origin of the kidneys used in the preparation of the 1957 vaccine is unlikely to ever be determined with any certainty." Another was that "the possible presence of SIV or related virus particles in the vaccine preparation cannot be discounted." Furthermore, one of the concluding recommendations was that "a limited number of samples of vaccine stocks available at the Wistar Institute could be tested for the presence of HIV/SIV viruses." The committee recommended that testing should be done by, or under the supervision of, the

CDC and the WHO, and should be conducted in at least two experienced laboratories, where "stringent measures should be adopted to avoid laboratory contaminations." Apparently just a single vaccine sample "possibly directly relevant to the Congo trials" had been identified.

The most intriguing recommendation was the final one. "In closing," the scientists wrote, "we feel compelled to mention that the current controversy highlights the problems and difficulties associated with using monkey tissue for production of vaccines administered in humans." Noting that most OPVs were still produced in African green monkey kidney cells, the panel concluded that although such vaccines could now be certified free of SIV, the possible contamination of polio vaccine lots with "other monkey viruses which have not yet been discovered . . . provides a powerful argument for the use of well-characterized cell lines for vaccine production." Noting that at least one major European manufacturer had recently abandoned the production of vaccines in monkey kidney tissue, the report ended with the bald statement that: "A serious effort is needed in the US and other countries to effect a switch to well-characterized cell lines for vaccine production."

Thus it was that the Wistar committee of 1992, in response to the threat posed by unspecified simian viruses, ended up recommending exactly the same action that Koprowski (and other scientists) had advocated after the SV40 scare of 1960. The clock had spun back thirty-two years, and seemingly nothing had changed. Of course, then it was the kidneys of rhesus and cynomolgus macaques that posed the potential risk; now it was perceived to be those of African green monkeys. But that was hardly the point. The committee was advising that monkey kidneys — of any variety — should no longer be used to manufacture vaccines.

Furthermore, although the expert committee was clearly skeptical about the OPV/AIDS hypothesis floated by Curtis, it had provided no evidence to repudiate it. As a later commentary put it: the committee "categorised the probability of SIV crossing to humans in the CHAT-1 polio vaccine as extremely low/extremely small/extremely rare, but it had failed to discover a single concrete refutation. In fact, on every scientific ground, it had acknowledged the potential of the polio vaccine theory."[37]

---

The new director of the Wistar Institute, Giovanni Rovera, noted the findings, thanked the committee, and announced that "in the interests of objectivity and scientific knowledge," he had contacted the director of the CDC and the co-secretary of the steering committee on hepatitis and polio at the WHO, offering to make available for testing the one sample that might be directly relevant to the Congo trials.[38] A few questions were asked from the floor, mainly by

Curtis, who agreed that the objections to his hypothesis made it unlikely, but added: "Look at the numbers. There were 300,000 people inoculated. Let's say fifty had sores in their mouths, or inhaled the virus deep into their lungs. If they get it [SIV/HIV] and each person passes it onto another person every year, that's all you have to do to get the current 6.5 million Africans [infected with HIV]."[39]

However, most of the journalists present concluded in their reports that the panel of experts had more or less knocked the OPV/AIDS hypothesis on the head.[40] Only Curtis remained fairly upbeat about the theory, quoting Raphael Stricker, who commented that the committee report had "recommend[ed] changing the way the world makes polio vaccines," and that this was "an astounding statement from an official body."[41]

———————

Hilary Koprowski, meanwhile, had clearly had enough of being the butt of speculation in the lay and medical press. One week after the expert committee announced its findings, his lawyers filed a $2.7 million damages suit against the Associated Press, for a wire service story that had claimed, quite wrongly, that one of Koprowski's vaccines had already been tested and found to contain "a type of AIDS virus found in monkeys."[42] Without prompting, AP withdrew the story a few days later, but the suit went ahead anyway, with Koprowski's lawyers attesting that he had "suffered severe mental and emotional distress," that he had been exposed to "public contempt and ridicule," and that his reputation had been "blackened and injured."[43]

Then in December 1992, Koprowski's lawyers sued Rolling Stone, its parent corporation, and Tom Curtis.[44] The complaint, which again centered on the issue of defamation, alleged that Curtis's article had destroyed Koprowski's reputation, "in that a reasonable reader could infer that [his] polio vaccine infected its recipients with the AIDS virus," a claim that was alleged to be libelous on the grounds that there was no scientific evidence to support it.

Several commentators, however, considered that the libel suit against Rolling Stone and Tom Curtis also addressed a far more basic ethical question — that of whether or not people had the right to express and freely debate controversial scientific hypotheses.[45]

# IV

## EUROPEAN FEEDERS

*No lesson seems to be so deeply inculcated by the experience
of life as that you never should trust experts.*

— LORD SALISBURY,
letter to Lord Lytton, 1877

# 19

AN UNTIMELY PASSING

It is best to be frank. The Belgians do not have a good reputation in Europe. According to legend, they have a capacity for inflicting boredom on almost any company, and a popular brainteaser in British pubs involves the naming of "three famous Belgians." The internal divisions between the French-speaking Walloon and Dutch-speaking Flemish areas engender an intensity that is quite baffling to outsiders, and the cuisine is supposed to rival that of the English for banality, even if it is grudgingly acknowledged that they do make nice chocolate and *pommes frites*.

I have to report that much of this is unwarranted. The fact that Brussels was awarded the European Community headquarters has meant that many of the gripes about bureaucracy and international ineptitude are laid, by association, at its door. But several of the cities (like Antwerp, Ghent, and Leuven) are full of character, beauty, and delightful surprises, and many of the people seem to be naturally imbued with kindness, consideration, and a lack of small-town pomposity. As teenagers, a friend and I used to arrive on the midnight ferry at Ostend, and hitchhike through the night toward sunnier climes, usually getting lifts with extraordinary rapidity. On several occasions we ended up in someone's home at three in the morning, being invited to take some food, or offered the spare bed.

Of more relevance to this book is the fact that Belgian scientists and medics, compared to some of those from other European nations, are usually commendably generous with their time and knowledge. Nonetheless, in the course of my Belgian researches I did detect a tendency, especially among those of the old school, to pine after colonial Africa and the wonderful freedoms (to live comfortably, to conduct experimental research) that it afforded. It was apparent that for some, at least, the sad tale of the flight from the Belgian Congo remained a jigger, burrowing away busily beneath the skin of the national psyche.

One to whom such a description undoubtedly did not apply was Professor Jean Sonnet. In December 1991, just as Pascal's working paper was being published in Australia, as Tom Curtis was phoning Hilary Koprowski in the course of researching his *Rolling Stone* article, and nearly a year before the Wistar's expert committee delivered its verdict and Koprowski began to sue, I wrote to Professor Sonnet. He was the Belgian physician who for ten years during the fifties and sixties, both before and after the Congo's independence, had headed the department of internal medicine at Kinshasa University Hospital, formerly known as Lovanium — which may well have been the very place where L70, the first HIV-positive blood sample, was taken in 1959. He was one of only a few dozen Belgian doctors who stayed on in the country through the political upheavals of 1960 and 1964, because he knew that the new nation was desperately short of trained medics, and he believed that the Hippocratic oath involved an obligation to provide service where it was needed.

During the early eighties, by which time he was professor emeritus at St. Luc's Hospital, another Leuven University offshoot situated at the northern edge of Brussels, Sonnet was one of the first Belgian doctors to become alarmed by the large number of AIDS cases he was seeing among black African patients. He continued to research AIDS for the last five years of his professional career and in 1987, the year of his retirement, cowrote a remarkable paper for the *Scandinavian Journal of Infectious Diseases,* entitled: "Early AIDS Cases Originating from Congo and Burundi (1962-1976)."[1]

I didn't encounter this paper until 1991, which was regrettable, because it contained some of the most compelling clues then published about the early epidemiology of the syndrome. But early in January 1992, my letter to the professor elicited a courteous reply, together with copious notes on the seven cases detailed in his paper, which provided a great deal of additional information about the patient histories and clinical outcomes. I wrote back with some observations and further questions, and enclosed a letter from Fergal Hill, offering to analyze by PCR the frozen tissues of two of the patients, which Dr. Sonnet had told me were still available.

One morning in early spring Professor Sonnet phoned me at home. He sounded gentle and kindly — but rather frail. He explained that he himself was just about to leave for the hospital, but as a patient, rather than a physician. He had to go in for a fortnight's observation, but told me that he hoped to be able to arrange something with regard to the tissue samples. We arranged that I would phone him a few weeks later, when he was back home.

This, however, was not to be. He remained hospitalized for several weeks, and his condition deteriorated. When I phoned his house in early April, his daughter told me that he had a fulminant cancer of the pancreas, and was fading fast. The following morning a letter arrived from his son, explaining that his father had come home to die among his children and grandchildren, and thanking me for my letters. Inside the letter was a brief note from Professor Sonnet, clearly written during one of his wakeful moments, and with some effort. He died a few days later.

What I did not know, however, until I phoned again some weeks afterward and spoke with his widow, was that Jean Sonnet had put all his AIDS research into boxes, and handed them to his successor at St. Luc, Bernard Vandercam, with the instruction that I was to be given access and allowed to photocopy whatever I felt to be of interest. Madame Sonnet told me that her husband had considered me "a friend of the last hour." Later, when I phoned Dr. Vandercam, he invited me to come and stay at his home while I looked through Dr. Sonnet's papers.

---

In the end, I was unable to get across to Brussels until the end of August 1992, and then only for a week's visit. Bernard Vandercam proved to be much younger than I had expected — still in his thirties — and a friendly workaholic, devoted to the patients on the AIDS ward. Later, he took me home, introduced me to his wife, his two children, his cat, and to the six large cardboard boxes containing Jean Sonnet's AIDS research. The next morning, armed with a dictionary and a large pot of coffee, I got down to work.

Over the next few days, by piecing together details from Sonnet's 1962–1976 article, his letters to me, the material in the boxes, and the various patient medical files, I built up a much clearer picture of the seven patients in question. Three of these had died from clinically defined AIDS, while four were sick with, or had died of, serologically confirmed AIDS. Four of the patients were Belgians, two were Congolese, and one Rwandan, but in each case exposure to HIV (if indeed it had occurred) seemed to have happened in the Congo or Burundi, in the fifties, sixties, or seventies.

By far the most controversial case was the first, involving a Congolese woman, Hélène, who had died in Kinshasa on February 25, 1962. She had spent the last twelve days of her life in the care of Dr. Sonnet and his assistant, Jean-Louis Michaux, at Kinshasa University Hospital. Her precise age was never established, but various medical papers suggest that she was between forty and fifty. In the few weeks before her death, Hélène had been living in Matete, a suburb of the capital, but Dr. Sonnet revealed that she had recently arrived there from Lisala, one of the major stops for the river steamers plying between Kinshasa (formerly Leopoldville) and Kisangani (Stanleyville).

I interviewed Dr. Michaux a few days later, and found him still emotional about his former colleague. He spoke warmly of his professionalism, the precision of his thinking, and the care he took about small details. And he still recalled Hélène — the fact that she was married, that she spoke little French, and was not very wealthy. Her profession was marked down as *"indepéndante,"* indicating that she was self-employed, probably as a petty trader, though whether one based in Lisala or a *commerçante* in the great floating market aboard the river steamers is not clear. Some of the women traders aboard the boats were known to augment their income by casual prostitution, though Michaux emphasized that there was nothing to suggest this in the case of Hélène.

He also remembered that she had appeared at the hospital in very poor shape. At eighty pounds, she weighed about two-thirds of normal body weight, and had a puffy face caused by chronic and purulent gingivitis, dental abscesses, and a large, painful fistula of the submandibular lymph node (below the jaw). The lymph nodes of her armpits and groin were greatly enlarged, as was her spleen, her legs were swollen, and she was having difficulty breathing. X rays revealed osteonecrosis of the lower jaw and a bilateral pneumonia; various bacteria were isolated from her mouth and from the pus oozing from the gaping wound below her jaw. Hélène failed to respond to treatment, and died a few days later of sepsis and respiratory failure. At autopsy, multiple lesions of Kaposi's sarcoma were found inside her body, particularly in the lungs, spleen, and several lymph nodes. This was something of a surprise, in that no skin lesions of KS had been identified prior to death.

During those last few days, the doctors managed to glean from the patient that she had been hospitalized at Lisala four years earlier because of swollen lymph nodes, breathing difficulties, and dental problems. She was diagnosed as having tuberculosis, but during the following years, she was readmitted and given "many injections" of streptomycin and penicillin, without any improvement. Her lymph nodes had continued growing, and she continued losing weight until finally she was put on the boat for Kinshasa, to seek help at the hospital there.

A few years after Hélène's death, Jean-Louis Michaux had written his thesis on the subject of immunoglobulin levels in healthy and diseased Bantu, and Helene's levels were by far the most abnormal of all the dozens of patients studied. He kept the sera from these patients in a deep freeze but, sadly, they were ruined by a power failure shortly before his departure from the Congo.

In his notes on the case, Jean Sonnet recorded that by August 1984 he was already convinced that Hélène had died of AIDS. Shortly afterward, he wrote to David Fluck, the American pathologist who had performed the postmortem, who wrote back to concur with Sonnet's retrospective diagnosis. In November of that year, Sonnet decided to fly to Kinshasa, in the hope of locating Hélène's autopsy samples for testing, but he found that all of them had disappeared. Nonetheless, when he got home, he and Michaux wrote a paper entitled "An Early AIDS Case in a Zairian Woman Presenting with an Aggressive Variant of

Kaposi's Sarcoma in 1962," and submitted it to the *Lancet* and the *Annals of Internal Medicine*. The paper documented Hélène's levels of lymphocytes (very low) and immunoglobulins (very high for both IgA and IgM; slightly below normal for IgG) and demonstrated, by means of a table, that these closely resembled those of three Congolese patients with confirmed AIDS from the early eighties.[2] Both journals rejected the paper on the grounds that because T-lymphocyte studies had not been performed on Hélène, the diagnosis of AIDS had to remain speculative. It was three years before Sonnet and Michaux's longer article was published in the Scandinavian journal.

Further support for an AIDS diagnosis was provided by an important paper on the natural history of HIV infection in adults, which was published by two Africa-based physicians in 1991 — but which I came across only after Dr. Sonnet's death.[3] The authors found that oral manifestations were common in African AIDS, with 19 percent of people with AIDS in Kigali, Rwanda, suffering (like Hélène) from ulcero-necrotic gingivitis, and with HIV-positive patients in Kinshasa presenting with submandibular swellings and mouth ulcers. Another article, from 1988, highlighted the importance of submandibular gland dysfunction as an early sign of HIV infection, and identified the oral cavity as a significant route of bacterial infection in AIDS patients.[4]

It is noteworthy that both doctors Sonnet and Michaux, with their considerable experience of African AIDS in Belgium, were convinced that Hélène had died of the syndrome.[5] However, there is also a viable alternative diagnosis. Sonnet and Michaux's investigations revealed the infiltration of the bone marrow with immature plasmocytes, which suggests that she may have been suffering from a B-cell lymphoma. Such a condition might itself have been the cause of immunosuppression, or might have been an opportunistic infection sparked by the presence of HIV. Since there are no longer any remaining tissues or sera, the diagnosis of AIDS can only be tentatively advanced.

---

One intriguing connection highlighted by Dr. Sonnet's notes was the fact that Hélène's hometown was Lisala. This lies just a hundred miles from Yambuku, where five villagers were found to be HIV-positive in Kevin De Cock's study of Ebola samples taken in 1976.[6] Three of these five had developed AIDS by 1986, with the serum of one providing the earliest sequenced isolate of HIV then in existence. Furthermore, Grethe Rask, the Danish doctor who died of AIDS in 1977, had worked at the mission hospital at Abumombazi, a further fifty miles up the same road, between 1972 and 1975.

So if Hélène really did have AIDS, there was now evidence of five cases of apparent AIDS and two further cases of HIV infection emanating from a 150-mile stretch of road in the heart of the Congolese rain forest — with all infections occurring in 1976 or earlier. Alone of the AIDS cases, Hélène was not serologically confirmed as HIV-positive, but with or without her, the existence of such an early cluster in a predominantly rural area was surely, I felt, significant.

Professor Sonnet commented on this in some notes written in 1988. The Yambuku study had just been published, and Sonnet proposed a refined version of Kevin De Cock's theory that AIDS might be an old, endemic disease that had remained stable in localized rural areas like that around Yambuku for a long time.[7] He proposed that a crucial change might have occurred after 1958 or 1959, when previous Belgian restrictions on travel by local people were eased. Previously, he wrote, in order to get a travel pass, an African had first to be tested for venereal disease.

More than ever, I wished Professor Sonnet were still alive, for this is one point I would have enjoyed discussing with him. I would have pointed out that much of the latest phylogenetic evidence suggested that HIV was not, after all, an ancient virus, and I would have asked him whether travel restrictions like those he described could really have kept a virus like HIV "locked up" in a place like Yambuku, just one hundred miles (on a serviceable road) from a major river port. After all, I would have argued, HIV infection does not usually present like a venereal disease; for most of its course it is asymptomatic, and only sometimes in the final stages does it cause genital infections. If AIDS were really an ancient condition, I would have asked, would it not therefore have emerged in a major city like Leopoldville much earlier than it actually did? I knew Jean Sonnet would have relished such a discussion, for he was so clearly a man for whom the truth took precedence over egotistical concerns.

———

Even though the other six cases in Jean Sonnet's paper relate to much later in time, they are still early enough to be significant. It is worth noting that none of them is known to have had any of the famous "risk factors" other than heterosexual activity. Case 2, Daniel, was a Belgian construction worker who had been based in Kinshasa between 1971 and 1976. The medical chart revealed that he first fell ill with shingles (a common AIDS prodrome) in 1974, and that he developed further symptoms suggestive of HIV infection (lymphadenopathy, facial eczema, weight loss, and exhaustion) in early 1976. He returned home for medical treatment, but after a year or so his condition improved, and in June 1977 he returned to Africa as foreman of a building project in Bujumbura, Burundi. Soon after his arrival, he met — and later married — "Maria," a twenty-year-old Tutsi refugee from Rwanda; they had their first child together in 1978, and another in 1979. The following year, he again returned to Belgium, this time suffering from fever and penile warts, and coughing up blood. He died in Brussels in November 1981 at the age of thirty-four, as a result of a massive pneumonia, and *Rhodococcus equi* and *Toxoplasma gondii* infections of the brain.

Although Daniel's tissues were never tested retrospectively, it is very likely that he was HIV-positive, because his wife Maria, Case 3 in Sonnet's series, was found to be infected when tested in 1984 and 1985. She was still alive (though showing some prodromal symptoms of AIDS) a decade later, and she informed me that she had only had one "low-risk" sexual liaison since her husband's death. It seemed probable that she had contracted HIV from Daniel, and that he became infected with HIV between 1971 and 1974 in Kinshasa where, Maria told me, he had had several girlfriends. Maria suffered her first symptoms of immunosuppression in 1978, early in her second pregnancy, which may well have represented a seroconversion illness, but none of her three children are HIV carriers.[8]

Case 4, Gilbert, was another Belgian expatriate, who worked for Gecamines (formerly Union Minière de Haut Katanga), the huge copper mining company in the southern Congo province of Shaba, between the years of 1964 and 1977. He was based in Likasi, a large town seventy-five miles north of the Congo's second city and mining capital, Lubumbashi. For the first few years he lived with his Belgian wife, but because of the uncertain political situation she returned home at the end of the sixties, after which it is suspected that Gilbert had a number of Congolese girlfriends. His first symptoms suggestive of immunosuppression occurred in 1975, and during the next two years he suffered partial blindness and deafness, weight loss, fever, and mouth ulcers, eventually dying in Brussels in November 1977, at the age of forty-four, from a *Toxoplasma gondii* infection of the brain. Gilbert's tissues have never been tested, but his wife — tested in 1986 — was HIV-negative.

Case 5, Yvon, was a Belgian man who did a two-year stint of voluntary overseas service in the Congo between 1976 and 1978. His medical records reveal that he was based in the small town of Lubudi (again in Shaba, two hundred miles northwest of Lubumbashi), and that he had frequent sexual encounters with local women (many of them prostitutes) in these two places. He was found to be HIV-positive in 1985. He denied any other risk factors, apart from occasional heterosexual activity in Belgium, and he died of AIDS in Brussels in September 1989.

In some ways, cases 6 and 7 in Sonnet's series, again a married couple, are perhaps the most intriguing of all. Louis was a Belgian cartographer, born in 1914, who married Veronique, a Congolese seventeen years his junior, in 1952. In the close-knit expatriate community of the Belgian Congo of the early fifties, mixed marriages were rare and uncelebrated events, but theirs was a happy and successful union, resulting in six children born between 1954 and 1974. Their place of residence is not known, though it seems to have been in Kikwit (three hundred miles east of Kinshasa) for at least some of that period. This is inferred from the medical notes that reveal that Louis had a hernia operation there in 1958, and contracted hepatitis there at a date unspecified. In 1968 the couple left the Congo for Belgium, never to return, but in December 1981, Veronique suddenly fell ill with lymphadenopathy and meningitis, attributed to a CMV infection. She was diagnosed HIV-positive in 1985, and eventually died of AIDS in May 1987. Her husband also tested HIV-positive in 1985, but only developed symptoms after his wife's death, dying in July 1988. All six children were found to be HIV-negative.

Before their deaths, Veronique strenuously denied any risk factors such as intravenous drug use or extramarital activity, while Louis testified that his only possible risk factor was "past heterosexual exposure" (presumably in the Congo). These claims are backed up by a logical examination of the timings involved. The first case of AIDS in Belgium was the Congolese airline secretary who displayed symptoms a few days after flying in from Kinshasa in 1977. A further two people contracted AIDS in 1980 and six (including Veronique) in 1981, all of whom were African, or who were thought to have contracted their illness in central Africa. The tardy occurrence of the Belgian epidemic (compared to that of the Congo) suggests that, even as late as 1975, very few people in the country — whether Belgian or African — were HIV-positive. In 1975, Veronique was a forty-four-year-old mother of six, and Louis a sixty-one-year-old, neither representing a likely candidate for promiscuous sexual adventure. One must conclude that the obvious scenario is probably the correct one — and that at least one member of the couple was infected in the Congo in 1968 or before. In all likelihood that person would have been the first in Belgium with the human immunodeficiency virus — and must have survived for some two decades with HIV-1 in the bloodstream.

---

I spent three days working my way through the six cardboard boxes and photo-copying relevant documents, but it proved to be time well spent — even if it was only later that the full significance of these seven cases of Jean Sonnet's would become apparent.

The other documents also had their own stories to tell about the further spread of AIDS in Africa in the early years of the eighties. They included detailed lists of AIDS cases from Congo, Rwanda, and Burundi seen in Belgium between 1981 and 1985, individual patient histories, and drafts and redrafts of papers read at symposia and conferences, or submitted to different journals. During the early eighties AIDS in Africa and Africans was still a controversial subject, and few of the articles had been published.[9]

One of the most striking things about the African patients who had ended up seeking treatment in Brussels hospitals during the early eighties was the sheer geographical spread within the former Belgian territories. Most, of course, came from Kinshasa, but there were others from Bujumbura, Kigali, Kisangani, Bukavu, and from the provinces of Shaba, Kasai, and Bas-Zaire. And small epicenters were visible, even at a range of several thousand miles. One early center of infection was the Gecamines company, and many of the personnel from mining towns in Shaba, black and white, feature among the patients. Gilbert was the first, but a black engineer developed symptoms in 1978, and others soon followed. Another early focus was a bank in Kinshasa, with several employees affected.

In one of Sonnet's articles, thirty-two of the forty-two patients analyzed had flown to Brussels specifically to seek treatment, while of the other ten, none had been living in Belgium for more than two years. The fact that so many arrived by air indicates that they were either rich enough to purchase their own air tickets, or were employed by a company that was prepared to do so. For a short while, this encouraged the perception that AIDS was primarily a disease of the African elite, when it was actually the case that "elite patients" were merely the most visible subgroup of all those affected in central Africa. The patients included diplomats and politicians, businessmen and bank officials, doctors and engineers, a priest and a missionary, a mayor, a jeweler, and a young female student who, after the university closed in 1980, had taken to providing sexual services for the Congolese army. Altogether, approximately 30 percent of the patients reported a past history of heterosexual promiscuity. By contrast, only one patient declared himself a homosexual.

---

Sometime after leaving Belgium, I began to draw up a chart to depict these earliest recorded African AIDS patients, those in whom first symptoms had appeared prior to 1980. Even if not all of these cases had been serologically confirmed from stored tissues and sera, I was surprised at just how many plausible cases there were. I was also impressed by the support the chart afforded to the concept of a new virus emerging in humans, causing sporadic cases of disease in the sixties, followed by a rolling epidemic from about 1975 onward — evidence of a virus that had gained strength and vigor, and was now starting to explore new directions and possibilities.

THE CONGO TRIALS

The "preliminary report" in the *British Medical Journal* of July 26, 1958, about the feeding of Koprowski's two new vaccines, CHAT Type 1 and Fox Type 3, in central Africa may have been only just over two pages long, but it was a key paper.[1] It included details of the first large-scale open field trial of an attenuated OPV anywhere in the world, and of the first vaccinations with such an OPV in response to a poliomyelitis epidemic.[2] However, the preliminary report was — it seems — never followed by a full report. It is a strange omission for such vitally important research.

Because of its historical significance, it is necessary to review this paper in some detail. It begins with a surprisingly specific piece of background information about the genesis of the project. Hilary Koprowski apparently participated in a WHO-organized workshop on rabies held in Muguga, Kenya, in 1955, and there met a member of the Belgian Veterinary Service, Dr. T. J. Wiktor — another Pole and one who would become, a few years later, an illustrious member of staff at the Wistar Institute. Wiktor put Koprowski in contact with Ghislain Courtois, the director of the Laboratoire Médical in Stanleyville, and Koprowski proposed to him "a programme of experiments for the evaluation of attenuated strains of poliovirus in chimpanzees." Once permission and financial support had been obtained from the Belgian Congo government, a chimpanzee colony was established beside the Lindi, a tributary of the Congo River close to Stanleyville.

Details of the polio work conducted at Lindi camp are sketchy, to say the least, though it is stated that results will be reported in another paper due to appear in 1958, a "manuscript in preparation" by doctors Courtois, Koprowski, Norton, and two other Belgians, Ninane and Osterrieth. What *is* detailed in the *British Medical Journal* paper is that (as a safety test additional to those already conducted in

America on rhesus monkeys) five chimpanzees were injected in the spine with undiluted CHAT vaccine, and a further five with Fox. None of the chimps showed signs of illness and, at autopsy, only one animal (injected with Fox) had "mild lesions of the spinal cord suggestive of poliomyelitis infection." The caretakers at Lindi were also vaccinated with OPV "in order to protect them against possible exposure to the virulent poliomyelitis used for challenge of vaccinated chimpanzees." (Vaccination and challenge experiments were standard practice at the time, and involved first vaccinating an animal and then, a few weeks later, challenging it with virulent poliovirus, to see whether or not it had been immunized.)

Other safety tests for CHAT and Fox involved injecting the vaccine viruses into rabbits, guinea pigs, and infant and adult mice, "to rule out the presence of other viral agents such as B virus, lymphocytic choriomeningitis and Coxsackie viruses"; filtering them through bacteria-retaining filters; and finally feeding them to a small group of infants and adults in the United States. No further details are given about these tests, but apparently "in no instance was there a reaction of any kind."

The report goes on to state that some of the rhesus monkeys injected intraspinally became paralyzed, though again no details are given of the figures. Presumably this applied to both vaccines, because the authors continue: "this, however, has not deterred us from using these strains for mass vaccination purposes, as there is no strain of attenuated poliovirus available anywhere in the world completely devoid of pathogenic properties when injected intraspinally into rhesus or cynomolgus monkeys."

It is noteworthy that the different monkey species (rhesus macaque and chimpanzee) used for safety testing the vaccines are mentioned specifically, whereas no information is given about the species that provided the kidney tissue cultures in which the relevant pools of CHAT and Fox were grown.

The vaccination of the caretakers proved to be doubly useful, because its "successful outcome . . . prompted us to undertake clinical trials in the Belgian Congo on a much larger scale than had been attempted so far." Authorization for these field trials was apparently obtained in the second half of 1957 from Dr. Charles Dricot, the chief physician of the colony. Some of the first feedings employed vaccines in gelatin capsules, but in the later vaccinations, vaccine was administered directly, 1 milliliter at a time, either on a spoon, or else by squirting it into the mouth of the vaccinee, using an automatic pipette.

After feeding of the Lindi caretakers, the vaccinations seem to have taken place in four separate stages. The first campaign described involves 1,978 schoolchildren in Aketi, an important railhead and river port on the Itimbiri River, two hundred miles northwest of Stanleyville, who were given CHAT in capsules. A hundred children were bled prior to vaccination, fifteen of whom were found to lack Type 1 polio antibodies; of these, only two still lacked these antibodies when retested two months later. During this period, "rigid clinical observations failed to show any signs of illness which could be attributed to the vaccine." Six months later, Fox was fed to the same population, and of 43 (of 100 tested) lacking Type 3 antibodies, 41 had developed immunity when tested two months later. It appeared, therefore, that the new Koprowski vaccines were both safe and effective in humans.

In Stanleyville itself, 4,228 individuals of all ages (including a group of European schoolchildren) were fed CHAT, and some 500 Fox, in the period from March 1957 to February 1958. Again, no ill effects were noted.

The next feedings came in response to polio epidemics. Between November 1957 and January 1958, eight cases of paralytic polio were apparently seen in infants and children from the town of Banalia, eighty miles north of Stanleyville, and toward the end of January, 21 more cases were reported from the towns of Bambesa, Watsa, and Gombari, between three hundred and four hundred fifty miles to the north and northeast of the provincial capital. All the outbreaks appeared to have been caused by Type 1 poliovirus. "Following the recommendation of the Expert Committee on Poliomyelitis of the World Health Organization and upon the request of the Medecin Provincial [chief physician] of Province Oriental," CHAT vaccine was given to "every inhabitant" of the four towns — a total of 22,886 persons. Apparently no further polio cases were seen after the fourth day following vaccination.

The final campaign, in the Ruzizi Valley, is described as "a mass vaccination trial," which was staged between February 24 and April 10, 1958. The report states that "immunization of the total population of the community was decided upon only if 12% or more of the sera collected were found to have no antibodies against a given type of virus," and reveals that exactly 12 percent of eighty-four serum samples collected at random from the valley showed an absence of Type 1 antibodies. A total of 215,504 men, women, and children were therefore vaccinated with CHAT in liquid form, at a rate of between three thousand and eleven thousand a day. "The native population were informed by their chiefs about the vaccination project and assembled daily at fixed rally points. . . . Medical authorities were asked to report any occurrence of illness which could be attributed to vaccination, but none was reported." For comparative purposes two mission schools were included in the trial, with the pupils of one being given the vaccine and those of the other school a placebo. Four hundred fifty additional blood samples were also taken from children just prior to vaccination to check antibody status, but the tests on these had not been completed.

Together with a large map showing the seven major vaccination sites, this was the sum total of information provided in this, the first-ever report of a mass vaccination with OPV. Authorship of the article was attributed to five scientists, with Ghislain Courtois afforded the honor of being first named. Also credited were Gaston Ninane (another member of the Stanleyville laboratory) and two Americans who had participated in the Ruzizi Valley vaccinations. These were

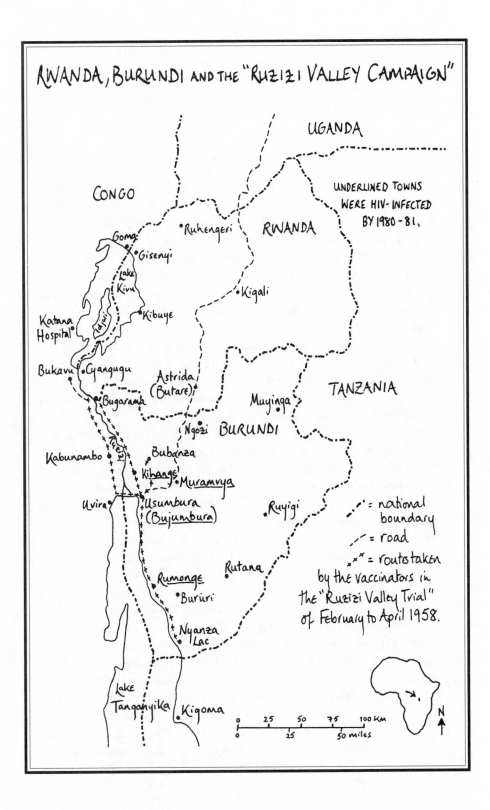

# RWANDA, BURUNDI AND THE "RUZIZI VALLEY CAMPAIGN"

UGANDA

CONGO

RWANDA

UNDERLINED TOWNS
WERE HIV-INFECTED
BY 1980-81.

•Ruhengeri

•Goma
•Gisenyi
Lake
Kivu
•Kibuye

•Kigali

Katana
Hospital•

Bukavu •Cyangugu

Astrida
(Butare)

TANZANIA

•Bugarama

Muyinga•

•Ngozi  BURUNDI

Kabunambo

Bubanza

Kibangs'
•Muramvya

Usumbura
(Bujumbura)

•Ruyigi

Uvira

Rutana

= national
boundary

= road

= routes taken

Rumonge
•Bururi

by the vaccinators in
the "Ruzizi Valley Trial"
of February to April 1958.

•Nyanza
Lac

Lake
Tanganyika •Kigoma

0    25    50    75    100 Km
0         25        50 miles

N

Agnes Flack, the medical director at Clinton Farms, a women's prison in New Jersey where some of the preliminary research on CHAT and Fox had been conducted, and George Jervis, the director of laboratories at Letchworth Village in New York, a center for mentally handicapped children, and the site of Hilary Koprowski's very first OPV feeding back in 1950.

---

Just before leaving for Belgium, I had been searching through *Index Medicus* for a more complete report of these vaccinations, and for the promised paper by Courtois, Koprowski, and others about the polio research conducted on the Lindi chimpanzees. I was unable to find anything further by Koprowski about OPV work in the Congo, apart from several very detailed reports from 1959 and 1960 about the vaccinations of children in the capital, Leopoldville. Neither could I find the promised paper about the chimpanzee work, even though it had been cited in the *British Medical Journal* article as being "in preparation." But while searching for this, I came across another article in a Belgian journal about the Ruzizi Valley and Province Oriental vaccinations. It was attributed to a single author, Dr. Courtois, the man who had directed the research at both the Laboratoire Médical and the nearby chimp colony.[3] His account (which was published in the same month as the Koprowski paper) is not mentioned or cross-referenced in any of Koprowski's articles.

This article by Courtois is important, for although rather discursive, and not — in any sense — a final report on the vaccination campaign, it does add several vital details to the original. It specifies the precise titer or concentration of the vaccine that was used in Ruzizi, and the fact that the vaccine was diluted sixtyfold with saline solution before feeding. And it mentions the specific pool of CHAT vaccine that was employed: 10A-11.

But the most important feature of Courtois's article lies in the clues it provides about where the vaccine was fed in the Ruzizi mass trial. Courtois gives exactly the same total number of vaccinees — 215,504 — as the original article, and he provides a detailed analysis of the lowland area that had been selected as a suitable site for the campaign. In the course of this, he describes not only the rice fields and meandering rivulets of the Ruzizi Valley, but also the region to the south of Usumbura (Bujumbura), along the eastern shore of Lake Tanganyika as far as the small town of Nyanza Lac. He does not specifically state that vaccine was also fed in this lakeshore area. But he does refer to Usumbura as lying roughly in the center of the vaccination region — and reveals that whereas 74,000 were fed on the Congo side of the border, nearly double that number (141,000) were fed in Ruanda-Urundi. All of this suggested to me that the people living alongside the huge expanse of Lake Tanganyika in what is now southwest Burundi had also been fed CHAT pool

10A-11 in early 1958. If correct, however, this raised the question of why only the Ruzizi Valley had been mentioned in Koprowski's report.

———————

To find out more, I needed to interview some of those who had been involved in the actual vaccination campaigns. However, soon after arriving in Belgium, I learned that Ghislain Courtois had died of cancer back in the early seventies, at the age of fifty-four. Since the two Americans who had helped with the vaccinations, Agnes Flack and George Jervis, were also dead, and since Koprowski had not himself been present, it seemed that there was only one of the major participants in the Ruzizi trial who might still be alive — Dr. Gaston Ninane.

He proved difficult to locate. I tried various numbers without success, but after four days managed to track him down to a hamlet in the Ardennes. He sounded friendly and courteous on the phone, and he agreed to an interview the following afternoon.

The small farming village where Gaston Ninane resided was set among rolling hills dotted with woodland and fields full of cows; he lived in a long, handsome house on the main street. He met me at the door and escorted me to the lounge, where his sister soon brought in biscuits and freshly brewed coffee. As Dr. Ninane poured, I was able to size him up. He was apparently in his mid-sixties — a slight man, below average height, who moved a little stiffly. He had a naturally serious face, but he seemed to be smiling a lot, and he spoke quickly, in bursts. There was something vulnerable and nervous about him, and already I found myself starting to like him, though as yet I had no inkling of what a revealing interview this would turn out to be.

We spoke in English, for Dr. Ninane's English was a lot better than my French. He told me that he had arrived in the Belgian Congo in December 1953, and had stayed until just after independence in June 1960. First he had been based at the medical laboratory in Leopoldville and later at the one in Stanleyville. He spent a lot of time working on rabies, and after an incident in which he was bitten by a laboratory mouse infected with the virus, was forced to undergo the full course of fourteen injections of vaccine in the stomach. In fact, he said, he had performed the injections himself — which sounded like the sort of experience that might predispose someone toward oral vaccination.

Later, in 1955, he was part of the Belgian team that attended the WHO rabies course at Muguga, Kenya, which was where he first met Hilary Koprowski, who was one of the course leaders. Koprowski had brought with him an experimental rabies vaccine, which required only a single inoculation. When he asked the fifty or so course participants if any of them would like to serve as guinea pigs, about half of them volunteered — and the first of these was Gaston Ninane. (This seems to have been partly prompted by bravado, and partly by the fact that the previous vaccinations had given him a very high level of immunity, so that he would almost certainly be protected even if the new vaccine should revert to virulence.)

Later, apparently, he and Koprowski had had a long talk, during which the American outlined his ideas about polio vaccination, and the Belgian suggested that he might like to try out his new polio vaccines on chimpanzees, which were readily available in the Congo. Two days after the conference ended, Koprowski apparently followed Ninane to Leopoldville to have further "intimate discussions" about the proposal. A few months later, Ninane says, he was moved to the lab at Stanleyville, and soon afterward the chimp colony was established. "If I'd stayed in Leo," explained Ninane, "maybe nothing would have happened."

Lindi camp became functional at some point during 1956. It was at an isolated spot, some ten miles west of Stanleyville (now Kisangani), on the north bank of the Congo River. Just before the camp was the Lindi tributary, which had to be crossed by a hand-operated ferry. The chimps were provided by a French hunter, who, with his team of fifteen Congolese helpers, went out into the forest to catch the animals. To begin with, Ninane said, they only had forty or so chimps, housed in cages inside two large hangars, but before long the operation was to get much, much bigger. At the height of the experiments, he had been in charge of about 140 chimps, which, he told me, probably made it the largest chimpanzee colony that the world had ever seen.

At this point, Ninane started to describe the actual vaccinations, and I was happy to sit back and let him talk. The first report of Koprowski's new vaccines, he told me, had been presented at the Geneva conference in July 1957, and soon after this he, Gaston Ninane, had "vaccinated the whole country." I asked him to be more specific, and he told me about the polio epidemics — how he had heard from a doctor in the forest about an outbreak of polio, so he and an assistant had driven up there with flasks of vaccine packed in ice. When they arrived, they informed the local people by means of tom-toms that the doctors had brought them *dawa* (medicine). When all the inhabitants had assembled, they got them into a long line and started vaccinating. He said that he counted everyone, and that the totals usually turned out to be higher than the official populations — perhaps because not everyone was paying their taxes! Within four or six days of each campaign, all reports of polio ceased. He could remember the location of only one of these anti-epidemic vaccinations, this being at a big military base not far from the Sudanese border, which we eventually decided must have been the army town of Watsa.

He went on to explain how he had taken prevaccination and postvaccination blood samples from several of the people around Stanleyville, to test for polio antibodies. Apparently this was a lengthy process, and he had a lot of difficulty tracing the individual vaccinees. Finally he had taken to handing out pieces of paper to certain people at the time of vaccination, with the instruction that they should be handed back to him when he returned. The laboratory had sent these bloods packed around with ice, he told me, on planes that flew from Stanleyville to Brussels, with just the one stop at a U.S. Air Force base in Libya. By this stage, several professors from Leuven were involved in the vaccine program, and one of these people would pick up the samples at Brussels, take them back to Leuven (presumably keeping some samples for the Belgian research), and then, after replacing the ice, put the remainder on another plane bound for Koprowski in Philadelphia. This happened ten or twenty times, he said.

I knew that Leuven, the ancient Catholic university in the town of the same name, some twenty miles east of Brussels, seemed always to be at the cutting edge of Belgium's academic and medical research, and that it was the parent institution for major Belgian hospitals such as St. Luc, and for foreign universities such as Lovanium outside Leopoldville. So I asked Gaston Ninane exactly what Leuven's involvement with the vaccination program had been — and he introduced a completely unexpected piece of information. To begin with, he said, the vaccines used in the Congo had been made in Philadelphia at the Wistar Institute, but later they had begun using versions made in Leuven. He subsequently explained that this was partly because of the distance from Philadelphia to Stanleyville, and the importance of keeping the vaccine at or below 4°C (or 39.2°F), and partly because the Belgians had wanted to be directly involved in the manufacturing process. Ninane thought that some time during 1958, Koprowski had started sending the Leuven scientists flasks containing the attenuated viruses and other flasks containing the monkey culture cells, so that the two could be combined and made into large pools of vaccine.

Ninane also confirmed other details from the preliminary report in the *British Medical Journal*. Yes, they had given some of the chimps intraspinal injections of the vaccines, to check that the attenuated viruses were safe, and did not cause paralysis. Then they had given a few nonvaccinated chimps virulent poliovirus, to prove that it did indeed paralyze. And finally they had done vaccination and challenge experiments to prove the vaccine really did protect against wild poliovirus. He said that to begin with the challenge poliovirus had been fed, but that later they had also injected it intravenously, intraspinally, or intracerebrally (into the bloodstream, spine, or brain, respectively). For the more difficult procedures, the chimp would first be anesthetized, or else fed barbiturates to make it dopey; for easier procedures (like taking blood), the animal could often be distracted with a banana while a couple of assistants grabbed it by the arms.

I asked him where else the vaccinations had been carried out. There had been lots of them, he said, including the mass vaccination in Ruzizi in 1958. In that campaign they had traveled north to south, stopping at fifteen to twenty different places over a period of some weeks. He added that they had started off using tablespoons, or mixing vaccine with a little milk for the babies, but found that this took a lot of time. It was he who had come up with the method of vaccinating by a pipette attached by a tube to the flask of vaccine. This made the vaccination technique a lot simpler, since all they had to do was make a quick squirt into each mouth in the line.

So who else had participated in these campaigns? He remembered working with George Jervis and Agnes Flack, the two American doctors whom Koprowski had sponsored to fly out and participate. There were also a number of locally based doctors and medical assistants, white and black, who helped for various periods. He recalled the Ruzizi plain, with its rice and sugarcane, as being a beautiful region with a moderate climate, containing several small hotels where they would stay at night. Everyone, apparently, had enjoyed themselves: not only were they pioneering a new medical procedure and helping the local people, but they were enjoying a real holiday besides. They traveled in two teams, each in its own car (with Flack, a committed nationalist, always insisting on riding in the Buick), and never stayed more than a couple of days in any one place. He remembered just three of the locations where they stayed: Kamanyola (a military base in the Ruzizi Valley), Bujumbura (then Usumbura, the capital of Ruanda-Urundi), and Nyanza Lac.

When I asked about the latter place, Ninane gradually recalled that he had been part of a team of three (himself, another white, and a black) who spent five or six days feeding the vaccine to people along the eastern shores of Lake Tanganyika. This seemed to have been after Flack and Jervis had left. He confirmed that they had vaccinated as far south as Nyanza Lac, a small town virtually on the border with what is now Tanzania. He recalled a particular incident around sunset, down by the lakeshore, at the end of a long day's work. While their African assistant cooked supper, the two whites stripped and jumped into the water, in the process disturbing a hippo, which had been lying submerged just ten meters away. All parties involved had moved with some speed from that point on.

I asked how they had checked on the future health status of the vaccinees, and Ninane confirmed that local doctors had been instructed to report to Stanleyville any subsequent cases of polio or unexpected disease, and that no such reports had been made. It seemed that this was the extent of the follow-up for the first mass OPV field trial in the world.

Ninane also recounted an incident in which he had flown in a light plane to a town in Equateur province, downstream of Stanleyville on the river Congo. He had spent a day or two vaccinating all those in the town — perhaps five thousand or so, but he couldn't remember the year. We examined the map, and Ninane decided that the town must have been either Bumba or Lisala. He knew that he had also vaccinated in several other places in both Province Oriental (the region to the north and east of Stanleyville) and in Ruanda-Urundi, but was unable to recall the specific names. He said that most requests for vaccine had come from areas where there was a large settler population, like Kivu district around Bukavu, and the agricultural land to the north of Stanleyville, around Isiro. The difficulty, he said, was that his papers had been left behind when he, together with many other Belgians, had been airlifted out of the Congo by military plane in August 1960, just two months after independence.

So how many further vaccinations did he think that he personally had carried out after the end of the Ruzizi campaign in April 1958? Dr. Ninane reflected and then said that he had probably vaccinated a further 250,000, making a total of half a million vaccinees in the years up to and including 1960. However, for the last year or so before independence, responsibility for the vaccination program had been transferred from the medical service to the *Hygiène* department. After this, the people from the Stanleyville lab no longer did the immunizations themselves, but instead responded to vaccine requests from specific towns by dispatching the appropriate number of doses — usually by air, inside small, portable fridges. He was a little uncertain about specific towns, but said that vaccines had certainly been sent to Ruanda-Urundi, and to other regions in the Congo, such as the province of Bas-Congo to the west of Leo.

It was perhaps two hours into the interview before Gaston Ninane mentioned Ghislain Courtois for the first time. Courtois had been his boss in Stanleyville from 1956 until 1959, he told me, and had then taken over as general director of the medical laboratory in Leo, after the previous director had fled across the river to Brazzaville during an early period of rioting. Ninane, in turn, took charge of the Stanleyville lab. "Courtois and I did all the work together," he suddenly told me, this being the first time that he had abandoned the role of prime mover in the vaccine program. "There were lots more vaccinations: Courtois would have the answer. But Courtois is now dead, I think."

He mentioned the vaccination of 75,000 children in Leopoldville, which had started in late 1958 and continued into 1960. He added that, just as in other towns in the country, CHAT had also been fed to adults in the capital, not just to children, but that he could not be sure when the adult vaccinations in Leo had started. Courtois was very much in favor of the complete vaccination of the white population, he added, and at one point — probably in 1959 — the governor-general had made a formal announcement to the effect that the vaccine was safe and available free of charge, and had advised all those in the colony to get immunized. Apparently the day after this decree was published in the local press, Ninane arrived at the laboratory to find a long queue of volunteers waiting to be vaccinated.

Later, he mentioned the visits made by various scientists from overseas. At one point, he said, perhaps half a dozen Belgian scientists, including Lise Thiry, the famous woman virologist who later became a member of parliament and who was then based at the Institut Pasteur in Brussels, had come out to Stanleyville for a conference. He also recalled a German, Friedrich Deinhardt, who had stayed in Stanleyville for some weeks, conducting hepatitis experiments on the chimps. I asked if he recalled the 1959 visit by Arno Motulsky, and Ninane promptly volunteered the information that Motulsky had heard about their operation from Hilary Koprowski, and that this was why he had selected the Belgian Congo for his blood studies. He added that the geneticist had remained for two or three weeks in Stanleyville and that they had gone out together on two or three occasions, with Motulsky taking blood at the same time that Ninane was vaccinating. Later, he recalled that one of the samples Motulsky had taken in Leopoldville had subsequently proved that HIV was already present in the Belgian Congo in 1959. This pleased him, he said, for it effectively disproved all the other theories that AIDS had come from Haiti, or had been made in an American military laboratory.

Finally I asked Ninane about CHAT: why was it called that? Some had suggested it might stand for CHimpanzee-ATtenuated — was this possible? He agreed that this would make sense. I asked Ninane if this would mean that CHAT had been attenuated through chimps, and there followed a most extraordinary five minutes. He replied: "Not through chimpanzees. The virus was cultivated in kidney cells, chimpanzee kidney cells, but the Italian [Renato Dulbecco] found a method to distinguish between different viruses [to select] the one which was not pathogenic. The kidney cell, the chimp kidney cell, multiplied easily, and it was a good substrate for the poliovirus." I asked him if he had supplied the chimps that were used for the substrate, and he replied that he had not; they had come from the Wistar. So I pointed out that the papers of the time talked of monkey kidney tissue culture as the substrate, and did not specifically mention chimpanzees. He replied "Monkey — *voilà*. It's surely *monkey* kidney cell; I'm not sure that it's *chimpanzee* kidney cell."

It was clear that this could have been a genuine mistake, a slip of the tongue, the use of a wrong word in a foreign language. On the other hand, it seemed that Dr. Ninane had suddenly realized the potential significance of the species of kidney — for he went away, and returned holding a copy of a letter published a couple of months before in the *Lancet*. This letter had mentioned the hypothesis that "poliovirus vaccine lots dispensed in [the Congo] from 1957 to 1960 and prepared in African green monkey kidney cell cultures" might have contained the precursor virus to HIV-1, but another part of the letter mentioned that the closest primate relative to HIV-1 was the SIV of the chimp.[4]

Gaston Ninane now seemed upset, and he stressed that "it's completely crazy to say that the Wistar vaccine was spreading AIDS." He started to provide reasons why it could not be so — that the vaccinations had happened thirty years before, while AIDS had only appeared recently, and so forth. After a while, I tried to reassure him that I understood what had happened, that he had muddled up two words, and he calmed down. "Excuse me. I don't know if it was a chimp, or a baboon or something like that [which supplied the kidneys]. *Monkey*. Excuse me; I am getting old."

It was now early evening, and it was clear that we were both getting tired, so we arranged to meet again the following afternoon. Dr. Ninane found a place for me in a small country hotel a few miles away, and as darkness fell, drove me over there in his car.

———————

In the morning, it was good to have a chance to review my notes, and to take stock. I was beginning to realize that although Gaston Ninane apparently had a good memory for certain details, that memory also tended to place him in the role of the main protagonist — even when, perhaps, his role had been less prominent. One of the many examples was his account of bringing Koprowski to the Congo. This differed from Koprowski's own account in the *British Medical Journal,* in which it is the vet, Dr. Wiktor (who also attended Muguga), who serves as the contact between Koprowski and Courtois, and Ninane is not even mentioned. Similarly, Ninane had described himself as the central figure in all the events at the Stanleyville lab, even though Courtois had been its director from 1956 until 1959. On the other hand, it did seem likely that he, rather than Courtois, had been actively involved in many of the actual vaccination campaigns. There was obviously a need to clarify certain details, but it was also obvious that for many of these topics, he was the best available witness.

When Gaston Ninane arrived at the hotel, he insisted on taking me for lunch at a restaurant in a medieval town nearby. This time, however, I was determined to get through the rest of my questions, rather than let him lead the conversation. It was tougher than I had expected. After lunch we walked alongside the river, which bisects the town, and sat down on a bench beneath the walls of the castle. I started off by asking him how the vaccine had been delivered to the Ruzizi Valley. He thought that it had probably come from Leuven; it had been delivered in several glass bottles, each containing half a liter or so of the fluid. These had arrived by air, packed in ice, and they had transferred the vaccine that was not to be used straightaway into freezers or fridges along their proposed route. One of these fridges, he concluded after looking at the map, had probably been at the Congolese village of Kabunambo, in the center of the valley, which was the headquarters of the Mission Médicale du Ruzizi.

I also asked him some more about the chimpanzees, and he told me that in 1957 a brand-new medical laboratory had been built in Stanleyville, and an animal house beside it, which had later allowed some of the chimps, especially the larger ones, to be moved in from the less accessible site at Lindi. It was not entirely clear what impact this had made on the polio work. I asked Gaston Ninane whether they had had facilities to manufacture vaccines in Stanleyville, and he replied that vaccine-making was far too technical an operation for a lab such as theirs — apart from which, the first deep freeze had not arrived in the lab until early in 1960. Apparently they had always received the vaccines already made up, never separately as concentrated virus and monkey kidney cells.

Whatever, the new facilities in Stanleyville clearly allowed the scale of the research to increase. After 1958, the polio work began to wind down, but a variety of other projects were launched — all in conjunction with American scientists, many of whom appeared to be friends or associates of Koprowski. First there had been Deinhardt's work on hepatitis, and later work was planned on artherosclerosis, various forms of cancer, and hormones — some of it, apparently, funded by the Rockefeller Foundation. Ninane particularly remembered a visit by two American dignitaries, whom he referred to as "senators," who were hoping to set up a study on heart disease. This study apparently did get started, with the hearts of wild chimpanzees (in fact, those animals that had been inadvertently killed during the capture operations) being compared to those of chimps that had lived for six months at Lindi camp, being fed a Western diet of butter and cream.

However, like all the research projects, these had to be abandoned at the time of independence. Ninane still spoke about this bitterly, about how these studies were potentially huge operations, which could have gone on for ten or twenty years. Everything, he said, collapsed because of the political situation, and the chaos that followed Belgium's sudden granting of independence, which had left the new nation so woefully unprepared.

The dénouement of this unique period of research was equally tragic. After independence, none of the Congolese came in to work anymore, and very soon there was no food left for the chimpanzees. So what happened to them when Ninane flew out in August 1960? "I left them there. Some were released by the blacks; some I asked to be shot by the soldiers. Probably they ate them."

At this point, I produced a paper by Koprowski showing his description of how CHAT had been made,[5] and we agreed that it was not clear exactly how he had attenuated the vaccine. But this did prompt Ninane to emphasize that he had not been involved in any way with the attenuation process. "I didn't *attenuate* the virus in Zaire," he said. "I *tested* different lots of the vaccine . . . in the chimps, to be sure that there was no pathogenic strain of the virus remaining," he explained.

Finally, I told him about Sabin finding a viral contaminant in CHAT in 1959 — something about which he apparently knew nothing. What if that virus had been an SIV, I asked. Was it possible that the vaccination campaign could have started the AIDS epidemic? Ninane took a long time to think about this, before saying: "Koprowski and Sabin hated each other. They were not very good friends. Yes — it's a worry. But we have vaccinated so many people, and nothing has happened. I first vaccinated myself, I drank the vaccine, and forty years afterwards I'm still living." I said that one would hardly expect every lot or pool of the vaccine to be contaminated. But, from the opposite perspective, could one be sure that every lot was safe? He acknowledged that there could have been a problem "in one lot, in some lots, possibly — but I cannot answer."

―――――――

Dr. Ninane drove me back to the station and offered to keep me company until the train came, but he looked exhausted, and I persuaded him to head off back home. Before he left, he told me, only half in jest, that I must be from the CIA or the KGB. I could hardly blame him, for it was clear that my questions about AIDS had deeply disturbed him, and upset the friendly atmosphere that had been established over the course of two days.

As the train rolled back through tightly wooded valleys toward Liège, I realized that Gaston Ninane was not the only one who felt shattered. The protracted interview had also involved quite a lot of tension for me, especially when it came to putting those final, blunt questions to this essentially kind and decent man. However, these were the questions that had to be asked.

It was clear that even before our interview, he had read about the hypothesis linking AIDS to CHAT vaccine. Nonetheless, something strange had undoubtedly happened toward the end of our first conversation, when he had started talking about chimpanzee kidney cells. It appeared that he had muddled the words for "chimpanzee" and "monkey," but was it possible that he had not realized the potential significance of chimpanzee SIV until I pressed him about the species that had provided the kidneys?

I had the sense that Dr. Ninane had generally answered my questions truthfully, even if there did seem to be certain anomalies. It was clear from the *British Medical Journal* article and Ninane's own account that prevaccination blood samples had been taken at Aketi (100), Ruzizi (450 to 500), and around Stanleyville. Postvaccination blood samples were a lot more difficult to organize, and apart from a few dozen at Aketi, they appear to have been taken only at Stanleyville, where Ninane was based. Yet Ninane had spoken of ten or twenty occasions on which refrigerated human sera had been flown back to Belgium and the United States.

Another mystery involved the sudden construction, in 1957, of the large modern laboratory and animal house in Stanleyville. Why had this huge investment been made if no freezer was installed until 1960? This was a detail that just didn't make sense. Furthermore, it suggested that perhaps other work and research might have been carried out there, over and above that which had been reported in the medical literature.

And there did seem to be a pronounced dearth of accurate published information about this crucial episode in medical history. Ninane said that as far as he knew the much-cited article by Courtois and others (including himself) about the chimpanzee work, variously described as being "in preparation" and "to be published, 1958,"[6] had never actually appeared. It was now becoming apparent that the Lindi research had been conducted on an unexpectedly massive scale, and that it had probably involved more than a hundred animals, many of which had died — or been sacrificed — in the process. Although animal rights were not considered a burning issue in the fifties, the chimpanzee has always held a special place in people's affections, so it seemed possible that the secrecy about the chimp work might have been prompted by concern about the reaction of the general public.

However, it was less easy to explain the revelation that the so-called Ruzizi Valley trial had actually extended twice as far as reported in Koprowski's article. Why had the Lake Tanganyika leg of the trial not been mentioned in that article, and only hinted at in the article in the Belgian journal, written by Courtois alone? The figures in the latter piece made it clear that the total of 215,000 must have included the lakeshore vaccinees, but Koprowski had quoted this same figure for the Ruzizi Valley alone. This suggested that he was keen to be the first to stage a mass OPV trial, and to have impressively large numbers of vaccinees to report but, inexplicably, was less accurate about the regions where the vaccinations were staged.

Coincidences had begun to crop up, too. Ninane recalled vaccinating in either Lisala, or in Bumba a hundred miles away, and Lisala was the hometown of Hélène, who had died of AIDS-like symptoms in 1962, after first falling sick in 1958. It was also apparent that many other vaccinations, unrecorded in the medical literature, had occurred in other towns in the Congo and Ruanda-Urundi. And in Leopoldville, where Ninane said that adults as well as children had been vaccinated with CHAT, there was this intriguing coincidence of an HIV-positive sample of blood dating from 1959, just a few months after the start of the vaccinations there.

What was abundantly clear was that the CHAT trials in the Congo merited further investigation.

———

A few months after our meeting, Gaston Ninane sent me a letter. Inside was an old clipping from a Belgian Congo newspaper, with a note attached reading: "Found by my sister in her 'Dinosaur Archives.' Don't remember the name, or the date, of the newspaper." The article in question, entitled "War against Polio in the Stanleyville Bush," described a visit by a local journalist to an isolated research center in the rain forest. The center was described as "Mission Koprowski," and was quite clearly the camp at Lindi, for it contained sixty chimpanzees housed inside two enormous hangars. It had been made available by the colonial government to facilitate various research projects, including the fine-tuning (*"mise au point définitive"*) of Koprowski's oral polio vaccine. At the time of writing, Koprowski and Norton were visiting from the United States, and were training doctors Courtois, Ninane, and Osterrieth in their methods of work. Gaston Ninane had not mentioned this visit during our two lengthy interviews, and indeed it was the first confirmation I had come across of Koprowski and Norton themselves attending the site of the chimpanzee research.

Ninane's letter also featured various skeptical clippings about the OPV/AIDS theory, and the overall tone indicated that he was keen to discourage any ideas I might have that the CHAT trials could be related to the outbreak of a new disease two decades later. By this stage, however, I was already far less inclined to agree with him.

This was largely because I had come across a remarkable 1989 article from a French journal, the *Bulletin de la Société de Pathologie Exotique*, which detailed a study of HIV prevalence in the very parts of Burundi where CHAT had been fed in early 1958.[7] The research had been conducted on 658 sera, which had originally been drawn as part of a study into arboviruses, conducted in 1980 and 1981.[8] After the Nahmias study from 1959, Desmyter's investigations in Kinshasa in 1970 and 1980, and the Nzilambi/De Cock paper about Yambuku in rural Equateur in 1976, this French paper represented the next earliest evidence of the presence of HIV in central Africa.

The article was by Jacques Morvan, Bernard Carteron, and colleagues from the Laboratory of Clinical Biology at the army medical school in Bordeaux, and it provided dramatic evidence of much higher HIV prevalence than any of the previous papers, including the 1980 study that found that 3 percent of young Kinshasa mothers were HIV-positive. Overall, 29 of the subjects tested (4.4 percent) showed evidence of HIV infection, although prevalence varied greatly from region to region. In the central plateau region, which makes up most of eastern Burundi, there was zero infection, whereas in the volcanic spine that runs north to south, which represents the watershed between the rivers Nile and Congo, 2.89 percent of the sera were positive. By contrast, in the capital Bujumbura over 8 percent were infected. A rural zone in the west, "the plain of Imbo" (consisting of the Ruzizi Valley and the shore of Lake Tanganyika) demonstrated an overall prevalence of 3.66 percent. However, all the positive sera came either from Gihanga, a village in the Ruzizi Valley some fifteen miles north of Bujumbura, or from Rumonge, a small fishing center and port on the lake, roughly fifty miles to the south. Prevalence in the latter place was exceptionally high, at almost 12 percent.

There were a number of dramatic inferences to be drawn. The first was that the study revealed an unexpectedly high prevalence in both urban and rural Burundi at the very start of the eighties, one that already exceeded that in the huge metropolis of Kinshasa, Congo — and that therefore suggested an early seeding of the virus.

Second, although there was a significant difference between urban (8.08 percent) and rural (2.82 percent) seroprevalence, this was less pronounced than might have been expected. (In 1986 in Rwanda, for instance, the urban/rural differential was over 13:1.)[9] Furthermore, the rural prevalence appeared to be concentrated in certain specific places such as Rumonge and Gihanga. Whereas the classic explanation of HIV epidemiology in Africa is predicated on urban-to-rural diffusion, this early snapshot of the epidemic could be interpreted in terms of either urban-to-rural or rural-to-urban spread.

Third, these early pockets of high seroprevalence were all in those places where CHAT vaccine had been fed in the Ruzizi/Bujumbura/Lake Tanganyika field trial in early 1958. In areas where the vaccine was not fed, HIV prevalence was markedly lower. Indeed, the only two positive sera from outside the vaccinated zone both came from places close to the main road running from Bujumbura through the mountains, toward Rwanda and Uganda. This tentatively suggested that HIV had arrived first in the western lowland strip of Burundi, which included Bujumbura, that it subsequently diffused northward toward Rwanda, and that it was a long time before it spread to eastern Burundi.

In particular, the high seroprevalence in the lake port of Rumonge suggested that the long, narrow shape of Lake Tanganyika, stretching more than four hundred miles from Bujumbura as far as southern Tanzania and northern Zambia, might have represented another important route of viral diffusion — a hypothesis that was afforded some support by the relatively early appearance of HIV infection in Zambia. Just as the steamers of the Congo River were thought to have facilitated the spread of HIV along an east-west axis, so the steamers plying to and fro along Lake Tanganyika may have served as a north-south conduit for the virus.

Correspondence with the authors of the article revealed three further important facts. The first was that the sera had been collected from people attending dispensaries and hospitals as out-patients; all had been "apparently in good health," except for a few who were feverish (possibly from malaria). Clearly this information, which had not been mentioned in the original paper, somewhat reduced the significance of the HIV-prevalence findings, in that the cohort was a population seeking medical care rather than a cross section of the general adult population (for instance pregnant women).

The second factor was that both of the doctors I questioned were confident about the veracity of their findings, and pointed out that the different test methods they had used[10] were considered more reliable than most. Indeed, in that they managed to isolate HIV antigen from two sera that they had previously defined as HIV-antibody-negative (which had tested positive on one assay and negative on another), they suspected that the real prevalences might have been even higher.

Third, seven of the positive sera came from foreigners (five Rwandans and two Zairois), all of whom were tested at Bujumbura hospital. This emphasized how already, in 1980/81, HIV was becoming seeded in an itinerant population, which had the capacity to spread it across frontiers — in whichever direction.

Even if the cohort tested was not a representative cross section of the population, the finding of 29 HIV-positive sera from as early as 1980 and 1981 was still highly significant. This was not least because, of the three places in central Africa for which I had now come across evidence of widespread HIV infection in 1981 or earlier, two (Kinshasa and western Burundi) were also places where CHAT had been fed, while the third (Yambuku) lay within one hundred miles of where, according to Gaston Ninane, CHAT had been fed at either Bumba or Lisala.

# 21

## PRIMATE IMMUNODEFICIENCY VIRUSES

As it happened, one of the more important details to emerge from the interviews with Gaston Ninane — that at the end of the fifties Koprowski's vaccines were given not just to young children in Leopoldville, but to all age groups — was confirmed almost immediately, and from an unexpected quarter.

I had been invited by Jean Sonnet's widow, Simone, to join her family for Sunday afternoon tea. It was a bright, fresh day, and as we sat outside on the patio with beverages and a variety of sumptuous cakes, I was quizzed by her daughters about my ideas on the origin of AIDS. I ran through most of the major theories, explaining why they did not work, and finished up with the classic theory of natural transfer, involving a hunter with cuts on his hands. But, I added cautiously, there was also the possibility that medical science had inadvertently played a role — and I began to explain the reasons for the concern about the oral polio vaccines that had been fed in the Belgian Congo. Madame Sonnet, who had been present for the latter half of the conversation, suddenly got up and went inside. When she returned, she was holding her vaccination certificate from the fifties.

The first vaccinations, against typhoid, were done in Brussels in 1957, and then in 1958 came three shots of IPV made by the Belgian vaccine company, RIT, and administered at Lovanium by her husband. Then came two further entries, both with their own official rubber stamps. On December 16, 1959, she had been given CHAT (though it was officially described as "Polio vaccine, Type 1, Koprowski strain"), and on January 20, 1960, she had been fed with Fox. Madame Sonnet added that she thought her husband had received the vaccines also, some time before herself.

The Institute of Tropical Medicine in Antwerp has a fine reputation, and one of its researchers, Martine Peeters, was leader of the team that had first identified a simian immunodeficiency virus, SIV, in sera from a common chimpanzee, *Pan troglodytes*. Of all the SIVs that had been discovered by 1992, this was the only one that appeared to be a really close relative of HIV-1.

Back in 1989, Peeters and her colleagues had produced a classic article announcing the discovery of SIV antibodies in two chimps from the west central African country of Gabon, and the successful isolation and sequencing of a virus (SIVcpz) from one of the animals.[1] Then just recently, in May 1992, they had published a second article about another SIV-positive chimpanzee, one that had been intercepted by Belgian customs officials after a flight from Kinshasa.[2] Dr. Peeters and her collaborator, Marleen Van den Haesevelde, had again managed to isolate and sequence SIV from the blood of this smuggled animal, and discovered that this latest isolate (SIVcpz-ant) differed greatly from the Gabonese isolate (SIVcpz-gab-1). Only about 70 percent of the DNA was the same, though it was nonetheless clearly from the same HIV-1/SIVcpz branch of the phylogenetic tree.

Dr. Peeters sketched a map to show the places of origin of the two Gabonese chimps described in her original article. The first, the SIVcpz-gab-1 animal, came from the jungle along the Gabon-Cameroon border near the main road from Libreville to Yaounde. When this animal was six months old, its mother had been killed by hunters, and the young chimp was brought to the Gabonese capital, Libreville, and purchased by a French family. They had passed it over to researchers when it became too big to keep as a pet, and in 1992 it was still alive and healthy. The second chimp, the animal that had shown evidence of HIV-1-like antibodies but had not produced a viral isolate, came from near Makokou in eastern Gabon. When about two years old, it had been wounded by hunters, and its mother killed. It spent two days at the hunters' village, and was then transported to a French research institute, the Centre International de Recherches Médicales, in Franceville. The animal died of its wounds a week later, but not before the people at CIRM had taken and frozen some samples of blood. Using the knowledge gained from the first chimp SIV sequence, the Peeters team intended to design more specific PCR primers, in a further bid to isolate SIV from the sera of this second animal. (Primers are short fragments of DNA used in PCR to locate the sequence one wishes to amplify, rather like using a teaspoon of yogurt to "seed" a new culture.)

I asked Martine Peeters why so few examples of SIV had been identified in wild chimpanzees. Dr. Peeters disagreed with the premise, saying that she had tested almost a hundred chimps (more than fifty from Gabon, ten from Ivory Coast in West Africa, and thirty-four from zoos in Belgium), and had found three that were SIV-positive. "I don't think that's little," she said.

Another intriguing possibility, one recently highlighted by Luc Montagnier, was that in the past, chimpanzees held by animal exporters in places like the

Cameroons had sometimes been injected with human blood in a bid to protect them from the human diseases to which they were likely to be exposed once they arrived in the United States and Europe. If some of these captured chimps had later escaped, or been released, then perhaps what was being seen here was not a true SIV at all, but rather an HIV-1 that had adapted to chimpanzees.

Although she was sensibly cautious, it was apparent that Peeters believed that the SIVcpz isolates were chimpanzee, rather than human, viruses. Of course, this debate made the provenance of the smuggled chimp, the one that had produced the new SIVcpz-ant isolate, all the more important. Peeters told me she thought it came from somewhere in the Congo, though nobody knew from where. A few months later, one of Dr. Peeters's coworkers wrote me a letter to confirm that this third chimp was a member of *Pan troglodytes schweinfurthi*, a different subspecies to the chimps found in Cameroon and Gabon (*Pan troglodytes troglodytes*).[3] SIVcpz was thus shown to be quite widespread, in that it had infected at least two of the three subspecies of *Pan troglodytes,* and the hypothesis that it might be a human virus artificially transferred to chimps no longer seemed tenable.

I asked Dr. Peeters what follow-up work her team was doing. "We are currently studying our [Gabonese] chimp to see if he becomes sick. People take time to do so, perhaps chimps do also," she observed. Apparently he was now six or seven, and not yet showing any signs of sickness or depressed immunity. "Even knowing why he is not sick is interesting," she said, adding that if he did fall ill with simian AIDS, he would be the first example of a wild African monkey or ape to do so. Of course, one of the chief inferences that might be drawn if the animal remained healthy was that it was infected with an "ancient" virus, which had been in chimpanzees for many generations. If, however, it suddenly fell ill with a form of AIDS, then it was probable that (like humans, and Asian monkeys such as the rhesus and cynomolgus macaques) it had recently become cross-infected with a virus from another species. Peeters added that in the wild, chimps could live to fifty or more. There was therefore no way to hurry the research; one simply had to watch and wait.

Indeed, she said, she was more cautious than Beatrice Hahn and her collaborators from Birmingham, Alabama, the team that had recently reported samples of HIV-2 that appeared to be virtually identical to SIVsm, the SIV from the sooty mangabey.[4] The Hahn group had concluded that, in all likelihood, HIV-2 was in reality SIVsm that had somehow gotten transferred to humans. Peeters made it clear that they were not yet ready to make the same assumption about SIVcpz and HIV-1, which had only about 80 percent homology (genetic similarity). Perhaps, I suggested, the group of chimps that was infected with the immediate precursor virus to HIV-1 had not yet been tested.

We talked briefly about "medical blunder" theories of origin, such as those proposed by Tom Curtis and Charles Gilks, but it was clear that Dr. Peeters had little time for these. So we returned to SIVcpz. Presumably, I asked, she was keen to test other chimps from other regions to see if they too were SIV-infected. To my surprise, she showed a decided lack of enthusiasm. She said that chimps were now a protected species, and it was not easy to find them in the wild. You had to know where to go, and primatologists were not keen to help, because they felt such an inquiry would result in increased research demands on a dwindling population, or else that the chimp would become a bête noire, bludgeoned to death not just as a food source, but because of fear of the viruses it carried. Besides, she said, "we'd have Greenpeace down on our necks." I got the feeling that somebody had possibly already fired a shot across her bows — and that this, perhaps, was why she was also being so cautious with me. Perhaps she suspected me of being an animal activist.

Before I left, I gave Dr. Peeters a copy of an article I had found, published in 1961, by (among others) Courtois, Ninane, and Osterrieth from the Stanleyville lab.[5] It was a breakdown of the blood groups of 175 of the Lindi chimps, the research having been conducted in Liège soon after the doctors' departure for the Congo. The article analyzed the bloods of 158 common chimpanzees (*Pan troglodytes schweinfurthi*) originating from various locations on the north bank of the Congo River and 17 pygmy chimpanzees (*Pan paniscus*), an entirely separate species that came from the south bank. It was an intriguing piece, in that it detailed remarkably wide-ranging differences in blood characteristics among *Pan troglodytes,* which had come from six different collection points, less than four hundred miles apart in the tropical rain forest. The most unusual group, apparently, consisted of apes from Mambasa (a small town in the heart of the Ituri Forest, which was home to a large community of pygmies — the human, not the chimpanzee variety). From a taxonomic viewpoint, the article was proposing that these Mambasa chimps should be considered as a new subspecies of *Pan troglodytes.*

Peeters had already proven that great diversity existed between different SIVcpz isolates, and I suggested to her that perhaps here, in the east of Congo, was a good place to look for an SIVcpz that was even closer to HIV-1. For the first time, she became animated, and even a little excited. Perhaps she was wondering whether any of the 1961 chimp sera were still available. For my part, I was thinking that putting chimps from widely different geographical sources and genetic types together in a chimpanzee colony might be a good way of encouraging a chimpanzee virus from one group to pass to another group, and perhaps to assume a different character. Perhaps this could make a virus become more pathogenic, or more transmissible. Maybe here, among the chimpanzees from Lindi camp and the Laboratoire Médical de Stanleyville, was where one could find the missing link, the SIV that had ended up being transferred across to *Homo sapiens.*

By the time I left, Martine Peeters was a lot more friendly. However, I didn't point out to her that the chimps from the blood group study had been housed at the same camp where Koprowski's OPV research had been carried out a few years earlier. I suspected that the implications might make her a little nervous.

---

The next day, I finally arrived in the ancient university town of Leuven. Despite being situated just inside the northern Flemish-speaking part of Belgium, the fifteenth-century university has, for many years, bridged the cultural and linguistic divide and is widely acclaimed as the country's foremost seat of learning. Indeed, a new campus has recently been built at Louvaine-la-Neuve, in the Walloon (French-speaking) zone. The town of Leuven is small, with narrow, cobbled streets, and boasts some famous breweries and a vigorous railway industry.

I was here to check a few facts with Professor Jan Desmyter, the virologist whose studies had provided two of the key reference points for the early history of AIDS. It was he who had led the team that tested the bloods, taken in 1970, of eight hundred prenatal and postnatal mothers from Kinshasa, and found two of them positive for HIV-1. And again, it was his team that tested another five hundred such mothers' bloods from 1980, and found fifteen positive.[6] These HIV-positive samples (originally taken as part of a hepatitis B survey) not only served, indirectly, to reinforce the plausibility of the many clinically defined AIDS cases seen in the city from the early seventies onward, but also strengthened the hypothesis that HIV had been circulating in the Congo from a relatively early date — as had already been suggested by the Leopoldville serum from 1959, and the sequenced Yambuku virus from 1976.[7]

Desmyter told me that both the 1970 and 1980 studies were absolutely watertight, having been confirmed by several different assays. The 1970 samples, he said, had been taken in Lemba, a new middle-class suburb of single-story concrete dwellings, which had been built near the university between 1967 and 1970. It was therefore quite possible that one or both of the infected mothers had been fairly recent arrivals in the city.

Equally, he said, the Nahmias serum from 1959 had been tested by so many different assays, and in different labs, that there was next to no doubt that it was a genuine HIV-positive sample.[8] (However, that sample had still not been sequenced, so one could not exclude the possibility that the original serum had been contaminated by a modern HIV isolate.)

The increase in prevalence in Kinshasa, from 0.25 percent in 1970 to 3.0 percent in 1980, was dramatic, and I asked if this twelvefold rise in the space of a decade, evidence of a fast-growing epidemic, was suggestive of a virus that was newly arrived in its human host. Desmyter responded that the speed of growth of the epidemic depended largely on the local situation. For instance, the Yambuku study, where prevalence had remained stable between 1976 and 1986, proved that in a rural area of Congo, if people didn't sleep around and didn't give blood, HIV did not necessarily gain ground.

Even in Kinshasa, the growth rate was not constant. Further bloods from pregnant women had been tested in 1986 and 5.6 percent found to be HIV-positive — a definite slowing of the growth rate.[9] He guessed that the current prevalence in Kinshasa adults might be around 10 percent, and said that it was impossible to know why the prevalences in east African cities like Kigali, Bujumbura, and Kampala had soared considerably higher. In the Congo, he said, HIV was not always where one would expect it, and he cited a range of unexpected prevalences (apparently rather high in certain rural areas, but remaining stable at around 4 to 5 percent in the mining towns of Shaba) to support the contention.[10]

I asked him how he thought the epidemic had got started, and he said that some time ago an SIV (probably a mutant, since SIVs and HIVs are especially prone to mutation) was transmitted accidentally from simian to man. It was not transmitted sexually, of that he was sure, though it could possibly have been transmitted through handling or butchering of monkeys. But as long as this had occurred in a village, and the infectee had had a relatively small number of sexual contacts, such an incident could have been confined. He did concede that there was a small problem with the theory, in that the only SIV close to HIV-1 was that found in the chimpanzee — an animal that is hunted and eaten only quite rarely. So what about the OPV/AIDS hypothesis, I asked. Desmyter replied that it simply didn't work: for one thing, the vaccines had been fed in other places apart from Africa. And although monkey kidney cells are used to grow enteroviruses, like polio, these viruses are much easier to grow than retroviruses, like SIV. He had to admit, however, that monkey kidney cultures will readily support spumaviruses, which are also types of retrovirus.

And this was the point, exactly on cue, that Professor Jennifer Alexander arrived in the room. It turned out that she had been working with Desmyter on hepatitis B for a number of years, and that she had decided, on a whim, to call by and see him on her way back from the United States to South Africa. I, however, knew Alexander from another context entirely, for she — together with Pascal in New York and Elswood in California — was one of the three researchers who, quite independently of each other, had come up with slightly different versions of the OPV/AIDS theory.

---

Professor Alexander, who headed the Department of Microbiology at Witwatersrand University in Johannesburg, became involved in the debate in 1989 when, together with another virologist, Gerasmos "Mike" Lecatsas, from the Medical University of Southern Africa (Medunsa) near Pretoria, she wrote a letter to the *South African Medical Journal*.[11] The letter was in response to an editorial published in 1988, which detailed the measures taken to protect South African oral polio vaccines (which were then being produced in the tissues of the local variant of the African green monkey, *Cercopithecus aethiops pygerythrus*) against contamination with SIV and other adventitious viruses.[12]

Lecatsas and Alexander made a number of salient points. Most important was their observation that quarantining donor monkeys for six weeks to check for signs of illness, and monitoring the tissue cultures made from their kidneys for one month for signs of cytopathic effect (CPE),* which might indicate a viral contaminant, were totally inadequate responses to the threat proffered by "slow viruses" such as SIV. Not only would SIV fail to cause visible disease in its natural host, but it would be unlikely to cause detectable CPE in such a short time period. They wrote that since the discovery of latent viruses such as retroviruses, "most virologists would agree that 'clean cells' are for practical purposes non-existent." They argued that merely testing tissue cultures for the presence of SIV was not enough. To attain acceptable levels of safety, it was also necessary to test lymphocyte cultures for SIV (since lymphocytes are the preferred target cells for SIVs, and are usually present in tissue cultures) and, because SIVs mutate so rapidly, to retest cultures "continually and consequently."

"While it would be simplistic to assume, and even more difficult to prove, that polio vaccine is the source of HIV infection in man, it would be equally naive to ignore the possibility," they wrote, adding that it might well prove necessary to change to a completely different method of vaccine production, such as subunit or recombinant vaccines, and to employ IPV as a stopgap. They concluded the letter unequivocally: "A reappraisal of safety testing of live human viral vaccines, not only here but also elsewhere, is now surely imperative."

An accompanying letter from another Medunsa virologist detailed the observation of 81 cultures of AGM kidney tissue for periods as long as two hundred days: 86 percent of them showed evidence of CPE caused by an adventitious agent, and 58 percent demonstrated contamination with simian foamy virus (SFV) — one of the spumaviruses that Desmyter had been discussing.[13] On average, it took fifty-four days for SFV contamination to become apparent (considerably longer than the standard observation period), and on occasions more than one hundred days. The author pointed out that no disease had yet been linked with human exposure to SFV, "but the high incidence of a retrovirus in these cells is disturbing."

In 1990, in response to these two submissions, the authors of the original editorial, Barry Schoub and two colleagues from the South African National

---

* Cytopathic effect: the visible impact of virus infection on cells in tissue culture.

Institute for Virology, replied with an angry letter that accused Lecatsas and Alexander of "recklessly wild and unscientific speculation," but failed to address most of the points that they had raised.[14] The letter mentioned, almost in passing, that the institute had now changed to Vero cells,[15] instead of MKTC, for OPV manufacture. This reaction presaged that of the Wistar expert committee of two years later: first the claim that the problem was exaggerated — and then, without fanfare, the adoption (or advocacy) of a different tissue culture system.

An accompanying note from Lecatsas and Alexander pointed out that Schoub's admission that the quarantine period for vervet monkeys was "not designed to detect latent infections" had effectively settled the issue.[16] They went on: "Current thoughts on the origin of HIV implicate chance infection of man in Africa with different simian viruses. To ignore the overwhelming statistical possibility of cross-species infection via millions of doses of vaccine over a 40-year period would be naive. We believe in the free expression and exchange of ideas as a necessary ingredient in scientific advancement. We also believe that sooner or later the questions we have raised will have to be addressed and, we hope, answered."

––––––––––

In June 1992, Alexander and Lecatsas had a further letter published in the *Lancet*.[17] Having initiated such a heated debate in South African virology circles, they had decided to check the African green monkeys at the Medunsa colony for SIV infection, and had promptly found an animal that was not only SIV-positive, but that — on Western blot — presented bands that were typical of HIV-1, rather than SIVagm. Apparently, the monkey in question had not been in contact with other animals, except for being gang-caged with other AGMs when it was brought to the colony. Alexander told us that her colleague Lecatsas was currently trying to get the results confirmed by the more sophisticated PCR assay but that, if correct, the implications were astounding. There could be an African green monkey SIV that was an even closer relative of HIV-1 than was the SIV of chimpanzees.

Desmyter was now in high spirits — clearly excited by the scientific implications, but nonetheless skeptical about the HIV-1-positive AGM. He said that atypical Western blot results were not unusual, and that he would be surprised if the virus did not show significant differences to HIV-1 when it was sequenced by PCR. No doubt, he added, SIV-positive AGMs *had* been used during the production of human vaccines, but it was unlikely, he felt, that any SIV would have survived the various manufacturing steps or, even if it did, that it could then have been taken up by humans through a vaccine given orally. Alexander replied that it didn't need to be a regular event — just one episode of someone being infected through an SIV-contaminated vaccine would do. Desmyter replied that he wouldn't be prepared to prove the point by drinking a culture medium containing SIV! I asked what the situation would be if a chimp, rather than an AGM, had been the kidney donor for the vaccine culture, and he conceded that this would make the chances of viral transfer much higher.

Before leaving, Desmyter made a last remark for the record. "I think that the odds that HIV has spread by means of a vaccine are vanishingly low, and that whatever merit there is to such a hypothesis should be weighed against the benefit of vaccines in general, especially in Third World populations, and the danger to those developing countries and peoples from these more or less intellectual games." He added that his belief was that the likelihood of HIV-1 being introduced through eating monkeys was infinitely higher than through vaccines.

---

By now it was getting late and our thoughts were turning to food, even if roast monkey meat is not a feature of Flemish cuisine. Desmyter had to leave, but Alexander and I found a brown café that was encouragingly full, and so we spent the next three hours eating and drinking and talking about hypotheses of viral transfer.

Jennifer Alexander appeared to be in her forties, but had the sort of openness that strikes years off an intelligent estimate. This was the first time I had spoken to a virologist who had looked into the OPV/AIDS theory seriously, and who had spoken out publicly in its support. She was especially intrigued by the performance of the people at the Wistar Institute. If, she asked, they had (as they had apparently admitted) several polio vaccine samples from the period,[18] then why did they not simply offer them for independent testing if they were as confident as they claimed about their purity? And what of the blood samples taken after the vaccinations — where were they now? Why not test these too?

During the evening, we also talked of many other things, such as the rumor that there had been a polio vaccine trial conducted by the Pasteur Institute in French West Africa (she suspected in Senegal) at around the same time as Koprowski's in the Congo, and that it had employed vaccine made in the kidneys of local monkeys. We talked of the differing abilities of simian viruses such as SIV, SV40, herpes B, and Marburg to grow and prosper in monkey kidney tissue culture. She told me a little about the SV40 debacle, and how there had been next to no systematic follow-up of those who were inadvertently given SV40 in their IPV or OPV. It was even rumored, she said, that at one stage the plug had been pulled on a freezer full of serum samples that were about to be tested. She added that one or two other viral vaccines (apart from those made in MKTC) were also made in rather "dirty" substrates.

Later, I showed her the only precise information that Koprowski had published about how he had made CHAT vaccine — which came in the form of a conference address, with charts, which had been inserted into the proceedings of the New York Academy of Sciences conference held in January 1957.[19] She perused the paper for some time, and finally confirmed my own impression: that on the most essential details, like the species of monkey used, and the number of passages used to produce the different vaccine pools, it simply was not clear.

Before she drove me to the station for the last train back to Brussels, Jennifer Alexander played devil's advocate with the OPV/AIDS theory. Having considered the main objections, however, she swept them aside. She said that most tissue cultures contained lymphocytes in which SIV could be present; the key question was whether the SIV would survive the process of vaccine manufacture. As for the oral transmission of SIV, this was no problem — apart from the realistic possibility of direct viral transmission through the mucosa of mouth and throat, how many out of 250,000 vaccinees would have sores in their mouths at the time of immunization; how many children would be teething?

And finally she told me about Dr. De Somer, who had been head of virology at Leuven for thirty years until he died in 1986 and Jan Desmyter took over. I told her about Gaston Ninane's certainty that Leuven had made OPVs for the Belgian Congo. If that was correct, she said, then it was De Somer who would have been in charge.

Perhaps it was the rich, brown atmosphere of the restaurant that evening, perhaps it was the congenial company, or the good Leuven beer, or the excitement after seven hectic days of interviews and meetings. But two days later, when I got back to England, I handed in my notice at the school where I worked. For the first time, I was convinced that as far as CHAT went, there was a genuine case to answer. From now on, I decided, I would need seven days a week to follow it up properly.

———

A few weeks later, I came across an interesting letter, which had been published by the *Lancet* back in 1986; it concerned the finding of HIV antibodies in one of the ninety-four chimpanzees housed at the Holloman Air Force Base in New Mexico.[20] The authors reported that this chimp, which had been born in the wild and imported from Africa in 1963 at the age of four years, had been inoculated with human blood products between 1966 and 1969, but that this was the "only significant experiment" in which she had been involved.[21] In 1986, shortly after giving birth to stillborn twins, she died from pneumonia, and from toxic complications relating to the birth. Blood taken both before and after death had tested strongly positive for HIV-1 on all five assays used, and the

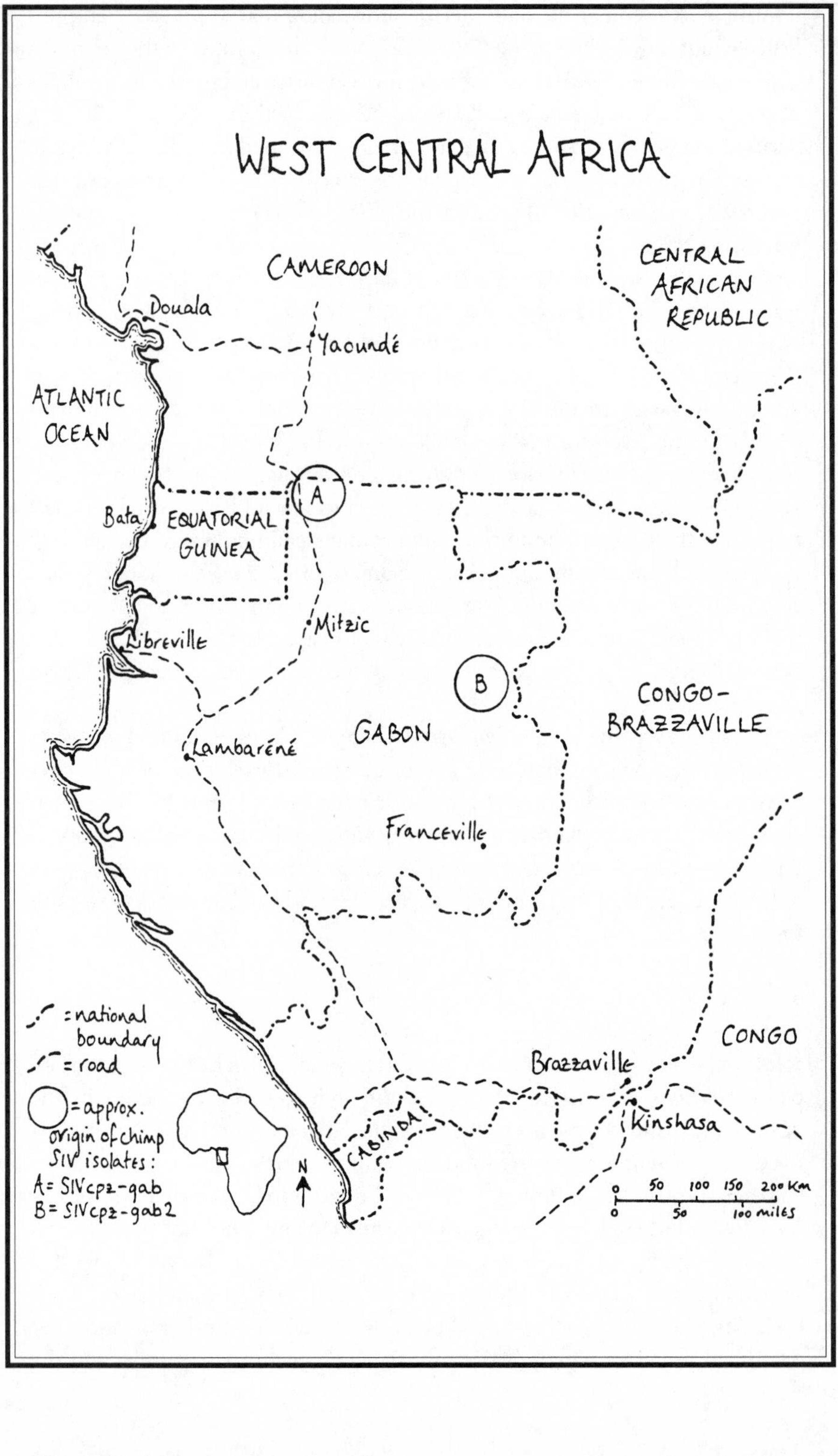

# WEST CENTRAL AFRICA

CAMEROON

Douala

Yaoundé

CENTRAL
AFRICAN
REPUBLIC

ATLANTIC
OCEAN

Bata

EQUATORIAL
GUINEA

(A)

Mitzic

Libreville

(B)

CONGO-
BRAZZAVILLE

Lambaréné

GABON

Franceville

CONGO

Brazzaville

Kinshasa

= national
boundary
= road

= approx.
origin of chimp
SIV isolates:
A= SIVcpz-gab
B= SIVcpz-gab2

CABINDA

N

0   50   100  150  200 Km
0        50       100 miles

virologists were apparently in the process of testing her six living offspring, and other chimps with which she had been housed. Certain of her symptoms at death (the pneumonia, generalized lymphadenopathy, and swollen spleen) seemed suggestive of simian AIDS.

Early in 1993 I wrote to two of the authors, asking whether they thought that the chimp might have been infected with SIVcpz infection, or even if she might have been infected with HIV-1, either via the blood transfusions at Holloman, or by being deliberately infected with human blood prior to her export from Africa. (By this stage I had confirmed that this was a "protective" treatment that many Africa-based primate dealers had adopted during the late fifties and early sixties.)[22] The replies I received revealed that none of the progeny or associates of the dead chimp had tested HIV-positive, and that it was now thought unlikely that she had died of simian AIDS.

During the following months, there were some interesting developments. Larry Arthur, one of the coauthors of the *Lancet* letter, contacted the laboratory of Beatrice Hahn in Birmingham, Alabama, and offered to supply frozen tissues from the chimp in question (known as "Marilyn 205"). Samples of brain, liver, lymph node, and spleen were sent to Hahn in August 1994, and SIVcpz sequences were detected in the latter two tissues, indicating that the chimp had almost certainly been naturally infected with SIV prior to its capture in Africa.

By this time Martine Peeters and her Antwerp team had already managed to obtain an isolate, SIVcpz-gab-2, from the second Gabonese chimp, the one that had died from its wounds at Franceville,[23] which meant that Marilyn 205 had provided the fourth chimpanzee SIV to have been isolated and sequenced (SIVcpz-us).[24] The proximity of the two Gabonese SIVcpz isolates, and their distance from the other SIVcpz isolates and those of HIV-1, made it virtually certain that the four chimps had not been independently cross-infected with HIV-1. It was now clear that a small proportion of wild-caught chimpanzees (roughly 2 percent of the 189 tested by the Antwerp and Holloman teams) were naturally infected with their own SIV variants.

However, in the light of the heterogeneity suggested by the Lindi blood groups paper, and the fact that chimps are notoriously unwilling to cross even small rivers, it seemed to me that certain isolated chimpanzee bands in the rain forest might prove to have much higher SIV prevalences than 2 percent. Indeed, they might turn out to be infected with viruses that were considerably closer to both HIV-1 Group M and HIV-1 Group O.

# 22

PIERRE LÉPINE

AND THE PASTEUR INSTITUTE

The circumstantial evidence favoring a link between CHAT and HIV-1 continued to accumulate, but meanwhile I was keen to follow up the hint, given by both Blaine Elswood and Jennifer Alexander, that trials of a French polio vaccine had occurred somewhere in West Africa at around the same time that CHAT was being fed in the Belgian colonies of central Africa. I ended up phoning the person whom Alexander had cited as the source of the rumor: Chuck Cyberski, a television producer from San Francisco who had AIDS. Cyberski confirmed that he had spoken informally with Leonard Hayflick, the man who had developed the human diploid cell strain, WI-38, for the Wistar Institute. Hayflick, he said, had told him that, back in the fifties, the French had tested one of their own polio vaccines "in the Congo area of Africa." He could provide no further details, but this sounded like the part of French Equatorial Africa now known as Congo Brazzaville, rather than the former Belgian Congo.

After a long search in the Keppel Street library, I came across an article that described just such an event.[1] It documented an outbreak of polio that had occurred in a group of villages near to the town of Mitzic, in what was then French Equatorial Africa, in 1957. Mitzic lies on the main road some 250 miles east of Libreville, the capital of present-day Gabon, and 250 miles south of Yaounde, the capital of present-day Cameroon. The College Normal du Gabon, a prestigious secondary school, was based there, so we can assume that it was home to a fairly large colonial population.

Between the months of July and November, ten cases of polio apparently occurred in one of the nearby villages, and another six in villages within a thirty-five-mile radius. Seven of the sixteen cases were fatal. So unexpected and virulent was this epidemic that two French doctors, led by L. J. André, a captain in the colonial medical service based at the Pasteur Institute satellite at nearby Brazzaville, decided to vaccinate the local population. He employed "the Lépine vaccine of the Pasteur Institute in Paris." Starting on November 1, 1957, a total of 2,100 of the children of the district (aged from six months to fifteen years) and 150 students from the college (aged eleven to eighteen) were injected with three doses of the vaccine at three-week intervals. Although participation was voluntary, there was an acceptance rate of over 95 percent. Only two further cases of polio were seen in the area after the campaign, both in nonvaccinees.

Although the vaccine was described as being injected, it was not specifically stated whether this was a killed or a live preparation. On the face of things, it appeared to have been an inactivated (or killed) vaccine — for at that stage I believed that all injected polio vaccines were of that variety. But, as I learned after some weeks of reading, this was not necessarily the case. In fact, 1957 was the very year when the maker of the vaccine, Pierre Lépine, was experiencing a series of changes of heart about the best approach to polio vaccination.

Lépine had been head of virology at the Pasteur Institute in Paris since 1941, and he was yet another iconoclast in a profession populated by iconoclasts. Like the other great vaccine-makers, he inspired great loyalty among his immediate colleagues, and yet was frequently mocked by opponents, especially for his long-winded conference addresses. He also had a singular approach to polio vaccination, which was quite different from those of Salk, Sabin, and Koprowski. Although for many years he favored an inactivated polio vaccine, he employed a two-stage process of killing the poliovirus, starting off (like Salk) with formalin, but then also exposing the virus to another chemical, beta-propiolactone.[2] But he kept abreast of the growing movement toward live polio vaccines, and at various times from 1955 onward appeared to be leaning toward incorporating a live virus component into his vaccination regime. I write "appeared" judiciously, for Lépine had a circumlocutory writing style, which does not always make it easy to divine his exact meaning.

In July 1955, Lépine was one of the six course leaders at the WHO workshop on rabies, held at Muguga, Kenya.[3] One of the other leaders was Hilary Koprowski, and we can be confident that the two men would have spent some time during the eighteen-day course talking about the pros and cons of different approaches to vaccination. In the same year, writing in the *Bulletin of the WHO*, Lépine discussed both killed and live polio vaccines, and stated that live, attenuated strains of poliovirus could be administered either orally or by injection.[4] (In this respect, he differed from all other contemporary polio vaccine-makers, and for this reason, one cannot correctly refer to his live polio vaccine by the normal acronym of OPV.)

By January 1957 he was attending the virus conference staged at the Waldorf Astoria by the New York Academy of Sciences, and was advocating a different regime again: this time a series of two or three injections with IPV to establish antibody protection, followed by a booster of live vaccine to establish more permanent immunity.[5] He stressed his belief that completely attenuated strains were of little use as a basis for live vaccine, since they were simply too weak to establish long-lasting, effective immunity. His idea, rather, was to use the immunity conferred by the IPV as cover for the administration of highly antigenic (that is less completely attenuated) strains of live virus vaccine. He stated that the live booster could be given either subcutaneously or orally, and that it should be administered between three and ten months after the initial IPV injections. However, in chimpanzee experiments, the booster had worked well when given orally just one month after the primary injections.[6]

This, then, was Lépine's declared position at the start of 1957. All seemed to be going well, because by June 1957, he was described by Agence France Presse as having granted a big American pharmaceutical company the right to manufacture his polio vaccine, which, "contrary to the Salk vaccine, employs preparations of live virus."[7] This was clearly the attenuated vaccine, but by July his position had apparently shifted once more, for at the Geneva polio conference he was declaring that an attenuated vaccine booster administered *orally* — after a course of IPV shots — seemed to be either too weak to augment the level of immunity, or else too immunogenic and therefore potentially dangerous. For the time being, he went on, they had given up experimenting in this area, although the work might well resume if attenuated strains were obtained that were so innocuous they could safely be administered *by injection*.[8]

A week later, he was one of the members of the WHO Expert Committee on Polio Vaccines, which decreed that live vaccines could safely be administered in certain circumstances — for instance, in the face of a polio epidemic.[9]

A polio epidemic was, of course, exactly what occurred around Mitzic over the next five months — from July to November 1957. It therefore seems possible that the three shots of Lépine vaccine to which André's article refers might have consisted of two shots of IPV to establish immunity, followed by a booster shot of live virus vaccine. There is nothing in the article to suggest that a new method of immunization was being used, but, then again, there was no technical reason why André, in Africa, would need to have been informed of the manufacturing details. If the vaccination using this method was a success, it could be announced to the world; if not, then perhaps the less fuss the better.[10]

The foregoing is pure conjecture, and there is no published record in any of Lépine's many papers from the fifties about *human* trials of a live polio vaccine. However, there is one further clue that lends real support to the scenario. In July 1958, the Tenth International Symposium on Virology was held in Lyon, partly in celebration of the opening of the new laboratories of the Pasteur Merieux for the production of Lépine's polio vaccine (presumably the IPV). Hilary

Koprowski gave a brief address about the Ruzizi trial and the vaccinations in response to polio epidemics in the northeastern Congo.[11] During the discussion that followed, Professor Lépine supported Koprowski's approach, stating that when faced by a menacing polio epidemic like that in the Congo, an appropriate method of reaching "almost 98% to 100% of the population" in a short space of time was the administration of a live attenuated vaccine, which, by spreading rapidly in the population, would protect it from infection with the more dangerous wild virus.[12] Outside the epidemic period, Lépine went on, it was easier to give primary vaccinations of IPV, which could be reinforced later with attenuated virus. "We have conducted experiments along these lines," he says, "and we continue them, but we can only proceed with very great prudence and much deliberation." This apparently circumspect reference, with its stress on prudence and deliberation, suggests that the experiments may have involved human trials, such as the vaccinations in response to the Mitzic polio epidemic of the previous year.

According to his published articles, it would seem that after 1957 Pierre Lépine returned to his preferred vehicle of IPV, which was injected into tens of millions of arms in France and Germany in the decade that followed its introduction in mid-1956. Only in 1966 did the numbers vaccinated with Sabin's OPV exceed those for Lépine's IPV in France. This was much later than in most other countries in the world.[13]

Pierre Lépine died in 1989, and there are few people who still recall his work in the fifties. One of them is Professor Pascu Atanasiu, a Romanian émigré who was appointed to Lépine's laboratory shortly after escaping to Paris at the end of the Second World War. In the course of a lengthy conversation in 1994, Atanasiu described Lépine as "a cultivated and brilliant man," and insisted that he was always opposed to the use of live vaccines until the Sabin strains were adopted in 1963. When pressed, he finally said that there had also been another team working under Lépine, coordinated by Valentine Sautter, which may have prepared live polio vaccine for use in trials. Later, however, he added that Professor Lépine would never have conducted field trials since, as he put it, live vaccines are impossible to control once introduced into the field. He mentioned, almost as an aside, that he felt Hilary Koprowski's approach to field trials in Africa and elsewhere to have been "dangerous," and added: "I have reservations about his honesty. . . . He is an *arriviste*." But those discursive papers written by Lépine between 1955 and 1958 suggest that Professor Atanasiu's recollections are far from complete.

Furthermore, there is evidence that other French researchers were far from cautious about conducting field trials in Africa. One of Lépine's papers refers in passing to a little-known oral polio vaccine that was developed in 1952 by two doctors from the Pasteur, Georges Blanc and Louis-André Martin. They injected virulent poliovirus into a rabbit, and created what they thought was an attenuated polio vaccine from its spleen and blood.[14] After safety tests in monkeys seemed to prove it innocuous, they staged an oral vaccination campaign on some 5,700 children in Casablanca, Morocco, after a small epidemic (involving five polio cases) had occurred there in early 1953.[15] Only in 1955 did Lépine discover that far from containing attenuated polioviruses, the vaccine actually consisted of a "parasitical rodent virus."[16] Fortunately, this virus appeared to cause no ill effects in humans. Nonetheless, these overhasty trials of an inadequately researched vaccine struck uncomfortable echoes of Kolmer and Brodie's campaigns in the thirties and, equally, were a portent of other African campaigns that would follow later in the fifties.

———————

Another aspect of Pierre Lépine's individual approach to polio vaccination involved the primates that he used for tissue culture work and vaccine production. For whereas in the fifties Sabin used cynomolgus macaques, Gear used African green monkeys, and Koprowski used — well, whichever primates he used — Lépine favored *Papio papio,* the Guinea or Western baboon.[17] The Pasteur Institute was supplied mainly from an animal station called "Pastoria," close to Kindia in French West Africa, which began operations in 1925 and continued to supply Paris with chimps, baboons, and other primates until 1958, when the country became independent Guinea Conakry.[18]

It therefore seems likely that Lépine's attenuated polio vaccines — which in 1956 and 1957 were being injected into chimpanzees (and perhaps into humans around Mitzic) — would have been manufactured in a substrate of baboon kidney tissue culture, just like his IPVs.

Some years later, in 1962, following the discovery of SV40 in the tissues of Asian monkeys, and the decision by other vaccine-makers to switch to using tissues from African green monkeys, three of Lépine's vaccine workers gave a lecture to the Académie Nationale de Médecine in Paris in which they indulged in a little unashamed flattery of their boss.[19] The French orientation toward Africa was fortunate, they said, because the French had always used African monkeys for their vaccine preparation, which species seemed to be less contaminated with latent viruses than Asian monkeys. In particular, these monkeys are not naturally infected with either herpes B or SV40.

In 1985, of course, things would begin to look rather different, when a new class of virus was discovered (the SIVs), which naturally infected African, but not Asian monkeys.[20] In the years that followed, more and more would be learned about these viruses — not least that many different African monkeys were host to their own SIVs, several of which were so different from each other that they

must have been evolving separately for thousands, if not millions of years: very possibly from the time of speciation.*[21]

Perhaps surprisingly, very little testing of *Papio papio,* the Guinea baboon, seems to have taken place, and certainly no SIV has yet been found in this sub-species.[22] However, in 1989, SIV was reported in the yellow baboon, *Papio hamadryas cynocephalus,* from central Tanzania.[23] Two of these baboons tested positive for an African green monkey SIV, which raised "questions about whether [they] may have been infected by green monkeys in their native habitat." In 1994 the baboon SIV isolate was finally sequenced — and confirmed as being virtually identical to the SIVagm found among green monkeys from this region.[24] The authors of the report note that in Mikumi National Park, Tanzania, troops of baboons and African greens are known to live in close proximity, and they hypothesize that one of the baboons (perhaps even the index animal, the one that had provided the viral isolate) might have attacked and eaten an African green, becoming cross-infected in the process.

The authors advance this as a model for horizontal transfer of SIV from species to species in Africa. In fact, however, there are only three primate species found in Africa that attack and eat other monkeys. One is the baboon. One is the chimpanzee. And the third is the human being. Anyone who has seen one of the films of chimpanzee troops hunting other monkeys, and the ferocious climax to the hunt — in which the victim, after attempting to defend itself, is literally torn limb from limb — can visualize the possibility of viral transfer occurring during such an orgy of bloodletting.[25] Baboon attacks on other monkeys are similarly gory affairs, so it is certainly possible that Guinea baboons, like yellow baboons, might have become cross-infected with SIVs from other local monkey species. Whether the horizontal transfer analogy holds for present-day *Homo sapiens* is more debatable, for human methods of catching monkeys do not involve tooth, claw, and direct hand-to-hand combat. Moreover, twentieth-century humans are in the habit of cooking monkeys before eating them.

---

From as early as 1986, there had been a series of reports of atypical HIVs, which did not give normal readings on HIV-1 or HIV-2 assays, being detected in west central Africa.[26] Some scientists began speaking of a possible "HIV-3" from that region. But it was not until the early nineties that the existence of a third strain of HIV was confirmed.[27]

---

* Speciation: the process by which new species are formed; *time of speciation* is effectively the moment when two related species (in this case, of monkeys) evolve from a common ancestor.

Although various genetic characteristics indicated that this strain belonged to the same branch of the family tree that included HIV-1 and the chimpanzee SIV, the pattern and sequence of chromosomes made it apparent that it was the result of a separate transfer of an SIV from nonhuman primates to humans.[28] Presently, the new HIV variant came to be known as HIV-1 Group O (for "Outlier" group), to distinguish it from the main group of HIV-1 viruses, which was now redesignated as HIV-1 Group M (for "Main" group).[29] Group O was found in roughly 6 percent of the HIV-1-infected people in southern Cameroon, in about 3 percent of those from Gabon, and in a handful of French people who had historical links with this part of Africa.[30] The earliest recorded case of Group O infection appeared to stem from the start of the eighties, and involved a Frenchwoman who had apparently worked as a barmaid in Reims, a garrison town where some of the recruits would presumably have served in Cameroon or Gabon.[31] She had one healthy child in 1972, but gave birth to another child in 1980 who died of typical neonatal AIDS the following year. She herself died of confirmed AIDS in 1992, at the age of forty-one.[32]

However, the resulting phylogenetic tree presented a fresh mystery, for the Group O isolates proved to be slightly more distant than the Group M isolates to the chimpanzee SIV sequenced by Martine Peeters.[33] This was despite the fact that the individual *Pan troglodytes troglodytes* that had provided the Peeters isolate, SIVcpz-gab-1, had come from the very same border region of Gabon and Cameroon that appeared to represent the epicenter of Group O. So although it appeared likely that HIV-1 Group O, like Group M, had evolved from a chimpanzee SIV, there was no evidence to suggest that it had emerged through human contact with *local* chimpanzees.

Interestingly, however, this apparent epicenter of HIV-1 Group O embraced the town of Mitzic in northern Gabon, just 130 miles south of the Cameroonian border, where Dr. André had vaccinated against polio in 1957.

I began to formulate a tentative hypothesis. More than two thousand people had been vaccinated in 1957 with a Lépine polio vaccine, which was probably grown in the kidneys of the Guinea baboon, *Papio papio*. Because this vaccination occurred in response to a raging and particularly virulent polio epidemic, one that had caused seven deaths, and because Lépine's own writings at this time period include references to the use of an attenuated polio vaccine administered either by mouth or by injection, there is a basis for suspecting that the final round of injections administered in the villages around Mitzic *may* have contained live, attenuated poliovirus. Even if the three vaccinations were all of IPV, it is still possible that the vaccine was incompletely inactivated, and that it contained contaminating viruses from the substrate.

Lépine believed that African monkeys were commendably free of latent viruses, but he did not know about the SIVs. One of the baboons used to make the vaccine may have been host to an SIV — either an SIV "naturally" found in *P. papio,* or else one acquired from another monkey species.

Apart from the Guinea baboon, the only other primate we know to have been present in large numbers at the holding center at Pastoria in Guinea, and to have been shipped from there to the Pasteur Institute, is the western subspecies of the common chimpanzee, *Pan troglodytes verus.* Only ten of these animals have ever been tested for SIV — and all were negative. It is entirely possible, however, that this subspecies of chimp is host to its own SIV, in the same manner as the other two subspecies of *Pan troglodytes.*

We can gain some idea about conditions at Pastoria from a lengthy newspaper report published in 1926, which details 195 primates being admitted to the center in that year, comprising 89 chimps, 80 baboons, and 26 other small monkeys.[34] Chimpanzee capture methods were primitive, and necessitated the slaughter of many of the adults, killed while trying to protect their young. Once inside Pastoria, disease outbreaks were rife, and nearly half of the chimps died within fifteen days of arrival, apparently from a variety of bronchial and diarrheal conditions. Many of the animals were used in experiments designed to test a vaccine against tuberculosis, in the course of which 15 chimps and 59 other monkeys (mainly baboons) were housed in two separate cages, each group being a mixture of TB-infected, vaccinated, and control animals. Viewed from seventy years on, it seems that experiments such as these must have encouraged interspecies and intraspecies infections with a variety of different simian pathogens, which is probably part of the reason for the very high initial mortality rates.

Another more scholarly report from 1957 records that, every year from 1950 onward, an average of 40 chimps and some 400 Guinea baboons were exported from Pastoria to Paris in one huge shipment.[35] By this time, the chimps were being kept in cages inside two long buildings, which sound not unlike the hangars at Lindi, but during the day adjacent pairs of chimps were allowed to spend time in larger cages in the open air. Chimpanzee mortality was only slightly better than three decades earlier, with 34 percent of all the chimpanzee "lodgers" dying, half within their first month at Pastoria.

The transfer of SIVs between different species at primate research centers is now well-documented from various episodes in America from the sixties onward, so it certainly seems possible that an SIV from *Pan troglodytes verus* could have been transferred to a *Papio papio* (or vice versa) either during initial capture, or at Pastoria, or else during the process of shipment to Paris.

If an SIV *was* found in either *Pan troglodytes verus* or *Papio papio,* and sequenced, and found to be similar to HIV-1 Group O, then I wondered what the advocates of natural transfer would make of that. In that case, there would certainly be a mystery to solve, because neither *P. t. verus* nor *P. papio* is found in Cameroon or Gabon, the Group O epicenter.

A few days after my discovery of the André paper about the vaccination campaign in Gabon, I got a letter from Blaine Elswood, showing that he too had
come across details of this, or a similar trial. The letter also referred to a
rumored meeting in Paris in the summer of 1992 between Leonard Hayflick,
Stanley Plotkin, and "a past head of the Pasteur Institute."[36]

If true, the story was intriguing, for although Plotkin was now the head of
Pasteur Mérieux (the vast French vaccine house allied to the Pasteur Institute,
which makes most of France's vaccines), he had — at the time of the Congo
trials — been a righthand man of Koprowski's at the Wistar. Furthermore,
the Pasteur Institute is the publisher of *Research in Virology,* the journal that
had undertaken to print Elswood and Stricker's long-awaited article on the
OPV/AIDS theory.[37]

As Elswood told it, during the Paris meeting Plotkin and Hayflick argued
that it could just as easily have been the Pasteur's vaccine trial in Gabon (rather
than Koprowski's in the Congo) that had sparked the AIDS epidemic. He said
that the source of this story was (once again) Chuck Cyberski, the San Francisco
TV producer, who had apparently heard it direct from Leonard Hayflick.

For many years, I was unable to confirm — or disprove — that such a meeting had actually taken place.[38] What I did learn, however, was that in September
1992, *Research in Virology* faxed Elswood and Stricker a request that they reduce
their article to only letter size.

This they did, and the letter was finally published in January 1993, after a
delay of thirteen months.[39] Though much reduced in size, it was considerably
more succinct than the first draft. Unusually, the letter was accompanied by a
"note from the editorial board," which publicly invited Dr. Koprowski to reply
to the letter. The note also stated: "It is legitimate to raise questions about the
still mysterious origin of the AIDS epidemic and not to exclude the role of
medical actions." It went on, however, to express skepticism — on the grounds
that up to 1961, rhesus and cynomolgus monkeys had been used to make the
tissue cultures for polio vaccines, whereas after 1961, vaccines had been made
in the tissues of African green monkeys and baboons. Although all four species
could be infected with SIV, these viruses were, it was claimed, "very distant from
HIV-1 and therefore could not be at the recent origin of the latter virus."

This direct reference to the use of baboon tissues was interesting, being the
first indication I had come across that the French had continued to use baboon
kidneys for making vaccines in the 1960s.[40] The failure to mention that the
Lépine vaccines (whether killed or live) had been made from baboon kidneys
from the mid-fifties onward was therefore all the more intriguing.

The editorial note ended with an even more interesting paragraph. "The
primate virus which is closest to HIV-1 is the [SIVcpz] virus isolated from

lymphocytes of a chimpanzee captured in Gabon. Since chimpanzee tissues have never been used for poliovirus production, it is difficult to imagine how massive contamination of polio vaccines by a virus rarely detectable in chimpanzees could have occurred." It was a most tellingly worded comment. For if, of course, it could be proven that such a vaccine *had* been made from chimpanzee tissues, then the concluding part of the statement could effectively be reversed.

They had had to wait a long time, but Elswood and Stricker had finally been allowed into the orchard to shake a few trees, and some nice ripe apples had fallen.

# 23

## THE NORWEGIAN SAILOR

In March 1993 I set off once more for Europe, to initiate several new investigations that might shed some light on the earliest traces of AIDS. One of my first calls was to Dr. Boris Velimirovic, who, in 1962 and 1963, had helped coordinate medical services for the WHO in the newly independent Congo. He had spent time in Kinshasa, and in the region around Bukavu in the east, where he had looked after Tutsi refugees who were sheltering on the Congolese side of the Ruzizi Valley after the first great wave of ethnic violence in Rwanda. Among other things, he organized vaccinations against smallpox, measles, TB, and polio (using the Sabin OPV). I was of course interested to learn whether he might have seen any AIDS-like illnesses in these places. He had not, he said, which was very much what I had expected. Although a positive sighting or two would have been powerful evidence in favor of the OPV/AIDS theory, it was also clear that even if the theory was correct, there would in all probability have been only a tiny number of AIDS cases occurring within four or five years of the vaccinations — with Jean Sonnet's patient, Hélène, as one possible example. The chances of any such patient having been seen by Velimirovic were slim.

However, Velimirovic did confirm something I had discovered from the medical literature:[1] that many of the Tutsi refugees fleeing Rwanda at this time were suffering from TB and other respiratory infections — which, in Africa, are two of the principal presentations of AIDS. However, he claimed that, rather than being a result of HIV infection, these illnesses were more likely to have been precipitated by hunger, poor living conditions, and the stress of flight.

Yes, he said, he had heard of the OPV/AIDS theory. He did not proffer a direct opinion about it, but said that in order to check it out, one would need to look at all the places where the vaccine had been fed, including, for instance, European countries. I told him that it seemed that different pools of vaccine might have been fed in different places. We discussed the findings of the Wistar committee, and he went on to make one very pertinent comment: "It would certainly be possible to locate more vaccines than that one found in the Wistar Institute freezers. There are obligations to keep samples of vaccines used." Velimirovic pointed out that a few samples of the CHAT pools used in the Congo, or of prevaccination and postvaccination blood samples, might even have been sent to the WHO. It struck me that, given the historical importance of this and similar early vaccine trials, such a procedure should have been a universal requirement.

Later, I asked him how one might try to monitor the spread of HIV in a place like the Congo. Here he proved to be really helpful. He explained that the WHO kept banks of stored sera at Yale, and in Tokyo and Prague, and that the latter center had lots of serum samples from tropical areas dating from the sixties and even earlier. He said that these included sera from the Congo, Uganda, Kenya, Senegal, and Somalia, and that, as far as he knew, they had never been investigated for the presence of HIV. He said that if one could get approval from the WHO hierarchy, it would certainly be possible to undertake a retrospective HIV survey. But, he added, there was another way to approach the problem — by checking whether any WHO personnel who had served in the Congo had gone on to die of mysterious diseases. At the end of a tour of duty, all WHO personnel had to return to Geneva for a medical check and, for insurance reasons, their health records continued to be kept up-to-date thereafter. Given the subsequent early emergence of AIDS in Haiti, he felt it would be especially interesting to examine the health records of the Haitians who had served in the Congo. He recalled some two to three thousand Haitians working there in the sixties; most of them, he said, used to spend their biannual leaves in the United States and Canada where, later on, many of them emigrated.

Velimirovic also gave a powerful insight into the less-than-optimal way in which mass vaccinations were sometimes carried out in Third World countries. He told me that he personally had witnessed smallpox vaccinations being conducted in the Ruzizi Valley with no attempt being made to sterilize the needles between jabs. He believed that unsterilized needles were a significant factor in the spread of infections like HIV in the tropics. It was not only poorly conducted vaccination programs; it was the fact that both qualified doctors and quacks tended to reuse needles far more often than was intended by the manufacturers, and that even after being consigned to garbage bins at the back of hospitals, needles were sometimes recovered and recycled by members of the public. Such factors could not have been involved in the initial transfers of the immunodeficiency viruses into humans, but they could have played a significant role in onward transmission thereafter.

During the previous three years, I had undertaken a library search for very early cases of some of the indicator diseases typical of AIDS, much as Robert Root-Bernstein had been doing at around the same period.[2] I had chosen four in particular: CMV infection, cryptococcal meningitis, Kaposi's sarcoma, and PCP, to see whether any of the case histories were suggestive of the type of immuno-suppression caused by HIV infection.

The first reports in the literature of these four conditions had all been fairly recent: 1925, 1894, 1872, and 1911, respectively. In his book *Rethinking AIDS*, Root-Bernstein had proposed many of them as early cases of AIDS. During 1990 and 1991, I had been thinking along similar lines, but the more closely I looked into some of these archival case histories, the less plausible the hypothesis of HIV involvement became.

My investigations into the first two diseases were fairly cursory. I found that the earliest example of fatal CMV infection in an adult, and the only recorded case in the world literature prior to that of Sadayo F. in Montreal in 1945, involved a thirty-six-year-old married engineer, Frederick S., who died in New York City in December 1924. At autopsy, "inclusion bodies" (typical signs of CMV infection) were found in the intestines, liver, and lungs, but there was also evidence of bacterial infections of the liver and abdomen, which had led to uncontrollable fever and septicemia.[3] In those preantibiotic days, it was these latter infections that seemed to have killed him. Frederick had had a venereal infection in 1915, but there was nothing to suggest that he had been infected with HIV.

Cryptococcal meningitis is also often suggestive of compromised immunity and is more easily recognized than CMV infection. The first report in the literature pertains to Germany in 1894,[4] but I was most interested in its emergence in the Congo, where the first clue that some people might be suffering from AIDS was a sudden exponential increase in this condition in the hospitals of Kinshasa. Forty-four cases were diagnosed between 1978 and 1984 — all of them fatal, and many featuring other opportunistic infections like TB. By contrast, only twenty-one cases had been diagnosed in the whole of the Congo in the previous twenty-five years, all of which appeared to be of the primary type, which does not involve an immunocompromised host.[5] Nearly 60 percent of these early cases recovered, especially those patients who were treated with the antifungal preparation amphotericin-B, after it became available at the start of the sixties.[6]

Dr. Jean Delville, who had seen two of the Congo's first three cryptococcus patients in Elizabethville (now Lubumbashi) at the start of the fifties, confirmed that the symptoms in these two cases were very specific, and did not suggest the general immunosuppression that is typical of AIDS. The different presentations of pre-AIDS and post-AIDS cryptococcal meningitis thus appeared well defined.[7]

I also investigated Kaposi's sarcoma, several of the aggressive, fatal presentations of which from bygone days had been proposed as possible cases of AIDS.[8] There was a wealth of literature on the subject, beginning with Dr. Kaposi's original descriptions published in 1872, and many of these cases entailed aggressive presentations.[9]

A little background is needed here. Moriz Kaposi arrived in Vienna as Moriz Kohn, but renamed himself after his hometown of Kaposvar in Hungary, in an attempt to distinguish himself from all the other Dr. Kohns then practicing in the city. He swiftly became a dermatologist of renown, and the eponymous sarcoma was only one of several skin conditions that he identified, and that would subsequently be named after him. Three of the six cases described in his first paper are intriguing, in that they bear similarities to the aggressive, disseminated form of KS, which would emerge a century later as one of the presentations of AIDS, especially in gay men. Indeed, a review article published in 1984 about this paper had been titled: "Did Moriz Kaposi describe AIDS in 1872?"[10]

The first of Kaposi's six patients was one Leonhard Kopf,[11] described as a mastersmith from Brodes in lower Austria. In 1867 Herr Kopf — then sixty-seven years old — began suffering from swollen feet and hands, and by the following year the lymph nodes of his armpits and groin swelled up, while his lower legs, arms, and face became covered in the plaques and nodules that would become familiar sights on television screens in the 1980s. On September 22, 1868, after two months in a Vienna hospital, he discharged himself explaining that "he wanted to die 'among his own people,'"[12] and Dr. Kaposi clearly felt that the condition would prove to be fatal.

Because, unusually, the patient had been named, I decided that it would be interesting to try to follow up this first recorded case of KS. First, however, I had to locate Brodes, and according to even the best gazetteers, there is no longer a town of that name either in Austria or in the old Austro-Hungarian Empire, which used to spread across a quarter of Europe. I did, however, locate a settlement called Prottes, twenty-five miles from Vienna, and on the off chance I wrote to the town clerk. A month later Herr Manfred Grunwald, secretary to the mayor, wrote back to tell me that I had identified one of the ancient names of the village,[13] but added that so far his searches of the archives had not managed to identify a Leonhard Kopf.[14]

It was Easter Sunday when I arrived in Prottes, and walked through rain-swept cornfields along the lane between the railway station and the town, to ask directions to Herr Grunwald's house. The family was getting ready for lunch when I arrived, but I was greeted warmly and invited to join them. Later, Manfred got out some of his local history books, which revealed that in 1866, following the defeat of 270,000 Austrians by the smaller but better armed Prussian army at the battle of Koniggratz, the Austrian army had been harried southward for a further month. Finally, Emperor Franz-Josef sued for peace just

as the Prussians were about to attack Vienna, an act that signaled the beginning
of the end for the Austro-Hungarian Empire. Between July and early August
1866, six thousand Prussian soldiers had occupied Prottes, eating sixty-two
cows and the entire potato crop — and introducing cholera, which killed 20 of
the town's 824 inhabitants. Whether the events of the war were in any way connected to Herr Kopf's falling ill the following year cannot be known, but their
proximity in time is at least suggestive.[15]

Later that afternoon, Manfred and I wandered round the village and he
pointed out the house that used to contain the smithy. At the fourteenth-
century church, a cassocked priest boasting a medieval beard showed us the
records of births and deaths for the parish, inscribed in copperplate in a huge
leather-bound book. Eventually, to my great pleasure, we found the registra-
tion of Leonhard Kopf's birth, on October 18, 1800. However, even though we
searched through the death records for five years starting in September 1868,
we could find no entry for Herr Kopf — who had not after all, it seemed, died
"among his own people" upon his departure from the hospital in Vienna.

This small negative result suggested that this case at least, despite the apparently aggressive presentation of the disease, had very likely involved the classic KS
that is unconnected to HIV infection. And although Kaposi had described some
of his other cases as "rapidly lethal, within two to three years," there had been no
other opportunistic infections to support the hypothesis that there might have
been an early outbreak of AIDS in central Europe in the nineteenth century.

Later, at the Institute of Tropical Medicine in Antwerp, I met with Professor
Paul Gigase, who, between 1955 and 1962, had been based at Katana Hospital,
some thirty miles north of Bukavu on the western shores of Lake Kivu, in the
Congo.[16] He had an especially good perspective on Kaposi's sarcoma in Africa,
because he had participated in two studies of the condition at Katana — one
between 1959 and 1961, and the other in the early eighties. Because of political
unrest, the first study had never been completed, but the researchers were able to
confirm that the incidence of KS in this part of eastern Congo — where it comprised more than 10 percent of all malignant tumors — was as high as anywhere
in the world.[17] Other studies demonstrated that KS incidence was only slightly
lower across the border in Uganda and Tanzania,[18] and so an epicenter of
endemic KS was identified around Lake Edward, Lake Kivu, and Lake Victoria.

When the AIDS epidemic emerged in America in the early eighties, with KS
apparently one of its most frequent presentations, some researchers wondered
whether this part of Africa might also turn out to be the source of the new epidemic. For this reason, Paul Gigase returned to Katana in 1983, as part of Bob
Biggar's ill-fated investigation into KS and AIDS. As has already been told, the
flawed study, with its false positives, led Biggar to conclude that HIV itself might
be endemic to the region,[19] and although he later admitted that he had probably been wrong,[20] not everyone noticed.

Gigase told me that he now believed that the KS around Katana in 1960 and in 1983/4 had been essentially the age-old benign condition, with occasional aggressive cases, which were, however, unlikely to have been HIV-related. In fact, he added, KS was a far less significant component of the African AIDS epidemic (about 6 percent of all cases) than it was of the U.S. epidemic, in which it occurred in 15 percent of all cases.

He ended by saying that theoretically there *may* have been some AIDS cases in central Africa prior to 1960, but that such cases certainly couldn't have been frequent, because otherwise they would undoubtedly have been documented as unusual presentations by the many experienced British, French, and Belgian doctors working there at the time.

Over a period of years I spoke with five such experienced physicians[21] who had helped organize two major symposia on KS in Kampala, Uganda, in 1961[22] and 1980.[23] Interestingly, none of the papers from either conference included any cases that were compellingly suggestive of generalized immunocompromise, and each of the doctors, in their different ways, expressed skepticism that KS as a presentation of AIDS had been seen before the late 1970s — in Africa or elsewhere. As they pointed out, any aggressive case of KS from 1868 onward could theoretically have been caused by HIV, but without a positive antigen or antibody test, this could only be speculation.

It was not until 1994 that virologists confirmed that a particular strain of herpes virus (which became known as HHV8 for human herpesvirus 8, or KSHV for KS-associated herpesvirus) is found in patients with Kaposi's sarcoma.[24] By this stage it was becoming apparent that the major reason why KS and AIDS have become so intertwined in the popular psyche was that the bathhouse culture of the 1970s encouraged both HIV and KSHV to increase exponentially among American and European gay men at almost exactly the same moment in time. Since both viruses are spread by sex (and, in the latter case, especially by oral-anal sex), many men became infected with both viruses; however, by the start of the nineties, some of the gays who contracted KS tested repeatedly HIV-negative. Presumably they had first been infected with KSHV, and only then had adopted safer sex procedures, which saved them from exposure to the more lethal virus.[25]

Because aggressive KS can occur with or without the involvement of HIV, it must be concluded that, on its own, the disease is not a good indicator for spotting potential pre-epidemic cases of AIDS.

---

By contrast, *Pneumocystis carinii* pneumonia, PCP, is still the classic opportunistic infection of AIDS patients in the Western world. *Pneumocystitis* infection seems to be quite common among small rodents,[26] and the majority of humans are exposed to the *Pneumocystis* organism at an early stage in life with-out any harmful impact.[27] The devastating pneumonia occurs only when the host becomes debilitated through other factors.

The first human infection of PCP was identified serendipitously during an autopsy by Dr. C. Chagas from Brazil in 1911; the patient was an adult male who had died of the unrelated parasitical infection that is now named after him (Chagas' disease).[28] The next reported adult case cropped up in a retrospective review of 104 autopsied lungs carried out at the Institute of Tropical Hygiene in Amsterdam at the start of the forties; one twenty-one-year-old man was found to have been infected with *Pneumocystis,* though his official cause of death was not detailed in the medical paper.[29] Over the next two decades, all adult cases of PCP reported in the literature involved patients suffering from systemic diseases like leukemias, cancers, or Wegener's granulomatosis, for which the treatments themselves tended to compromise immunity. The only apparent exceptions were those mysterious cases already reported — such as Sadayo F., George Y., Ardouin A., Alice S., Dick G., and Dave Carr. As already explained, it now appeared that in many of these cases some other factor, unidentified at the time, might have been involved — but that this factor was unlikely to have been HIV.[30]

However, it was also important to look at the PCP outbreaks that had occurred among European infants, starting in the 1930s but increasing expo-nentially in the fifties and sixties. My research led me to the Czech parasitolo-gist Kamil Kucera, one of the great experts on the disease. I first met Dr. Kucera in 1991 at his tiny apartment in a bleak housing complex on the edge of Prague. It turned out to be a Tardis, the rooms overflowing with velvet drapes and huge oil paintings, rescued from his ancestral home. Professor Kucera, who was already in his eighties, was inordinately kind and, despite his faltering English, spent many hours discussing his researches with me.

In the years that followed, Kamil Kucera posted me over 250 minutely scripted, tissue-thin pages, these being translations into English of long sections of his doctoral thesis. They included lists and maps of all the PCP clusters he had studied in Czechoslovakia, and further lists of all recorded cases of PCP in the medical literature, most of which involved infants and children.

When I next visited Kamil, in 1993, I told him about my researches into sev-eral of the earliest PCP cases in adults, none of which — with the possible excep-tion of the Manchester sailor — seemed likely to have been presentations of AIDS. He in turn was dubious about the several PCP epidemics that had occurred in Czech orphanages and children's homes in the 1950s and 1960s (which some 1980s and 1990s commentators believed to have been HIV-associated).[31] He said that a natural reservoir of *Pneumocystis carinii* (whether it be in rodents, as he believed, or in the soil) was clearly present in Czechoslovakia, but that these outbreaks of disease seemed to have been prompted by the poor hygiene and medical conditions obtaining in the children's homes, which had lowered the resistance of several of the inmates, especially the infants.

At this point, I decided to tell Kamil Kucera my own pet theory about what might have been responsible for these PCP epidemics.

It was the retrospective identification of fifteen cases of *Pneumocystis carinii* infection among autopsy specimens from infants who had died of pulmonary diseases at Kilo, a gold-mining town in the northeastern Belgian Congo, between 1941 and 1944,[32] that first alerted me to the possibility of another possible cause of immunosuppression, which had not been identified in the literature. Gold and uranium-bearing ores are often found in close association in hydrothermal veins (as, for instance, in Colorado),[33] which led me to wonder whether there might be a correlation between PCP and mining activities, particularly those involving uranium-bearing ores such as pitchblende. If the waste materials from the mining operations at Kilo were indeed rich in uranium, this could have represented a real health hazard to the fifty thousand inhabitants of Kilo township, especially its infants, through contaminated air and water.[34]

Historical events provided some support for this hypothesis. First, there was the case — detailed previously — of George Y., whose sudden development of PCP unassociated with any other disease came a few months after he moved to Northwest Territories to work at what may well have been a uranium mine. A second and similar case, again apparently linked to radiation exposure, involved a British naval officer who died in 1985 of PCP and non-Hodgkin's lymphoma, twenty-nine years after serving on board H.M.S. *Diana,* a ship that twice "sailed through the cloud" within an hour or two of atomic explosions.[35] A friend of the deceased told me that with his weight loss, ulcers, and other skin problems, he had resembled an AIDS patient by the time he died, but his doctor told me informally that he had tested negative for HIV.[36]

The third piece of supporting evidence was also the most substantial. One of the major uranium mining regions of the world is situated in southern Germany and the northwest of the Czech Republic, particularly in the Erzgebirge Mountains, which separate the two. In places like Jachymov, silver mining has been going on since 1515,[37] but it was only at the end of the nineteenth century that rich deposits of pitchblende were identified in the same lodes. These contained not only uranium, but also the radium used by the Curies in their famous experiments of the early 1900s. There had always been high levels of pulmonary disease (known as "Ore Mountains Miners' Disease") among the Erzgebirge miners, but not until 1926 was an association with lung cancer established.[38] By this time, it was reckoned that the average Jachymov miner was dying after ten to fifteen years' labor in the mines, largely because of the inhalation of uranium dust and radon gas.[39]

In October 1938, the German-speaking Sudetenland in Czechoslovakia — which includes the southern part of the Erzgebirge Mountains — was occupied by the Nazis. One of the reasons for this early move toward war was the necessity for the Third Reich of controlling the rich uranium deposits at Jachymov, so that it could proceed with its plans to manufacture an atomic bomb. German miners from all over the country were moved to the Czech mining town, although much of the dirty work was carried out by Czech, Soviet, Polish, and French prisoners of war. A regime of hectic extraction continued at Jachymov until late 1944, under often inhuman conditions, and even though the German A-bomb never materialized, uranium ore was shipped all over Germany, both to the bomb project headquarters, and to various chemical and dye companies.

Something very similar happened in Czechoslovakia in 1948, after the Communists seized power. For the next fourteen years, uranium mining was pursued on a massive scale, with 1.5 million tons of ore being shipped to the Soviet Union for its atomic and nuclear bomb projects — an annual production rate one thousand times higher than during the prewar period. Mines were opened all over the ore-bearing region in northern Bohemia and western Moravia, with the rock being trucked to two refineries just to the south of Jachymov for processing, before being forwarded to the Soviet Union by rail.[40]

Since there were not enough miners to maintain this rate of production, Paragraph 231 was enacted, whereby a court no longer required proof of guilt in order for persons suspected of opposing the regime to be imprisoned as spies or subversives.[41] Some 50,000 political prisoners — including farmers, soldiers, and professors — were thus forced to work in the new mines. The Jachymov area, which was merely the worst of many, was closed off to the outside world between 1948 and 1962; inside the wire were ten concentration camps with names like "Equality," "Concord," and "Fraternity," each sited around the head of a mine.[42] Food was withheld if the men failed to meet their quotas; those caught attempting to escape were summarily shot. Only slightly less inhumane conditions obtained from 1946 onward in the uranium mines of East Germany, where up to 300,000 men are reported to have been involved, some as prisoners, some as mining employees.[43]

The significance of all this for PCP is that the first major proven outbreaks of the disease among European infants and premature babies parallel the exponential increase of uranium-related activities in these two countries.[44] During the early forties, cases of PCP were recorded at Halle-Wittenburg in Germany, a transport hub halfway between the A-bomb factories at Stassfurt and Stadtilm. After the war, the first confirmed German outbreaks of PCP occurred in 1952 and 1953 in places like Jena, Leipzig, and Dresden, the major towns close to the uranium-producing region of the Erzgebirge.

The first large-scale clusters of cases in Czechoslovakia occurred in the western part of Bohemia, where twenty-four infants and prematures with "interstitial plasma-cell pneumonia" were identified in the hospital at Pilsen (the large town nearest to the uranium mines of Jachymov and Pribram) by the pathologist Josef Vanek between 1945 and 1952, most cases being identified in the final three years.[45] In 1951 Vanek's colleague, the great parasitologist Otto Jirovec, was the first to identify the causative agent of this pediatric pneumonia as *Pneumocystis carinii*.[46] Further clusters of cases were seen in Prague, Most, and Olomouc (1952), and at Gottwaldov, Novy Jicin, and Opava (1953), all of which are towns close to the labor camps and uranium mines of Bohemia and Moravia.[47] From the early fifties onward, PCP outbreaks begin to crop up elsewhere in Czechoslovakia and Germany, and then further afield in Europe, like ripples radiating outward. By 1958, reports of the disease among infants had emerged from fourteen other European countries, as far apart as the United Kingdom and the Soviet Union.[48] Many of these reports involved institutional epidemics in hospitals and nurseries.[49]

Infants do not frequent uranium mines, but those living near poorly maintained tailings dumps or processing plants may well be exposed to harmful radiation and radionuclides through wind-blown dust and contaminated water, and become immunosuppressed, and infected with PCP, as a result. Further PCP infections could then take place in state-run nurseries and hospitals where infants and premature babies are kept in close proximity, and where the standards of nutrition and hygiene are less than optimal.

Kamil listened to my exposition, and said he was impressed by the basic hypothesis, but felt that even closer epidemiological links might exist between PCP cases in infants and the thousand-kilometer rail route along which the ore was transported in open wagons to the Soviet Union. The likeliest rail route from the Jachymov processing plants would have been via Most, Prague, and Olomouc, and then on to Lvov in the U.S.S.R. — either via Ostrava and Krakow (Poland), or via the armaments town of Vsetin and Kosice. This correlates extremely well with the second batch of PCP outbreaks in Czechoslovakia.

What we were proposing, in effect, was that PCP, the great opportunist, could take hold under several conditions and situations — including exposure to radioactive gas, dust, and water, and being raised in the unhealthy conditions that obtained in the state-run orphanages behind the Iron Curtain. Kamil Kucera was confident, moreover, that these PCP outbreaks in the fifties and sixties were not early instances of HIV infection and AIDS in central Europe. This conclusion was strengthened when he sent me a slide and a smear from the lungs of two Czech infants who had died of PCP in 1955 and 1962, both of which subsequently tested negative for HIV-1 on PCR.[50]

---

Having now looked at several examples that certain commentators had hypothesized to be examples of archival AIDS, and having found them to be implausible, I made my next visit to follow up on an early AIDS cluster that seemed very likely to be genuine. The index case was the Norwegian sailor mentioned earlier, who, together with his wife and youngest daughter, had died in 1976 — though the sailor's first symptoms of immunosuppression had appeared a decade earlier.[51] All three patients had had clinical courses typical of AIDS, and all three had tested HIV-positive on at least two different assays, even if these findings had never been confirmed by PCR.[52] Such a triumvirate of family members could not easily be explained away by coincidence or contamination.

I had already been in contact with the lead investigator on the case, Stig Frøland. When I first phoned him in 1990 he had seemed friendly, and promised to discuss the medical histories with me if I came to Oslo. But when I eventually arrived there in April 1993 he was less than cooperative and proved to be unavailable for a meeting throughout the time of my stay in Norway. Some of his colleagues later told me that he was not eager to share information about the famous sailor and his family with anyone else.

Fortunately, others proved more willing to talk about the case. Thomas Bøhmer had treated the sailor in the Oslo *Rikshospitalet* at various times during the final seven years of his life, and he remembered him well. He told me the man's name, "Arvid Darre Noe,"[53] and how he had first attended hospital in the port of Kristiansand, at the southern tip of Norway, in 1966, with a wide range of symptoms, including muscle pains, rashes, and lymphadenopathy. By chance, Stig Frøland had at the time been an intern at this very hospital, and had apparently helped to treat Arvid. By the time that Dr. Bøhmer first came across him in Oslo in 1969, he was suffering from general lassitude, respiratory problems, a small but persistent ulcer on the leg, and swollen lymph nodes in the groin. Arvid failed to respond to a variety of different treatments, but eventually felt well enough to return to work.

The youngest of Arvid's three daughters was born in 1967, but by 1969 she too was suffering from recurring ailments. These included a strange bacterial arthritis of the knee, respiratory problems, and a condition resembling septicemia, which affected her whole body. In 1971, the doctors treating father and daughter (including Frøland, who was now an Oslo-based immunologist) got together and did an exhaustive immunological workup. Both patients reacted strangely to a battery of different skin tests, and their lymphocyte counts appeared to be falling. The possibility of an inherited disorder was considered, but abandoned when it was subsequently discovered that Arvid's wife had been suffering similar problems — including persistent thrush infections and episodes of pneumonia — since 1967. She too was carefully reexamined, and it now became clear that all three family members were suffering from some sort of immune abnormality involving not only B-lymphocytes (which produce antibodies that circulate in the bloodstream) but also, more unusually, T-lymphocytes (which control the immune response within cells).

By 1975, Arvid was suffering a *Candida* infection of the lungs; he later became incontinent and mentally disorientated, and developed paralysis of the lower limbs. His daughter, having suffered a series of bacterial, viral, and fungal infections, eventually died in January 1976 from a generalized chicken-pox infection, which spread to her central nervous system. Arvid died three months later. In May of that year, his widow developed acute leukemia, and she then suffered dramatic mental and nervous system impairment; she died in December 1976. The two elder daughters remained physically healthy, but the events of that dreadful year caused deep emotional trauma for both.

The many common factors, especially the defects in B- and T-lymphocytes, clearly demonstrated that there was a link between the three deaths, but the doctors had little idea what it might be. What clues there were afforded little help. Arvid, who was just twenty-nine when he died, had been a drinker, but not a heavy one, and he had been the responsible breadwinner for his family for nearly fourteen years. His sexual history appeared unremarkable, although he had been a sailor during his teenage years, and had sailed all over the world, during which time he had contracted venereal diseases on at least two occasions. They had never, as far as Dr. Bøhmer recalled, gone into details about the specific ports that Arvid had visited, but he had certainly been to Africa, and almost certainly, he said, to East Africa. These events might have been connected to his illness, but there were also other possibilities, which the doctors had pursued with equal vigor. One of their main concerns, apparently, was that the family might have contracted something infectious — perhaps from the rather dirty well-water on the farm where they lived. The doctors became further alarmed when they discovered that the wife's sister, who lived in another village forty miles away, had developed cancer, but relaxed again when the cancer went into remission. The whole affair was shrouded in mystery, and it was because of the lack of substantive answers that they did not rush to publish details of the case.

When a report of the cluster did finally appear in a Scandinavian journal in 1986, it featured an unfortunate error, because serum samples from all three patients were found to be negative for HIV.[54] It was only later, in 1988, that sera taken in 1971 for father and daughter and in 1973 for the wife were found to be HIV-1-positive on two "second generation" ELISA assays and a Western blot. The familial connection, and the fact that all three had died of AIDS-like diseases, made it virtually certain that these serological results were reliable.

It occurred to me that since neither the Manchester nor the Leopoldville isolates from 1959 had so far been sequenced, these sera from 1971 could yet provide the oldest HIV-1 isolate, supplanting the Yambuku sample from 1976.[55] I asked Bøhmer whether there were any plans to amplify and sequence the viruses on PCR. He told me that all the tissues and medical notes were now held

by Dr. Frøland, and that he had no idea of his plans. But he added that Dr. Karl
Wefring, the consultant pediatrician who had cared for the youngest daughter,
could perhaps tell me some more about the case. Dr. Wefring worked at Tønsberg,
sixty miles south of Oslo, and Dr. Bøhmer provided a note of introduction.

Founded in A.D. 871, Tønsberg is the oldest town in Norway, and like the whole
western shoreline of the Oslofjord, it is steeped in associations with the sea. A
few miles to the north lies Horten, the naval headquarters of eastern Norway
since 1818, and a little to the south is the town of Sandefjord, where much of
Norway's huge merchant fleet is based. But Tønsberg itself, after a millennium
of prosperity, is a town in decline. The last shipyard closed down in 1992, and
now the only real links with the days when goods were shipped in from around
the world and forwarded by road to the rest of Europe are the two large trucking companies that are still based there.

   Dr. Wefring was out of town, so I went down to the local library, and looked
through some back numbers of the *Tønsberg Blad,* to find the obituary notices
of the various family members. They had all, it seems, been buried at an
eleventh-century church a dozen miles away. It seemed like an appropriate way
to spend the afternoon, so I took a bus, getting off at Asgardstrand, where
Edvard Munch had, for many years, lived and painted in a small, yellow, clapboard dwelling, which he later described as "the only house where I have been
happy." From there, I walked for several miles on springy turf through birch
woods full of white spring flowers, past Viking burial mounds, small jetties, and
the blackened steel surface of the fjord. Finally, in the late afternoon, the stone
tower of the church appeared in the distance. It took only a few minutes to
locate the graves of Arvid's family. An old woman saw me writing down the text
on the tablets, and led me a few rows away to another set of tombstones bearing the same surname, all dating from 1984. It transpired that Arvid's brother,
a military airman, had crashed into high-tension wires on a training mission;
his parents, unable to bear yet another tragedy, had died of broken hearts a few
months later.

   The next morning I met Dr. Wefring — a large, gentle, dignified man with a
shock of white hair, whom I liked immediately. It emerged that he had spent
some considerable time tracking down the details of Arvid's naval career, and
that he still had the information on file. We ended up striking a deal. I gave Dr.
Wefring my word that I would not contact either of the two surviving daughters, who had apparently been assailed with requests from journalists over the
past few years, and in return he brought out the file and related the details of
where Arvid Noe had sailed and when.[56]

   His first trip abroad, of some nine months' duration, had apparently begun
in August 1961, just a few days after his fifteenth birthday. Arvid started on the
lowest rung, as a kitchen hand on board the *Høegh Aronde,* but within a few

months had been promoted to deckhand. The ship traveled to and fro along the West African coastline, from Cap Vert to the Gulf of Guinea and the Bight of Benin, calling at most of the harbors in between: Dakar in Senegal, Conakry (Guinea), Freetown (Sierra Leone), Monrovia (Liberia), Abidjan in Ivory Coast, Sekondi-Takoradi (Ghana), Lagos and "several [other] harbors in Nigeria," and finally a port in Cameroon, probably Douala. Dr. Wefring told me that Arvid Noe had been sexually active from a young age, and that he seemed to contract a venereal disease every time that he ventured abroad; on this occasion it had been gonorrhea. It was significant, however, that although the *Høegh Aronde* visited many of the countries where HIV-2 is now widespread, the ship did not venture as far as Matadi, the marine port of the Congo, where Arvid could conceivably have been exposed to HIV-1, which had already appeared a few miles inland, at Kinshasa.[57]

When he got back from West Africa, Arvid was still just a lad of fifteen, and he stayed in Norway for the next seventeen months. During that time he married a woman three years his senior and then, when she was six months pregnant, he set sail once more. While she completed her term in Norway, Arvid experienced his own nine months of labor, down in the engine room of an oil tanker, the *Thorshall.* In June 1964 he was back home for two months' leave, seeing his infant daughter for the first time, and then in August he reembarked from Sandefjord with the *Thorshall.* This time he was employed as a stoker, and once again the ship traveled between the great oil terminals of Saudi Arabia and Iran, harbors in the United Kingdom, Holland, Malta, and Sicily, and the southern hemisphere ports of Dumai (Sumatra), Singapore, and Sydney. There was also one other place that the *Thorshall* visited, which, according to hints given by doctors Bøhmer and Wefring, might have been where Arvid had his second gonorrheal infection. That place was Mombasa in Kenya, where the ship was berthed for just two days in the December of 1964.

Arvid returned home at the end of May 1965 and, once again, his wife swiftly became pregnant, with their second daughter being born in March 1966. But by July 1965, Arvid was already at sea again, this time as a *motormann*, working in the engine room on the *Sundove.* He was away for less than four months, traveling first around northern Europe and then to Puerto Rico, Barbados, Trinidad, and Guyana, whence his ship ferried bauxite to various ports in Canada.

The *Sundove* returned to Europe in November 1965, and Arvid went ashore for the final time. By the following year he was already sick, and he sought treatment at the hospital in Kristiansand — which, intriguingly, was 150 miles from his home. Dr. Wefring recalled that by this time he had a positive Wassermann reaction for syphilis, so it seemed possible that Arvid was trying to conceal this information from his wife. If so, this was a sad irony for, given his symptoms, Dr. Wefring was certain that by 1966 Arvid Noe was already HIV-positive.

Further proof was provided by the fact that in December 1967 his third daughter was born — the girl who some nine years later would die of AIDS.

Karl Wefring and I spent some time discussing the possible sources of Arvid Noe's HIV-1 infection. The medical history apparently revealed that he had never had a transfusion, and he appeared not to have been bisexual. It seemed most likely that he had become infected during his overseas travels, and probably after a sexual encounter with a female prostitute in a port, but this scenario still embraced more than four years and dozens of ports. We talked about the evidence offered by the dates of birth of the two seronegative daughters, in January 1964 and March 1966 — and debated whether or not this indicated that he had become infected during his final trip in late 1965 to northern Europe, the Caribbean, and Canada. I argued that this was unlikely, for — apart from this case and that of the Manchester sailor — there were no confirmed sightings of HIV in any of these three regions before the 1970s. Furthermore, Arvid's shore leave in the middle of 1965, after his second voyage on the *Thorshall*, had been only seven weeks, so it is quite possible that he was already HIV-positive by then, but did not infect his wife. Certainly, even if she was infected, she did not transmit the virus to their second daughter, who was conceived at this time.

---

After I returned from Norway, I spent some more time pondering what might have happened to the Norwegian sailor. HIV is not very easily transferred during heterosexual sex, but one thing that does facilitate its transmission is the presence of genital ulcers.[58] It was notable that Arvid's syphilis infection (a disease that follows an indolent course, and which therefore may have been contracted during any of his journeys) only became apparent in 1966. Perhaps this was the time when he began suffering from genital lesions, which, in turn, facilitated the onward sexual transmission of HIV. Sadly, there was only one person who had access to the precise medical history and that person, Dr. Frøland, was not telling.

Arvid Darre Noe had traveled to each of the six major continents, and since a prostitute community in any port city would clearly afford a good pool for the virus, and since that virus could have been introduced to the port by any of the thousands of sailors arriving from other ports, it was clearly possible for him to have been infected anywhere. However, the scenario was clearly far more straightforward if Arvid had been infected in central Africa — the place with the earliest evidence of AIDS, and the home of the chimpanzees that appeared to be natural hosts to the precursor of HIV-1. At its simplest level, such a process needed to involve just two people — the source prostitute and Arvid. If, however,

Arvid was infected in Singapore, Australia, or Holland, then at least four people had to have been involved in the transmission chain — which would make it all the more remarkable that others did not become infected, thus triggering a worldwide AIDS epidemic in the sixties.

Only twice had Arvid Noe traveled anywhere near the hearth of HIV-1 infection in central Africa. The first was either late in 1961 or early in 1962 — when he visited harbors in Nigeria and Cameroon; unfortunately, this was the least precise section of Karl Wefring's researches, with the information apparently having been gleaned from a series of phone calls. But shortly after my visit to Norway, it was revealed that a small proportion of HIV-1-positive people in Cameroon and Gabon were infected with Group O viruses,[59] so it was certainly possible that Arvid had gotten infected in Douala (Cameroon's major port and commercial center), or even nearby Lagos. However, there was no evidence that HIV-1 Group O had been responsible for any clinical infections before 1981, when the French baby from Reims died of AIDS caused by this variant — so the hypothesis appeared unlikely.[60]

A much likelier venue for Arvid to have contracted HIV seemed to be Mombasa in Kenya, which he visited in late 1964. Although the port lies some 750 miles from one of the mooted early centers of HIV-1 infection (Rwanda and Burundi), there was one piece of strong supporting evidence, provided by one of Arvid Noe's brothers. This man said that another brother (who refused to be interviewed) had joined the merchant fleet in 1964, and that he subsequently bumped into Arvid in a port in North America (which seemed likely to have been in Canada during Arvid's final trip in the fall of 1965). Arvid, apparently, was feeling unwell, and traced his illness back to an injection he had received some months earlier — very possibly in Africa. It seemed that Arvid could have been referring to a penicillin injection, administered after a brush with gonorrhea in Mombasa. However, the idea that the needle was to blame seemed implausible, because his venereal symptoms would not have developed for four or five days — by which time he would have been back on board ship where, presumably, the sick bay had a supply of clean needles. In all likelihood, therefore, it was the episode that led to his needing an injection that was significant.

At this stage it seemed probable that Arvid Noe had contracted gonorrhea and HIV-1 at the same time — and that this had occurred in the port of Mombasa on either December 5 or December 6, 1964.

There was one other thing that Karl Wefring told me that day which seemed important. He said that later, when Arvid's health recovered, he worked for some time as a long-distance truck driver, transporting goods down to central

Europe, to Germany and beyond. First a sailor and then a trucker. This information had appeared nowhere in the literature, and it struck me that from the point of view of HIV-1 spread, there could have been few combinations of professions with as much potential for disaster.

Of course, if Wefring was correct, and if Arvid *had* traveled down to Germany as a truck driver in the seventies, and had had sex with women he met on the way, then the cases of the two German men who had died with AIDS-like symptoms in January 1979 took on a new significance. Of particular importance was Herbert H., the bisexual violinist from Cologne, who had sometimes hired female prostitutes for his parties. This meant that — theoretically at least — Herbert might have represented the point at which HIV-1 crossed over from the straight to the gay community.

However, Dr. Wefring did not know which trucking company Arvid had worked for, and in any case I had to leave Norway the following day. It was clear that certain details about Arvid Noe would have to wait for another visit.

# 24

SWITZERLAND AND SWEDEN

Geneva is a strange town. It serves as global headquarters to several organizations, including the World Health Organization, so — like New York and Brussels — it is home to large numbers of rather well-paid international experts. And yet it possesses an uncertain personality, having nothing of the glitzy, self-possessed assurance of Zurich, or even the patrician stolidness of the state capital, Bern.

The WHO headquarters are equally unimpressive, comprising a large rectangular block of fifties concrete and steel on the hillside overlooking the lake of Geneva. It is here that many of the far-reaching decisions about global medical policy, vaccination campaigns, and the responses to new disease threats are made. It was here, in the early eighties, that the director-general, Halfdan Mahler, was — as he later confessed — slow to respond to the threat posed by the AIDS epidemic. And it was here, between 1986 and 1990, that the much-lauded American doctor Jonathan Mann, formerly head of Projet SIDA (the American-backed AIDS program in Kinshasa), took over as the first director of the newly convened Global Program on AIDS (GPA), which he handled with an exemplary blend of urgency and political acumen.[1]

My first task at WHO headquarters was to try to track down the sample of CHAT vaccine, which, according to the Wistar expert committee and the Wistar Institute president, Giovanni Rovera, had been offered to the WHO for testing some seven months earlier, in October 1992.[2] Nobody seemed to know anything about it, but as I was dispatched from one department to another, I did get the chance to speak to a number of interesting people in related fields. David Heymann, head of the Office of Research at the GPA, told me that "I understood that they had not found any specimen [of CHAT vaccine] left over from the studies." When I told him that one vaccine vial relevant to the Congo trials had apparently been located and made available to the WHO, he said, "I think you can be pretty sure that if there was this one vial left that there was nothing in it." At another point in the conversation he said that, in any case, the origin of AIDS was "certainly of no interest today." He added that various departments at the WHO had prepared a joint statement on the OPV/AIDS controversy some time earlier.

I later obtained a copy of this statement, which turned out to be an internal memorandum on the "Safety of Oral Poliovaccines," dated May 8, 1992, and addressed to the six regional WHO directors.[3] The paper was intended to provide them with "information which may be helpful . . . in answering questions which may arise," and contained the following sentence about the OPV/AIDS theory, underlined, in the first paragraph: *"This speculation is without scientific basis."*

After stating that "OPV is one of the safest vaccines known," it went on to claim that "the polio vaccine strains used by Dr Koprowski in central Africa . . . are being tested by sensitive techniques for any evidence of SIV contamination." The lack of any reliable information about this alleged testing suggested that this statement was incorrect when written in May 1992, and that it was still incorrect eleven months later. There again, if the claim was correct, and CHAT vaccine samples *had* been tested for SIV, then why had no results been announced?

The memorandum ended by giving four reasons why, even if testing revealed that SIV sequences *were* present in early vaccine preparations, the implications for the *"Rolling Stone* hypothesis," or for the safety of OPV, would be "virtually none." These were that

> (1) It is virtually impossible that HIV could have evolved from hypothetical contamination with SIV within the time period postulated, given the genetic differences between them and the epidemiological data on the length of time the major HIV subtypes have been in existence. (2) No known human virus is closely related to SIV. . . . (3) Experiments at several laboratories . . . indicate that attempts to deliberately infect primary monkey kidney cells with SIV under the conditions used for production of OPV were unsuccessful (SIV or HIV *cannot* replicate on kidney epithelial cells), showing that significant amounts of SIV could not possibly be present in OPV. (4) Transmission of other viruses, for example to animal handlers, is well documented. Extensive testing of animal handlers for antibodies against SIV has been negative, showing that this particular virus passes only with great difficulty from monkeys to humans.

In fact, the second and fourth of these claims had both been comprehensively disproved by several detailed scientific papers published between 1987 and 1992,[4] while the third was true only if one ignored the fact that most OPVs contained lymphocytes and macrophages, which were the natural host cells to SIVs and HIVs.[5] Furthermore, the first claim was highly contentious, and was to be put in proper perspective by Simon Wain-Hobson in Paris only a few weeks later.[6]

The memorandum was, in short, a defensive and entirely inadequate response to the OPV/AIDS hypothesis, one that had clearly been drafted in haste. One could perhaps understand the political necessity of preparing such a memorandum back in May 1992, in a bid to dampen down the latest vaccine controversy until a more reasoned response could be made. I was astonished, however, that I should have been handed a copy of this memo nearly one year later, as if this was the definitive response of WHO experts to the OPV/AIDS theory. If this was the best riposte that the WHO could manage, then Jennifer Alexander was right: the powers that be were either not taking this business seriously, or else they were very worried indeed.[7]

I was reminded of a similar internal statement that had been released soon after the *Rolling Stone* article by the U.S. Food and Drug Administration in the form of an "FDA Talk Paper" entitled "No AIDS Risk from Polio Vaccines," by one Brad Stone.[8] This single-paged typed document observed, *inter alia:* "The Public Health Service has seen no convincing evidence to support this alleged connection, or even indicate that it is remotely possible." At another point, the FDA paper asserted that "There are no reliable scientific data which indicate that the AIDS virus originated from monkey retroviruses." In fact, by April 1992, when this was written, virtually every piece of reliable scientific evidence indicated that HIV had originated from monkey retroviruses.

What was clear was that papers such as these were able to deliver official-sounding denials without possessing any legally or scientifically binding official status.

---

Fortunately, my peregrinations around the WHO building also led me to the office of Dr. Victor P. Grachev, an elderly Soviet scientist from Biologicals, the WHO unit responsible for maintaining the safety standards of viral vaccines. Dr. Grachev had worked with the great Soviet vaccinator Chumakov, as part of the team that had organized the vaccination of 92 million people with Sabin's OPV in the space of three months in 1960. He told me that in 1961, after the discovery of SV40, the Soviet scientists had tested the sera of scientists and technicians involved with OPV production, and had found very high levels. Victor Grachev was one of those who tested positive, and although neither he nor his colleagues had fallen sick, this had clearly awakened him to the dangers of simian contaminants. In the end, Dr. Grachev proved to be a wonderfully frank source of information about the dangers of viral vaccines.

He began by telling me that an informal meeting of WHO experts had been held in Geneva in July 1985, to discuss the then recent discovery of SIVs in Old World primates, and the implications this had for vaccines made in the tissues of such monkeys. I told him that I found it immensely reassuring that such a meeting had been held so promptly (to some extent, this showed that Louis Pascal was incorrect when he claimed that nobody had responded to the threat of SIVs in vaccines). The experts had tested twenty vaccine lots and 250 vaccine recipients, and failed to find any evidence of SIV. They had further concluded that "Monkey kidney cell cultures would be expected to contain few, if any, T-lymphocytes" (the cells most likely to be infected with SIV).[9] Nonetheless, in November of the following year a "WHO Study Group on Biologicals" (which had included Hilary Koprowski) had recommended that banks of continuous cell lines be developed for the future manufacture of viral vaccines, in preference to monkey kidney tissue culture (MKTC).[10] It seems that such recommendations were frequently made — and frequently ignored.

The study group, of course, is significant, because it shows that in November 1986, at the very latest, Dr. Koprowski was aware of the theoretical possibility that his CHAT vaccine — along with other vaccines prepared in MKTC — could have been contaminated with SIV. If he had any concerns on this score, then this was both the time and the opportunity to address them — or, alternatively, to alert a fellow scientist who could then have mounted a careful and impartial investigation.

I asked how many polio vaccine production centers were now using continuous cell lines (CCL), or human diploid cell strains (HDCS) like Leonard Hayflick's WI-38,[11] and Victor Grachev started doing sums. He concluded that of the 24 polio vaccines being made around the world (6 IPVs and 18 OPVs), which were listed by Biologicals, only one (the IPV made at the Pasteur Mérieux in Paris, now headed by Koprowski's former assistant, Stanley Plotkin) was made in CCL, and one other (the OPV made by Wellcome in the United Kingdom) in HDCS. He added that two labs (Lederle in the United States, and Barry Schoub's lab in South Africa) were thinking of changing to CCL, and that two others, in Iran and China, were thinking about using HDCS.[12]

I was intrigued by the fact that all three organizations that were using, or thinking of using, CCL — the vaccine houses headed by Plotkin and Schoub, and Lederle — had previously been involved in the OPV/AIDS controversy — either in their own right, or through past association with Koprowski. I asked Grachev why 22 of the 24 major polio vaccine laboratories were still using MKTC, and he made it clear that it was largely for reasons of commercial viability. Primary monkey kidney cultures were, it seems, easier to make and produced higher vaccine yields.

I asked just how high such yields were, and Grachev calculated that using modern methods a single pair of monkey kidneys could produce up to 20 liters of concentrated vaccine. I worked out that if the same tissue culture yield had been obtainable in 1958, for the CHAT preparation used at Ruzizi, which had been diluted sixty times,[13] then the kidney tissues of a single monkey would have provided enough vaccine to feed over a million people: more than four times as many as were fed at Ruzizi. Even as early as 1955, when less sophisticated primitive tissue culture techniques were in use, between three thousand and ten thousand doses of vaccine could be produced from a single pair of kidneys.[14] This meant that even if these early methods of making monkey kidney tissue cultures had been employed, then the kidneys of just twenty-two monkeys could have been sufficient to provide vaccine for the Ruzizi trial.

Grachev returned to his theme of the relative safety of different tissue cultures. "Our aim in the WHO," he told me candidly, "is to push . . . continuous cell lines, because primary [monkey] tissue culture is very danger[ous. It has] viral contaminants." Between 30 percent and 50 percent of all monkeys had to be rejected because the tissue cultures made from them contained one of the eighty-odd known simian viruses, he told me, and if wild monkeys from Africa (rather than those bred in captivity) were used, the figure grew as high as 60 percent. This was the result if monkeys were quarantined for six weeks to see if they showed signs of illness, and the control bottles containing tissue cultures made from their kidneys were observed for a total of twenty-eight days — which was current standard practice. (Guidelines in the fifties, of course, had been much more relaxed.) However, even higher percentages proved to be contaminated if the tissue cultures were checked over a longer period, like two months, he said. Of course, some of the adventitious agents had been identified only with the passage of time: SV40 in 1960, the highly virulent Marburg virus in 1967, SIV in 1985, and Ebola (a close cousin of Marburg) in monkeys housed at a facility in Reston, Virginia, in 1989.[15] "Really," he concluded, "we ought to stop production using primary tissue cultures." For a senior international health official, this was a remarkably bald statement, and indicated just how dangerous he felt the situation to be.

So we got to the bottom line, and I asked whether we could be confident that a monkey that was host to the simian ancestor of HIV-1 had not been included among the animals that had provided tissue cultures for vaccine production back in the fifties. Since the HIV ancestor was a slow-acting virus, a lentivirus, which was apathogenic for its natural host, it would have produced no visible signs in the monkey itself, and might well not have caused any visible effect in the tissue culture control bottles during the observation period. In response, Victor Grachev sighed a long, drawn-out sigh. Eventually he said that at the WHO meeting in 1985, they had concluded that the SIV from African green monkeys was an "absolutely different virus" from HIV. Seeing that I was not very impressed by this, he went on to draw an analogy with the outbreak, beginning in the mid-eighties, of bovine spongiform encephalopathy, BSE, in British cattle that had been fed material derived from the ground-up body parts of sheep, which had probably contained the sheep pathogen scrapie. "You know," he said, "we [didn't have] any *in vitro* diagnostic test for these diseases. Absolutely nothing. It's only clinical [signs that indicate whether or not an animal is infected]." It was clear that he was bracketing the lentiviral diseases with the prion diseases, and saying that prior to the discovery of AIDS-like diseases and BSE, neither of the slow-acting causative pathogens could be detected in the test tube.[16]

As I was leaving, Dr. Grachev made one final comment. "In Russia we have a very good [proverb]. You should seven times . . . check [whether] it's good or not. And only one time cut. Because after you cut, it's impossible to [stick it back together]." I also thought the proverb well tailored, and wondered whether — had seven careful safety checks been performed before certain cattle feeds and polio vaccines had been released — some of the disease outbreaks of the late twentieth century, such as BSE and AIDS, might have been prevented.

---

There was also another important matter that I wanted to follow up in Switzerland. A careful perusal of the medical literature relating to CHAT vaccine, including the reports of various polio vaccine conferences, showed that it was one of two European countries in which pool 10A-11 had been fed in small-scale trials. (The same pool of CHAT, 10A-11, had been used in the Congo and Ruanda-Urundi in early 1958.)[17] Between November 1957 and the end of 1960, CHAT 10A-11 had been given to some 400 people in Switzerland, and to about one thousand individuals in Sweden.

I met Dr. Fritz Buser (who had personally administered many of these early Swiss feedings of CHAT) in a large old-fashioned restaurant full of crystal and brass in the center of the state capital, Bern. He was now eighty years old, a small man who was polite and gentlemanly and smartly dressed. Following the great traditions of polio vaccine research, we settled down with a large pot of coffee and several interesting selections from the *patisserie* counter.

Dr. Buser began by explaining how, between 1957 and 1959, over four million doses of Salk vaccine had been given in Switzerland, but that there was little enthusiasm for the shots among the general public.[18] At this time, Buser had been working as a pediatrician in the capital, and he was approached by Dr. Meinrad Schar, who was chief of sera and vaccines at the Swiss Public Health Department. In the early fifties, Schar had been based in San Francisco working on plague organisms, and he had got to know Hilary Koprowski through Karl Meyer, a Swiss-born doctor who had supported Koprowski's OPV trials at Sonoma through the George Williams Hooper Foundation, of which he was director.[19] Later in the fifties, said Buser, it was not possible to conduct open trials in the United States, but after hearing about Koprowski's apparently successful feedings in the Belgian Congo, Schar agreed to conduct a carefully supervised trial of his new vaccines in Switzerland. Buser was enlisted to provide the pediatric patients.

Thus it was that, in 1958, Koprowski sent Schar supplies of CHAT pool 10A-11 (for Type 1 polio) and Fox (for Type 3 polio).[20] The vaccinations were given by dropper, direct into the mouth, and mostly took place in Buser's own office in Bern.[21] Dr. Buser recalled that "prominent people in Switzerland said 'Please leave your hands off that dangerous vaccine. If you don't, the media will ruin your reputation.'" But by that time they had already "secretly vaccinated" 400 infants and children with CHAT, 90 of whom were also fed Fox.

Blood tests were taken before and after vaccination, as were stool samples, both from the index children and from family members, to check whether the virus had spread from vaccinees to close contacts. Immunity, especially with CHAT, was "excellent," being successfully established in 99 percent of the children and all the infants, and with antibody levels remaining high in the two years following. In about a third of the families there was intrafamilial spread of the CHAT vaccine virus, but it showed no tendency to revert to virulence. The less stable Type 3 vaccine (in this case Fox) was always more of a risk, but Buser commented: "We were lucky; we had no case of paralysis. If we'd had just one case, important people would have cut our throats."

The literature records that Switzerland went on to mount larger, open trials of CHAT on 40,000 children from the cantons of Basel and Aargau (around Zurich) in 1960, and of CHAT and Fox on 320,000 children from Bern, Luzern, and Aargau cantons in 1961.[22] Apparently there were two cases of polio in CHAT vaccinees, and six in Fox vaccinees; interestingly, Dr. Buser added that, in reality, cases of vaccine-associated paralysis "may have been more" than the reported figures, but would not give further information. The details of the specific pools of CHAT and Fox used for these large trials appear nowhere in the literature, and Buser could not recall the details, save for the fact that they had not been the same pools as those used in 1958.

Later, in 1962, Buser and colleagues staged a field trial of three Koprowski OPVs (CHAT, W-2, and WM-3) made in Hayflick's human diploid cell strain (HDCS), which were successfully tested on 800 infants and children.[23] By then, however, other Swiss doctors had also tried out the Lederle and Sabin strains on hundreds of thousands of youngsters,[24] making Switzerland the only country in the world to stage mass trials on the vaccine strains of all three major OPV manufacturers. By the end of 1962, Sabin's Type 1 (LSc) and Type 2 (P-712) vaccines were adopted throughout Switzerland, although Koprowski's WM-3 was preferred to Sabin's Type 3 vaccine, Leon. This unique combination of vaccines continued to be fed until 1970, when Sabin objected and the Koprowski Type 3 strain was dropped from the schedules.

Dr. Buser, for his part, was still an unashamed fan of these final Koprowski polio vaccines made in HDCS. CHAT, he said, was if anything slightly more immunogenic than LSc; P-712 and W-2 were equally effective; while WM-3 was safer and more stable than Leon. He told me that whereas there had been no cases of polio in Switzerland between 1962 and 1970, there had been a handful of cases of paralysis (both in vaccinees and in contacts) after 1970. Sera from these cases had been analyzed in Germany and found to be related to the Leon Type 3 vaccine, which apparently had the potential, on very rare occasions, to revert to virulence. Nothing had been written about this in the literature, Buser explained, because they had not wanted to damage the vaccination program.

Dr. Buser described Dr. Koprowski as a "*bon vivant* . . . very clever, but also a very efficient and very productive brain." He was not indiscriminate in his praise, however. He recalled one occasion when Koprowski had invited him to lunch in Philadelphia, and had ended up giving him a cold drink and a sandwich. Another time, he told me, Koprowski had taken him for supper at the Schweizer Hof in Bern, and Buser had ended up paying. Fritz Buser was clearly a man who enjoyed eating out, and these incidents had stuck in his memory. By contrast, he recalled that on the one occasion Albert Sabin had invited him for lunch, Sabin had taken care of the bill.

It struck me that, for someone who was trying to promote his vaccines in Switzerland, Koprowski had on these occasions employed poor tactical skills. Later, I made sure that the *patisserie* bill ended up on my side of the table.

---

Shortly afterward, I interviewed the other leading figure from the time of the OPV trials in Switzerland, Professor Meinrad Schar, at his office in Zurich. He was then seventy-two years old, and although his recollection of these events started slowly, he remembered more and more as the interview progressed. Furthermore, he demonstrated that he was both a shrewd and an uninhibited analyst of the period. He described Koprowski as "hilarious . . . very open-minded . . . very friendly and ingenious, and he also knows how to raise money for his institute." Although he made it clear that he still kept in contact with Koprowski, seeing him every few years, he was not afraid to relate episodes that did not reflect so well upon the man and his vaccines.

After the small trials in 1958, Schar became a supporter of Koprowski's vaccines, and in 1960, when a group of private physicians in Bern, Basel, and St. Gallen began a trial feeding of the Cox/Lederle vaccines, Schar intervened. He convinced the Federal Office of Public Health that these strains had already been proved unsafe in other trials (such as those in West Berlin and Florida), and that the Swiss feedings were taking place without any proper follow-up. Later, Schar phoned Koprowski, and asked if he could provide Wistar Institute vaccines to replace the Lederle strains in a twenty-thousand-person trial, which was scheduled to take place in Basel. Koprowski apparently flew over himself to visit officials at the Swiss Federal Office of Public Health, and subsequently supplied one million doses of CHAT and W-Fox for feeding at canton level in 1960 and 1961.

Two years later it was Schar (who by then was in charge of vaccine testing at federal level) who finally decided on the Sabin strains in preference to Koprowski's. Unlike Buser, he felt that Sabin's strains were "definitely better," including the Type 3 strain, Leon. Another significant reason, he told me, was that Koprowski had never really developed a successful Type 2 strain. Indeed, Schar recalled that in both 1958 and 1960, Koprowski had argued that it was only really important to possess a good Type 1 vaccine, since this protected against the most virulent poliovirus, and also, he claimed, offered a degree of protection against the other poliovirus types.

I asked Schar what substrate Koprowski had used to make his vaccines before 1962, and he replied that he was unsure, but that it was "probably rhesus monkey" kidney. But then he added an interesting comment. Joseph Melnick, he said, had discovered in 1960 that the addition of magnesium chloride to polio vaccine eliminated the threat of SV40, and had patented the technique. Albert Sabin's vaccines, thenceforward, had always incorporated magnesium chloride, but Koprowski apparently "never used" the salt, so "perhaps he could have had SV40 in there," Schar hypothesized.

I wondered whether there could have been another interpretation of this story — that Koprowski could have been using the kidneys of a simian other than the rhesus macaque, one that was not known to be susceptible to SV40. (Intriguingly, a report published years after the initial SV40 scare, in 1967, included a section that detailed the testing of sera from 85 chimpanzees resident in three different U.S. labs: not one was found positive for SV40.[25] Another article published that same year, however, reported the isolation of seven new simian viruses from chimp tissues, including two foamy viruses — or retroviruses — both of which were isolated from the kidneys.[26]) Professor Schar seemed to feel my hypothesis was viable, so I went on to outline the OPV/AIDS theory to him. He listened carefully, and then, to my surprise, commented: "If it would be true that [AIDS] was found in areas where the CHAT strain had been used, then [the theory] could be true." I pointed out that for central Africa at least, this appeared to be the case. I asked whether his safety tests would have shown up a lentivirus, had one been present in one of the vaccines, and after some thought, he answered: "I'm sure we wouldn't have found a lentivirus, because of the short observation time." When I asked if chimpanzee kidneys could have been used as the substrate for CHAT, he replied, "Yes, it could be."

Earlier, he had told me that samples of all the vaccines used in Switzerland, including at least fifty milliliters of the concentrated CHAT pool that

Koprowski had delivered in 1960, had been stored at the Swiss Federal Office of Public Health. However, he said, he did not think that it was still held nowadays. I asked if he would check for me, especially to see if any of the pool from 1958, 10A-11, remained, and he agreed to do so.

In the course of the conversation, Professor Schar mentioned that he had once found a viral contaminant in Lépine's inactivated polio vaccine, something that had sparked a huge row with the Pasteur Institute. Schar reported this finding to Lépine, and then sent a sample of the vaccine to Robert Hull, a Canadian expert on simian viruses.[27] Hull eventually found "a pox virus never before seen in rhesus monkeys," which he thought must originate from the African green monkey (though it would seem more likely, given that Lépine was using baboon kidney for his tissue cultures, that *Papio papio* was the source). Whatever, the Pasteur apparently accused Schar of damaging the reputation of Lépine's vaccine, but Schar stuck to his guns, and even insisted on the Pasteur paying the bill for the Canadian testing.

For almost the first time, I began seriously to consider whether not only Lépine's attenuated polio vaccine, but also certain batches of his IPV, could have contained other contaminating viruses — such as an SIV. At the end of our conversation, I asked Meinrad Schar whether it were possible that Lépine's vaccine had ever been tried out in West Africa. "It's quite possible," he answered promptly, "and if they had a bad experience, nothing more would be heard about it." If Schar was right, then it seemed that modern medicine might also, inadvertently, have sparked the sudden cataclysmic emergence of HIV-2. Without doubt, I needed to look further into the origins of the second AIDS virus also.

———————

Like Switzerland, Sweden is another country with fine public health services and, consequently, a high level of hygiene. Because of this, Sweden was, by the 1940s, experiencing frequent polio epidemics, especially among adults who lacked naturally acquired antibodies. These culminated in the epidemic of 1953, in which more than five thousand people were paralyzed.[28] Nowadays, it is almost the only country in the world to have remained completely loyal to IPV, in the form of a "Super-Salk" vaccine, inactivated at a lower temperature; this takes longer to kill the virus, but results in better immunogenicity than Salk's version. This Swedish IPV was the brainchild of Professor Sven Gard.

In 1959, Professor Gard spent some eight months on sabbatical at the Wistar Institute, during which he helped defend Koprowski against Sabin's charge that CHAT was contaminated. Since then, he has become one of the grand old men of virology, respected throughout the world for the clarity and wisdom of his speeches and articles. I found him living in a sheltered community for the elderly, situated among pine woods a few miles north of the Swedish capital, Stockholm. He came down to the foyer to meet me, a dignified individual of eighty-seven years, tall and slender, with the hard, chiseled features that ennoble some men of that age. His grasp was dry and very firm, and he kept hold of my hand for some seconds, leaning forward to look closely into my face with strong, gray, serious eyes. Then he turned and led me to the library.

He started by explaining to me how he and his colleagues had never seriously considered using OPV in Sweden. "We had excellent results with our own inactivated virus," he told me. "The last domestic case in Sweden was in 1961; after that we haven't . . . seen a single case of poliomyelitis in properly vaccinated individuals."

I asked him about the various experiments with CHAT that he and his colleagues at the Karolinska Institute, most notably Margerete Böttiger, had conducted between 1957 and 1962. He explained that in every case, the subjects had first been vaccinated twice with IPV to confer protection, before the OPV had been fed — first to infants and then to other family members. This research, he explained, had been staged in order to study the spread of the live vaccine within the family setting; it had never been an attempt to establish immunity with OPV.

The first of these trials was of CHAT pool 10A-11, and involved eight-five persons from twenty Stockholm families — the infants being fed in November 1957, and the remaining family members some ten months later.[29] Further trials were staged in the winter of 1958/9 on 675 family members from Stockholm and nearby Eskiltuna,[30] and in early 1960 on another thirty-two families, and 150 children from a boarding school for the blind. These trials, involving about a thousand subjects, had all employed CHAT pool 10A-11. In March 1961, another thirty-six hundred primary schoolchildren from the northern suburbs of Stockholm, aged between seven and fifteen, were fed with CHAT 10A-11, which had been passaged once more in cynomolgus kidneys at the Karolinska.[31] At this stage, after almost five thousand experimental feedings, it was concluded that although CHAT was safe, there was as yet no live Type 3 strain safe enough to use in Sweden. Plans to follow two IPV injections with an OPV booster therefore had to be abandoned, and it was decided instead to give IPV boosters at five-year intervals.[32]

"We don't use live virus. We don't have to," Gard went on. "With the inactivated virus properly produced, we achieve immunity levels much higher than you ever get with . . . attenuated strains." I asked if he was totally opposed to OPVs. "Yes," he answered. "With attenuated virus, you introduce millions of infection sources into the community each year. . . . The so-called attenuated virus strains — we know that they are not stable." I could see his point, but it occurred to me that whereas IPV could work well in an orderly country with a strong tradition of communal responsibility, such as Sweden, it would be far more problematical in other countries that enjoyed less than 100 percent vaccination cover. Gard added that he was suspicious about the safety of other attenuated virus vaccines (such as, for instance, that against measles), which perhaps, he felt, had the potential to "go underground" and then re-emerge in virulent form many years later. Some people, he added, suspected that multiple sclerosis might be a rare late effect of the measles vaccine virus, because monoclonal antibodies against measles appeared in the spinal fluid of many MS cases.

Later, I asked about the controversy between Sabin and Koprowski about the safety of CHAT and, in particular, Sabin's finding of a viral contaminant. Gard replied that while working in Koprowski's lab, he had repeatedly tested the CHAT strain and had not been able to repeat Sabin's results, which is why he had argued on Koprowski's behalf at the Washington conference. I explained to Gard that the pool of CHAT that Sabin had tested was in fact 10A-11, and was therefore different from the pools (13 and 18) that were fed in Leopoldville and Poland during 1958 and 1959.[33] Was it possible that Sabin had found the adventitious agent in one pool, while he and the others who had tested CHAT for Koprowski and found it contaminant-free, had examined another pool? "That's quite possible," Gard replied, after some thought.

———————

The following day, I interviewed another of Gard's former colleagues at the Karolinska, Margerete Böttiger. Dr. Böttiger, who was fondly recalled by colleagues from the fifties for her perspicacity and beauty, had subsequently been responsible for identifying the first AIDS case in Sweden — the young Congolese boy born in 1975 who had displayed unusual symptoms in 1976, and had become seriously ill soon after arriving in Scandinavia in 1978.[34] She told me that she had joined the Karolinska Institute in 1957, and had helped to organize most of the OPV trials, eventually writing her Ph.D. thesis on the subject of polio vaccination in Sweden.[35]

Toward the end of our conversation, Professor Böttiger mentioned two very important details. She said that the protocols for CHAT (detailing how it had been made) probably still existed — at least for the Swedish version. Then I asked if she still had samples of the original vaccines. She replied: "I can't tell . . . but it might be possible." When I pressed her, she said that they certainly still had the version that had been passaged in Sweden, but she couldn't tell if they still had the original 10A-11 from Koprowski. "It could be stored somewhere . . . [in] one of the three hundred freezers," she conceded, finally. As I got up to leave, I asked how one would go about applying to test a sample from this CHAT pool. Dr. Böttiger now seemed agitated, and her previously very competent English was becoming ragged. She explained that any decision about sending vaccine samples abroad would have to be taken by someone at a higher level, probably by her current boss, the head of the National Bacteriological Laboratory (NBL),

Professor Hans Wigzell. And even then, she added, they would probably want to test it themselves first. The Swedes are notoriously careful about preserving materials, and I suddenly got a powerful hunch that samples of CHAT pool 10A-11 would prove to be still in storage at the NBL.

Before leaving the NBL, I also interviewed Dr. Carl-Rune Salenstedt, the director of vaccine production. Like Gard and Böttiger, he was unable to recall which monkeys Koprowski had been using to make his vaccines, but he did have a clear memory of what they had used in Sweden. He said that when he first arrived at the institute, in 1955, they had been using rhesus macaques to make vaccine for the early IPV trials, but that they had changed to using cynomolgus macaques from Indonesia in around 1957; at some point in the sixties they had switched to the African green monkey. I asked about the current substrate, and he told me that as of July 1994, they would be changing to the use of Vero cells — a continuous cell line. The reasons, he said, were partly ethical (because of heightened sensitivities about killing monkeys to make vaccines), and partly because of the threat posed by monkey viruses, which, he acknowledged, had been more substantial than they, the virologists, had realized during the fifties and sixties. He added that if they had just quarantined their monkeys for three months instead of the standard one-month period, the threat would have been all but eliminated.

Dr. Salenstedt also mentioned that in his early days at the institute, he had participated in a "very intensive discussion" about whether to launch trials of IPV in northern Sweden and OPV in the south of the country. The idea had never been implemented, he added.

This reminded me of something that Sven Gard had told me: that although officially during the fifties, all vaccines should have been imported through the medical authorities and the state pathology laboratory, "it was easy to circumvent the regulations and [import] limited amounts of vaccine; there was no strict control on such business." I wondered if it was possible that, in the early days, an oral polio vaccine might have been brought in and tried in a southern town like Goteborg or Malmo, and Gard replied that yes, it was possible. In fact, he believed that a few physicians had imported Sabin's OPV during the early sixties, even though it was not licensed in Sweden.

This brought me back to David Carr's visit to Malmo in the first six days of June 1957. I wondered whether it was conceivable that a Swedish doctor who knew Koprowski might have been sent an early version of CHAT, and tried it out in Malmo even before the start of Sven Gard's Stockholm trials in November. Gard had told me that he certainly didn't know of any such event, but had then given me the name of Lars Kjellen, who had been head of the virology department in Malmo during the fifties. Kjellen was away from home when I visited the city a few days later, but there were other interesting leads to follow.

There was, for instance, fat King Karl the Tenth, sitting astride his horse, Hannibal, in the central square, the *Stortorget* — the same statue featured in the background of that faded 1957 snapshot of Dave Carr and his two shipmates. There was a photo shop on the edge of the square and, on the off chance, I showed the photo of the sailors to the elderly proprietor. He looked at it for a few seconds, and then said that he knew the man who had taken it — a photographer whom he described as "a real original," who used to snap tourists in the square every summer, using a big wooden box camera. To the rear of the camera was attached a black hood, into which was sewn a pair of gloves; beneath the hood were two bowls, of developer and fixer. On this occasion, I was told, the photo had not been left long enough in the fixer, because the tops of the sailors' heads (and that of good King Karl) were all rather faded.

I also called in at the offices of the local newspaper, the *Sydsvenska Dag-bladet,* where a helpful journalist translated various articles from June 1957. Here, indeed, were reports of the visit from Londonderry of the frigates *Zest* and *Whitby* ("boats which smell of gunpowder"), and the fact that "wide trousers are a common sight in Malmo these days" as the four hundred British sailors enjoyed a summer break after their winter maneuvers in the North Sea.[36] Here too were accounts of the traditional contacts that occur when young men arrive in a new port. There was a snapshot of a happy group of sailors and local women in the *Kungsparken,* and a commentary piece lightheartedly declared that "we hope our British guests liked the Malmo girls just as much as the girls like them."

Some time after this, I managed to track down Dr. Kjellen, who wrote me that he himself had never been involved in any Swedish OPV trials, and that, having made inquiries among Malmo colleagues of that era, he had come across no information to suggest that any OPVs, "either of Koprowski's or of Sabin's products," had been used in the city.[37]

Just as in Northern Ireland, there was an intriguing coincidence between a Koprowski vaccine having been fed, and a visit to the same country in the same year by the "Manchester sailor." But that seemed to be as far as the coincidence extended. There was no evidence to suggest that any CHAT vaccine had been fed in Sweden until the first Stockholm trial on infants in November 1957 — which was five months after David Carr's visit. And without such evidence, any hypothesizing about sexual contacts between Malmo women and their British guests was merely idle conjecture.

---

Altogether some fourteen hundred people in Sweden and Switzerland, mainly infants, were fed the original CHAT 10A-11 pool from the Wistar between 1957 and 1960. Was it possible that there had been early cases of AIDS in either of these two countries? The only clinically plausible case of which I knew was Huminer's case of the twenty-three-year-old woman from Goteborg, Sweden, who died in 1969, after a two-year illness caused by an atypical and disseminated mycobacterial infection, *Mycobacterium kansasii.*[38] I therefore traveled to Goteborg to speak with Jack Kutti, one of the woman's physicians, who reviewed the case with me, concluding that his patient had had an unexplained immunodeficiency, possibly congenital, which would probably have been successfully treated with a drug like rifampicine, had one been available in the sixties. It seemed probable that, had she experienced the same symptoms in 1993, her diagnosis would have been one of idiopathic CD4+ lymphocytopenia (ICL).[39]

In conclusion, I found no evidence to suggest that AIDS had emerged prematurely among the populations of Sweden and Switzerland, the two European countries where CHAT pool 10A-11 had been fed in the fifties. A vaccine pool is supposed, by definition, to be homogeneous, and provided this was the case, and that there was no difference between the batches of pool 10A-11 fed in Africa and those fed in Europe, then the finding appeared to weaken the hypothesis that this particular pool of vaccine might have contained an SIV contaminant.

AN INTRODUCTION TO HIV-2

Apart from following up on the Norwegian sailor and the early CHAT trials in Sweden, there was one other major reason for my visit to Scandinavia: to undertake some further research into HIV-2, and its extraordinarily high prevalence in the West African state of Guinea-Bissau. Both Sweden and Denmark have provided relief and medical assistance to Guinea-Bissau since 1974, when the local liberation movement, the PGAIC, finally succeeded in driving the Portuguese from the country.[1] These countries have also been involved in many of the better studies of "the second AIDS virus."

Ever since the existence of HIV-2 was first reported in 1985, and the virus was formally identified as another cause of AIDS in 1986,[2] certain crucial differences between it and the original HIV, now renamed HIV-1, had been apparent. First, the area where HIV-2 was found was so clearly focused in West Africa, with secondary foci emerging in countries that had formerly had colonies in West Africa — notably Portugal and France — that most scientists felt it was legitimate to speak of the virus as being endemic in that region, and of West Africa representing its hearth (or geographical source).[3] Second, when HIV-2 was sequenced, it was found to be only 40 percent to 50 percent homologous (genetically similar) to HIV-1, although it was subsequently found to be extremely similar to the SIV found in the sooty mangabey, *Cercocebus atys* (the range of which also embraces West Africa). This strongly suggested that the two HIVs had evolved independently of each other, and that HIV-2-related AIDS represented a separate zoonosis (human disease acquired from an animal).[4] Third, HIV-2 seemed to infect people at a later age than HIV-1, and the evidence suggested that it was a less transmissible virus.[5] Fourth, HIV-2 appeared to take longer than HIV-1 to cause AIDS; the usual estimates for

# GUINEA-BISSAU (Showing areas of HIV-2 prevalence over 5% circa 1987, superimposed on Portuguese and guerrilla-held areas circa 1969)

Ziguinchor ×

SENEGAL

Kabrousse ×

● São Domingos (7.5%)
● Ingoré (16.0%)
● Pirada (6.3%)
Pauna (5.4%)
Sonaco (8.7%)
● Gabú (5.1%)
● Bafatá (7.0%)
Bambadinca (9.1%)
● Galomaro (26.8%)
◉ Xitole (8.8%)
Caió (7.9%)
BISSAU (7.0%)
● Bubaque (19.2%)
Catió (8.0%) ◉

GUINEA

**Legend:**

- ·–· = national boundary
- ◯ (hatched) = liberated region
- ◯ = Portuguese-held & contested regions
- ● = Portuguese-held towns
- ◉ = Portuguese fortified camps in liberated zones
- × = other town

N ↑

0    25         50 miles
0  25    50    75 km

Every area of high latter-day HIV-2 seroprevalence appears to have been a Portuguese-held area or garrison town during the Liberation War.

The data from Bissau, Bafata, and Caió derive from precise cluster sampling conducted in 1987 or 1989. The remainder of the cohorts studied are less precise, being of "general population and patients" (1986/7).

SOURCES: B. Davidson, "The Liberation of Guiné" (Penguin, 1969). HIV/AIDS Surveillance Database.

latency being about twenty years for the former virus and ten years for the latter.[6]

During my visit to the State Bacteriological Laboratory in Stockholm, I spoke with Dr. Gunnel Biberfeld, the leader of a team that had conducted a detailed investigation into HIV-2 in Guinea-Bissau, which lies to the south of Senegal and has a population of less than a million. She told me how, in 1985, the SBL team had first begun isolating an unusual virus — typical of HIV in its core proteins (*gag* and *pol*) but differing greatly in the envelope protein (*env*). Then Max Essex and Phyllis Kanki published their paper about HTLV-IV,[7] and Biberfeld's team thought that they had probably found the same virus. (In fact they had not. Essex and Kanki's team had been dealing with a lab contamination caused by an SIV from a rhesus macaque;[8] it was Biberfeld's team that had actually isolated the new human virus.) At this point, Biberfeld recalled that a young Swedish doctor, Anders Naucler, was still based in Guinea-Bissau, and he became her student, producing his Ph.D. thesis on HIV-2 in 1991.

The key question about Guinea-Bissau, she told me, was why the prevalence was so high in that country — dramatically higher, even, than in other West African countries, although Casamance, the most southerly province in Senegal, where many Guinea-Bissan refugees lived or had lived, was also badly affected.[9] The most plausible explanation, she said, was that HIV-2 "would seem to have emanated from there." As for the HIV-2 age-prevalence curve, with its gradual initial rise, followed by a much higher level of infectees aged forty and above — this, she said, was probably a function of the fact that HIV-2-infected people survived much longer than those having HIV-1. But why were so few persons in their teens and twenties infected? She said that recent research seemed to indicate that there was a much lower titer of virus present in asymptomatic HIV-2-positive (as compared to HIV-1-positive) people, so that the risk of others being infected after a single sexual or parenteral exposure to an HIV-2-infected person was probably that much lower.[10] It was, in short, more difficult to get infected with HIV-2 than HIV-1, so that even "high-risk" persons tended to be older by the time they seroconverted.

I asked her about sooty mangabeys, the putative source of the virus that had become HIV-2 in humans, and Dr. Biberfeld told me that she didn't know how common they were in Guinea-Bissau. But she said that once the virus had become established in humans, for spread to occur you needed the right number of people living in close contact, including sexual contact (such as occurred in towns), and you needed people to travel from one area to another. She further explained that even if there had been a few sporadic AIDS cases in rural areas before the recognized HIV-2 epidemic, there would probably have been little or no onward transmission, provided those persons remained in their villages.

When I asked her if there was any evidence of HIV-2 existing in Guinea-Bissau before 1980 (the date of the earliest retrospectively HIV-2-positive blood samples from that country),[11] she said there was not, because frozen blood samples from before 1980 were not available, due to the frequency of power cuts. As for her ideas on origin: "I haven't been so interested in that aspect, because it is a sensitive topic, and the Africans feel it is stigmatizing them." Dr. Biberfeld was clearly a sensitive and caring woman, but some of her replies were as dry as those of a seasoned politician.

Finally, she told me that her team were now looking at potential killed and live vaccines against HIV-2. In an animal model (using cynomolgus monkeys), they had demonstrated protection against challenge using inactivated virus, and had also successfully immunized three out of four monkeys that had been given an attenuated strain of HIV-2, and then challenged with SIV — thus demonstrating at least partial cross-protection against a closely related virus.

Dr. Biberfeld gave me a copy of Anders Naucler's thesis, a wide-ranging review of the prevalence and clinical impact of HIV-2 in Guinea-Bissau.[12] In terms of seroepidemiology, he had found that in the city of Bissau in 1987, 0.05 percent were infected with the principal AIDS virus, HIV-1 (one person out of two thousand tested, including patients with AIDS), while 8.6 percent of antenatal women, and 36.7 percent of female prostitutes were infected with HIV-2. By contrast, only 1.4 percent of stored sera from 1980, taken from rural adults living close to Bissau, were HIV-2-positive, which, he wrote, "suggests that the spread of the virus has increased significantly during the last decade." He also found that twenty of the HIV-2-positive patients hospitalized in Bissau had progressed to AIDS during a six-month period, a finding that differed significantly from those of Phyllis Kanki's group, which had reported finding no clinical signs of immune suppression in a group of HIV-2-infected prostitutes in Dakar, Senegal, after a year of follow-up.[13]

———

The researcher whom I was most interested to meet, however, was a Danish doctor, Anne-Grethe Poulsen, from the Statens Seruminstitut in Copenhagen. Poulsen was the coauthor of some very interesting seroepidemiological papers about HIV-2 infection in Guinea-Bissau, and had encountered a surprisingly high level of HIV-2-positivity in elderly people, including those in their seventies. (In this, she differed from Anders Naucler, who had not detected HIV-2 infection in Guinea-Bissans aged over sixty.)

Dr. Poulsen turned out to be unexpectedly young and disarmingly attractive, in the classic Scandinavian manner of fair hair, pale skin, and lithe good health. She had promised to share some of her HIV-2 data with me if I visited her in Copenhagen, and I started off by asking her about prevalence levels in different parts of the country: in which places was HIV-2 especially common? She knew of three regions, she said — these being Bissau (the capital), Bafata (a provincial town about one hundred miles inland), and the semirural area of Caio (some sixty miles northwest of Bissau on the coast), in all of which adult prevalence levels of between 6 percent and 9 percent had been detected.[14] Elsewhere in the country, Poulsen said, HIV-2 prevalence appeared to be much lower. For instance, in parts of the Biombo region, to the west of the capital, prevalence was only about 1 percent.

She thought that ethnicity might be partly responsible for these differing prevalences. In Biombo most of the people were Papel, whereas in Caio they were largely Manjaco, and Poulsen said that some Manjaco women seemed to become "nomads" for a while, either before they got married or after they divorced or separated, and that many seemed to work as casual prostitutes in "houses with high verandahs" in Bissau city.[15]

I told her that the various serological studies contained in the HIV/AIDS Surveillance Database suggested that more than 5 percent of Guinea-Bissan adults were infected in seventeen different places, both urban and rural, located in six of the country's eight regions.[16] Anne-Grethe Poulsen was skeptical, observing that "the Portuguese did [HIV] studies all over the country in a very unscientific way." They had employed no epidemiological techniques, she claimed; they had merely rounded people up and taken their blood.

Then we got on to the subject of the high seroprevalence of elderly people in Guinea-Bissau. Poulsen and her colleagues had recently produced a report about a group of nearly four hundred people aged 50 and over living in Bissau city.[17] Nearly 20 percent of the people aged between 50 and 60 were HIV-2-positive, as were 12.4 percent of those aged 60 to 70, and 8.7 percent of those aged 70 to 80. No HIV-2-positivity was detected in eleven subjects aged over 80. The overall positivity in the over-50 group was slightly higher for women than men.

A previous seroepidemiological study, which she and colleagues had carried out on more than thirteen hundred persons of all ages living in three suburbs of the city of Bissau had detected less than 1 percent prevalence for the age-bands up to 25, rising suddenly to 7.5 percent among 25- to 30-year-olds, 14.7 percent among 30- to 40-year-olds, and plateauing at around 20 percent among those aged between 40 and 60.[18] This plateau, she said, indicated either that old people were surviving with HIV-2, or that a roughly equal number of people were getting infected and dying (thus removing themselves from the study population). The latter scenario seemed unlikely, given that one would expect sexual transmission at least to decline with increasing age.

She thought that most of the HIV-2 transmission was occurring among those in their thirties, with forty years representing the age of greatest risk. As for perinatal transmission, from mother to baby, they had not detected a single case of infantile AIDS, and only four of more than six hundred children aged one to fourteen whom they had tested were HIV-2-infected — with the histories indicating that some may have been infected through transfusions.

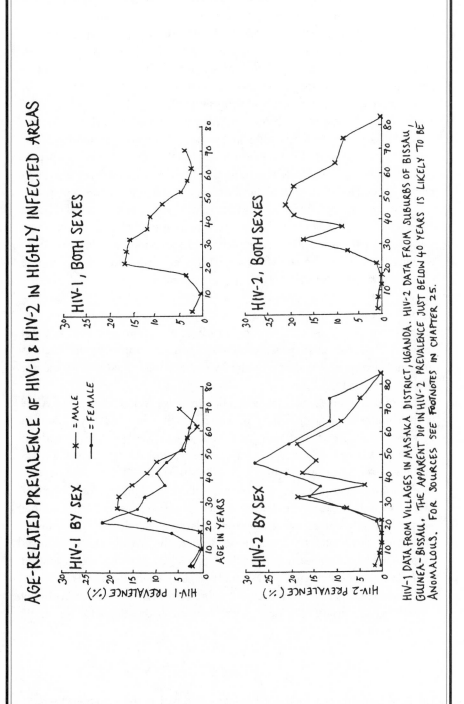

## AGE-RELATED PREVALENCE OF HIV-1 & HIV-2 IN HIGHLY INFECTED AREAS

HIV-1 BY SEX

— ✳ = MALE
—•— = FEMALE

HIV-1 PREVALENCE (%)

AGE IN YEARS

HIV-1, BOTH SEXES

HIV-2 BY SEX

HIV-2 PREVALENCE (%)

HIV-2, BOTH SEXES

HIV-1 DATA FROM VILLAGES IN MASAKA DISTRICT, UGANDA. HIV-2 DATA FROM SUBURBS OF BISSAU, GUINEA-BISSAU. THE APPARENT DIP IN HIV-2 PREVALENCE JUST BELOW 40 YEARS IS LIKELY TO BE ANOMALOUS. FOR SOURCES SEE FOOTNOTES IN CHAPTER 25.

However, she added, researchers working in Banjul in the Gambia, just north of Guinea-Bissau, had apparently come across eight pediatric cases.

The Guinea-Bissan HIV-2-prevalence figures were considerably higher than those for any other population group tested anywhere in the world, and I asked Dr. Poulsen what she made of them. She said that when she and her colleagues first gathered the data, they began thinking that HIV-2 must be much less pathogenic than HIV-1, and not especially transmissible — that it typically required a lot of potential exposures before someone became infected. But then they realized that they were seeing old people who had probably been infected for decades, and who were still quite healthy, and that it was only younger people (mostly in their thirties, forties, and fifties) who were actually dying of HIV-2-related AIDS. The youngest case they had come across, she said, was a man who had died at age twenty-five. They began to think that there were several versions of the virus, some of which were of very low pathogenicity, but others of which caused a fatal disease, sometimes only a few years after infection. She wondered whether the original crossover had involved a less pathogenic virus, but one which had since passed sexually through many humans and started to cause disease. She noted that life in Guinea-Bissau had changed in the last few decades — that nowadays the young moved around after dark in the capital, behavior that would not have been allowed in olden days and that was still frowned on even today in rural areas. Basically, she was proposing that changes in human sexual behavior had caused the virus to change its nature, and become more dangerous to its host.

Dr. Poulsen pointed out that even today, there was still relatively little AIDS in the country. Most people, she said, had not even seen an AIDS patient, and very few Guinea-Bissans believed that the disease really existed. She pointed out that it was debatable whether doctors would have noticed HIV-2-related AIDS had it not been for the model provided by HIV-1-related AIDS, and the fact that from 1985 onward, medical people were specifically looking out for a "new disease." She added that the predominant feeling, even in Bissau itself, was that people had only started dying of chronic diarrhea and similar symptoms in about 1987. From what I had read, it seemed that the first Guinea-Bissan cases might have begun appearing sporadically some ten years earlier, in around 1978.[19] But whenever these first cases had occurred, Dr. Poulsen reiterated once again her belief that HIV-2 was an older virus than HIV-1, one that had only recently become visible in epidemic form, probably because it had only recently become pathogenic.

---

During the months that followed, I spent a lot more time trying to track the early history of HIV-2. I followed up on the earliest recorded cases of HIV-2-related

## HIV-2/SIV PHYLOGENETIC TREE,
## SHOWING FIVE SUBTYPES OF HIV-2

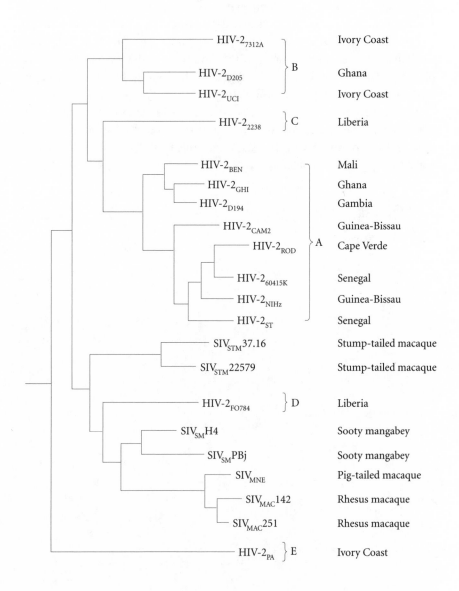

| | |
|---|---|
| HIV-2₇₃₁₂ₐ — B | Ivory Coast |
| HIV-2_D205 | Ghana |
| HIV-2_UCI | Ivory Coast |
| HIV-2₂₂₃₈ — C | Liberia |
| HIV-2_BEN | Mali |
| HIV-2_GHI | Ghana |
| HIV-2_D194 | Gambia |
| HIV-2_CAM2 | Guinea-Bissau |
| HIV-2_ROD — A | Cape Verde |
| HIV-2₆₀₄₁₅ₖ | Senegal |
| HIV-2_NIHz | Guinea-Bissau |
| HIV-2_ST | Senegal |
| SIV_STM37.16 | Stump-tailed macaque |
| SIV_STM22579 | Stump-tailed macaque |
| HIV-2_FO784 — D | Liberia |
| SIV_SM H4 | Sooty mangabey |
| SIV_SM PBj | Sooty mangabey |
| SIV_MNE | Pig-tailed macaque |
| SIV_MAC142 | Rhesus macaque |
| SIV_MAC251 | Rhesus macaque |
| HIV-2_PA — E | Ivory Coast |

SOURCES: F. Gao et al., "Genetic Diversity of Human Immunodeficiency Virus Type 2: Evidence for Distinct Sequence Subtypes with Differences in Virus Biology," *Journal of Virology,* 1994, 68(11), 7433–7447. Not to scale. The right-hand column shows the country of origin of each HIV-2 sample and the species of monkey from which each SIV strain was isolated.

AIDS, which had occurred in the 1970s, and the majority of which seemed to involve Portuguese soldiers who had served in Guinea-Bissau (or Portuguese Guinea, as it was formerly called) during the 1960s. I followed up on the history of that war, and of the other campaigns — vaccination campaigns — that the Portuguese had conducted. I investigated the vaccinations that had been carried out elsewhere in West Africa, notably those against yellow fever, measles, and smallpox. I researched the history of the slave trade in the region, and the role played by Portugal and former Portuguese colonies, like Brazil. And I began studying West African primate populations.

Eventually, I discovered that there were certain strange anomalies in the data. Once again, it seemed, the classic theory of natural transfer was not enough, at least by itself, to explain why the HIV-2 epidemic had started. These anomalies will be analyzed further, later in this book.

# 26

PAUL OSTERRIETH

AND FRITZ DEINHARDT

Dr. Paul Osterrieth was not one of the authors of the original *British Medical Journal* paper on the Congo and Ruzizi vaccinations,[1] but I was gradually coming to realize that he was one of the key participants in the various research projects that had been conducted at the chimpanzee camp at Lindi. He was co-author on five such papers, including the manuscript that was referred to as being "in preparation" in the polio articles by Koprowski and Courtois — the one that had never appeared.[2]

One of these five papers involved attempts to transmit hepatitis to chimpanzees,[3] and contained an intriguing piece of information. A single paragraph toward the end of the paper revealed that six shipments of chimpanzee kidneys had been sent by air from Stanleyville to a research team based at the Children's Hospital of Philadelphia (CHOP). Upon arrival, the kidneys had been made into tissue cultures. Five of the six shipments produced viable cultures, which appeared not to be contaminated with either foamy agents or other latent viruses. These tissue cultures were then used, it seems, in unsuccessful attempts to grow infectious hepatitis virus — *in vitro* experiments, following the *in vivo* research that had previously been conducted on the chimps at Lindi. The lead author on this paper was a German doctor, Friedrich Deinhardt.

I had managed to locate only three references to chimpanzee kidney tissue cultures in the entire medical literature, and this was one of them. The inference was obvious. If tissue cultures originating from the kidneys of the Lindi chimps had been successfully grown in Philadelphia and used for hepatitis experiments, perhaps they had also been used for other research in the same city — research by Hilary Koprowski and his colleagues at the Wistar Institute, relating to their development of polio vaccines.

I had traveled overnight on the train from Prague, and Dr. Osterrieth — a tall, rather handsome fair-haired man in his sixties — met me at his small local station in southeastern Belgium. We drove up to his farmhouse, situated on the top of a ridge looking out over the rolling hills of the Ardennes, where his wife, Odette, had already prepared a sumptuous breakfast of various breads, meats, and cheeses. As the coffee bubbled in the percolator, I explained in greater detail just why I was so interested in his Belgian Congo work, including the experiments on polio. One of them — Odette, I think — mentioned the controversy in the medical press about CHAT and the AIDS epidemic, and inquired whether I was going to be asking questions about that. I confirmed that I would be, and added that if the hypothesis was false, then it was surely vital that the relevant evidence should be produced to prove just why it was false.

After breakfast, Paul Osterrieth led me through into the lounge and we began the formal interview. He started by telling me his history in the Congo. He had arrived in 1954, spending his first two years working as a general practitioner at the hospital at Basoko, farther down the Congo River, and in October 1956 he was promoted to the microbiology section of the Laboratoire Médical de Stanleyville. Soon after this, he told me, he was awarded a WHO fellowship, which enabled him to spend four months in the United States, to get some virology training at the Centers for Disease Control satellite in Montgomery, Alabama. Ghislain Courtois had been keen for him to get more experience, so that he could head the virology department in the new lab, which was just then being built. His job, he said, had essentially been to hunt for insect-borne viruses like yellow fever and Chikungunya, and to search out new viruses. As an example of the importance of the latter work, he cited the outbreaks of the deadly Ebola virus in Sudan and the Congo in 1976. "What I want to stress with Ebola virus is that it is not unusual to get viruses from the wildlife [leading to] human epidemics."

He went on to tell me that an important part of his job was to find systems in which viruses could be tested. Sometimes they injected blood from patients into mice, but more often they used tissue cultures in order to grow and examine the viruses or bacteria. When I asked which tissue cultures, he told me monkey kidney, and also HeLa, but seemed unwilling to provide further details. I asked him which types of monkey had provided the kidneys and, again after a lengthy pause, he replied that he couldn't remember. I pressed him, asking if it would have been African green monkeys or chimpanzees . . . and he immediately replied: "No, no, not chimpanzees." So I asked him which were the commonest monkeys around Stanleyville, to which he answered "*Cynocephalus,* baboon." This surprised me, for I knew that baboons were mainly found in the open savanna regions, and the nearest savanna region to Stanleyville was in

Uele region, at least three hundred miles to the north. I let it pass, however, and presently Dr. Osterrieth added that "We were not making a lot of tissue culture, just a little."

I next asked him to tell me about the polio vaccinations, and he pointed out that it was Courtois who had been more closely linked with the chimpanzee camp and the polio work. He went on to say that he used to inspect Lindi camp from time to time when Courtois was not available, and that the only vaccinations with which he had lent a hand had been those in Stanleyville itself, where he and a nurse had fed the vaccine at one of the dispensaries. "In my memory, it's a very short episode. We worked a lot on the chimps, and then it was decided to begin the vaccination, and very quickly it was stopped." He gave two reasons for this. The first was that when Koprowski began vaccinating in Poland, the Stanleyville vaccine was transferred there. The second reason was that the Congo was not an ideal population in which to study vaccination: most Africans already had antibodies to polioviruses, and antibody detection in vaccinees was often hampered by interference from other viruses. He said that his recollection was "that Koprowski wanted very badly to test the vaccines . . . as quickly as possible . . . because there was some sort of competition between himself and Sabin. [He] got an opportunity to do it in Stanleyville, but as soon as he got [a more] suitable population, he switched."

I was again surprised by one aspect of what Paul Osterrieth was telling me, for I was almost certain that the pools of CHAT vaccine used in Stanleyville and in Poland had *not* been the same. Even pool 13, which had been used for the vaccinations in Leopoldville, had been fed to fewer than three thousand individuals in Poland,[4] so it seemed unlikely that any CHAT vaccine had actually been transferred there from the Congo. I said nothing, but wondered whether Osterrieth's comment was linked to the fact that no cases of AIDS had been seen in Poland before the mid-eighties, and to an understandable desire to prove the safety of the African CHAT pools by association.

I asked what specific work had been done with the chimps, but Osterrieth's memories of this proved to be patchy. He recalled only that he had taken blood from chimps at various times, that they had vaccinated some of them and then later challenged them with wild virus mixed with cream, so that it was not destroyed too quickly by the gastric juices. For these experiments, the scientists would transfer the chimp from its normal wooden cage into another cage containing a movable iron grille, which allowed the animal to be forced forward and immobilized.

Later, Dr. Osterrieth fetched his photo albums, and as we began to look through the pictures from the Congo period, his memories started flowing more freely. There were pictures of the Wagenia fishermen on the rapids just above Stanleyville, and of elegant colonial houses on tree-lined streets. Osterrieth explained how Stanleyville had "developed fantastically" in the years between

1957 and 1960. Economically, he said, it was a very important place, acting as an entrepôt between the river and the rain forest road system. One of the leading employers was OTRACO, L'Office de Transport Congolaise, which operated the huge river barges and ferries plying between Stan and Leo, a thousand miles downstream, and there were also large offices for the companies and parastatals dealing with cotton, wood, coffee, and mining.

As regards air transport (significant, of course, both for humans and for human viruses), there were several internal Sabena flights a day, notably to Leopoldville, Elisabethville, Bukavu, and Usumbura, and by the late fifties there were six semidirect Sabena flights a week between Stanleyville and Brussels, which called variously at Khartoum, Cairo, Tripoli, Athens, and Rome. Osterrieth said that the crews would change around at Stanleyville, where there was a famously comfortable Sabena guest house. A private company, Sobelair, also operated a Johannesburg–Stanleyville–Juba/Khartoum–Cyprus–Brussels flight, with a one- or two-day stopover in Cyprus for the crews.

Dr. Osterrieth also had pictures of the chimp camp — of the doctors, the African workers, of Norton taking blood from a chimp, and of another chimp in chains, sitting on top of her cage. Slowly, he began to recall the names of some of those who had worked at Lindi — such as Daenens, the bald Belgian who had been in day-to-day charge, and Rollais, the French hunter who had headed the capturing team. He recalled the small hand-drawn car ferry across the river Lindi just above the point where it entered the Congo from the north, a mile or so before one arrived at the camp. He also recalled that some of the chimps had names, and were allowed to move around the camp more as pets than as experimental animals. There was Djamba (literally "the bush"), who would wash his hands with soap, just like the scientists, but who liked to eat it afterward. And there was Marie-Paulin, who always shook hands with visitors; the only exception being King Leopold, on whom she turned her back with considerable hauteur.

When I asked how many chimps had been used in the research, he replied "There was a turnover." Did he mean that they had forwarded some of the animals elsewhere? No, he replied, but sometimes some of them died. I pressed further. Osterrieth said there had been a big problem with pneumonia, an epidemic more or less, and one of the germs involved had been *Klebsiella*. They were unable to determine if the deaths had been caused by the *Klebsiella* bacterium alone, or because a primary virus had allowed the *Klebsiella* to prosper as a secondary invader. He was unable to give even an approximate idea of the number of chimps that had died as a result, but I later discovered that he had written a paper on the subject in mid-1958, which reported the analysis of 142 different strains of the bacterium.[5] There was no precise numerical breakdown, though the isolates were said to have come mainly from patients suffering urinary infections and fatal pneumonias at Stanleyville hospital, but also from chimpanzees and small laboratory animals.

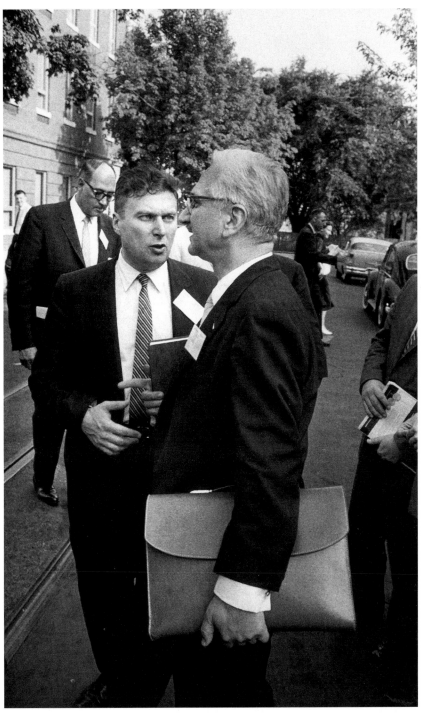

Hilary Koprowski and Albert Sabin in conversation at the
First International Conference on Live Poliovirus Vaccines,
Washington, D.C., June 1959. *(Credit: R. Phillips)*

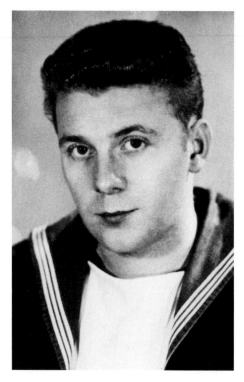

David Carr, the "Manchester sailor," in Royal Navy uniform, circa 1957. *(Credit: M. Carr)*

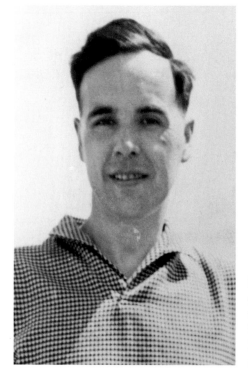

Dr. Trevor Stretton, circa 1960. The previous year, Stretton was senior house officer on Ward M4 at the Manchester Royal Infirmary, where he helped to look after David Carr during his final months. *(Credit: T. Stretton)*

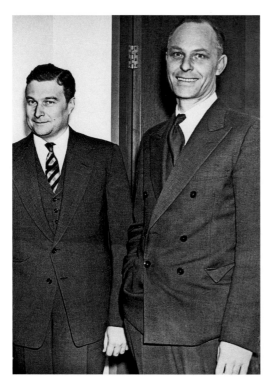

Hilary Koprowski and George
Dick in Belfast, 1956.
*(Credit: B. Dick)*

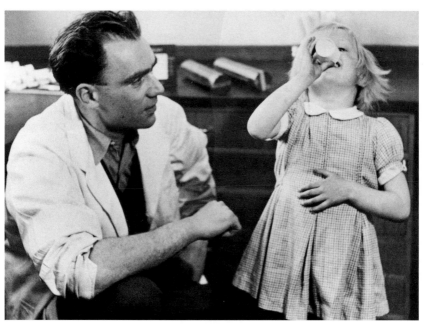

David Dane pictured feeding George Dick's daughter with
Koprowski's first Type 1 polio vaccine, SM, in 1956.
*(Credit: B. Dick)*

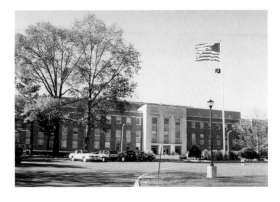

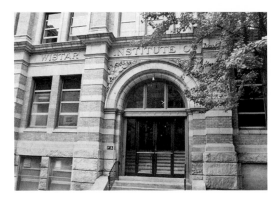

Lederle Laboratories, Pearl River, New York, 1993. *(Credit: E. Hooper)*

The Wistar Institute, Philadelphia, 1993. *(Credit: E. Hooper)*

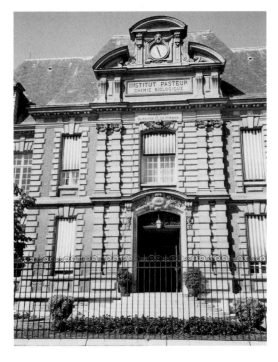

The Pasteur Institute, Paris, 1997. *(Credit: E. Hooper)*

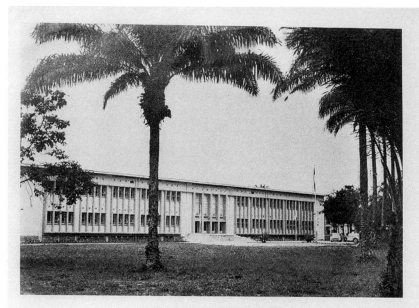

Stanleyville. — Laboratoires.

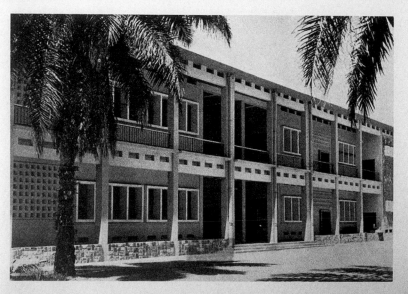

Stanleyville. — Animaliers.

The new medical laboratories (including the virus labs),
and the animal house at Stanleyville, Belgian Congo, 1957.
*(Credit: Prins Leopold Instituut voor Tropische Geneeskunde, Antwerp,
Belgium; photo published in* Annales de la Societé Belge de Médicine
Tropicale, *1958, 38, 240)*

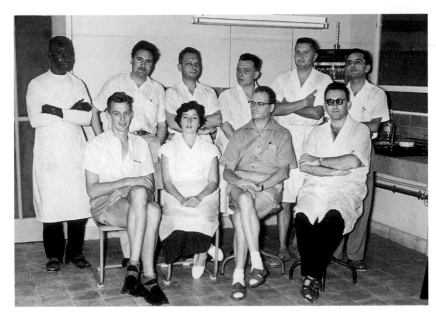

Staff of Stanleyville Medical Laboratory in mid-1958. BACK ROW: unknown African assistant, M. Hendrickx, Dr. Ninane, M. Brakel, M. Doupagne, M. Poffe. FRONT ROW: Dr. Osterrieth, Mme. Dherte, Professor Welsch (sabbatical visitor), Professor Vandepitte. Doctors Courtois and Mangen, and Mme. Liegeois are absent, perhaps on leave. *(Credit: J. Brakel)*

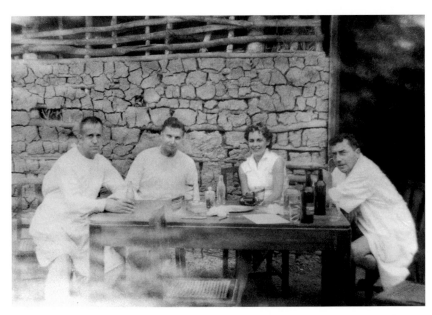

Norton, Koprowski, Sabena stewardess, Courtois, pictured at Camp Lindi, 1957. *(Credit: Gail N. R.)*

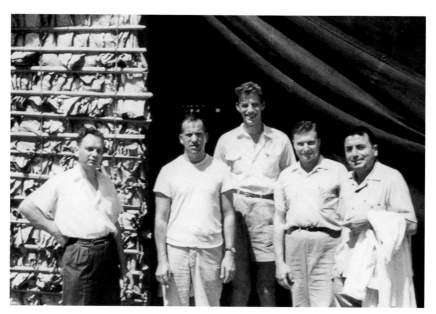

Gaston Ninane, Tom Norton, Paul Osterrieth, Hilary Koprowski, Ghislain Courtois. The Belgian-American team of chimp researchers outside one of the hangars at Camp Lindi, 1957. *(Credit: Gail N. R.)*

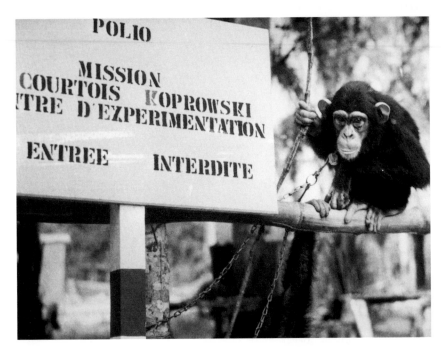

Djamba and Camp Lindi sign. *(Credit: G. Rollais)*

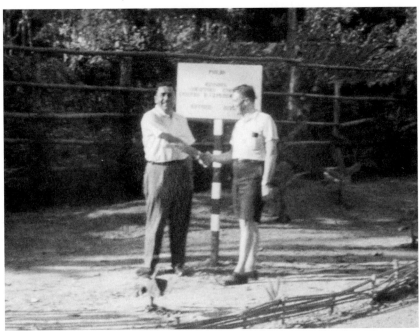

Hilary Koprowski and Ghislain Courtois shaking
hands at Lindi, 1957. *(Credit: Gail N. R.)*

The fact that both humans and chimps were dying from *Klebsiella* infections in Stanleyville in 1957/8 was remarkable information, for *Klebsiella pneumoniae* is one of the classic opportunistic infections of AIDS.

---

Later, Osterrieth told me about Tom Norton, Koprowski's technician, with whom he had clearly got on very well. He recalled an evening in which scientists from several nations had been dining together: Belgians, Spaniards, and Americans (including Koprowski with his heavy Polish accent), and Norton had announced that he might not be fluent in other tongues, but that he understood English in every language! Osterrieth said that the laboratory technician had been "elegant" in comparison to his boss, who went in for more flamboyant attire, including a notorious ensemble of a "very funny" black-and-white shirt and long black shorts, which were too tight for his rather generous waistline. He described Koprowski as being "very bright, very dynamic," but it was clear that he had liked him much less than his assistant. Later, over lunch, Odette Osterrieth confided that Koprowski had been "very sure of himself, very bossy ... very much a *patron.*" Her husband thought that Koprowski had visited Stanleyville several times, but Odette recalled that she had seen Koprowski there only twice — the first time in early 1957, when he had arrived with Tom Norton, and the second in October 1957, when he had spoken in halting French at the symposium on viral diseases, which was held to coincide with the opening of the newly built laboratory and animal house. Both of them agreed that although Norton had visited Stanleyville only the once, he had stayed on for several weeks after Koprowski left.

Osterrieth's visit to America, between October 1957 and January 1958, was mentioned on several occasions. It soon became clear that as well as working in Montgomery, Alabama, he had spent some time in Philadelphia, where he had first met Friedrich Deinhardt and his bosses at the Children's Hospital, Werner and Gertrude Henle. He revealed that during this visit he had stayed at the Wistar Institute, Koprowski having expressly asked Courtois that his assistant should spend some time working there, because of the polio work. Osterrieth added that he had received training in tissue culture techniques.

Later, he said he had had "a very funny time at that lab, because I never knew exactly why I was there." Altogether, Osterrieth said, he had not spent long at the Wistar, "maybe one or two weeks," and he saw very little of Koprowski during this period, although on one occasion the two of them did travel together on a train up to New York. All this did indeed seem rather strange, given Koprowski's previous insistence that Osterrieth should be trained at the Wistar.

Eventually, I asked Osterrieth the key question — whether or not he had sent chimpanzee kidneys to Philadelphia as part of the hepatitis studies. There was a long pause, and he didn't answer. I pointed out that this fact had been mentioned in Deinhardt's paper, and he began laughing. "Then I did," he said, holding up his hands, "yes, I think I did." I asked him how they had been sent, and he said that he didn't remember well, but that they must have been cut into tiny pieces and put into nutrient solution. Then he changed the subject, and began telling me about the time that he had shipped a pair of owl-faced monkeys to America, and how they had arrived in perfect health.

I steered him back to chimp kidneys, and asked how many such shipments had been sent; he replied that it was "not many." "We were sending a lot of things all around," he added. "Since we had the chimpanzees, we were bleeding them also for blood group studies, and sending the blood to Liège." (The paper in question showed that a total of 175 chimp sera had been sent to Belgium in a single shipment.)[6] The sera had been sent in small containers, other materials had been sent in thermos flasks, and he eventually confirmed that the chimpanzee kidneys had been dispatched in large metal flasks, hinged at the top, roughly eight inches in diameter and sixteen inches high. The minced-up kidneys had been packed around with ice, the hinges were forced home to keep the whole flask airtight, and a screw valve allowed the air to escape as it warmed and expanded. These flasks were dispatched on a plane to Brussels, and then on to Philadelphia where (as reported in the hepatitis paper) they were opened three to six days later, and found to contain viable chimpanzee kidney tissue.

I told him I really wished that I could still speak with Tom Norton, to find out which kidneys had been used to make the tissue culture for the polio vaccines. He said that at that time there had been only two types of culture — HeLa and MKTC, the latter made first from rhesus macaques and later from African green monkeys. I told him that AGM kidneys had not been used until the early sixties, but pointed out that Pierre Lépine had used the baboon for his tissue culture work at the Pasteur Institute. "I would say that if Pierre Lépine would use it [baboon tissue], it's probably likely we did," he responded. "It was easier and less costly to get baboon [locally] than to get rhesus from India." I asked why not use chimpanzee kidneys, if they were available and were being exported to Philadelphia at that very time. "No, certainly not," was the response. I asked why not. "Because . . . I think . . . if I remember, I think the few kidneys that were sent . . . were sent to Deinhardt" at the Children's Hospital of Philadelphia. "I don't know, but my impression is that there were not many close contacts between the two labs," he added; "Fritz was working with Henle, but not at all with Koprowski."

I also asked Osterrieth about the promised paper about the polio work on the Lindi chimps, which had been referred to by Courtois and Koprowski in their polio articles, and he said that he thought it had never been published, but that I could try contacting André Courtois, Ghislain's son, who still held many of his father's papers. Once again, one of the supposed coauthors on this "manuscript in preparation" was confirming my suspicion that no such paper had ever appeared — a state of affairs that clearly left a huge gap in the published information about Koprowski's polio work in the Congo.

Later, I asked about how they had actually obtained the kidneys for the hepatitis studies: had he and his colleagues perhaps removed single kidneys from different chimps? "Certainly not," he replied. Well, had they killed them especially for their kidneys then? To this, Osterrieth sighed a sigh. Were they the kidneys of dead chimps then, perhaps brought back by the hunter, for I had heard that sometimes adult animals had to be killed in order to capture the young?[7] "No, no, no, no, no. They were from the camp," Osterrieth answered, but did not provide any further information. It sounded quite possible that the animals in question *had* been sacrificed for their kidneys.

I returned to the question of quantities, and this time Osterrieth acknowledged the figures in the original paper, saying that yes, they must have sent five or six shipments, and that each shipment would have comprised "not more than two kidneys. . . . It's a lot; for tissue culture it's already a lot." He went on to say that after trypsinizing (further breaking down the tissue by addition of an enzyme), a few of the cells could be used to seed new cultures in hundreds of roller tubes, each of which would produce a continuous monolayer of new cells within two or three days. I pointed out that, according to a recent interviewee at the WHO, one normal pair of monkey kidneys could produce between fifty thousand and a million doses of polio vaccine, and that a chimp kidney would certainly be larger than that of a normal monkey.[8] "I'm almost sure that the kidneys from the chimpanzee were not used for vaccine production," he commented, before reiterating that "I don't think that there was a close cooperation at all between the two labs" in Philadelphia where the hepatitis and polio research had been conducted.

This time, I pointed out that as far as I knew, this was not correct. Joseph Stokes Jr., the Quaker doctor who was head of the pediatric department at (and later director of) the Children's Hospital, had been a major collaborator and coauthor on Koprowski's polio vaccine studies in New Jersey between 1956 and 1958: those at Clinton Farms (the women's prison), Woodbine (a home for mentally handicapped children), and Moorestown (an affluent community just across the river from Philadelphia).[9] Furthermore, the virologist Klaus Hummeler who, like Deinhardt, was then a research fellow in the Henles' lab, collaborated with Koprowski on two of his Clinton papers and on the key report of the Congo trials in the *British Medical Journal.* In the latter, he had been thanked at the end for his "valuable help in the testing programme."[10] Since the first of these coauthored papers was read at a conference in May 1956,[11] exactly a year before Koprowski moved from Lederle to the Wistar, it was clear that Koprowski had been collaborating on polio studies with Stokes and Hummeler from the Children's Hospital for a considerable time before he joined them in Philadelphia.

Toward the end of the afternoon, Paul Osterrieth and I both relaxed. I sensed that had he chosen to do so, he could have provided more information on certain issues (such as his U.S. visit in 1957, the tissue culture work at Stanleyville, and the Lindi chimpanzee research), but knew that — for all the gaps — he had still told me a great deal. Furthermore, he and his wife had been inordinately kind, keeping me fed and watered throughout the day, and sharing such personal items as photo albums and home movies. One of these latter was especially interesting, showing Koprowski, Norton, and Courtois strolling around outside the mud walls of one of the chimp hangars at *Mission Koprowski*, together with Ninane, Daenens, and Djamba the chimp. It was while we were watching this that Paul Osterrieth told me the tragic story of his son. In 1957, in Stanleyville, he had fallen ill with a fever, and although they thought he had recovered, he later developed a persistent autoimmune disease. He died in 1968, in his early teens, in the middle of a kidney transplant. I did not ask whether the boy was ever fed CHAT vaccine. Osterrieth himself was fed CHAT, so it is possible that others in his family were fed also.

Later, I outlined the CHAT/AIDS theory, and while Osterrieth listened with an open mind, he finally raised three counterarguments. He conceded that most tissue cultures did contain lymphocytes, but felt that the chance of their surviving through to the final vaccine was small, and that it was therefore unlikely that SIV could have survived either. Second, he reckoned that the risk of an SIV infecting someone by mouth via an oral vaccine (as compared to through the skin, by means of an injected vaccine) was minimal. I gave the examples of gay men who practiced only oral sex contracting HIV from a partner, and of babies becoming infected from breast milk, as two instances which disproved his hypothesis. All right, he said, but he doubted that even as many as 2,000 people had received the vaccine in the Congo. I answered that it was actually more than 300,000, meaning that if just one in 25,000 persons was vulnerable to infection by the oral route, then a hypothetical SIV contaminant could have been transferred to a dozen humans in the course of the vaccinations — enough, I suspected, to kick-start the epidemic. In response, he conceded that such a scenario was "not ridiculous."

In the early evening, just before driving me back to the station, Paul Osterrieth sat me down in the lounge and gave me a pep talk. "If the conclusion of your book is going to be that CHAT vaccination is involved in the origin of AIDS," he told me, "then it's a political time bomb." I told him that I hadn't come to any conclusions yet, but added that I had not yet come across a convincing argument to disprove the theory. "On the principle, I agree," he continued, "but not on the details. I think there is no need for CHAT to be involved.

And there is no evidence — I mean hard facts. The only good way would be to prove that there is a virus in CHAT vaccine. All the rest is coincidental, and is very dangerous."

Why was that, I asked. "Well," he explained, "if you publish a book that shows a lot of coincidence, it will make a lot of noise, it will be heavily attacked by scientists, and it will be used by African politicians to extract money from Western governments and will encourage them in the very, very bad feeling that their misfortune can be laid at our door, and in the feeling that all their wrongs can be solved by our money and not by their own efforts. I would say," he concluded, "that if you're not 100 percent sure, don't publish."

We parted twelve hours after we had met, back on the railway platform, and I assured Dr. Osterrieth that I would bear his warning in mind.

---

When I reviewed the day's discussions, I was once again struck by the extraordinary fact that not one of the participants in the vaccine research and trials could recall which tissue culture had been used to make the vaccine. Osterrieth had eventually said that they had probably been using baboon kidneys to make tissue culture in the Stanleyville virus lab, since they were cheap and available — but he was unable to say for certain. There was, however, another species of simian kidney that was cheap and locally available in Stanleyville, and this was the same species of kidney that was being flown, at this very time, halfway around the world to Philadelphia — in order to make tissue cultures.

I also thought further about Paul Osterrieth's attempt to persuade me not to publish unless I was "100 percent sure" of the facts. It seemed to me that as long as the Wistar failed to release its vaccine samples for testing, and as long as Koprowski resorted to the law in response to attempts to investigate the hypothesis, then one was left with little alternative but to amass as much evidence as possible, and then publish — in the hope that other witnesses from the fifties would thereby be persuaded to make their own contributions to the debate. As it was, the historical evidence already provided a highly plausible scenario for how a vaccine such as CHAT might have become contaminated.

I was also bothered by Osterrieth's insistence that there were no close links between the Wistar Institute and the Children's Hospital of Philadelphia, (CHOP), where the six shipments of chimpanzee kidneys had been converted into tissue culture. By contrast, Sven Gard had told me that the two labs were closely affiliated, and this was further confirmed a fortnight later, when I arrived in Munich to visit Professor Jean Deinhardt, Friedrich Deinhardt's English widow.

She explained that she and her husband had met in 1959, when she was working on inbred rats at the Wistar, and he was in the virus lab at CHOP.

Hilary Koprowski acted as matchmaker, and it was a whirlwind romance, with the wedding following just three months later. Her husband, whom she called Fritz, had died only recently — in April 1992.

She went on to provide some detailed background to the hepatitis research. There was a close-knit medical community in Philadelphia, she told me, and Hilary (whom she rated "a very good virologist") was friendly with Gertrude and Werner Henle, who had set up one of the first virology departments in America at CHOP, staffed by talented research fellows such as Fritz and Klaus Hummeler. There was a great deal of interchange between the two institutions, she told me, with collaborative studies, the sharing of equipment, and the staging of open seminars, attended by staff from each. "People spent a lot of time in each other's laboratories learning techniques and so on," she added. Both the Henles' department and Hilary's institute were geared toward pure research, and all three of them plus Deinhardt and Hummeler were, in addition, professors at the University of Pennsylvania just up the road. In all likelihood Hilary would have talked about his chimp camp at Lindi, which had been deliberately sited "outside civilization" so that the chimps used in the polio studies were less likely to be infected with human viruses. The idea of inoculating these same chimps with the stools of human hepatitis carriers probably first came about at one of the joint seminars, she said.

Since Fritz was still a bachelor, he was the member of the Henles' team best able to take off to Africa for a few months. Jean Deinhardt told me that he assembled a boxful of fecal specimens from Willowbrook, a home for handicapped kids on Staten Island, where children had been experimentally exposed to hepatitis,[12] and that he flew out to the Congo early in 1958. (It subsequently emerged that he set off in late January, and returned at the end of April.)[13] He booked two seats: one for himself, and one for the "box of shit."

The work was highly experimental. There was at that time no means of testing for the presence of hepatitis virus, so Deinhardt was using fecal material that he hoped would contain the virus, and inoculating it into creatures that he hoped would be susceptible. The only way to establish whether or not the chimps actually were infected was to make carefully recorded clinical observations, and to run weekly or biweekly liver function tests. In the course of three months, Fritz Deinhardt staged experiments involving a total of thirty chimps, five of which died in the process. Another seventeen were used in two further experiments conducted after his departure. Jean Deinhardt commented that the work was "theoretically very interesting," but that the results were inconclusive, even if, in retrospect, human hepatitis almost certainly was transmitted to the animals.[14]

She also said that although chimps were too strong and vigorous to make good lab animals, you could get a lot of materials from a chimp — such as blood and stools. I asked her about the use of chimpanzee kidneys for tissue cultures, and after an initial hesitation, she acknowledged that some had probably been sent back. "I don't think that they cared very much about conservation considerations in those days — there were no ideas about what the population sizes were," she added. She spoke of this time, the late fifties, as being the Gold Rush period of virology, when scientists were "trying out lots of tissues in the lab . . . looking for susceptibility. If you could [find] a tissue culture which was susceptible to a virus, you could study *in vitro*, rather than *in vivo*. . . . After Fritz's return, the Belgian Congo started breaking up, so the use of the chimps had to stop."

Later, we discussed the OPV/AIDS theory, and she told me she herself had not followed it closely, but that in the opinion of people she knew and respected, the hypothesis was very unlikely. She was, however, consummately fair in her analysis, and many of her subsequent comments ran counter to this conclusion. She said that she doubted that an SIV could survive the various preparation stages of a vaccine, but then conceded that a lentivirus "would be the most likely [virus] to have slipped through and remained undetected" by the safety tests of the day. Furthermore, she felt that the mouth was a very easy place for viral infection to occur. She added that the case of the Manchester sailor constituted "no evidence at all" against the hypothesis, and that the eight-page publication by the Wistar committee sounded like little more than a pre-liminary report. Presumably, if the Wistar was going to have the vaccine sample examined at the CDC and elsewhere, a fuller report would appear in due course.

Furthermore, she stressed that "it is *very important* [which] monkey kidneys were being used. . . . As a zoologist, it has always shocked me how sloppy labo-ratory scientists have been in the past with the definition of their materials, when they obtain them from species like nonhuman primates. . . . Even today, you see papers which are published which say 'monkey kidney' instead of 'rhe-sus monkey kidney' or whatever." I asked whether, since the chimp kidneys had been brought all the way from Africa to Philadelphia, any of the virologists would have tried growing poliovirus in them. "It would have been logical to try that," she answered, "and there would have been no contraindication to doing it." She confirmed that chimpanzees would probably have been sacrificed espe-cially to provide the kidneys, and that it was unlikely that kidneys from "overtly unhealthy animals" would have been used. She was unable to tell me whether or not Fritz had sent the kidneys back himself, though later I was told by Gertrude Henle that he had been responsible for sending some of the shipments, while reports prepared by the Henles for the Armed Forces Epidemiological Board, who sponsored the hepatitis research, made it clear that at least two shipments were not dispatched until the following year, 1959.[15]

Jean Deinhardt added that somewhere she had her late husband's photos, some old movies that had been transferred to video, his personal diary, and a lab book of his experiments — but that I would have to come back again if I wanted to see these. All in all, she had proved to be one of my frankest and most helpful informants — and she was to help still further. I told her how important it was that I got to interview Hilary Koprowski. Did she have any ideas about how best to approach him? She told me that he felt very threatened after the Curtis article but advised that if I showed an interest in the history of polio vaccine development, then he could hardly fail to grant me an interview. It proved to be excellent advice.

---

I also called once more on Gaston Ninane, who was as kind and helpful as ever. It was fortunate that I did so, for he had remembered some further details about the vaccinations in Ruanda-Urundi. He was now certain that after the end of the main Ruzizi Valley vaccination he had returned to Stanleyville, and that he later flew back to Usumbura, carrying more vaccine. It was then that, with another Belgian doctor, he completed the vaccination down the east side of Lake Tanganyika as far as Nyanza Lac. He also insisted that the vaccine used in this campaign had come from Leuven, and not Philadelphia, though he was unable to specify whether this applied to the whole campaign, or just the latter part of it. Since the *British Medical Journal* paper (which referred only to the Ruzizi Valley) had clearly stated that "the large pools representing each strain were prepared in the Laboratories of the Wistar Institute,"[16] it seemed possible that only the Lake Tanganyika part of the trial had used the Belgian version of the vaccine. Six months earlier, Ninane had told me that Koprowski had supplied Leuven with both the vaccine virus and the tissue culture cells in which to grow it, but now he said that he had no idea how the Belgian vaccine had been made — whether they had employed Koprowski's tissue cultures or their own.

Ninane told me that he had also vaccinated in Ruanda, along the eastern shore of Lake Kivu (to the north of Bukavu), though he could not recall the names of individual towns and villages. Apparently this vaccination was the only time he had visited this region, and he remembered it clearly for three reasons. The first was that Lake Kivu was unusual in African terms, for it had no crocs or hippos, so one could swim there in complete safety. The second revolved around the temperature gradient — in the small hotels where he stayed, they would serve locally produced strawberries after dinner, and yet they would eat them in front of a roaring log fire, because the nights were so cold. The third was his memory of clouds passing over the Virunga volcanoes, away to the north, and changing from white to red and back to white as they moved above the glowing craters. It was hard to estimate from how far away one could witness such a spectacle, but it suggested that he might have vaccinated around the northern end of the lake, perhaps around the present-day towns of Gisenyi and Kibuye.[17]

———————

I also interviewed Professor Jean Vandepitte — an especially interesting witness, in that he had appeared at various different times and places in the course of the events that I was researching. It was he who had helped Arno Motulsky collect the blood samples from around Leopoldville in early 1959 — including L70, which was still the earliest HIV-1-positive sample known.[18] It was he who had investigated and reported one of the first recognized cases of AIDS from the Congo — that of the Air Zaire secretary who had fallen sick in Belgium in 1977.[19] And it was he who had taken over as temporary director of the Laboratoire Médical de Stanleyville when Ghislain Courtois was on leave between late March and early September 1958, a period that had included the latter part of Fritz Deinhardt's visit and the end of the mass vaccination in Ruzizi and Ruanda-Urundi.

SEROLOGICAL EVIDENCE SUGGESTIVE OF HIV-1
INFECTION IN CONGO UP TO 1970

|    | Sex | Age | Date by which infected | Likely place of infection | Suggestive evidence | Died of AIDS? | Reference |
|----|-----|-----|------------------------|---------------------------|---------------------|---------------|-----------|
| 1  | m   | ?   | February–April 1959    | Leopoldville/ Kinshasa    | HIV+ serum          | n/a           | 1         |
| 2  | m   | 0   | 1967–1969 (if perinatally infected) | Yambuku      | Boy, aged 7 to 9, gave HIV+ serum in 1976 | 1985 | 2 |
| 3  | m   | 54  | 1968                   | Kikwit                    | Tested HIV+ in 1985, left Congo in 1968 | 1988 | 3 |
| 4  | f   | 37  | 1968                   | Kikwit                    | As above; wife of (3) | 1987        | 3         |
| 5  | f   | ?   | 1970                   | Kinshasa                  | HIV+ serum          | n/a           | 4         |
| 6  | f   | ?   | 1970                   | Kinshasa                  | HIV+ serum          | n/a           | 4         |

REFERENCES
1. *Lancet,* 1968, 1(ii), 1279–1280.
2. *N. Engl. J. Med.,* 1988, 318(5), 276–279.
3. *Scand. J. Infect. Dis.,* 1987, 19, 511–517.
4. 1st Int. Conf. AIDS Assoc. Cancers in Africa (Brussels, 1985), poster P12.

Vandepitte acknowledged that the Congo seemed to be the breeding ground for AIDS, and said that Congolese and Belgian doctors like himself had seen cases of unrelenting diarrhea and fatal cryptococcal meningitis from the country "many years before" the recognized epidemic. "I believe the first cases were already [occurring] in 1975," he went on. "By then, AIDS was already endemic on a massive scale. [It] coincided with a period of relaxation of traditional family mores."[20]

We spoke of the OPV/AIDS hypothesis, and he said that he himself had not been involved in any of the polio research, but that in any case he did not believe in the theory. However, when I asked whether there had been a Belgian version of CHAT made at Leuven, he answered that if such a vaccine had been made then it would have been the work of Professor De Somer, "who was very interested in live vaccine." De Somer, he explained, had headed the virology section at the university (being succeeded upon his death by Jan Desmyter), but had also worked at the Belgian vaccine house of RIT. It was RIT that had produced most of Belgium's inactivated vaccine at this time, but Vandepitte said that RIT might also have prepared some pools of OPV for De Somer during this period.

I was already scheduled to leave Belgium the following morning, but realized that I would need to make yet another visit, in order to follow up further on the Belgian vaccine.

---

On the way back to London at the end of the trip, I had arranged a one-day stopover in Paris, in order to interview Stanley Plotkin, Koprowski's former collaborator at the Wistar, who was now medical and scientific director of the vaccine house Pasteur Mérieux, and Luc Montagnier, the head of virology at the Pasteur Institute. I was disappointed to learn, just a couple of days before the meeting, that Plotkin would have to cancel. Nonetheless, I was pleased to be getting an hour with Montagnier, the discoverer of HIV-1 (and, many would say, the codiscoverer of HIV-2).

As it turned out, because he had to rush to catch a plane, the hour turned into rather less than half of that. I was shown into a huge, ornate room, and a few minutes later a public relations official came in, closely followed by Professor Montagnier, to whom I was then formally introduced. The niceties over, we sat down on a long sofa and began talking, and Montagnier proved himself to be reassuringly friendly and uninclined to stand on ceremony. I was impressed by his keen intelligence, his apparent lack of intellectual pride, and by his surprisingly open adoption of controversial positions.

In 1988, Montagnier had written an article in which he suggested that the beginnings of the two AIDS epidemics had come about as a result of changes in civilization during the last few decades, especially the seventies, and in which he identified "the massive use of blood transfusions, the trade of blood and blood products, an increased sexual promiscuity [and] intravenous drug abuse" as likely factors.[21] But now he told me that he had changed his mind, and that he currently believed that a more convincing explanation for the genesis of AIDS was provided by his "mycoplasmal co-factor" hypothesis. This proposed that HIV required the presence of a co-factor, such as a mycoplasma (one of the tiniest known microorganisms, smaller even than a virus), before it could cause AIDS. He felt that a crucial event might have been when the intensive use of antibiotics in the fifties, and in particular of tetracycline, led to the development of new, antibiotic-resistant strains of mycoplasma. According to this scenario, HIVs might have been present in man for a very long time before AIDS emerged. He proposed, for instance, that a harmless, nonpathogenic HIV-1 might have been endemic not just in Africa, but within small population groups in several parts of the world (such as on the east and west coasts of America, in India, and in Thailand), with the situation changing only when the new resistant strain of mycoplasma entered the equation, increasing the virulence of HIV-1 by a factor of several hundred, and sparking the epidemic emergence of AIDS in various different places. Similarly, he said, HIV-2 might have crossed harmlessly from mangabey to human countless times in the past, with HIV-2-related AIDS emerging only after the arrival of the mycoplasmal co-factor in West Africa.

When I asked him his views on the OPV/AIDS theory, Montagnier said that he had followed the situation carefully, and what different people like Koprowski had said about it, and he felt that since only tissues from macaques and African greens had been used for polio vaccine production, the theory was "very unlikely." I pointed out that Koprowski himself could not recall which species of monkey had been used, and Montagnier swiftly responded that it was "for sure not chimps. Chimpanzees were not used." I pointed out that chimps had been used extensively for testing the vaccine, and might somehow have contaminated the tissue culture, and Montagnier admitted that the chimp SIV was the only known monkey virus that *could* be the source of HIV-1. However, he proposed that a likelier explanation for the origin of AIDS was that SIVcpz and HIV-1 had diverged at the point of primate speciation (in other words about four million years ago, when chimpanzees and humans are thought to have evolved from a common ancestor). This, of course, tied in with his mycoplasma theory and the concept of small, ancient pockets of HIV infection scattered around the globe.

Montagnier did add one other important point, when he said that it would be wrong to believe that two cycles of freezing and rethawing (like those to which CHAT had apparently been subjected) would kill off any simian lentivirus in a vaccine preparation.[22] He said he thought this would reduce the titer of any simian contaminant, but would not kill it completely.

However impressed I was by Luc Montagnier as a man and as a scientist, I found that I was far from persuaded by either his mycoplasma theory, or by his proposal that chimp SIV and HIV-1 might have diverged some millions of years ago. As regards the former theory, all the available seroepidemiological evidence suggested that it was *HIV* (rather than Montagnier's posited antibiotic-resistant mycoplasma) that had not been present in places like the Belgian Congo prior to the fifties, North America prior to the mid-seventies, or in India and Thailand prior to the mid-eighties. With regard to the latter theory, most virologists and phylogeneticists were now confident that HIV-1 and SIVcpz had diverged between forty and seven hundred years ago. To propose a period of several million years required a dramatic resetting of the molecular clock.

———

Plotkin's cancellation meant that I had a few hours to spare in Paris, and I was lucky enough to get to see Simon Wain-Hobson who, despite his very English manner, had also developed the reputation of being the enfant terrible of the Pasteur's virology labs. It was he who had sequenced the first chimpanzee SIV isolate of Martine Peeters's group, three years earlier.[23] He proved to be much younger than I had expected, lean and fit, possessor of a full mustache and a certain "in-your-face" vibrancy in his manner of speaking.

A couple of months earlier, I had heard on the virology grapevine that, after the Wistar committee had delivered its report, committee member David Ho had contacted Gerald Corbitt at his lab in Manchester, and persuaded him to send some samples of the Manchester sailor's tissues for further testing. Corbitt and his technician, Andrew Bailey, had been having problems sequencing the virus through most of 1992.[24] The latest rumor was that Ho had come up with a sequence of a "typical yet unique" Euro-American isolate . . . whatever that meant.

My first question to Simon Wain-Hobson, therefore, was about the Manchester sailor sequence, and I quickly realized that here was no craven flunky, concerned not to say anything out of turn. Far from it, in fact. "It's like a normal North American or European isolate," he exclaimed. "It doesn't fit, doesn't make sense. I haven't seen the data, I've only heard about it . . . [but] the feeling is it's a little too close for comfort [to modern HIV strains]." Later, we turned to the 1969 "Robert R." isolate from St. Louis, which had first been reported as positive by ELISA and Western blot fully six years before, in 1987 — and Wain-Hobson was equally skeptical. "Why haven't we seen data?" he asked. "There's a simple thing: Robert R.'s been around [for several years] and we've not got any published [PCR] data. To me that smells, OK? It's as simple as that. . . . And I would say, in the age of PCR, even the Manchester seaman stuff smells. I could [ask] my student, give him a sample, and he could give me sequence data within probably two weeks. So don't mess around. Don't tell me I need three years. It doesn't make sense."

Next he spoke about the chimpanzee SIV isolates. He said it was important to understand some things about chimps: that they live in troupes that don't mix one with another, that they don't like water, and that they don't swim or cross rivers. So, he said, it was possible to have a virus in chimpanzees living in one small area, but not in the area adjacent. He pointed out the difficulties that emanated from the fact that chimps were rare and a protected species — how in their sequence paper they had backed away from emphasizing that HIV-1 had probably originated from SIVcpz, for fear that people might start chimp-bashing. As for how SIVcpz might have gotten into humans, he (like Montagnier) was confident that natural crossover was not an adequate explanation for the twin epidemics of HIV-1 and HIV-2. "It seems to me that to have two distinct viruses going by two different zoonotic routes is far more improbable than an explanation which unifies the two epidemics. And I would say that I like dirty explanations — which involve human frailty, failure. Simply because humans are that way. . . ."

It seemed clear that Wain-Hobson would have no problems with a hypothesis of iatrogenic origin for AIDS — one in which medicine was mooted as the cause — so I asked him about the OPV/AIDS theory. He told me that it was "a theory which merited discussion" and that he had been surprised to find out that "they hardly knew which [species] of animal they were using" to make the vaccine. "Why not discuss it?" he asked. "I would have thought only those people who've got something to hide don't want to discuss it."

I gave him quite a lot more background, and explained that there seemed to be a possibility that chimp kidney might have been used to make some of the vaccine, and he responded: "If there was a chimp connection . . . then that becomes fascinating. You've just given me even more ammunition for my belief in the human foibles theory. And just hearing that, and knowing Koprowski a little bit, I mean . . . I must confess that I am not surprised." I asked what he meant, and he told me of an episode in which Koprowski and other researchers (including Robert Gallo) had announced a link between "Gallo's human retrovirus" and multiple sclerosis,[25] when it was "obvious from the outset they had PCR contamination." (He went on to tell me that in virology circles the joke was that PCR stood for "Probably a Contaminated Reaction.")

As for the possibility of SIVcpz transforming into HIV-1 between the late fifties and the present day, he felt that was no problem at all. "If we were to talk about HIV-1, or . . . about HIV-2, can we get all that variation in thirty, forty years? It would not shock me. [In fact], I put it the other way round. I would *expect* all that divergence to have arisen in thirty to forty years." I asked him about the scientists who proposed that it must have taken hundreds of years, or even millions of years, for such divergence to occur, and he replied: "I think . . . my colleagues are wide of the mark. They haven't understood."

Later, we talked about the possibility of locating and testing some CHAT samples. Sure, said the enfant terrible, he'd be happy to do the PCR work if I could locate any samples, "but the answer is that you're probably not going to find the samples in freezers." Given that the samples in the Wistar's freezers seemed to be no nearer being tested than they were when Curtis published his article fifteen months earlier, I was inclined to agree with him.

## THE QUIETING OF LOUIS PASCAL

It was not until February 1993 that I finally sent a detailed response to Louis Pascal's immense letter of the previous September. At the end of March, just as I was about to set off to Europe, another of the now familiar express packages arrived by courier. It was good timing, for I was able to take a copy of the contents with me, and to read it at my leisure on transcontinental trains traveling between Vienna, Oslo, Brussels, and points in between. During the course of that trip, I was to discover that the latest sheath of papers from the founding father of the OPV theory was as fascinating as the first, but sometimes for rather different reasons.

As before, there were the generous batches of articles, and copies of his correspondence with various scientists (notably Bill Hamilton, an evolutionary biologist from Oxford University, and Brian Martin, an expert on science policy and sociology, based at Wollongong University in Australia), together with others such as Blaine Elswood and Tom Curtis. I was interested to see, in one of these letters, that Pascal acknowledged that he was probably best defined as a philosopher. But it mattered little how he was categorized, for the extent of his knowledge about AIDS clearly surpassed that of most scientists, of whatever level and discipline.

The main item in the package was a long, friendly personal letter to me, in the middle of which were two remarkably well-honed extended metaphors. The first of these likened reality to a huge boulder that topples from a cliff and shatters into a thousand pieces. He compared the unraveling of the history of the origin of AIDS to an attempt to reconstruct the boulder, piece by piece, which reveals that a large fragment from the core of the rock is missing. As the other pieces fit into place, one slowly becomes able to identify the shape of the bottom part of the missing fragment, and also to advance a hypothesis about the shape of the upper part — perhaps even to draw a picture of what one feels it might look like. As one adds further pieces, more of the shape of the missing fragment is revealed. If one's basic hypothesis (or sketch) is wrong, one will realize this fairly quickly. By contrast, it will only be possible to prove that the missing fragment conforms exactly to one's picture of it once the last of the surrounding pieces is slotted into place. But as soon as the first of the pieces surrounding the core, representing say 10 percent of the adjoining area, is joined to the reconstructed boulder and shown to match one's sketch of the fragment, one already knows that one's hypothesis is at least somewhere close to the truth, "because there is no way that a random guess or badly false theory would produce a result that matched perfectly even over one tenth of the missing area."

His theory of origin, he implied, was like that — every time a new piece of data was added to the reconstruction, it matched the picture he had hypothesized. Other theories, by contrast, were quickly shown to be impossible. With these, a piece of broken boulder would emerge that showed the missing fragment had to be a completely different shape to that visualized, or that undermined the whole exercise by demonstrating that two or more boulders must have crashed down from the cliff above, rather than one.

His other metaphor was even more elegant. This is what he wrote:

> In any moderately complex situation, there are always so many individual events that some of them must represent improbable occurrences. Say you do 100,000 things in a day. It is easy to get numbers this large if you break things down finely enough. You just took a step: that is one thing. You just blinked your eyes: that is one thing. You just took a breath: that is one thing. You just turned your head to the right: that is one thing. Well, what are the chances you would take a step, take a breath, blink your eyes and turn your head to the right all at the same time? . . . [W]ith all the step-taking and eye-blinking that you do in a day, it wouldn't surprise me to learn that you do this improbable combination of things several times in a day. And if you do 100,000 things in a day, then events so "rare" that they occur only one time in 10,000 must be occurring ten or so times every day.

This is similar to what the Wistar committee has done in its report. But there is an even worse fallacy they committed. Let us ask what are the chances that you will take a breath precisely at 5pm, blink your eyes precisely fifteen seconds later, take a step precisely 8.15 minutes later, receive a phone call precisely 1.02 hours later, etc. If you multiply enough such occurrences together, it does not take long to reach improbabilities so large that they will verge on impossibilities no matter how many individ-

ual actions you may perform in a day. But suppose your whole day has
been put on video tape. . . .

Pascal went on to reason that one could easily argue (as he claimed the Wistar
committee had done) that the odds against such a series of occurrences happening at such precise times were astronomical, and yet there was the videotape,
which, if genuine, proved that they actually had happened. "After something has
occurred, the chances that it occurred automatically go to 100%, no matter how
remote might have been the odds beforehand," he wrote.

The implications for the Wistar report, with its conclusion that, because of
the various improbabilities, "it can be stated with almost complete certainty
that the large vaccine trial begun late in 1957 in [the Belgian] Congo was not
the origin of AIDS," were obvious. Pascal's example might also be applied to
the early CHAT vaccination campaigns involving some 250,000 people, a few of
whom — say, for argument's sake, twenty-five, or one in 10,000 — might for
particular reasons have been more vulnerable than others to becoming orally
infected by a virus. Perhaps some were already immunocompromised, or had
bitten their tongues just before being vaccinated; perhaps a boy had a mouth
ulcer or a baby was teething.

Pascal's videotape metaphor was a neat way of illustrating that apparently
unlikely combinations of circumstances can, in fact, occur. But for one to be
able to *prove* that they have occurred, one has first to locate the videotape, and
to establish that it is not a fake.

---

These were wonderful images, and they seemed to me to emanate from the
mind of an exceptionally logical thinker, and one who had the great gift of being
able to present ideas in a clear and easily digestible manner. However, there were
other aspects of this latest letter of Pascal's that I found distinctly disturbing.

For one thing, the faint whiff of paranoia that had been apparent in September
1992 had now grown considerably stronger. Since that first letter, Koprowski had
initiated his defamation suit against Tom Curtis, and Pascal was deeply concerned
by the fact that Curtis had turned over all of his, Pascal's, letters to the *Rolling
Stone* lawyers, raising the possibility that they might in turn be revealed to the
other side's attorneys. He was also now discussing such possibilities as letters
being intercepted in the mails, and scientists being paid millions of dollars to fal-
sify archival samples, on the basis that one authentic-looking sample of HIV-1
originating from before 1957 would effectively scupper the CHAT theory. I had
to admit that it was only sensible to think through the worst-case scenarios, but it
seemed to me that Pascal was being overly fearful.

Then there was the hubris. The man was in many ways a genius, to be sure, but sometimes this arrogant insistence on his own intellectual superiority, and his characterizing of others as fools, was a bit hard to take. A fairly typical example was the claim he made for his hypothesis, that there was "no example in the history of science, or of any other field, of a theory that [has] had as much evidence in its favor and as little evidence against it that [has] ultimately proved importantly wrong." Pascal challenged me to refute this. I was left with the feeling that here was a man who loved to argue a theoretical point such as this, who relished the cut-and-thrust of debate, and who was absolutely confident of his ability to come up with a compelling counterargument to any alternative that one might propose. I suspected that what was actually at issue here was not the merit of the OPV/AIDS theory, but rather the confirmation of Louis Pascal's rational preeminence.

Such a declamatory stance becomes even more difficult to take when one is on the receiving end. In "What Happens When Science Goes Bad," Pascal had discussed the two major CHAT vaccinations in Leopoldville and Ruzizi, and concluded that the two campaigns must have used the same pool of vaccine.[1] In my previous letter, I had told him that this was one small point on which he was incorrect, in that I had discovered that two different pools of CHAT had been used. His response was strange, in that he told me that he doubted my claim, and "would be surprised if I could disprove" his logical deduction. I found it worrying that his first response to being told that he might have made a small error was to question the validity of my research.

Not knowing that I had already done so, Pascal suggested that I might like to follow up one of his leads by interviewing doctors Dick and Dane about the Belfast vaccinations. Furthermore, he claimed that somewhere in his papers he had seen an article or report that mentioned that the Manchester sailor had at one time been based in Belfast during his time in the navy. He was normally very careful with papers, he told me — especially important ones such as these — but this one item had inexplicably been mislaid.

Having gone through the logbooks of David Carr's ship H.M.S. *Whitby* and discovered that it had never visited Belfast during the time that he was on board, and knowing that nobody else bar David's family and the Ministry of Defence could have followed up (for nobody else had access to his service history), I suspected that Louis, having discovered that Koprowski's previous Type 1 vaccine SM had been fed in Belfast in 1956, and that the city had then housed the biggest shipyards in the world, had put two and two together and made an informed guess. Having followed this up on the ground, I felt that the more likely explanation was that of a fairly mundane coincidence.

Pascal was intent on having this putative "Belfast connection" investigated, and the lengths to which he would go were illustrated when I delved further into the package and found copies of three letters that had been sent to David Carr's physician Trevor Stretton. Clearly Pascal wanted to get information from Stretton, but without alarming him with an account of George Dick's polio vaccinations, so instead he seemed to have concocted a complicated story. He told him that he had come across evidence that a "cell therapist" had conducted several unconventional experiments in Belfast in 1956, involving the injection of chimpanzee cells into at least fifty human beings, and that the experiments had been stopped only after several of the subjects came down with a mononucleosis-like condition, which Pascal suggested might have been an HIV seroconversion illness. Details of these procedures had never been published, he went on, but the cell therapist had written two letters to someone who had then passed them on, in confidence, to him (Pascal). He asked Stretton whether the patient who had died in 1959 could conceivably have been involved, and whether this could have been the source of his AIDS infection. A female colleague, he added, was "adamant" that she had seen an article stating either that the sailor originated from Belfast, or that he had been based there while in the navy.[2]

These letters to Stretton bore a different name and address, and a note to me implied that he had persuaded a friend to write them on his behalf — although it was also possible that he was adopting a pseudonym, a device he appeared to favor.[3] As it happened, Dr. Stretton had mentioned on the phone a few months earlier about getting some strange letters "from a chap in New York who appears to know quite a lot about cell work," and had sent me a copy of one of them. It came as something of a shock to discover that this had actually been written by Pascal, and to realize that his desire to establish a "Belfast connection" was leading him to concoct one story for Stretton and a conflicting version for me.

I began to feel that, despite Pascal's generosity with source materials and ideas, and his tremendous desire to get at the truth, there were occasions when his sure touch and sense of direction deserted him. Not for the first time, I had the sense that he liked to view himself as the puppeteer, tensing the strings of the protagonists and, alone among them, able to view the entire stage.

Or perhaps a better analogy was that of the grand-master, who saw his various collaborators and sources as pawns, to be moved to and fro across the board as he deemed fit. "Not counting me," he wrote elsewhere in the letter, "you have a better mind than anyone else actively looking into this disease. Take care of yourself. There are many, many lives depending on you." I knew he had written in similar terms to Tom Curtis — so it seemed that he viewed the two of us, at least, as his knights, or rooks. He seemed unable, however, to see that intended compliments such as this one might come across as somewhat manipulative and condescending.

He had started off this letter by explaining that his self-imposed isolation, and his inability to talk directly to Curtis, myself, and the various scientists involved, meant that he tended to bottle things up, and this led to his letters becoming inordinately long, and to his using them as a sort of therapy. To some extent, therefore, he was bouncing ideas around. But some of these ideas were, to my mind, far less impressive than the initial OPV/AIDS hypothesis. He now proposed a convoluted scenario of origin that involved the ancestor of HIV-1 contaminating a culture of HeLa (the immortalized human cell line), which in turn had become superinfected with another retrovirus called Mason-Pfizer Monkey Virus. This doubly contaminated HeLa culture, he suggested, might then have contaminated the monkey kidney tissue cultures used by Koprowski to make his Type 1 vaccines, SM and CHAT,[4] thus introducing the AIDS virus to people in both Belfast and the Congo — and explaining, in one fell swoop, both the case of the Manchester sailor and the AIDS epidemic in Africa. Pascal rather sardonically referred to this series of propositions as his "Grand Unified Theory." To me, this complicated sequence of events seemed entirely unnecessary if, as experienced scientists like Jennifer Alexander and Cecil Fox had suggested, many of the early monkey kidney tissue cultures (such as those made in the fifties) were likely to have contained lymphocytes, which could readily support HIV or SIV growth.

Another example of Pascal's less-compelling hypotheses was his blithe claim that "I am pretty sure I have found the source of HIV-2," when the limited details he provided, involving a vaccine campaign in Brazil, were far from persuasive. Overgrandiose claims such as these tend to end up having the opposite effect, and I found that the small, niggling doubts about Pascal's style were multiplying.

His level of secrecy and inaccessibility only added to these reservations. In my February letter I had told him that I would be flying across to the United States some time in 1993, and that I would very much like to arrange a meeting, partly so I could bring him up to date about my own research. He now replied that this would not be possible for a number of reasons, some of which he explained. He said that he was a semi-underground person, who operated better by working on his own, and that he feared the sort of revelations that a writer or an investigative reporter would be certain to make. He also suggested that it was safer for someone like him to communicate only by letter — hinting that otherwise it would potentially be all too easy for certain of his opponents to rid themselves of their "turbulent priest."

On one level I could understand Pascal's desire for anonymity, and I could also see that his status as a mystery man lent a certain excitement to proceedings. Nonetheless, I was uneasy. Having a clandestine figure so deeply involved in the hypothesis, and masterminding much of the strategy, was in some respects a boon, but it demanded that the figure in question be above suspicion. And while he did indeed seem to be an honorable man and a seeker after truth, the fact that he was unwilling to give any but the most basic details about his own background, and that he apparently had manipulative tendencies, gave me pause for thought. Just as Pascal had done when reviewing the possibility of deliberate attempts to discredit the OPV/AIDS theory, I decided to consider the worst-case scenarios.

Was it conceivable that he was providing snippets of information and a lot of hypothesis in a bid to tease out far more in return? Or even that he was a fifth columnist, working for those who would prefer to see the role of polio vaccines exonerated, and those who questioned their safety discredited? (This seemed absurd, but it still bore thinking about, in that it is a classic counterintelligence technique.)

None of these suppositions struck me as being very likely. However, I was reminded of one of Pascal's own central premises — that the real sin of omission by the vaccine-makers of the fifties was to fail to consider the disastrous consequences if there was even a 1 percent chance that the contaminating viruses in their live vaccines were not, after all, innocuous. On the same basis, if there was even a tiny chance that Pascal was less trustworthy than he seemed, then it could well be disastrous were I to tell him all about my research by letter.

There was another point to consider, also. If things went wrong; if those who proposed the OPV theory of origin ended up (as they seemed to be doing) facing million-dollar lawsuits, then it was unlikely that Pascal himself would be among the defendants. This, of course, was also true of other celebrated orchestrators of the past, such as Deep Throat in the Nixon debacle. But Deep Throat had at least been physically present in the shadows of the underground car park, so that Bob Woodward had the opportunity to see his outline, to hear his voice.[5] With Pascal, even this was denied.

Some real seeds of doubt had been sown, and I decided that before sharing the fruits of three years of research with him (including such details as what had happened to David Carr, and the important clues that were emerging about the events at Ruzizi and at Lindi), I really did have to have the reassurance of meeting Louis Pascal in person.

---

I got back from the Europe trip in May, soon after which another letter from Louis arrived, this time containing a stunning refutation of a letter in *AIDS* by a Japanese team under Dr. Y. Ohta.[6] Ohta's team had previously tested various organs from two SIV-positive African green monkeys and found that although some of these organs contained detectable virus, the kidneys did not. Furthermore, they were unable to find detectable SIVagm in oral polio vaccines made in the kidneys of African green monkeys, or find SIVagm antibodies in 190 children who had been fed the vaccine. This letter had assumed particular significance because of the stress placed upon it by the Wistar committee in its debunking of the OPV/AIDS theory.[7]

Ohta's letter concluded: "From these results, poliomyelitis vaccines may be considered not to be contaminated with SIVagm, even though they are prepared in primary kidney-cell cultures from SIVagm-infected [African green monkeys]." But Pascal claimed to have detected eleven "fatal errors" — eight in the paper itself, and three arising from the fact that the Wistar committee had used the paper in an inappropriate manner. The foremost of these shortcomings was that, in exonerating OPVs, Ohta's team had tested the kidneys of only two monkeys, when many other experiments have demonstrated that it is possible to isolate SIV from one antibody-positive animal, but not from another, or from one organ of an infected animal and not from another.[8] Other objections included the fact that nobody could be sure which monkey species Koprowski had used; that Ohta's team had not employed PCR, by far the most accurate test for viral presence; that the cultures had not been superinfected with poliovirus or other viruses (as those used in the Congo presumably had been); and, perhaps most tellingly, that the experiments to detect SIV growth after the virus had been inoculated into AGM kidneys were "for no scientific reason" halted after four weeks, just as reverse transcriptase levels (indicating SIV growth) appeared to be rising. For these and other reasons, Pascal concluded that "The piece by Ohta et al. cannot be used to support the contention that Koprowski's monkey kidneys did not transfer AIDS' ancestor into human beings."

A few days later, I wrote back to Pascal with a lengthy reply. I complimented him on the Ohta piece, and explained that I felt that he was by far the most incisive thinker I had come across on the subject of origin. However, I added, I believed that I had probably now overtaken him in terms of primary research, including the interviewing of several of the central figures — something that he was prevented from doing. I told him that I did indeed know quite a lot more about many of the subjects in which he was interested, and said that we could potentially help each other a great deal more. But I said that I was uneasy about trusting such confidential information to the mails or the phone lines, and felt that the matter could only really be handled were we to have the chance to discuss in person.

I expected either a positive response, or a friendly declining of my request. I had no idea of the furies I was unleashing.

———

Three months later I received another long letter from Louis, which featured at its core an absolutely furious tirade. He lambasted me for what he later called my "demanding to meet . . . and refusing to take no for an answer," and then accused me of "playing some kind of game," without, however, giving specific instances of what he meant. He further accused me of manipulating him, saying that there were many lives depending on his concealing his identity, and that if I did somehow discover who he was, then probably many lives would be lost. The only concrete reason he would give for this reluctance to meet was that governments and other organizations would kill in order to cover up embarrassing stories, and that "there is even the possibility that the only reason you are still alive is that they cannot make a move against you until they have located me."

This seemed not only vague, but heavily paranoid. However, a few paragraphs later, he did become a little more specific — and personal to boot. "Your overall understanding of AIDS is rather poor. This is not so much because you are ignorant, but because much that you know is not so: you are too dependent on the establishment, and they are at least as incompetent as they are evil, and vast portions of their AIDS knowledge is false, and you have believed many of these things. Moreover, there are many important things about AIDS apart from its origin that the establishment has not perceived, and you have missed these things too. And your overall understanding of how AIDS fits into the larger picture is even more poor. And these are critically important deficiencies which will lead you into many errors in your decision making. Consequently, I do not trust your judgment and am not about to give you the power to ruin everything when you do not perceive either the reasons or the danger."

This was not exactly the end of our correspondence; we did exchange a couple more letters, but it was clear that the chance of real collaboration had gone. I began to realize that despite Louis Pascal's great mind, and his great generosity with information and ideas, he was prepared to deal with people only when they played according to his rules. Sooner or later, almost everyone who dealt with him (including Tom Curtis, myself, and even Brian Martin) somehow incurred his wrath. In my case, I had dared to ask a second time for a meeting; in Brian's, he declined to publish another paper of Louis's unless he was willing to make some revisions for legal reasons.

In the end, we were all exposed to Pascal's great, self-righteous anger, and to accusations, for instance, that by our actions we were probably causing the deaths of others, sometimes in large numbers. For many of us, personal assaults such as this (combined with Pascal's insistence that he — and only he — should be protected by a cloak of anonymity) became so off-putting that they negated the many remarkable benefits of working with the man. Finally, the tension and mounting paranoia involved in this sort of contact reached such a pitch that I had few regrets when communications with Louis Pascal, the father of the OPV/AIDS theory, finally ceased.

---

Sometimes the light changes and, before one knows it, one's perspective has shifted also. There were always times when, despite my exasperation with Louis for his intransigence, the positive things about him remained in the foreground.

These were the times when I could see that Louis Pascal, as well as other skeptics like Tom Curtis, Blaine Elswood, Jennifer Alexander, Mike Lecatsas, Bill Hamilton, and, indeed, myself were perhaps all cast from the same mold. We were all, to differing degrees, feisty iconoclasts, quick to doubt the veracity of official pronouncements, but perhaps also a little too ready to doubt each other. In some brooding lights, I could see us suddenly as a cast of oddballs from a Beckett play, doomed forever to circle around each other muttering of collaboration, but never quite achieving it.[9] Instead, we seemed to be forever waiting for . . . the final proof, the final reassurance.

Sometimes the shadows would shift again, and I would wonder whether we were, in fact, so very different from those iconoclasts of yesteryear — the Sabins and Koprowskis, the Coxes, Salks, and Lépines. Had not they started off, just like us, as questioners of received wisdom, as challengers of convenient assumption?

# V

## THE PASSAGE THROUGH THE POOLS

*If you're anxious for to shine in the high aesthetic line as*
  *a man of culture rare,*
*You must get up all the germs of the transcendental terms,*
  *and plant them everywhere.*

— W. S. GILBERT, Patience

*In skating over thin ice, our safety is in our speed.*

— RALPH WALDO EMERSON, Prudence

# 28

A MAN OF MANY IDEAS

As anyone who has ever completed a careful piece of research — be it a school project or a Ph.D. thesis — is aware, the process of investigating a subject in some detail, the process of gradual discovery, can be both seductive and intense. At times it transcends both of these and becomes truly inspiring. And it is during these latter times that, just occasionally, one gets to experience one of the most joyous events human beings are capable of experiencing. It's right up there with watching your first child being born, the best of lovemaking, or the week-long trek through the mountains. It is the moment when gray cells collide, and the researcher claps hand to forehead in dawning certainty and wonder. It is the moment when Archimedes forgets his towel — the *Eureka* moment.

After the trip to Europe in the spring and early summer of 1993, and partly on the basis of advice given me by Jean Deinhardt, I began a far more detailed investigation into Dr. Hilary Koprowski's polio work. As the months passed, my collection of Koprowski reprints grew. Now, in addition to the key papers published in mainstream medical journals, I began locating his addresses to different conferences, and his off-the-cuff comments made in conference discussion sessions. I also located his polio texts in other languages, as well as a wide range of articles by his erstwhile collaborators from such countries as Belgium, Poland, Croatia, Switzerland, and Sweden.

By late summer, I had assembled not only a comprehensive set of Koprowski's sixty-odd polio papers published between 1946 and 1963, but also a wide selection of his other articles on subjects as diverse as rabies, SV40, multiple sclerosis, and the presence of latent viruses in tissue culture.

I began drawing up a chart of Koprowski's various polio vaccine trials conducted between 1950 and 1961 (the year when he last prepared polio vaccines in

KOPROWSKI'S HUMAN POLIO VACCINE FEEDINGS
RECORDED IN THE SCIENTIFIC LITERATURE

| | Date fed | Vaccine used | Nos. fed | Place of feeding (U.S. unless stated) | Ages | Reference |
|---|---|---|---|---|---|---|
| 1 | Feb. 27, 1950– Mar. 12, 1951 | TN | 22 | Letchworth Village, NY | 20 children +2 adults | Am. J. Hyg., 1952, 55, 108–126 |
| 2 | Jul. 1, 1952 | TN | 61 | Sonoma | 8 months– 8 yrs. | Proc. Soc. Exp. Biol. Med., 1953, 82, 277–280 |
| 3 | 1953 | SM | 3 | Letchworth | Children | Proc. Soc. Exp. Biol. Med., 1954, 86, 238–244 |
| 4 | 1954–1956? | SM N-90 TN | 20 12 | Woodbine | 6–12 yrs. | Am. J. Med. Sci., 1956, 232, 378–388 |
| 5 | Apr.– Jul. 1955 | SM TN | 38 32 | Sonoma | 6–15 yrs. | JAMA, 1956, 160, 954–966 |
| 6 | 1956? | MEF1 | 18 | Sonoma and Woodbine | 2–12 yrs. | J. Immunol., 1956, 77, 123–131 |
| 7 | Aug. 1955– June 1956 | SM N-90 TN | 22 8 | Clinton | Infants up to 6 months | JAMA, 1956, 162, 1281–1288 |
| 8 | Feb.–June 1956 | SM N-90 | 14 | Belfast (N. Ireland) | 11 adults, 2 infants, 1 girl of four | BMJ, 1957, i, 65–70 |
| 9 | Feb.–July 1956 | TN | 190 | Belfast (plus N. Ireland towns and Oxford, U.K.?) | 21 adults, 159 children, 10 infants | BMJ, 1957, i, 59–65 |
| 10 | Up to Aug. 1956 | SM N-90 | 94 | Not revealed | Adults (Clinton) and children | Spec. Publ. N.Y. Acad. Sci., 1957, 5, 128–133 |
| 11 | Oct. 1956– June 1958 | CHAT Fox P-712 | 41 35 22 | Clinton | Infants (plus a few adults) | Pediatr., 1959, 23, 1041–1062; 4th Int. Conf. Polio, July 1957, 112–123 |
| 12 | Mar. 1957– Feb. 1958 | CHAT Fox | 4,228 533 | Stanleyville (Congo) | All ages | BMJ, 1958, ii, 187–190 |
| 13 | May 1957 (CHAT) and Dec. 1957 | CHAT Fox | 1,978 | Aketi (Congo) | School- children, mostly 5–15 yrs. | BMJ, 1958, ii, 187–190 |
| 14 | Starting Nov. 1957 | CHAT 10A-11 | 85 | Stockholm (Sweden) | 20 families (children plus adults) | PAHO1, 350–354; PAHO2, 187–190 |

| | Date fed | Vaccine used | Nos. fed | Place of feeding (U.S. unless stated) | Ages | Reference |
|---|---|---|---|---|---|---|
| 15 | Jan.–Feb. 1958 | CHAT 10A-11? | 22,886 | Banalia, Gombari, Watsa, Bambesa (Congo) | All ages (in response to epidemics) | *BMJ,* 1958, ii, 187–190 |
| 16 | Feb. 24, 1958– Apr. 10, 1958 | CHAT 10A-11 | 215,504 | Ruzizi Valley and Ruanda-Urundi | All ages | *BMJ,* 1958, ii, 187–190 |
| 17 | Jan.–June 1958 | CHAT 4B-5? P-712 Fox | 89 84 84 | Moorestown, NJ | 36 adults 53 children (1–15 yrs.) | *Acta Paed.,* 1960, 49, 551–571 |
| 18 | 1958 | CHAT 10A-11 Fox | 400 90 | Bern and Geneva (Switzerland) | All ages | *PAHO2,* 322–323 |
| 19 | Aug. 18, 1958 –April 1960 (CHAT); Sept. 1959 (Fox) | CHAT 13 Fox | 76,400 ? | Leopoldville (Congo) | 0–5 yrs. | *Bull. WHO,* 1961, 24, 785–792 |
| 20 | Starting Oct. 20, 1958 | CHAT 13 | 2,920 22 | Wyszkow Warsaw (Poland) | 6 months– 16 yrs. | *PAHO1,* 497–507; *PAHO2,* 522–531 |
| 21 | Winter 1958/9 | CHAT 10A-11 | c. 400 | Sweden | 107 families | *PAHO1,* 350–354; *PAHO2,* 187–190 |
| 22 | Dec. 1958– Mar. 1959 | CHAT Fox | 96 | Clinton | Infants | *N. Engl. J. Med.,* 1961, 264, 155–163; *Lancet,* 1960, i, 1224–1226 |
| 23 | Jan.–July 1959 | CHAT Fox P-712 | 850 805 335 | Philadelphia | 445 infants plus 405 children | *PAHO2,* 277–287; *JAMA,* 1960, 123, 1883–1889 |
| 24 | Jan. 1959– Apr. 1960 | CHAT | 65 | Philadelphia General Hospital | Premature infants | *Pediatr.,* 1962, 26, 794–807 |
| 25 | June 1959– Mar. 1960 (CHAT); Nov. 1959– May 1960 (Fox) | CHAT 18 Fox | 7,130,000 6,250,000 | Poland | 6 months– 14 or 15 yrs. | *PAHO2,* 522–531 |
| 26 | Winter 1959/60 | CHAT 10A-11 | c. 500 | Sweden | All ages | *PAHO2,* 187–190 |

## KOPROWSKI'S HUMAN POLIO VACCINE FEEDINGS
## RECORDED IN THE SCIENTIFIC LITERATURE (*continued*)

| | Date fed | Vaccine used | Nos. fed | Place of feeding (U.S. unless stated) | Ages | Reference |
|---|---|---|---|---|---|---|
| 27 | 1960/1? | WMIII (in MKTC) | 9 | Philadelphia General Hospital | Infants | *Proc. Soc. Exp. Biol. Med.,* 1961, 107, 829–834 |
| 28 | 1960/1 | CHAT 23? W-Fox | 360,000 | Aargau, Basel, Bern, Lucern (Switzerland) | Children and infants | *Am. J. Publ. Health,* 1962, 52, 959 |
| 29 | Feb.–Apr. 1961 | CHAT 23? W-Fox | 1,340,000 1,288,000 | Croatia | 3 months– 20 yrs. | *Am. J. Publ. Health,* 1962, 52, 958–959 |
| 30 | 1960–1962 | CHAT 10A-11 (Swedish version) | 4,212 | Sweden | All ages | *European Assoc. Against Polio,* 1962, 140–144 |
| 31 | 1961/2? | CHAT 24 WI-2 WMIII | 46 45 44 | Philadelphia General Hospital and Clinton | Infants | WHO document; "Virus Diseases/WP/6," July 5, 1963 |
| 32 | Apr. 4, 1962 | CHAT 24 | 123 | Uppsala (Sweden) | 8–13 yrs. | *Am. J. Hyg.,* 1964, 79(1), 74–85 |
| 33 | 1962 | CHAT 24 WI-2 WMIII | 800 | Switzerland | Infants and children | *Proc. Symp. Characteriz. & Uses of HDCS* (Opatija, 1963), 381–387 |
| 34 | 1962/3 | CHAT 23? 24? WI-2 WMIII | 2,238,000 1,272,000 640,000 | Croatia | All ages | *European Assoc. Against Polio.,* 1964, 196–199 |
| 35 | 1963 | WMIII | 11,000 (half each in MKTC and HDCS) | Croatia | Children | *1st Int. Conf. Vaccines Against Viral & Rickettsial Dis. Man.,* PAHO Sci. Publ. 147, 1967, 185–189 |
| 36 | 1964–1966 | CHAT 24 WI-2 WMIII | 25,600 17,400 23,100 | Croatia | Children | Ibid. |
| 37 | 1964 | Trivalent | 117,300 | Croatia | Children | Ibid. |

— Over 9.1 million people were fed vaccine in MKTC (30 trials)
— At least 1.3 million were fed vaccine in HDCS (last 7 trials)

monkey kidney tissue culture, MKTC), and between 1961 and 1966 (involving polio vaccines made in human diploid cell strains, HDCS). More than nine million people had been vaccinated in total. I was able to identify thirty-seven different trials, the first twelve of which seemed to have been conducted (or at least initiated) while he was at Lederle, and the remainder during his directorship of the Wistar. Some of the details of the smaller trials were unclear — often there was no indication as to when or where a trial had taken place. Furthermore, it seemed that not all the vaccinations had been recorded in scientific papers, for in the early days, on the occasions when he gave running totals of vaccinees, they often exceeded the totals that had been formally reported. Nonetheless, as the months went by, I managed to build up an increasingly accurate version of events.

The trials had apparently been conducted in four main stages. The majority (especially in the early days) were small affairs, staged first in the United States and later in Europe — and involving as few as three, or as many as a few hundred, vaccinees. A total of twenty-one such trials occurred between 1950 and 1962, involving a total of about 7,000 individuals. (In modern parlance, these would probably be defined as Phase One trials, staged to check the safety of experimental vaccines on small numbers of subjects, and Phase Two trials, staged to assess the immunogenicity of the vaccines — their ability to immunize and protect against disease.) Second came a group of five trials conducted in central Africa between 1957 and 1960, which, according to the records, had involved a total of 321,000 people, plus a Polish trial on almost 3,000 people in 1958. Then, between 1959 and 1961, came the three mass feedings in Poland, Croatia, and Switzerland, which had involved a total of more than 8.8 million individuals, mostly children, and most of whom were fed with more than one vaccine strain.[1] (The latter two groups were effectively Phase Three trials, designed to check the efficacy of the vaccines on a large scale.)[2] Lastly came seven further trials (Phase 1 to Phase 3 inclusive) of Koprowski polio vaccines grown in HDCS, which were conducted between 1961 and 1966. Over a million persons were vaccinated, almost all in Europe and mainly in Croatia.

These thirty-seven human trials represented the visible product of a massive body of research conducted over many years, during which Koprowski and his major collaborators — such as Norton, Jervis, and Plotkin — had devoted much of their time and intellectual energy to the challenge of conquering polio.

Much of the account that follows was put together in the course of midnight study sessions, during which I first experienced the occasional *Eureka* moment. Some of the technical details may be difficult to absorb at first reading, but they are important, in that they provide vital background evidence about the history of CHAT oral polio vaccine, and the context within which that history needs to be viewed.

Throughout his career, but particularly after his arrival at the Wistar Institute, Hilary Koprowski has demonstrated a predilection, in his conference speeches but also in his written articles, for classical, literary, and philosophical quotation. He has also proved himself to be a specialist in the humorous (and sometimes the scurrilous) aside. This is such a contrast to the dry and sometimes impenetrable prose of many of his fellows (such as Albert Sabin), that it frequently affords welcome refreshment, even to the most sober-minded listener or reader.

Certain of his quotations, however, be they from American limerick writers, German philosophers, French poets, or ancient Greek soothsayers, would seem to be of questionable relevance to the subject at hand. One example features in an article from 1981, which ends as follows: "While exploring all these wonderful (in my opinion) ideas about the future of biology, I always, however, keep in mind the words of Francis Picabia, 'The thing about ideas is to change them as often as you change your shirt.'"[3] Here, one feels, is a man who changes his shirt with alacrity — and a knowing smile. One senses a love of peacock display, and of the swish and rush of Science as fashion show.

And as one reads on through the articles of Hilary Koprowski, this line of Picabia's keeps returning, as an eerie refrain. On one level, one can see that open-mindedness and fluidity of thinking are wonderful qualities in a scientist, and ones that are especially admirable when — as here — they are still apparent in someone in his late sixties. Here, one feels, is a man who loves the intellectual thrill of pitting his wits against Nature, a man with tremendous energy and an impressively quick inquiring mind. And yet here too lies the problem of the man: the dragonfly inconstancy that runs as a vein throughout his work. He flits from idea to idea, from flower to flower, supping from all — yet dwelling on none.

––––––––––

But what of the actual content of these sixty-odd papers? Koprowski's very first article on poliomyelitis, published in 1947, four years before his first publications on polio vaccines, reveals that he is already collaborating with two establishments that would feature prominently in his subsequent polio research: Letchworth Village (a home for mentally handicapped children at Thiells, New York, where George Jervis headed the research department), and the Children's Hospital of Philadelphia.[4]

Several of Koprowski's papers about the early work on his Type 2 vaccine, TN, are remarkably detailed. They record, among other things, the first trial feedings of children, chimpanzees, and (at the suggestion of Albert Sabin)[5] cynomolgus monkeys. They also contain, however, several rather intriguing discrepancies and anomalies, none of which appear to have unduly alarmed the authors, or other polio researchers of the era.

For instance, the very first paper on OPV feeding, published in the *American Journal of Hygiene* in 1952,[6] reveals that it was pool 16 of TN that was fed (in February 1950) to the very first vaccinee, and to another nine of the original twenty child "volunteers" at Letchworth Village, who are described as "non-immune."[7] It also records, however, that twenty-two of the forty-four rhesus monkeys injected intracerebrally with this same pool 16 went on to develop either moderate or severe clinical signs of poliomyelitis, and that ten of them died. In fact, of all the five pools of TN discussed in this paper, pool 16 was far and away the most virulent, being the only one to cause severe clinical symptoms or death in the monkey safety test. The fact that it was used so prominently in the first human trials is remarkable, and would seem to bring into question the most basic principles of safety testing.[8]

And there was more. A paper by Koprowski, Norton, and George Jervis published in an Austrian journal in 1954[9] reveals the exact dates between 1949 and 1952 when various early pools of TN and virulent poliovirus were fed experimentally to sixteen young chimpanzees. The article explains, quite correctly, that the first feedings of TN to chimps occurred in September 1949, five months before the first human feeding of TN. It also claims that TN pool 16 was fed to two chimpanzees *before* it was fed to humans. However, the accompanying tables reveal the exact opposite — that pool 16 was first fed to chimps on July 27, 1950 — which is *after* the first seven Letchworth Village children were vaccinated with the same pool.

What this shows is that the first humans to be fed OPV used a pool of vaccine that had proved highly virulent in the monkey safety tests of the day, and one that (despite claims to the contrary) had not been tested by prior feeding to chimpanzees. These would have been remarkable errors at the best of times, let alone when reporting the first human trials of a new vaccine.

In spite of these errors, this lengthy account in the *American Journal of Hygiene* of the first human feeding of OPV, with its dates of feeding, specific pool numbers, and so forth, is in other respects one of the most impressive of all Koprowski's polio articles.[10] It is clearly written, impressively detailed, and unadorned with the flourishes and sideswipes that characterize some of his later publications. And unlike those subsequent papers, difficulties in the manufacturing process are freely admitted.

The authors report, for instance, that TN pool 16 involved seven passages in mouse brain, and thirty-five passages in the brain of the cotton rat. Later pools (like pool 31) actually involved fewer cotton rat passages, since passages in this substrate were — rather alarmingly — discovered to increase the virulence of the attenuated virus.[11] This demonstrates that backtracking and trial and error were — at this stage anyway — part and parcel of the attenuation process.

For whatever reason, Koprowski and Norton were never again to be so precise. In subsequent work they only very rarely recorded the exact dates when individuals (either humans or simians) were fed vaccine, and they often neglected to identify the specific pool of vaccine used in a particular trial. Indeed with one of their vaccines, CHAT, they never properly documented the pool-by-pool passage history.

———

Koprowski's sometime failure to record events accurately was further revealed at a conference entitled "Biology of Poliomyelitis," held in January 1955 and organized under the auspices of the Section of Biology of the New York Academy of Sciences. As chairman of this section, Hilary Koprowski was called upon to deliver the opening address, in which he pondered whether the French poet Paul Valéry's comments about history might not also apply to the field of polio research. Koprowski explained that Valéry had deemed history to be "the most dangerous product that the chemistry of the intellect has invented. It engenders dreams, it intoxicates the workers, it begets false memories, . . . and makes scientists bitter, arrogant, insufferable and vain."

In 1955, with virology still in its infancy, there was still great uncertainty about the best method of growing vaccines, and of assessing the virulence of those vaccines, and a large part of the conference was concerned with the varying susceptibilities of different animals and tissue culture systems to poliovirus. Albert Kaplan of Yale reported that the kidneys of the newborn rabbit, the baby hamster, the capuchin (a South American monkey) and the rhesus macaque from Asia were susceptible to polio in ascending order, but that only the rhesus macaque kidneys could actually grow poliovirus, and then only *in vitro*. (His attempt to inoculate kidneys with poliovirus *in vivo*, in live macaques, failed to produce detectable virus.) Sidney Kibrick of Harvard proposed human kidney as the best tissue culture for detecting poliovirus, claiming that it was even more susceptible than monkey kidney. The great bacteriologist S. E. Luria, meanwhile, made the seemingly obvious, but highly significant point that if a virus were grown in a number of different cells, it was the *last* host cell in which it had been propagated that was crucial, and that determined its host range thereafter.

Koprowski, for his part, stated that his own preferred approach to attenuating a virus was to propagate it in an "unnatural host" (one like rodent brains or chick embryo, which was not susceptible to the virus under normal conditions) rather than to adopt "the demanding and often controversial" method of trying to change the virus by applying certain genetic principles — such as subjecting it to rapid passages in monkey kidney tissue culture, which was what Sabin was by then doing.

However, elsewhere in the conference proceedings, Koprowski and his collaborator from Letchworth Village, George Jervis, reveal that they too have been experimenting with monkey kidney as a substrate. In one discussion session, Koprowski casually mentions that a version of TN has been passaged forty-seven times in monkey kidney tissue culture (MKTC),[12] while Jervis reports that two of the other Lederle vaccine viruses, SM (Type 1) and MEF1 (Type 2), have also been subjected to multiple passages in MKTC, before being adapted to other substrates.[13]

These scattered clues indicate that by January 1955 Koprowski and Jervis — just like Sabin — were experimenting with growing attenuated polioviruses in monkey kidney. And clearly the experimentation continued, for according to Koprowski's published accounts in the literature, the SM vaccine he used in trials in 1955 and 1956 was prepared by multiple passages in chick embryo, followed by five or six alternating passages in monkey kidney tissue culture and chick embryo tissue culture (CETC). He makes it clear, however, that the final host cell was chick embryo.[14] In particular, this claim features in his table documenting the "History of Attenuation of SM Virus (Type 1)," published in December 1957, after he had left Lederle for the Wistar. Here he reports that SM N-90, the variant that had been used in the trials at Sonoma, Woodbine, Clinton, and Belfast, had been "made into a large chick embryo pool."[15]

As I read and reread the relevant articles, I began to suspect that Koprowski's assertions about the final host cell (the one that, according to Luria, would determine the host range of the poliovirus strain thereafter) did not quite add up. There were various clues that fueled my suspicions. There was the decided ambivalence about the final substrate that was apparent in some of the articles — especially those reporting the SM trials at Woodbine and Clinton. Then there was the fact that the reported passage history of SM N-90 changed between Sonoma (fourteen CETC and five alternate MKTC/CETC passages) and Belfast (thirteen CETC and six alternate MKTC/CETC passages), and the realization that this could easily mean that one extra passage had taken place, and that MKTC (instead of CETC) had now become the final substrate.[16]

Finally I found the proof in an article by Victor Cabasso, whom Herald Cox appointed to take charge of polio vaccine research at Lederle after Koprowski's departure. In 1959, Cabasso published a superbly detailed paper entitled "Cumulative Testing Experience with Consecutive Lots of Oral Poliomyelitis Vaccine."[17] And there, in the chart depicting the passage history of the SM strain, was the revelation that SM pool N-90 had not been made in chick embryo tissue culture, as Koprowski had claimed, but instead in monkey kidney tissue culture.

It was this discovery — that Koprowski had been preparing his vaccine in one way, and reporting something quite different in the literature — that constituted the first of my "Eureka moments."

I could think of only two possible reasons for his lack of candor. One, perhaps, was the desire to conceal details about his approach to vaccine development from rivals such as Sabin. Another could have been the opposition of

HISTORY OF THE ATTENUATION OF SM AND CHAT VIRUSES (TYPE 1),
AS GIVEN BY KOPROWSKI

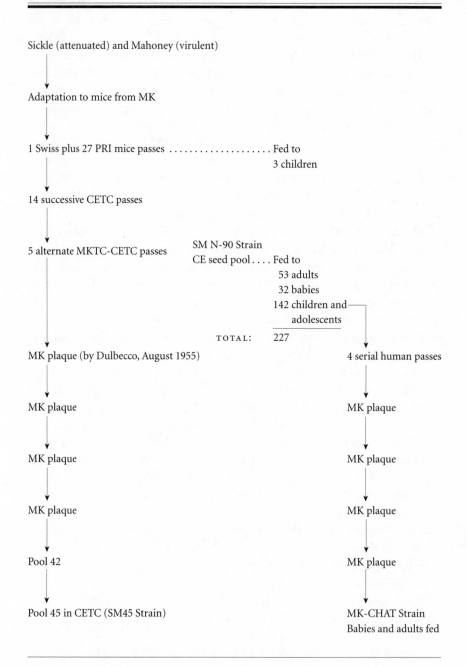

Sickle (attenuated) and Mahoney (virulent)

Adaptation to mice from MK

1 Swiss plus 27 PRI mice passes . . . . . . . . . . . . . . . . . . . . Fed to
                                                                      3 children

14 successive CETC passes

5 alternate MKTC-CETC passes        SM N-90 Strain
                                    CE seed pool . . . . Fed to
                                                         53 adults
                                                         32 babies
                                                         142 children and
                                                             adolescents
                                    TOTAL:    227

MK plaque (by Dulbecco, August 1955)                     4 serial human passes

MK plaque                                                MK plaque

MK plaque                                                MK plaque

MK plaque                                                MK plaque

Pool 42                                                  MK plaque

Pool 45 in CETC (SM45 Strain)                            MK-CHAT Strain
                                                         Babies and adults fed

KEY: MK = monkey kidney; CE = chick embryo; TC = tissue culture.
SOURCE: Special Publication, N.Y. Acad. Sci., 1957, 5, 128)

his boss at Lederle, Herald Cox, to the use of MKTC, because of his fear (well justified, as it turned out) of contaminating monkey viruses.

Whatever, Koprowski's basic attitude toward the issue of substrate seemed to be that it was of little relevance. Just how lightly he treated it can be gauged by the penultimate paragraph of his 1956 article in the *American Journal of Tropical Medicine* in which, for almost the only time in the fifties, he discussed his choice of polio vaccine substrate.[18]

This was what he had to say:

> The source of material used for virus cultivation cannot be disregarded altogether. It should be represented by tissue which is least apt to harbor human pathogens — although the dilution factor which can be applied to a poliomyelitis virus suspension may be beneficial for the elimination of other "passenger" viruses.

And that was it. His failure to record that he was using a monkey kidney substrate meant that there was no discussion of the dangers of contaminating monkey viruses, but merely a vague mention of unspecified "passenger viruses."

He concluded this paper in vigorous mood, as follows:

> The progress of research on live virus immunization is slow but steady. Its tempo depends unfortunately less and less on the actual achievements in the laboratory and in clinical trials, and more on the turbulent state of emotionalism which reigns at present in this field. . . . It is understandable that in such an age, the scientist bears an even greater responsibility than ever. It is hoped that his voice will be listened to and that his judgment will prevail.

Koprowski was of course right when he opined that the scientist involved in preparing polio vaccines bore an exceptional degree of responsibility. One wonders, however, how he squared that statement with his own misrepresentation of the species used to provide the host cells for the SM substrate.

Since it is now clear that some of the human trials of SM pool N-90 involved a preparation made in MKTC, this begs exactly the same question as does the controversy about CHAT, thirty years later. Precisely which species of monkey was employed?

————————

The importance of the latter question can be highlighted by certain other developments in the field of polio vaccination during 1955. The question of the host cell, of the species used to make the vaccine, took on a new significance when the Indian government halted the export of rhesus monkeys, after an incident in which four hundred of them were found suffocated at London airport. Faced by the prospect of a complete shutdown of vaccine production, the manufacturers of IPV (which was just then moving into the mass-production stage) were thrown into panic, as were their colleagues working on OPV. By April 1955, the Indian ban had been partially lifted for monkeys that were to be used by bona fide medical institutions,[19] but by then the seeds of uncertainty had been sown, and various initiatives had already been launched in order to find an alternative source of primates.

Since the organization of shipments of live monkeys from another country took time, a lot of interest was shown in a new technique proposed by Joseph Melnick, and backed by Dr. Payne of the WHO: that of extracting and trypsinizing the kidneys in the country of origin, and then shipping the resultant cells — rather than the whole monkey — by air.[20] Trypsinization is an important technique, which involves the use of an enzyme, trypsin, which partially digests the kidney tissue into a soup containing individual cells and very small clumps of cells. First described by Renato Dulbecco in 1954, this technique allowed a greater yield of tissue for poliovirus cultivation.[21]

Meanwhile, at the start of May 1955, Dr. Kingsley Sanders, representing the Medical Research Council of the United Kingdom, flew out to Fajara in British West Africa (in what is now the Gambia), where he obtained kidneys from four different monkey species — the Guinea baboon (*Papio papio*), the African green monkey (*Cercopithecus aethiops sabaeus*), the red monkey (*Erythrocebus patas*), and an unspecified colobus monkey. Four of the six kidney shipments he sent proved to be usable on arrival in the United Kingdom, and the kidneys that had been trypsinized in West Africa prior to dispatch proved to be the most usable.[22]

The July 1955 meeting of the MRC's Committee on Laboratory Investigation of Poliomyelitis duly recommended that a team be sent to West Africa to explore the possibility of establishing a local supply of monkey kidney tissue, and, if appropriate, to undertake trypsinization of kidneys. "To make it a more attractive proposition," the minutes go on, "this work should be combined with virus studies in what is likely to prove a hyperendemic area for poliomyelitis." Unfortunately, the minutes for the next meeting of this particular committee are missing, and there is no record of whether this experimental scheme actually proceeded as planned.[23]

By the time of the WHO meeting on poliomyelitis vaccination, held in Stockholm in November 1955, the interest in African monkeys as a tissue culture source had intensified. Dr. James Gear from the Poliomyelitis Research Foundation of South Africa reported that his institution had been using trypsinized kidney cells from the local subspecies of the African green monkey for IPV production since 1954. Pierre Lépine announced that a specially equipped laboratory for vaccine production had been set up at the Pasteur

Institute more than a year earlier, and that they had been studying the use of kidneys of different African monkey species, as well as human fibroblasts, in order to make polio vaccine. Production had been raised to one hundred liters a week, and vaccine had been stockpiled for future use.[24]

Eventually, the Pasteur would select the kidney of the Guinea baboon from West Africa as its preferred substrate for polio vaccines. However, the famous institute had also investigated the possibility of using the tissues of monkeys from *central* Africa and, to this end, had been collaborating since 1953 with a Polish vet based in the Belgian Congo. His name was Alexandre Jezierski, and he comes into the story a little later.

----

The two key Koprowski papers about CHAT vaccine were both published in the form of transcripts of speeches, which were delivered to conferences held in New York and Geneva in January and July 1957.[25] In fact, the transcript of the New York speech was altered later to incorporate details about CHAT and Fox, and so his first public announcement about these new vaccines was actually made place at the Fourth International Poliomyelitis Conference in Geneva, just ten weeks after he took over as director of the Wistar.

Free at last of the inhibiting influence of Cox, Koprowski was now his own boss, in charge of a research institute and able both to set the agenda and to raise his own funds. Furthermore, he had managed to persuade several of his supporters from Lederle to join him in Philadelphia. The speech that he delivered was a *tour de force*. The most important new scientific information was that his latest vaccines, CHAT and Fox, had been made in monkey kidney tissue culture, employing the plaque purification technique of Renato Dulbecco, which Sabin had been successfully using for nearly two years.[26]

Plaque purification represented a huge leap forward in terms of ensuring the purity of viruses used in vaccines. A plaque was presumed to represent the impact of a single virion, or viral particle — in this case, of poliovirus — on MKTC grown on a gel. (The virion would replicate inside a kidney cell and then break out, destroying the cell in the process. Over time, a clear circle, or plaque, would be produced denoting where the kidney cell had been destroyed and the virus remained.) "Triple plaque purification," which quickly became the byword for purity in OPV production, therefore involved carefully extracting material containing poliovirus from the center of a plaque, inoculating it into another monkey kidney culture, allowing it to reproduce, and repeating the process twice more.

In his Geneva speech, Koprowski first reviewed the history of the SM vaccine (including N-90, which he continued to claim had been made in a chick embryo seed pool), and then described how, after four human passages (feeding the virus to humans and extracting it from their stools) and several further plaque purifications in monkey kidney, it had been transformed into CHAT. Now that CHAT had superseded SM N-90 at the Wistar, he was not afraid to observe that his former Type 1 poliovirus strain was perhaps not ideal for use as a vaccine, having been insufficiently purified. (Perhaps this was hardly surprising, given that the original SM isolate had been a mixture of the attenuated Sickle and virulent Mahoney strains.)

He described CHAT as a "substrain" of SM N-90,[27] and presented a detailed diagram of what he termed the "SM CHAT plaque line," showing how different plaques of CHAT had been safety tested intraspinally and intracerebrally in monkeys, and how certain of these plaques (not always the least virulent) had been selected to seed further cultures.[28]

There was one very important piece of information that emerged from this diagram. This was the identity of the CHAT strain that the two researchers

SM CHAT PLAQUE LINE, AS REPORTED BY KOPROWSKI

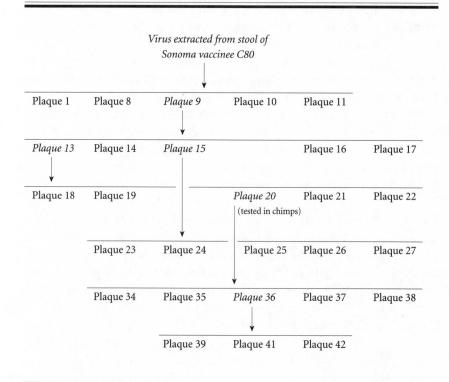

SOURCE: Special Publication, N.Y. Acad. Sci., 1957, 5, 129. (For reasons of space, details of the monkey safety tests have been omitted. It is unclear which plaque or plaques were used to manufacture the different pools of CHAT vaccine virus.)

had injected into the spines of the five chimpanzees at Lindi camp, without ill effects. This was shown to be a triple plaque purified virus, which was identified in the diagram as Plaque 20.

However, what may not have been immediately obvious to those who attended this impressive presentation at Geneva, or who read the subsequent paper, was that certain of the crucial details were missing.

The most important omission from the Geneva paper involved the description of how CHAT had been made. The plaque line diagram for Fox (Koprowski's first Type 3 polio vaccine), which featured in the same paper, not only included details of the various plaque purifications, but also clearly indicated which plaques had been made into which MKTC pools. By contrast, the equivalent diagram for CHAT provided no details at all about the links between plaques and pools. In other words, it failed to reveal which specific plaques had been selected, and then grown out in monkey kidney, to produce pools of CHAT vaccine, such as pool 10A-11 and pool 13.

What the CHAT plaque line diagram did reveal was that just one further plaquing could substantially increase or decrease the virulence of the virus. The failure to identify which plaque or plaques had been used to make up the actual vaccine pools was therefore both surprising and disturbing.

Koprowski had provided information (albeit not always entirely accurate) about the passage history of all his other polio vaccine strains — TN, SM, and Fox. But for CHAT vaccine, this essential information was never vouchsafed.

This, of course, only served to encourage speculation. Could it be that the plaque that represented the actual source of the CHAT vaccine fed around the world was a relatively virulent one (like Plaque 35 or 38)? Or was it that, for whatever reason, the real provenance of the CHAT strain was rather different from the account that Koprowski had provided — just as there seemed to be a crucial discrepancy in his description of SM pool N-90? Whatever, his failure to provide accurate and essential information about the provenance of the CHAT pools was a notable omission.

There were also other unexplained details about CHAT. Early in the process of developing the new vaccine, Koprowski had used virus originating from the stool of the fourth human vaccinee in the Sonoma serial passage study, code-numbered C80 — a virus that had produced lesions and paralysis in several of the safety test monkeys. He had used this excreted virus from C80 in preference to that from the sixth vaccinee (C82), which was, as he himself pointed out, "innocuous" in monkeys.

Once again, this highlighted the fact that the process of vaccine development was a delicate balancing act. If the vaccine-maker used virus that was too attenuated, that failed to cause any lesions in monkeys, he risked failing to immunize the human vaccinee. If he went to the other extreme and used virus that was insufficiently attenuated, he risked paralyzing his human subjects. Looked at from this perspective, the monkey safety test was useful only in indicating which virus strains fell in the middle ground — strains that did not paralyze *all* of the monkeys, but that equally did not paralyze *none* of them.

Despite this lack of clarity and transparency about the history of CHAT, Koprowski was to launch into a remarkable harangue against his fellow scientists at the end of the Geneva address. He told them that there was an urgent need to begin mass field trials of OPVs, concluding as follows:

> Strains available today for large-scale clinical trials may be as good as they probably ever will be. . . . The time has come when a careful and patient evaluation of the attenuated viruses as immunizing agents against poliomyelitis may lead those who have a sense of proportion to the conclusion that the price one has to pay today for the comfort of future generations is indeed negligible.

A similar speech to that delivered at Geneva appeared in December 1957, in the published version of the conference held at the New York Academy of Sciences.[29] It ended, however, not with a polemic (as in Geneva), but with a flourish that is pure Koprowski. He quoted from Bertrand Russell's essay "Knowledge and Wisdom" as follows: "'There are, I think, several factors which contribute to wisdom. Of these, I should put first a sense of proportion: the capacity to take account of all the important factors in a problem and to attach to each its due weight.'"

This was excellent, but Koprowski could not resist adding a final throwaway line for good measure: "As for the rest, 'you pays your money and you takes your choice.'"

Koprowski had certainly done that, for by the time the piece was published open trials of his vaccines in the Belgian Congo (as yet unreported) had already taken place at Aketi and Stanleyville; two months later the mass trials would begin in Ruzizi.[30] Just as Koprowski had been the first scientist to feed OPV to a human, so he was clearly eager to be the first to conduct successful mass trials of OPV. Once again, it was he who had the courage to take the leap across the void. But, one must ask whether, by so doing, he was really demonstrating the wisdom and sense of proportion that he and Bertrand Russell apparently so valued.

In 1959, in a paper published in a journal of genetics, Koprowski provided a rather different analysis of his polio work from those he was in the habit of delivering at polio conferences, or submitting to scientific journals.[31] Throughout this wide-ranging review of virological theory and technique, he is not only characteristically charming, but also uncharacteristically self-effacing. He even admits that the "historic" approach to attenuating poliovirus, similar to those approaches used for smallpox and yellow fever — in other words, attempting to adapt the virus to a "seemingly unsusceptible host and then waiting for the grace of God to take the teeth out of [it]" — had been wrong. He further concedes that "this author was one of the early culprits," having adapted both Type 1 and Type 2 poliovirus to the brains of laboratory rodents. He explains that although these early polio vaccines had caused humans to develop antibodies, and had triggered no visible illness, the use of monkey kidney tissue cultures and the invention of the plaque purification system had since permitted a far more precise search for avirulent strains.

In the concluding section of the piece, he asks: "What is adaptation, virulence, attenuation? Answers to these questions are either unavailable or within the realm of delightfully speculative hypotheses, indicating that, wise as we may seem to be, there still remains much to be learned." With this commendably humble acknowledgment of human and scientific frailty, Hilary Koprowski shows that, at least when addressing geneticists, he can admit that he and his fellow vaccine-makers are still tentatively feeling their way through the uncertainties of the attenuation process.

However, in another speech delivered in October 1959, the Alvarenga Prize Lecture given to the College of Physicians in Philadelphia, we see a very different side to Koprowski's nature. Entitled "Historical Aspects of the Development of Live Virus Vaccine in Poliomyelitis," it is an unashamed panegyric to his own achievements in the field. At the outset, Koprowski expresses his intention of attempting to trace the origin of poliomyelitis vaccine, and says: "In doing so I shall be obliged occasionally to dispel certain myths and make sure that the legends and parables surrounding these myths are not substituted for history." Nonetheless, several sections of the address are named after various of the labors of Heracles — the overall attenuation process, for instance, to the taming of "The Ceryneian Hind," and viral purification to the cleaning of "The Stables of Augeias."

He is not slow to acknowledge his own primacy in the field, observing: "It was . . . not too easy to bring over to our side the indifferent and the undecided, since my associates and I were alone in this field when the work began, and remained so for several years. Gradually, however, other scientists became aware of this problem and joined us in this field of endeavor, which by then was developing rapidly." He ends even more pointedly, quoting Schopenhauer's aphorism on merit: "There are two ways of behaving with regard to merit: either to have some of one's own, or to refuse any to others."

In this speech, Koprowski displays few doubts about his own merit, and he makes some rather inflated claims about the use of his own vaccines. He states that "ten million children and adolescents in Poland are being vaccinated now," even if the true figure was then around seven million.[32] And he adds: "More vaccination campaigns organized in several provinces of the Belgian Congo are raising the number of vaccinated individuals into the millions." In fact, even if the actual vaccinations in the Congo were many more than officially reported, "millions" is an exaggeration.[33]

---

Koprowski had the honor of giving the opening address at the Second International Conference on Live Poliovirus Vaccines, in June 1960, and he entitled his speech "The Tin Anniversary of the Development of Live Poliovirus Vaccine," in commemoration of his first feeding of TN on February 27, 1950. He ended the speech with a story that gently mocked alarmist talk about the dangers of contaminating monkey viruses. "The greatest detective of them all, Sherlock Holmes," he said, "was less impressed by the mysterious stranger on the premises than by the failure of the dog to bark in the night. Perhaps in *The Case of the Spiked Potion* too, the mysterious agents encountered in our laboratories are less significant than all those healthy children who never complain! As Holmes himself remarked: 'In solving a problem of this sort, the grand thing is to be able to reason backwards. That is a very useful accomplishment, and a very easy one, but people do not practice it much.'"

That same afternoon, Ben Sweet and Max Hilleman made their sensational announcement about the dangers of the "vacuolating agent," SV40, in cultures of monkey kidney, and it appears that Koprowski himself quickly did some backward reasoning. Before the year was up, he too was voicing loud concern about the dangers of MKTC, and advocating a wholesale changeover to human diploid cell strains for vaccine production.

However, it was not until 1962 that Hayflick and Koprowski published their seminal paper about the adaptation of CHAT to human diploid cell strains.[34] Many of Koprowski's collaborators, such as Joseph Pagano and Fritz Buser, are still of the opinion that these final polio vaccines made in HDCS were more stable and efficacious than the Sabin strains — and they may well be right. But by this stage, Sabin had already won the polio race, and although Koprowski's erstwhile collaborators, like Böttiger in Sweden, Buser in Switzerland, and Ikic in Croatia, subsequently wrote enthusiastic reports of their trials of Koprowski HDCS vaccines, nobody took very much notice.[35] Koprowski's name no longer appeared on the papers, and he had already switched his attentions to perfecting a rabies vaccine. It seems that he had lost the stomach for the fight — and it is hard not to feel some sympathy for the man.

---

Probably the most interesting paper of all with regard to the history of CHAT was one of the last to appear. It was published late in 1961 in *Virology,* with Stanley Plotkin (now employed by the Wistar rather than the Public Health Service) as lead author, and Hilary Koprowski as last, and it described the intratypic serodifferentiation test (IST), a technique for distinguishing virulent from avirulent strains of poliovirus. In one of the paper's tables, the IST values of seven different pools of CHAT are compared. They are identified as 4B-5, 10A-11, 13, 18G-11, 23, 24, and DS. I had come across all of these, apart from 23 and DS, and it seemed likely that they represented the major pools of CHAT that had been prepared for vaccine trials.[36]

The paper explains that the seven pools include two prepared at the Wistar, three (identified as 4B-5, 18G-11, and DS) prepared in other laboratories, and one (pool 24) that was made in a human diploid cell strain, rather than MKTC. Despite the infuriating failure to identify which two pools out of 10A-11, 13, 23, and 24 were made at the Wistar, and where the other two of these pools might have been prepared (perhaps partly at the Wistar and partly elsewhere), this table still provides far more information about individual pools of CHAT than any other paper ever published by Koprowski and his collaborators.

By this stage, I had some of the details of which pools were fed where. Pool 10A-11 had been fed to hundreds of thousands in Ruzizi; it had also been used in the small-scale early trials in Switzerland and Sweden. Pool 13 had been fed to 76,000 children aged up to five years in Leopoldville, and 2,888 villagers living around Wyszkow in Poland. Pool 18G-11 (or 18) had been fed to over seven million people in Poland; it later emerged that this pool had been prepared at the Wyeth Laboratories in Radnor, Pennsylvania. Pool 23 appeared to have been the last pool of CHAT made in monkey kidney tissue culture. Feedings with this specific pool had not been identified in the literature, but the timings suggested that it might well have been used in the large trials in 1960/1 — involving 360,000 people in Switzerland and 1,340,000 in Croatia, Yugoslavia. Pool 24 was the first trial pool of polio vaccine to be made in Hayflick's original human diploid cell strain, WI-1, and is only known with certainty to have been fed to six infants, at the Harrison Department of Research Surgery, at the University of Pennsylvania Medical School in Philadelphia.

Pool 4B-5 was more of a mystery. There was just a single reference to pool 4B in the literature, and various clues suggested that it had probably been fed to roughly a thousand people in the trials at Moorestown, New Jersey, and Philadelphia.[37]

Pool DS was even more problematical, although its significance was eventually revealed in a paper submitted by Stanley Plotkin in October 1960 to the WHO Study Group on Requirements on Poliomyelitis Vaccine.[38] This is a superbly detailed thirty-seven-page review of the latest developments in OPV research at the Wistar, and it includes an early version of the table in Plotkin's serodifferentiation paper — but the letters DS do not feature. Instead, the pool is described in full, as "De Somer." So here was official confirmation in a publicly available document of what Gaston Ninane had already told me — that the Belgians had prepared their own version of CHAT. It had clearly been made (as Jean Vandepitte and Jenny Alexander had surmised) by Pieter de Somer of Leuven University and the RIT vaccine house.

———————

After four months of research into Hilary Koprowski's polio vaccines, I felt ready. I wrote to his office at Thomas Jefferson University, explaining that I was writing a book about the history of polio vaccination, and requesting an interview. When a month had passed and there was no reply, I decided to phone him. I was put through straightaway.

"Let me describe to you the situation," Koprowski told me in a rather heavy accent. "There is a case, a court case, against *Rolling Stone* for defamation, dealing with polio — that I spread, through polio vaccination, AIDS. Therefore the interview which we can have here . . . may have to take place in my lawyer's office, which wouldn't be bad."

I said that was absolutely fine, and asked how long he could spare for the interview. Koprowski explained that he was recovering from an operation, and would probably find it difficult to sit for several hours at a stretch. Nonetheless, he made it clear that, provided he took the occasional break, we could have as long as I needed.

Back in 1992, he had said he was refusing further interviews on this subject,[39] but a year and a half had now passed since the publication of the Curtis story and, though I didn't realize it, the lawsuit against *Rolling Stone* was about to be resolved. I booked a transatlantic flight and then, feeling excited and a bit nervous, began drawing up a long list of questions.

# 29

My first interview with Hilary Koprowski, professor of microbiology and immunology at Thomas Jefferson University in Philadelphia, took place at the offices of his attorney, Mr. James Beasley, on the morning of October 20, 1993. This was just over two years after his departure from the Wistar Institute, where he had been director since 1957.

I had slept badly the night before and arrived early, feeling nervous, to wait on one of the well-padded sofas in a foyer of mahogany and Laura Ashley pastels. After a few minutes, a strangely familiar figure eased his way through the tall entrance doors. I knew Hilary Koprowski only from the various photographs taken in the fifties, and despite realizing intellectually that he would look much older, I was still somewhat taken aback by the impact that thirty-five years had had. He did not look unwell as such, but he did look gaunt, with sunken cheeks, and there were liver spots on his face and hands. He walked with a slight stoop, and supported himself with a stick. He was wearing a well-cut and expensive overcoat and, as he unbuttoned it, a pair of braces of vivacious design (decorated, it appeared, with pale, pre-Raphaelite beauties clad in lustrous reds and blues) peeped through from beneath. Still life in the old dog, then.

I rose from the sumptuous sofa, and Dr. Koprowski shuffled toward me, an appraising look on his face. "You have kind eyes," he said, as we shook hands. "Are you a kind man?"

There was no doubt about it. It was the opening move of a game of chess.

As we traveled upstairs together in the tiny wooden lift, Dr. Koprowski explained that he was still recovering from the effects of an abdominal operation a few weeks earlier. His problems, he told me, probably stemmed from an episode when he had swum off the Galapagos. Before I had the chance to ponder whether this frail old man was actually a latter-day Darwin, prepared to brave the vicissitudes of foreign travel and an indigenous flora and fauna in the pursuit of science, we were ushered into James Beasley's capacious office.

Koprowski's attorney asked a few brief questions (notably whether I had anything to do with *Rolling Stone* or its lawyers), and then he told me that while the court case was still under way, I would not be allowed to ask any questions about "that controversy." He would sit in on the interview, he said, at which point I was allowed to switch on the recorder and start in with my questions. In fact, as the morning progressed, Beasley became visibly restless, and by noon (by which time it was clear that I was not subjecting his client to too severe a grilling), he began leaving the room to attend to other matters.

First I asked Dr. Koprowski what he considered to be his major contribution to medicine, and he answered, rather formally: "My major contribution to medicine was development of the live oral polio vaccine, and massive vaccination [with] that vaccine. Mass vaccination." Even after living for nearly half a century in America, his Polish accent was still very pronounced, and his grammar somewhat uncertain. I was somewhat taken aback, especially in view of his reputation as a linguist.

I inquired about his early years, and he answered in some detail. He started playing piano with his mother at the age of five, he told me, and at the age of twelve won a scholarship to study at the Warsaw *conservatoire*. The next four years were hard, for he had to study at school during the morning and early afternoon, before moving to the *conservatoire* at four o'clock each day, and completing his piano practice and two lots of homework during the evening. It seems likely that his mother was a driving force during these early years in his life, and by his mid-teens he was already playing with considerable flair and authority, and was spoken of as something of a prodigy.

Then, from age sixteen to twenty-two, between 1933 and 1939, he attended medical school in Warsaw, graduating just before the September invasion by Germany, which marked the start of the Second World War. "I was always interested in . . . what then was called basic biological phenomena, rather than practical aspects of medicine," he added. During his third year of study, he became a volunteer assistant at the Department of Experimental Pathology of the University of Warsaw, and he spent the following summer at University College, Dublin, working on blood ammonia. This was also the subject of his first published paper, which appeared in the *Biochemical Journal* in 1939.[1] By this time he was already married, to Irena, a fellow scientist whom he had met at university.[2]

Shortly before the German invasion, the Koprowski family fled to Rome. He stayed there until 1940, receiving his full music diploma from the local *conservatoire* and, in a "completely illegal operation," acting as a physician for the Polish draft board, working out of the embassy and giving medical examinations to those volunteering for the Polish army in exile. Koprowski told a story of a man who came in to renew his passport, but who ended up in a line of naked medical examinees. It was a good tale, and I found myself beginning to respond to his undoubted charm. As he relaxed, it was clear that the years had lent his face (with its gray eyes and long, curved nose) a handsomeness that was perhaps less evident when he was younger. Those eyes were the clincher, for they could twinkle conspiratorially or cut right through you, according to mood.

In June 1940, just before Italy joined the war, the Koprowski family had to flee ahead of the fighting once again, this time traveling to Portugal and then to Brazil. Koprowski ended up in Rio, where, walking disconsolately through the city one day, he came across an old friend from Warsaw who advised him to try for a position at the local branch of the Rockefeller Foundation. The next day he went along for a chat with the director and, despite having rather poor English, was pleasantly surprised when he was offered a job.

He spent the next four years working with the virologist Edwin Lennette at the Yellow Fever Research Service, funded jointly by the Rockefeller Foundation and the Brazilian Ministry of Health. Part of the work involved investigations into encephalitis (which sometimes used to occur after yellow fever vaccination), which stood Koprowski in good stead for his subsequent research into other neurotropic viruses (those which affect the central nervous system), like rabies and polio. In 1943 they conducted a contact experiment with Venezuelan equine encephalomyelitis virus (VEEV), in which they injected a large number of laboratory mice and put them in boxes with some uninfected mice. A few hours later, several of the lab staff experienced severe flu-like symptoms, including fevers and headaches of shattering intensity. Lennette and Koprowski then conducted a second, similar experiment, in the course of which they themselves became infected. All eight VEEV infectees were able to return to work within a fortnight, though both of the chief researchers reported the continuance of such symptoms as shaking hands and insomnia for a longer period. The investigators later isolated this "very, very volatile" virus from six of the eight patients, thus proving that the equine virus could be transmitted to humans, and their results were swiftly published by the prestigious *Journal of the American Medical Association*.[3]

Koprowski added that about three years later the U.S. army developed a successful vaccine against this virus, with which it immunized its soldiers. This indicated that its potential as a biological warfare agent was swiftly recognized, but I didn't ask whether there was any direct link between his own research into VEEV and the development of the military vaccine.[4]

In 1944, many of the American research personnel in Brazil began moving out of the country, and Hilary was awarded a United States immigration visa. He arrived in his newly adopted home in November of that year, and immediately gravitated toward the headquarters of the Rockefeller Institute in New York, where he began writing up several papers based on his and Lennette's Brazilian data.

He clearly hoped to gain full employment with the institute, but in this he was disappointed. Nonetheless, while there, he got to know both Peter Olitsky (Albert Sabin's boss) and the virologist Max Theiler. It was apparently Olitsky who suggested to Koprowski that he should consider working for one of his former pupils, Herald Cox, at Lederle Laboratories, part of American Cyanamid. Koprowski explained that he had great reservations about joining a commercial institution, but that he was eventually won over by another great virologist, George Hirst (the later director of the New York Public Health Research Institute), who assured him that working commercially was fine, provided one maintained one's standards.

He joined Lederle as a research associate under Herald Cox at the end of 1944, after which he continued to visit Theiler to discuss the possibility of developing a live attenuated viral vaccine against polio — just like Theiler's 17D for yellow fever, which was the first truly successful attenuated vaccine. The great man was apparently very interested, and he encouraged Koprowski to continue this line of research. Koprowski said that more than that, Theiler gave him his chief technician, Thomas W. Norton, as well. Norton played an enormously important role in the early work on polio because, after spending so many years with Theiler, he was "an extremely skillful lab worker . . . [a] very talented man." This, Koprowski explained, was why he subsequently named his first attenuated polio vaccine (TN) in Norton's honor. Meanwhile, Lederle had acknowledged Koprowski's potential by appointing him, in 1946, as assistant director to Cox in the Section of Viral and Rickettsial Research. He was to remain in that position for the next eleven years.

Why, I asked Koprowski, did he believe from the very start that the best approach to immunization was with live attenuated vaccines? He told me he felt that such vaccines could provide lifetime immunity, and that attenuated viruses might eventually replace virulent wild viruses in the environment. He also felt that for the developing world, killed vaccines were expensive and impractical, compared to a single dose of live vaccine (which could often be administered by mouth, as in the case of polio). He added that he had seen someone in Cairo receiving rabies shots after being exposed to the virus, and had wondered then how many people would be likely to continue with the full course of fourteen or twenty-one extremely painful injections of killed rabies vaccine. How much better it would be if someone could develop an attenuated vaccine that required only a single shot — like the Fleury rabies vaccine, which he later developed.

Koprowski then gave me a little background to the development of TN Type 2 polio vaccine. It had been reported some years earlier that the cotton rat was susceptible to injections of poliovirus, and so they had taken virulent Type 2 virus, and passed it first through Swiss albino mice and then through cotton rat brain, using the technique of limited dilution, whereby each passage would be diluted down to the minimum concentration at which infectious particles could still be detected. Eventually, it was assumed, all the virulent strains of poliovirus would be weeded out of the preparation, and it would be attenuated. They then tested the virulence of the preparation by injecting it into the brains of monkeys, the principle being that if it caused paralysis, it was insufficiently attenuated. After this, they made a larger pool of the vaccine, checked it for possible bacterial contamination, tested it again in monkeys — with the result, he stressed, that "again all monkeys survived"— and finally fed it to humans. He added that he and Tom Norton were the first two humans to be fed the virus. Apparently they already had the appropriate antibodies, but "we wanted to know whether anybody would swallow such a horrid mixture. And luckily it tasted like cod-liver oil."

What Koprowski was now telling me conflicted with what is to be found in his own published papers in two important ways — first, as regards the safety testing in monkeys. In reality half of the forty-four monkeys injected with TN pool 16 (the pool fed to the first Letchworth Village children) became paralyzed, and ten of them died. Second, according to his own papers, it was *not* he and Norton who were the first to be fed TN. It was actually the Letchworth children who were first, and the two adult volunteers fed were Tom Norton and Herald Cox, who were vaccinated nearly a year later.[5]

During this part of the discussion, there was a particularly significant moment. As soon as monkeys were mentioned for the first time (in the context of safety testing the trial vaccine by injecting it into monkey brains), Koprowski volunteered the information that these had been "rhesus monkeys — there are no others." This again was incorrect, for in a later paper Koprowski and Norton reported that both chimpanzees and cynomolgus monkeys had also been used at Lederle at this very time, beginning in 1949, in vaccination experiments with TN.[6] The question of monkey species was indeed a key issue, but it was one that I did not wish to broach until later in the interview.

When I asked Koprowski when he had first tested TN in chimpanzees, he answered that "strangely enough, the chimps came later than the humans." This appeared to be commendably candid, but I quickly realized that Koprowski had apparently completely forgotten his own trials of TN in chimpanzees between 1949 and 1952. "No chimps," he went on. "This went first in humans. There were no chimps available then in U.S."[7] He continued: "Of course the chimp work — let me jump to the Congo — was based on whether the chimp reacts to the vaccination and to the challenge the same as humans. You couldn't challenge humans [with virulent virus, to check if the vaccination had worked], but you could challenge chimps." He later added that "a relatively large colony of chimps" was needed to carry out vaccination and challenge experiments, and that they didn't at that stage have such a colony. The clear inference was that this was why they had created the colony at Lindi in the Congo.

This was intriguing. In his one published paper on Lindi, Koprowski had recorded injecting both CHAT and Fox into the brains of five chimpanzees, as an extra safety test for the vaccines in addition to the normal monkey safety test. He had also mentioned vaccination and challenge work, but only in a passing reference to "virulent poliovirus used for challenge of vaccinated chimpanzees." No further details of this research had been provided in the *British Medical Journal* paper. And neither, when I questioned him now, was he able to provide any further information, though he did say if I wrote such questions down, he would try to check for me.

Once again, I had to wonder why the chimpanzee experiments, which Koprowski had considered so vital for the development of his polio vaccines, had been so poorly documented — and why, even now, he was apparently so forgetful (or was it reticent?) on this subject.

———————

Hilary Koprowski's account of the first human feedings of TN vaccine at Letchworth Village, a large center for mentally handicapped children near Thiells, on the west bank of the Hudson in upstate New York, was far more straightforward. He explained that George Jervis, who was the director of laboratories at Letchworth, used to come and visit them at Lederle, which was the nearest scientific institution, just a dozen miles away. They discussed a variety of research matters, and Jervis said how afraid he was that an outbreak of polio might occur among the Letchworth children, since many of them were in the habit of throwing feces at each other, and sometimes eating them too. Eventually it was decided that the two institutions would help each other. Koprowski would supply them with the new vaccine, TN, and Jervis would take responsibility for feeding it to the children. The only things that the Lederle team requested in return were serum samples, taken before and after vaccination, to check the polio antibody levels, and stool samples, so that they could check for how many days after vaccination the vaccine virus was excreted through the alimentary tract. Koprowski described it as a "good bargain. . . . The deal was made, and he fed, on February 27, 1950, the first child in the world [with] live poliovirus."

This was one date, it seemed, that Koprowski would never forget. Although he had apparently been present,[8] he did not provide any further details about the actual mechanics of the feeding. This was perhaps because (according to his own paper in 1952) the first vaccinee, a six-year-old boy, was so handicapped that he had to be fed the vaccine through a stomach tube.

Koprowski told me that this research "was kept quiet" for a year, until the Hershey conference convened by the National Fund for Infantile Paralysis in March 1951. He had been invited to talk about approaches to rabies vaccination, and instead staged a coup de théâtre by announcing the first successful human feedings of OPV, to the consternation of Tom Francis (Salk's mentor from Pittsburgh, who would later organize the first IPV trials) and the concern of Albert Sabin about the potential implications. His comprehensive account of the experiment, with dates of feeding, specific pool numbers, and so forth, was published a year later.

The next major development, Hilary Koprowski told me, was that tissue culture techniques became available, following the pioneering work by John Enders and colleagues in 1949. By this time, he explained, his Type 1 strain, SM, had been developed, and news of his OPV research had spread around the world. Two important people had become interested, these being Karl F. Meyer, the director of the George Williams Hooper Foundation, based at the University of California in San Francisco, and Joseph Stokes Jr., the professor of pediatrics at the Children's Hospital of Philadelphia. And it was under their auspices that the feeding trials were enlarged, so that TN and SM were fed at two other homes for mentally handicapped children — the Sonoma State Home just north of San Francisco, and the Woodbine facility in southeastern New Jersey. He was unsure of the precise dates, but thought that these trials had mainly occurred in 1954 and 1955. At both homes, local physicians took on the job of monitoring the clinical status of each vaccinee, and obtaining serum and stool specimens, while Koprowski and Norton took care of the lab work.

Koprowski explained that SM, his Type 1 vaccine, had been prepared in monkey kidney tissue culture, again through limited dilution techniques, "collecting the material which was *barely* passable, *barely* infectious, making another pool," and so on. He added, however, that "if I remember correctly — you have to check on reprints — there was also a passage in an unusual host, like chick embryo." Later, he explained that these were the two essential methods of attenuation: terminal dilution, and the passage of the virus through unusual hosts — like cotton rat brain or chick embryo — which served to modify the virus to a point where it was still able to infect, but was almost completely apathogenic. "My views were the following," he summarized. "Whatever it needs . . . to get to nonparalytic strain for monkeys, use that. It doesn't matter which."

Even if he was unsure about the various stages of preparation of SM, he was certain about one thing — that the final substrate had always been monkey kidney tissue culture. "Never chick embryo?" I asked. "No, the pool of feeding always was monkey kidney," he replied. "The chick embryo was too low a titer to make any pool in the world."

So it was that Hilary Koprowski confirmed my suspicion that from 1955 onward he had been using monkey kidney as the final vaccine substrate. It seemed that he had forgotten that in his published articles of the time, he had claimed to be using chick embryo.[9]

When I asked how he procured the monkeys, he told me that Lederle had had many; "remember we worked for a commercial institution and money didn't matter as far as buying monkeys." They used hundreds of monkeys every year, he told me, and then added swiftly: "all rhesus monkeys." No cynomolgus? I asked. "No," he answered, "and the tissue cultures which we used were rhesus monkey kidney." This was intriguing. During 1992 he had been remarkably equivocal, claiming at different times that he had used tissue cultures derived from African green monkeys, rhesus, cynomolgus, and already excised kidneys from an unknown source. But now, it seems, the ambiguity had been replaced by certainty: he had used rhesus and only rhesus.[10]

We discussed some of the specifics of the Sonoma vaccinations with SM and TN — how he and Norton had carried the vaccine strains across to San Francisco in two thermos flasks; how they had first had to seek permission for the trial from the local commissioner of health; how Norton and another technician, Doris Nelsen, had investigated the serum and stool samples at the Hooper Foundation labs in San Francisco. And what had been the main findings that came out of Sonoma? He answered this one readily. "That Type 1 and Type 2 [vaccines] do produce protective antibodies, that you have excretion of virus, and that it is not transmitted to contacts." I pointed out that in fact the vaccine virus had been transmitted to five of fifteen potential child contacts, but Koprowski replied that "it was limited to those who throw feces . . . but not those who take care of the children." This was a fair distinction, although it was not entirely accurate. Three of the five contact infections occurred among children who were deemed to be at only "slight" or "moderate" risk of reception or ingestion of feces, while elaborate precautions (the changing of shoes, the donning of gowns, and the disinfecting and frequent washing of hands) were taken to prevent infection of the nursing staff.[11]

I asked him about the controversial serial passage experiment at Sonoma, in which virus excreted by one child was passaged in monkey kidney and then fed to another child, up to a total of six human passages. It was an important experiment, he said, in order to check that the vaccine did not revert to virulence after passing through the human gut; he himself had not been involved, but Thomas Nelson, the Sonoma superintendent, had fed the passaged virus to the children, and must have sent the resulting stools across to Tom Norton to evaluate in monkey kidney tissue culture.[12] Within the context of the era, this was a vital test to carry out, and indeed Smorodintsev in the Soviet Union went even further, completing a series of eleven or twelve human passages of all three of Sabin's strains.[13]

We talked some more about the problems of live virus spreading (which, he said, was no problem, in that it was now accepted as beneficial if attenuated viruses replaced wild ones in the environment) and of reversion to virulence (he said that there was no evidence that any of his vaccines had reverted, and that, in any case, the safety tests used to pick up reversion were so sensitive that they erred on the side of safety). I asked whether this had not been, in many respects, the dark age of virology, with scientists moving around blindly, feeling their way as they went. He said that it was easy to look back from the vantage of today and to ask "why didn't you do this and that?" but that the necessary knowledge and technology simply hadn't been there in the fifties. He added that nowadays it wouldn't even be allowed to safety test vaccines by inoculating them into the brains of monkeys. "So it had a little advantage, the 'dark age,'" he concluded.

I asked about the Cutter incident, and whether it had not given a great boost to the cause of OPV, at a time when it looked as if IPV was about to win the race. He replied that IPV only gave short-term immunity, and that it was useless as a global vaccine. Furthermore, he added, he had always maintained that "you are in better shape using a known live virus which you check for safety," than to have surprises caused by a virulent virus that has been improperly inactivated. The Cutter incident "was one of many incidents, of many incidents" caused by inactivated vaccines, he said, and he gave other examples, such as a poorly prepared rabies vaccine that had started killing children in Fortaleza, Brazil, in 1963. He made it clear that the only inactivation procedures he felt were fully adequate were those proposed by Sven Gard ("an excellent scientist") in Sweden, before adding that in Sweden they "*never* use live virus [OPV]." Once again, he had volunteered a piece of information that I knew to be wrong. In fact, more than five thousand doses of live vaccine had been fed in Sweden, and the OPV in question had been CHAT, his own strain.

He then spoke a little about Albert Sabin, reminding me of how originally, in 1951, Sabin had had "a great deal of reservations" about OPV, but that he had later acknowledged that it was Koprowski's pioneering work which had given him the idea of pursuing the OPV approach. In the end, Koprowski said, "it was proven a number of times that there was no difference" between his strains and Sabin's. He realized, however, that he was "working against the odds" when the National Foundation for Infantile Paralysis shifted its support from Salk to Sabin, and when he, because of his commercial backing, received nothing from the NFIP.

In the course of the day, there were many, many times when Koprowski simply answered "I don't remember"; "I don't recall." On several occasions he explained that some time before he had undertaken a spring-cleaning of his memory banks. "I frankly tell you," he said, "that there are things which I try to clear from my memory. I can give you the principles and I have a very good recall memory for the important things. But the details [of] how many pools are prepared, the titers of each pool, I have no knowledge. And I don't think that knowledge is recoverable, because of death of Mr. Norton."

Hilary Koprowski was getting tired, and when I asked him what he recalled about the vaccinations at Clinton Farms, the women's prison in New Jersey, he seemed happy to return to the sort of anecdotal memories that had clearly not been discarded during the spring-cleaning. He told me that the thing about Clinton was "there were no guards. If there were guards, they were inconspicuous. The only problem with these women was that Route [78] passed next to Clinton Farms. They used to go up and stop a truck, climb next to the driver, have an intercourse within the next mile, return to the prison, and often became pregnant. Therefore Miss Mahan [the prison governor] was on hand with newborn children, and she again was afraid if there would be an epidemic of infantile paralysis." This struck me as being pleasingly colorful, but a most unlikely account of how the Clinton prisoners came to conceive their children — however radical and trusting Miss Mahan's regime might have been. I mentioned this, and Koprowski responded: "If you write that down, can you imagine what you will get from the feminist organization? . . . Enormously furious."

He told other tales of Clinton, too, funnier and less fanciful ones. These featured several colorful characters, such as the prisoner who used to cook excellent dinners for Koprowski, Stokes, and Norton when they visited — and who turned out to be serving a life sentence for poisoning her husband; Agnes Flack, the prison medical officer, who ended up flying out to the Congo to help with the vaccinations there; and Mrs. Roosevelt, the president's widow, who used to attend the graduation ceremonies. Most of the prisoners, he told me, ended up with some form of professional training, as accountants, cooks, beauticians, or whatever. What was abundantly clear, however, was that Edna Mahan was a remarkable woman, and an inspired prison reformer, and that many of the inmates would have followed her through fire. Koprowski himself was clearly impressed. "Feeble-minded homes I would like to forget. But these [were] unforgettable experiences. . . ."

As lunchtime approached, I realized that there was no chance that I could complete the rest of the interview in the time remaining, and we began making arrangements for a continuation the following week. I did, however, ask him one last question, about his first attempts to stage vaccine trials in Africa, in places like Tristan da Cunha and South Africa. Koprowski eventually acknowledged that the planned trials had probably never taken place — "for whatever reasons I don't remember." He said that he had recently received a letter from the South African James Gear, and that it had mentioned these planned trials. He would look up the letter, he said, before our next appointment.

He asked me to jot down any particular points that I wanted him to check, including such details as dates. He also hinted that his wife might be willing to let me see the scrapbook of newspaper clippings that she had kept over the years. I was impressed by the amount of time he seemed prepared to spend with me, and by his willingness to cooperate. Eventually a time and place were agreed for the continuation of the interview, and we parted on good terms.

Like so many of the best-laid plans, however, this one was about to go spectacularly awry.

———

When I arrived at his office in Thomas Jefferson University a week later, I knew straightaway that something was wrong. I suspected that it might be something to do with James Gear, and I was right. At the start of 1993, I had written Gear a letter, asking a number of questions about Koprowski and his polio research in Africa. The information I had been seeking included the dates of his visits to South Africa, whether any of his OPVs had ever been fed there, and whether there were any significant differences in manufacture between CHAT and the South African oral polio vaccine. Gear had written back to state that no Koprowski vaccines had ever been used in South Africa, but for most of my remaining questions, he had advised me to contact Koprowski. As I had feared when Koprowski mentioned having recently heard from Gear, the two men were friends, and Gear had sent him a copy of my letter. I found him at his desk, with the copy in front of him.

He explained that both he and his attorney had had copies of the letter for some months, but that both of them had overlooked it when I requested an interview. It was only yesterday, when his secretary was searching out the letter from Gear, that it had come back to his notice. He was sorry, he said, but he would not be able to continue the interview until I had spoken with Ellen Suria, an associate of James Beasley's.

Up to this point, he had been pleasant and controlled, but now suddenly he became angry. He told me that he thought my questions about him to Gear were "an interrogation," and added that even if he did end up completing the interview, he would probably not now answer any questions about Africa. In any case, he said, he might have to take advice about whether or not my letter was actionable. Now it was my turn to become demonstrative. I told him he must be joking if he thought he could take me to court for asking legitimate questions. I said I was sorry that my letter had upset him, and that I would set off immediately to see Ellen Suria. As I walked the few blocks to her office, I realized that in all likelihood this would mark the end of my interview with Koprowski — just as it was getting to the interesting bit.

Ms. Suria was a lot more pleasant than I had expected. I told her that I appeared to have upset Dr. Koprowski with my letter, and that I was dismayed because it seemed to have scuppered the rest of the interview. She replied that they had been a bit shocked at first when they read it, and that they couldn't allow him to answer my questions right now. But, she added, she could tell me in confidence that *Rolling Stone* was about to publish a retraction and apology, probably next week. Once that was in print, she said, it should be possible for me to finish the interview. She advised me to go back right away and tell Koprowski the result of our discussion.

Before I left, however, she showed me two brief articles about Raphael Stricker, Blaine Elswood's coauthor on his articles about CHAT and AIDS.[14] They demonstrated that several years earlier, Stricker had falsified and suppressed data that was later included in a paper published in the *New England Journal of Medicine*,[15] that the paper in question had subsequently been retracted by its other authors,[16] and that Stricker had had voluntarily to refrain from receiving federal grants or funds for a period of three years.[17] I was shocked by this revelation, which could obviously damage not only Stricker's credibility, but also — by association — that of Elswood and his hypothesis.[18] I was impressed, however, by Suria, and her combination of gentle and tough.

I went back to Koprowski's office, and he was in a far sunnier mood. Yes, he said, if I kept in contact with his secretary, he would finish the interview after the *Rolling Stone* settlement had been completed. He began telling me about the settlement, and about how it would bring an end to this awful matter. The wording of the retraction had been agreed, he confided, but they were still involved in final negotiations about where and when it would appear. *Rolling Stone* wanted it to be on the letters page, which, Koprowski added sourly, was entitled "Love Letters and Advice." He was having none of that. He wanted it published in as prominent a position as the original article, if not more so. In fact, he said, with rising excitement, he felt that to guarantee getting the attention of the readers, it should be published over the picture of a beautiful woman, one who was "naked from the breasts to the genitalia." With his hands, he demonstrated which parts of the body this would involve.

---

In the days following this first interview with Koprowski, I went through my notes of the meeting on several occasions. I was struck first by how selective his memory seemed to be — just as he had explained on several occasions. It appeared that he was well able to recapitulate anecdotes and vignettes, but that he unfortunately had poor recall for his various polio experiments — save, perhaps, for the very first one at Letchworth.

By this stage, I had probably interviewed more than a hundred scientists and doctors in their seventies, eighties, and nineties, and from that perspective, I felt that Koprowski's inability to recall any details at all about certain parts of his research was unusual. It was early days yet, but it seemed that two of the problematical areas involved his work with chimpanzees, and the work carried out in Africa.

The other striking thing about the first interview was that there were several quite significant errors, or inconsistencies, in what he had told me. Some of these I had realized at the time, but had not challenged for fear of jeopardizing the rest of the interview. Others I confirmed only when I got back to my hotel room and had the chance to review the relevant papers. First, there was the claim that he and Tom Norton had been the first humans to be fed TN vaccine, even before the first child "volunteer." Second, there was his insistence that the monkeys used for the safety tests of the first-ever polio vaccine given to humans had all survived. Third were the claims that the only primates he had used at Lederle had been rhesus monkeys, and fourth, that the substrate he had used to manufacture TN and SM had been MKTC (once again derived from rhesus). A fifth instance was his claim that OPV had never been used in Sweden. In each case, the account that Koprowski had given me contradicted reports published in the contemporary literature, or else his more recent statements (for instance about the CHAT/AIDS controversy).

It was notable that all these five statements had been volunteered, unsolicited, in the course of the interview. Sometimes they had popped up unexpectedly — not out of context, exactly, but at the first mention of some related matter. Whatever the vagaries of his memory on other issues, it seemed that these five pieces of information, at least, were details that Koprowski had now placed on the record.

---

A week or so later, I flew across to California to spend some days with an old friend from Africa, while I completed my West Coast researches. He lived in a clapboard house in Berkeley, and I slept on a soft and ancient mattress, which prompted strangely evocative dreams. Three of them were memorable enough to write down upon waking, and all of them contained multiple images of the AIDS investigation.

The last of these dreams took place in what seemed to be a Middle Eastern police station (possibly inspired by the film *Midnight Express*). I parked my car, went inside, and asked to speak to the man in charge. I was told to sit down and wait. Lots of others were waiting also. The man in charge seemed to be feared. Suddenly, however, he strode in and, in contrast to his reputation, he seemed friendly. After a while, he led me out to the back of the police station, where there was a large, deserted garage full of oil drums. I started asking questions, but he cut me short by asking if I wanted to see the vaccine. I was surprised, but answered that yes, I did want to see it. With a smile, he produced a small vial, and I thought I could see "10A-11" written on it. I asked if I could examine it more closely, and now I could see the "10," at least, quite clearly. He handed it to me but, as I held it up closer, the numbers disappeared. Instead, printed vertically on the side of the vial, below a treble clef, was a five-note musical phrase. I knew that these five notes were familiar, but couldn't quite make them out.

At this point I woke, and there was a tune playing in my head. It was the "uh-oh" motif from stage and screen melodramas, the one that ends with a *fortissimo* piano trill as the villain flings open a door at the back of the set and, swirling his black cape around him, advances onto center stage.

# 30

## THE WEST COAST TRIALS

One of the things that most fascinated me about CHAT was the name. Nowhere in the literature was its origin explained. Sometimes Koprowski and his Wistar colleagues wrote it as "CHAT," in capitals, as if it were a set of initials or an acronym; other times as "Chat," as in an abbreviation. Certainly it was an intriguing departure from the two letter titles of the first two Koprowski vaccines, TN and SM, and from Fox — named after John Fox of Tulane University, who provided the original Type 3 isolate from a symptom-free poliovirus carrier.[1]

There were no further clues in the scientific literature, but there was a single reference in a *Time* article about the Ruzizi vaccinations, dating from August 1958, which claimed that CHAT was named after "the initials of the child from whom it was taken," which presumably meant the fourth child in the human serial passage study at Sonoma, whose stool had contained the appropriate virus.[2] The *Time* reporter had not specified a source, though it may well have been Koprowski himself, for the tone of the report was one of glowing praise, and the reporter appeared to have had access to inside information.[3]

However, there were also other possible interpretations, some of which highlighted the importance of the role played by chimpanzees in the development of CHAT. The full name of Sabin's Type 2 vaccine was "P-712 Ch 2ab," with the "Ch" indicating that the vaccine virus had been passed once through the alimentary canal of a chimpanzee. If the "Ch" in CHAT or Chat was also taken to represent "chimpanzee," then the name could indicate that the vaccine was "chimpanzee-attenuated" (perhaps meaning, as with P-712, that it had been passaged through the gut of a chimp or chimps), or else "chimpanzee adapted and tested" (perhaps meaning that it had been adapted to the chimpanzee host by single or multiple passage, and then tested for virulence in the same species). The latter was the version tentatively suggested by Louis Pascal in "What Happens When Science Goes Bad."[4]

Then I came across an article by Renato Dulbecco and colleagues, published in 1957, which compared the virulence of various poliovirus strains.[5] They had tested several wild and attenuated polioviruses, including OPVs supplied by Sabin and Koprowski. The latter had supplied one Type 3 strain — "Fox, pool 12" — and two Type 1 strains — "SM N-90, pool 21" and "Charlton, plaque 20." Given the fact that Dulbecco gave a preliminary discussion of this work at the New York Academy of Sciences conference early in January 1957, the research seemed likely to have been conducted in the latter half of 1956.[6] It seemed almost certain that Charlton plaque 20 equated with CHAT plaque 20, which was the variant of CHAT that Koprowski and Norton had tested in early 1957 in the spinal cords of the five Lindi chimpanzees.[7]

This still did not explain why the name had been abbreviated from Charlton, although one possible explanation might have been to avoid confusion with a naturally attenuated Type 1 poliovirus that had been christened "Charleston" after the town in which it was isolated.[8] This was incorporated as the Type 1 component of an IPV manufactured in Belgium,[9] which had already been tested on humans by June 1957.[10] Another reason might have been that Koprowski felt the need for a new name for a Type 1 strain that had been largely developed at Lederle, but on which he now intended to base his polio vaccine work at the Wistar Institute. However, it was also not impossible that the name "CHAT" had been chosen for more than one reason. Perhaps it represented the initials, or the abbreviated name of a child, but also contained an allusion to the chimp work — one which could be revealed in the fullness of time if it proved a successful vaccine, and if the climate of public opinion allowed.

---

The Sonoma Developmental Center, as it is now called, is claimed by some of its staff to be the largest such facility in the world. When the institution was founded in 1891, it was known as the California Home for the Care and Training of Feeble-Minded Children. By the 1950s it was called simply the Sonoma State Home, and housed thirty-seven hundred mentally handicapped children, together with the fifteen hundred staff members who cared for them. Nowadays, this is home to some thirteen hundred developmentally disabled child patients from all over northern California; they suffer from a range of largely congenital conditions, including cerebral palsy, Down's syndrome, and hydrocephaly.

During the First World War, Jack London, who lived near the valley, wrote a short story entitled "Told in the Drooling Ward," which described Sonoma from the perspective of one of its patients.[11] Although the title is ironic, the story is unusually sentimental for London, and carries more than a hint of shocked sensibilities. Hilary Koprowski was also disturbed by the condition of some of the children, and would later attempt to put a romantic — even a heroic — gloss on his experiences here. In his Alvarenga Prize lecture of 1959, in which he reviews his own achievements in the field of polio vaccination, he refers to his work at Sonoma in the context of Greek mythology. He describes the "fateful meeting" that took place in New York, in January 1952, between Joseph Smadel (who Koprowski identifies as a later associate director of the U.S. Public Health Service, though he was then a senior scientist at the Walter Reed Army Medical Center),[12] Karl Meyer (director of the G. W. Hooper Foundation at the University of California), and himself, as follows: "I was looking for counsel from Nereus and Prometheus. Dr. Smadel was familiar with our work on the immunization of man with living poliomyelitis virus and suggested to Dr. Meyer and myself that we establish a co-operative study. This led to prolonged and fruitful collaboration, when the search for the golden apples of the Hesperides was conducted near the Golden Gate, more precisely, in Jack London's *Valley of the Moon*. . . . Plucking of the golden apples in this eleventh labor of Heracles took several years, but the results . . . of the investigations were very gratifying."

---

Koprowski's main collaborator at Sonoma had been a young pediatrician with a growing reputation by the name of Thomas Nelson. By the time of my visit to California in late 1993, Dr. Nelson was seventy-two years old and retired. When I requested an interview, he suggested that we should meet at Sonoma itself, which seemed an excellent idea. One morning in late fall I drove up from San Francisco along Route 12, past vineyards, groves of redwood, and piles of boulders clustered in open fields, turning off along the scenic route for the Valley of the Moon. As I rolled through the main gates of Sonoma, and over the speed bumps, I was struck by how few of the children were to be seen. Presently, I arrived at a large grassy rectangle lined with palm trees, around the edges of which lay the various administration blocks and the hospital. Away to the north, spaced along wide, deciduous avenues, were dozens of single-story cottages housing Sonoma's children.

I was led up to a conference room and there introduced to Dr. Nelson and to various current members of the staff. It was apparent that things had been arranged ahead of time, and we sat around a large table, while Dr. Nelson delivered what appeared to be a semirehearsed speech about his ten years at Sonoma, and the polio trials. Interestingly, none of the present staff seemed to be aware that such research had taken place forty years earlier.

The background to the trials was interesting. In 1951, after graduating in pediatrics from the University of California–San Francisco, Nelson was appointed chief pediatrician at Sonoma — a position that appealed to him partly because of the tremendous potential it afforded for research. At this time the state home was essentially a self-contained village of some five thousand souls; it was spread over sixteen hundred acres, and had fruit orchards and farms that kept it supplied with dairy produce, poultry, and pork. It also had its own fire and police departments, a railway station, and a post office. Dr. Nelson effectively became the chief physician for all the nurseries, and of the acute-care hospital, which had one hundred beds and was staffed by various full-time specialists, ranging from surgeons and radiologists to psychiatrists and pediatricians. He immediately began doing epidemiological and clinical research into the various parasitic diseases that used to plague the crowded cottages where the children resided.

Some time early in 1952, soon after the "fateful meeting" in New York, Karl Meyer asked Thomas Nelson if he was interested in staging trials of Koprowski's vaccines at Sonoma. Meyer told him that "money's not a problem . . . Koprowski's got the money . . . he said you just develop a budget." The cash was to be channeled through the Hooper Foundation, so that from the perspective of the state of California, the trial was being funded by academic rather than commercial sources. Nelson was happy to accept, not least because his uncle had died of polio, and he himself had been partially paralyzed by the virus at the age of five, leaving him with one leg shorter than the other.

There was less red tape in those days, and with Meyer's assistance the appropriate clearances (up to the level of the state departments of mental hygiene and public health) were swiftly obtained. So it was that in July 1952 they test-fed TN vaccine to 61 Sonoma children aged from eight months to eight years. Tom Norton flew to California to oversee the experiment, which seemed to go successfully, for 52 of the 61 children showed a significant rise in antibody levels and were considered to have been immunized. Dr. Nelson told us he thought that this early trial was conducted in the rear of Cromwell cottage, but that he recalled very few of the details.

The success of that first trial encouraged the collaborators to proceed further. In March 1954, following a meeting between Karl Meyer, Koprowski, and George Jervis, a draft protocol for a second set of Sonoma trials was sent to Nelson for information and comment. Essentially, what was being proposed was a joint trial of TN and SM, and a separate trial of MEF1, the Lederle Type 2 strain adapted to chick embryo by Manuel Roca-Garcia.

By 1954, Tom Nelson was assistant superintendent, and once again it was made clear to him that no expense should be spared. In November of that year, the sera of about five hundred Sonoma children were evaluated at Lederle, since only those children who lacked antibodies to one or both of Type 1 and Type 2 polio would be included in the experiment. Nelson then hired a team of pedi-atric social workers, who were given vehicles and sent out around Northern California in order to explain the trial to the parents of potential participants, and to obtain their written consent.

A newly built cottage, Lathrop, containing two open wards and a group of isolation rooms, was used for the trial. Thirty-two registered nurses were spe-cially hired and installed for the duration (April to July 1955) at a "very plush hotel" in a local resort.[13] Led by the redoubtable Kate Smith, a former pediatric nurse and administrator from the University of California Hospital, their job was to provide round-the-clock supervision and care for the 70 children aged between six and fifteen who had been selected as vaccinees.[14] In practice, this meant that about eight nurses worked each shift. This was a very different level of care to that which typically obtained at Sonoma where, Nelson explained, three nurses per shift might be employed to look after the 150 residents in a single cottage. A young clinician, Dave Chadwick, was hired to oversee the oper-ation and to check on the clinical status of all the participants.[15]

The children were fed the SM vaccine in gelatin capsules, and the TN in the form of a raspberry milkshake. Later, the nurses had to obtain the many blood and stool samples that were required by Tom Norton, whose whole life, accord-ing to Nelson, "seemed devoted to the study. [He was even] more compulsive than I was." Norton and Doris Nelsen had flown in from Lederle, and were based in the Hooper Foundation labs in San Francisco, testing the stool samples to see how long the different polioviruses were being excreted, and the postvac-cination blood samples to evaluate antibody levels.

Before entering Lathrop, the special nurses (and the few visitors who were admitted) had to don caps, gowns, and booties, which were to be removed on leaving. The two wards and the isolation wing were separated by a central hall, and to reduce the risk of cross infection, it was forbidden for anyone to travel from one experimental area to another without first washing and changing. "This was very, very strict isolation, because we were terribly afraid that the virus would get out . . . into the community," Nelson explained.

One of the things that the researchers wished to establish was whether the vaccine viruses could spread from one child to another under various condi-tions. In one ward they placed vaccinees and nonvaccinees in neighboring cots, to see whether nonvaccinees became infected. (Two out of seven did, and it was presumed that this was related to the fact that feces-throwing was a popular form of interaction for some of the children.) In the other ward they put "the intimate contact group"— children who were encouraged to play together each day on the same plastic mat — touching each other, sharing toys, and so forth. This time, three out of eight nonvaccinees became infected. They also used ten isola-tion rooms, in each of which two children were put in cots in opposite corners, as part of a titration study to determine the ideal concentration of the vaccine.

Later that morning, Nelson took me on a tour of the grounds, where the streets were wide and gracious and planted with dozens of different exotic trees. At one point he told me that there had in fact been an outbreak of polio at Sonoma shortly after one of the studies ended: four children had become paralyzed in a hut close to where the trial had been held. Because of the crowding and hygiene problems, polio epidemics were not uncommon in institutions like Sonoma, and it may well be that the cluster of cases was entirely unrelated to the vaccinations. Nelson was not entirely certain when this had happened, but later he sent me a newspaper clipping, which revealed that the outbreak had occurred four months after the TN trial on 61 children, which places it in October or November 1952.[16] The article ended by reporting that Koprowski and Meyer had "made a series of tests to find whether the outbreak could possibly have been connected with the experiments. They found, to their relief, that it couldn't have been." Why the details of this investigation did not feature in their medical paper on the trials, published in 1953, is not apparent.[17]

Tom Nelson escorted me around Lathrop, where the 1955 trial had been staged. Although the small cell-like isolation rooms had been replaced, much of the rest still smacked of the fifties — the long corridors, the locked doors, the smell and colors of an institution. At last I got to meet a few of the more mobile children, many of whom were disarmingly trusting and affectionate. I was also reminded of just how severe some of their disabilities were, and of the enormous strains that caring for them must engender. I wondered what it must have been like back in the fifties, when there were more than twice as many children in a ward, and the conditions were far more basic.

Dr. Nelson also showed me the isolation room in the infectious-disease ward of the hospital, which is where the third and final part of the Sonoma trials was staged. Although it had only involved the feeding of four children, this was by far and away the most controversial part of the trials — the serial passage study, staged to see whether or not SM reverted to virulence after human passage. Virus was obtained from the feces of four of those children who had been infected by contact (presumably fecal-oral contact) with SM vaccinees. These viruses, which represented the second human passage of SM, were pooled, checked for virulence by being injected into the brains and spinal cords of cynomolgus monkeys, and then fed to a child who represented the third human passage, and so on until six human passages had been effected. The virus from the last child's stools proved to be innocuous for the eight monkeys tested.

Nelson admitted to me straightaway that such a study could not be carried out today. Although Koprowski, in his New York Academy of Sciences address of 1957, had referenced a paper about the serial passage work by Nelson, Meyer, Norton, and himself, which was apparently "to be published," Nelson told me that no such paper had ever appeared, and added: "I think part of the reason . . . was that we were afraid of criticism." Nelson, however, had himself written up the experiment, and presented his findings to the annual general meeting of the Western Society for Pediatric Research in October 1957.[18] He told me that when he read his paper ". . . there was a great deal of interest. Someone from the audience said that this was a study which shouldn't have been done." Koprowski was not present, and Nelson added that he had been "a little disturbed that he didn't come to answer questions about the lab part of the study."

The society itself has never formally published the text of the speech and does not possess a copy, although Dr. Nelson did manage to locate one for me in his loft. This revealed that the fathers of three of the last four children involved in the trial were physicians, and the fourth was a dentist. They had been deliberately selected on the grounds that they would be able to understand the importance of the study, and the possible dangers of the vaccine reverting to virulence.

Much of the relevant lab data (such as the results of the monkey safety tests) was included in the published version of Koprowski's address to the January 1957 conference in New York.[19] A table in that article showed, intriguingly, that the excreted viruses from some of the last four vaccinees in the trial (coded as C79, C80, C81, and C82) were rather virulent for monkeys. For vaccinee C80, the child whose stool provided the source of the CHAT strain, two of the eight monkeys injected intraspinally with undiluted fecal virus became paralyzed, and three showed lesions of the spinal cord.[20]

Thomas Nelson made it clear that he himself assumed full responsibility for the serial passage study. He said it had almost certainly been staged in 1956, the year he was appointed superintendent at Sonoma, and long after Koprowski and Norton had returned east. It was actually he who had suggested to Koprowski that they should conduct the trial, rather than vice versa; in fact, he said, Koprowski "had had to be persuaded." He explained that since the earlier tests had shown that SM vaccine virus could occasionally infect nonvaccinees, it was important to check whether it was "going to spread from patient to patient, [and revert] back to a street virus," which might then be transmitted among the community at large.

He had personally interviewed the parents of the last four vaccinees, in order to obtain signed consent, and had also set up very strict rules for the trial, to ensure that poliovirus could not escape from the isolation room where it was staged. He oversaw it too, helping to monitor the clinical status of the vaccinees; apparently none showed any evidence of illness related to the vaccine feeding. Nelson reckoned that the entire experiment, involving the feeding of the last four vaccinees and the testing of their fecal viruses by Norton in Pearl River, had probably taken about ten months.

By this stage, we had finished our tour of the hospital block, and I asked Dr. Nelson why it was that the fecal virus of child C80 — a fairly virulent virus — had been chosen by Koprowski as the basis for CHAT vaccine, in preference to the innocuous virus from C82. "I'm curious, too," he answered; "I don't think I ever got an answer from Koprowski about that." But he told me that the father of the C80 vaccinee (a child with multiple abnormalities) had been a doctor, a classmate of his at UCSF, and that the first four letters of his surname had been "C-H-A-T." He supposed, he said, that this was why the vaccine had been so named.

This, combined with the Dulbecco paper's mention of "Charlton plaque 20," served to identify the family of C80. Although "Charlton" did not quite begin with the letters "C-H-A-T," it was close enough to suggest that this must be the name to which Nelson was referring — and this was confirmed when I looked in the U.S. Medical Register, and located a Dr. Francis Charlton, who seemed to have been a contemporary of Nelson's at medical school. He was retired and living in San Francisco, and I phoned him that evening to arrange a meeting.

---

Frank Charlton turned out to be a handsome, affable man, and since it was a couple of days before Thanksgiving, his household was hectic with friendly, noisy grandchildren. He led me upstairs to the relative calm of his study, and I broached the subject of polio vaccinations. It was clear that he was a little surprised that I should have asked to interview him on this subject, and he spent ten minutes or so telling me about the Cutter incident and the Sabin Sundays, back in the fifties and sixties. He told me about his four children — how the older ones had received the Salk shots, while the younger ones had been fed Sabin's sugar cubes.

Eventually I asked, tentatively, if he had had any other children. He told me that his wife had caught rubella early in one of her pregnancies and that yes, they had indeed "lost two family members." Their last child, a boy, had been born at the end of the fifties with a severe case of Down's syndrome, while in 1952 their third child, a daughter, had been born with multiple congenital abnormalities, including skull defects, hydrocephaly, club feet, a cleft palate, and problems with her circulatory system. In 1955, they had bowed to the inevitable, and agreed to move her to Sonoma State Hospital, where she eventually died — as a result of complications from her several acute illnesses — in 1969. Her initials had been AAC.[21]

I asked whether the girl had been vaccinated against polio while at Sonoma, and he said that in a lot of state hospitals vaccinations are given routinely — that it is not deemed necessary to check every time with the parents. Could she, I asked, have been included in a trial of an experimental vaccine? Now that I had jogged his memory, Frank Charlton began to recall some details. He remembered that Thomas Nelson had been a classmate at UCSF, and eventually he came to the conclusion that he may well have agreed to his daughter's participation in a polio vaccine trial. Later, I showed him the Dulbecco paper, and asked if he had ever been approached for permission for a vaccine to be named after him, or his daughter. On this point he was quite certain. He had not been.

Before I left, Frank Charlton gave me a brief letter addressed to the Sonoma administration, authorizing them to send me a copy of his daughter's medical records. They arrived soon after my return to England, and confirmed all the information that Frank Charlton had provided, including the fact that "immunization with live polio vaccine" had occurred during 1956. The month was not detailed.

---

This apparently solved the mystery about the name of CHAT vaccine. It seemed that at some time during 1956 (almost certainly after May),[22] Koprowski and Norton had decided to begin plaque-purifying the excreted virus from Frank Charlton's daughter, vaccinee C80 in the serial passage study, and that after three plaque passages in MKTC they came up with Plaque 20, which had a very high titer (log 8.2, or roughly 15 million viral units per cubic centimeter) but which was only of moderate virulence for monkeys. It seems that they were so pleased with this plaque that they prepared a small trial pool from it, which they both sent to Dulbecco for inclusion in his comparative study of OPV strains, and took with them to Africa, for further testing in chimpanzees.

What was still unclear was why, in 1956, when they sent this Plaque 20 material to Dulbecco, they decided to call it Charlton, instead of categorizing it as a new pool of SM. It seemed possible that they were already planning their move to the Wistar, and sensed that Plaque 20 might be usable as the basis for a "new" Type 1 vaccine, one that could be further manipulated after they left Lederle. Hence the need to distinguish between the two strains. Whatever, by July 1957 and the Geneva conference, they had decided to rename the vaccine CHAT.

Why did they choose "CHAT," rather than "CHAR" or any other derivation from Charlton? Perhaps, simply, CHAT seemed catchier, more memorable. Or perhaps the reason was that CHAT had an additional resonance, a hidden meaning for those in the know. Was CHAT a bilingual play on words — a phonetic version of C80 put into French?[23] Or did CHAT also mean "chimpanzee-attenuated," or "chimpanzee adapted and tested"? Only two, or perhaps three people, would have known the answer to these questions: Hilary Koprowski, Tom Norton, and possibly Ghislain Courtois.[24] Only one of these three men was still alive — and he, apparently, was unable to remember.[25]

# 31

---

THE EAST COAST TRIALS — AND THE QUESTION OF

INFORMED CONSENT

---

In his initial report of the feeding of the twenty children with TN at Letchworth Village, Hilary Koprowski explained the process whereby he and his colleagues decided to feed oral polio vaccine to humans for the first time. "[The] gaps in knowledge," he wrote, "concerning the mechanism of infection and immunity in poliomyelitis are obviously due to the fact that, as far as is known, human beings have never been exposed to actual administration of living poliomyelitis virus for clinical trial purposes. Such considerations, as well as the availability of an attenuated strain of poliomyelitis virus (as evidenced by its lack of pathogenicity for monkeys), prompted the authors to feed a non-immune human volunteer on February 27, 1950."[1]

Somebody, he was saying, had to be the first to take the plunge. His group had what they felt was a suitable vaccine strain, and they also had the courage to leap into the unknown.

Let us leave aside the fact that they took that leap with a vaccine strain that had signally failed to exhibit a "lack of pathogenicity for monkeys," in that it paralyzed half of them and killed nearly a quarter. Let us instead look at the use of that word "volunteer."[2] In fact, "Volunteer No. 1" was a six-year-old boy so severely handicapped that he had to be fed the vaccine through a stomach tube, which suggests that he himself was most unlikely to have volunteered for this or any other experiment. The other nineteen volunteers were similarly handicapped, but there is no mention, anywhere in the article, about permission being either sought or granted from the respective parents. This anomaly was lampooned in the *Lancet* editorial that appeared shortly afterward, with its sarcastic reference to "twenty volunteer mice."[3]

The medical historian Allan Chase has written that "The prevailing and very eugenically oriented American medical ethics of the first half of this century considered mentally and physically handicapped children to be the subjects of choice for medical experimentation."[4] The mood of scientists and public alike changed quite swiftly as the fifties progressed, however, and Koprowski was one of the few who continued to use handicapped children in his vaccine trials — at least until 1956. (By comparison, Sabin used prisoners, while Dick and Dane tended to seek participants from among their own families and those of their university colleagues.)

Koprowski did not respond immediately to the criticism of that first report from Letchworth. But by the 1955 Sonoma trials, he was taking care to ensure that appropriate permissions had been obtained from the state departments of mental hygiene and public health and from the parents of each child — and that this fact was well documented.[5] Thomas Nelson's memories of the trials, and the internal papers from the era that he provided, confirm that — within the context of the times — the second Sonoma trial was conducted ethically, and that parents were appraised of the potential benefits and risks. But this of course begs the far more basic question of whether it is ethical to use severely disabled people for medical experimentation in the first place.

---

Roughly contemporaneous with the 1955 Sonoma trials on the West Coast were two further trials of Koprowski vaccines on the East Coast at Woodbine, New Jersey, a "state colony" for handicapped children similar to that at Sonoma.[6] As with Karl Meyer in California, the process was facilitated by the good offices of a "broker"— a respected senior doctor who was able to recommend Koprowski and his vaccines to some of his own acquaintances and colleagues. In this case, the broker was Joseph Stokes Junior, the revered Quaker pediatrician who was physician-in-chief at the Children's Hospital of Philadelphia (CHOP). Stokes helped establish Koprowski at three of his future vaccination venues: Woodbine state colony; the women's penitentiary at Clinton; and Moorestown — a small, middle-class town in New Jersey, just across the river from Philadelphia, which was also Joe Stokes's birthplace.

Stokes himself is long dead, but I spoke with Elizabeth McGee, a clinician from CHOP who helped with the Woodbine trials. She told me of the physical arrangement of the study area, and of the very strict isolation procedures that they followed. And she spoke warmly of Dr. Stokes: "He was very intuitive — he really knew how to handle people and to bring out their feelings, to bring out the core of the problem."

She also explained how the collaboration between Koprowski and her ex-boss had worked. She told me: "He [Dr. Stokes] was used, poor thing. I mean, he thought [Woodbine] was a good project; he liked these guys and they came to him, they wanted help, and he helped them set it up. He had influence in New Jersey, everybody respected him." Dr. McGee confirmed that there had been close links between Hilary Koprowski, Joe Stokes in the CHOP pediatric department, and the Henles, Hummeler, and Deinhardt from the CHOP virology department. All the aforementioned were part of the facility at the University of Pennsylvania and, although she did not know whether the CHOP virologists had played an active role in the Woodbine trials, she felt confident "that they were very aware of what was being done."[7]

---

The Woodbine trials were the last that Koprowski conducted in homes for mentally disabled children. From late 1955, the main venue for his U.S. trials shifted to the women's prison at Clinton, in the agricultural heartland of New Jersey; again, Joe Stokes was the facilitator. These days it is known as the Edna Mahan Correctional Facility, but back in the fifties it was known as Clinton State Farms.

It took several phone calls and a formal letter to the New Jersey Department of Correction before I was allowed to visit the prison, and once at the gatehouse there were detailed forms to be filled out, and an impressively exhaustive search was made of myself and my bag. It was clear that the "prison without bars" ethos of the fifties, from the days of Edna Mahan and Agnes Flack, no longer obtained.

I was taken to meet a surprisingly young superintendent, Mrs. Blackwell, and her deputy, Pat Christie, who was nearing retirement and seemed to be a representative of an older-style approach to prison management. Both were clearly more than ready to be of assistance, but seemed surprised at my interest in the trials. Mrs. Blackwell, a brisk, efficient woman, was able to provide some general background history.

The women's prison at Clinton first opened in 1913, and for many years was the only state prison in New Jersey for female offenders serving sentences of a year or more. Because of changing sentencing policies, its population fluctuated over the years; at one time in 1953 (two years before the Clinton polio trials began) there were 370 inmates and 158 staff. In those days, most of the prisoners had been incarcerated for crimes such as prostitution, property offenses, arson, and murder; there were also a few drugs cases, mostly relating to heroin. Girls aged less than eighteen were also incarcerated in Clinton if they had committed serious offenses — or if they were pregnant they would be transferred to Clinton shortly before delivery.[8]

During the fifties, approximately sixty infants were born to Clinton prisoners every year.[9] They were delivered inside the prison at Stevens Hospital, and then kept for some time in the nursery, which contained a small dormitory, a quarantine room, a play area, and a "formula room."[10] This was staffed by the medical director, Dr. Agnes Flack, and by several nurses; a local physician made frequent visits. Under normal circumstances, the babies spent only a few weeks with their mothers. After this, some would be "released" to family members; more often, however, they would be fostered, or sent to a home run by the State Board of Child Welfare.

Mrs. Blackwell told me more about Edna Mahan, "a very strong-willed person with her own set of [principles]," who served as superintendent of Clinton from 1928 until her death in 1968. During those four decades, she initiated reforms that had far-reaching consequences right across the U.S. penal system. She stopped the use of handcuffs and initiated the concept of a "prison without fences," building up a community based on an honor system, whereby those who had shown themselves worthy of trust were identifiable by the wearing of different color dresses, from blue through gold and cerise to a senior echelon of "student officers," who had to wear "a rather ghastly shade of institutional green." Many of the prisoners went out into the relatively wealthy local community to work as domestics, maintenance workers, or farmhands. Mrs. Blackwell added that as far as she knew none of the prisoners had ever got pregnant *during* their period of incarceration, thus undermining Hilary Koprowski's dinner-party tale of impregnations by passing truckers.

By this stage, the two women were rummaging through books and folders of newspaper clippings, and each in turn began to find items relevant to the polio trials. They found information about the feeding of polio vaccines to the women in 1966, which surprised me, for I had not been aware that the OPV trials had continued for a whole decade. One came across an article in a local paper from February 1958, about Agnes Flack setting off for the Belgian Congo (in "the Dark Continent") in order to help vaccinate seventy-five thousand people from Stanleyville, Elisabethville, and Costermansville (now Kisangani, Lubumbashi, and Bukavu).[11] The other suddenly came in with a large book that carefully detailed all the infants born in Clinton since the fifties: their names, dates of birth, and into whose care they had been "released." Without even having to ask, I was provided with a photocopy of the Clinton birth records from 1955 to 1960, omitting only the surnames.

———————

That evening, back in Philadelphia, I began searching through the various documents relating to Clinton. These included various published papers about the vaccine trials,[12] the birth records I had just been given, and a brief note about the Clinton feedings that had been lodged with the WHO.[13] This was essentially a two-page submission made by Hilary Koprowski, newly arrived at the Wistar, to the WHO Expert Committee on Poliomyelitis, sitting in Geneva in July 1957, which reported that since September 1955, "all infants born at Clinton Farms" to the prison population of roughly 500 had been vaccinated with OPV in formula. The vaccination of 33 infants was described. Three had been fed Koprowski's new Type 3 vaccine, Fox. Another 30 infants had been fed with what was described as "three sub-strains of SM virus": 22 with SM N-90, two with SM-45, and 6 with CHAT. In addition, 64 prisoners and 38 staff who lacked Type 1 antibodies had been fed SM N-90 in capsules — something that is not mentioned anywhere else in the literature. Apparently all the infants and adults tested were found to have developed the appropriate antibodies, and "no signs or symptoms of illness were noted" among vaccinees.

The published scientific papers on Clinton had identified each infant by a number, and provided details of their ages, in days, at vaccination. By comparing this with the birthdates in the nursery records, I was able to piece together most of the rest. It was possible to deduce which infants had been fed, and when, and thus to discover when the different variants of SM, TN, Fox, and CHAT were first administered at Clinton Farms.

It took several hours to unravel the first eighteen months of the trials, but a number of important things were revealed. First, roughly half of the infants born at Clinton during this time had been fed OPV — not all of them, as was claimed in the submission to the WHO. Second, those children who had not been vaccinated stayed at the prison roughly four to six weeks before being released into care; the vaccinees, by contrast, stayed an average of four to six months, presumably so that their health and antibody status could be monitored. Thus, although no financial reward was offered to participating mothers, the potential of spending longer with one's child may well have represented an incentive, as may the impact that participation might be expected to have on a parole board. Third, one of the infants living at Clinton at the time of the first SM trials subsequently had to go to the local medical center for a ten-day cardiac evaluation, and was then "released" three weeks later to the Crippled Children's Hospital.[14] One plausible explanation would be that he was suffering from polio. At this stage, I could not be certain whether or not this infant had been vaccinated with SM, or included in a contact experiment, but (just as with the polio outbreak at Sonoma) the episode should surely have been mentioned in the published reports of the trials — which it was not.

Fourth came some illuminating discoveries about the timings of the experiments, which were never specified in Koprowski's published papers and yet are very relevant to an understanding of his research program. During the first stage of the trials, which lasted from November 1955 to June 1956, a total of 25 children were fed either SM N-90 (Type 1), TN (Type 2), or else both vaccines in sequence. The first three experimental feedings of Fox, Koprowski's Type 3 vaccine, occurred in October and November 1956, (although in each case, at least one further feeding was needed before the infant was immunized). The numbering system indicates that there were a further eleven vaccinations between June 1956 and January 1957, but these are not identified in the papers.

A degree of certainty returns on February 27, 1957, when six infants were fed CHAT. It is clearly significant that this — the first multiple feeding at Clinton for several months, and the first official trial of the new Type 1 polio vaccine — occurred on the seventh anniversary of his first feeding of an OPV to a human subject, on February 27, 1950. Koprowski had a particular fondness for this date, as evidenced by his many references to it in his papers, and the occasions when vaccinations occurred on its anniversary.[15]

The confirmation of the dates of the first official feedings of Fox (October 1956) and CHAT (February 1957) were important, for they proved beyond doubt what had seemed likely for some time — that both vaccines had been developed by Koprowski and Norton some months *before* they left Lederle and joined the Wistar Institute, in May 1957.

Although at this stage I did not yet have enough information to work out the exact dates, it was clear that later in 1957 and early in 1958, Koprowski and Plotkin began trying out three other vaccines at Clinton, in addition to CHAT and Fox.[16] One was P-712, Sabin's Type 2 vaccine, a sample of which he himself had given Koprowski. The second was "Jackson," another Type 2 vaccine, which was essentially Roca-Garcia's MEF1 adapted to MKTC instead of to CETC. (This proved to be unsuccessful as a vaccine, with only one of four recipients excreting virus, and none developing antibodies.) The third and most extraordinary strain was "Wistar," a Type 1 vaccine that, according to the description, was "provisionally regarded" as an isolate from the stool of a calf that had developed Type 1 antibodies.[17] The trials of these two latter vaccines confirm that Clinton State Farms had now become the major venue for Koprowski's group to field-test their new experimental strains.

---

Dr. Andrew Hunt, who had regularly visited Clinton during the first feedings of SM and TN in 1955 and 1956, is now retired and living on an island off the coast of Georgia. Having worked for Joe Stokes at CHOP between 1946 and 1952, he moved north to run the Hunterdon County Hospital in Flemington, New Jersey — a job that also entailed visiting Clinton State Farms. During the SM/TN study, Dr. Hunt took stools and blood samples, and checked on the physical health of the infants, both before and after they were fed the vaccine.

His brother George, a departmental editor for *Life* magazine, heard about the trials from Andrew and sent down a photographer. An upbeat feature piece about Clinton duly appeared in October 1956, based around a series of excellent photos.[18] Dr. Hunt gave me some large prints, including one of Hilary Koprowski measuring vaccine into a baby's bottle, and another of him leaning solicitously over a crib, feeding one of the babies vaccine mixed in formula.

And yet now, it seemed, Dr. Hunt viewed the trials from a slightly less rosy perspective. Between 1964 and 1977 he had been dean of the medical school in East Lancing, Michigan, where he initiated a medical ethics program that dealt with, among other things, such issues as informed consent, and the use and misuse of power by physicians. Looking back on his involvement in the Clinton trials, he admitted that "these were the days before they thought much of medical ethics in research. We just used them . . . babies in this situation were [viewed as] research subjects." A caption on one of the *Life* photos stated that "mothers permitted the tests." Nevertheless, Andrew Hunt's account suggested that he had real doubts about whether the permission had constituted *informed consent*.

––––––––

The next major trials to be held in the United States were in the form of a household study conducted in Moorestown, New Jersey, where Joe Stokes's brother, Emlen, shared a practice with three other Quaker physicians in the Joseph Stokes Memorial Building (named in honor of their father). One of these doctors, Edmund Preston, told me of the very careful way in which the trials had been staged. Apparently he himself had been recruited during 1957 by Stanley Plotkin, who seemed to have taken over responsibility for vaccination trials soon after he arrived at the Wistar on secondment from the Epidemiology Intelligence Service (the EIS, the epidemic "firemen" of the CDC and the U.S. Public Health Service). As devised by Plotkin, the Moorestown trial had three main objectives: to evaluate the effectiveness of vaccines representing the three polio types (CHAT, P-712, and Fox) in subjects of different ages; to see whether there was contact spread of these vaccines in a family setting; and to establish whether the vaccines changed in character after passing through the human gut.

Dr. Preston told me that in the fifties Moorestown was already a dormitory suburb of Philadelphia, which he described as a "community of educated people": professional people with degrees, many of whom had married each other and produced sizable families.

The Quaker physicians wanted to identify large, intact families whose youngest members (the index children) had not previously received shots of Salk vaccine. They came up with a total of eighteen such families, consisting of thirty-six adults and fifty-three children. The parents attended a meeting at Emlen Stokes's house in November 1957, where the nature of the trial was explained in detail.[19] Many of the volunteers were personal friends of the physicians, and Dr. Preston remembers telling them that this was their "chance to participate in making medical history." He added that they had to be convinced that nothing dreadful would happen to their children — that they would merely become immune to polio before other families in the area.

The vaccine was administered in either a fruit-flavored milk drink or in gelatin capsules, and a project nurse took blood samples from the volunteers at four different stages of the study, and called twice a week over a period of six months to collect stool samples from each of the family members. One of the participating mothers recalls that she was teased for years afterward about the containers of stools that used to reside in her Frigidaire.

Plotkin's remarkably detailed paper on the trial was published in June 1959, and revealed, among other things, the timing of the feedings. Just before the trial proper, those index children who were aged six months or over were given two shots of IPV at fortnightly intervals, to confer baseline protection. They were then vaccinated with CHAT in mid-January 1958, followed by Fox and P-712 at three-week intervals. Nine weeks later, vaccination of the entire family began with the same order of vaccines, and the final stool collections occurred at the end of July. Monkey safety tests and dates of seroconversion showed that virus that represented the first, second, and third human passage strains of the vaccine within the families did not show a "significant degree of neurovirulence." Surprisingly, despite its twenty-one pages of text and twenty tables of data, the paper does not reveal the pool of vaccine used in the trials.

The Moorestown trial, which at the time was clearly the most exhaustive piece of research to have been conducted into the properties of CHAT and Fox, was put into perspective by a contemporary news clipping, which reported that it had been organized "in conjunction with a team of epidemiologists representing the USPHS [United States Public Health Service] Communicable Disease Center* field post that is located in Wistar."[20] This gives a new insight into the presence of the EIS officers at the Wistar, suggesting that they were not simply there on secondment, but as part of a formal collaboration between the Public Health Service and the research institute.

---

As well as Stanley Plotkin, the other EIS officer involved with the Wistar's polio research was Joseph Pagano, and it was he who took charge of the final (and largest) stage of the U.S. trials of Koprowski's polio vaccines. Dr. Pagano now lives near Chapel Hill, part of the "research triangle" in North Carolina, and with his vigorous mustache and full head of hair, does not look like a man approaching retirement.

---

* Communicable Disease Center: The old name for the Centers for Disease Control (also CDC), of which the Epidemiology Intelligence Service (EIS) is a part.

Pagano told me that he had trained with the Epidemiology Intelligence Service in Atlanta in June and July 1958, and had gone to the Wistar in August. To begin with, he helped Plotkin at Clinton and Moorestown, but he organized the feedings in Philadelphia himself. Eight hundred and fifty children originating from "lower-income groups" were vaccinated between January and July 1959, being divided almost equally between infants (aged up to six months) and children of up to five years. All were fed with CHAT and some 805 returned for the Fox vaccination, but only 335 received the Type 2 vaccine, P-712, apparently because Sabin stopped supplying it.[21]

The Philadelphia trial was an important new development in the ever-enlarging OPV program, being the first large field trial to be staged in the open community in North America. Pagano was at first a little surprised when I proposed this to him, but then conceded "I never thought of it that way. Yes, I suppose that's right."

Pagano recalled that the trial had been conducted in the part of Philadelphia where "there were poor people living in crowded conditions, where there really was a big hazard of polio." Later, he added that it had involved the "mostly black section" of the city, but was unable to identify which districts of Philadelphia this meant.[22] Pagano added that "follow-up was important . . . I think we had good control," but again was unable to recall the details.

From early 1959 until the spring of 1960, Pagano was also involved in the feeding of 65 premature infants at Philadelphia General Hospital,[23] which he described as a "big city hospital . . . more for indigent people who couldn't afford hospitalization." He added that "the thinking in those days was probably to study the vaccine in the population that most needed it. . . . If you could improve immunity in this high-risk population, you'd be achieving a great deal. The other reason was the accessibility of these people."

He did not recall which pools of vaccine had been used in Philadelphia. It seemed logical to assume, however, since both the trials in the open community and the premature nursery started soon after Moorestown ended, that the same vaccine pools (ones that had been very closely monitored in the American environment, and found to be safe even after three serial passages through the human gut) might well have been used again. 4B-5 had probably been used in Moorestown, so this was probably the CHAT pool used in Philadelphia as well.[24]

Pagano also spoke about the Croatian trial of CHAT made in human diploid cell strain, which he helped Drago Ikic (from the Institute of Immunology in Zagreb) set up in the early sixties. Pagano told me that Ikic appeared to be mainly interested in manufacturing the new vaccines himself, and that he (Pagano) had repeatedly to stress how vital it was to include controls. "I always had a sneaking suspicion that when they actually did the trial, they probably didn't pay too much attention to the control group," he confided.[25]

As my research into Koprowski's trials continued, it was becoming increasingly apparent that a host of random human factors could play a part in even the most carefully controlled trials. Even in the superbly detailed Plotkin papers about Clinton and Moorestown, there are small discrepancies — inaccurate dates, numerical totals that do not add up correctly, ages that are given as one thing in the text, as another in a table. Usually such errors or inconsistencies were of minor import, and made little or no impact on the overall findings. But not always. If there could be uncertainty about something as basic as the inclusion of a control group in the first-ever mass trial of oral polio vaccine made in human diploid cell strains, what other mistakes might have been made; what other omissions might have occurred?

Sometimes, of course, potential errors were picked up in time; on occasion, even, they were reported. For instance, one of the papers presented at the second Washington conference on OPVs by Koprowski's Polish collaborator, Przesmycki, related the story of a mistake made by a nurse involved in the mass feeding of Koprowski strains in Poland. She had previously been administering Salk vaccine, and she mistakenly injected thirteen children with CHAT pool 18, instead of giving it by mouth. Apparently none suffered any ill effects, and three of the four children who were tested later proved to have developed Type 1 antibodies.

One wonders, however, whether this small and (as it transpired) harmless error would have been reported if one of the children *had* fallen ill, or if the outcome had not turned out to be interesting from a virological viewpoint. We know that at least one infant born at Clinton in late 1955 (during the early trials of SM and TN) developed heart problems, and later had to be sent to the Hospital for Crippled Children — but that this fact is nowhere mentioned in the report of those trials. We also know that four children developed polio at Sonoma, four months after the 1952 TN trials, and that although the outbreak was apparently found to have been caused by a "street virus" rather than the vaccine virus, nothing was ever written about this episode in the medical literature.

Of course, all medical interventions are liable to mishap or accident. I was reminded of Boris Velimirovic's story of smallpox vaccine being administered in Ruzizi in the early sixties, and of a needle being passed from one arm to the next with no sterilization in between. What is clear is that the further away from the cloistered environment of the laboratory such research is staged, the more the scientist relinquishes control, and the more chance there is that human frailty and imperfection may play a role. A trial held in an institution like Sonoma or Clinton is one step away from the lab environment; a trial staged in local households or city health care clinics a further step. But how much control is lost when one moves the trial not dozens but thousands of miles away — to Poland, perhaps, or to the Belgian Congo? What happens when a remote trial is staged and an error occurs that is not picked up — or that somebody decides it might be politic not to report?[26]

And, to return to the starting point of this chapter — what of the people who stand to lose when an oversight does occur, when scientists make a blunder — what of the "volunteers"? Even when consent was obtained, were those who gave their consent (for instance the parents of the vaccinees) really aware of the potential risks? Indeed, were the scientists themselves fully cognizant of the dangers to which they might be exposing their research subjects as a result, for instance, of contamination of the materials used to make a vaccine? Andrew Hunt's obvious concern, when looking back at the Clinton trials almost four decades later, is illuminating. Even if consent had been obtained, was this really *informed* consent as we understand it nowadays?

---

As it happened, this very same question was addressed in August 1960, when a Manchester physician, Dr. D. E. Jeremiah, wrote to the *British Medical Journal* about Koprowski's historical review of the first ten years of oral polio vaccination, which the journal had published the previous month.[27] Jeremiah was horrified by the fact that Koprowski's first trial of TN at Letchworth had been kept secret by the investigators for over a year, until it was apparent that it had caused no ill effects. "In view of the large number of so-called experimental trials of various kinds at present being undertaken, is it not high time that some control be placed on individuals carrying out such trials on people who have not volunteered?" he asked.

Koprowski responded in the same journal, two months later. "Because of the discovery which my colleagues, Dr George Jervis and Mr Thomas W. Norton and I made 10 years ago," he wrote, "85 million people throughout the world have now been effectively vaccinated against poliomyelitis. It therefore seems rather pathetic to find that to-day there is still a voice crying out (in the wilderness, we hope) for 'protection' against 'individuals carrying out such trials on people who have not volunteered'. . . it would have been catastrophic indeed if it had been Dr Jeremiah whose permission was sought in 1950 for vaccinating the first group of children with live attenuated poliomyelitis vaccine. . . . Even though Dr Jeremiah might think he was chosen, as was his glorious namesake, to be 'battle-ax and weapon of war', what he is attacking in his letter is not the depraved Babylon but the windmills of La Mancha."

Koprowski's jeremiad is, as ever, festooned with quixotic literary allusion. But he had failed to address the English doctor's central point. Indeed, in a conference speech delivered in 1980, Koprowski admitted that he had known he "would never get official permission from the State of New York" to stage the original 1950 trial at Letchworth, but had gone ahead nonetheless.[28]

Dr. Duncan Jeremiah died in 1979, but his son and namesake is still alive. He wrote me, explaining that his father had been in charge of several vaccination campaigns in Manchester, over a period of more than a decade. He recalled that a central feature of the original draft of his father's letter to the *BMJ* had been Koprowski's huge vaccine trials in the Congo, but that this section was omitted from the published version at the request of the journal. Apparently his main concern about the Congo vaccinations had been that they "involved children, whose medical history was not fully known, receiving a substance which had not previously been exhaustively tested for unwanted and possibly damaging side-effects. . . . My father in no way would have objected to either informed consenting volunteers, ie adults, taking part in such trials or in principle to mass vaccination of children where such vaccinations had been proven to be safe."[29]

Informed consent is a tricky subject. But one wonders to what extent, especially in the fifties, dependent people — like prisoners, attendees at state-run institutions, or colonized Africans — were either prepared or equipped to question the apparent certainties of the men in white coats. How many, in reality, would have been willing to ask one of these men of vision and good intent about the safety of his procedures?

# 32

## AT THE CDC

James Curran, the longtime head of the Division of HIV and AIDS at the Centers for Disease Control,[1] has piloted his ship on a long and arduous voyage through turbulent waters. During that voyage, some of his crew may have become emotionally overwrought and even, on occasions, mutinous — but Curran has held steady at the helm.[2] This says much for his political skills and, perhaps, for his willingness to be ruthless when the occasion demands. He is a good public relations man, who often finds time to give interviews to visiting writers and journalists, and he has the sort of frank, slightly amused face and manner that are hard to dislike. He is, however, somewhat easier to tie down to a desk than he is to tie down to a definite answer. One comes away from a meeting with Dr. Curran feeling good about him and good about oneself, but less certain that what one has just been talking about really had a great deal of significance.

I asked Curran a series of questions about possible and confirmed American AIDS cases from the fifties to the seventies, but he was unable (or unwilling) to provide any details beyond those that can be obtained in the literature. But as I was packing up to leave, I asked what had happened to the Koprowski sample, which, according to the Wistar committee, had been about to be tested at the CDC a year earlier. He told me I should speak with Dr. Brian Mahy, director of the Division of Viral and Rickettsial Diseases at the CDC's Center for Infectious Diseases. Curran added that from what he knew of the arguments, the hypothesis was not that plausible. I suggested to him that the hypothesis would become more tenable if it turned out that chimpanzee kidneys had been used to make the vaccine. He didn't comment directly on this, but he did make one very practical suggestion, saying that "a careful understanding of how the vaccine was produced, [and where] the various lots of the vaccine . . . were used — if that could all be tracked down — would be useful. Which populations received which lots, where they were, things like that." He mentioned the fact that some had claimed that the vaccine lots used in Poland and the Congo were the same, adding that researchers would need to check that, and to document where in Africa the vaccine had been given. So, finally, Dr. Curran did come up with one practical suggestion that transcended the dictates of official caution and expediency. It seemed a good note on which to end the interview.

———————

As luck would have it, I was able to speak with Dr. Mahy straightaway to clarify the situation about the Wistar sample. He told me that contact had been made between Dr. Giovanni Rovera (the current Wistar director), Dr. Walter Dowdle (the current acting director of the CDC), and himself just before the Wistar report was released in October 1992, and that Rovera had written a letter to them on October 8, formally requesting that the CDC be one of two laboratories to test the polio vaccine sample. There had been further contact by phone a month later, and a letter of response from Dowdle to Rovera on November 20, 1992,[3] in which Dowdle formally offered the services of the CDC "as one of the two independent laboratories selected by the Wistar AIDS/Poliovirus Advisory Committee, to test the sample of seed virus used in the 1957 polio vaccine trials."

I asked what had happened in the eleven months since then. "I think you must appreciate that . . . any lab which gets involved in this activity is going to have to feel able . . . to make a reasonable contribution, and I think even the committee themselves were very, very dubious as to whether sufficient sample material really was available to do a proper analysis," Mahy explained. His department had the materials and technical ability to test even a small sample of virus, he said, but "I would agree with the committee, that the chances that we will get an unequivocal result are probably relatively small because, unless it was overwhelmingly obvious what happened, the interpretation might be difficult, particularly given the fact that we can't [have] further material." In any case, he added, "I think it would be quite wrong to proceed with this unless there [are] two independent labs" to undertake the study. Why was that? I asked. "Because . . . what we're looking at here is material that, frankly, a not very reputable scientific magazine [meaning *Rolling Stone*] has claimed contains material which is responsible for the spread of AIDS. Now . . . if the CDC pronounces one way or another on this . . . opposing groups will challenge the CDC to prove the veracity of their finding."

The WHO (as originally suggested by the Wistar committee) was not appropriate, he said, because it did not have the laboratory facilities to be able to conduct the testing. He himself had suggested the lab of Beatrice Hahn in Birmingham, Alabama, but since nothing had come of that, he assumed that she had not wanted to get involved. Ronald Desrosiers of the Wistar committee had been delegated to organize the testing, Mahy told me, but there had been no further news in recent months.[4]

---

The person whom I was most keen to see at the CDC was the polio expert, Olen Kew, the youthful director of the molecular virology section in Mahy's Division of Virological Diseases, who proved to be an unashamed advocate of the benefits of vaccination.

Dr. Kew first provided a very helpful broad history of IPV and OPV. He explained that Sabin's rapid passage approach to attenuation was probably more sophisticated genetically than that of his OPV rivals, but that even in the nineties it was not exactly clear how rapid passage resulted in the attenuation of virulent strains. "Maybe he was a genius," he said at one point. "The more we know about his work, the more respect there is in the scientific community." There was, however, a downside, he added, because all three of Sabin's vaccine strains had a tendency to revert to virulence. "There is a problem with vaccine-associated polio," admitted Kew; "it definitely does exist. Sabin never really wanted to confront this problem, and perhaps rightly, because the main problem is wild virus." He added that Sabin came from the generation when the Kolmer and Brodie vaccines were being tested in humans, and perhaps tended to feel that vaccine-associated polio was a minor problem in comparison to those disasters of the thirties.

I, however, was still a little shocked by this revelation, even when he placed it in perspective by asserting that today, throughout the whole world, there are some 120,000 cases of paralytic polio, of which only about 500 are vaccine-related, including four to six cases a year in the United States, and perhaps one to three in the United Kingdom. He added that litigation related to vaccine-associated polio had so frightened the polio vaccine labs that six of the seven OPV manufacturers had voluntarily withdrawn, leaving Lederle the sole remaining OPV producer in the States.

To give some idea of the recent impact of vaccination, he said that there had been roughly 400,000 polio cases in 1980, which was before polio vaccine had been used on a worldwide basis, meaning that the current incidence of paralytic polio was just 30 percent of its incidence a dozen years ago. Nowadays, he said, the disease had been eradicated in the Americas, and the hope was to eradicate it globally by the year 2000, making it only the second disease, after smallpox, to be eliminated by human intervention. The first or second decade of the next century, he added, was probably a more realistic target.

I asked about the library of polio vaccine strains that his predecessor, Jim Nakano, had collected over the years. Kew told me that the library was expanding all the time, and that it might now comprise more than forty thousand samples of poliovirus, including viral isolates from clinical and asymptomatic cases. These samples included many of the original vaccine seed strains, though not the actual production lots that had been fed to, or injected into, vaccinees.

Part of the collection was there in the freezer at the end of his lab. It included samples from Sabin, Salk, Koprowski, Cox, and so forth, but not all were the original strains; some had been passaged again at the CDC, using the original substrate (normally MKTC) in order to boost the titer, or concentration of virus, because frozen seeds have a tendency to lose their strength with the passage of time.

The entire collection was carefully indexed. Dr. Kew told me that CHAT was included in the collection, and he found what appeared to be four entries for pool 13, representing a series of passages at 37 degrees centigrade, performed at the CDC, beginning on August 16, 1960.[5] He also found other examples of Koprowski vaccines — such as Fox pool 12[6] and WM3 pool 17, both Type 3 strains. Neither SM N-90 nor TN was represented, and Kew admitted that he had a much better collection of the Sabin strains than the Cox or Koprowski ones.

We got to talking about the history of the different strains, and Kew told me that Sabin's strains were clearly recorded in the literature; in particular, there was a review article written by Sabin and Boulger that had been published in 1973, and that clearly documented the full passage history of his three polio vaccines.[7] As far as the Lederle-Cox strains went, he agreed that the Cabasso's "consecutive lot" paper of 1959 provided impressively detailed passage histories. On the other hand, he said, Koprowski's passage charts were broken up into several different papers, and he had never managed to track down the history of his strains "in any clear way." He went on to say that "there are some interesting genetic relationships between the Cox and Koprowski strains." When prompted, he conceded that the seed lots of CHAT and Lederle's SM vaccine were genetically very close, but declined to comment further.

Later, we discussed the comparative characters of the poliovirus and HIV. Both have an RNA genome. This, he explained, makes them probably ten thousand times more mutable than DNA viruses (like, for instance, the yellow fever virus), which means that attenuated polioviruses are far more likely to revert to virulence than attenuated yellow fever viruses. HIV, which not only has an RNA genome but is a retrovirus (or to be strictly correct, a lentiretrovirus), has even fewer structural constraints restricting the types of mutation that can occur, and the most flexible areas of HIV mutate perhaps a million times faster than normal DNA viruses. Olen Kew added that the V3 loop of HIV's envelope gene (part of the surface of the virus) contained the most rapidly evolving series of

amino acids that virologists had thus far discovered, and it was this unprecedented ability to change shape that allowed the HIVs to evade the immune system. The variability of these segments of virus actually conferred selective
advantages for the virus, so that evolution would tend to encourage further
variation.

The poliovirus also evolves quickly, but not so quickly as to allow the virus
to evade the immune system. So the good news for human beings is that polio
vaccine of a certain type (be it OPV or IPV) is effective against any poliovirus
of that type encountered anywhere in the world. By contrast, HIV demonstrates
the phenomenon of immune escape, in which mutants become so different
from the original virus that they are no longer recognized (or controlled) by the
immune system. By corollary, no single vaccine against HIV is likely to be able
to offer universal protection against such a cloud of mutant strains.

When we got to talking about the OPV/AIDS hypothesis, Olen Kew pronounced himself a skeptic. "It can't be mathematically proven, by strict deduc-
tive logic, that it couldn't happen, but there are many reasons to disbelieve it and
no reasons to believe in it," he claimed at the outset. But he had other, powerful
reasons also for opposing any rocking of the boat. "We now have a successful
polio eradication initiative. And what concerns us is the raising of issues that
might discourage people from taking the vaccines — which have been exhaustively tested and evaluated and used now for more than thirty years. . . . If the
public were to think that these vaccines are unsafe, it might undo thirty years of
progress."

I argued the opposite line — that if mistakes had been made along the way,
it was surely better to confront them honestly and learn from them, than to pre-
tend that they hadn't happened. Kew agreed with this, but still said that "one has
to keep in mind the larger picture, [which] is that polio immunization has been
one of the great medical success stories of the twentieth century. . . . The great
plague of the 1950s, which really has been with us throughout this century,
is on its way out. . . . There's no evidence [of] any complications associated
with polio immunization, except for the very rare cases of vaccine-associated
poliomyelitis. And if polio is eradicated, we won't even have to deal with *that*
problem any longer. . . . That is a story I would like to see come out." It was not
just defeating polio, he added. It was the question of having the confidence to
take the next step and to tackle other killer diseases — such as measles, which
kills two million children throughout the world every year, and then neonatal
tetanus. Later, if the right vaccines became available, then perhaps they might
be able to beat hepatitis B and even AIDS.

Later, however, he conceded that there had been a number of experiences in
the history of immunization that raised "very legitimate concerns." He cited the
contaminated yellow fever vaccine given to Allied troops during the Second
World War, which had resulted in tens of thousands of cases of hepatitis B. It

was experiences such as these, he said, that resulted in the setting up of rigid guidelines to control methods of vaccine production. It struck me that although such production guidelines were indeed being established in the fifties, they were still just that — guidelines, rather than requirements — with regard to unlicensed polio vaccines. It was only those polio vaccines that had received official licenses in the United States, namely Salk's IPV and Sabin's OPV, which had ever been governed by legally enforceable requirements.

We discussed the ways in which polio vaccine contamination could theoretically occur. Olen Kew pointed out that developing the vaccine virus is a small-scale operation, even if the attenuation process may involve using cells from different types of animal (such as rodents, chicks, or monkeys) that support passage of the poliovirus. However, tissues (usually kidneys) from a far larger number of animals are used during the process of vaccine production, when a seed pool is made up into large pools of vaccine. So if contamination were to occur, it would be far likelier to happen in one of the vaccine production steps than during the initial poliovirus attenuation steps. This is especially true if the contaminating agent is very rare (if, for instance, it was present only in the kidneys of a single primate, which happened to provide tissues for the final substrate).

I asked about the advisability of using human tissues for the final substrate, and Olen Kew told me that whereas continuous human cell lines (like HeLa) had never been used for vaccine production, due to the risk of transmitting cancer-causing units such as oncogenes, a human cell strain like WI-38 now looked "pretty attractive," because by 1993 it had been studied for more than thirty years, without any safety problems becoming apparent.

It was getting late, and I felt the time had come to tell Olen Kew a little more about my researches into the Congo polio vaccine trials. I started by explaining that by early 1958 at the latest, chimpanzee kidneys from Lindi were already being used to provide tissue culture material in a virology lab (that of the Henles, at CHOP), which frequently collaborated with Koprowski. I explained to him that in the only scientific paper I had come across that referred to the experimental use of chimpanzee kidney tissue cultures for growing polioviruses, those cultures had proved just as susceptible to poliovirus as rhesus monkey kidney tissue cultures — if not more so.[8] Since Luria and others had emphasized that the final host cell was crucial in determining a virus's host range thereafter, and since chimps were the animals genetically closest to humans, might it not have appeared reasonable to incorporate chimpanzee kidney tissues into the vaccine-making process, perhaps as the final substrate?[9] Olen Kew conceded that such cells would probably provide a high yield of poliovirus, but pointed out that they would be very expensive.[10]

Kew was firmly convinced of the capacity of vaccines to save millions of lives — a proposition with which I wholeheartedly agreed. But as we carried on talking, and I explained more about the epidemiological and historical evidence that supported the OPV/AIDS theory, I could see a change come over him. He would still say nothing on the record that might be construed as support for the hypothesis (which, given his position, was entirely understandable), but the real emotion, and even shock, that registered on his face at certain points in the conversation told a different story.

But now he returned to his earlier theme — that this was a cost-benefit issue. What were the benefits of having such information revealed, and how did they balance the costs that might be incurred? "There's a number of things that we learn in the course of our work that we don't suppress, because that [would be] unethical, but we do not emphasize. . . . We will not be very vigorous in promulgating this information to a broader audience, which may not be easily able to interpret it. . . . What's of great concern to us in the public health service, certainly me personally, is that a balance of accurate information be given, but that people [should not become] frightened about the safety of the current vaccines used, which have a tremendous safety record." It was vitally important, he said, that people around the world should not become afraid that they might get AIDS from polio vaccine.

I agreed with him that all polio vaccines are now tested for retroviruses like SIV and HIV, and that the possibility of SIV being transferred to humans through today's polio vaccines was therefore near to zero. My interest, however, was to establish whether an ancient polio vaccine, one about which we have much less accurate data with respect to safety testing and mode of preparation, could have sparked an even more serious disease than the one it was meant to eradicate.

"Some," he said, "might ask [you] to give this successful [polio eradication] program a bit more time before it has to contend with controversies which could be disruptive." I told him that I understood his concerns, that I would write what I had to write as responsibly as I could, but that I could not delay publication of the book because of the perceived possibility that some readers might misconstrue the message. However much I sympathized with his position, it was finally up to the public health service to assure people that the vaccines produced today are exhaustively tested and absolutely safe.

He in turn revealed that his perspective on the hypothesis was less clear-cut than it had been when the subject was first mentioned several hours earlier. He said he believed that the logic of the case I had presented to him was "much tighter" than that displayed in previous articles on the subject, and that although he did not accept the theory, it had been rendered "much more plausible." He added that it would be necessary to get some "really precise epidemiology — and retrospective serology if that's available — to evaluate this hypothesis in an unbiased and critical way."

Finally, we talked about the lessons that could be learned, whether or not the hypothesis was proved to be right. He said that one lesson that had already been learned with the passing of the old colonial world was that everybody had to be treated in the same way — that you could not act as if colonized peoples were research subjects. The same, of course, applied to handicapped children and women prisoners. And from a scientific perspective, he conceded that the desire to be first and to get recognition sometimes created problems. "So if the lesson [of your book] is to be careful — that getting your name on the paper first is not the most important thing, but to be right is the most important thing, that to have as accurate a picture of nature as you possibly can is the most important thing — then that is a fair warning." History, he acknowledged finally, had a nasty way of repeating itself.

By the time we parted it was getting on for midnight. I felt that of all the interviews that I had conducted over the course of three years, this had been one of the most beneficial. There were several specific subjects on which I did not agree with Olen Kew, or he with me. But on the important issues, we did concur. More to the point, he was one scientist about whose integrity and motivation I had no doubts whatsoever, and for whom I felt unqualified respect.

---

I had now been following up potential American cases of archival AIDS from the fifties and sixties for more than three years — and there did seem to be a common theme, in that the closer I looked, the more these cases receded into the realm of the improbable. However, it was still clearly very important to try to establish just when HIV and AIDS had arrived in North America, and to this end, I began looking at three intriguing case reports from the seventies, all of which provided suggestive evidence of AIDS from before 1978, which had now become widely accepted as the start of the U.S. epidemic.

The first of these cases involved a woman from New York City who had been an intravenous drug user between 1975 and 1977. She and her then-husband, who also injected drugs, had one healthy son born in 1973, but their second child, a daughter born in December 1977, was found ten years later to be HIV-positive. Three clues — the fact that the mother separated from her husband before the daughter was born, the lack of evidence of sexual abuse, and a strong HIV sequence similarity between daughter and mother (who herself tested HIV-positive in 1988) — suggested that the girl had been perinatally infected (either in the womb, during delivery, or from breast milk in the months immediately following). This meant that the mother herself had probably been infected by 1977. I phoned the lead investigator, Harold Burger, a clinician from the Department of Medicine at the State University of New York at Stony Brook, and he told me that the daughter had since died of AIDS and that the mother was still alive, albeit immunocompromised, in 1993. This meant that she had been infected for at least sixteen years, which, said Burger, made her the longest documented survivor with HIV-1 on record.

There were five other children born in New York City in 1977 who later tested HIV-positive, but none prior to that year. Furthermore, the earliest evidence of HIV infection in a gay New Yorker also pertains to 1977 — all of which provides a telling clue about the date of arrival of HIV in the nation's largest city.

The second possible case of AIDS was the least certain of the three. It involved a forty-three-year-old man who presented at Philadelphia General Hospital in the seventies with a history of weight loss, respiratory infections, cyst-like growths on hands and thigh, and a positive tuberculin test. Over the next thirty months, he continued to lose weight, and a liver biopsy showed highly unusual enzymes, together with granulomas and giant cells. An initial diagnosis of Wegener's granulomatosis (as in David Carr's case) was later changed to disseminated actinomycosis, after the fungus *Actinomyces israelii* was cultured from a biopsy specimen, but there were still uncertainties about the underlying process, and no details were known about the final outcome.

I interviewed both of the authors of the short paper on this case.[11] The younger, Robert Smith, recalled the patient as an unemployed black male, an indigent, who had originated from "one of the ghetto areas" of Center City, Philadelphia; he calculated that his symptoms must have begun in 1974, and continued until 1976 or 1977. There was a possibility that the man had been a drug user. "A lot of things we saw at Philadelphia General . . . like fungal infections, you'd wonder how they got immune-suppressed. In retrospect . . . I think it's possible that this gentleman had AIDS," he told me. He also recalled another AIDS-like case from the mid-seventies involving a female prostitute who had extensive *Granuloma inguinale* of the groin, persistent fevers, and bacterial superinfections — none of which responded to a wide range of treatments.

Smith's older colleague, Charles Heaton, also recalled these two cases, and though somewhat more skeptical than Smith, agreed that both patients could have had AIDS. The woman, he remembered, had eventually died of gram-negative sepsis, sometime before the closure of the Philadelphia General in 1977. During the mid-seventies, Heaton had also been working at CHOP, and remembered seeing a number of children with immune abnormalities, adding that "several of these might have [had] HIV." When asked how HIV might have been present at such an early stage in Philadelphia, he responded that it was of course a huge seaport.

The third case that I followed up was by far the most intriguing. It involved a five-year-old black girl who died of sepsis in 1979 in Newark, New Jersey. Autopsy demonstrated a deficiency in T-lymphocytes and LIP, a type of childhood pneumonia that is a classic marker of immunosuppression. She had been born in 1973 or 1974 to a promiscuous sixteen-year-old who was an intravenous drug user. The mother was suffering from thrombocytopenia at the time of delivery, which could be indicative of early symptoms of HIV infection. Six months later the daughter fell ill with anemia, hepatosplenomegaly, thrombocytopenia,

*Salmonella,* and pneumococcal sepsis, and she was treated with multiple blood transfusions.

I went to see the author of the paper, a pediatrician named James Oleske, and he told me some of the background to the case. Dr. Oleske is a large, soft, gentle man, who clearly has a profound love of children, and has been deeply moved by the many young AIDS patients whom he has had in his care. He told me that he moved to Newark to head the Division of Immunity and Infectious Diseases in 1975 and that it was some two years later that he began seeing kids with unusual immunodeficiencies. "I was in the wrong place at the wrong time," he explained.

Oleske reckoned that from the perspective of HIV, Newark was the perfect place to invade. There was a lot of drug use, and this formed a bridge between the heterosexual and homosexual populations. New Jersey was the first state to feature drug users rather than gay men as the major risk group, and also the first to experience a large number of women and children with AIDS. Oleske believed that many of the earliest AIDS cases in Newark involved drug users who needed cash, and who prostituted themselves in New York bathhouses and other gay venues. When they returned, they spread the new virus to partners of both sexes, and to those with whom they shared needles. He told me that he first realized that GRID, the newly reported disease of gay men, was also occurring in other groups in late 1981. This was when he was asked by a colleague to draw blood from a drug addict who had immune problems (pediatricians are famous for their ability to "find a vein"), and he realized that this same man was the father of a young girl who had died mysteriously of PCP six months earlier.

In 1982, he wrote an article describing eight unusual cases of immune deficiency in children; patient No. 6 was the girl who died in 1979, while the remainder had fallen ill since 1980.[12] In six of the eight cases, at least one of the parents was a drug user; the parents of the other two children came from Haiti and the Dominican Republic. One of the children had a twin who was unaffected, and this convinced Oleske that what he was seeing was not a congenital immunodeficiency, but rather a new disease in children. When the article was published in May 1983, some of his colleagues apparently accused him of sensationalizing and poor investigative technique. In fact, Oleske reckons that by the end of 1982, he had already seen thirty-two further cases of pediatric AIDS, but he wrote up only those eight cases on which he had comprehensive data.

Later, Oleske confirmed certain key details about the history of his Patient No. 6. He said that she had first been brought to his attention in about 1976, by a gastroenterologist working in Livingston, about five miles west of Newark. Much later, he said, in 1984 or 1985, a sample of the girl's serum, originating from 1978, tested HIV-positive on an early ELISA test. Even though many of these early assays were unreliable, this result, combined with her highly suggestive clinical history, persuaded Oleske that she had indeed died of AIDS. He also confirmed that she had already experienced typical symptoms of immunosuppression *before* her first transfusions at the age of six months. Considering the mother's thrombocytopenia at the time of birth, this strongly suggested that the daughter had been vertically infected, and that the mother had herself been HIV-positive when giving birth in 1973 or 1974. The mother, Oleske said, had refused to have blood drawn or to have any medical follow-up after the child died.

James Oleske told me that he would be willing to give me further details about the case once he had located the original medical chart. During a second meeting with him a few weeks later, he read one or two details from the girl's chart (details that had already been published), but when I asked about the mother, he was unwilling to vouchsafe any further details, except to say that he had seen her again at one of his pediatric clinics only about eighteen months ago. He did not say whether this was because she had another child with symptoms of immunodeficiency. I commented that if she was still alive, and if she had indeed had HIV infection in the early seventies, then she must have been infected for at least two decades, which would be of considerable interest from a virological viewpoint. But Dr. Oleske was now vacillating, almost by the minute, about whether or not he could show me the chart with the names blacked out.

Eventually, in desperation, I decided to tell him about the work done at Clinton, and the importance of discovering whether any of the babies born there and fed with trial polio vaccines might conceivably have become HIV-positive as a result. I said that if he could tell me just the mother's Christian names (a device commonly used by doctors as a way of identifying a patient without breaking confidentiality), I could see if these names matched those of any of the Clinton infants born between 1956 and 1958. Dr. Oleske said that if HIV had been introduced as a result of a polio vaccine, he would have expected to have seen HIV-positive children being born to all types of mothers, including those in the affluent suburbs. "Unless," he continued, "you could tell me that the [vaccine] lots were only given to inner-city kids." I said that he appeared to have hit the nail right on the head, for in America, at least, the suspect pools had been fed almost exclusively to mentally handicapped children, infants born to female prisoners, and inner-city infants and children. "*That* would tie in," he commented.

Oleske eventually told me that he needed to check with his attorney on the legal implications of furnishing further information, and he promised to let me know the result by the end of the month. James Oleske is a fine and caring pediatrician, but despite my dispatching a number of reminders over the next two years, he never got back to me.

---

It was, of course, intriguing that both the last two proposed cases, from Philadelphia and Newark, involved persons who had lived either in, or close to, places where Koprowski's polio vaccines had been fed in the United States. The actinomycosis case from Philadelphia was questionable, but if Oleske's pediatric case of AIDS had, as seemed very likely, acquired HIV perinatally, then one had to ask how a sixteen-year-old girl (even if she was a promiscuous intravenous drug user) came to be infected in 1973 or 1974, at least three years before the first confirmed instance of HIV infection in North America.

She must have been born sometime between late 1956 and early 1958, the very years when the first experimental pools of CHAT were being fed to the infants at Clinton, some forty miles west of Newark and Livingston on Highway 78. Could she have been a Clinton baby?[13] If she was, and if Oleske did indeed see her at a clinic in 1991 or 1992, then one has to conclude that she may have been infected with HIV for some thirty-four years — the longest of all the long-term survivors. Despite this, she appears to have been able to infect others, like her daughter, with a strain of HIV of sufficient pathogenicity to cause AIDS.

If this hypothesis holds water, could this be what happened in Africa as well? Could a small group of infants have been infected with a minute dose of SIV back in the fifties, and have become subclinically infected with the virus — effectively as silent carriers? And did they begin infecting others — such as their sexual partners and babies — with human-adapted SIV (effectively the first HIV) only when they themselves achieved sexual maturity in the 1970s?

It is doubtful whether pertinent records on such issues can be gathered in Africa. But if James Oleske would be willing and able to share information about the mother of Patient No. 6 — perhaps with an investigator from the NIH or CDC — we might be able to learn more about where and when the initial introduction of HIV into North America actually occurred.[14]

# 33

TOM NORTON

It was only at the very last minute that I managed to locate Tom Norton's daughter, Gail, whose address and phone number had been given me by Paul Osterrieth. I had been phoning her number for three days without success, and was heading westward from New York when I decided to stop at a shopping mall and try one last time. There were a few rings and then I heard Gail's rather reedy voice.

She sounded intelligent and friendly, and immediately I found myself liking her. Yes, she said, she would be happy for me to drive up to Maine to talk with her about her father's work. But had I spoken with Hilary Koprowski yet, and did I know that Hilary had all her father's records? She went on to explain that about eighteen months earlier, Hilary had phoned her mother in Florida to ask if she still had Tom's papers. My quarters were running out, so we had quickly to finalize arrangements, and so it was only after I had put down the phone that I realized that Hilary Koprowski must have obtained his former lab technician's papers just a couple of months after the *Rolling Stone* controversy broke.

Despite the lovely rolling hills of New Hampshire, where the trees were still decked in the foliage of fall, it was a long, tough drive up the coast to Maine. I arrived at the turnoff from the highway late the next evening, and found a western-style motel, which provided a good night's sleep. The following morning I drove the last twenty miles through squally showers down toward the coast and over the causeway. The pines dripped, the windshield wipers slapped, and the day felt distinctly mournful.

Gail met me at the door of her cleverly designed wooden house, which over-looked an inlet of the sea. She had a gentle manner, and the way she acted and spoke was more redolent of a child of the sixties than one born during the Second World War. She sat me down at a table by a huge window and provided some very welcome breakfast. And then she started to tell me about her dad.

The Norton family, she said, had originally arrived in North America in the seventeenth century, and her father had been born in 1909, in Wellsville, New York. Tom's own father had died when he was sixteen, and it fell to him to take care of his two sisters and a brother. He was accepted at Syracuse, but financial concerns prevented his attending. Although he had neither a degree nor a doc-torate, he went to the Rockefeller Institute and worked under Max Theiler, con-ducting much of the laboratory work on the yellow fever vaccine for which Theiler won a Nobel Prize in 1951. During his free time he liked to paint and to write detective stories, some of which had been published. He was both well read and open-minded, and on one occasion went along to a Communist party meeting, just to see what it was like. "He wasn't afraid at all," said Gail, "and that's borne out in his polio work."

It was while he was at the Rockefeller, toward the end of 1944, that Tom first met a Polish refugee named Hilary Koprowski. Hilary was still finding his feet in his new country, and, like everyone else, he found Tom Norton to be kind and affable. "He felt that my dad was a regular American who could help him," Gail added. When Hilary got the opportunity to start doing polio work at Lederle, he asked Tom to join him, and her father swapped jobs. Gail told me that Hilary's immediate boss at Lederle, Herald Cox, was a man with problems — a manic-depressive, whose behavior was unpredictable and often bizarre. Appar-ently he once threatened Tom with a paper knife. As the years went by, things became ever more polarized between Hilary and Tom and their coterie on the one side, and Herald Cox and his supporters on the other.

Gail recalled the early vaccine trials at Letchworth Village, Woodbine, and Clinton — and she also recalled that she and her two sisters — and Koprowski's elder son — had been either the first, or among the first, to be fed with one of the polio vaccines. By this stage, Tom had purchased David's Island, a small island off the coast of Maine, as a vacation home. Gail remembers the fear that polio engendered in those days, and the long summer drives from New Jersey up to Maine, rendered longer by the fact that they always avoided the major cities. On this particular occasion, Tom had brought some doses of the vaccine with him, and he fed it to the girls, and to four local children who used to play with them on the island.[1]

Gail also recalled the trip that her father and Koprowski made to Africa — she thought in 1956, though it could have been later. By the time that they left, she told me, both men knew that, upon their return, they would be leaving Lederle for the Wistar Institute — but they still had to keep it a secret. When

they eventually announced their impending departure, there was open resent-
ment. Gail could not remember the exact circumstances of their departure, but
did recall that it had been abrupt. "Did they leave in the middle of the night?
Did they take all their papers and stuff with them, and leave nothing behind?"
she wondered rhetorically. "My father must have had regrets," she concluded.
"He didn't like to hurt people."

The Wistar, however, was a whole new ball game. In 1957, when they arrived,
it was old, dreary, and run-down, and was known as "The Morgue" by local college students. The first thing Hilary did was to take Tom out of the lab and
appoint him assistant director. Then he employed an architect, built new laboratories, and hired bright young scientists to work in them. The Wistar Institute
and Hilary Koprowski became synonymous, and before long, he had made it
into an international research institute; at one stage, apparently, Tom was the
only native-born American on the staff. Gail recalls meeting brilliant scientists
from all over the world: men like Vittorio Defendi, David Kritchevsky, and
Tadeusz Wiktor. "I loved it," she said. "It was like a little United Nations. What a
contrast to the tight, rigid society of New England!"

The Wistar is affiliated to the University of Pennsylvania and is sited on campus, with almost all of its scientists having teaching positions at the university.[2]
It was a cozy relationship, and had fringe benefits also, such as the fact that all
three Norton daughters got free tuition there — providing an education that
might otherwise have been difficult financially. The arrangements were made
by Hilary, who was a past master at arranging such deals. He was always being invited (and paid) to speak at meetings in exotic places, or else arranging
for up-and-coming scientists, or old associates, to take up short consultancies
at the Wistar, or to attend conferences that he himself was convening. Tom,
meanwhile, would mind the home front. "I honestly don't think he could have
done it without my dad," Gail commented.

Gail was very frank about the dynamic between the two men. She told me
that "Koprowski is a Pole: very emotional, but also tough. He got to the top by
stepping on people." She said she felt that Hilary lacked social skills; that he
always felt isolated among the Quakers and bluebloods of Philadelphia. "He was
the foreigner, the refugee," she said, "and he needed an 'in' . . . he used my
father's background to get through to these people." She told me that from 1957
until 1973, when Tom retired, he acted as a mediator between Hilary Koprowski
and the rest of the world. "Everything in the institute, every piece of mail, went
to my father first, and then to Hilary. . . . Hilary was so temperamental that this
avoided many unpleasantnesses," she added. "My father was always the human
relations person. Hilary was making the contacts — but then my dad was sent
in. That's why Hilary always stayed with my father — he really did need him.
And my father needed him [too], for credentials and money." It had been a
strange and powerful mutual dependency.

"My father always said that Hilary was a great grant-writer; this was his real forte," she went on, adding that her dad had believed that other scientists, such as Sabin, "had more creative ability, but [that] Hilary was a great promoter."

Gail was also quite forthright about the "set of problems" from which Koprowski suffered. At different times, she said that he was self-centered, that he had an explosive temper and a big ego, and that he could be theatrical and very childish. It all added up, she said, to his having a "ghastly personality." On the other hand, he was able to recognize these shortcomings in himself, and to value the important role that Tom played in shielding him from some of the fallout. "Part of his problem is that he's a genius," she added. "He's a concert pianist, [as well as a great scientist]. Anyone who can do more than one brilliant thing has to be a genius."

Strangely, Gail said, she was the member of her family who had always liked Hilary the most, the one who would stick up for him. Certain of her relatives saw him as an opportunist, or felt that he used Tom, being far too ready to over-load him with work. Whatever the truth of that, matters came to a head for her father all too quickly after his move from the comfortable lab environment at Lederle to his administrative post at the Wistar. Just after Christmas 1957, seven months into his new job and aged just forty-eight, he suffered his first coronary. Perhaps this was why it was Agnes Flack and George Jervis, rather than Tom Norton, who participated in the Ruzizi mass trial in February 1958. Gail freely acknowledged that there were other factors that contributed to the heart attack, such as his smoking of sixty cigarettes a day and his high cholesterol level. But afterward, even though he stopped smoking and changed his diet, he was an altered man.

Later in the day Gail phoned her big sister, Ann, to find out more about her father's documents — the ones her mother had posted to Hilary after his phone call the previous year. Ann told her that as soon as she heard from her mom what had happened, she had written to Hilary, and that he had replied with an unusually friendly letter, saying that he would return the papers as soon as he had finished with them. But Ann also reminded Gail that she herself had copies of many of the documents, adding that if I came down to see her in New York, then I could photocopy whichever pages were of interest. "But are these the same as the papers which Mom sent to Hilary? And will my mom even remem-ber which things she sent?" wondered Gail, after putting down the phone. She also wondered why Hilary didn't have his own papers, and why he needed to have her father's.

The only document of her father's that Gail possessed was an impromptu nine-page account of the first feeding of TN at Sonoma, in 1952, which Tom had written on the plane home from San Francisco. It provided a fascinating insight into the vicissitudes of scientific collaboration, revealing that from the outset, there had been a remarkable degree of friction between Tom on the one hand and Thomas Nelson and Karl Meyer on the other. "Was it just a hot summer?" mused Gail, "or did Hilary promise something and didn't deliver?"

Presently, Gail got out the photo album that depicted her dad's trip to Africa in a hundred-odd snaps, some of them ill-focused and now quite faded. She said that her father, who had loved the idea of travel, always thought back to this Congo journey as his trip of a lifetime. Here were photos of Stanleyville — the Sabena guest house where Tom and Hilary had stayed; the new medical laboratory, its construction almost complete; and the remarkable Wagenia fishermen by the rapids in the Congo River. Here was a group shot featuring Ghislain Courtois, Hilary, and Tom, together with a strikingly pretty woman who, according to Gail, was a Sabena stewardess with whom Hilary made friends during his visit. (He is wearing comically ill-fitting shorts, she a dirndl skirt, and they are standing side by side rather stiffly, their arms just touching.) Here were shots of Camp Lindi — the entrance arch of bamboo, with the large flags of Belgium and the United States fluttering to one side; a sign announcing that this was the *"Centre Courtois Koprowski,"* with the eponymous scientists shaking hands in the foreground; Courtois vaccinating a baby; and a group shot of the Lindi scientists in front of one of the great hangars: Osterrieth, Courtois, Koprowski, Norton — and Ninane, standing slightly to one side. Another shot featured a posed ensemble of a dozen or so of Lindi's African staff. One was standing on his head, while another lay propped on the ground with beer bottle poised.

Here too were the chimpanzees . . . Djamba, the tame chimp, sitting on a table; and two other animals being lifted aloft to demonstrate the paralysis of a limb. (Gail confirmed that her father had been giving virulent poliovirus to some of the chimps.) Also included was a rather gory shot of two of the African workers, in aprons and rubber gloves, using a hammer and chisel, apparently to remove a chimp's spinal cord in what looked like a makeshift lab in the camp itself. (I later showed a copy of this photo to a virologist, who attested that material removed in this way would be almost unusable for sectioning and the assessment of spinal lesions.)

Then came a large group of photos of Tom and Hilary (motion picture camera poised) with the pygmies of Camp Putnam, or Epulu, in the Ituri Forest of the eastern Congo.[3] There were further photos of Lake Albert and of Usumbura (the latter featuring Tad Wiktor — the man who had introduced Koprowski to Courtois), and finally a few shots featuring a meeting of government officials and scientists in Nairobi. Although unsure when the trip had taken place, Gail recalled that her father had been away for more than a month, and that he had returned at some time in the spring.[4] Of one thing she was certain, though — this was the only time that her dad had been to Africa.

---

Gail had, of course, read the article by Tom Curtis, and was unimpressed, though she did concede that "it was perhaps not so far-fetched." She said that it did highlight the shortcomings of vaccine research in the fifties, and the fact that they were not aware of all the viruses that might have been present in the monkey kidneys they were using. But in order to develop something as important as a vaccine, she said, "it's absolutely necessary for someone to take the risks. And that's why it's absolutely necessary for the scientific world to come together to defend Hilary after the *Rolling Stone* article." This, she added later, tended in any case to be what happened — because most professors tended to feel they were a "common group working towards a common goal."

Gail was, however, surprised that the Curtis article had not included an episode from the mid-eighties, in which Hilary and colleagues from the Wistar had used an experimental rabies vaccine on some cattle in Argentina, without the prior permission of the proper authorities. "It was a dishonest way of doing research," she observed, adding that the resulting furor had been much publicized; "all [the people] in the field know about it and are embarrassed by it." (I later discovered that this episode, involving one of the first-ever field trials of a genetically engineered vaccine, had indeed prompted widespread outrage, including a leading article in the London *Times*. One of the most disturbing aspects was that milk from the vaccinated cows had apparently been drunk by local people.)[5]

Gail also told me about Gertrude Henle, a former friend and scientific colleague who would no longer have anything to do with Hilary, or even with those whom she considered his friends. In 1991, a year before the *Rolling Stone* controversy broke, there had been another intriguing episode, she told me, when the Wistar trustees had effectively sacked Koprowski as director, after thirty-four years at the helm.[6] Nobody knew the full story, but apparently it had come as a dreadful shock to Hilary. He sued the Wistar on grounds of age discrimination, and the matter was eventually settled out of court.[7]

Later in the afternoon, Gail took me in a rowboat across to David's Island, where her father had vaccinated the child population some forty years before. The shutters of Tom's cottage were now boarded up, it smelled musty inside, and the small building was starting to be overgrown by foliage. But back in the fifties, she said, when the place had had no running water or electricity, it had been "a magical place for a kid." It was here, on the porch, that her father had died "a perfect death," not so long after his retirement from the Wistar. He had been reading a story to his grandchildren, and had turned his head to look at the sunset. Then, without a sound, he passed away.

I spent the whole day with Gail, and by the end of it we were both exhausted. She had provided a completely new insight into the birth of CHAT, and the stresses and tensions that had been its labor pains. In the early evening, she began giving me the names and addresses of other Wistar scientists, whom she said I should try to contact — and I began to tell her something more about my researches, and the fact that I suspected that there might have been a problem with one of the Wistar vaccines. She accepted this, I thought, with surprising equanimity, saying that if my suspicions were right, then she would prefer that it came out into the open, rather than be brushed under the carpet.

Despite her natural candor, it was not until just before I left that she really spoke her mind about Hilary Koprowski. She told me that he was an only child, and she thought that he had probably "needed a good spanking" in his earlier years. Then, just as I was packing up, she said what was really in her heart. "He embellishes a lot," she warned me. "You can't believe anything he says."

---

Gail's elder sister, Ann, lives on Long Island, and I visited her two days later. To begin with, Ann asked me to enlarge on what I had mentioned at the end of my conversation with Gail, about the possibility that something might have gone wrong with one of the vaccines. She listened carefully to what I had to say, and then began telling me the story of her father's papers.

Sometime in June or July the previous year, she told me, Hilary had phoned her mother and asked whether she still had any of Tom's documents. Her mother had originally thought that she had not, but later she searched around and found several files, which she duly posted off to Hilary. Ann said that she and her sisters were quite upset when they heard about the episode, and she showed me the draft copy of a letter she had written Hilary in mid-July in which she asked him to return the documents "when you are finished with the information they contain." Hilary had written back a week later, to explain: "As you probably know, one of the fondest dreams of your father was to write with me a book about the discovery of the oral polio vaccine." He said that his wife had now elected to take on this task, including all the "nonsense" that had been written about the relationship between AIDS and the polio vaccine — and this, he said, was why he had requested her father's papers. "I do not see much sense in making Xerox copies of all his papers and return to you now the originals. We will return all the materials, if you agree, after the last draft of the book is completed." Ann wrote back in August 1992 to agree to his proposal. Since then fifteen months had passed, and she had heard nothing more from Hilary. Her mother apparently had little recollection of what she had posted to him.

Later, Ann showed me a file of her father's clippings and memorabilia. This included some of his early work on a book which, according to the title page, was by Thomas W. Norton and Hilary Koprowski, and which went under the working title of *Polio — An Adventure*. There was an outline, which explained that the book would be written from the perspectives of the two authors in turn, and a list entitled "Sequence of Events," detailing the years in which the principal trials and research breakthroughs had occurred. There was also a proposed "jacket blurb," which included the following: "The authors . . . tell their story with refreshing candor and humor, and the layman is given the opportunity to be in on the day-to-day struggles that confront a scientist, on his thinking processes, and in the case of a disease like polio on the political ramifications which evolve often to the point of hysteria."

There was also a rough draft of the first chapter, in twenty-nine pages. Although this mainly dealt with Koprowski's first research into poliovirus, in 1946, it started with a scene that took place some four years later. This was the opening passage:

> It was the evening of February 27, 1950. For the three men in the room it was perhaps the most momentous time in their lives. In a few minutes they were about to do something that might be a cause for controversy for years to come, yet in their minds it had to be done beyond any reasonable doubt.
>
> A door opened and a nurse wheeled the boy in. His emaciated figure was pathetic even in that place. The limbs were rigid. He had never been able to bend them from birth.
>
> One of the men stepped forward and spoke to the boy kindly. The boy knew him well. He was the doctor who came to see him often. When he was asked to drink a cup of chocolate milk, which the doctor held to his lips, he drank it eagerly. He smiled goodbye as the nurse took him away again.

---

Ann told me that she preferred not to compete in the memory stakes, and that her own recall was not as good as that of Gail. But later that afternoon she phoned her younger sister Susie in Colorado, so that I could speak with her as well. With regard to the events surrounding the departure from Lederle, Susie told me that she distinctly remembered "some slight scandal regarding whether Dr. Koprowski was actually allowed to take research with him — [it was] almost a legal case . . . there was some discussion about whether you can or cannot take viruses with you." She told me that Koprowski "will be extremely annoyed with all of us for speaking to you," and added that she had recently been discussing the polio/AIDS hypothesis with a cell biologist, who had stressed to her that a lot of things could have gone wrong back in the fifties, when scientists were taking organs from one animal, grinding them up in a blender, and then introducing them into other animals. The risks of viral transfer to the new host were substantial. If my book was to demonstrate that something like that had happened, "my sisters and I have all agreed that of course we would be sad, but . . . we would all want it to come out."

Ann, for her part, told me some of the good things about Hilary Koprowski — that he was "a larger-than-life character," funny and very alive, a great speaker and joke-teller. "He was a pragmatic man," she added. "He wouldn't have cheated on a trial. If he had to bend a couple of rules to make a trial happen, he would have done that."

In the afternoon, Ann left me to look through the clippings and other papers, which provided several more pieces of the jigsaw. An article from the *San Francisco Call-Bulletin* in March 1956 reported the beginning of the Belfast trials and commented: "It is all in line with Dr. Koprowski's desire to proceed cautiously, with the emphasis on being sure rather than being in a hurry, despite the vital need for the 'final answer'."[8] An article that had appeared two days earlier in the *San Francisco Examiner,* however, quoted him as having told scientists and physicians: "Gentlemen, we're living in the era of live polio virus vaccine. You don't have to wait for it another ten years or more. It is here already!"[9]

Probably the best of the articles in regional papers was one by Bruce Hotchkiss, which appeared in the *Newark Evening News* toward the end of October 1956.[10] It was a detailed report of the early Clinton trials, and included the information that two Clinton infants had been fed the new Type 3 vaccine, Fox, the previous week, although "Lederle first fed [the vaccine] to human volunteers in June."[11] The article mentioned that thirty-four infants had participated in the vaccine testing program thus far, nine of whom were still involved in the current study taking place in the nursery.[12]

The Hotchkiss article, with its announcement of the first feeding of Fox vaccine, marked an important watershed for Koprowski, for this was the last time that he publicly presented his research findings to the news media as a representative of Lederle Laboratories. The next time he made a public statement to a newspaper was just over three months later, by which time he was beginning to seem less keen about identifying himself as a Lederle employee.[13]

This next article also put a definite date on the trip to Africa, for on February 1, 1957, the *East African Standard* ran a long front-page piece about Koprowski and Norton's arrival in Nairobi, Kenya.[14] Intriguingly, the two men are described merely as "leading workers in the field of anti-poliomyelitis research"; there is no mention of their representing any organization or company. Koprowski had apparently addressed a local meeting of the British Medical Association in Nairobi two days earlier, after which the two men had discussions on the possibility of introducing a pilot immunization scheme in Kenya. No decision had been reached, but Koprowski stressed that the production costs of his vaccine were "infinitely lower" than those of its rivals, and computed that "a liter, sufficient to immunize 1,000,000 people, can be produced for little more than £1,000." He added that for the purpose of the pilot scheme, the vaccine could be supplied free by Lederle Laboratories of New York (the only mention of Lederle), "where most of the research has been done."

Koprowski went on: "For the past seven years we have carried out only small, limited trials in institutions. That stage is now over. We are not yet ready to put the vaccine on the commercial market, but we feel we have now reached the point where large-scale clinical trials should be attempted." Three trial schemes were being discussed with the Kenyan authorities — an immunization of all children aged below two months in localities where polio was prevalent, the vaccination of the entire population in such areas, or the vaccination of a small number of volunteer families.

It was also reported that "[c]arrying supplies of their vaccines, Dr Koprowski and Mr Norton leave today for Stanleyville. There, in collaboration with the Medical Director, Dr G Courtois, they will carry out experiments in chimpanzees." Afterward, they intended to fly on to South Africa, to discuss possible pilot schemes there. "Dr Koprowski's vaccine," the text went on, "has no name."

In fact, of course, the new vaccine did have a name, which at that time was "Charlton."[15] Perhaps the reason why Koprowski preferred not to identify a vaccine on which "most of the research [had] been done" at Lederle, was that he and Norton were clearly considering taking this new vaccine with them to the Wistar Institute, where they would formally move three months later. By the time of their arrival, of course, the vaccine would be called CHAT.

It is also remarkable that Koprowski should be claiming that his nameless vaccine was ready for large-scale field trials, when it was in reality an entirely new preparation that, at that stage, had been tested on only two infants.[16]

Koprowski had told the local reporters that: "Mr Norton and I would be delighted if an immunization scheme could be started in Kenya. We feel that the Colony has an excellent Government medical service and careful public health authorities. Results of a scheme here would really mean something."

In fact, those public health authorities were perhaps more careful than Koprowski envisaged, for an accompanying editorial provided a very balanced appraisal of the present situation regarding OPV.[17] The writer had clearly read Dick and Dane's articles about TN and SM in the last edition of the *British Medical Journal,* and retained no illusions about the potential dangers of OPV reversion, commenting that "professional bodies remain to be convinced that the degree of safety recommends its universal use." On the other hand, the commentary continued, OPV was cheap, provided very good immunity, and was easily administered in epidemic conditions. It went on to say that until now, only vaccines approved by the Medical Research Council in London had been used in the colonies. However, since the MRC had no powers of veto, "conceivably the vaccine could be used for clinical trials. Its use in the pilot schemes suggested by Dr Koprowski is at the discretion of the [local] medical authorities, and, in any event, the vaccine must be given under the supervision of responsible practitioners and restricted to volunteers."

As I was later to discover, Koprowski's address to the local branch of the BMA and his public announcement about the vaccine did generate some real interest. Before he departed Nairobi, he left several hundred capsules of Charlton (or CHAT) Plaque 20 with the senior government doctor, who had written that editorial — and who, by coincidence, was also George Dick's brother-in-law.

There was just one postcard from Africa that had made it back to New Jersey and survived down the years. It had been written by Tom to his daughters, was dated the same day as the newspaper article, February 1, and was apparently posted from Uganda. It reported that the two men had spent the previous night with Howard Binns at Muguga, Kenya (the same place where Koprowski had attended the WHO rabies workshop eighteen months earlier), and that they were now on their way to Usumbura.

Apart from these clippings, there were surprisingly few further clues to be had from Ann's folder of her father's papers. There was a small section of a large scale map featuring the town of Bomili, which lay some two hundred miles northeast of Stanleyville. There were various inscriptions made on the map by hand, and its presence in Tom Norton's papers suggested that it might conceivably have represented a capture zone for chimpanzees, or even a vaccination test site. There was also a single photo of the two scientists and Courtois and the Belgian stewardess at Lindi, but that made up the entire memorabilia from the Congo. There was nothing to indicate whether Hilary or Tom had continued to South Africa, though it seemed likely that if Tom had gone, his daughters would have remembered the fact.

An American newspaper clipping from April 11, 1957 provides an outer parameter for the date of Tom Norton's return.[18] The article reported that the Radrock Association (based near Fair Lawn, New Jersey) had heard a talk from Tom Norton, "recently returned from the Belgian Congo," where he had been doing experimental work on chimpanzees. The paper appeared to be a local weekly, which suggested that Tom was back home by the end of March or the start of April. There was also a postcard sent to Koprowski and Norton after their return to Lederle, which had been signed by several of the scientists at Stanleyville — Courtois, Osterrieth, Ninane, Rollais (the Frenchman who captured the chimps), and three others: Van Oye, Brutsaert, and Stijns. Osterrieth had written "See you later, alligator" beneath his name.

Apart from this, there was also Tom's farewell card from Lederle, signed, it seemed, by everybody in the lab save for Herald Cox. And there was one other newspaper article, which included some intriguing information. It was from the *Boothbay Register*, Tom Norton's local paper in Maine, and it reported that the experimental work at Lindi had been carried out on "a rare species of chimpanzee called *paniscus*, the blood of which is near that of man in its chemical constituents."[19] *Pan paniscus* is the name of the pygmy chimpanzee, found only to the south of the Congo River, whereas the common chimp, *Pan troglodytes*, is found exclusively to the north. Although I knew that some pygmy chimps had been present at Lindi, I had had no idea that much of the early experimentation had involved this species. It was not difficult to see that this could be a very important detail in the CHAT story.

---

Toward the end of the afternoon, Ann and I went down to the local library to photocopy some of the papers, and I asked whether she would be making any further attempts to recover her mother's documents from Hilary. She replied that she would do whatever was needed to get the papers back. "I'm prepared to tell him that I'll take out a suit and let the press know if he doesn't return [them]," she concluded.

Her resolve was encouraging and yet, as I drove away that evening, I still felt concerned. I kept thinking back to what Gail had told me a couple of days earlier: "We've no way of knowing what it was my mom sent him." What if, among the papers that had been posted to Hilary, there had been lab notebooks, or a detailed account of the research at Lindi?

# 34

HILARY KOPROWSKI — END GAME

In its issue of December 9, 1993, *Rolling Stone* published a "clarification" entitled "'Origin of AIDS' Update."[1] In this, it was stated that Tom Curtis's article of spring 1992 had merely raised "the theoretical question" of whether the precursor virus of AIDS could have been introduced to humans during Koprowski's OPV campaign in the Belgian Congo between 1957 and 1960.[2] Furthermore, it went on: "[T]he editors wish to clarify that they never intended to suggest that there is any scientific proof . . . that Dr. Koprowski, an illustrious scientist, was in fact responsible for introducing AIDS to the human population or that he is the father of AIDS."

The piece continued by emphasizing that Koprowski had "conducted his work in a manner wholly consistent with the available medical information at the time," that his work had saved thousands of people from polio, and that he had been a forthright advocate of human diploid cell strains instead of monkey kidney tissue culture for human vaccines since 1961. The clarification also referred to the conclusions of the Wistar committee, and its citing of the case of the Manchester sailor as proof that the CHAT vaccinations in the Congo could not have been the origin of AIDS.

Although it had not been published over the body of a naked woman (as Koprowski had wished), the disclaimer ended: "*Rolling Stone* regrets any damage to Dr. Koprowski's reputation that may have been caused by the article and believes this clarification sets the record straight."

In reality, the clarification withdrew little, if anything, from the content of the original article. Although it contained an expression of regret, it was in no way a retraction.

The resolution of the dispute, though far from satisfactory, had an additional significance for me. It meant that, if Hilary Koprowski kept his word, I would get to complete my interview with him.

---

I was back in Philadelphia once more. There were still three weeks to go before the Christmas release of Jonathan Demme's acclaimed movie about AIDS and the law in that city of brotherly love,[3] but the papers were full of excited pre-publicity. And as it happened, my second meeting with Dr. Koprowski would, as before, involve his lawyer — but this time a different one. We met at Koprowski's rooms at Thomas Jefferson University, and were taken by chauffeur-driven limousine to the offices of the new attorney, Richard Sprague. During the journey, Koprowski told me that he was pleased with the *Rolling Stone* "retraction," and claimed that the final version had been much stronger than the initial draft.[4]

Presently, we were escorted into Sprague's office (which I noted to be even larger than that of the other lawyer, James Beasley), and at the doorway an assistant handed me a piece of paper concerning an award that had just been made to Dr. Koprowski. I sat down on the chair to which I was directed, near the back of the room, and then Sprague, seeing me reading the paper, suddenly barked: "What are you doing with that? You shouldn't have that." And he thrust out his hand, waiting for me to bring it up to his desk. I stayed put, regarding Sprague as levelly as he was regarding me. For a few seconds there was an impasse, and then Koprowski leaned around in his chair, smiling, and took the paper from me. I couldn't be sure, but this felt very much like a piece of theater — a put-up job intended to gain ascendancy at the start of the meeting.

In the end, I was invited to bring my chair up closer to Sprague's desk, and he began in a brisk and business-like manner. I asked if I could tape-record the meeting, so I had a record of what was said. He refused. Instead, he told me that his client wanted the opportunity to correct any "mistakes" (the quote marks were indicated by his tone of voice) that he might make during the forthcoming interview. He was apparently asking to be sent a draft of the relevant passage, so that he and Koprowski could vet the text.

I told Sprague that this would be tantamount to forfeiting editorial control of the book, which I was not prepared to do. If that was his client's condition for granting the second interview, then I had better leave there and then. The lawyer suddenly became more conciliatory, and after some further discussion we agreed that I would send him a copy of the interview tapes, so that Dr. Koprowski could check through these, and add any comments he wished, or correct any factual errors.

Sprague said that he wasn't going to ask to sit in on the interview, but that he did want to add one more thing for both of us to consider. If Dr. Koprowski said "Eisenhower" when he really meant "Roosevelt," or if he told me that a vaccine trial had taken place in 1951 when it had really been in 1952, and if he didn't qualify that with "as well as I recall," or "to the best of my recollection," then he had only himself to blame if what I eventually reported was incorrect. He was giving a pretty clear message to both of us about how he felt this second interview should proceed.

As we left, however, it seemed that Koprowski was not entirely happy about something, because he returned to Sprague's office, staying there for ten minutes or more. Eventually he re-emerged, but he still seemed uneasy throughout the drive back to his office. I got the impression that perhaps the doctor had expected the lawyer to strike a tougher deal.

---

Back in his office, I noticed that this time he had dressed rather more eclectically, in a navy blue silk shirt under a red and gray golfing pullover. He also looked less gaunt than when I had seen him six weeks earlier. The office itself was bright and open, featuring a number of modern paintings on the walls. I got out my recorder, and this time Koprowski had one too — a small dictaphone.

Before I could begin my questions, Koprowski indicated that he wished to make a formal statement to the tape. "I am going to make an introduction now," he said. "I can talk to you the best way I recall, but I am talking from memory and memory is fallible, and moreover some of the things I will not remember, because you are speaking now about almost forty years — correct?"

I started off by asking about his ill-starred collaboration with George Dick in 1956. Koprowski gave a lengthy account of how he had met Dick and provided the SM and TN vaccines for him to test, how they were supposedly collaborating, how he had provided Dick with a technician, Doris Nelsen, "paid for by ourselves," to lend a hand, and how the next thing he knew was there had been a big splash in the "yellow press" in Britain about a doctor who had fed his own children polio vaccine, and who was now afraid for their health.[5] When I asked what might have caused the difference between the results in Dick's laboratory and his own, he told me "there are a million explanations," but cited just one. He told me that Dick must have regrown the vaccine viruses that he (Koprowski) had supplied, employing a further passage in monkey kidney.

This was an awkward beginning. Over the years, I had several conversations with doctors Dick and Dane about this point, and both were absolutely clear — that the SM and TN vaccines they fed in Belfast and Oxford were exactly as supplied by Koprowski, without further passaging.[6]

Koprowski recalled flying to Belfast in the very early days of the trial, but had no recollection of any later meeting in London with Dick and Dane, when the negative findings from Belfast were discussed.[7] What he did remember was that Dick had attended a large polio conference in New York in 1957, and had "made a big hullabaloo" about the results. This was clearly the New York Academy of Sciences conference that Koprowski — as chairman of the NYAS section of biology — had organized, but when I asked him about his own speech at that conference, he said he recalled nothing about it.[8]

This was unfortunate, for I had been planning to ask him about the difference between the speech he delivered at the conference, and the text of that speech which later appeared in the conference proceedings. By this stage, I had deduced that most — but more likely all — of the text and charts about CHAT and Fox (which made up almost all of the published version of the speech) must have been introduced into the records of the conference which were published in December 1957, eleven months later.[9] What was published, in effect, must have been virtually an entirely new speech.[10] It was this published version which was cited as the key source for CHAT and Fox in almost every article which he wrote about the vaccines thereafter.

Later Koprowski added that at the time that Dick made his address at this conference, he (Koprowski) had been sitting with Albert Sabin, and both of them had been concerned that Dick's report would damage confidence in OPV. "It took the late John Fox and me to persuade him [Sabin] not to throw in the sponge . . . not to give up," he told me.

I asked if it was correct that after Dick and Dane's reports in the *British Medical Journal* in January 1957, and Dick's address at the New York conference, he had never used these versions of SM (pool N-90) or TN again. Koprowski said: "Now, my recollection would be that SM N-90 was already being supplanted by CHAT at that time, unrelated to any Belfast situation. Finally, you know, neither I nor other people paid great attention to [the] Belfast studies." Which other people did he mean? "Well, about four million Russian citizens. We [had] requests from Poland, requests from Yugoslavia, requests from Switzerland for vaccine." He was now talking about the demand for the plaque-purified strains produced by Sabin and himself, which had been used in European trials from 1958 onward. By contrast, it seemed pretty certain that nobody had requested SM N-90 or TN after the Belfast debacle.

When I asked Koprowski to tell me again about the final substrate used for the feeding pools of SM N-90, he answered very precisely: "Monkey kidney — rhesus monkey kidney." Later he told me that "the only choice [was whether] we made in chick embryo or in monkey kidney, and I don't think in chick embryo we got a titer big enough. So we probably used in every case rhesus monkey kidney." There seemed little purpose in pointing out that in the scientific papers written at the time, he had claimed that SM was prepared in a final tissue culture of chick embryo.[11]

At this stage of the interview in particular, I was acutely aware of the importance of not challenging Koprowski too directly, for I felt it was vital not to jeopardize my chance of questioning him about his experiences in the Congo. I was mindful of the fact that during our altercation about Gear's letter a few weeks earlier, he had already said that he might not answer any questions about Africa.

I next asked Koprowski one of the key questions, namely in which lab CHAT and Fox had been developed, and he replied: "I don't know. I have no idea." I pressed him: were they developed at Lederle or the Wistar? In reply, he began by confirming that he had taken over as director of the Wistar on May 1, 1957 — but then he began to meander. "Some strains of virus were also sent to South Africa," he continued, "they were sent to RIT company [in] Belgium, and probably some other place . . . I don't remember . . . this was for production." Then he added that the "RIT vaccine may have been used in Leopoldville, and RIT also may have been supplied to Switzerland. This is all recollection — nothing certain."

I persisted with my original question. Presumably, I said, CHAT and Fox had been developed at Lederle; was this not correct? "Ninety percent correct," Koprowski answered. When asked to expand, he told me that perhaps some of the people he had mentioned had returned to him one of his own strains that had been passaged, or plaque purified. I asked what difference there was between the two techniques, and he explained that when one passaged a virus, one took a large dollop of material comprising millions of virions and introduced it into a new tissue culture. By contrast, plaque purification involved taking what was hoped to be a single virion and producing progeny from that.

So I asked again what the 10 percent of the work that had not been carried out at Lederle had involved. "I can't tell you," he replied. "I tell you that there is a possibility that maybe one of these organizations, or maybe a scientist, would have plaque purified. We collaborated with a large number of people."

I decided that it might be better to approach this from another perspective, and asked him to tell me about the rabies workshop at Muguga, Kenya, in 1955, the one where he had first met the workers from the Belgian Congo. He told me about Tadeusz Wiktor, a fellow Pole whom he would later employ at the Wistar, who spent most of his life working on the development of rabies vaccine. It was Wiktor who, according to Koprowski's *British Medical Journal* article, had put him in touch with Ghislain Courtois, so I asked him to tell me about the setting up of the chimp colony at Lindi. I noticed that sometimes Koprowski would speak as if reading from text, and this was one such time. "Dr. Ghislain Courtois, who was director of . . . the colonial laboratories . . . at Stanleyville . . . had established a chimpanzee colony. . . . He approached me, [asking] whether we would like to use his facilities . . . to undertake some research." I asked where exactly this had happened, and he answered that he could not recall. However, this directly contradicted his own account in the *BMJ*, which stated that it was he, Koprowski, who had suggested the chimp experiments to Courtois.[12]

I asked Koprowski how he had responded to the Courtois approach. "We said that we were very interested to have the possibility of finally observing, in an animal closely resembling [a] human being, in relation [to] polio, secretion of the attenuated virus after feeding, antibodies formed et cetera after feeding . . . whatever was in the paper. You have the paper?" I told him that I didn't. He was incredulous. I asked him which paper he meant, and he said he thought it had appeared in the *Proceedings of the National Academy of Sciences*, and that the title had been something like "the comparative susceptibility to attenuated polio of man and ape." I realized that the paper he was speaking about had actually been published in 1954, long before the Lindi research, and that it described the first experimental feeding of chimps with TN between 1949 and 1952.[13] When I told him this, he responded: "I had no access to chimpanzees. . . . I don't remember one experiment in chimpanzees done before Congo, but it is possible."

I spent the next half hour or so trying to elucidate exactly what work had been carried out at Lindi camp. He told me that it was important to carry out tests "in large animals, in large numbers." All the work, he explained, had been financed by the Belgian government; he had paid only the travel expenses to and from the Congo for himself and Tom Norton, nothing more. So what work had been done? Well, they had fed the attenuated viruses to the chimps, and checked for antibodies in the blood. In addition to this, he thought that perhaps Courtois on his own had been checking the susceptibility of the chimps to wild poliovirus, but he couldn't recall the details. Courtois, he said later, had been in charge of the camp, and had been very interested in the chimp work, visiting Lindi most days. All the follow-up work, he added, had been done in his laboratory in Stanleyville. Once again, this contradicted other accounts, which had it that most of the follow-up laboratory work was done in Philadelphia and Leuven.

We were interrupted by Koprowski's secretary, announcing a call from Dr. Gallo. "Close it," he snapped at me, nodding at the tape recorder — one of the few occasions that day that I saw a less polished side of Koprowski's personality. He elected to take the call in his secretary's office, and this gave me the chance to take a look at some of the paintings on the walls. On the far wall was a depiction in black and white of a woman, naked and crouching on the ground, head downward, with long black hair straggling across one shoulder and breast. Only one hand was visible, and the knuckles were arched — apparently in ecstasy or pain. If this piece was highly erotic, the others were more esoteric. There was a small Russian icon of a Madonna figure in golds and crimsons, below which, on top of the bookcase, was a photo of Koprowski shaking hands with his compatriot the Pope. Over to the left were two unmistakable Neanderthals pedaling

busily round and round on snow-white bicycles. On the far wall was a painting
of a harlequin sprawled on the ground, and another — which dominated the
room — of a monkey adorned around head and shoulders in white lace. I was
studying this one when Koprowski came back in, and told me that it was called
"Monkey as a Cardinal," and was by a Slovenian artist, Ciuha.

The one common factor that I could detect in the paintings was that of a certain jokiness and irreverence about the machinations of the human ape — a
healthy disrespect for pomp and circumstance, for the more obvious trappings
of power — including, perhaps, religious power. Otherwise, few clues emerged
about the identity of their owner, apart — possibly — from a certain evasiveness, a desire not to be pigeonholed or tied down, a concealing rather than a
revealing of the inner self.

―――――――

When we resumed, I asked Koprowski to describe the camp at Lindi, near
Stanleyville. It had been built in 1956, he thought. He described the bamboo
arch of the entrance, and the fact that inside the camp there had been "a lot of
cages — comfortable cages, big cages" for the chimps. One interesting point, he
told me, was that most of the chimpanzees at Lindi were *Pan paniscus*, a type
that — he said — was only rarely seen in zoos in the West, because it was so difficult to keep. This species was a hairier, blacker animal than *Pan troglodytes*, the
common chimp, "the one which looks like a clown"— and at one point there
must have been thirty or forty *Pan paniscus* at Lindi. It was good to have confirmation of this important detail, which had not been mentioned in the scientific literature of the time (even if it had featured in Norton's local newspaper).[14]

So we got back to the central question — the work he had done with the
chimps. They had wanted, he said, to vaccinate the chimps, keep them for several years, and test for duration of immunity, but this idea had to be abandoned
when the Congo became independent. This was an entirely new claim — that
they had wished to see for how long the chimps had remained protected — and
so I inquired what the response to vaccination had been. "As far as I know they
were superbly immunized," Koprowski replied.

Again he said that he couldn't remember which vaccines had been used. I
reminded him that his *BMJ* paper had reported that he had been testing CHAT
and Fox, and added that presumably he had been evaluating different pools of
the vaccines. He burst out: "Please, stop pressing me . . . I can tell you things
about the principles. Most of the other things have data and publications, [but]
if there are no publications . . ." He broke off, and then suddenly said: "My
records, as I told you, from 1956 or '57 to 1970 . . . well, I can't find." I had no
recollection of his telling me anything of the sort, but he continued: "When we
moved to Wistar, my records from '57 to '67 or '68 . . . they were gone. So I have

no access to them, because they are not there. These people from Wistar . . . Inadvertently probably, while they were transferring all my records, [they] disposed of them somewhere. So even if I would like to go back, I have nowhere to go back."

This was very strange. Koprowski stated quite clearly that this loss had occurred while moving *to* the Wistar, which must have been shortly before or after May 1957 — and yet it was records from *after* that time that had apparently been lost.[15]

Records or no records, I was amazed that he and Courtois could have gone to such lengths to test his vaccines in a chimp colony in the heart of Africa, and yet now, thirty-five years on, he should apparently have forgotten the reasons why. So I decided to change tack, and asked Koprowski directly about the two procedures that had been mentioned — albeit briefly — in the *BMJ* paper about Lindi: intraspinal inoculations of chimps with the vaccine strains (to test safety), and vaccination and challenge (challenging vaccinated chimps with wild, virulent poliovirus, to ensure that they really were immunized).

With regard to the vaccination and challenge, he said that although he recalled the chimps being vaccinated, he didn't remember any challenge with wild poliovirus. (Afterward I realized that he was probably not present when any of the chimps was being "challenged," which perhaps helps explain the confusion.)[16] But when I mentioned intraspinal inoculations, he started slowly piecing that part together. "What I do remember is that the vaccine was checked for safety in chimps. . . . Oh yes, that's something different. That means that [the] vaccine, before immunization of people in the Congo, was checked . . . which never before had been done intraspinally in chimps, which [had] only been intraspinally tested in monkeys. You see you have a very good memory," he went on with a twinkle. "You should be asking yourself questions rather than me."

He was wrong, however, about the intraspinal inoculations. By this stage, Albert Sabin had been reporting for two years on the gradient of susceptibility of various primates to poliovirus,[17] and had inoculated the spines of sixty-two chimpanzees with his different vaccine strains.[18] None developed paralysis. Koprowski would certainly have known this, since Sabin announced these findings at the New York conference in January 1957, just three weeks before Koprowski's departure for Africa.

Indeed, later on Koprowski added that if a vaccine did not paralyze monkeys by the intraspinal route, then it would not cause paralysis in chimpanzees. This was exactly what Sabin had reported, and it made me wonder what he had to gain by inoculating the spines of the Lindi chimps, when he had already done this in monkeys. I asked how many Lindi chimps had been injected intraspinally. "Well, if there were two pools, that would be ten chimps," he said.

After half an hour of questioning, I had established what had happened to ten of the Lindi chimps — which was exactly where I had started from, in that this was the sole statistic included in the *British Medical Journal* paper. Koprowski said he remembered nothing of the vaccination and challenge work, which had also been mentioned in that paper, and I was left to wonder just why he and Norton had gone out to Lindi in the first place. In retrospect, I wish that I had put this to him, there and then.

––––––––––

We moved on. I asked Hilary Koprowski to recall some of his other experiences in Africa. He told me the tale of having to make a speech in French while in Stanleyville, and of first taking a drink of *mazoot* — a local concoction combining whisky and Coke ("It's horrible to think about") to steel his nerves. Stanleyville, he went on, had been a "delightful town . . . we were away from all the . . . tensions and everything else; we did our work in this chimpanzee colony." Then suddenly, in midsentence, he recalled another episode. "There came a veterinarian, Jezierski, who took us to the pygmies." I asked if Jezierski was a Polish name, and he confirmed that it was, but that he had been an officer in the Belgian veterinary service. Jezierski had taken them to Camp Putnam, and Koprowski went on to recount the visit — the same visit that Tom Norton's daughter Gail had mentioned — and explained that they had spent about three days together. He continued with tales of the Putnams' disastrous marriage and adventures with the pygmies, but I was only half listening. I was still recovering from the news about Alexandre Jezierski.

Jezierski, I knew, was a vet who had been based at Gabu-Nioka, across in the far east of the Belgian Congo, close to Lake Albert. He had spent years working in his small laboratory in the heart of the African bush, and in addition to his formal work, he had tried to develop a set of attenuated polio vaccines. One of the key elements of his research was that he had tried growing poliovirus in a number of completely novel substrates, such as testicles, lungs, and spleens from lizards, turtles, and pangolins, and the kidneys of elephants. None of these experiments had met with success. But, rather more hopefully, he had also tested the kidneys of several different African primates, including chimpanzees, before finally settling on three different species of colobus monkeys as providing the best substrates. And now Koprowski was telling me that it was Jezierski who had taken them to see the pygmy camp at Putnam (or Epulu, as it is now called).

Tom Norton's photo album confirmed that the safari must have taken place during that first trip to Stanleyville in early 1957. I recalled that there had been a cluster of photos of Epulu and the Ituri Forest, which were mixed in with others of Lake Albert. If Norton and Koprowski had visited Epulu with Jezierski, then they probably traveled to Lake Albert on the same occasion. This might well mean that they also visited Jezierski's lab at Gabu-Nioka, which was just a few miles from the lake.[19]

Perhaps unwisely, I decided not to question Koprowski further about Jezierski, lest he recognize the direction that my thoughts were taking. But the fact that the three men had spent several days together during that first African trip was a revelation. It made it that much more likely that, following Jezierski's lead, he and Norton had also decided to try growing their vaccines in the kidneys of locally available simians. The most readily available simians to Koprowski and Norton would, of course, have been the chimpanzees housed in their "comfortable . . . big cages" at Lindi camp.

Koprowski, meanwhile, was reminiscing about the Congo. "I don't know Leopoldville; I only went there two or three times for a short period of time. I was there in Stanleyville myself several times with Norton." When I pressed him to be more specific, he told me that he and Tom Norton had been there maybe five or six times, and that Norton had gone to the Congo once or twice more on his own.

By contrast, Gail and Ann, Tom Norton's daughters, as well as Ninane and Osterrieth, were all quite certain that Norton had visited Stanleyville just the once. As for Koprowski, the collective memories of others placed him in Stanleyville on two (or possibly three) occasions.[20] This latter squared reasonably well with Koprowski's own account, but his claims about Norton were wildly inaccurate.[21]

I wanted to find out more about how CHAT had been prepared, and decided to ask Koprowski specifically about CHAT plaque 20, the isolate that had been tested in the spines of five Lindi chimps, apparently causing neither paralysis nor lesions. He explained that plaque 20 had more value than other plaques (because it had been tested in both monkeys and chimps rather than in monkeys alone), and that he therefore decided to amplify it into a large pool, or seed-lot. In other words, Koprowski seemed to be saying that it was actually Plaque 20 (from one of the third plaque lines) that had been used as the basis for the CHAT vaccine, rather than one of the plaques from the fourth (or even the fifth) plaque line, as suggested by the text of his New York Academy of Sciences paper. But when I tried to put this to him, the portcullis slammed down, and he told me that what I was suggesting was "all pure conjecture."

Nonetheless, if his original comment was correct, and if it was indeed Plaque 20 that had been amplified (passaged once or twice more in monkey kidney) to produce the original CHAT poliovirus seed pool, then one important new detail of CHAT's passage history was now known. What was still not known, of course, was the order of passages and plaque purifications that had been carried out later, to produce the later pools of CHAT poliovirus.

Next I asked about the source of the name, CHAT; I told him that some observers had suggested that it might stand for "CHimpanzee-ATtenuated." "No, no, no," he replied, "this I know. It was named after the donor of this strain." And was this CHAT, in capitals, or Chat in little letters? "Capitals

CHAT," he said. I pointed out that in his own papers he used both versions of the name, as if they were interchangeable, and he replied, a little gruffly: "It's the same strain, however you spell it."

Turning to the vaccination campaigns in Africa, he said that he remembered nothing of the vaccination of nearly two thousand schoolchildren at Aketi, but that he himself had been present at some of the vaccinations in Stanleyville, which had been organized by Courtois. Koprowski said that it was Courtois who had decided to vaccinate the caretakers at Lindi camp, as well as the various scientists who regularly visited from Belgium. He remembered that he had left "about five hundred" vaccine capsules behind with Courtois, and said he suspected that he might have used them for his own vaccinations. "We were not checking whether he fed more people. That I cannot tell you" was how he put it. But it seemed very possible to me that he had actually left behind some two thousand capsules, which were then used for the Aketi vaccination.

From here, we moved to the subject of the mass trial in Ruzizi, and Koprowski seemed both irritable and defensive throughout this part of the interview. To start with, he reemphasized that it was Ghislain Courtois who had got permission from the colonial authorities to conduct the mass trials. "Then we gave the material and said to Jervis and Flack: 'Vaccinate,'" he added. "And make no mistake of the map as made Curtis," he added, suddenly referring to the author of the *Rolling Stone* article. "This is highly rural area. His map is big mistake."

He then showed me a letter sent him in May 1992 by a Belgian physician, Philippe Van De Perre, who was working for the National AIDS Control Programme in Kigali, Rwanda.[22] Van De Perre had written that the Curtis hypothesis was "certainly not supported by our regional [HIV] epidemiology findings," and made a number of other observations that countered the arguments in the *Rolling Stone* article. Koprowski was later to cite much of Van De Perre's information almost verbatim in his riposte to Curtis in *Science*,[23] including certain errors (like those relating to the location of the Ruzizi trial, and the claim that Kinshasa and Shaba province are "several thousand kilometres" from the Ruzizi area).[24]

We returned to the trial itself: why had Flack and Jervis been chosen to attend? "When we discussed with them, they were both very happy. They both wanted to go," said Koprowski. I asked if they had volunteered to go and supervise, and he replied, "Feed, not supervise." Who, then, had supervised the trial? I asked. Koprowski had been getting increasingly defensive over the previous few minutes and now, for the second or third time that day, he lost his temper. "Nobody supervised," he almost shouted. "They feed the children. They feed the infants. They supervised the whole thing and fed 256,000 in six weeks."[25]

It seemed that whatever command structure there might have been for this, the first ever mass-feeding of OPV, Koprowski was not aware of it. He was, however, able to recall some of Flack and Jervis's stories about the trials, such as the fact that "the call to mass vaccination was made by . . . drums, drums, drums, drums. . . . And it was a heroic undertaking, 256,000 in six weeks. They were on their feet for a long time. And every day a new wave, a new wave, standing. They finished always with darkness." Both Flack and Jervis were now dead, he added.

I asked what the importance of the Ruzizi trial had been, and he declaimed rather loudly, as if from a script: "To demonstrate that you can mass-vaccinate by oral route a large population in a short period of time. This was the purpose of the trial." So at the end of the day, that was what it was all about. The first mass vaccination against polio in the world had been carried out — in order to test whether large numbers of people could be vaccinated quickly. If nothing else, this was disarmingly frank.

Had there been any follow-up of the vaccinees? I asked. "The follow-up was arranged by Courtois to check on the occurrence of paralytic polio and infantile paralysis and things like that — which was a very difficult task, because it was a highly dispersed rural area. And everybody was told by native translators that if any child showed signs of illness following vaccination, it should be reported." And had there been any reports after the mass feeding? "No . . . no untoward things reported."

Back in Philadelphia, it was time for a feeding on a rather smaller scale. It was time for lunch.

---

We carried on for a further two hours in the afternoon. In the main, Koprowski seemed calmer now that we had finished with Ruzizi, and his answers became more precise. We started off by discussing the feeding of CHAT pool 13 to most of the under-five population of Leopoldville between August 1958 and April 1960, and he explained that the vaccine had been supplied on the request of Courtois, because there had been an epidemic of polio under way, and added that the "vaccination replaced the epidemic," meaning that the vaccine virus had replaced the wild polioviruses in circulation. But this too was incorrect, in that the polio epidemic actually began two months *after* the beginning of the vaccination.[26]

I asked next about the statement he had made in 1959 — that campaigns then under way in several provinces of the Belgian Congo "were raising the number of vaccinated persons into the millions." Koprowski confessed that he was "completely blocked." He continued: "You see . . . the vaccine was prepared in large supply for the Congo, and probably was vaccinated by the local authorities. They would inform me by letter; they informed me of everything but, as I say, I have no records of that." OK, I said, but who was supplying the vaccine used in the other Congo campaigns apart from Ruzizi and Leopoldville? Koprowski told me that "the original vaccine was, I think, prepared by the Wistar Institute. Subsequent vaccines were, I think, prepared partially by the Wistar and partially by RIT, a Belgian firm, which was supplied with seed-lots and which was preparing vaccines and these vaccines were put in the hands, I presume, of the medical officers of the provinces." This correlated precisely with what Ninane had said. Koprowski added: "I have my doubts that it reached a million people. It is my feeling — nothing else." But did he know where else the vaccines had been fed? "The only town vaccination was Leopoldville. All the rest were highly rural areas," he answered.[27]

---

The rest of the interview went a lot more swiftly. Koprowski told me that the main reason for his departure from Lederle was that under a new president, the company seemed to be more market oriented, and less geared toward giving a free rein to research initiatives. He decided to leave before it was too late, and to search for an institution that he could build up from the beginning, according to his ideas of how a research institution should function. I asked him how he had got on with Herald Cox, and he said: "Friendly; sometimes not friendly — but passable." When I said that others had mentioned big clashes between himself and Cox, he said "there were not big clashes, there were different viewpoints." Then he switched off the recorder and gave me his viewpoint.

How was it, I asked, that Lederle had allowed him to take the vaccines with him to the Wistar if they had been developed at Lederle? "Well, there was no question of *taking* vaccines, because the vaccines actually could be obtained from fifty other sources spread around the world. There was no proprietor. As far as I know there was no patent." I asked about these fifty sources, and he said: "Congo, South Africa, Switzerland, everywhere there were vaccines around the world. Living vaccine — this is not a dead preparation." Clearly he meant that a vaccine virus could be recovered from the blood, or stools, of a vaccinee, so in real terms one could not lock up live vaccines inside a laboratory. He went on to state that "in the end, it became a moot point," because Lederle's vaccines weren't licensed — and instead they had to produce the Sabin strains. Of course, several observers felt that it was Koprowski's arrival at the Wistar with the unpatented vaccine strains that had dealt the mortal blow to Lederle's vaccine development program.

Then I asked about the NIH polio research grant, number E-1799, which Koprowski had received at the Wistar for many years. To my surprise, he told me that because he felt that the polio work had the highest priority, he had applied for this grant when he knew he was going to leave Lederle, so that it became operational as soon as possible after his arrival at the Wistar. This provided confirmation of what many had said anecdotally — that he had been preparing for his move to the Wistar for some time before he actually left Lederle. He told me that I would laugh at the sum of money involved (which had actually been $66,000 in 1958, rising to $187,000 in 1964).[28]

When we got around to the controversial keynote speech he had made at the Fourth International Poliomyelitis Conference in Geneva in July 1957, just two months after his arrival at the Wistar, Koprowski gave a very frank response. "This speech," he told me, "was prompted by . . . the fact that everybody was asking 'Have you tested the vaccine for this?'; 'Have you removed this, removed that?' Now if that [had been] done at that time, we would delay the vaccination for ages. And my interest was to move on with vaccination — polio was a plague throughout the world — and we should not be distracted by everybody putting his nose in." So, I said, you were basically saying that the time has come to move against . . . "To move against and *vaccinate*," said Koprowski, completing the sentence. Quite without trying, he had recaptured the tone and urgency of the original speech, tuning back into his mood of four decades earlier.

In many ways Koprowski's speech at the Geneva conference, which immediately preceded the deliberations of the expert committee on large-scale OPV trials, constituted the key public moment of his polio work. After years of frustration at Lederle, he had moved to a new institution, and he had in his possession the new plaque-purified CHAT and Fox vaccine strains, which by then had been tested in monkeys, chimps, and humans with apparently minimal ill effects, and that he felt confident were safe. Koprowski was now neck and neck with Albert Sabin, who had started so long after him, and so he didn't want to delay any further — he wanted to try out his vaccines en masse. And this, one presumes, is why, toward the end of the speech, he said the following: "The advocates of 'safety' do not want to pay any price for immunization; yet exactly what are the costs one might have to pay for a method of immunization which would not only protect the vaccinated subject against the disease but also may lead to elimination of poliomyelitis. . . ?"

He ended his Geneva address by calculating that the price was "negligible." Some might feel that, over the years that followed, SV40 and SIV were to prove otherwise.

---

From here, we moved on quickly to Koprowski's native land, Poland, where the huge vaccinations of CHAT and Fox had begun in 1959. He recalled nothing about the initial 1958 trial of CHAT pool 13 (the same pool used in Leopoldville), involving some three thousand persons, mainly from the small town of Wyszkow.[29] What he recalled was that Dr. Przesmycki (or "Smithy," as he was apparently known), director of the State Institute of Hygiene in Warsaw, had

approached him during a conference to ask if he would like to conduct a clinical trial in Poland "in face of epidemics." Koprowski recalled that some sort of
support (presumably financial) had been available from the U.S. government,
and Przesmycki had gone on to request that the Wistar supply vaccine for the
entire child population of the country, from six months to fifteen years. Large
pools of CHAT and Fox were made by Wyeth Laboratories, put in glass containers, and shipped free of charge to Gdansk by the Moore McCormack Lines;
between June 1959 and April 1960, the Poles vaccinated seven million with each
vaccine. There were no reports of any ill effects after the vaccination, he said,
and the vaccine proved "*surprisingly* preventative . . . there were 630 cases of
paralytic polio when [the trial started], and the number of cases dropped to
three after vaccination."[30] He told me that at some stage the Institute of Hygiene
had started producing its own version of the vaccine (presumably CHAT,
though he didn't specify), though he was not sure if the Wistar or Wyeth had
provided a seed-lot, or if Smithy had carried out a further passage in Warsaw.

At this point, something rather strange happened. Koprowski had started
coughing, and so I offered him a Fisherman's Friend. This is a long-established
British brand of throat lozenge, the impact of which resembles that of a fresh
herring slapped smartly across the cheek. At first Koprowski refused, but I
insisted that he try one. A few moments passed and then, as with Marcel
Proust's *madeleine*, sensory stimulus invigorated the memory. "Aah — these
I like," he said. "You know, my father lived in England. These I know from
this time. Nineteen fifty-four, fifty-five. He was a textile manufacturer in
Manchester." Of all the towns in England, and all the years, this was the combination most likely to activate my own memory banks. For this was the place
where David Carr lived, and the time just before he began his national service
in the Royal Navy. I popped a Fisherman's Friend myself, and invited him to
continue.

Koprowski told me that his father, Pawel, had had a textile converting and
import-export business based at 5 Beaver Street in central Manchester. He did
business with many of the big cotton manufacturers in that city, and he lived for
many years at an apartment block called Didsbury Court, on Wilmslow Road
in the south of Manchester.

"It's superb," Koprowski said presently, pointing to his cheek, where the
lozenge bobbed around inside. "It's revived my spirit and memory." I reached
across and gave him the packet — and he spent the next fifteen minutes
recounting a detailed history of his father, with names, dates, and places.
Toward the end of this, he told me that after his father died in 1957, he had
wanted to commemorate his life and his attachment to Manchester in some
way. He eventually decided to set up the Pawel Koprowski Vacation Fund. Every
couple of years, a Manchester student would get two or three hundred pounds
for a holiday, the only condition being that the recipient should send Koprowski

"a postcard or some communication" describing his or her trip. Most of them, he said, elected to write a lot more than a postcard and so, in 1991, Koprowski had arranged for several of their descriptive essays to be published in book form. He went to his bookshelves, and then handed me a copy of the Pawel Koprowski Memorial Vacation Awards — a rather splendid-looking paperback printed on thick hand-made paper.

---

We got back to the subject of the trials. He had already briefly mentioned those in Croatia and Switzerland, and also the plans to vaccinate in Tristan da Cunha and East London (South Africa), although according to the published records, neither of the latter trials had actually taken place. He then added that there might have been a small-scale trial in Belgium, among "some children of friends, something like that," perhaps organized by De Somer and Courtois, but he could not recall for certain. I asked whether he had ever vaccinated in England — during his visits to Manchester, for instance? He looked at me a bit strangely and didn't answer, but shook his head.

At this point I got out a copy of the "serodifferentiation" paper written by Plotkin and himself in 1961, in which seven different pools of CHAT had been compared, three of which were described as having been "made in other laboratories."[31] I asked if he could tell me any more about the different pools. Koprowski looked at the paper and eventually acknowledged that DS probably stood for "De Somer," which would mean that it had been made at RIT in Belgium, and that 18G-11, the pool fed in Poland, had been made at Wyeth. As for 4B-5, he agreed with me that it might have been fed at Moorestown. I observed that this was the earliest number of the seven pools, and had therefore presumably been developed at an early stage — a proposal that he rejected. 4B-5, he said, could indicate a production lot made at Wyeth or even in Croatia, with the Wistar electing to use the same numerical designation. "This may be anything. This [pool number] does not refer to any information about passage or origin," he said finally. I suspected that this was wrong, and that the pool numbering *had* proceeded in chronological sequence. In the end I asked whether he had a passage chart for CHAT. "No," he answered. "It would be in the . . . detailed records which I don't have."

But this did lead us on to something rather more interesting. A few minutes earlier, he told me that he had already looked through "all the records" in an attempt to find the answer to how the pools had been prepared, but without success. Now he added that he had viewed all of Tom Norton's records also, and that they had revealed "a measly situation." What did he mean? Norton, he said, had "wanted to write history, [or] *attempt* to write history. . . . I thought he would give the detail about pools, but there were none." He went on to say that

he had only managed to identify "the pool which Wyeth made," which was presumably pool 18. He added that he had also searched through the freezers at the
Wistar Institute, but had managed to locate only one ampoule that might relate
to the work done in the Congo. It had the number "13" written on it, and he suspected that it represented a seed-lot of virus rather than an actual sample of
vaccine.[32]

So, had this ampoule been tested for HIV, I asked, deciding it was time to
grasp the nettle. "I wouldn't even inquire or ask about it," he replied, "for the following reason. What would it mean testing half a ml of virus when you use
100,000?" I digested this one for a while, and then proposed that surely a pool
is homogeneous, meaning that any part is representative of the whole. He
agreed with this, but then launched into a halting explanation that brought him
back to where he started: if you tested one ampoule for HIV, critics might say
that you had not tested the entire pool. Koprowski was growing extremely exer-
cised, and it was becoming harder and harder to follow what he was saying. "You
can't win," he exclaimed, finally. "So [there's] no sense in doing test, when all the
time they claim it's a nonsense."

Later I put it to him again that if he was confident that the sample did not
contain HIV or SIV, then to have it tested would surely provide a strong argument in favor of his rejection of the CHAT/AIDS theory. "No, no," he repeated,
"because I think [even if it tests negative, the] argument goes on *ad infinitum*. . . . I am not objecting against testing. Go ahead and test it. [But] I think
[if] these people want to hypothesize, use my hypothesis." It was a strange kind
of logic, in that the argument was likely to go on *ad infinitum* for the very reason that the Wistar Institute, after having initially offered to have a sample of
CHAT vaccine tested in order "to leave no stone unturned," had then signally
failed to do so.[33]

---

Having ascertained that I was now allowed to talk about the *Rolling Stone* article,
I asked for his response to the CHAT/AIDS hypothesis. He did not mince his
words. "It is nonsensical, unproven, invented — based on nothing." So on what
grounds did he reject it? First, he said, because his polio vaccines were made in
rhesus monkey kidney, and HIV had never been isolated from this substrate.
Second, because if you had initiated an epidemic of AIDS through vaccination
in central Africa in the fifties, "by now [the] population would be completely
decimated — or you would have a tremendously high rate [of HIV]." Third,
because the same vaccine pool had been used in Leopoldville and in Poland.
And fourth, because the vaccination "was done in rural areas of Rwanda and
Burundi," where HIV infection was now only "about 3.7 percent or 5 percent."
He paused. "I think it's enough," he said.

I said nothing, but I did not agree. Frankly, I was surprised that, a full year and a half after the Curtis article, his grounds for rejecting the hypothesis should still be so flimsy. His second, third, and fourth arguments were of dubious validity. As for the first, key argument . . . this was quite possibly unprovable if, as he claimed, all the relevant records had been destroyed.

------

Toward the latter stages of the interview, Koprowski said some other fairly remarkable things. With regard to the nonpoliomyelitis contaminant that Sabin claimed to have found in CHAT, Koprowski told me: "I remember that he did not test the strain that I sent him, but the strain after passage in his own monkey kidney culture, which quite obviously was contaminated with SV40 and other at that time unknown cytopathic agents. And that's what he was recovering." This conflicted entirely with Sabin's own account of how he ran the tests[34] and was an exact parallel of the argument he had used to counter Dick's findings on SM and TN.

He further explained that he had changed his mind since the late fifties, when he had complained about the use of "hundreds and thousands of monkeys and chimpanzees" for the assessment of vaccine safety,[35] and he now once again felt that this was the most important safety test. Even if, for "reasons of conscience," you could no longer use chimps, he now preferred *in vivo* tests in monkeys to *in vitro* tests carried out in tissue culture as an insurance of the safety of a vaccine.

So, I asked, if you were trying to test polio vaccines today, how would you go about it? "I would have absolutely not the slightest idea," he said. "[In] conditions today, I may not have permission to have my trials. Neither I, nor Sabin, nor Salk. Or we [would] have been so discouraged that we may give up the project." All right, I said, but how would you approach developing and testing a vaccine against AIDS, for instance? "I don't know. I am always a bit perturbed about the mutation of the virus — whether we will ever catch up." But, he added, if a vaccine were to be developed today, it would have to be for the developing countries, and such a vaccine would have to be an oral vaccine, like that against polio.[36]

He was clearly proposing a live attenuated AIDS vaccine — a highly controversial idea, largely because of what could happen if the vaccine reverted, or recombined with an existing HIV variant and introduced new HIV strains into the human population. One of the few to have openly advocated such an approach was Ronald Desrosiers of the New England Regional Primate Research Center. Desrosiers had also served on the Wistar expert committee, and had apparently been the man delegated to get the Wistar's CHAT sample tested.

So what, I inquired finally, would he like to have written on his gravestone? This one he answered promptly. "Probably the same as what is written on a slab

[in] Toledo cathedral [over] an unnamed cardinal or archbishop. . . . Here lies powder; nothing more." And if somebody was writing his obituary in *Nature,* as he had done for Sabin, what one comment would he be most happy to see? This time he had to think a little longer, but then he had it. "Hilary Koprowski liked life," he said. I had little doubt that this was true.

Presently I got up to go, and we stood in front of the painting of the monkey dressed as a cardinal and shook hands. He looked me full in the eyes, and his eyes twinkled. I recalled the feeling at the start of the first interview that I was engaged in a chess game — and I had to concede that Koprowski, at least, would probably feel that he had forced a draw. I saw it differently, for the second part of the interview, even more than the first, had been full of inaccuracies, contradictions, and failures to recollect key pieces of information. However, in addition, one or two fascinating details had been confirmed, or revealed.

Nonetheless, as I left the room and walked along the corridor, I began to realize that to some extent, I too, like others before me, had slipped under the spell of this extraordinary character, this man of many parts.

---

Toward the end of this second interview, Hilary Koprowski had the opportunity, on the record, to rebut the OPV/AIDS hypothesis, and his response involved four separate arguments. Because this issue is so important, I shall now respond in full to each of those four arguments, the arguments that Koprowski apparently felt were "enough" to consign the hypothesis to the rubbish-bin.

Let us start with his second argument, which was that if CHAT had been contaminated, AIDS and HIV infection would by now have spread to much of the general population of the Congo, Rwanda, and Burundi. This is based on a doubtful premise, for some of the places where CHAT was fed (such as Bujumbura) now have among the highest rates of HIV infection in the world.[37] Furthermore, other vaccination sites (such as Leopoldville/Kinshasa) displayed an unexpectedly high prevalence of HIV in the early days of the epidemic, between 1959 and 1980 — and Kinshasa in the seventies was the first place in the world to experience an epidemic of AIDS.

His third argument, that the same pool 13 of CHAT was used in Poland and the Congo, is again dubious, for pool 13 was fed to at least 75,000 in Leopoldville/Kinshasa, but to fewer than 3,000 in Poland. Because of this disparity in numbers, if pool 13 was contaminated with SIV, it could quite possibly have infected a handful of African children (sparking an epidemic), but no children in Poland — or else one or two who failed to infect others. Alternatively, it might be that it was not pool 13, but another pool of CHAT, that was "the problem pool." 10A-11 was apparently fed to several hundred thousand in Africa, but elsewhere to only about 1,500 in Sweden and Switzerland. Pool DS, it seems, was probably fed only in Africa. Furthermore, I later learned that different batches of the same CHAT pool were sometimes prepared at different laboratories and in different substrates — a detail that completely invalidates Koprowski's argument.[38]

His fourth argument, that CHAT was only fed in rural areas of Rwanda and Burundi, but that nowadays HIV prevalence in these areas is low, is not only incorrect (for the vaccine was also fed in the city of Bujumbura), but also based on a false premise, for HIV prevalence of up to 5 percent is in fact worryingly high for a rural area. Furthermore, one of the villages where CHAT was fed, Rumonge, had HIV prevalence of nearly 12 percent in 1981 — an extremely high infection rate for so early in the epidemic.[39]

As for Koprowski's first, key argument about using rhesus kidneys, this is not, as far as I can determine, supported by a single piece of documentary evidence — and, of course, the relevant papers have apparently been lost. Furthermore, his newfound certainty that only rhesus macaque kidneys were used to make his polio vaccines conflicts with the several accounts he gave earlier in the controversy, which variously suggested that he had used kidneys from African green monkeys, rhesus macaques, cynomolgus macaques, and unknown primates (already excised). Later I learned from a member of the Wistar expert committee that Koprowski had told another committee member that he simply couldn't remember which monkeys he had used.[40]

The Wistar committee was probably correct when it concluded: "Unfortunately, the origin of the kidneys used in the preparation of the 1957 vaccine is unlikely to ever be determined with any certainty." There is, however, one ray of hope — though it depends on a sample of some of the CHAT vaccine that was fed in Africa being located and released for independent testing. If that ever happens, then modern methods of PCR analysis may be able to establish the species of monkey kidney that was used to produce the vaccine.[41]

# 35

OTHER VIEWS,

OTHER VOICES — FROM LEDERLE

TO THE WISTAR

During the rest of my seven-week trip to the States in the winter of 1993, in the days before and after the second interview with Hilary Koprowski, I spoke with several other virologists and research scientists who had been colleagues of his during his thirteen years at Lederle Laboratories and his thirty-four years as director of the Wistar Institute. Many of these men and women gave detailed interviews, which provided fascinating historical and scientific background to the story of the development of OPVs and, in particular, CHAT.

It took some time to set up a formal interview at Lederle Laboratories, but I was eventually able to have two meetings with Stewart Aston, the former head of the virus and rickettsial production lab, a courteous, thoughtful man of seventy-four years whom Lederle often employed as a spokesperson during legal actions. At the company's insistence, the interviews were also attended by the then head of viral vaccine research, Caroline Weeks-Levy, and, on one occasion, by the head of public relations, Craig Engessor.

In the course of some eight hours of answering my questions with great precision and unfailing charm, Aston did make a few departures from official company pronouncements — but only a few. One was to concede that the original TN vaccine, fed in 1950 and 1951, was "not sufficiently attenuated," as indicated by monkey safety tests. Another was his admission that he had always wondered why SM, the first Type 1 vaccine, was a mixture of two different isolates, the attenuated Sickle and the virulent Mahoney; he pointed out that it was strange to plaque-purify a virus when you were unsure of the parent characteristics.[1] But despite his key position in the manufacturing process, he could not remember what the final substrate for SM N-90 had been, whether monkey kidney or chick embryo. "They were using all sorts of different substrates," he conceded. Both Cox and Koprowski were praised unstintingly, on one occasion as "colleagues that I almost revere," and it took a lot of questioning before Aston eventually admitted that they were "two strong divergent personalities who just couldn't get on under the same roof."

When the conversation turned to CHAT, Mr. Aston did on one occasion state that he "had always felt that it was an isolate which he [Koprowski] had got in the Belgian Congo." On another occasion, he said that the virus was something that Koprowski had "arbitrarily picked out of a freezer" at Lederle, and then worked on further after he left. Why, then, had he changed the name to CHAT? Eventually, Weeks-Levy suggested that the "AT" part could mean attenuated, and then Aston added that "CH" could stand for chimpanzee, just as Sabin had used "Ch" to indicate a passage through a chimp in his P-712 Ch 2ab strains. There was a pause, and then I eventually asked the question that we all knew was hanging in the air: "So 'CHAT' could mean chimpanzee-attenuated?" "That's your words," replied Aston quickly. Later, Weeks-Levy pointed out that such a phrase could mean attenuated for chimpanzees (safety tested in chimps), rather than attenuated in chimpanzees (passaged through chimps). Later again, Aston pointed out that since any primate is a natural host to polio, you could put a poliovirus into any species — marmoset, African green monkey, rhesus, cynomolgus, chimpanzee, or gorilla — and get back a different (mutated) virus.

At the end of these two lengthy meetings, my knowledge of virology and the principles of attenuation had undoubtedly improved, but I was left with the strong impression that a policy decision had been made to give me a noncontroversial interview. (As the only remaining OPV manufacturer in the United States, Lederle was also the only pharmaceutical house still faced with vaccine-related polio suits, so sensitivity on this subject was perhaps understandable.) In addition, it seemed to me that Lederle (albeit unnecessarily) might be feeling somewhat uneasy about the fact that the parent strain of CHAT poliovirus (SM N-90) had been developed in-house, even if the final key manipulations that produced CHAT vaccine (the human passages and plaque purifications, which led to Plaque 20, and the MKTC passages that followed Plaque 20) had apparently been conducted independently by Koprowski and his associates.[2]

---

A considerably different view of Koprowski's Lederle years was provided by Dr. Victor Cabasso, a past Lederle employee, now retired and living in California. An Egyptian by birth, Cabasso arrived at Lederle in 1946 at the age of thirty-one as a research virologist, and has been involved with OPVs for most of his working life.

He was extremely forthright about Koprowski's first feeding of OPV in 1950/51. According to him, the source strain of TN had indeed been brought to Lederle by Tom Norton when he arrived from Theiler's lab at the Rockefeller Institute,[3] and that Norton and Koprowski had manipulated the virus in rodents, and tested it intracerebrally in monkeys, and "then decided that the time had come to cross [the Rubicon]," by feeding it to twenty children at Letchworth Village.

"It was a very foolhardy thing, in retrospect, to do," commented Cabasso. "Of course, ignorance is bliss." He explained that it was subsequently discovered that "even if you doused a thousand completely seronegative individuals [persons lacking natural immunity] with a fully virulent [Type 2] virus, you [would] have [only] one case of paralysis." So Koprowski's first OPV trial "was heroic in one way, but in retrospect . . . was probably insignificant." I had never viewed the 1950 Letchworth feeding from this perspective before, but had to admit that Cabasso was probably right. It did, however, establish an important precedent in that it was the first live human polio vaccine trial since the disastrous Kolmer affair of the thirties — and an apparently successful one, in that none of the vaccinees fell sick or died.

Cabasso said that from about 1952 onward, the strains between Herald Cox and his deputy started becoming apparent. Cox, he said, was a driven character who lacked self-confidence, and who tended to veer from back-slapping elation to a depression so profound that he would have to take days at a time off work. According to some, he kept a loaded pistol in his desk. By this stage, Koprowski and Norton were producing their first versions of TN and SM made in suspensions of rodent brains, while Cabasso and Roca-Garcia were working with the Type 2 strain, MEF1, which they seemed to have adapted to chick embryo. As Cox associated more and more with the latter group, so the Lederle lab began to split into two opposing camps.

Thereafter, relations between Koprowski and Cox deteriorated quickly. As director, Cabasso said, Cox should really have had his finger on all the projects that were taking place in the lab, "but Koprowski . . . went around the country and the world talking as if the project belonged to him, and that Lederle had nothing to do with it." When I asked him about the final substrates used to grow TN and SM, Cabasso said he was unsure, and that "his publications are extremely difficult to interpret, because the details are not there." He did mention, however, that primates had not been in short supply at Lederle, in that there had been a huge animal house containing between 600 and 1,200 rhesus and cynomolgus monkeys, up to a dozen chimps, plus assorted chicks, rabbits, and rodents. He added that during Koprowski's final two years at Lederle, Cox had had "absolutely no control over him anymore," adding that by this stage, "nobody knew what he was doing. He was keeping things very much to himself, and was making all sorts of commitments outside. This was probably what brought . . . the whole thing to a head . . . the fact that he acted as a free agent, no longer as a person responsible to. . . . Lederle."

Eventually, he said, the stresses became so great that Koprowski was asked to leave by the Lederle management. He apparently attempted to stage a counter-coup by suggesting that they should instead appoint him over Cox's head as director of virology, but the managers held firm. "But then, when he left, he took with him the [vaccine] strains which had been developed with company money. . . . He took the TN, he took [SM N-90]. . . . And then as soon as he got [to] the Wistar, he started churning out vaccine, and he [followed up] connections which he had [established while] at Lederle, particularly with the Belgian Congo. . . . He had [already] arranged all of these things and then, as he left, he took with him all of these arrangements and made them part of his program at the Wistar Institute. It was a very, very bad period for Lederle."

Not only this, but Tom Norton and four or five of the Lederle scientists decided to accompany him to the Wistar. "He was able to persuade a number of people to leave with him . . . to make it a little bit more dramatic," Cabasso explained. "It was . . . a slap in the face of Cox. Here is a man who is leaving . . . but to show his worth, he [is] taking with him some very promising young men." It was at this point, Cabasso added, that he had been appointed to take over as head of viral immunology research, and because Cox hated to travel, it was often he who represented Lederle at polio conferences around the world.

I asked him for more specific details about the history of the CHAT strain, and Cabasso said that Koprowski had worked on it while he was at Lederle, but that it had never been called CHAT in those days, and that the other Lederle scientists never worked with it after his departure because he had taken it with him. "In totality the strains were Lederle strains, and then all of a sudden, there was a set of strains called the Koprowski strains after he left. Now certainly . . . he didn't get them out of thin air, but he manipulated them enough to change [their] names . . . a passage or two here, a different name there." It was clear that Cabasso was still outraged by what Koprowski had done, and he added that when he left, the Lederle management had considered suing him for appropriation of private property, but eventually decided against it because "they thought that they would just get into a [legal] morass."

I asked Cabasso to sum up his feelings about Koprowski, and this is what he said: "Koprowski was a man of extreme ambition. Koprowski was a man of very limited conscience. Koprowski didn't care how he hurt people as long as he could [achieve] his ends. And he could be an extremely ruthless adversary if he was impeded in any way."

Even more tellingly, Cabasso detailed three instances in which Koprowski had reported lab contaminations as real phenomena.[4] One of these,[5] he said, caused a lot of problems for other researchers, "but he never came out to disprove, to say 'Sorry, I was wrong, it's not true.' . . . It took us one hell of a long time to straighten [it] out," said Cabasso. "And it was not the first time that he was taking a lab contamination for a fantastic discovery, not the first time."

---

From a skeptic to an unashamed fan. I next spoke to David Kritchevsky, who worked at Lederle from 1952 to 1957, and who was one of the half-dozen scientists who joined Hilary Koprowski when he relocated to the Wistar in 1957. In 1993, he was the only one still working there. Dr. Kritchevsky is one of the world's leading experts on cholesterol, and a personal friend of Hilary Koprowski. He is also an extremely funny and acerbic man.

Herald Cox, said David Kritchevsky, "was the most insecure person I've ever known. I mean the guy would ask the janitors: 'Do you think I'm doing a good job?'" By contrast, the management apparently loved him: "Cox was one of the boys, he used to tell bad jokes, he used to describe himself as a 'Hoosier.'[6] ... And Koprowski ... I mean to them, the abstract idea of a short, fat guy with an accent who plays piano is reprehensible. They're glad to have his ability, but they don't want to have dinner with him. ... [Koprowski] knows wines, he knows music; I've never seen anybody like this, I have to tell you. So he even makes them feel bad about that, because they say: 'Hey, did you hear Rachmaninoff's concert last night?' and he says: 'Yeah, and he missed the G flat in the Second Movement.'"

So, he went on, Koprowski realized that his chances of promotion at Lederle were minimal, and he decided to move to a place where he could be the boss. In late 1956, six months before the actual move, he told Kritchevsky that he was to be made director of the Wistar, and invited him to come and join him; Kritchevsky accepted. How come the Lederle vaccines went with him? I asked. It was a live attenuated vaccine, answered Kritchevsky — you put it in eggs, or tissue culture, and you've got something new. He added that he had an idea of how Koprowski might have transported the strains in a different form, because at one time at Lederle, "we had freezers full of baby shit from all of his ex-trials." From a virological perspective, baby shit represented vaccine virus plus one human passage.

Kritchevsky's basic line was that the great polio vaccine developers of the era despised each other, but that Koprowski was by far the best of the bunch. Sabin, for instance, he characterized as "A pure son of a bitch, but a bright guy. The guy did great things, [but] just because someone does great things doesn't mean that he's a great person." He mentioned Koprowski's obituary of Sabin, and the fact that it gave a misleading impression that the two men were intimate. He said he'd like to see these two plus Cox and Salk in a tag-wrestling contest.

"To my mind," he went on, "one of Koprowski's great scientific gifts is being able to smell what's going to be important." He told a story about Koprowski coming back from a meeting in early 1952, and raving about "a paper by John Enders, about a new technique called tissue culture, and [how] that's going to be the way to grow viruses." Cox, he went on, had insisted that nobody in his department would ever use monkey kidney, but "Koprowski clandestinely ordered the equipment, and clandestinely began to do it." He said he could remember Tom Norton ordering the roller tubes for making the MKTC, even while Cox remained committed to chick embryo as a substrate. So, I said, in the papers they published, Koprowski and Norton had to conceal the fact that they were using monkey kidney as a substrate. Kritchevsky agreed. In the space of half a minute, he had confirmed my deduction that, with respect to the SM trials in 1955 and 1956, Koprowski had been reporting one thing in the scientific literature, and doing another.

Kritchevsky described their arrival at the Wistar in 1957: there were, he said, fixtures and fittings from the 1890s, a skeleton hanging in a corridor, and perhaps a dozen people in total in the building. "And suddenly Koprowski comes in. He brings in a bunch of people, everyone starts running for grants, everybody starts looking for renovation money — and in a relatively short time, the place is clean, there are a lot of labs, and there's an awful lot of work being published. . . . I think it was Emerson in an essay said that every institution is a reflection of one man, and I think the Wistar is a reflection of him." He explained that the Wistar developed a very, very good scientific reputation, and that there were never any factions, like at Lederle, "because there's nobody to have a faction against. He's running it." Apparently over the years Koprowski appointed certain individuals, Kritchevsky included, as associate directors. "And I must say, with Koprowski if you're an associate director you do a lot of association and not a lot of direction."

So, I said, a benevolent dictatorship. Did Koprowski have any faults at all? Kritchevsky told me that he was arrogant, that he was short-tempered, that he didn't suffer fools gladly. "He has a personality that's very powerful, and there are a lot of people who just get nervous in the presence of people like that." But apart from that, he had done some remarkable things scientifically. Did he consider his former boss a genius, then? "He's not always right," said Kritchevsky. "If he was, I'd take him to the track with me. But by and large, his gambles usually pay off."

This seemed an appropriate moment to ask about the events in Africa. Kritchevsky knew little about the actual vaccinations, although he had seen the photos on Koprowski's wall of a crowd of blacks, and one of them having vaccine squirted down his throat.[7] As for the *Rolling Stone* article, he said: "I can see that he would be a little bit snake bitten. This thing with *Rolling Stone* was a real traumatic experience for him. . . . As litigious as American society is, I can see some lawyer getting everyone with AIDS to sue him."

Neither could Kritchevsky tell me much about the chimp colony at Lindi. But he did relate a story about how he, Koprowski, and Courtois had planned to establish a chimp breeding colony and research station on a nearby island in the Congo River. This home-grown colony would have been quite different from the Lindi setup, he said. He tried to illustrate the difference. "For instance," he said, "in Johannesburg, they were still making polio vaccine in 1965 using monkey kidney. And they would bring in . . . a hundred African green monkeys, and . . . would keep them in this cage and hope they're all OK. What Courtois had in mind was breeding them right there, so then you know that they haven't been exposed to other viruses or anything else." He added that if monkeys are brought in from the wild, then you have to throw away half of them because of viral infections.

This was an intriguing explanation, for it linked the idea of a chimpanzee breeding colony to the use of clean primate kidneys for polio vaccine manufacture. I asked him if he thought that the chimps, like the AGMs, had been used to *make* polio vaccines. "I know they were used to test it," replied David Kritchevsky, "but I don't know anything else about that."

---

A few days later, I was able to follow up the links between Koprowski, the Lindi chimps, and the CHOP virology team from another angle. Unfortunately, both Fritz Deinhardt (the man who had done hepatitis studies at Lindi in early 1958) and his former boss, Werner Henle, were now dead. But Werner's wife and long-time colleague in the virology department, Gertrude Henle, was still very much alive. I located her in an old people's home set among the wooded acres of Delaware County, to the west of Philadelphia. Although in her eighties, she seemed to have lost very little of her renowned shrewdness and intelligence.

Because she and her husband had been such towering figures in the world of American virology in the fifties (as brilliant as Albert Sabin, in the opinion of many contemporaries), I first asked Gertrude Henle to tell me something of their background. She explained that she had met Werner in Heidelberg in 1932, and that they got married in New York in 1937. By this stage, both had been given posts at the University of Pennsylvania, where they began a working relationship that would last over half a century. In those early years Werner attempted — unsuccessfully — to make a vaccine against sperm, while Gertrude concentrated on saliva studies, and developing an inactivated mumps vaccine. Later, at the beginning of the war, they both moved to CHOP, and developed a vaccine against flu, which is basically the same one used today. The virus diagnostic lab opened in 1945, and they opened another virus lab in CHOP soon afterward, where they took on a steady trickle of young German scientists, including Klaus Hummeler at the start of the fifties, and Fritz Deinhardt in 1954.

Soon after the start of our discussion, Gertrude Henle embarked on a story about an argument she had had with Hilary Koprowski, but then suddenly she stopped, saying that she had better not go into the details, adding only: "He is one of the worst persons I have ever met in my life." Later in the interview, however, she explained a little more. She told me that she had liked him very much when they first met, but that soon after this "he was very nasty to me." The argument had apparently had something to do with her checking some of Koprowski's results and finding that they were not repeatable in her own lab, and a counteraccusation by Koprowski that she had stolen some of his work from the Wistar. More than that she would not say, but it became clear that she had never forgiven Koprowski for what had happened, and had had no contact with him since.

We turned now to the subject that really interested me, namely the visit by Fritz Deinhardt to Lindi camp between January and April 1958, to study the effects of infectious hepatitis virus in some thirty of the chimpanzees.[8] Dr. Henle confirmed that the hepatitis research had been funded by the Armed Forces Epidemiological Board, and that this included the Congo study. She added that Deinhardt had gone to the Congo just the once, at the time that Koprowski was working on his polio vaccine, and said that it was possible that Koprowski had helped set up the visit. She admitted that she had not been too keen on Deinhardt's going; again she was not certain of the specific reasons, but suspected that it might have involved her personal feelings about Koprowski.

In the early fifties it was considered that *Homo sapiens* was the only "susceptible animal" to hepatitis, and Dr. Henle conceded that another of the reasons for her lack of enthusiasm about the study might have been that two prisoners had met their deaths while taking part in human hepatitis experiments — though these were apparently not from the group with which she and her husband had been working.[9] However, by the late fifties there was a growing suspicion among virologists that infectious hepatitis virus might be transmissible to chimps. Deinhardt's Congo work was one of the first attempts to test this experimentally, and Dr. Henle confirmed that the research had been inconclusive. Many of the chimps showed evidence of slightly altered liver function (suggesting that they might have been infected with the virus), but only one demonstrated symptoms typical of human hepatitis.

Next I asked about the chimpanzee kidney tissue cultures that are mentioned, almost in passing, at the end of the article. To refresh her memory, I showed her the relevant paragraph of the paper, which described the dispatching by air, from Stanleyville to Philadelphia, of six shipments of minced chimp kidneys.[10] Despite the fact that a lot of time (from three to six days) passed between kidney excision and tissue culture preparation in the Children's Hospital virus lab, five of the six shipments produced good cultures after trypsinization (the addition of the enzyme trypsin, which helps break down minced tissues into individual cells and clumps of cells).[11] Gertrude Henle scanned the paper and read aloud the sentence about not finding any latent or adventitious viruses in the chimp kidney tissues.

Monkeys, by contrast, "are loaded with latent viruses," she commented. I did not bother to point out that in the years following 1958, several researchers had reported that chimpanzee tissues were similarly riddled with contaminating viruses.[12]

I asked if Fritz Deinhardt had sent the six shipments of kidneys back himself, and she agreed that he had dispatched them by air during his time in Stanleyville.[13] Had chimpanzee tissue cultures been sent before from there? I asked her. There was quite a long pause. "Well, of course, they had tissue cultures from the monkey kidney for making polio vaccine," she answered, carefully. Was that chimpanzee kidney, I asked, in an attempt to confirm the key point. Again there was a pause. "I have no idea what that one was," Gertrude Henle replied.

Sometimes, in the course of an interview, one comes to an important junction and makes the wrong choice. Relistening to tapes months or years later, it is easy to see that one should have abandoned a certain path much earlier than one did, or else followed up an avenue of questioning much more promptly or vigorously. This was one of the latter times, for this was clearly the moment to establish exactly what Gertrude Henle meant by these apparently carefully weighed comments. She appeared to be saying that primate kidneys had been sent out from Stanleyville before Deinhardt's visit at the start of 1958, and that they had been used to manufacture polio vaccine. If Gertrude Henle was correct, then it is hard to imagine that the vaccine in question could have been other than Koprowski's CHAT or Fox, or that the monkey kidneys could have been other than chimp kidneys.[14]

Even in her eighties, Gertrude Henle was still a very precise and careful scientist, and her unwillingness to specify the vaccine or vaccine-maker, or to identify the monkey, suggests that the information was based on hearsay — that she had not witnessed the process herself. And who might have been the source of such a story? The most likely candidates would presumably have been her husband, together with Fritz Deinhardt, and even Tom Norton or Hilary Koprowski, before she and Koprowski fell out. Among that group of Philadelphia-based scientists — the ones who might have been privy to such important information — she and Koprowski were the only ones still alive.

But unfortunately, instead of pressing Dr. Henle for further details straightaway, I decided that it was only reasonable to provide some background information about CHAT vaccine, including the fact that certain aspects of its provenance were not entirely clear. "Who is interested in all that now?" she asked. I told her that I was, and why, and she said: "But, you know, the deed is done. . . ." So I explained further about the potential significance of this information, including a mention of the close relationship between HIV-1 and chimpanzee SIV. "I have never heard anything [about that]," Gertrude Henle muttered under her breath.

Later, I asked her again whether shipments of chimpanzee kidney might have been sent from Stanleyville to Philadelphia before Deinhardt's visit, and whether these might have provided material for the manufacture of polio vaccine, for instance at the Wistar Institute. But by now Gertrude Henle was wary of making any further comment on the subject. She made no attempt, however, to deny or withdraw the initial statement.

I asked if she thought it was wrong to follow up events such as these. "I don't say you are wrong, but it might be futile," she said. "The trouble is, what can you do about it? Something has happened, yes, but what can you do about it?" I explained the reasons why I thought it was important to investigate such matters — one of the most important being that if mistakes had been made, then perhaps similar mistakes might be avoided the next time around.

"But you don't understand," said Dr. Henle, "that this was an era when we didn't know that monkeys [had] these other viruses. . . . What shall I say? It would be very difficult to prove. You know, you work at a certain time, and something explodes. But there will be other things exploding, what with the molecular business [genetic engineering] that they are now doing. . . . The trouble is . . . it's always something new which happens. . . . Do you think this doesn't happen all the time?" A little later she warned me: "If you are fighting Hilary Koprowski, God help you. . . . He is very vicious."

She also offered some parting advice. "Don't forget that I'm an awful lot older and wiser. I know a lot more about life than you do, because you're very much younger." It was said kindly, with a smile, and yet as I drove away, I was thinking to myself that on this occasion I was happy to be bracketed with the younger and more naive.

---

Other voices produced other opinions about Koprowski. He had clearly made a strong impression on many of the women whose paths he had crossed — and not always negatively, as with Gertrude Henle. I met Mrs. Anna Wiktor, the widow of Tadeusz, the Polish vet whom Koprowski had first met at Muguga, and whom he later employed for some thirty years at the Wistar Institute, during which they collaborated on developing a rabies vaccine. She told me: "I was always scared of him. He [has] such a brilliant, intelligent, sparkling personality that when you talk with him, you feel like . . . a little ant someplace on the ground — even though he is not such a tall man. His personality gives you this impression of greatness. [He] was like that from the moment I met him, and is like that today."

Another Polish woman with whom I spoke was Dr. Zofia Wroblewska, again a longtime employee of the Wistar Institute, who described him as "a man of the

Renaissance. He's very interested in anything human — medicine, human art, human love. He's got a beautiful collection of art, he's interested in crime stories and the history of the church. He even wrote a novel not long ago — about a painting discovered on a yacht. He's a very polyvalent man. . . . He [was] really a very efficient director of this institute." But just as I was beginning to wonder whether Dr. Wroblewska was being a dutiful employee, for Koprowski had, after all, suggested that I interview her, she remembered some less idyllic qualities. "We all complained about him being merciless. If he wanted us to do something, we had to do it, no matter our opinion on it. Sometimes in the middle of the night we [had] to take tissue after a multiple sclerosis patient had died. We had instantly to go, whatever the weather. It was like in the army."

She said that she thought the CHAT/AIDS hypothesis very unlikely, but added that some in the Wistar had been rather taken aback by certain elements of the controversy. "We were surprised he didn't know which tissue culture he had used for CHAT," she said, getting right to the nub of the problem. "And why not test the vaccine? It would show good motivation."

---

A different perspective again was provided by Leonard Hayflick, the developer of WI-38, the human diploid cell strain. Hayflick had done his doctoral dissertation at the Wistar between 1952 and 1956, before Koprowski's arrival, during the years that, he said, marked the beginning of the "golden era of virology," when the ability to grow viruses in tissue cultures rather than in live animals opened up vast new possibilities for research. He had been away from Philadelphia for two years when he learned from Werner Henle that Koprowski was looking for a tissue culture specialist. Hayflick jumped at the chance of returning to Philadelphia, where he headed the Wistar's tissue culture laboratory for the next ten years.

When he started working for Koprowski in 1958, Hayflick's job was to supply cells of various types to the Wistar Institute's new team of researchers. At the time, there was great interest in the possibility of using normal human tissue as a cell culture medium. Although cancerous tissue is easy to procure from hospitals, normal human tissue is more problematical, in that most people prefer not to part with it. In any case, adult tissue is frequently host to viral flora including adenoviruses, so Hayflick began investigating the potential of human fetal tissue as a source of "clean" cell cultures.[15] At the time, Sven Gard was on sabbatical at the Wistar, and he was able to arrange a supply of such tissue from abortions conducted in Stockholm. When Hayflick began growing this tissue in the lab, he found that fibroblasts (the cell type which holds tissue together) were the cells most easily cultured, although they died after a finite number of divisions: normally about fifty. However, fifty population doublings produces a massive number of cultured cells. Hayflick decided to characterize this new type of culture as a human diploid cell strain (HDCS).[16]

At the end of the fifties, when Hayflick was developing WI-1, his first experimental HDCS, all polio vaccines were still being manufactured in monkey kidney tissue culture. This was largely because polio will only grow in primate cells,[17] because monkeys are the cheapest available primates, and because the kidney is one of the largest discrete and easily removable organs. However, it was becoming widely realized that there were inherent problems with this tissue culture system. As Hayflick put it: "Monkey kidneys, as you will recall, were notorious for their content of unwanted viruses — potentially dangerous viruses, maybe even [the simian precursor of] HIV, who knows?" This was, to say the least, a remarkable aside.

His human diploid cell strain, by contrast, was capable of growing every single human virus, and could be frozen at different passage levels and studied for years, if one wished, to ensure that it was free of adventitious viruses. Whereas, he said, every individual monkey kidney (or pair of kidneys) is "a universe unto itself [with] respect to virus contamination," a human diploid cell strain like WI-38 represents a single universe — one that can be checked for viral surprises and that had proved itself, he claimed, to be an "absolutely clean" substrate. And, he went on proudly, "that single WI-38 universe can be used to produce all of the world's human virus vaccines this century . . . theoretically 20 million metric tons, whereas one monkey kidney can only produce a few thousand doses."[18]

Hayflick's enthusiastic advocacy of WI-38 was understandable, given the scandalous way in which it had been ignored by governments and vaccine manufacturers down the years. The corollary of this frank advocacy was that he was also uninhibited about the dangers of monkey kidney. He pointed out that although SV40, for instance, was a contaminant of the seed strains used to make all three types of Sabin's polio vaccines, it was in reality the final substrate that presented the real problem in terms of contamination. "Triple plaque purification tells you nothing about the substrate, just [about the attenuated polio] virus. The final substrate [for polio vaccine] was constantly contaminated monkey kidney," he said. Once again, he mentioned HIV-1, but quickly added that "as far as we know" the virus does not replicate in a substrate of rhesus and cynomolgus kidney.

Later, however, when I pointed out the uncertainty about the species used to make the final CHAT vaccine strains, and the lack of details about the derivation of the different pools, he said: "In retrospect, we can be very critical about these things, about things that seem so obvious today. But even if you make the worst case out of it, the worst case being that the CHAT pool was contaminated with HIV [or SIV] — even if that were true, there is nothing that was known at that time which could have prevented that from happening. Nobody was doing things at that time ... which were devious." To support his last statement, Hayflick pointed out that he had vaccinated his own children with CHAT.

What I found refreshing was that here was a long-term Wistar employee, a close colleague and in many ways an admirer of Koprowski's, who — even if he did not believe that the CHAT/AIDS hypothesis was true — was not afraid to address the possibility rationally and without hysteria.

Hayflick was interesting in his analysis of Koprowski. On the one hand, he thought him "a brilliant, marvelous personality; an excellent scientist; a tough leader." On the other, he conceded that Koprowski "frequently did things ... which made me very unhappy." Although unwilling to be absolutely specific, Hayflick did say that Koprowski had done "things behind my back that I didn't appreciate," which included "something that I thought was underhand." He also mentioned an episode about which I hadn't heard, which had involved Koprowski's patenting of the hybridoma process for making monoclonal anti-bodies — a technique that is "a major, major aspect of the biotechnology indus-try today."[19] This process, he explained, had actually been discovered by two British scientists, but they had failed to patent it, leaving Koprowski free to reg-ister his own patent. "I suppose it wasn't illegal," said Hayflick, but it was prob-ably "unethical in the eyes of many people."

In many ways, Leonard Hayflick was perhaps the most even-handed of all the one-time associates of Hilary Koprowski whom I interviewed. In his final assessment, he was apparently equivocal. Like so many, he was amazed — even seduced — by the man's Renaissance qualities, by his enthusiasms, by his mul-tiple talents. But he was also aware, sometimes painfully so, of his shortcomings, of his cavalier treatment of people, of his dilettantism, of his occasional bend-ing of morality to his own ends, and selectivity about the information that he imparted.

# 36

DAVID HO

The very last meeting I had scheduled during this seven-week American trip was with Dr. David Ho, the director of the Aaron Diamond Center in Manhattan, which was already — in late 1993 — regarded by many as the leading center of HIV research in the world. I wanted to see him for two reasons. First, he had been one of the six members of the Wistar's expert committee, which had pronounced that CHAT vaccine had almost certainly not been the source of AIDS. Second, it was Ho who had then contacted the Manchester team, and persuaded Gerald Corbitt to send him samples of David Carr's tissues for further PCR analysis. Although he had published nothing on his findings, he had spoken to several reporters during the course of 1993, and had stated on the record that the HIV-1 in the Manchester sailor's tissues appeared to prove that the AIDS virus had been in existence for "many decades — or even perhaps centuries."[1] The inference was that this disproved "a whole bundle of origin theories," most notably the CHAT hypothesis.[2]

The only time Ho could spare was on my final afternoon in the States, so we arranged that I would meet him for an hour on my way to the airport. I arrived well ahead of time at the Aaron Diamond Center, loaded down with bags packed with papers and cassette tapes. I did not yet know it, but another *Eureka* moment was looming.

———

David Ho was entirely different from how I had imagined him. With his round, boyish face and pudding basin haircut, he could easily have passed for a man in his twenties, although he was actually forty-one. I soon realized, however, that he was a remarkably astute, clear-headed thinker, with the capacity to cut right through to the heart of a problem, and to adapt quickly to a situation as it developed. He had a reputation for getting things done, and even for being rather ruthless — which reputation, as I later came to realize, was perhaps not entirely unjustified.

He started by telling me some of the background to his collaboration with Corbitt and Bailey on the PCR work. He explained that during the deliberations of the Wistar committee the previous year, they had dug out some of the old reports of cases likely to be examples of archival AIDS, including several articles in the *Lancet* (almost certainly the letters from Germany, Belgium, and Denmark, relating to cases in 1976 and 1977), and the St. Louis case from 1969. But the most important report they investigated, he told me, had been that of the Manchester sailor who had probably become infected while traveling abroad in the navy between 1955 and early 1957. "That may or may not be true, but we think that's true. And if so, he acquired the virus before the polio vaccine trial, which started in late '57," Ho explained, "so that simply says, well, the polio vaccine cannot be the origin of AIDS or HIV."

It was when Ho realized that Corbitt and Bailey had still not obtained the full sequence of the HIV that they had managed to amplify on PCR, that he suggested to Corbitt that his own lab might be able to help. Andrew Bailey had been struggling with the work for over two years, sequencing a few fragments here and there in between other bouts of lab work. Ho's scientists, by contrast, using DNA that the Manchester team had already extracted, managed to sequence the entire HIV genome, all ten thousand or so nucleotides, in the space of a few months. "You've got the whole sequence?" I exclaimed. "Yes," answered Ho, "but" (and now he started laughing) ". . . from a kidney tissue." Clearly the fact that HIV had been isolated from the kidney was somewhat embarrassing within the context of the CHAT/AIDS hypothesis, for it appeared to support the concept that HIV could survive in kidney cells.

Ho went on to say that they had used their own conserved primers (suitable for all known variants of HIV-1) and had managed to get the whole genome out in five easy pieces. He added that the small portions of sequence that Bailey had obtained matched up nicely with their longer sequence.

I said that they must be very excited about all this. "Oh, we're still very excited," he said. "The thing is the sequence we obtained has very important implications for the evolution of these viruses." He went on to say that there was only one hitch — that they needed additional tissue materials from Manchester, in order to be able to confirm their results.

So far they had examined DNA that had been extracted in Manchester from the kidney and bone marrow, together with several other examples of DNA, which had been amplified in the course of Bailey's PCR work. Although they had found HIV in the kidney DNA, they had failed to find any in the bone marrow DNA or in the amplified PCR products. For this reason, they had asked George Williams, the retired pathologist who was in possession of several of the tissues, to provide some more of the original material. Despite stating several times that he was on the point of sending more tissue, Dr. Williams had apparently still not done so, and finally David Ho had even offered to go and collect it himself. It was clear that he was now losing faith in Williams. He said that until he did get more tissues and could confirm the presence of HIV, he was not prepared to talk about his findings at big meetings, or publish any papers on the subject.

He told me that they had also spent a lot of time on phylogenetic analysis, comparing the sequence that they had got with other sequences of HIV-1, and had found that the "virus is not all that different in sequence from the viruses we have today in our population. Even though there's a space of thirty years or more." He confirmed that the sequence was that of a subtype B virus, the subtype that predominates in North America and Europe and that is causing the greater part of the worldwide pandemic of AIDS. "We know it's not exactly identical to any known virus. So we're comfortable that it's not a lab contamination by a known isolate," he replied. The back of my neck was beginning to tingle.

He went on to say that a lot of virologists had expected that the sequence would prove to be quite close to the SIV found in chimpanzees (SIVcpz), which was presumed to be the ancestral sequence for HIV-1. He himself, he admitted later, had expected greater divergence from modern sequences. However, the sequence they eventually obtained was actually a "run-of-the-mill subtype B."

There used to be people, he added, who felt that HIV-1 and SIVcpz had only diverged on the phylogenetic tree perhaps fifty or so years ago. I asked him to name some of these people, and he mentioned Gerry Myers, head of the HIV Sequence Database. If their Manchester sequence was confirmed, however, then this interpretation of events went out the window.

Ho quickly sketched me out a sample tree, to demonstrate what he was talking about. He drew five major divisions of the primate immunodeficiency virus (PIV), all of them diverging from a central node. Three of the branches represented the SIVs of the African green monkey (SIVagm), the mandrill (SIVmnd), and the Sykes' monkey (SIVsyk). Off to the left was the HIV-2/SIVsm branch, toward the end of which there was a cluster of sub-branches representing HIV-2, the SIV of the sooty mangabey (SIVsm), and that of the macaque (SIVmac). Away to the right was the HIV-1/SIVcpz branch. Some way before the end of this, the chimpanzee SIV (SIVcpz) split away, and then, further along, the HIV-1 branch divided into smaller branches representing the different subtypes, or clades: A, B, C, D, E, and F. On the branch marked B, he drew a thick growth of twigs, representing the different isolates of the Euro-American AIDS epidemic, and on one of these twigs he wrote "1959."

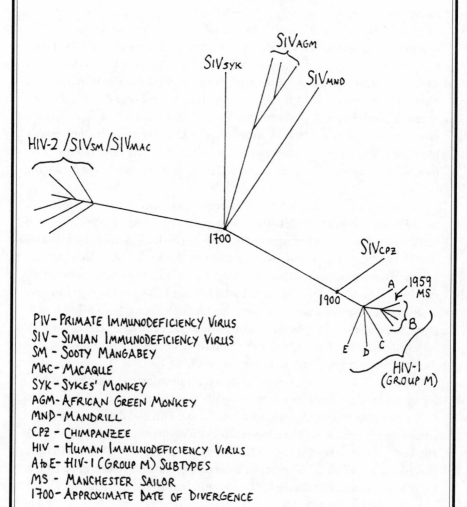

PIV PHYLOGENETIC TREE,
AS SKETCHED BY DAVID HO IN 1993

SIVagm

SIVsyk

SIVmnd

HIV-2 /SIVsm/SIVmac

1700

SIVcpz

A    1959
       MS
1900          B

E   D   C

HIV-1
(GROUP M)

PIV— PRIMATE IMMUNODEFICIENCY VIRUS
SIV— SIMIAN IMMUNODEFICIENCY VIRUS
SM — SOOTY MANGABEY
MAC— MACAQUE
SYK— SYKES' MONKEY
AGM— AFRICAN GREEN MONKEY
MND— MANDRILL
CPZ — CHIMPANZEE
HIV — HUMAN IMMUNODEFICIENCY VIRUS
A to E— HIV-1 (GROUP M) SUBTYPES
MS — MANCHESTER SAILOR
1700— APPROXIMATE DATE OF DIVERGENCE

Then he circled the subtype B branch, and wrote "30" underneath it, indicating that if the Manchester sequence was genuine, then this branch must have started to bush out about thirty years ago. He was now able to work backward and date the other major nodes, starting with the divergence between the HIV-1 branch and the SIVcpz branch, which, according to this scenario, must have occurred approximately one hundred years ago. As for the initial node, where the five major branches split one from another, he wrote "300" against that. He explained that these were the *minimal* number of years ago that divergence had occurred, based on the Manchester sample, because the tree he had drawn assumed a linear rate of growth. But if, as some people thought, the HIVs had been evolving much more quickly in the course of the current AIDS epidemic (in other words in a nonlinear manner), then this effectively pushed the earlier nodes even further back in time.[3] Some people, he told me, had even suggested that you could multiply the ages of the nodes by a factor of ten.

Ho said he was shocked that the British had not done more to find out about the travels of the sailor, and he started to tell me about a British TV producer who had apparently found out more about the man's movements, in the course of a few days of phoning around, than had any of the Manchester scientists.

At this point, I was unable to restrain myself any longer. I knew that Ho seemed to believe that David Carr had traveled to Africa, and that this was probably based on some of the erroneous press reports that had appeared in the United Kingdom at the time that Corbitt and Bailey announced their initial PCR findings in 1990.[4] I told him that I had found out sometime ago where David Carr had traveled while in the navy. His whole demeanor changed. He said: "Maybe you could tell me a few details about this man."

I told him that I would, but the hairs on the back of my neck were standing up again, and this time I knew what was going on. All sorts of stored information and memories were being processed — including my several rather unsatisfactory contacts with George Williams, his unwillingness to release tissue samples for confirmatory testing, Simon Wain-Hobson's skepticism about the lack of progress on sequencing, the fact that David Carr had probably been no closer to Africa than Gibraltar, the fact that he had not been promiscuous. Added to all this data was David Ho's own visible unease about the case, despite his understandable desire to believe that the Manchester sequence was genuine (and thus momentously important). Quite suddenly, a circuit was completed and there was a read-out.

A moment of time had passed, and now I was certain, without a shadow of doubt, that the Manchester sailor sequence had been a contamination. I put the question to Ho — could there conceivably have been cross contamination in one of the Manchester labs? He paused for a second or two, and then said quietly: "Yes." Then he added: "That's what we're afraid of. That's why I want confirmation."

Ho told me that Corbitt had written to him, detailing the precautions they had taken, including taking the sample to a lab that had never previously been used for HIV work, but he still wondered if something might have gone wrong. "If PCR technology has a flaw, it's that it's too sensitive, and could pick up contaminations from the environment," he observed.

I needed to leave this subject for a few minutes, so I began to tell him some more about my own researches — how I had got hold of tissues from two AIDS-like cases that were even earlier than that of Carr, and how both had been PCR-tested by Fergal Hill at the Department of Haematology at Cambridge University, who had failed to detect any trace of HIV. Then I related some of my own dealings with George Williams. I told Ho that after I discovered that he (David Ho) was also working on the case, I had gone back to Williams and asked him again whether he might be able to supply some tissues for Fergal Hill to test. Initially he had said that he would be happy to cooperate,[5] but when I followed up by phone a few weeks later, he had changed his mind. Now he told me that he would be unable to help because David Ho had asked for further tissues, and there was very little material left on the blocks; they would get destroyed, he said, if he attempted to slice away any more. (And yet, when I first interviewed him in 1990, he had told me that he had taken about fifty blocks at the autopsy in 1959.)[6] In other words, Williams had rejected my request on the grounds that he was helping Ho, but had still not supplied Ho with the promised tissues.

David Ho echoed my concerns, though some of what he said next was off the record. He also told me that John Crewdson had looked into this case, and had walked away from it, saying that he did not trust certain parties. Ho repeated that Williams "knows the kind of investment we made already. We just need to sequence a tiny bit, and if they match up, we're done." He explained that although the sequence they had obtained was that of a fairly typical subtype B, "it doesn't match up identically to any known virus. All we're trying to say is that it's not a contaminant of any known virus."

I asked Ho if there was any possibility that there might have been deliberate contamination of the samples. He told me that they had matched up the human DNA from the kidney with that from the bone marrow, and proved that they were almost certain to have come from the same individual. In the HIV DNA from the kidney, he added, they had encountered what is called a "quasispecies phenomenon" — they had found not just one sequence, but a mixture of closely related sequences, which is exactly what one finds *in vivo*, in HIV-positive individuals.[7] However, with a laboratory contamination, you normally find just a single sequence — that of the HIV isolate that is being used (perhaps as a positive control) in the lab. Suddenly, without warning, he cut to the chase.

"The only type of contamination that would account for this is if somebody added some cells from a modern AIDS patient to the DNA extraction process," he said. "So if this is a contamination, we feel that it's a deliberate one."

I was aghast. I told him that right from the beginning, George Williams had been absolutely tight-lipped about where the samples were being held. Suddenly David Ho broke in. "His home," he said.[8]

When asked to sum up where he stood on the case now, Ho put it succinctly: "I'm very concerned that we've spent a lot of time and energy working on something that may have a big hole somewhere at the other end. I am absolutely confident about what we have done here, but I'm concerned about my interaction with the people at the other end, particularly Williams."

———————

Later, we got back to the subject of David Carr's travels. I told Ho that it seemed likely that Carr had never traveled outside Europe. Ho sounded disappointed, but then asked if he had ever been to Eastern Europe. Again, I told him no. The furthest confirmed place that he had visited was Gibraltar. "Ah, Jeez," said Ho. "We said northern Africa; Gibraltar doesn't even count as northern Africa."

I added that there was still a possibility that David Carr might have made a day trip to Tangier.[9] But even if he had made that trip, and even if he had had sex in a brothel there, it would still signify very little, in that the first evidence of any form of HIV being detected in Morocco stemmed from the period 1984 to 1987. In 1991, almost three hundred persons from the general population of Tangier had been bled, and none had tested positive.[10] Just as tellingly, HIV infection among female prostitutes in Andalucia, the region of southern Spain that surrounds Gibraltar, was zero in 1985,[11] and continued to be relatively low five years later.[12]

Ho asked if the patient had been gay, and I told him there was no evidence to suggest that he had been. He then observed that Carr had had biopsy-proven perianal herpes at the end. My understanding, I told him, was that although the huge anal sore had very likely been herpetic, this had not been clinically diagnosed. In any case, perianal herpes did not constitute proof of a homosexual lifestyle.

Ho stressed again that the geography was important, "because you could [ask]: 'Was there an earlier epidemic that occurred in Europe that was missed?'" I asked if he was thinking of the PCP epidemics that had swept across Europe (but especially the eastern states like Czechoslovakia and East Germany) in the fifties, and he agreed that he was. So I told him about my contacts with the Czech PCP expert, Kamil Kucera, who was convinced that HIV had not been involved. Apart from PCP, hardly any of the other normal presentations of AIDS — such as wasting, skin lesions, unbridled fungal infections, and so forth — had been identified among the children and infants involved in these Eastern European outbreaks, and the tissue samples that Kucera had provided for PCR analysis had not contained any detectable HIV.

When I told Ho that Sweden was the only other place outside the United Kingdom that David Carr was known to have visited, I could see that he too was reaching a turning point, and finally admitting to himself that the case of the Manchester sailor was almost certainly not a genuine case of AIDS. He in turn confirmed an interesting rumor about the St. Louis case from 1969, saying there were widespread misgivings about the original Western blot results,[13] and that autopsy material had been extensively tested by the Cetus Corporation and found to be PCR-negative for HIV.

Later, Ho explained his other reasons for having suspected that the Manchester sailor case might be genuine, which centered on the apparently slow rate of evolution of certain SIVs. He told me that a colleague of his had sequenced ancient materials from mangabeys in museums, and found that they contained SIV isolates that were very similar to modern isolates of SIVsm.[14] (In fact, this research would also subsequently turn out to be flawed — again, in all likelihood, as a result of PCR contamination in the laboratory.)[15] Ho also pointed out that SIVsm had been transferred to macaques in primate centers in America in the sixties, resulting in the new macaque virus, SIVmac, and yet there was little evidence of divergence between SIVsm and SIVmac. It occurred to me that one factor here might be that sick macaques had generally been removed from holding pens, or else sacrificed, and so the macaque epidemic of SIV had perhaps not had the same opportunities for onward spread as the human epidemic of HIV.

---

I had just a quarter hour left before I had to leave, so I finally got on to the subject of the Wistar expert committee. I said that I had to be frank — I had been surprised by the report, and felt that the reasons expressed for rejecting the OPV/AIDS hypothesis had been insubstantial. The one exception, of course, had appeared to be the Manchester case — and even that now appeared to be dubious. What did he feel now?

Ho told me that when you make a monolayer (a single cell layer) of monkey kidney tissue culture, you lose most of the lymphocytes and macrophages, "and you basically end up with epithelial type of cells which do not carry HIV [or SIV]." So, he said, if they had passaged these a few times and then grown the poliovirus, it would be extremely unlikely for any SIV to have survived — especially since they were also freeze-thawing the cells. "We actually took Koprowski's protocols and [went] through [them] step by step, and tried to say what is the chance of a tiny amount of SIV surviving all of those steps, and to [be transmitted] to a human. . . . And these were their original protocols." He conceded that the Manchester case had also "played a role." Not just a role, I pointed out, but the clinching role.

Ho said that there was only one CHAT sample from this period left, "and they want to get it into the right hands, done properly. And I don't think anybody wants that assignment." I said that from what I'd heard, the Wistar considered that there was too little material left to divide it into two, so that two different laboratories could test it. I said that this sounded very strange — surely you only needed just one drop for PCR work? Ho agreed. "I think that [the Wistar claim] is probably not true," he said. "The Wistar would be perfectly happy just to bury the whole thing anyway."

Later, Ho volunteered the fact that "those people really don't know what type of monkeys they used to get the kidneys" for making tissue culture, adding that Koprowski had admitted this to Frank Lilly of the expert committee.[16] I just had time to propose that if one of the CHAT pools used for feeding people in Africa had been made out of chimpanzee kidneys, "there would be considerable grounds for concern, would there not?" Without elaboration or qualification, Ho simply said, "Yes."

As I was packing up to go, I asked David Ho if he still had some of the Wistar committee documents, or any of the background materials that had contributed to its deliberations and findings. He said that he still had a file "this big"— holding his hands quite wide apart — and he agreed to send me copies of the key documents. He also promised to keep me posted on developments on the David Carr case and, indeed, suggested that we collaborate on this topic.

Clearly the most important information to come out of the meeting with David Ho was that the finding of HIV in the tissues of the Manchester sailor had been flawed. This, of course, overturned the key item of evidence offered by the Wistar expert committee to support its dismissal of the CHAT/AIDS hypothesis. There might be other reasons (like whether SIV/HIV could survive the vaccine-making process, as mentioned by Ho) for doubting that hypothesis, but these would be far less persuasive if the repeated hints that chimpanzees or their organs had been involved in the manufacture of at least one batch of CHAT could be substantiated. Once again, the game was on.

In the end, matters did not work out quite the way that we had planned. Apart from sending one brief letter in March 1994, telling me that he had finally received further tissues from George Williams, David Ho did not communicate with me again until after the story that the Manchester sailor case was false had been broken by the British science journalist Steve Connor, fully fifteen months later, in March 1995.[17] A few months after this, however, David Ho did eventually send the documents that had been viewed by the Wistar expert committee — documents that were to prove extremely significant for the OPV/AIDS hypothesis.

# VI

## WHIRLPOOLS AND SINKHOLES

*What was he doing, the great god Pan,*

    *Down in the reeds by the river?*

*Spreading ruin and scattering ban,*

*Splashing and paddling with hoofs of a goat,*

*And breaking the golden lilies afloat*

    *With the dragonfly on the river.*

— Elizabeth Barrett Browning,
"A Musical Instrument"

# 37

BILL HAMILTON

My first meeting with William D. Hamilton, the Royal Society research professor[1] in evolutionary biology based at Oxford University, took place in September 1993, shortly before my departure for the States. I contacted him mainly because, of the several eminent scientists to whom Louis Pascal had sent his OPV articles, he was one of the very few to have replied encouragingly,[2] and to have continued to correspond thereafter. It was clear from the text of that correspondence (copies of which had been sent me by Pascal), that Hamilton had immediately grasped the import of the central hypothesis, which he considered far more important than Pascal's emotive tone of delivery, or his lack of formal scientific qualification. It was also clear that Hamilton was an exceptionally open-minded scientist, one who was unfettered by concerns about funding and establishment approval.

Professor Hamilton invited me to visit him at his cottage in a small village near Oxford. It turned out to be old, entwined by ivy, and conveniently attached to the back of the local pub. As he answered the door, he cut an impressively professorial figure, tall enough to have to stoop slightly at the threshold, with a head of thick, curly silver-gray hair and a serious face, which had vertical lines etched into it. He spoke little, and when he did it was slowly and quietly, on occasions even hesitantly. However, it soon became apparent that what he had to say was well worth listening to.

He made some coffee, and we sat down on ancient armchairs afloat in a small sea of papers and books. We started out by discussing the mysterious author of the OPV/AIDS hypothesis. I explained that Pascal and I had had something of a falling-out, and Bill Hamilton said that he was little surprised, in that Pascal clearly had a cantankerous streak, and very easily became upset with people. However, he added, his theory was impressive, and he could see no flaw with the central arguments. "He understands the evolutionary implications better than most natural scientists," he continued, which, coming from one of the world's leading evolutionary biologists, was an impressive testimonial. "I also think he has been very badly treated by the medical establishment," he added, referring to the rejection of Pascal's several important articles on the subject by a series of journals.

Hamilton went on to say that the assumptions made by medical scientists, that species jumps are very unlikely, were quite wrong. He pointed to the fact that none of the African monkey species infected by SIVs seemed to get disease — in these species, at least, the virus had apparently evolved long enough to have a minimal impact on its simian hosts. For a sexually transmitted virus, this was doubtless adaptive: sick monkeys cease to copulate and transmit, so it is the less pathogenic viral strains that develop an evolutionary advantage. In Asian monkeys and humans, by contrast, the pathogenic impact of the virus showed that it was newly introduced, and not yet adapted. This was borne out by the phylogenetic trees, which demonstrated that the branching of the HIV lineages, and the divergence of the SIV lineages found in Asian monkeys from those in African monkeys, had occurred very recently, over a time scale of tens or (at most) hundreds of years. By contrast, the various primate species that played host to these viruses had clearly evolved from each other over a time scale of millions of years. A species jump was the only rational explanation for the evolution of the HIVs and the Asian SIVs, and the synchronicity of emergence of these viruses suggested that human hands (perhaps even those of the medical scientist) may well have played the crucial role.

Hamilton's work on sex as a driving force in evolution meant that he was fascinated by AIDS, and especially by the very small proportion of people who might turn out to be resistant to the disease. He surmised that it would perhaps take "many hundred of years before we can all be descended from the one percent who [might be] resistant." At the same time, however, the mutability of the virus had other, more negative implications for *Homo sapiens.* "There's likely to be a very wide divergence of this virus in the human population," he added. "It's certainly possible that it will change its mode of transmission." This, of course, is one of the greatest concerns about a volatile virus like HIV-1 — that a variant might emerge that is transmissible by insects, or by aerosol means: through coughs and sneezes. Similarly, a new variant of the dreaded Ebola virus — one that became epidemic among monkeys at a holding center in Reston, Virginia, in 1989 — was thought to have been transmitted by the aerosol route, since the infection spread not only to monkeys in different cages, but also to those in different rooms (presumably via the air-conditioning system). Fortunately the Ebola Reston variant proved not to be transmissible to humans but, as Richard Preston pointed out in *The Hot Zone,* we may not be so lucky the next time around.[3] Hamilton observed that the sudden epidemic outbreaks of Ebola virus in southern Sudan (near the Congo border) and northern Congo (around Yandongi and Yambuku) in 1976[4] had all the characteristics of zoonoses — diseases that have jumped from animals to man — and wondered whether Ebola, also, might have emerged as a result of vaccination campaigns.

Like myself, Hamilton was convinced that the key part of the HIV-1 story was the connection with chimpanzees, which are the only animals to carry a closely related form of SIV. He noted that there was still a minimum 20 percent difference between HIV-1 and the known isolates of SIVcpz, but suggested that this could be bridged in a relatively short period of time. He gave the example of the serial passage of human poliovirus in simian tissue culture, which was known to be a good way of encouraging genetic mutations (such as those causing attenuation), and said that the serial passage of the even more mutable SIVcpz in humans could quite swiftly cause that virus to become HIV-1. Alternatively, he said, there could be a wide divergence of SIVcpz strains present in different races of chimps — and perhaps a group of chimps infected with a strain that was genetically close to HIV-1 happened to be in the right place at the right time (or the wrong place at the wrong time, from a human perspective).

Hamilton's theorizing on this topic tied in so closely with what I had already learned about the activities at Lindi that I was quite taken aback. I decided, however, not to lay all my cards on the table at once, but instead asked him about the hypothetical potential of a vaccination campaign to spread an SIV contaminant. Yes, he said, the monkey kidneys used to make the vaccine could easily have contained lymphocytes, which, in turn, could have contained an SIV. Infants, with their immature immune systems, would undoubtedly have been the most vulnerable to infection with tiny amounts of such a virus, but children also might have been more at risk than adults — especially in a mass vaccination such as that in Ruzizi. "I just bet that one in a thousand kids, in the agitation, would bite its cheek or tongue, especially when confronted by a white man," he mused. This, of course, would provide an even more accessible portal of entry for the hypothetical viral contaminant to the human bloodstream.

Shortly before I left, I asked Bill Hamilton what would be required for him to be convinced by the OPV/AIDS theory, and he listed three factors. These were that a virus even closer to HIV-1 be found in a chimpanzee; that chimps be implicated in the tissue culture used to grow batches of the CHAT vaccine; and that the Manchester sailor case "could somehow be dismissed."

His parting words were ones of encouragement. "I hope you and Pascal get a fair hearing," he said. "I think it's very important, both for future generations of humanity, and for the future of medical science. So many mistakes have been made, and we need to examine the process, and see what's going wrong." We arranged that I would call on him again after my return from America.

When we next met, on New Year's Eve 1993, at least one of Bill Hamilton's three requirements had been met, in that the Manchester sailor case now appeared to be unsound. By this stage, I had already decided that I could confide in Hamilton, and spent most of the afternoon and evening describing the results of my researches in America and Europe. His comments and feedback were invariably pertinent and valuable, and at the same time he was clearly excited by what I had managed to discover.

With respect to the *Rolling Stone* clarification and the continued hostile reception afforded the OPV/AIDS theory, he said that "a lot of people in virology may believe that the story could be true, but see their world crumbling, and are afraid for the story to get out." He went on to surmise that in the late fifties, most virologists would have been more concerned to keep human cancer genes out of their vaccine substrates than about the many simian viruses they were discovering — most of which then appeared to be harmless.

But what interested Bill the most was the news that the pygmy chimp, *Pan paniscus* (also known as the bonobo) as well as the common chimpanzee, *Pan troglodytes,* had been heavily involved in the vaccine research at Lindi. For one thing, the presence in a single chimpanzee colony of two species, which have been naturally segregated for tens of thousands of years by the Congo River, raised fresh possibilities of cross-species viral jumps — in either direction. (Although nobody had yet discovered an SIV in *Pan paniscus,* only very few of the creatures had been tested.) For another, the pygmy chimp, he told me, is "notorious for its sexual promiscuity."[5] One of the pertinent questions that all this raised was whether a pygmy chimp and a common chimp, if left alone in a holding pen, would have sexual contact with each other (Bill had read somewhere about the two species interbreeding).[6] Another was whether the two animals would fight. Either activity could result in viral transfer.

Bill also floated a pet theory of his own, one that raised some very interesting possibilities. Although as a hypothesis it was new to me, something rather similar had crossed my mind after the discussion with James Oleske about the case of the New Jersey teenager who appeared to have infected her infant daughter with HIV perinatally, but who was herself still apparently healthy at the age of thirty-six. What, he said, if a small inoculum* of SIV (as, according to Pascal's hypothesis, might be contained in a polio vaccine) had — because of the tiny amount involved and its as yet imperfect adaptation to the human environment — the effect of immunizing some of its recipients against HIV, just as the deliberately maladapted virus in a live polio vaccine immunized against

---

* Inoculum: A biological material that is introduced into a living organism or substrate.

poliomyelitis? And what if such "HIV vaccinees" entered a silent carrier state, similar to that exhibited by some persons with syphilis, so that they themselves showed no symptoms of disease, but had the capacity to infect others, such as sex partners or children? According to this scenario, the first appearance of AIDS might not be among those fed the vaccine, but rather among their primary contacts. Indeed, as the epidemic progressed, and more and more HIV variants, specially adapted to humans, emerged through mutation and recombination, it was even possible that the only people immune to these new wild HIVs would be those who had received the contaminated vaccine.

In fact, he went on, it was probable that a vaccine contaminated with SIV would actually elicit a wide range of host responses. Some recipients might end up immunized against HIV. Others, such as normal healthy adults, might remain entirely uninfected, for the simian contaminant was, after all, not yet adapted to humans. A third, smaller group of recipients — consisting mainly of infants and the already immunocompromised — might become infected and go on to get disease.

It was a fascinating hypothesis. We both agreed, however, that for the present at least it was entirely conjectural and would be extremely difficult either to prove or disprove. Instead, we set to thinking about practical ways in which to investigate some of the remaining missing details about CHAT. Clearly it was vital to find out more about what had happened at Lindi and, to this end, I told Bill that I would be going back to Belgium some time in the new year. The other, even more important, avenue to pursue involved trying to track down a sample of the original CHAT vaccine.

I brought Bill up-to-date on the follow-up that I had done so far. In the summer of 1993, I had made several phone calls to the Wistar Institute, and ended up inquiring of Martha Lubell, a public relations representative, about progress on the testing of the CHAT sample. She told me that it seemed to be at a standstill, in that the CDC had agreed to test the sample, but only if one or two other organizations did likewise. "My understanding was that there were two problems," she had added. "They do not have a large enough sample for it to be tested more than once, and also there were no [other] organizations that wanted to do it." When I suggested that this was effectively a Catch-22 situation, she replied: "Yes, I was just going to say the same thing."[7]

Information gathered since then — from David Heymann at the WHO and Brian Mahy at the CDC — suggested that Catch-22 still applied, and that the Wistar sample was not about to be tested. There was, however, one other possible avenue to follow. I told Bill about my conversations a few months earlier with Margerete Böttiger and Carl-Rune Salenstedt of the Karolinska Institute in Stockholm, and the strong suggestion that they still had samples of Koprowski's CHAT pool 10A-11 in their freezers, together with the appropriate protocols. We talked about this for a while, and then Bill told me that he had to attend a three-day conference in Scandinavia in late January. If I liked, he could meet with me in Stockholm after the conference, and we could make a joint visit to see Hans Wigzell, the director of the Karolinska, to seek his permission to have a sample of the vaccine released for testing.

This seemed an excellent idea, and we talked for a while about the scientific methodology such a study would involve. Clearly it would be preferable to include control samples of other polio vaccines (like another OPV, and perhaps the Swedish IPV made by Sven Gard), so that the tests could be conducted in the context of a double-blind study, and ideally the vaccines should be tested independently, in two separate labs. Bill further proposed that as well as having the vaccines tested for the presence of HIV and SIV, it might well be possible to check the mitochondrial DNA of the host species, to determine which species of primate had provided the tissue culture cells in which the vaccine had been made. This was an entirely new idea to me, and it offered a realistic technique that might finally establish the substrate that had been used for CHAT vaccine.

After years of sometimes painfully slow research, it was a joyous experience to meet with someone who believed in the importance of examining the OPV/AIDS theory properly, who agreed that it might very well have merit, and who was fully prepared to lend his considerable weight and experience to further the investigation. And there was more to come. Before I left that evening, I explained to Bill that my funds were now all but exhausted, and that without taking out a substantial bank loan, I would be unable to complete the remaining European research. I knew that during 1993 he had won two prestigious and lucrative prizes for his work in evolutionary biology — the Crafoord Prize from the Swedish Academy of Sciences, and the Kyoto Prize from the Inamori Foundation, based in Japan. Would he be willing, together with the intellectual and moral support he was already providing, to lend me enough cash to complete the research?

Without further ado, Bill produced a checkbook. He told me that one of the conditions of the Kyoto Prize was that some of the money, at least, should "be used for the good of mankind," and that he could not think of a better project to support. He told me to consider the check as a grant, rather than a loan.

Driving homeward, shortly before midnight, I knew that there could not have been a better way to end 1993.

---

The meeting in Stockholm was arranged for January 24, 1994, and involved Bill Hamilton and myself on the one hand, and Hans Wigzell and Carl-Rune Salenstedt (respectively the general director and the head of vaccine production at the State Bacteriological Laboratories) on the other.[8] Salenstedt came across — as before — as being kindly and rather avuncular; but Wigzell was altogether a different character — dapper, courteous, and clearly very sharp, but with a discernible streak of coolness and control. After Wigzell had given a brief but elegant opening speech, he turned the floor over to Bill, who explained the potential importance of the sample and the reasons why it was vital to test it. I followed with a brief review of the evidence that suggested that there might be merit to the OPV/AIDS theory, including the fact that the Wistar appeared less than keen to test its own Congo vaccine sample.

In response, Salenstedt confirmed that Margerete Böttiger did still have samples of CHAT vaccine, which had been stored at minus 70°C since being received from the Wistar in 1957 or 1958. She also had sera from the Swedish vaccinees, taken before and after vaccination. He went on, however, to say that Böttiger was uneasy, because it was unclear to whom the vaccines belonged, and she did not recall the terms of the initial agreement. She knew only that Koprowski had originally given the vaccines to Sven Gard, to be used in small-scale trials in Sweden. Salenstedt had already asked Gard for his advice, which had been that they had best consult Koprowski direct.

Now Wigzell entered the debate for the first time. He said that Koprowski was very intelligent and a good scientist, but added that he was a "big cat," and one who "always land[ed] on his feet." It could be a very fussy legal matter to determine to whom the vaccines now belonged — whether it be the Karolinska, the Wistar, or Koprowski himself. Just as I was visualizing Koprowski's likely reaction, and beginning to think that we had come all this way for nothing, Wigzell added that there might be another alternative — to test the vaccines in Stockholm without informing Koprowski. But because of the legal difficulties, they wouldn't be able to pass on samples of the vaccines to anyone else.

Wigzell proposed that the samples should be checked for the presence of HIV-1, HIV-2, and SIV, using PCR. Bill interjected to say that we would also very much like to know the species in which the vaccine had been manufactured, to see whether chimpanzee tissues might have been involved. But Wigzell replied that it would probably be very difficult to determine the host species, since it would require the use of specific primers, and that it would be best to establish first whether an immunodeficiency virus was present. If one was, it would then be appropriate to try to establish which host cells had been used for the substrate. He added that the monkey used should have been documented in the protocols, and that they would "dig out all the papers" that were available. However, all written materials were stored in the archives, which now occupied over a mile of shelving, so that might not be easy.

Wigzell acknowledged that if there was any truth to the OPV hypothesis, then they would need to test "a lot of worried people" in Sweden who had been fed the vaccine, but that to undertake such tests was justifiable from their point of view. "Let's assume I find the [vaccine] sample is positive," he went on. "I [would] then have to sort out the legal situation with the Wistar Institute, and then I'd have to check with the Ministry of Health. But I'll not run away. Being a director of a large government institute, I have to take good things, but bad things as well. I will not be gagged. I wouldn't like it, but I wouldn't duck it."

He added that if their testing revealed nothing, then this would argue against the likelihood that this batch of vaccine was contaminated. In that case, he said, the title of my book could be "A Close Shave." It was said with humor, but it seemed to me to be a little premature for anyone to be thinking of potential book titles.

Wigzell said that we should get back to Salenstedt by the middle of February, by which time they should have located the protocols, and might even have started testing the vaccine samples. When asked once again whether the vaccines could also be tested independently, by a neutral third party, which would render the results less of a political hot potato if they did turn out to be positive, he said that he might be willing to send samples of the vaccine to the National Institute for Biological Standards and Control, in Potters Bar near London. "We'll think about it," he added.

Outside, as Bill waited for a taxi to take him to the airport, he and I discussed the import of the meeting. Bill was encouraged, feeling that Wigzell had been sincere, albeit worried, and that he genuinely wanted to test the vaccine. I, too, was very pleased, in that for the first time an agreement had been struck to test a sample of CHAT vaccine for the presence of lentiviruses. However, I was a little less sanguine than Bill, in that the agreement seemed to be hedged around with a number of caveats. In particular, I was concerned that Wigzell had not agreed to release any sample of vaccine for independent testing or, indeed, to test the vaccines for host DNA.

And as it turned out, the testing procedure would go far from smoothly.

---

From Stockholm, Bill returned home to England, while I took a train north to Lapland. At Abisko, a village near the Norwegian border, I found the perfect place to stay — a converted wooden cabin with a sauna. Outside, it was 35°C below, the coldest weather for ten years, and there were just a few hours of daylight before the great arctic darkness took over, interrupted only by the northern lights, which bounced and danced in the frozen sky. The cabin was surrounded by fields of unbroken snow, like blank sheets of paper awaiting the first line of text. A week went by, and I mapped out a plan and synopsis for the present book.

Back in Oxford, Bill had also been busy. Toward the end of the week, a lengthy communication from him juddered forth from the fax machine at the local railway station. It contained the draft of a follow-up letter to Wigzell and Salenstedt, informing them that he had contacted Dr. Wesley Brown, chair of the department of biology at the University of Michigan, an expert in mitochondrial DNA work, who would be willing, if required, to test the vaccine samples to establish host species. He also argued forcefully that the vaccine samples should be tested in two laboratories, writing: "Mr Hooper and I both feel that it is extremely desirable, both to cover your lab and to arrive at facts believable by all, that the vaccine be tested, preferably simultaneously, for both viruses and host DNA *in some other lab in addition to yours.*"

Also included in the fax was the text of a letter entitled "AIDS Theory vs. Lawsuit," which Bill had just submitted to *Science.*[9] This letter highlighted the freedom of speech issue that had first been raised by Brian Martin from Wollongong University,[10] and emphasized that it was vitally important that the OPV theory of origin be given a fair hearing. In particular, it contrasted the "good science journalism" of the original *Rolling Stone* article with Koprowski's reply to *Science* (in which he had represented the Curtis article as "idle, unresearched speculations by a reporter") and the subsequent defamation lawsuit, which had been withdrawn only after *Rolling Stone* had agreed to publish its clarification. Hamilton admitted that the Curtis article had featured a couple of small errors (which he identified), but added that apart from these "it is hard to see what . . . Koprowski considered unfactual, unreasonable or unduly *ad hominem* in the matters described." He also pointed out that there were snags to the OPV/AIDS theory, and carefully analyzed five such snags, to each of which he also provided answers of varying persuasiveness.

He went on to explain that he was not advocating the theory as the most likely explanation for AIDS. "My object is simply to emphasize that every theory has snags and ways round, and that the proper course of Science is to allow *all* theories to be discussed so that their critical points can be focused and tested. It is certainly not the way to use lawsuits to terrorise individuals and journals that try to promote discussion." After comparing such an approach to that of burning heretics alive, he asked: "Are we starting this all over again with a Medical Establishment now in the robes of a universal Church? . . . The overcrowding of humanity plus its fluid mixing means that *in respect of future human epidemics,* failure to heed lessons before launching new public health campaigns has a potential to result in hundreds of millions of deaths. Nor is it just potential if the AIDS-polio connection turns out to be right: the above rough estimate is then certainly an under-estimate."

After highlighting the pioneering work on the theory done by Louis Pascal, but also by others like Blaine Elswood and by Lecatsas and Alexander in South Africa, Hamilton added that the OPV/AIDS theory "seems to have stirred action in a half dozen or so . . . scattered, diverse, well-informed people." He went on to point out that the panel convened by the Wistar committee, after six months of deliberation, had produced a strongly dismissive report, but that "several items in that report [seem] weak"; and he added that the failure to test the one vaccine sample identified by that panel, even though so many months had elapsed, "seems extraordinary." Curtis, he wrote, "has summarized the outcome as like a jury bringing a verdict of not guilty when an obvious key witness is still waiting in the court to be heard."

Hamilton concluded strongly, pointing out that the continued use of monkey kidney tissue to make vaccines and the increasing use of organ transplants from primates to humans were increasing the likelihood of future species jumps by pathogens, which "may be very dangerous for human future, indeed could conceivably deny humans having a future. Scientists should listen to and investigate with due care all hypotheses, including common sense suggestions and warnings from outside their ranks; they should not endeavour to suppress them. In the face of overbearing professional mystique, disregard, and now even litigation, the public becomes justified in its growing disillusion with science and in some of its deepest fears."

Hamilton also submitted a covering letter to the editor of *Science,* Daniel Koshland, in which he added further supporting evidence, including a point-by-point refutation of Koprowski's letter to *Science*[11] published in August 1992.[12] He pointed out that the subject of his letter "has a long history of rejection and even near ridicule in *Science,*"[13] and said that he expected it "to be given a rough ride by most referees." But he urged Koshland to "consider the issues concerned, and why such rejection might be strongly expected from such sources." He ended this covering letter by gently reminding the editor of his qualifications for making the submission, including the several articles he had had published in *Science* over the years, and the fact that within the course of twelve calendar months in 1992 and 1993, he had won three large international prizes for his work in evolutionary theory. Two of these, he pointed out, "are intended to fill subject gaps between the Nobel prizes and to be equivalent to them."

Less than three weeks later, a brief communication from Christine Gilbert, the letters editor of *Science,* acknowledged that Hamilton was "superbly qualified to comment," but informed him that she had discussed his submission with Dan Koshland, "and he believes that it would not be appropriate for *Science* to publish it at this time, as we have devoted considerable space to the topic you address." A further extremely eloquent letter by Hamilton to Koshland, requesting him urgently to reconsider, met with a similarly negative response.[14]

Later, Hamilton redrafted and reinforced the text of the *Science* letter, and submitted it to *Nature,*[15] again enclosing a covering letter for the senior editor, John Maddox, which explained why he felt the issue was so important and outlined the history of its rejection by scientific journals, including a mention of Louis Pascal's own rejection by *Nature* itself. The journal submitted the letter to one referee, and then it too rejected it, principally on the grounds that "it doesn't contain any substantially new revelations." Hamilton was, however, invited to submit a commentary piece, which could examine the various different theories of how the virus arose.[16] He declined, feeling that such a huge subject could not usefully be reviewed in the two pages offered.

Bill Hamilton may be one of the leading evolutionary biologists of his times, but he was discovering for himself, and for the first time, how the dead hand of inertia tends to fall on a theory that seriously threatens the central tenets and self-esteem of the scientific world. Once again, major journals had stonewalled a statement urging that the OPV/AIDS theory should be taken seriously. Later, Bill told me he felt that he was "swimming in treacle."

At the start of the 1990s, the Vatican issued a belated apology to Bruno and Galileo for the treatment it had afforded them four centuries earlier.[17] It may be that in years to come, the spiritual and technological descendants of Dan Koshland, John Maddox, and other pillars of the current scientific establishment will find it in their hearts to apologize retrospectively to William Hamilton, Louis Pascal, Tom Curtis,[18] and others, for the failure to publish their warnings about the origin of HIV-1, and about the risks to humanity of further unintended microbial gifts from medical science.

# 38

## THE TWO SAILORS

At this point, a brief update is required on the European mariners — David Carr and Arvid Noe — who, rightly or wrongly — have become the two persons most closely associated with the early course of the AIDS epidemic.

———

Although it seemed clear that what the Manchester doctors and David Ho had sequenced was a contamination with a modern HIV strain, I was still not yet *convinced* that David Carr had not had AIDS. What if he had after all been infected with HIV, but the broken strands of ancient viral DNA had not been picked up by PCR, in contrast to the more readily detectable "modern" HIV DNA from the contamination? I decided that I would be remiss if I did not at least look into what had happened to David in those last two years of his short life, and the surprising link between Dr. Koprowski and the city of Manchester.

The Pawel Koprowski Memorial book that Hilary Koprowski had given me during our second interview made it clear that the renowned virologist had idolized his father;[1] the introduction was full of tales of treacle and derring-do. It also contained details of how and when his father had died, and the fact that the last time Hilary had seen him alive was on February 25, 1957, when Pawel was recovering from surgery in a London hospital. Hilary had apparently flown back to America, only to be informed by telegram of his father's death shortly afterward.

This was strange timing indeed. Only days before this, Hilary Koprowski had been on his way back from that fateful trip with Tom Norton to the Belgian Congo. It seems that he must have stopped in England, spent some time with his father, and then flown back to the States on February 25 or 26. It may be that one reason for the timing of his return was an understandable desire to participate in another important event. This was the first "official" feeding of CHAT vaccine to the six infants at Clinton, which occurred on February 27, 1957, the seventh anniversary of his first-ever use of oral polio vaccine. His father died in his adopted hometown of Manchester just hours later, and Hilary once more crossed the Atlantic to attend the funeral on March 1.[2]

The memorial book makes it clear that he stayed in Manchester for a further two weeks. I wondered if it was possible that during this fortnight he offered his newly developed vaccine, Charlton — or CHAT — Plaque 20, to local clinicians, just as he had offered it to doctors in Nairobi and Stanleyville a few weeks earlier. Alternatively, this could have happened later, if he returned for a memorial service, which, in Jewish tradition, is often held a year after the burial. By March 1958, of course, David Carr was out of the navy, and was once again working in central Manchester at the Kemsley House printers.

The other important lead that I wanted to pursue was the possibility that Dave Carr might have paid a visit to Tangier in Morocco. After many disappointments, I managed to track down "Kevin," a self-employed builder, who had been Dave's best friend for the final years of his life. He recalled that ever since they first met in 1954, Dave had always had pallid skin and trouble with his gums, which he thought was termed "pyorrhea." He told me that yes, Dave had been to Africa, but then spoiled it by saying that the place he recalled was Istanbul. When I prompted him with Tangier, he told me that that too rang a bell. He recalled nothing about visits to brothels, but added that Dave "could easily pull a bird. He was a good-looking lad."

Another friend, "Clive," at whose wedding in September 1958 Dave had been best man, told me not to believe everything Kevin said, and that as far as he knew, Dave — despite being popular with women — had not been very experienced. "It was different in those days," he added. "Nights out didn't end up between the sheets as they seem to these days. Many virgins went to the altar in the fifties. It was a different ball game." He vaguely recalled that Dave had once bragged about going into "some sort of brothel, a sleazy sort of place [where he'd] taken advantage of the local facilities." Clive conceded, however, that Dave might have borrowed someone else's story in order to impress his mates over a few pints.

Finally, I managed to trace someone who had been on the *Whitby* during her Gibraltar visit of February 1957, and who had even been on a day trip to Tangier with about a dozen other ratings, including a larger-than-life figure recalled only as "Big Robbo." Apparently the sailors had spent the afternoon wandering around the bazaars and markets of the Old Town. When shown a photo, my informant said he did not remember Dave Carr as having been on the trip — and added that in any case, they had never gone to a brothel. They had all

DAVID CARR'S TRAVELS ABOARD HMS WHITBY,
NOVEMBER 1956 TO AUGUST 1957

returned in the late afternoon, save for Big Robbo and one of the others, who were arrested for drunkenness and had to be escorted back to Gibraltar the following day.

Another man from the *Whitby,* a petty officer, did recall Dave's face from the photos, but said he thought that he had worked as a steward rather than a stores assistant. He thought that the Big Robbo episode had been the only time that any of the crew had visited Tangier that February of 1957, and that further visits had been banned after Robbo's arrest and disgrace. He added that the Spanish brothels of La Linea and Algeciras had been off-limits at that time, owing to a border dispute, and that prostitution was strictly illegal in the small British dependency of Gibraltar. The brothel hypothesis, therefore, was becoming less and less plausible.

Around this time, a third approach to the Royal Navy produced some important documents — among them a complete, dated record of the ships on which David Carr had served during his period of National Service. This gave a rather different version of events to those previously provided by naval records. Dave had apparently spent his first month of National Service, November 1955, doing the basic training course at H.M.S. *Drake* in Devonport,[3] and had then moved to H.M.S. *Ceres,* the Royal Navy Supply and Secretariat School, where he appeared to have trained first as a steward, and then as a victualing stores accountant. Between May and November 1956, he had served at H.M.S. *Harrier,* a "stone frigate" in Pembrokeshire, South Wales, which served as the navy's weather forecasting school. (It appeared that the previous claim that he had served on H.M.S. *Warrior* — the headquarters ship for the 1957 nuclear tests — had been mistaken, the result of a careless reading of a handwritten entry on his file.) It was confirmed that between November 1956 and the end of August 1957, Dave had been based in Northern Ireland with H.M.S. *Whitby,* before returning to H.M.S. *Drake* for the final two months of his service.

For the first time, it was possible to come to certain firm conclusions about the travels of David Carr. First, it was clear that the only time he left Britain was during his two years in the Royal Navy. His union records showed him to have been working in Manchester throughout the rest of the fifties, so he certainly did not (as some have hypothesized) do an extra stint in the merchant navy after his National Service. Second, his naval records and the appropriate ships' logs show that the only two places he visited outside the British Isles were Sweden and Gibraltar. The logs make it clear that the *Whitby* was either moored in Gibraltar or on maneuvers in the Mediterranean throughout that fortnight in February 1957, which proves that the ship did not call at any other Mediterranean or African port.[4] Third, eyewitness accounts suggest that David was not a member of Big Robbo's raiding party on Tangier.

In short, it seemed that David Carr had probably never visited Tangier, let alone visited an African brothel or had sex with an African woman.[5]

However, I was still determined to try to find out more about Hilary Koprowski's visit to Manchester after his father's death, and to this end I located the exclusive apartment block where his father, Pawel, had lived, and the office and sweatshop in a now-deserted building beside the canal, from where he had run his import-export business in the forties and fifties.

Although I was unable to trace any of Pawel's friends from the cotton industry, I did manage to locate the ninety-seven-year-old Dr. John Wilkinson, who had signed Pawel Koprowski's death certificate on February 28, 1957, ascribing the death to a heart attack. He was also, at that time, head of the Department of Haematology at the United Manchester Hospitals (which included the Manchester Royal Infirmary, where David Carr died).

Dr. Wilkinson still recalled Pawel Koprowski, and the fact that he used to visit him in his rooms at Lorne Street, behind the MRI, for checkups after his cotton-buying trips to Europe and the Americas. He remembered meeting the son, Hilary, on two occasions — once at the funeral, and once when they discussed the idea of creating some sort of memorial for his father. It was Dr. Wilkinson who had suggested making it a vacation award, and who then agreed to serve as head of the board of trustees. I asked Dr. Wilkinson if he and Dr. Koprowski had spoken about polio vaccines, and he told me they had never discussed his work.

As far as I could determine, and despite the fact that CHAT had been tested in humans for the first time just before his father died, there was no evidence to suggest that Hilary Koprowski had brought his polio vaccines to Manchester, or that he offered them to local physicians for trials. If he had done so, then Dr. Wilkinson would surely have been among those invited to participate.

Pawel's grave is situated in the Jewish cemetery in south Manchester. It is a beautiful memorial — a simple black marble headstone, rough-hewn around the edges, bearing inscriptions in English and Yiddish.

And even here there is a strange coincidence. For just over the wall behind the memorial stone is the crematorium where, thirty months later, the ashes of David Carr were consigned to the earth beneath a simple rosebush. The last resting places of the two men are barely seventy yards apart.

But if not AIDS, then what did cause Dave Carr's death? Later in 1994, I asked Val (as next of kin) to write two more letters to the navy, seeking further information about Dave's medical history. As a result, she received a photocopy of his medical records for the period of his National Service. They revealed a lot more than anyone had anticipated.

In particular, they showed that Dave's health problems had begun in February 1956, while he was training at H.M.S. *Ceres,* at Wetherby on the North Yorkshire moors. A medical entry on March 19, 1956, revealed that he had been suffering for a month or so from "an irritating rash over both legs"; various medicaments had been tried, without success. By the end of March, Dave was back in Devonport, where he was found to be suffering from two boils on his thigh, and excema on his calf. These were treated with massive penicillin injections and a further range of creams and lotions.

By August 1956, Dave was in South Wales, where he had a sebaceous cyst removed from the back of his neck, causing him to take eleven days off active duty. And by June 1957, just after the visit to Malmo, he was back in the sick bay, this time with a rash on the buttocks, which was treated with "little response." A further medical examination detected a nonfungal rash in the groin and armpits; it was noted that he had been suffering from such symptoms for the past year. Apparently, several treatments had been tried without effect.

What this clearly reveals is that Dave Carr was suffering chronic and wide-ranging skin infections for all but the first three months of his two-year National Service, and that these began in February 1956, fully a year before the visit to Gibraltar. We know that these problems continued after his naval discharge at the end of 1957, because his civilian medical records attest that he began attending Christies Radium Hospital in Manchester on a monthly basis from the start of 1958, to get radiotherapy and steroid treatment for rashes on his back and shoulders. They also reveal that he had been suffering from gingivitis since early 1957, and from hemorrhoids and *pruritis ani* (an itchy anus) "for many years."[6]

There was also one further intriguing clue in the medical records. In November 1955, upon his induction into the navy, Dave had received the full regime of vaccinations, including a tetanus shot. And, at some time in January 1956, at H.M.S. *Ceres,* he had been "pretreated," and was then given an "ATT" injection on the final day of that month.

I was unsure what the latter two entries might mean. However, I was eventually able to interview a senior officer of the Institute of Naval Medicine in Gosport, who told me that the ATT entry could have referred to a booster of antitetanus toxoid. But he too was uncertain what "pretreatment" might indicate, saying only that "it sounds like he was being pretreated for something he was going to be exposed to," such as malaria. I pointed out that members of the armed forces had also been used as guinea pigs in germ warfare experiments during this period, and the officer agreed that such trials had taken place. He promised to investigate discreetly, but he never got back to me with any results.

Was it just coincidence that Dave Carr's first skin problems started during February 1956, a few weeks after these vaccinations and the "pretreatment"? In 1984 it was reported that tetanus boosters given to healthy people can cause a temporary but significant decline in CD4/CD8 ratio (the ratio between two different types of lymphocytes, the T-helper and T-suppressor cells), for a period of up to a fortnight. To some extent, this mimics the impact of AIDS, although in the latter instance the decline is usually permanent.[7] Quite apart from this, occasional cases have been reported in the medical literature in which people respond badly to vaccinations, especially the multiple immunizations that are often given at the start of a military career — when they tend to coincide with a period of heavy physical exertion and emotional stress.[8] For example, the "vaccine cocktail" given to many Gulf War combatants prior to their departure or during their presence in the war theater, is now being associated in many quarters with Gulf War syndrome.[9]

In conclusion, we can only say that David may have been immunocompromised even before the start of his National Service in 1955, or he may have been one of those unfortunate few for whom the administration of a series of vaccines triggers a significant decline in health. This process may well have been exacerbated by the radiotherapy and steroid treatments he received during 1958. Whatever, it seems very probable that David Carr finally succumbed not to AIDS, but to what doctors would now define as ICL, or idiopathic CD4+ lymphocytopenia — which the press sometimes calls "AIDS without HIV."

---

Even as one postulated case of archival AIDS in a sailor seemed less and less plausible, another similar case — that of the Norwegian sailor — became ever more credible. Given the fact that sera taken in 1971 and 1973 from three members of the same family (Arvid, his wife, and his youngest daughter) had all tested HIV-positive — and that all three had died with symptoms typical of AIDS — the case seemed incontrovertible. After the David Carr debacle, the case of "Arvid Noe" had taken on the mantle of the earliest instance of AIDS on record.

Accordingly, after my visit to Stockholm and Abisko, I took the train west to Norway, and spent two more days following up the story. This time, apart from the doctors, I also interviewed two of Arvid's former bosses at the trucking companies where he worked in the early seventies, during the time of his apparent remission from AIDS.

I discovered a lot more about Arvid's history. After he recovered from his first bout of illness in 1966, he worked for a couple of years in the big marine shipyard in Horten. Then, in July of 1969, the year when his youngest daughter first fell sick, he started working for a long-distance haulage firm. In October, he and a colleague broke new ground by driving down to Bandar Abbas in the Persian Gulf with spare parts for the Norwegian merchant fleet; the round trip took nineteen days, and was later described as "the world's longest truck route."[10] Arvid never traveled that far again, but for the next four years he made weekly runs down to central Europe, delivering ship paints, waxes, and polyesters, and returning with raw materials for the Norwegian factories.

Although his destinations included Rotterdam in Holland, Liège in Belgium, Lyon (France), Basel (Switzerland), Milan (Italy), and Vienna (Austria), 70 percent of these trips had been to West Germany. He delivered to factories throughout the country, but mostly to the industrial area of the Ruhr, where he apparently visited "almost every town." One of the delivery points was Cologne, and the major pickup point for return cargo from Germany was a factory making polyester powder in Wesseling, which lies just ten miles south of Cologne.

The transport manager of one haulage firm gave me some background about the lives of the drivers. Usually they drove alone, and slept in their cabs in truck parks. Since there were no black boxes in those days, it was up to them how they scheduled their trips; they had only to arrive back in five days or seven days, depending on the destination. In those days, truck drivers were among the best-paid workers in Norway and many, he said, had girlfriends in different towns, or would pick up prostitutes when they stopped for the night. His guess was that Arvid was one of those who did so, and this was confirmed by one of his former drivers, who told me that Arvid had often bragged about his sexual adventures — both as a trucker and during his time at sea.[11]

---

Knowing what we do now about the early appearance of AIDS in West Germany — a phenomenon that is at first sight surprising, given the lack of colonial links between that country and Africa — it is hard not to look at the long journeys of Arvid Noe in the early seventies, and to posit a connection. It is certainly possible that the young soldier from the Koblenz area would have visited prostitutes, especially during his time of National Service.[12] And the fact that Herbert H., the bisexual violinist from Cologne, liked busty women for his orgies suggests that he and his bisexual friends may have hired female prostitutes with the desired physical attributes. The musician first fell sick with the symptoms of AIDS in late 1976,[13] and so he may well have become infected during the early seventies, when Arvid was driving to and fro across the Ruhr. It may even be that the musician and the truck driver had sex with the same woman, and that Herbert's bisexuality denoted the point at which HIV-1 crossed from the heterosexual to the homosexual community. Furthermore, just forty miles north of Cologne (and close to yet another of Arvid's factories) lies Gelsenkirchen, the family home of the gay German chef who left to work in Haiti in 1977, before succumbing to AIDS in New York in 1980.[14]

At this point in my researches, in early 1994, it began to seem that far from being a link in a broken chain, Arvid could conceivably have been the point-source of the Euro-American epidemic, the carrier who brought the ancestral strain of HIV-1 subtype B out of Africa to the industrialized world.

Of course, in order to prove this hypothesis, it would be necessary to confirm that both Arvid and Herbert had been infected with HIV-1, and then to sequence their viruses, to determine whether or not they came from the same clade, or subtype. Around this time, Dr. Mike Tristem, head of the virus laboratory at the Imperial College campus at Silwood Park, just outside London, twice wrote to the Norwegian and German doctors who held sera from Arvid Noe and tissues from Herbert H., formally offering to undertake PCR analysis on the samples. A sample from a KS lesion on Herbert H.'s leg was repeatedly promised, but never arrived. Dr. Frøland, by contrast, simply ignored the correspondence. Later on, Karl Wefring told me that "Dr. Frøland is very firm: he will do the PCR screening himself."[15]

So we sat back and waited for news from Oslo.

---

I was also looking further back in the mooted transmission chain, and by this time was all but convinced that Mombasa was where Arvid had become infected with HIV. He had shown his first symptoms of prodromal AIDS in 1966, and was therefore almost certainly infected during his time in the merchant fleet. His younger brother (on the basis of Arvid's own comments) believed that an episode in an African port had been responsible for his illness;[16] Dr. Wefring reported that he caught gonorrhea during both his visits to Africa; and Mombasa was Arvid's only African port of call during his final two ocean voyages.[17]

If I was right, then two big questions remained. Who had been the carrier who infected Arvid? And how had an HIV-positive person come to be in Mombasa in 1964 — so long before the beginning of the recognized AIDS epidemic?[18]

The first hypothesis that had to be examined was that Mombasa might have been the very place where the crucial transfer of SIV into humans occurred. And, as mentioned earlier, there had indeed been an OPV field trial that had taken place at the right place and the right time to fit with such a scenario.

Between December 1959 and December 1960 more than 1.7 million Kenyans, including 55,000 from Mombasa, were vaccinated with a South African Type 1 OPV made by James Gear.[19] The vaccine was based on Sabin's LSc strain, and was prepared in a tissue culture made from the kidneys of the South African subspecies of African green monkey, *Cercopithecus aethiops pygerythrus*. This, it may be recalled, is the same species of monkey in which

Mike Lecatsas later reported finding a virus that showed "HIV-1-like" bands on Western blot.[20]

Could it be that James Gear's OPV was contaminated with the simian precursor of HIV-1? Frankly, this seemed implausible, for had this been the case, one would have expected cases of AIDS to have begun appearing in places where the vaccine was fed — such as Kenya, Mauritius, South Africa, and Kampala in Uganda[21] — by the late sixties, or certainly by the seventies. Public health was well monitored in those countries during these years, and yet there is no evidence of AIDS emerging until the start of the eighties, long after the first cases had begun appearing in the Congo and Rwanda.

Furthermore, labs like those of Fergal Hill in Cambridge and Beatrice Hahn in the United States subsequently conducted PCR tests on sera from Lecatsas's African green monkeys, and failed to obtain any convincing HIV-1-like sequences. In short, there was no persuasive evidence to suggest that the strange results on Western blot were anything more than nonspecific reactions, perhaps lab contaminations.[22]

This brought me back to a second possibility, one that was raised — and then casually dismissed — by Robert Gallo in the Tom Curtis feature in *Rolling Stone*.[23] Was it plausible to suggest that an HIV-1 newly arrived in humans could have traveled from the area of the large-scale CHAT vaccinations, for instance in Ruzizi in early 1958, to the city of Mombasa in late 1964?

A brief glance at the transport connections between Rwanda and Burundi and the Kenyan coast suggested that, contrary to Gallo's conclusion, the hypothesis was eminently reasonable, and that a single infected person could readily have carried the virus from one place to the other. Thirty-five miles south of Nyanza Lac, the most southerly CHAT vaccination site in Burundi, is the Tanzanian lakeport of Kigoma — which is also the western terminus of the railway from Dar es Salaam. From Dar, the next major seaport to the north — just 200 miles distant — is Mombasa. Alternatively, the road connections from Rwanda through Uganda to Kenya could have brought a traveler to Mombasa in just a couple of days.

In short, if Arvid Noe had indeed been infected in Mombasa, then it was certainly conceivable that a single individual who had been infected with HIV through a polio vaccine trial in the late fifties could have been the source of his infection. One could imagine, for instance, that a young Rwandan woman who had lost her husband in the ethnic violence of the early sixties might have fled Rwanda for the Kenyan coast, where she was forced into prostitution in order to support her children. Perhaps Arvid was one of her first customers, but then — after a few weeks or months — before any others had been infected with HIV, she went back westward, disenchanted, to rejoin her fellow-refugees. And perhaps a few years later, in a camp somewhere in Tanzania or Uganda, this woman fell sick and died, to be buried quietly beneath foreign soil — just another sad statistic in a continent that gets more than its fair share of tragedy.

---

It would have been remarkable if my various transmission hypotheses had hit on the exact route taken by HIV-1 on its travels from central Africa to Europe, the Caribbean, and America. However, they did provide a plausible scenario for how the virus *might* have spread — one that did not conflict with the historical evidence, and that correlated with the travel history of Arvid Noe, the man who was now the earliest clinically and serologically confirmed case of AIDS in the world.

# 39

The *Bibliothèque Royale* — or Royal Library — in the center of Brussels is an impressive building, approached via two lengthy flights of stone steps and entered through a neoclassic vestibule of vast proportions. It houses the best collection of Belgium's colonial newspapers and magazines — including, of course, the provincial publications from the Belgian Congo and Ruanda-Urundi.

I returned to Brussels in the spring of 1994 and spent the first week at one of the benches in the reading room, while porters ferried leather-clad volumes from Stanleyville, Leopoldville, Elisabethville, Bukavu, and Usumbura to and fro on mahogany trolleys. I flicked through these ancient journals page by page, day by day, looking for entries relating to vaccinations, polio, Koprowski, Plotkin, chimpanzees, monkeys, or other topics of interest. It was achingly slow research, but every day revealed some new items of interest, and gradually a fuller picture of life in the final years of Belgium's African colonies, and of the vaccination program, began to emerge.

The first reference I was able to locate to the Courtois/Koprowski collaboration appeared in an edition of *Le Stanleyvillois* from November 1956. A general article on polio featured a passing reference to a group involving Dr. Courtois and some American researchers, which would shortly begin conducting "purely experimental" studies of live polio vaccine administered to "monkeys."[1]

Further perusal of the two Stanleyville papers (*Le Stanleyvillois,* and *L'Echo de Stan*) revealed that Koprowski had apparently paid only two visits to the city, both in 1957. There were several articles about Koprowski and Norton's visit in early February, the first of which[2] was an account of an open lecture about polio vaccination, which Koprowski had delivered at the nursing school in Stanleyville on the evening of February 7 (six days after the two men left

Nairobi).[3] In this report, Koprowski is described as being a professor from "the University of Philadelphia,"[4] the vice-president of the New York Academy of Sciences, scientific expert of the World Health Organization, and head of its mission to the Belgian Congo. The reference to his WHO expert status is misleading, in that this title pertained to his work on rabies, not polio, and the claim that he was head of a WHO mission to the Congo is simply incorrect.[5] Even more significant is the fact that no mention is made of his being a Lederle employee, even though he continued to be one until the end of April.[6] In all practical senses, Koprowski was acting as if he had left Lederle and was already at his director's desk in the Wistar Institute.

In his introduction to Koprowski's speech, Ghislain Courtois points out that "for a while now, the services of the Stanleyville laboratory have had a zoological center where tens of chimps have been collected in order to conduct polio experiments." The nature of the work is described, rather vaguely, as "the development on chimpanzees of criteria showing the efficacy of the attenuation of live vaccines"; apparently "once these attenuation criteria and the absolute efficacy of oral vaccination have been shown, it will be possible to proceed to mass-vaccination on a world scale."

Koprowski then delivered his speech, which mainly concerned the history of OPV. He said that in the United States some seven hundred people had been vaccinated against Type 1 and Type 2 polio "and not a single accident or failure has been recorded." Recent research, he went on, had allowed the development of a vaccine against Type 3. Experiments were currently under way to see if the Type 1 vaccine was capable of immunizing humans against "other viruses" (meaning, it seemed, Types 2 and 3 polioviruses), and these experiments could only be conducted on chimps, the species closest to man — hence the research in Stanleyville. This suggested that the vaccination and challenge work had actually been designed to test cross immunity between polio types. Of course, if CHAT could protect against Type 2 poliovirus, then Koprowski no longer needed to develop a Type 2 vaccine.

Both the Stanleyville papers also featured eyewitness accounts of visits to Lindi camp, where the reporters were shown around the "Mission Courtois-Koprowski" by the two polio researchers.[7] The reports describe the warning signs reading "Danger," "Polio," and "No Entry," and explain that "behind the barricades are some of the commandos fighting against one of the most distressing diseases of the twentieth century." There is a sentry post, a residential area for the camp workers (who have apparently already been vaccinated against polio), a brick building that is intended to house the offices and laboratory, and a prohibited area containing "two vast hangars sheltering 60 chimpanzees," which are to be used for the perfection *("mise au point définitive")* of a vaccine discovered by Dr. Koprowski. Apparently "no other experiment has involved such a large number of chimpanzees," and assisted by Mr. Norton, Dr. Koprowski is initiating doctors Courtois, Ninane, and Osterrieth into his methods of work. Koprowski is said to need "as many people as possible to lend themselves for trials in all countries in the world." In the Congo itself "a large-scale vaccination of the population" is foreseen.

Another article revealed that Koprowski was due to leave Stan on February 11 for Leopoldville "to meet with the colonial authorities, and to submit a program of research and permanent collaboration between the Laboratoire Médical and the group of American scientists in charge of the development of this vaccine." Norton, meanwhile, would be staying in Stanleyville "for a good while" to continue the research.

Similarly, the Stanleyville newspapers featured several reports about the Symposium on Viral Diseases in Central Africa, held in late September and early October 1957, to celebrate the opening of the brand-new Laboratoire Médical building, which contained a fully equipped virus laboratory.[8] These were rather haphazard summaries by news reporters, but the photographs of the new laboratory and animal house revealed them to be impressive two-story buildings, with frontages of perhaps fifty and twenty-five yards, respectively.[9] This represented an enormous financial investment for a colonial regime that was often referred to as being strapped for cash, and indeed for the Laboratoire Médical de Stanleyville, which was then manned by just five doctors, two auxiliary doctors, two nurses, and two sanitary agents.[10] Once again I found myself wondering whether the collaboration between Belgian and American scientists on the polio and chimpanzee research was in any way linked to the construction work; and whether any American money had been quietly deployed to assist the project.[11]

In addition to Koprowski, there were several other distinguished speakers at the conference. The Belgian attendees included Lise Thiry (who was later to become a well-known socialist politician), and Pieter De Somer from RIT, who spoke on the IPV campaign then under way in Belgium. De Somer's presence was interesting, given that soon after this his laboratory apparently started making a version of CHAT. And from the Congo, the attendees included the medical directors of the four other medical laboratories — those of Leopoldville, Bukavu, Elisabethville, and Luluabourg.

Two other intriguing attendees were Dr. M. Vaucel, inspector-general of the overseas branches of the Pasteur Institute, and Dr. J. Heuls, the director of the Pasteur Institute of Brazzaville, in French Equatorial Africa. These are the very men who — just one month later — would presumably have been responsible for ordering the mass vaccination of more than two thousand children living around Mitzic, in present-day Gabon, with Lépine's polio vaccine, in response to a raging polio epidemic.[12]

As explained earlier, the last of the three injections at Mitzic may have been of IPV, or it may have been an experimental booster of live vaccine. Lépine had spoken and written favorably of such an approach during 1957, and in June the Pasteur Institute had apparently granted a manufacturing license for a live polio vaccine to "a large American pharmaceutical company."[13] If the two senior Pasteur representatives were impressed by Koprowski's live vaccine ideas as outlined at the Stanleyville conference, and felt that this was the way forward for polio vaccination, perhaps they decided to take advantage of the Mitzic polio outbreak in order to stage a field trial of Lépine's version. Certainly the American drug company would have required evidence that Lépine's live vaccine had been proved safe in humans before proceeding to large-scale manufacture.

The first reports about the mass vaccination in the Ruzizi Valley appear in the Congo papers in early March 1958, with an article about Jervis, Flack, and Courtois vaccinating 150,000 with Dr. Koprowski's vaccine, "which has already been adopted in Switzerland."[14] Two further reports published in Bukavu and Usumbura in the first half of April — at around the time that the vaccination campaign was finishing — revealed that it had indeed covered an area much larger than the Ruzizi Valley.[15] The vaccination was now said to have involved "all those populations on the plain bordering the northern part of Lake Tanganyika, at least 80,000 in Kivu and 140,000 in Ruanda-Urundi," and to have extended from Bugarama (at the southwestern tip of present-day Rwanda) to Nyanza Lac (at the southwestern corner of Burundi). The campaign had apparently been placed under the control of two men: Dr. Gillet, the director of the medical hygiene service for Kivu province in the Congo, and Dr. Meyus, the equivalent official in Ruanda-Urundi.

These two reports constituted the first documentary confirmation of the area covered by the so-called Ruzizi trial. And the contrast between the newspaper reports from March and April provided the first hard evidence to support my growing suspicion that the so-called Ruzizi Valley vaccination documented in the British Medical Journal had occurred in two stages: a vaccination of some 150,000 (attended by Flack and Jervis) on both sides of the Ruzizi Valley (presumably with CHAT 10A-11 made at the Wistar), and a secondary vaccination of 65,000 to 70,000, conducted by Meyus and Ninane along the eastern shores of Lake Tanganyika, which may well have involved a different batch of vaccine (the Belgian-made version of CHAT, if Gaston Ninane's memories were correct).

In addition, one of these two newspaper articles contributed a fascinating, and remarkable, piece of information. It stated that "experimentation on some four hundred chimpanzees" captured in Province Oriental (the province surrounding Stanleyville) had contributed greatly to the perfection of the polio vaccine formula.[16]

The Belgian Ministry of Foreign Affairs, on the rue Quatre Bras opposite the Palais de Justice in Brussels, has a large African archives department, and a small room where scholars and researchers may view files on request. Unfortunately, much of the material concerning the polio vaccinations appeared to have been filed under Service d'Hygiène, the department that assumed responsibility for the vaccinations during 1959 — and these Hygiène files are, with a few exceptions, officially closed to the public.

Nonetheless, the archives still contained many fascinating references to the vaccinations. I started by reviewing the annual reports of the Laboratoire Médical de Stanleyville, though these were available only up to 1958. These were important with regard to personnel, for they listed all those who had worked at the lab during that period, with exact dates. Otherwise, however, the lab reports were a disappointment, for references to the chimpanzee work were remarkably few and far between. The report for 1956 stated that polio trials were under way in collaboration with Dr. H. Koprowski, "vice-president of the New York Academy of Sciences" (no mention of Lederle), and that sixty chimps had already been used for the first tests. The 1957 report, which should have covered the greater part of the polio work conducted at Lindi, mentioned it only in the final paragraph of the report, as follows: "Chimpanzees: The experiments being conducted at Lindi camp are proceeding successfully. With some histopathological examinations missing, it is difficult at this time to give the precise figures. As soon as we know them, we shall communicate them."

The 1958 lab report began by asserting that activity in the lab had been particularly intense, and went on to explain that the study of the Koprowski strains of OPV in the chimpanzee was practically finished, and would be the subject of a paper that was being drafted. It went on to explain that the results of the vaccinations in the Ruzizi plain, and in response to four epidemics, had been published in the *British Medical Journal,* and promised that within months "other results will be published, and we look forward to the results of the vaccination campaigns which have been conducted all over the colony, and especially in Leopoldville."

This was the third published reference I had come across to a formal scientific report of the chimp work, a report that had previously been referred to as "in preparation" or "to be published 1958."[17] It seemed increasingly probable, however, that in reality no systematic account of the polio work at Lindi, apparently so vital in terms of the safety testing and, indeed, "perfection" of the Koprowski vaccines, had ever been published. It was now apparent — if it had not been before — that this vital research had, for some reason or other, been shrouded in secrecy from the very first.

Elsewhere in the 1958 report it was mentioned in passing that at the start of the year, the polio work conducted on the Lindi chimps had consisted principally of infection trials, studies of effectiveness, and intraspinal studies of attenuation.

Such experiments on polio Types 1 and 2 had apparently been completed, and during 1959 the researchers proposed to carry out the same work on polio Type 3.[18] The information seemed deliberately vague. By contrast, ten sentences are devoted to Fritz Deinhardt's hepatitis work, which was a far smaller project.

The biochemistry section of the lab made a very precise list of more than 2,100 biochemical tests carried out on the chimps, most of which seemed to relate to the hepatitis studies. The virology department, meanwhile, reported tests on seventy-four chimps for the presence of five human viruses. This department had also prepared two hundred tubes and ten bottles of tissue culture in baboon kidney, most of which had been used for adenovirus research, which proved futile, in that the unrefrigerated adenovirus samples turned out not to be viable upon arrival from the field. This is the only specific reference to tissue culture work contained in any of these annual reports, and although the quantities were small, it provided evidence that tissue cultures were being prepared in the Stanleyville lab by 1958 at the latest. It also supported Paul Osterrieth's belief that some tissue culture work had taken place in baboon kidney.

One of the Hygiène files that had not been closed contained a fascinating three-page document, written by Ghislain Courtois and dated October 1, 1957, which coincided with the virus symposium in Stanleyville. The first page consisted of budget forecasts for the future experimental work to be conducted at Lindi, and revealed that the researchers expected to handle one hundred chimpanzees a year for the next five years. It was anticipated that Lindi camp would cost just over two million Belgian francs ($40,000 U.S. at that time) per year to run, with expenses ranging from the cost of a truck for the chimp capture team ($6,000) to the wages of the members of that team (60 cents per day) and those of an assistant nurse who would be resident at the camp ($1 a day).[19] The next two pages detailed the collaborative research, which, it was hoped, would be carried out by the lab and the Wistar Institute, and began with a summary of work already completed — namely, intraspinal safety tests and "demonstrations of the efficacy of the vaccine." Because of this research, the paper went on, it had been possible to vaccinate twenty-five hundred people, mainly natives. "We . . . believe," Courtois continued, "that it is absolutely necessary to proceed to mass vaccinations. This presumes that the vaccine continues throughout to be tested on chimps . . . and that the Stanleyville lab can have a significant stock of these animals at its disposal."

This last comment was the most interesting, because of its casual assumption that the only way to ensure the "perfection," safety, and efficacy of CHAT vaccine was to test every single batch in chimpanzees. In fact, shortly before this,

Albert Sabin had demonstrated that chimps were of only limited usefulness for safety tests and infectivity studies. In two articles published in January 1957, Sabin reported that only "large doses of fully virulent poliovirus," when injected intraspinally, would paralyze chimpanzees (thus showing that Asian macaques were far more sensitive barometers of vaccine safety), and that humans were far more easily infected than chimps when attenuated polioviruses (like vaccines) were administered by mouth.[20] Sabin's articles (which both appear to have been familiar to Koprowski and Norton by the time of their departure for Africa in January 1957)[21] thus raised questions about what crucial role it was that the Lindi chimps were intended to play in the perfection of CHAT vaccine.

The Courtois document went on to state that Wistar Institute scientists were proposing further studies on hepatitis and arteriosclerosis in chimps, and that Professor Henle of the University of Pennsylvania would personally direct the hepatitis research. As regards arteriosclerosis, Courtois wrote that long-term studies in chimps would be possible, because the other research studies "will leave a stock of live chimps in a good state of health at the Stanleyville lab."

This is an important point. Intraspinal safety tests involve sacrificing chimpanzees, but at least the numbers are normally limited to five chimps per pool of vaccine tested. By contrast, vaccination and challenge (provided it works, which it should do) leaves a large number of healthy animals.

The document ends by pointing out how much the Stanleyville lab has gained through its collaboration with the Wistar — especially in terms of learning new techniques and establishing a modern virology service. "We can count on this collaboration continuing over the coming years because the work described above is supported by the US Public Health Service. . . . The American government has just given permission for Dr. Koprowski to visit Stanleyville with members of his staff every year for the next five years," Courtois concludes. (This casual reference to American government backing for the research is intriguing, and will be further discussed later.)

This document demonstrates that by October 1957, although Ghislain Courtois had already vaccinated some twenty-five hundred individuals (mainly Africans), he was still seeking permission to carry out a mass vaccination among the general population — a permission that, according to the *British Medical Journal* paper, was given by the director of medical services of the Congo, Dr. C. Dricot, "in the second half of 1957." It may, therefore, have been this very submission by Courtois that prompted Dricot to approve large-scale trials with the Koprowski strains.

Lindi camp was clearly felt to have extraordinary potential for medical research, and Koprowski and Courtois continued to push for an enlargement of the program. Ten months later, in August 1958, the minister of colonies in Brussels wrote to the governor-general of the Congo to tell him of a meeting he had had with the two men, in which they had told him of the Ruzizi mass trial and of forthcoming trials in Leopoldville and Bukavu, and had requested that the chimpanzee camp at Lindi be maintained for the continuance of collaborative U.S.–Belgian studies into hepatitis, arteriosclerosis, and cancer.[22]

---

Another open Hygiène file entitled "Poliomyelitis: Correspondence" provided a fuller picture of the history of IPV and OPV use in the Congo, mainly through the letters that passed between public health officials in Belgium and the colony. They revealed that in the second half of 1956, approximately ten thousand doses of South African IPV, made by James Gear's laboratory, were imported by the Leopoldville authorities; they had apparently decided that American IPVs were either insufficiently inactivated, or else inactivated to the point where they were useless. Interestingly, the shots were to be given exclusively to European children, and to those few indigenous children who attended European schools. It was apparently considered that a mass vaccination of the general population would not be effective, and that it might even "disturb the equilibrium of the poliovirus" in nature.[23]

However, the copious entries in this letters file suddenly stop in October 1956, and there is nothing more until July 1958 — a gap that coincides exactly with the period when one might have expected material relating to the Koprowski strains to feature prominently.

One of the first entries thereafter appears to have been prompted by the preliminary report of the Congo trials in the *British Medical Journal* a few days earlier. Dr. P. de Brauwere, the inspector general of hygiene in Brussels, writes to Charles Dricot, the director general of medical services in Leo, to note that by July 12, 156 cases of polio had occurred in Province Oriental since the start of the year, out of 445 in the whole of Congo. "Compared to the situation in 1957 (72 cases in twelve months), the epidemiological pace seems a little worrying, and since it is in this province that vaccinations with *live* virus have been carried out on a large scale, we are entitled to ask ourselves whether there might be some connection," he wrote. He requested a thorough inquiry, to establish whether there had been any polio cases among vaccinees, or whether any had come from communities living near to vaccinated areas. When he got no reply, he wrote again at the start of September, seeking an urgent response.

He was not the only one to be concerned. On September 6, 1958, a letter by an Oxford virologist, Margaret Agerholm, appeared in the *British Medical Journal* in response to the Courtois/Koprowski article of July.[24] She pointed out that the polio epidemic that had raged across the northeastern Congo in late 1957 and early 1958, had "occurred in close time and geographical location to a trial of oral polio vaccine which preceded it." In effect, she was suggesting that the polio outbreaks in Banalia, Gombari, Watsa, and Bambesa might have been caused by the migration of CHAT vaccinees from Stanleyville and Aketi to unvaccinated areas, and a reversion to virulence of the vaccines.[25]

Before the end of September, Dr. Wilfrid Bervoets, the Congo's inspector of hygiene, wrote back to De Brauwere providing more precise details of the vaccinations in Province Oriental, including numbers of vaccinees and exact dates.[26] The letter revealed that by July 1958 a further two vaccination campaigns had taken place at Rungu and Kilo, both in response to incipient epidemics.

The two campaigns are intriguing, for Rungu lies midway between Gombari and Bambesa, which had been vaccinated (or, in Bambesa's case, part-vaccinated) in January.[27] As for the vaccination of the gold miners of Kilo, Bervoets notes that the vaccination at the nearby town of Watsa in January 1958 had included fifteen

PROVINCE ORIENTAL CHAT AND FOX VACCINATIONS, 1957–1958 (AS REVEALED BY LETTER FROM BERVOETS TO DE BRAUWERE DATED SEPTEMBER 17, 1958)

| Location | Number | Vaccine | Date |
| --- | --- | --- | --- |
| Aketi schoolchildren | "Around 2,000" (1,978) | CHAT | May 1957 |
| Aketi schoolchildren | "Around 2,000" | Fox | December 1957 |
| Banalia | 3,798 | CHAT | January 8–12, 1958 |
| Kole | 384 | CHAT | January 8–12, 1958 |
| Gombari | 2,925 | CHAT | January 27, 1958 |
| Watsa | 14,569 (1,500 from Kilo-Moto mines) | CHAT | January 29–31, 1958 |
| Bambesa | 2,350 | CHAT | February 1, 1958 |
| Stanleyville military camps | 3,102 | CHAT | February 27, 1958 |
| Stanleyville military camps | 3,102 | Fox | May 27, 1958 |
| Rungu | 4,000 | CHAT | June 1958 |
| Kilo-Moto gold miners | 5,000 | CHAT | July 1958 |

These figures differ slightly from those in *BMJ* 58; only for Aketi can we be confident that the *BMJ* figure is more accurate.

hundred of the miners, but that twenty-eight further paralytic cases had then occurred between April and July in the mining camps and in the region bordering the town.

It was debatable whether the latter Watsa/Kilo outbreak was a continuation of the original outbreak of January 1958 (which had affected just two persons from Watsa) or represented a reversion to virulence of the type mooted by Dr. Agerholm. Had she known of these additional polio cases in the months following, in areas close to places like Bambesa and Kilo, where only part of the population had been immunized in January and February,[28] she might have been even more forthright in her claim that the vaccinations had raised "a number of problems, both epidemiological and ethical."

In his September response to De Brauwere, Bervoets merely noted that during 1958 there had been "flaming epidemics" in nonvaccinated areas close to vaccinated towns, resulting in 120 polio cases being reported from regions that "normally [experienced] only a few sporadic cases." Since these represented more than three-quarters of all the cases seen in the province up to August 1958, it is quite remarkable that he reported this fact without further comment. Instead, he blandly concluded that "the risk appears to be minimal. The medical service of the Province Oriental holds the view that the live Koprowski vaccine is a vaccine to use on a large scale in towns."

In his reply, De Brauwere apparently accepted the verdict of Bervoets, and concluded that "the information does not lead to the conclusion that live vaccinations and polio frequency are related." This, to say the least, is puzzling. De Brauwere had asked the right questions in the first place, and Bervoets had provided very complete documentation, which revealed that the vaccine virus could indeed have been spreading to neighboring areas and then reverting. But both men then drew surprisingly optimistic conclusions from the data.[29] Perhaps they had never read Dick's articles of a year before; perhaps they had little appreciation of the potential of polio vaccine to revert. Or perhaps they never seriously considered that the American vaccines could be less than safe.

---

The risk of reversion was highlighted once again after the vaccination of under-fives in Leopoldville with CHAT pool 13 began in August 1958. More than 76,000 children were vaccinated during the next twenty months, in a campaign that was extremely well monitored by the local medical services, as is documented by papers published in medical journals, and by detailed plans and protocols held in the archives. But once again, things ran far from smoothly. An epidemic of Type 1 polio began in October 1958, just two months after the inception of the program, in suburbs neighboring those where CHAT had been fed. The archives show that between January and early August 1959 there were 115 polio cases in Leo, and De Brauwere once again wrote nervously from Brussels that "this cannot plead in favour of the vaccine."[30]

A large gray area of uncertainty surrounds the Leopoldville polio epidemic. In 1960 and 1961, a series of extremely precise reports by Plotkin and Koprowski appeared in the *Bulletin of the WHO*, in the course of which they sought to demonstrate that the paralytic cases in Leo had been infected with wild virus rather than vaccine virus, including the thirty-nine vaccinees who developed polio (twenty-six of whom were infected with Type 1 poliovirus).[31] One of their arguments was that, because only 60 percent of the CHAT vaccinations in Leopoldville were successful, those vaccinees who became paralyzed were probably those for whom the immunization had failed. However, in an accompanying article that analyzed polioviruses recovered from CHAT vaccinees and nonvaccinees in Leopoldville, the United States, and Sweden, Sven Gard came to very different conclusions, namely that there had been reversion to virulence after human passage.[32] (During 1959, Gard had been a visiting professor at the Wistar, and it seems significant that soon after his return to Sweden he abandoned his work on OPV in order to concentrate on the perfection of a safe and effective IPV.)

Other letters in the archives indicate that the attitude of the Belgian authorities to IPV and OPV were very different. With IPV, the approach was to protect Europeans, especially children, living in the Congo, but not to disturb the equilibrium of the virus in the native population. By contrast, with the oral vaccine the approach was apparently to immunize the Congolese population en masse, but to be much more cautious with Europeans.

This was dramatically highlighted by a letter written in August 1958 by De Brauwere to a Brussels-based pharmaceutical company that had made inquiries about CHAT. He explained that the new polio vaccine "is actually still in the experimental stage," and that Koprowski was busy with the *mise au point*, the development process. This is absolutely remarkable, for by this point in time more than 300,000 Africans had already been fed CHAT. Apparently the *mise au point* was felt to be complete by September 1959, which is when Europeans living in Leo were first given CHAT vaccine.[33]

There was an interesting postscript to the Leo vaccinations. In mid-1961, there was a fresh outbreak of polio in Leopoldville, which by August of that year had caused 175 cases in Leopoldville province, mostly in the city itself. De Brauwere in Brussels wrote to Dr. Hector Meyus, the Belgian who had vaccinated along Lake Tanganyika with Gaston Ninane in April 1958, and who was now working as a medical hygienist in postindependence Leopoldville. The inspector general of hygiene pointed out that "the majority of people in that agglomeration had been vaccinated with the Koprowski strains," and said he would like to have details of the number of vaccinees among the polio cases. In a separate letter, he told Meyus that Courtois had assured him that there were still one million doses of the Koprowski vaccines in the freezers of the Leopoldville lab, which could perhaps be used to fight the epidemic. Meyus wrote back to say that all the relevant documentation had disappeared; he suggested that André Lebrun (the former head of the colony's hygiene service), might have taken it with him when he left. Neither, he added, was there any trace of the vaccine. If nothing else, this highlighted the haphazard manner in which the Belgian authorities took their leave of the Congo, and the way in which important materials and medical papers vanished in the process.

---

What of the other vaccination campaigns that were reported to have been staged, bringing the numbers of vaccinees in the Congo "into the millions"?[34] Here, the archives contain very little information — other than the fact that all vaccination activities were transferred from the authority of the medical service to the hygiene service, probably in April 1959.

A lengthy exchange of letters between Belgium and the Congo revealed that the intended mass vaccination in Bas-Congo, the province lying between Leopoldville and the Atlantic, had probably not taken place on the scale intended. Ghislain Courtois and André Lebrun proposed that some 200,000 from the province should be fed with CHAT, and in January 1960 the Ligue Nationale Belge Contre le Poliomyélite, a Belgian voluntary organization, signed an agreement with King Baudouin to meet the costs of the campaign. However, there were by then only months to go before independence, and the scheme fell victim to the political unrest that was sweeping the country. The inhabitants of Bas-Congo were some of the most politically active Congolese, and after years of enduring the paternalistic attitudes of the authorities in Leopoldville and Brussels, were apparently suspicious of the motives of the outgoing Belgian doctors. In one of the letters Lebrun writes sadly that "it is very difficult to make the Congolese of the Bas-Congo come to the vaccination sessions."[35]

In the course of this correspondence, in September 1959, Lebrun writes to the Ligue to inform their officials of the potential costs of the Bas-Congo campaign, and those for the other provinces, if the Ligue intends to help vaccinate the whole of the Congo. However, he adds, "we can exclude Ruanda-Urundi, where the administration has already done the necessary." This is one of several references to vaccination in the Belgian-administered territory to the east of the Congo, several of which mention the figure of one million vaccinations.

Astonishingly, the campaign in the Ruzizi plain, the first true mass vaccination in the world, was not referred to in any of the open files in the archives, save for one brief mention in a December 1958 letter from Bervoets, who claimed that 200,000 OPV doses had been given in the area "without causing any post-vaccinal accident." As for the further vaccinations in Ruanda-Urundi, there were no details to be had — until, that is, my last day in the archives section, when I was finally given the annual reports of the medical services of Ruanda-Urundi, which confirmed the total number of polio vaccinations that had taken place there each year. These rose from zero in 1956 to 758 (quite possibly of IPV) in 1957, to 215,504 (the exact figure recorded in the *British Medical Journal* article for the Ruzizi vaccination in both Congo and Burundi) in 1958.[36]

However, it was the reports of the next two years that were the most interesting, for they revealed 137,790 vaccinations in Ruanda-Urundi in 1959, and 382,638 in 1960. This went at least halfway toward confirming what others had been saying anecdotally — that a million doses of CHAT had been fed in the territory. There were still no clues as to *where* these feedings had taken place, but those half-million doses in 1959/60 meant that roughly one-sixth of the total population had been vaccinated in those two years alone. There were no further annual reports after 1960, even though Ruanda-Urundi was not granted full independence until 1962, so it was at least possible that further polio vaccinations could have taken place in the final eighteen months before decolonization.

Slowly by slowly, a more accurate picture of what had really happened in the Congo and Ruanda-Urundi at the end of the fifties was beginning to emerge.

---

At the end of my research in the African archives at the Ministry of Foreign Affairs, I went in to the office of one of the archivists, to express my thanks; she was busy talking with a colleague. By this stage I had got to know the archivists quite well, and I decided to try to explain something about my research — the fact that something might have gone wrong with the vaccination program, although I was still not sure about the details. I was not, I assured them, out to sensationalize the story, and if I found out that my suspicions were after all wrong, I would wash my hands of the whole affair.

The two archivists looked at each other, and then one of them told me that I was not wrong. She added that another researcher, a Belgian professor,[37] was also looking into the same story, but that he had not managed to find all the information that I had located. She would not go into further details — but as I left, the other archivist said quietly: "I am sure you will find what you are looking for." It was an eerie moment, for I had not the slightest doubt that they had monitored which files I had been reviewing, and that all three of us knew exactly the significance of what we had just been discussing.

# 40

GHISLAIN COURTOIS

It was time to try to find out more about some of the central figures in the story, in particular Ghislain Courtois, the debonair scientist who had been in charge of the Laboratoire Médical de Stanleyville until late 1959. I had been given the name and address of his son, André, some time before, but waited until the summer of 1994 to get in touch. This was partly because he was known to be a good friend of Hilary Koprowski, who apparently visited him whenever he came to Belgium.

André, who had followed his father into the medical profession, turned out to be a charming man. Although Ghislain had died of lung cancer back in 1971, at the age of fifty-nine, André still clearly missed him. He spoke with unalloyed warmth of his father's character. He described him as a "child of the village," and recalled that he had always won the archery contest at the annual festival. He was apparently a Catholic "with a big sense of duty . . . very kind, but firm." But he was also, André explained, a gregarious man, one who was a popular guest at parties because of his gifts as a raconteur; "it was never possible to stop him when he talked, and he told and told stories, always with humor." He also, however, had a very private — almost introverted — side to his character, and would happily spend his evenings alone with his history books and classical records. Apparently he "liked simplicity, discretion," and André added that women found him seductive.

Ghislain had arrived in the Congo in 1936, and between 1939 and 1959 he worked at the Laboratoire Médical de Stanleyville,[1] for the last nine years as its director. However, for the final year of Belgian rule he moved to Leopoldville, where he took over as *"Médecin-Inspecteur,"* or second in command to Charles Dricot in the hierarchy of doctors in the colony. A great source of pride to

Ghislain, André told me, was the fact that he had gone a long way toward eradicating yellow fever and polio from the Congo, and one of his greatest disappointments was the fact that the health-care system collapsed so quickly after independence. "He was a big lover of Africa. Africa was truly in his heart — even the population, the blacks," André explained. "And after '60, when the Congo completely broke down, he was very sad that all his life's work was destroyed."

André's own recollections of the Congo were rather more limited. He had visited there only once during his father's tenure in Stanleyville, and that between July and September 1956, when he was fourteen. He clearly recalled the chimp colony at Lindi, which had then just opened: "the camp was all new . . . it was really very handsome." He also recalled the two pet chimps that used to wander freely round the camp — Djamba and Marie-Paulin. At this time Ghislain was at Lindi almost daily, and Djamba used to jump up and down with excitement when he arrived: "he was like his son; it was magnificent."

André Courtois told me that Lindi camp, with its two large hangars, had been custom-built for the polio experiments, and that he had always thought that Koprowski had footed the bill.[2] He recalled that about thirty chimps had been present in the camp that summer of 1956, caught by Rollais the hunter. But later his father told him that altogether two hundred chimps had been used on the polio experiments over a period of several months.[3]

When I asked whether he recalled anything about pygmy chimps, *Pan paniscus,* André Courtois said that he had been too young then to tell the difference between them and *Pan troglodytes,* but that his dad "often spoke about *Pan paniscus,* I've got that in my ear. When I heard my father speak about chimps, almost every time he spoke about *Pan paniscus.*" Ghislain apparently used to say that the pygmy chimp had feelings and a soul, "just like a man."

André recalled nothing about the nature of the experiments: "a little boy wasn't told that sort of thing." Neither did he recall seeing any vaccinations. But his father did feed him some polio vaccine on a sugar lump during that summer in the Congo. Given the timing, this would probably have been either SM or TN. Ghislain apparently gave him some more OPV when he came home to Belgium on leave at the time of Expo 58. Presumably this was either CHAT or Fox.

Apparently when Koprowski had last visited André Courtois in Belgium, in 1993, he had spoken with him about the mass vaccination in Ruzizi. "He said: 'This thing that I did with your father, the vaccination, it was something completely historic for medicine, because it's the only time that so many people have been vaccinated so easily. . . . It wasn't necessary to have a list of the vaccinees and all that. . . . At that time it was just a trial, an experiment. You can't do trials of vaccines [now]; it could never be done again.'"

When I asked André Courtois to tell me about Koprowski, he became unashamedly sentimental. "I can just tell you that he was a good, kind man. He's maybe the most intelligent man I know, with extraordinary culture. He's truly an extraordinary man. . . . I can't speak about my father and Koprowski without damp eyes." Apparently whenever Koprowski came to Belgium, André Courtois would pick him up by car from Brussels. The other person he would always see was Lise Thiry, formerly the head of virology at the Pasteur Institute in Brussels, and more recently a socialist senator in parliament.

André himself clearly had some of the qualities of Ghislain. He had found some reprints of his father's papers to give me, and he also volunteered the names and addresses of several of his former Stanleyville colleagues. He particularly recommended Pierre Doupagne, a technician who had worked at the lab for many years and who, he assured me, would be able to answer all my questions. In addition, he phoned his sister Ann, a graphologist, who promptly invited me to dinner the following evening.

---

Ann Courtois turned out to be as helpful and charming as her brother. The dinner was superb, and throughout the evening she regaled me with tales of her father. She emphasized the "great mutual liking and admiration" that Hilary and Ghislain had had for each other, and showed me three Christmas cards from the Koprowskis, each with a photo on the front — Hilary dancing a waltz with his wife; Hilary astride a scooter; Hilary in shorts, holding an umbrella, with marabou stork in attendance. She too gave me addresses of Ghislain's former colleagues, and copies of several newspaper articles from the period. And as I left, she pressed into my hand a small ivory tortoise with three legs, which Ghislain had apparently kept on the desk in his office, as a symbol of the African virtues of patience and fortitude.

Both André and Ann, with their memories and gifts, had been extraordinarily kind. However, I was mindful of the fact that I had perhaps been exposed to something of a charm offensive. Hilary had apparently told André about the *Rolling Stone* article, which, André said, contained a "silly explanation" for AIDS, one that was "medically not possible." But it would have been naive to ignore the fact that the two elder children of Ghislain Courtois might well have deduced that this was the main reason why I was so interested in their father's work.

---

A couple of days later, I paid a visit to André's estranged Swedish wife, Berit. She recalled family trips to see Hilary in Philadelphia, when he would play Rachmaninoff on the grand piano and regale his guests with wonderful stories. "We laughed so much . . . we talked about everything and nothing," she said. Like her husband, she had clearly been captivated.

After a while, I told her that I too had met Koprowski and been charmed by him, but that I had also had some misgivings about some of the things he had told me (and some that he appeared to have forgotten). Berit explained that after the *Rolling Stone* article was published, Hilary had wanted André to write something in support of his work for the newspapers. She went on: "Perhaps he [Hilary] has blocked it out, because he was so shocked by the claims. He's very, very afraid that it will be some big black page in his life [at the end]. . . . He's been studying all his life; he really wanted to find remedies for everything. Now they're going to ask: 'Has he done something good, or something horrible?'"

This was one of the best analyses I had heard of how this whole affair must have affected Koprowski, and Berit went on: "If you don't take risks, you can't go further. He can't be judged if he did something a little bit 'non-Catholic.' [Anyway], they couldn't prove anything."

Berit then revealed that André had a great quantity of his father's papers. She explained that after they had argued one day, she had loaded up her car with twenty or thirty boxes of documents, and had driven them over to André's house, where he now kept them stored in his garage. She was surprised that André had not mentioned them to me, and she rang him at his home. Before long, I was given the phone. André, clearly put out, told me that he had never looked in the boxes, but that if I wanted to visit him the following afternoon, he would go through them with me.

This was clearly extremely kind, but by the time I arrived the next day, André was almost beside himself with rage. He spat out some bitter words, which, though aimed at his wife, were clearly meant for me as well. I felt embarrassed at the situation, but was not about to forgo the opportunity to view Ghislain Courtois's documents. André, still fuming, fixed up a lamp and led me down to the garage, where we spent most of the afternoon rummaging through the boxes. We never found the much-cited 1958 article about the chimp research at Lindi, which I was now almost sure had never been written. Nonetheless, we found several other papers of interest, together with letters and notebooks, and various technical volumes that his father had used in the Stanleyville lab. By this stage, André was back to his charming, generous self. He lent me several of the books, and drove me up to his office in the local hospital to photocopy the relevant letters and articles.

———————

I stayed up most of that night going through the papers. There was much of interest here, but there were also disappointments. The only letters were those dating from after Ghislain Courtois's return from the Congo in 1960. It was greatly to André's credit that he was prepared to give me copies of these — even if there had been a couple of occasions when he had not let me examine a particular letter. However, the copies in my possession showed that his father had written to an African at the institute of tropical medicine in Leopoldville in October 1961, asking him to help recover some documents about the Lindi experiments. At other times he wrote to European colleagues, asking them to send back his trunk, a box of blood samples taken after the CHAT vaccination in the town of Coquilhatville (now Mbandaka), and certain important books, including the New York Academy of Sciences volume featuring Koprowski's article on CHAT and Fox. It was not clear if these items were ever returned to him.

From his curriculum vitae and various other documents, it was possible to piece together Ghislain's activities in the fifties, when he was most active as a laboratory scientist. Interestingly, he had had links with the Pasteur Institute in Paris, where he had spent two sabbaticals in 1951 and 1954. In the latter year, he had been lead author on a paper about fungal diseases found in the Guinea baboons from Kindia, the kidneys of which were already being used by Lépine's virus department for tissue culture material.[4]

Between February and May 1955, Ghislain went on a three-month study tour of the Americas, starting at the Rockefeller Institute in New York and continuing to Rockefeller-sponsored labs in Trinidad and Rio. I had borrowed a copy of his bound notebook for this trip, which showed that he had been taught by some eminent scientists, including Jordi Casals in New York and H. A. Penna, the director of the Oswaldo Cruz institute in Rio (the same place where Koprowski had worked in the forties). The notebook contained a lengthy section on preparing tissue cultures, and another on the preparation of vaccines. The methods were relatively primitive, for these were early days for monkey kidney tissue culture, just before Dulbecco's plaque-purification technique and trypsinization became widely accepted and revolutionized the process.

1958 was revealed to have been a really hectic year for Dr. Courtois. Having helped with the Ruzizi vaccination in February and the first part of March, he then began his triannual leave — with Jean Vandepitte taking over as temporary lab director in Stanleyville. Ghislain flew to America, where he attended a training course at the Wistar, and another at Tulane University in New Orleans.[5] At the end of July the *British Medical Journal* report of the Ruzizi vaccinations was published, and less than a week afterward he and Koprowski were delivering speeches at the Brussels conference on viral diseases in Europe and Africa. Ghislain's address concentrated on the large-scale field trial in Ruzizi, and was later published in the *Annales de la Société Belge de Médicine Tropicale.*[6] Then in September he attended the Sixth International Conference on Tropical Medicines and Malaria, in Lisbon. This time he did not give a formal address, but one wonders whether any of his ideas about live polio vaccination might have been picked up by the Portuguese, for use in their African colonies.

The papers also included a copy of the minutes of an important meeting on cell cultures that had taken place in September 1967, in the wake of the Marburg virus outbreak. This appeared to be perhaps the first meeting at which the potential dangers of the vaccine substrate were addressed by scientists whose eyes were fully open.[7] The "Statement of the Cell Culture Committee," which ends this booklet, details the sort of undetected agents that the attending scientists were worried about. A paragraph on the dangers of agents such as scrapie in sheep pointed out that slow viruses from animal substrates might be present in human vaccines. "Furthermore, 'slow viruses' are known to cross species barriers," it ended laconically. In fact, most scientists would nowadays characterize the scrapie agent as a prion rather than a slow virus. But the significance is exactly the same, for both prions and lentiviruses such as SIV are hard to detect, and both jump species barriers.

Among the ten members of the committee who had prepared this statement were some well-known names, including Sven Gard from Stockholm, and Hilary Koprowski from the Wistar Institute.[8]

---

As for Ghislain Courtois's published articles, I had seen some of these before, but others were entirely new. They showed that during his twenty-odd years in Stanleyville, he had produced an impressive body of work on yellow fever (for which disease he was designated an official expert of the WHO), plague, tuberculosis, malaria, salmonella, rabies, and hepatitis. He had unwittingly discovered a hitherto unknown arbovirus, through the traditional method of becoming accidentally infected with it in the laboratory.[9] In addition, there was the polio research, which culminated in his helping to organize the vaccination of Belgian children with Sabin's OPVs, beginning in March 1963.[10]

Three of his papers described at some length the polio work carried out in the Congo or else the management of chimpanzees at Lindi. However, none of the three provided any detailed information about the actual polio work conducted on the chimps. Given the frequent contemporary references to the "perfection of," or "putting the finishing touches to," the vaccine by experimentation on the chimps, where were the published reports of this work?

The first of these three papers represented the text of an address that Courtois had given to a conference about endemic diseases in Africa, held at Lovanium University just two months before Congolese independence.[11] Most of the address dealt with polio, but it was confusingly arranged and expressed, and the English version suffered from Courtois's lack of dexterity in that language. I was reminded of Joseph Pagano's rather harsh opinion of Courtois: "I don't think he understood very much about vaccines. He was a typical colonial doing God knows what out there."

Nonetheless, the paper contained some important details, not divulged elsewhere. Courtois's brief discussion of how the attenuated strains had been obtained was interesting. He stated that, to begin with, the polioviruses were combined with "uncustomary living substracts" such as mouse tissues or chick embryos, which served to decrease their pathogenicity, and that they were then grown "on a culture of tissue in monocellular layer" to ensure that they were genetically pure (presumably a reference to the plaque purification of Dulbecco). "Two obstacles must be avoided," he went on: "that . . . the strain is so 'stable' and well adapted to its new artificial living substract that the titer may remain high but the strain is no longer antigenic for man. Otherwise, this antigenic power is real, but the strain is 'unstable' and a return to a state of virulence is to be feared." Clearly Courtois had thought at some length about the question of the final "substract" (or substrate), even if he conspicuously failed to provide any clues about the substrate that had been used for the Koprowski vaccines, for which he had helped "the final point to be made."

Another section of the speech quoted extensively (but without citation) from a 1956 paper by David Bodian about the dissemination of poliovirus in different chimp tissues.[12] This was an important discovery, for it demonstrated that Courtois was familiar with this paper, which demonstrated, *inter alia*, that poliovirus did not enter the kidneys of live chimpanzees, even when they were infected with polio. Clearly this had important implications for the potential use of kidneys from experimentally infected animals that had to be sacrificed.

Toward the end of this speech, Courtois revealed that "at this moment" the number vaccinated in the Congo and Ruanda-Urundi "is not far from a million." Courtois added that research conducted in Kivu province had revealed that "paralytic polio is eleven times less in those vaccinated than in those non-vaccinated." Again this was a significant detail, documented nowhere else; perhaps because it was alarming to have *any* cases of paralysis among vaccinees.

The other two papers were about Lindi, and although they revealed next to nothing about the research, they did provide detailed information about the setup at the camp. This topic had assumed increasing importance during the sixties, as ever larger chimpanzee colonies were established elsewhere in the world (such as at Holloman Air Force Base in New Mexico).

The first of these papers was delivered before an international symposium on the future of laboratory animals, held in Lyon in 1966, and was illustrated by several photos of the Lindi chimps and the wooden cages inside the hangars.[13] It began by explaining that the captured chimps were to be used for the development of a polio vaccine, and that the experiments allowed them to proceed at the start of 1958 with the first mass vaccination with OPV anywhere in the world. This, Courtois wrote, was intended as the first campaign of many that would benefit the infant population of the Congo, but circumstances prevented the greater part of these campaigns from being staged. In the end, they proceeded to the second stage of their projects, which involved establishing a chimpanzee breeding colony. After contacts had been made with the U.S. Public Health Service, a delegation led by Karl Meyer visited Leopoldville early in 1960, to meet with representatives of the Belgian Congo government. Again, however, the events of that year caused the abandonment of these projects.

It was Koprowski, he said, who had originally proposed the setting up of Lindi camp, in order to vaccinate the chimps, check their immune response, and then challenge them with wild virus, and in order to check the neuroviru- lence of vaccine strains and excreted vaccine viruses by intraspinal injection. "The entire program," he wrote, "involved the use of a considerable number of chimps." He did not specify how many.

Koprowski's initial idea had apparently been to use the chimps as soon as pos- sible after their capture, and he had thought it would suffice to attach each ani- mal to a post, under a roof to protect them from the rain. Officers from the hunting department made it clear that chimps needed a great deal more care than that, and so they decided to construct two metal hangars, fifty yards by ten, one as a quarantine station for the newly arrived animals, and the other for the experiments. In order to discourage casual visitors, they erected these hangars at an isolated spot ten miles from the laboratory, and on the far side of the Lindi River. The camp was sited a few hundred yards downstream of a village (which provided many of the workers), and was served by two streams, one of which was blocked to provide a reservoir. An electric pump provided a water supply and allowed for the hosing away of sewage; a generator provided light and heating.

The hangars were erected on a concrete floor, and had fenced sides, to moder- ate the temperature inside. The chimps were placed singly or in pairs in wooden cages, each about a meter square, with three sides of solid board (one of which contained a sliding door) and one side, plus ceiling and floor, constructed of a strong metal lattice. This arrangement allowed excrement to pass through into a disinfected zinc channel below. Every day the cages were cleaned, and a fresh lit- ter of dry grass provided. To keep the chimps warm at night, infrared heating was provided, and sometimes wood fires were lit in the alleys between the cages.

Guards were positioned at the entrance to the camp, and strangers were for- bidden to enter. Any visitors had to be vaccinated against polio before they arrived. A small village was constructed inside the camp for the workers and guards, and a European overseer lived onsite; the chimp hangars were segre- gated from the human living quarters by a second barrier, and all entering this inner compound had first to disinfect their hands.

The article went on to explain about the chimpanzee species found in the Congo: *Pan troglodytes* (the common chimp) on the right (or north) bank of the Congo River, and *Pan paniscus* (the pygmy chimp) on the left bank. The former was divided into subspecies: *P. t. troglodytes* and *P. t. schweinfurthi*. The areas in which these three types were located were, said Courtois, absolutely separate, probably a function of the fact that the chimpanzee, unlike other monkeys, hates — or is unable — to swim. The two types of chimp present at Lindi were *Pan paniscus* and *Pan troglodytes schweinfurthi*, for Stanleyville was situated in the middle of the two ranges.

To begin with, the scientists chose *Pan paniscus* for their experiments. Courtois reported that the pygmy chimps seemed to lose their defense mechanisms quickly and were therefore easier to capture; and that once in the camp they lost their aggressiveness "after being forced just the one time." But, he wrote, "events proved us wrong — for although we were swiftly able to collect dozens of pygmy chimps, we had the greatest difficulty in keeping them alive." To begin with, half of the *Pan paniscus* died within fifteen days of arrival. Most, it seemed, simply lost the will to live, and retreated to the back of their cages, refusing to eat or drink. Effectively, they committed mass suicide. The dead animals were autopsied, and examination of the adrenal gland* suggested that they had died of stress. The scientists tried several remedies: injecting anabolic steroids, isolating individuals in cages outside the main hangars, or "grouping several [chimps] together in one big cage." Nothing worked. Eventually it was decided to "use up" the remaining pygmy chimps and to restrict future captures to *Pan troglodytes schweinfurthi*. Courtois did not explain in what manner the pygmy chimps had been "used up," but it was unlikely to have involved vaccination and challenge or intraspinal inoculation, since no such data would have been comparable to data gained from *Pan troglodytes*.

The passage revealed the fascinating information that sometimes several chimps were housed together in a single big cage. This means that if SIV *was* present at the camp, then it could have been onwardly transmitted (by fighting or by sex) both between individuals of different species and between those of the same species.

The Courtois article also featured a brief account of the technique of capture of the common chimp, which, it was acknowledged, involved more than a little trauma and sometimes fractured limbs; such fractures usually led to death shortly afterward. The question of diet and the problems inherent in providing foods that the chimps would naturally find in the forest were discussed, as were the diseases to which they were prone, the most prominent of which was *Klebsiella pneumoniae*. Courtois wrote that they were astonished to find that a germ that was so common in man could cause such ravages in chimps — perhaps there was prior infection with another virus? They tested, but were unable to find any evidence of same.

In a speech given at the same conference the following year, this time with the primatologist, Joseph Mortelmans, Courtois enlarged on some of these

---

* The adrenal gland is situated on top of the kidney.

subjects.[14] He described the unsatisfactory methods that were nowadays employed for procuring apes, which, he said, involved suppliers with "a high-sounding name but less impressive qualifications," and he quoted a Dutch primatologist who reckoned that "for each young chimpanzee exported . . . between four and six females would have to be killed."[15] He contrasted this situation with the very strict rules about chimpanzee capture and export, which, he said, had obtained in colonial times (rather an ironical comment, given his account of a year earlier). He also claimed that the many companies that were now specializing in catching, housing, and transporting the many thousands of smaller monkeys needed for preparing and testing vaccines provided better care for their charges than did chimp exporters.

He added that chimps were now being smuggled out of central Africa, and were commanding prices of $400 a head once landed in Europe. "A little nearer the source of supply," they could be procured for $140 to $200 from sailors on board ships. In Africa, apparently, nobody had much idea of the scale of the problem, and if nothing was done, the great apes would soon be exterminated. It was for this reason, Courtois wrote, that he strongly suggested the establishment of an international body (perhaps under the aegis of the WHO) to set tight controls on the use as well as the capture of these animals. Even if he was blasé about the responsibility that the ex-colonial powers bore for the situation, his conservation ideas were ahead of his time.

As for diseases, he claimed that most of the enteric and respiratory diseases found in chimps were of human origin, acquired after capture. He pointed out that some infections that are benign in humans are lethal in chimps, although, he added, "this unfortunate relationship sometimes goes the other way," as evidenced by the then-recent Marburg outbreak. "Consequently everyone in contact with chimps, particularly with new arrivals, must take maximum protective action, something which has not so far been given sufficient attention," he concluded.[16]

There were several remarkable revelations in these two chimpanzee papers. One was the acknowledgment of the very high death rates involved in the capturing process, before the animals even arrived at Lindi. Another was the fact that the dead *Pan paniscus* had had their kidneys removed at autopsy so that the adrenal glands could be examined. If those glands showed signs of stress, and the rest of the autopsy showed no sign of a pathogen, then this would demonstrate that the animal had died of shock and misery, following its capture. Under such circumstances, would there be any reason for the virologists not to cut their losses by making the best use they could of the animal's tissues?

---

Several of the newspaper articles provided by Ann and André Courtois also proved interesting. One was a report of a press conference attended by their

father, André Lebrun, and Stanley Plotkin in May 1959, in which five new vaccination campaigns were listed, together with three others that were planned.[17]
Another, for which the main source appeared to be Ghislain Courtois, referred
to the deaths of "a score or two" of the pygmy chimps soon after their arrival at
Lindi, and went on: "[T]hey refused to eat anything but sugar cane until they
learned new eating habits from other, less shy, monkeys kept in the same
pens."[18] This strongly suggested that Courtois and his colleagues had decided to
use *Pan troglodytes* as trainers for *Pan paniscus,* and that during this period they
had caged the two species together.

If correct, this could be enormously important. For while the researchers
"used up" the remainder of the *Pan paniscus* chimps, many *Pan troglodytes*
started dying unexpectedly of *Klebsiella pneumoniae.*[19] This organism is a well-
known opportunist, frequently encountered both in simian and human AIDS.[20]
This suggested that when the two species had been caged together, something
more than survival instinct might have passed from one to the other. Perhaps
pathogens might also have been transferred in either direction across the species
barrier — pathogens such as *Klebsiella,* or, more crucially, SIV.

I realized that I needed to try to track down more of those who had been
involved with the chimp camp — such as Rollais the chimp catcher, and Daenens
the Lindi camp manager. Various reports had it that both were dead, but it was
clearly worth checking. But first I had a more pressing engagement. After two
disappointments, I finally had a firm appointment to see Dr. Stanley Plotkin,
the head of the Pasteur Mérieux vaccine house in Paris, and the former right-
hand man of Hilary Koprowski at the Wistar.

# 41

Toward the end of April 1994 I took a train to Marnes-La-Coquette, near Paris, where the Pasteur Mérieux, the Franco-American pharmaceutical giant that is one of the largest vaccine houses in the world, has its headquarters in a sprawling wooded estate. Although I ended up spending three hours with Professor Stanley Plotkin, its managing director, it was nowhere near long enough, and when I listen back to the tapes I realize that I was rushing throughout. I also realize that it was in some ways a strange and unsatisfactory meeting.

Plotkin was just as one of his members of staff had described him on the phone: "bald, a little large, five foot three." He was also pleasantly unassuming and matter-of-fact, and one could imagine that — like Tom Norton — he would have provided an excellent foil to his flamboyant former boss at the Wistar Institute. Certainly the best and most meticulous of Koprowski's polio papers were those on which Plotkin had been lead author. Altogether he had spent over thirty years holding positions (often simultaneously) at the Wistar, the Children's Hospital of Philadelphia, and the University of Pennsylvania, before moving to his present position with the Mérieux in the nineties.

He started by telling me something about his background. Having gone to medical school in New York City and completed his internship in Cleveland, he had intended to join the air force, but then he heard about a newly formed unit at the CDC in Atlanta, which, he felt, "offered an opportunity . . . to do some research while fulfilling a military obligation." He went to Atlanta in 1957, and at the end of the training period applied for an assignment at the Wistar Institute. "I fought to get that assignment, which I'm sure puzzled a lot of people, because nominally it was an assignment in anthrax," he told me, before explaining that once appointed, it was easy to see Koprowski and arrange to join his

OPV team. "With the impudence of youth, I proposed myself as a researcher, and I then immersed myself for several years in oral polio vaccine studies."

I asked Plotkin whether this CDC assignment at the Wistar had been part of the training process. "No, no," he replied. "It was part of my military service in a sense. The Public Health Service . . . for reasons which escape me, it's attached to the U.S. Navy, and the service that I joined at the CDC . . . called the Epidemi[ology] Intelligence Service . . . was funded by Congress when they were concerned about bacteriological warfare — but, of course, [it] rapidly expanded in the direction of public health, and is now . . . the premier epidemiological organization in the world. There's nothing that compares to it anywhere."

He explained that at that time the Wistar was "a very informal place. . . . It was a kind of a golden age because everything was sort of free and easy and . . . aside from the fact that Koprowski was director, there weren't any real hierarchies." He told me that he basically had had two roles, which involved his doing lab work on polio (studying various aspects of the attenuation of the viruses in cell culture) and helping to conduct clinical trials in the United States and overseas.

As a physician, he fitted naturally into the latter role, but his involvement in the lab work was intriguing, in that he had already made it clear that his only formal training in virology had been a (presumably brief) element of his medical degree. It seemed remarkable that a man with such little practical experience should have effectively taken over responsibility for the laboratory work at such a crucial time. Koprowski had started as director of the Wistar in May 1957, Plotkin arrived in August, and by the end of the year the young EIS officer appears to have been effectively running the Wistar's OPV research program. If this testified to Plotkin's intelligence and speed of assimilation, it also indicated the extent to which Koprowski was willing to back his judgment.

I asked him about his involvement in clinical trials and field trials of the Koprowski strains. He explained that this was thirty-odd years ago, and that he couldn't swear to the accuracy of his answers. Then he told me about the first clinical trial in which he had been involved, which was the feeding of infants at Clinton. "Those were . . . the good old days when people were deciding themselves what was ethical . . . rather than referring them to a committee," he admitted candidly, before adding that the aim of the research had been to study the immune response of infants to various doses and sequences of polio vaccination. They eventually decided that it was best to lead with the Type 1 vaccine, followed by the Type 3, and then Type 2; this was because the Type 2 vaccine virus "would crowd out the others if you administered it first," and as the least dangerous, it was also the least important to protect against.

When I asked about some of the unusual vaccines that had been tried out at Clinton, he admitted that he was never sure whether the alternative Type 1 strain, Wistar, which was allegedly a calf-adapted version of poliovirus, was actually "a fluke . . . or the real thing." Further discussion made it clear that he suspected that the vaccine virus might actually have been an attenuated Type 1 poliovirus, which had been passed mechanically through a cow's gut, but which had emerged pretty much the same as it went in.

Later, when I asked about the origin of the Wistar Institute polio vaccine strains, he told me he knew that there was a dispute about their ownership. I said surely they belonged to Lederle. "Certainly *some* of the work belonged to Lederle," he replied instantly. "I think the dispute probably lies in the area of who did what and when and where. And questions of intellectual property." I pointed out that if he, Plotkin, were to leave Pasteur Mérieux in the morning, taking samples of their vaccine strains with him, then Pasteur Mérieux would presumably not be happy; wasn't that effectively what had happened? Plotkin replied: "I don't know what arrangements were made and so I can't comment. When I arrived, there was no doubt at the Wistar to whom the strains belonged. That is to Koprowski. I am not aware of any legal action on the matter."

We moved on to the Moorestown trial, which had been set up to study the spread of poliovirus in families. "The spread of OPV is of course a double-edged thing," he went on. "On the one hand it clearly promotes the effectiveness of the vaccine in a public health sense. On the other hand, the spread of a virus that's already mutated creates some danger for the contact."

This was good, and clearly had implications for the far larger studies that were being simultaneously conducted in Africa. But when I asked Plotkin about the extent of his involvement in the Stanleyville and Ruzizi Valley trials, he told me that these had been done just before he arrived at the Wistar. I pointed out that most of the feedings in Stanleyville, Province Oriental, and Ruzizi had occurred between six and eight months *after* his arrival in August 1957, and he said, "Well, I won't argue the point — but it's funny, it's not my recollection."

When I asked about the work conducted at the Lindi chimp colony, Plotkin told me that he had not been involved directly, but the idea once again was to test the virulence of the vaccine in a susceptible animal. But on this subject, he was prepared to be far more forthcoming. "The difficulty with that approach is that . . . since even at the worst polio only paralyzes a small percentage of infected people, it would take a lot of chimps to show whether a virus was really attenuated. I mean, you could take a virulent strain like Mahoney and feed it in large quantity and paralyze chimps, OK. But if you were trying to distinguish between a very attenuated strain and a moderately attenuated strain, chimps would not do the job. Personally, I don't think a lot of real importance came out of those studies." Something that I had been suspecting for some time had just been confirmed, and by the closest colleague of the man who set up the studies.

I told him that I had always wondered about this, and why chimps were considered worth testing at all when reliable genetic markers had already been developed, and when macaques were already known to be more susceptible than chimps to poliovirus by intracerebral and intraspinal injection. Plotkin argued that everything needed to be viewed in its historical context. "The idea of using a local resource, that is chimpanzees . . . had some basis. In retrospect, of course, now that we have problems with preservation of species et cetera, it seems wasteful — but I think that at the time the idea was that this was the closest model, and therefore we could learn something useful." He pointed out that despite the invention of PCR, the FDA still required a monkey safety test for polio vaccines, and other vaccines as well.

I asked Plotkin how many chimps had been involved in the polio work at Lindi, and he said he really had no idea. "Except that I do know that there were at one time as many as thirty, forty chimps in the colony, and that at the time of independence, they were essentially killed and eaten. That's what I heard."

After some time, I asked whether it would not be logical, after having attenuated the vaccine virus through an unnatural host, to adapt it to a tissue culture from a host as close as possible to *Homo sapiens*. Until the advent of human diploid cell strains in 1961, that would surely have been not just monkey kidney tissue culture, but chimpanzee kidney tissue culture.

"That would have been a stupid idea," Plotkin responded. Why? I inquired. "Because to do that would have required a large supply of chimps." What about secondary and tertiary passages, I asked — surely that would produce enough tissue culture material? "You can do that for two or three passages, but [if] you're talking about producing vaccine for the world, it's simply not a starter," said Plotkin. I told him that Courtois had said that it would only require two thousand liters of polio vaccine to immunize the whole world,[1] and then I asked Plotkin again: Did it not make sound virological sense to use chimp tissue culture?

"No," he replied, with some finality. "You can grow virus just as well in monkey cells and, as it turned out, in human cells, as you can in chimp cells. I've never personally worked with chimp cells. I have no doubt that they can grow poliovirus, but you can produce extremely high titers in rhesus monkey kidney without any problem whatsoever."

But in fact, Koprowski wasn't trying to feed the whole world; he was experimenting, trying to develop the best set of vaccine strains. They wouldn't have needed a lot of chimps to produce enough vaccine for, say, 200,000 people — according to most commentators, just a few animals would have sufficed. In any case, the whole point about the chimps in the Congo, and at Lindi, was that from the perspective of the experimenters there *was* a large supply of them. They had been viewed, as Plotkin had just put it, as a "local resource."

And how *had* CHAT been made? I asked finally. "Well, the virus we used was produced in rhesus monkey kidney cells. And eventually [WI-38] diploid cells, later on," said Plotkin.[2]

Later, we turned to his own experiences of the Congo. He had visited just once, he said, in 1959. He told me something about the careful conduct of the vaccination in Leopoldville, how they had made estimates of population for each of the districts and kept accurate records of the number vaccinated and, of course, the number who developed polio. All this was possible only because of the highly developed medical services that the Belgians had set up, and the work of Ghislain Courtois and André Lebrun in particular. As had everyone else, he had appreciated Courtois. He described him as "a diamond in the rough; an old Africa hand [who did] virology by . . . the seat of his pants."

We talked some more about the vaccinations. "Of course," he volunteered at one point, "it was much more successful in the major cities than in other places we tried. . . ." He paused, as if deciding whether or not to tell me something, and then said: "I remember one place where we were even chased out of town. The rumor started that we were unsexing the African children by taking blood, and even though we bled some Belgian children, that didn't seem to satisfy things. . . . The parents stopped bringing their children for vaccination, and since we were surrounded by an angry crowd and had to be rescued by the army, we had to beat a hasty retreat." He told me this had happened in the town of Kikwit, and that they had vaccinated only "a couple of hundred" there.

I asked him in which other places in Africa they had done trials, and he told me that although he had visited other places like Ruanda-Urundi and Bas-Congo where vaccinations might have taken place later, he himself had been involved in vaccinations only in Leopoldville, Stanleyville, and Kikwit. Although he did not specify the month of his visit, I knew that he had been out in central Africa for at least the month of May 1959, since he had attended a press conference with Lebrun and Courtois on the first of the month,[3] and had sent a letter from Stanleyville to Fritz Deinhardt about the Lindi hepatitis work on May 28.[4]

I asked him about the polio epidemic that had started in October 1958, shortly after the beginning of the vaccination in Leopoldville. How could he be sure that the outbreak was caused by wild polioviruses, and was not linked to a vaccine virus that was starting to spread through the community and was reverting to virulence in some infectees? Plotkin said that he could not be certain, but that it was "highly improbable." For one thing, there had not been any clustering of cases, such as one might expect if the outbreak was linked to the vaccine. Also, *in vitro* tests, and later experience in Poland, showed that CHAT was well attenuated.[5] I asked how long after vaccination one might expect to see vaccine-associated cases, and he told me from seven to thirty-five days later, this being the incubation period of the disease.

I kept pressing, asking what was to prevent a hidden chain of infection, with a vaccinee passing on an excreted vaccine virus to another, who then passed on a slightly less attenuated virus to a third party, leading eventually to a vaccine-associated outbreak some months later? He agreed that intellectually this was possible, but that it was likely that lab strains did not propagate as well as wild viruses in nature. In any case, one did not see vaccine-associated epidemics in other countries in which OPV had been widely fed, such as the United States. I felt like saying that countries such as the U.S. had fed Sabin's strains, not Koprowski's, and pointing out other episodes (such as Sonoma and Province Oriental) in which there seemed to have been a polio outbreak a few weeks or months after a vaccination with Koprowski's strains. I decided, however, to keep my own counsel on this one.

I asked him what had been the purpose of the Ruzizi vaccination, and he said he thought that it had been a demonstration of feasibility, an "attempt to put OPV on a footing as a public-health technique. But of course the criticism could be leveled — and was leveled at the time, that you couldn't extract much useful information from it since it wasn't really controlled in any way. . . . [We] didn't know exactly whom we were vaccinating."

Next I asked Plotkin one of the questions to which I most wanted an answer, about the seven different pools of CHAT (4B-5, 10A-11, 13, 18G-11, 23, 24, and DS) mentioned in his 1961 paper.[6] To my great disappointment, he said he had no recollection whatsoever about these different pools, about how and where they had been prepared. In the end, he told me his best guess was that the numbers indicated plaque isolates of CHAT, as shown in the plaque chart, and that the letters indicated the plates in which he had grown out different samples of the same plaque. He added that the terms "lot" and "pool" were not very precise. He preferred to talk in terms of a "seed pool" containing "seed virus," this being what you started with, from which further passages would produce a "production lot," this being a quantity of vaccine prepared for human use.[7]

---

Plotkin spoke of Sabin and Koprowski as "extremely talented and brilliant people, both of whom I have known well," and his descriptions of them justified that claim. He spoke of Sabin as "a consummate general. He knew where to pick a battle and where to put his troops. . . . By going to the Soviet Union, he was able to validate his strains on a scale that was extremely impressive." He added that Sabin perhaps deserved to win the OPV race because of all the hard work he put in, and the degree to which he concentrated his research purely on polio vaccine, over a period of several years.

Koprowski, by contrast, "was a multisided individual who had many different interests . . . including administering the Wistar Institute . . . and his whole life was not committed to polio vaccine." Plotkin said that many people spoke of him as a "real Renaissance person," what with his background in music, and his knowledge about literature and art. "On the scientific side," he went on, "he has an extremely fertile mind . . . and the ability to arrange facts in such a way that ideas emerge." While Sabin had focused himself on polio, Koprowski had worked more or less simultaneously on polio, rabies, cancer, and various different viruses that were of interest as immunological models. Was it possible to spread oneself too thinly? I asked. "I don't think anyone has seen any thinness in Hilary," said Stanley Plotkin.

When we turned to the problem of contaminating simian viruses in tissue culture, Plotkin responded very much as Koprowski had done before. Once they had recognized the risk they responded sensibly by moving away from monkey kidney tissue cultures to human diploid cells. But, he added, the pathogenicity of SV40 was never really established, and "there was not a point at which it seemed like a catastrophic problem that was going to sink the whole venture."

He told me that the substrate they were currently using for both IPV and OPV at Pasteur Mérieux was the Vero cell, a well-characterized cell line. He explained that the problem with human diploid cell strains was that the yield of virus was not very high; human diploid cells were "more finicky" and harder to cultivate than monkey kidney cultures. The reason why most vaccine houses continued to use monkey kidney for polio vaccines was therefore partly economic, but also partly that monkeys could nowadays be raised in colonies, making it easier to produce kidneys that were free of viral contaminants.

As for the contaminating virus that Sabin had apparently found in CHAT, Plotkin said he didn't think that Sabin "stuck to that statement." Certainly he had never sent the virus in question to other people for testing. And Hilary, he said, had given him to understand that Sabin had retracted that statement before he died. Apparently Sabin had been appalled by the *Rolling Stone* article and "essentially could not believe that there was any such virus [SIV] in any of the polio preparations."

With regard to Tom Curtis's article, Plotkin had volunteered quite early in the interview that he had "a whole bunch of things" that Koprowski had written on the controversy, which he could pull out for me. However, when he checked, it turned out that all he could find were early drafts of Koprowski's letter to *Science*. "I considered writing a response myself, but I felt it was getting too much attention for something that's literally just . . . ," Plotkin said, his voice tailing off.

He gave me one of Koprowski's drafts: it was similar to the published version, but rather more angry and carping in tone, referring for instance to Elswood and Stricker (whom he called "Stickler") as "a layman and a doctor of medicine from San Francisco," and to Curtis as "a journalist who has no training in either biology, epidemiology or medicine." All the wounded pride, and the many errors and false assumptions of the final published letter were already there, though the footnotes were not yet out of sequence.

---

One of my last questions to Stanley Plotkin concerned vaccines against AIDS. A few months earlier, he had been quoted in the papers as saying that Pasteur Mérieux had begun human trials of a genetically engineered vaccine that consisted of gp160, one of the envelope genes of HIV, which had been introduced into a canary pox virus that was harmless for man. "If these approaches fall flat," Plotkin had apparently told the man from the *Observer*, "then the world is in big trouble. I don't see any other solution to halting the disease's spread."[8]

But Plotkin now seemed far less gung-ho on this topic. He told me that, in trials, monkeys had been protected against SIV and chimps against HIV-1 — but not every animal had been protected, and the scientists weren't really sure what, if anything, had provided the immunity. Was it antibodies, or was it some other function? (AIDS, of course, is different from other diseases, in that the presence of antibodies is normally taken to indicate that a person is infected, rather than protected.) This uncertainty made people nervous about trying out vaccines in humans, because any failures would cast a pall over the whole field of AIDS vaccine development. There were various candidate vaccines with differing degrees of promise, but none had all the desired properties. He personally was not pessimistic, but he did not think that the first vaccine tried would provide the final answer. I began to get the sense that the human vaccine trials had perhaps not been as successful as he had hoped.

Was he more hopeful for killed or live AIDS vaccines, I asked. Mostly he had been talking about killed vaccines, he said, but he had been interested in the prospect of a live vaccine before he left Philadelphia in 1990. At that stage, however, it had been considered a stupid idea, and he couldn't get funding. Now other groups (like that of Ronald Desrosiers) were attempting to develop live vaccines, but Plotkin counseled caution. "They run up against the very great problem that . . . if you induce AIDS instead of preventing it . . . that is obviously a major disaster," he said. "I don't think it's beyond reason to think that if everything else fails one might, in certain high-risk groups, try a live vaccine on the grounds that it's not likely to be worse than nature. Be that as it may, it's still an idea which is [a long way off]."

It was a frank appraisal of the dangers inherent in such an approach. But, I wondered, as I sat on the train speeding through the flatlands of Picardy back toward Brussels, what if there was spread of the AIDS vaccine virus and reversion to virulence, just as had occurred on certain occasions with live polio vaccine back in the fifties? What if a live AIDS vaccine experiment actually spawned a new strain of HIV that was, for instance, more transmissible? Could the vaccine-makers guarantee that such a thing would not happen? And in reality, how many people would wish a live vaccine against AIDS to be given a field trial in their community on the grounds that "it can't be worse than nature"?

It occurred to me that one of the things I had discovered over the previous two years was that on occasions well-intentioned scientific experiment *could* be worse than nature, but that sometimes scientists did not realize why until it was far too late.

———————

Some time after our meeting, I recalled the strange feeling I had had at the beginning of the interview, when Plotkin had been telling me about his arrival at the Wistar Institute in August 1957. I recalled that Joseph Pagano had also spoken about working on anthrax vaccines in his early days at the Wistar. Further reading demonstrated that during the fifties anthrax — like the Venezuelan equine encephalitis virus Koprowski had stumbled across in Rio — was one of the major preoccupations of the U.S. Army Chemical Corps,[9] because of its potential as a biological warfare agent. I decided to see whether Plotkin and Pagano had published anything on the subject.

What I found was rather shocking. First I came across an article by Stanley Plotkin and others on an epidemic of inhalation anthrax that, as the title revealed, was "the first in the twentieth century."[10] Philip Brachman, the lead author, and Plotkin were listed as being from the Anthrax Investigations Unit, CDC, Wistar Institute, Philadelphia, and the work had been supported by a contract with the U.S. Army Chemical Corps, based at Fort Detrick.[11]

The revelation that with Koprowski taking over the directorship of the Wistar, the institute began accepting contracts from the principal biowarfare unit of the U.S. Army was an unexpected discovery. So was the realization that this was perhaps what Plotkin had meant when he spoke about the "opportunity . . . to do some research while fulfilling a military obligation." But what was really striking was the content of that research.

Plotkin's article revealed that on August 27, 1957, a man from a goat hair–processing plant at a mill in Manchester, New Hampshire, fell sick with inhalation anthrax. During the next two months, there were eight further cases of anthrax at the mill, four involving inhalation anthrax and four cutaneous anthrax. The latter group survived, but four of the five inhalation cases died.

Cutaneous anthrax is a moderately rare and not especially dangerous skin disease affecting those who handle animal hair or its derivatives. During the previous sixteen years, there had been 136 cases of cutaneous anthrax at the Manchester mill, which turned goat hair and wool from southern Asia into lining material for suits. Only one case had been fatal. By contrast, there had been no previous cases of inhalation anthrax at the mill — and only twenty-three isolated cases had been reported in the world medical literature since 1900.[12]

The article presents a marvelously cool, clear historical and scientific analysis of the epidemic. It is written in typical Plotkin style, and one suspects that he may have been responsible for much of the work. The introduction states that the outbreak "presented an unusual opportunity to study both the epidemiology of this disease, and the effectiveness of an anthrax vaccine that had been given to some of the workers several months before the epidemic." A later article by the same authors reveals that 300 of the Manchester mill's 630-odd employees volunteered to be vaccinated with this live anthrax vaccine, although the remainder refused.[13] Beginning in May 1957, approximately half of the 300 were vaccinated with three primary injections at fortnightly intervals, while the other half received three injections of a placebo.[14]

The vaccinees had been due to receive three booster shots at six monthly intervals, but the anthrax outbreak in August caused the trial to be terminated. Of the five cases of inhalation anthrax, four had not participated in the vaccine program, while the fifth had received only the placebo. Although the abandonment of the Manchester trial did not allow statistically valid conclusions to be made about vaccine efficacy, calculations that also incorporated data from other mills where earlier vaccine trials had been staged led the authors to conclude that the vaccine was 92.5 percent effective. On this basis, the entire staff of the Manchester mill was immunized with the same vaccine during 1958.

But what had caused the unprecedented epidemic? The authors looked at various possibilities, and concluded that one particular batch of black goat hair from India might have been responsible. The evidence supporting this conclusion was, however, rather vague and inconclusive. Furthermore, the epidemiologists noted that detergents used for scouring the hair had been shown to enhance the virulence of anthrax spores, and that a new detergent had come into use during this period.

It is striking that these papers about the Manchester outbreak do not contain a single reference to the extraordinary coincidence whereby the first inhalation anthrax epidemic of the century occurred within three months of an experimental trial of a live anthrax vaccine. Also striking is the fact that one of the papers cited in the endnotes, produced by a member of the U.K.'s Microbiological Research Department (and major biowarfare research center) at Porton Down, deals with methods of infecting animals with airborne anthrax, and is largely concerned with the massive increase of infectivity of anthrax spores — by a factor of at least ten — when they are contained in a spray based on a commercial detergent.[15] The first inhalation anthrax victim in Manchester fell ill on the same morning that a new commercial detergent replaced the traditional scouring agents of soap and soda ash, but he was working in a different part of the mill from where the new detergent had been introduced.[16] Nonetheless, the authors comment that "an hypothesis which presents itself is that this particular batch [of goat hair] contained an unusual number of highly virulent anthrax spores to which was added for most of the epidemic a virulence-enhancing substance (the scouring detergent)."

The only reference to the implications for biowarfare research in these two lengthy reports comes in a single sentence at the conclusion of one of them, which reads: "The potential civil defense problem posed by anthrax aerosols is also emphasized."

---

Why were commercial detergents introduced at this particular moment at the Manchester mill? And why did this happen just three months after an experimental vaccination, on the very same day that the worst outbreak of inhalation anthrax of the twentieth century began?

It may of course be that the Chemical Corps scientists were simply very lucky from a research perspective, and that Mother Nature started an epidemic of inhalation anthrax at just the right moment to test their vaccine under field conditions. And yet, of course, there is another, more ominous possibility. This is that, unbeknownst to the Wistar team of Plotkin and Brachman, humans played a conscious role, and that a decision was made by the Chemical Corps to subject the vaccine to the ultimate field test — that of challenge with virulent anthrax organisms.

Such an experiment, if it occurred, could have involved the introduction of a single lot of goat hair that was known to be contaminated with virulent anthrax spores. In addition, it might have involved the introduction of a commercial detergent, which would have effectively exposed certain populations in the mill to a challenge roughly ten times as virulent.

These appalling possibilities may sound far-fetched, and yet the hypothesis is supported by internal army reports from the period. The 1959/60 annual report for the Commission on Epidemiological Survey (CES), part of the Armed Forces Epidemiological Board, contains the minutes of a meeting held on March 23, 1960, which was largely devoted to anthrax.[17] Dr. Harold Glassman of Fort Detrick (whose assistance had been acknowledged at the end of each of the Brachman/Plotkin papers) was the main speaker, and he opened his address with a review of the anthrax organism, including "ease of preparation and stability in storage and as an aerosol." He was especially interested in air-sampling studies at the Manchester mill, and with the case of a young military volunteer who had died of inhalation anthrax at Fort Detrick in 1958 after receiving a series of inoculations of killed and live vaccines, including one against anthrax. He stressed the fact that the Soviets appeared to have recently developed an attenuated anthrax vaccine for humans, and said that there was an urgent need from the U.S. side for "an examination of the protective properties of various vaccine preparations." Clearly the Manchester vaccine trial had not provided all the answers. A portion of Dr. Glassman's presentation was omitted from the minutes, presumably for security reasons.

Just in case anyone is in doubt about what the military and civilian members of the CES were talking about, this is made absolutely clear by the minutes of the executive session held on the same day. The main address was by General McNinch, who spoke on "The Philosophy of B.W. [Biological Warfare] Research 1960–65." The minutes record part of his speech as follows: "The army is interested in determining whether an agent is potentially effective or not effective. . . . Moreover, a vaccine program cannot be separated from the immediate fields of interest. In other words, effective prophylaxis comes within the scope of the program." Later in the meeting, General McNinch revealed what "the immediate fields of interest" were, when he "emphasized that high level committees consider biologic agents as good weapon systems and that the United States is presently poorly prepared defensively and offensively." The forthright general went on to say that the budget for the Chemical Corps would be quadrupled or more for 1962, that a pharmaceutical company should be contracted to "carry the vaccine program to a successful conclusion . . . and that the government should subsidize the program with respect to buildings, equipment etc."

―――――――――

Let us review briefly the links between the Wistar Institute and the anthrax research program. It seems that the Anthrax Investigations Unit at the Wistar was established primarily in order to monitor the vaccinations, and there is no suggestion that the unit was itself responsible for the turn of events that resulted in four tragic deaths. However, the Wistar's association with the Chemical Corps seemingly started as soon as Koprowski took over, and it may be that the acceptance of this contract with the military was linked to the sudden upturn in the institute's fortunes, which so many observers have said occurred thereafter. The Wistar was apparently a moribund institution before Koprowski's arrival in May 1957 (without even a proper director since 1938, according to the *New York Times*),[18] but within two years of his accession to the director's chair, he had apparently completely renovated the institute, increasing the staff to fifty and staging a major symposium, which was attended by more than five hundred biologists.[19]

It is unclear how long the collaboration continued, but worth noting that in 1958, Chemical Corps scientists exposed four young chimpanzees to anthrax spores of different sizes, and three of the test animals appear to have been pygmy chimps.[20] Given the limited availability of that species, it seems very possible that the apes would have been obtained through Koprowski from the team at Stanleyville.

In fact, the U.S. Army Chemical Corps and the air force were *clandestinely* funding a much larger CBW research program ("Big Ben") at the University of

Pennsylvania during this period. It received $2,900,000 in military funds, and was a "study of biological and chemical warfare from all standpoints — social, political, technological, scientific." In 1954 the "Institute of Cooperative Research" was established on campus to house this and similar projects. One specific example was "Project Summit," which, from 1958 onward, involved "analysis of air-delivered CBW agent-munition combinations in counterinsurgency situations,"[21] and included "research into the inducement and epidemic spreading of . . . anthrax."[22]

It must be stressed that despite the fact that both the Institute of Cooperative Research and the Wistar Institute are known to have been receiving Chemical Corps funds during the period 1957/8, and the fact that they were situated one block apart on Walnut and Spruce in Philadelphia, there are no documented links between the two institutes. It must also be stressed that whereas the army's funding of the Wistar research was publicly documented, its funding of research at the other institute (as far as is known) was not.

---

The anthrax episode provides important context to the Wistar's experimental research into polio vaccines. The key issue is that Plotkin, the Epidemiology Intelligence Service officer who virtually took over the Wistar's OPV program from late 1957 onward, and Joseph Pagano, the EIS colleague who followed him to the Wistar in 1958, were initially delegated to that institution by the U.S. Public Health Service to participate not in polio vaccine development, but in biological research that was funded by the military.

This is not to imply that the CHAT vaccinations in Africa were part of some biowarfare experiment — they most certainly were not. But they were effectively a biological experiment, and one that, just like the vaccine trial in the Manchester mill, involved far greater risks to participants and nonparticipants than would be considered acceptable nowadays. Both carry the heavy, sour smell of an era that believed that great problems like polio or the "Red Threat" required drastic solutions.

## LE LABORATOIRE MÉDICAL DE STANLEYVILLE

At this stage it was clearly important to find out more about those early Congo vaccinations, starting with the CHAT trial at Aketi in May 1957, the month of Koprowski's accession to the Wistar throne. Aketi was important, in that it represented the moment when the number of Koprowski's oral vaccinees suddenly jumped by two orders of magnitude. Previously, the largest feeding of a Type 1 OPV had been to thirty-eight children at Sonoma in 1955; now that figure suddenly increased to almost two thousand. The Aketi trial was, furthermore, the first large-scale trial of OPV in the open community anywhere in the world.

The only clue as to who might have been directly involved with the trial lay in the Belgian article by Courtois, which mentioned that the vaccinations had taken place at two schools, and had been carefully monitored by "Dr Forro, doctor of the local railways." Apparently "rigid clinical observations failed to show any signs of illness which could be attributed to the vaccine."[1] Some research in Brussels revealed that there was only one Dr. Forro working in Belgium — Dr. Alex Forro, living in a small provincial town. I phoned, and discovered that this was indeed the right family, but that the man I was seeking was his father, Michel, who had died two years earlier. Nonetheless, in 1957 Alex had been seven years old, and had spent part of the year in Aketi. He invited me over for a chat.

It transpired that Michel Forro, a Hungarian by birth, had been employed by Vicicongo, a transport company that had its headquarters at Aketi, and that dealt with most of the road and railway construction and haulage in Province Oriental. Aketi is an important port on the Itimbiri River, and in those days it rivaled Stanleyville as an entrepôt; a narrow-gauge railway served the wealthy agricultural towns to the east, and Vicicongo's large truck fleet transported

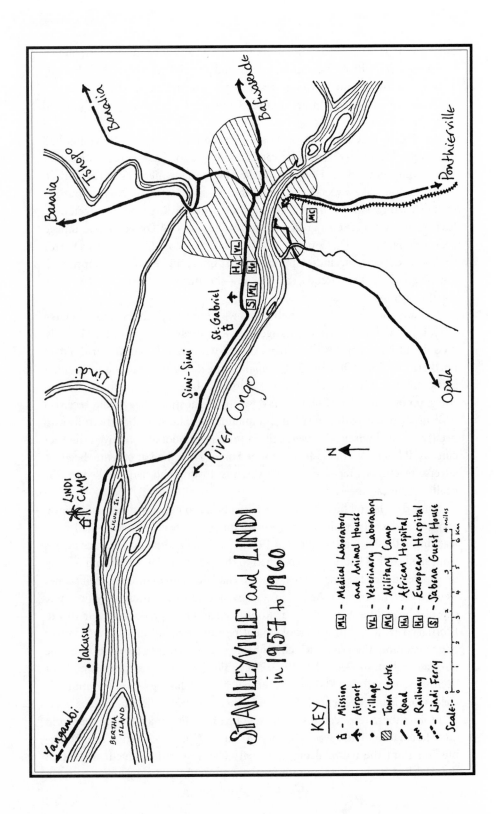

other goods as far afield as Usumbura in Urundi, and Juba in southern Sudan, returning laden with coffee, cotton, rubber, and palm oil. Aketi effectively became a company town, with Vicicongo assuming responsibility for the schools and hospitals, which served three hundred Europeans and about five thousand Africans.

Alex Forro had been away at boarding school for much of 1957, and had no recollection of any large-scale vaccinations. Neither did he recall his father ever talking about them. However, he did have a vague memory of being given some "samples like sweets" and being told to swallow them. And he put me in touch with Madame Bossut, the widow of one of the former directors of Vicicongo, who recalled a great deal more. She said that Dr. Forro had indeed been approached by Dr. Courtois, who asked if Aketi could be used as a zone for testing some new vaccines supplied by an American researcher, Koprowski. Forro agreed, and apparently that was it — no further permissions had been sought or granted.

Madame Bossut said that Aketi had a white primary school, and two large schools for African boys and girls aged between twelve and eighteen. The girls' school had been run by missionary sisters, who were based at Turnhout in northern Belgium. She added that apart from the school vaccinations, other black children were rounded up by the local police, who went from street to street announcing that if they went down to the hospital they would receive a *bonbon*. Apparently this ensured full attendance. She said that the fifteen to twenty white children who were still in primary school also received the vaccine, as did her own daughter, and Alex Forro. There had apparently been no adverse reactions afterward, though she was unsure who had checked on the health of the vaccinees.

Some days later, I had to travel past Turnhout, so I dropped by the medieval convent and spoke with two sisters — Emilia and Severia — who had been teaching at the Aketi girls' school in 1957. They recalled that two or three nurses from the hospital had been dispatched to the school by Dr. Forro, and had set up a table outside the classrooms. The girls had lined up in the sun, their names were written down, and then each was given a capsule (presumably the same capsules brought to Stanleyville by Koprowski and Norton during their visit in February 1957). The process took an entire morning, and they thought it had happened more than once, which probably meant that they also witnessed the Fox vaccination in December 1957. They said that Dr. Forro himself had not been present, and they did not remember his ever taking blood for antibody checks, or visiting the schools later on to check on pupils' health.

I found these recollections of the staging of the first mass trial in the world quite fascinating. There was no evidence that Dr. Courtois had first sought permission from the national or provincial government. It seemed rather that the trial had been staged quite informally, through an arrangement between friends, one of whom was the chief medic in a company town. Apparently a few whites as well as blacks were vaccinated, but the two thousand African school-children clearly had little option but to accept their *"bonbons."* I failed to find any evidence to support the claim that the "rigid clinical observations" referred to by Courtois had amounted to anything more than monitoring for major diseases. Interestingly, the sisters said that they had seen further cases of polio among Aketi children later on, which they thought was probably because not all had been vaccinated.

Alex Forro had told me that his father had left Aketi in late 1957 or early 1958, in order to build his own hospital at Angodia, an idyllic spot on the Uele River. Later, when I checked a map, I found that Angodia was just three or four miles from Bambesa, where there had apparently been six cases of polio in January 1958. This was just as Dr. Courtois was on the lookout for outbreaks that might allow him to test Koprowski's OPV "in the face of an epidemic," and Bambesa was duly vaccinated at the start of February.

———

Next I followed up with the man who had been recommended so warmly by both André and Ann Courtois as a potential source of information: Pierre Doupagne. Although not trained as a doctor, Doupagne had worked as a sanitary officer for the laboratory between 1949 and 1960, rising to the position of principal medical auxiliary for the last of those years. He clearly had an immense knowledge of the local conditions, and was a very kindly man as well.

Soon after my arrival, Doupagne fetched a document that I had never seen before — the 1959 annual report for the Stanleyville medical laboratory. Remarkably, no copies of this existed in the Belgian government archives, or even in the library of the tropical institute at Antwerp; I had even begun to suspect that no report had been issued for that year. He left me to peruse it while he went off to make coffee.

This report had been compiled by Gaston Ninane, who had taken over from Courtois after his departure for Leo in September 1959, and unlike any of the previous annual reports, it contained a few precise details about polio vaccinations. Apparently some 2,500 children had been vaccinated at Bafwasende, a small town to the north of Stanleyville, and a further 15,000 children in the campaign with which Plotkin had helped, in Stanleyville itself. (By 1959, the Ruzizi approach — vaccinating the entire population — had apparently been abandoned, because it was recognized that virtually the entire African population had acquired polio antibodies naturally by the age of five.)[2] This latter campaign had been carried out in collaboration with the Hygiène service, which, the report noted, had assumed responsibility for immunization during the course of the year — just as Ninane had told me in interview.

But what was really fascinating was that 250,000 doses of the vaccine had been "*conditioné*" (which in this instance apparently means transferred from large flasks into small vials)[3] at the Stanleyville lab, and then forwarded to Usumbura. This not only seemed to confirm that the second major vaccination campaign in Ruanda-Urundi had gone ahead, it also suggested that there was a possibility of contamination, if chimpanzee autopsies had been taking place in the vicinity of the processing of the vaccine.

The report also contained an interesting summary of the 1959 Lindi research. Five chimpanzees had been used to establish "the innocuity of a vaccine strain"; this sounded like a new OPV (perhaps the WM-3 Type 3 strain, which Plotkin had developed as a further attenuation of Fox). And 36 other chimps had been used in research into measles, encephalitis, and diabetes. This total of 41 chimps used for experimentation was a considerable reduction on the numbers that had passed through the camp at the height of the polio research in 1956–1958. It seems that the polio work was virtually completed, and that the association with the Wistar Institute and the Children's Hospital of Philadelphia, which had obtained throughout the work on polio and hepatitis, was perhaps winding down, with the camp now accepting research offers from other investigators.

Last, experiments proposed for 1960 were listed. These included three cancer experiments, innocuity tests on a Type 2 polio vaccine, and a study of poliovirus in the bloodstream after *injecting* with attenuated poliovirus (which appeared to pursue a line of thinking similar to Lépine's). But when Pierre Doupagne returned, he told me that there had been a lot of pre-independence unrest in Stanleyville in March and April 1960, so it seemed unlikely that these final experiments had actually taken place.

I commented to Doupagne that the 1959 report was considerably more detailed in its account of the polio work and the Lindi research than the previous annual reports had been. He had copies of these also, and began looking through them to see what I meant. "I'm astonished not to see more information about polio," he said finally. "Koprowski must have the notes." I told him that apparently he didn't, and he continued to express amazement. "It's not enough," he admitted, with a sigh.

Doupagne explained that he had been in charge of the bacteriological research and had carried out many of the examinations of the chimps. He said that many of those that died had had "tropical depression" as a result of their capture and incarceration; later, others died of pneumonia. The researchers began to realize that they knew very little about the habits of chimps and what they ate in the wild, so they commissioned the hunter to make a survey, so that they could improve the animals' diets.[4] They also arranged for each black worker to take special responsibility for two or three infant chimps. Doupagne said that steroid injections had helped (although it later occurred to me that if the chimps had been given steroids as Courtois reported, then this could have suppressed their immune responses and exacerbated the *Klebsiella* problem).

Doupagne added that at any one time, they had kept at least a hundred chimps; fifteen or so at the large animal house next to the medical laboratory, which had opened in October 1957, and the rest at Lindi. "It was a very big experiment," he went on. "Sometimes we were a little ashamed to see so many chimps destroyed like this." In addition, he said, a large proportion of the chimps (especially the older ones) died even before they got to Lindi — "half, surely."

Around this point in the conversation, there was a phone call from André Courtois, and although Pierre Doupagne continued to be friendly and helpful, I got the impression that he was less forthcoming thereafter. But he did go on to explain that when a chimp died, an autopsy would be done by Ninane, and that autopsy materials would be sent to either Philadelphia or Leuven for testing. On the other hand, he could remember nothing about where or how the vaccine had been made, or even the fact that there had been a Belgian version.

He did remember, however, that at one stage they announced that any doctor in the colony who wished to have vaccine "just had to ask" the Stanleyville lab. "Oh yes," he added, "many asked." Apparently they would surround the vaccine with blue freezer bags, of which they had a large supply, and pack it in metal flasks, which were then dispatched by air. He was unable to recall any of the places where the vaccine had been sent.

A couple of weeks earlier, I had come across a fascinating paper, which Doupagne had written just two months before his departure from Stanleyville in May 1960.[5] The report explained that in the course of bacteriological investigations in Stanleyville, yeasts of the *Candida* species had been encountered more and more frequently. One hundred and thirteen isolations were listed, apparently from the first three months of 1960, which represented a dramatic increase over the previous five years, when there had been an average of twenty-two isolations annually. Most of the isolates were of *Candida albicans,* which when it appears in atypical sites, like the throat or esophagus, is one of the most common opportunistic infections of humans with AIDS, and of monkeys with simian AIDS.

The source of the bacteriological samples was not cited, and so I asked Doupagne whether they were all from humans, or if some had come from the Lindi chimps (just as Osterrieth's *Klebsiella* isolates in 1958 had come from both humans and chimps). His reply was equivocal, and he could not say for certain that they were all human samples. What he did recall was they had identified an increase in pathogenic *Candida* infections — in the vaginas and around the breasts of women, especially those who wore bras, and in and around the mouths of small children. He added that once they started testing specifically for *Candida,* they found it in more and more of the samples.

Doupagne also mentioned that the members of the Laboratoire Médical de Stanleyville were organizing a reunion, the first since they had all departed the Congo back in 1960. The idea had started a few weeks before, during a phone conversation between himself and Jean Vandepitte (who had run the lab for that six-month period in 1958), and he, Doupagne, was making the arrangements. Apart from these two, Paul Osterrieth, André Courtois, and one or two others had agreed to attend; Gaston Ninane, however, had declined. He told me that they were due to meet in a restaurant (which he named) in Liège, and I asked if there would be any chance of my joining them. I was hardly surprised when he turned me down, for I suspected that my investigation might be one of the items on the agenda. It was clear that my questions about the Stanleyville research were beginning to make waves.

This feeling was confirmed a few days later, when I made contact with Jean Vandepitte and Paul Osterrieth, both of whom had been so friendly when they had spoken with me the previous year. Vandepitte was cool on the phone, and said he was too busy to see me. Osterrieth, by contrast, said he had an hour to spare, but sounded distinctly gruff.

When I arrived at his house a few minutes late, he scowled at me from the doorstep, and told me that since he had to collect his wife from the station, he had only forty minutes to spare. It appeared that he was regretting having agreed to see me again. I began by telling him about some of my research of the last year, but when he realized that I still thought that CHAT might be implicated in the origin of AIDS, he snorted derision. My impression was that he now felt that he had been far too candid during our first meeting, and having had time to reflect, realized that even if he had not been directly involved with the polio research, the fallout from a scandal might do him considerable damage. He responded to a few of my questions, but it was noticeable that some of his answers had changed. He now said he couldn't remember whether or not Stanley Plotkin had come to Stanleyville. And, more important, he denied that any chimp kidneys had been sent to America. When I pointed out that last time he had told me differently, he replied: "That might have been a slip." In the end, his greatly altered manner and revised version of events were too much for me. Before I had asked even half of my questions, I realized that the process was pointless, and so I thanked him and took my leave.

That same afternoon, I went to see Dr. Armand André, the former director of the blood bank in Liège, to ask him about the paper on chimpanzee blood groups that he had cowritten with Courtois, Ninane, and Osterrieth.[6] One hundred and seventy-five chimpanzee blood samples, including seventeen from *Pan paniscus,* had been air-freighted to Liège from Stanleyville, and although Dr. André could no longer remember the date, he confirmed that the sender had been Paul Osterrieth.[7] He could recall very little about the work, or about the interesting conclusions concerning the very different properties evident in bloods from chimps originating from different regions.

But when I asked him the key question — whether he still had the remainder of the chimpanzee blood samples in his freezers — he gave an interesting set of responses. First, he told me that he still had the blood samples stored. Then he changed his mind and said that he didn't, after which he said that he couldn't remember. Finally, he said that they had done so many tests that they had used everything up. At any rate, this seemed to scupper my best chance of locating some of the Lindi chimp bloods to have them tested for SIV.

It was a disappointing end to a disappointing day. Furthermore, although I was pretty sure that André's reaction was not connected to those of Vandepitte and Osterrieth, I had the strong feeling that doors were beginning to slam shut. There seemed to be a general closing of the ranks among the scientists who had served in the former Belgian Congo.

---

I did, however, attempt to get some perspective on the events in Stanleyville from a different angle, by speaking to Stéphane Pattyn, a member of the medical laboratory at Elisabethville between 1955 and 1960, and one who, together with his director, Jean Delville, had mounted polio antibody studies in Elisabethville, Leopoldville, and Bukavu.[8] Even as a young man, Pattyn had earned a considerable reputation for the clarity of his research. He was one of those who had attended the 1957 virus symposium in Stanleyville, and was now a highly respected virologist based at the tropical institute at Antwerp.

Dr. Pattyn told me that they had never fed "the famous CHAT strain" in Elisabethville, mainly because it was an experimental vaccine, and they felt that its safety and efficacy had not been proven. I showed him a newspaper article, which showed that in May 1959 a mass vaccination was scheduled to take place at Lubudi, two hundred miles north of the Katanga capital, and he said that he could not confirm whether or not it had actually gone ahead.[9] But he added that by the time CHAT had been approved for general use in the Congo, independence was only a few months distant.

I asked him to explain why they had not used the vaccine, when it was freely available in Stanleyville, just a couple of hours away by plane. He and Delville, he told me, had been very skeptical about the fact that in places like Ruzizi it had been given to large numbers of adults, when they knew from their antibody studies that African adults were already almost 100 percent immune. "Even if [CHAT] had been a virulent strain, it would not have caused any paralysis in these people," he added. Later, among the children of Leopoldville, it proved to have a very high failure rate, with only about 60 percent being successfully immunized. In those days E'ville (as it was known) had good rail connections with Johannesburg, so those whites who wanted to be vaccinated tended to travel south for inoculations with the South African IPV. Apart from that, he said, the lab team kept monitoring the polio situation by testing for the presence of virus in local sewage, and in the stools of children and infants who developed paralysis or meningitis.[10]

I asked whether they would have used Koprowski's strains in E'ville if a flaming epidemic had started, like the one that had swept the city in 1954/5, and he said he could not be sure, but he thought probably not. He added that there were still a lot of fears about the safety of OPV, even in the late fifties when CHAT was being fed widely, and the way in which he spoke of the chimp research at Lindi showed that he was little impressed by that as well. "Ask Osterrieth," he told me. "He was implicated in this whole thing." He declined to make any further comments. Even allowing for the fact that there might be a temptation for Stéphane Pattyn to be wise after the event, his conspicuous lack of support for the Koprowski strains and the CHAT vaccination program in the Congo was clear.

————————

There remained certain important details that I needed to check, and the only person I knew to check them with was Gaston Ninane. At the outset of our interview, I told him that in the last year I had found out a lot more about the Congo vaccinations and that I now believed it to be very possible that there was an association between some of these vaccinations and the first appearances of AIDS. He expressed incredulity, but agreed once more to do his best to help. I said I would like to show him some of my evidence and ask for his comments and, as it turned out, this approach successfully jogged his memory on a number of important points.

Among the points he was able to confirm was that he had vaccinated the population of Lisala (not Bumba), that in April 1958 he and Herbert Meyus had vaccinated down the eastern shore of Lake Tanganyika, from Usumbura to Nyanza Lac, and that at a later date he had fed CHAT along the eastern side of Lake Kivu. It was, he said, only in 1959, around the time that Courtois moved to Leopoldville, that the clinical trial period was deemed to be over, and the vaccine was approved for use in the whole of the Congo and Ruanda-Urundi.[11]

He also reconfirmed that the initial vaccine came from Koprowski, but was soon replaced by vaccine made in Belgium. "In my memory it was quite impossible to send vaccine in [any] volume from the United States. But . . . it was easy by plane from Brussels to Stanleyville." He said that the only two places in Belgium where the vaccine could have been made were the virology department in Leuven, or else RIT at Rixensart, both under De Somer, and added that they would have used the same production techniques as the American lab.

We talked for some time about how many chimps were used in the polio program, and Ninane was clearly very uneasy about the high numbers involved, but when I showed him various papers indicating a figure of four hundred, he eventually acknowledged that this could have been the total. He confirmed that when a chimp died, he would do a postmortem "almost every time," and that this would involve all the pulmonary and abdominal tissues, but usually not the brain or spinal cord. Yes, he said, this had included the kidneys — but no, he had never sent kidneys to the United States or to Belgium.

Later, I showed Ninane papers that proved that not only had chimp kidneys been sent from Stanleyville to Philadelphia, but that kidneys of some variety had been sent by Courtois to Europe in 1957 or earlier.[12] He first said that he didn't remember this, and that he was really "quite astonished." Then he said Koprowski already had chimps and other monkeys in America, which he could use to make tissue culture if he so wished. I pointed out that if Koprowski had decided to try an experimental pool made in chimp kidney, then it would clearly be easier to send kidneys direct from Stanleyville, where they were cheap and available, than to slaughter expensive animals in the United States. And how else could he explain the enormous number of chimps used in the space of some eighteen months? "Yes, yes," he agreed finally, "it is possible. Maybe he had to be first in the race."

But he continued to insist that he himself had not dispatched kidneys overseas. The Belgian Congo, he said, had been just like an army. The general (who, he said, was Ghislain Courtois) knew all, while he, Gaston Ninane, had been just the sergeant. He freely admitted that he had been responsible for the postmortems, for extracting the kidneys, but said that perhaps other researchers had taken kidneys back home with them, or air-freighted them across to the U.S. or Belgium.

Ninane claimed that he, and not Osterrieth, had tried to make tissue culture in the Stanleyville lab, which meant that, strangely, each man now claimed that he was the only one to have worked with tissue culture there. Ninane said that in the early days he had tried unsuccessfully for four or five months to make a tissue culture in which he could isolate viruses like yellow fever; then he had given up. At one point, he said that he had used tissue from chimpanzees; this being the first time that anyone had admitted making chimp kidney tissue culture in the Stanleyville lab. He said that he had been employing techniques he had learned in the early fifties from Professor Chevremont, a histologist at the University of Liège, and had used Maitland suspended cell cultures, which did not require the use of trypsin to break up the cells. He reiterated, however, that he had never produced any successful cultures.

He also acknowledged — albeit reluctantly — that in the final year, after he had taken over from Courtois, live chimpanzees had been sent from Stanleyville to the States. One of the recipients had been Fred Stare, a nutrition expert at Harvard, but at least half had been sent to other researchers, including, perhaps, scientists at the Rockefeller Foundation who were interested in studying arteriosclerosis. He could not recall the numbers, or whether Koprowski had been one of the recipients.

Before I left, Dr. Ninane mentioned that he had been phoned by Pierre Doupagne some three weeks earlier and invited to the Stanleyville doctors' reunion at the end of May, but that he had refused. He explained that it was actually being held at the Catholic university town of Leuven, and that he wouldn't go near the place.[13]

As I left, I thanked Gaston Ninane, once again, for his kindness and help. There was something about his jagged nonconformity, his crusty refusal to respect the pomp and circumstance of powerful individuals and institutions, that I found rather refreshing. Of all the doctors still alive from the Laboratoire Médical de Stanleyville, Ninane perhaps had the most reason to refuse to answer any more questions — and yet he was the only one who had always kept the door open.

# 43

By this stage, I had been investigating the OPV/AIDS theory for more than two years, and although I had managed to unravel many of the details, there were certain elements that seemed to shimmer backward whenever I reached out, like the grapes of Tantalus. Partly this was a factor of passing time, of the civil wars and unrest that the Congo, Rwanda, and Burundi had experienced since 1960, and the deaths of many of the central protagonists. But there seemed something vaguely sinister here too, like the fact that the most relevant period from the key file at the ministerial archives in Brussels had simply disappeared, and that the promised article about the polio research on the Lindi chimps had never been written.

The fate of that huge body of chimpanzees troubled me more and more. It was now clear that they lay at the very heart of the story, a point reinforced by the apparent unwillingness of those involved to talk in any detail about what had happened at the camp.

There seemed to be little more that I could learn from the medical men at Stanleyville, those who had run the laboratory and organized the chimp experiments. But perhaps I could find out further details from some of the animal specialists — the primatologists and vets — who had had dealings with the camp. In addition, there were two men — Daenens the camp administrator, and Rollais the chimp hunter — who would be able to provide a lot of information if they were still alive.

I started off with another huge slice of luck, when I contacted Joseph Mortelmans, the primatologist who cowrote the "Apes" article with Ghislain

Courtois in 1967. Until his retirement a couple of years earlier, he had been jointly based at Antwerp Zoo and the nearby Tropical Institute. We met at the zoo gates, and he steered me across to a café where we found a table away from the rest of the customers.

He surprised me by saying that he himself had worked in Stanleyville, between December 1955 and June 1956, when he temporarily took over the veterinary laboratory after the previous incumbent committed suicide. The vet lab was situated on the edge of the main town, while the medical lab of Ghislain Courtois was a mile or so to the west, out by the airport. Not surprisingly, the two directors quickly became friends.

At the start of the fifties, the Stanleyville vet lab had been run by Tad Wiktor, the same Pole who had got to know Hilary Koprowski at the Muguga rabies conference in July 1955. Mortelmans confirmed that it was there that the two men had discussed the idea of an experimental farm where Koprowski could carry out polio experiments on chimpanzees, and where Wiktor suggested Dr. Courtois as a man who might be able to help Koprowski conduct trials in humans.

It became clear that in early 1956, when Mortelmans was in Stan, the camp at Lindi had not yet opened. But as he recalled, Courtois was already keeping a number of *Pan troglodytes* chimps at the medical lab for research purposes. In those days, he said, the animals cost about fifty francs (one dollar) each, and there was an unlimited supply. Courtois he described as a great bon vivant, one who liked friends and conviviality. "He was not especially interested in this polio and rabies," said Mortelmans; "he was interested in them because they were new, they were in progress. . . . He wanted to be always one step [ahead]."

I asked Mortelmans whether he knew that Courtois had sent kidneys from Stanleyville back to Europe during the fifties. He said that he doubted that they could be kept sufficiently fresh. So I showed him the remark that Courtois had made in a discussion session at the Lyon conference in December 1967, where he and Mortelmans had presented their paper on apes.[1] Replying to a question about whether it was wasteful to send refrigerated kidneys from lab to lab, rather than purchasing live monkeys and sacrificing them, Courtois had responded: "More than 10 years ago we sent kidneys from the Congo to Europe and they were quite satisfactory." Mortelmans agreed that this could only have meant chimpanzee kidneys. Furthermore, it was clear that Courtois had been referring to 1957 or earlier.

For a moment, Mortelmans had a problem because, he said, jet planes like the 707s had not come in till 1959 or 1960, but I pointed out that even before that, it only took eighteen hours to travel between Stanleyville and Brussels.[2] Furthermore, in 1958 unrefrigerated chimp kidneys had been sent from Stanleyville to Philadelphia, and were still viable even three to six days after they left Africa.[3] Finally, he had to agree that the process was possible if one sent sterile kidneys, either whole or minced, and if the cell cultures were then prepared at the other end.

Despite his apparent skepticism, it was around this point in the interview that something happened. Until then, Professor Mortelmans had been a busy man, taking time out from his schedule to meet with me. But now suddenly he was fully engaged with the subject. I asked him what the chimp kidneys could have been used for. He paused for a while, before saying that in Stanleyville there was no problem of supply ("you could [just] ask for twenty-five chimpanzees"), and chimps were generally considered to be the last experimental animal before man. "So," he mused, "as it was not difficult to get them, why not use chimpanzees, and eventually chimpanzee kidneys?"

Was it possible that the kidneys were used for the final passage of the vaccine? I asked. "I think that that was the reason," he replied quietly. After all these months, someone had finally acknowledged this one simple fact: Chimpanzee kidneys could well have been used to prepare the vaccine.

I asked if Courtois had ever talked to him about this, and he told me he had not. "At that time," he went on, "people dealing with such topics were so automatically convinced that the easiest, the shortest way to get results was to use chimpanzees and chimpanzee cells and everything — and they were available. There were not the same problems of protection of wildlife . . . thirty-five, forty years ago, it was completely different."

Nowadays, he said, people would first ask whether it was possible, instead of chimpanzees, to use another monkey, like an African green or a macaque, or to use a cell line. But in the fifties "nobody doing the work was taking into consideration all these different steps. 'Let us go straight to wherever we have to go.' It's a question of mentality. You also have to take into consideration that all these people — Courtois, myself, even Koprowski — we were very young people. We had not the same philosophy as we have now. We hadn't the same experience as we have now. The general opinion in the world is not the same as now. . . . We asked our black collaborators — 'Next week we need five young chimpanzees,' and next week there were five young chimpanzees. That is no more possible. From an ethical point of view."

I told him that some four hundred chimps appeared to have been used for the polio work, and he was clearly shocked. He explained that in those days, because technology was less sophisticated, you needed a lot more animals to get the same result. "Now," he said, "when you use chimpanzees, you go to think at least three times about [using] one chimpanzee; forty years ago when you needed a chimpanzee, you said, 'Let's start with ten.'" He pointed out that in the fifties, the children of rich American families were falling ill with polio, and there was no problem about raising millions of dollars for research. "Everybody was wild about the fact that the solution was very close." Similarly, if today you said that there could be a safe vaccine against AIDS in two or three years, but that it would require four hundred chimps to obtain it, then you would get your four hundred chimps.[4] It was a powerful analogy, and I had to agree that this was probably true.

This was the first time that somebody close to the heart of events had had the courage to acknowledge the likelihood of what had taken place. Professor Mortelmans spent much of the rest of the interview giving me advice on who else I should try to contact. Every few minutes, he would reach across to my notebook, and write down another name, sometimes adding a phone number from his own address book. He told me about another of his friends, Pieter De Somer, who had been the first director of Recherche et Industrie Thérapeutif, or RIT, after the war, and about one of his (Mortelmans's) students, Constant Huygelen, who had taken over from De Somer in the sixties. And he told me about Mademoiselle Lamy, "a wonderful, beautiful young lady," who had lost a leg in an accident, and who had been in charge of the lab at RIT in the mid-fifties. He added that RIT had since been bought up by Smith Kline Beecham, and was now said by some to be the biggest vaccine house in the world.

He also told me about other vets whom I should try to see. One was Louis Bugyaki, a Hungarian by birth, who had taken over the Stanleyville veterinary lab from him when he left in 1956 and who stayed on until its closing at the end of 1959. And another was Alexandre Jezierski, the Pole who had run the small veterinary laboratory at Gabu Nioka, near the border with Uganda. I was already very interested in Jezierski, for I knew that he had had close contacts with the Pasteur Institute, that he had met up with Koprowski and Norton when they visited Stanleyville in 1957, and that he too had been developing an OPV — one made in the kidneys of African monkeys. Mortelmans said he thought Jezierski was still alive, and told me that as a past government employee, he should still be receiving a state pension. He wrote down the address of the pensions department in Brussels where I could perhaps locate his address, but added that it might be difficult because a confidentiality law had been passed in Belgium a few months previously.

I pointed out that there were remarkable similarities between what Jezierski had been doing in Gabu Nioka, and what Koprowski may have done at the Wistar, or De Somer at RIT. "The big problem, when you see it now," replied Mortelmans, "is that at that time there was no contact, no coordination. People were working in different places. And that may be one of the big merits of Koprowski. . . . So many people were doing work in small places, in small laboratories. But Koprowski realized that he had to go and see these people and . . . he tried to coordinate a little bit the efforts . . . and ideas of the different people. You need someone like Koprowski to have the benefit of the different work of different [researchers]. That is the admiration I have for Koprowski."

This struck me as a marvelous piece of analysis: Koprowski as the supreme synthesizer. Even if he had had no formal collaboration with Alexandre Jezierski, Koprowski had a habit of tapping into the genius of brilliant, difficult men like him, to extract the riches within. All his life he had had an eye for talent, and an instinct for how best to exploit it.

———————

The Hungarian, Louis Bugyaki, was not difficult to locate at his apartment in central Brussels. He had the slow, rather sad air of a man recently widowed, who found that time hung heavy on his hands. He was also courteous and gentle, and he proved just as willing to help as his predecessor at Stanleyville. He explained that he had arrived in the Congo in 1949, and had directed various veterinary labs before taking over from Mortelmans at the end of June 1956; he stayed till the lab closed at the end of 1959.[5]

He thought that Lindi camp had opened shortly after his arrival, and apparently "some sickness, at the beginning, eliminated a few animals." At some point between April and June 1957, Ghislain Courtois asked him if he would take charge of the medical surveillance of the chimps. At the time of Bugyaki's first visit, there were 100 to 120 chimps on site, mostly *Pan troglodytes,* but a few *Pan paniscus* also, and mostly aged two or less. In the wild, young chimps would still be held by their mothers, and would sleep huddled up with each other, but these animals were in individual cages, and several of them suffered from pneumonia. Bugyaki gave them some injections of penicillin and other antibiotics, and the death rates fell. He also advised the doctors to buy some kids' shirts from the local markets, to keep the chimps warm. "They had blue, red and all the . . . different colors. [It was] very amusing!" he told me. He visited every three or four weeks thereafter.

The medical doctors, he explained, gave the chimps the vaccine, and took blood, which was sent off to the States for analysis. He said that he hadn't seen the intraspinal testing, but that he had heard about it, and when I asked if they had also taken kidneys from the chimps, he said yes, he thought that they had, and that while some had been tested in the Stanleyville lab, "mostly they sent [them to] the United States, [to] Mr. Koprowski." He added that they were also sent to Belgium, to the university at Leuven.

When I asked why they had sent kidneys, he said it was for "tissue cultures and histopathological examination, certainly," and added that "I heard about this experimentation [from] Ninane and Osterrieth and Courtois." This was powerful testimony, because the dispatching of chimp kidneys so that tissue cultures could be made was the key point that Ninane and Osterrieth now denied.[6] When I asked directly whether the kidneys could have been used to grow vaccine, he said: "Maybe, maybe."

In all, he said, the polio program had gone on for about a year and a half and during the time that he attended the camp, the death rate from natural causes had been about 10 to 15 percent.[7] I said that I had heard that in the early days there had been higher death rates, especially among *Pan paniscus,* and he confirmed that they had refused to eat. He thought that because they were used to living in family groups, they could not bear being isolated in cages. Yes, they had also tried caging *Pan paniscus* and *Pan troglodytes* together — but that was only at the beginning, before the experimentation began.

I left Bugyaki's apartment feeling that at long last the various elements of this story were falling into place. In particular, Bugyaki believed that chimp kidneys *had* been sent to Koprowski in Philadelphia, as well as to someone in Leuven. And his predecessor in Stanleyville, Jos Mortelmans, believed that if chimp kidneys had been sent to these places, then they must have been used to grow the vaccine.

---

It turned out that Robert Daenens, the camp supervisor, had died back in the seventies, but after a few phone calls I managed to locate his widow, Godelieve, who had reverted to her maiden name and now occupied a prime apartment in Ostend, overlooking the casino and the beach. She told me that her late husband had been a big timber merchant in Belgium, and had decided to set up a wood manufacturing business at Basoko on the Congo River. He drove across the Sahara with five trucks full of equipment, but there was deceit and double-dealing by the drivers, and finally none reached its destination. So it was that in early 1956 Robert Daenens pitched up in Stanleyville, seeking a job.

Ghislain Courtois was just then searching for someone with good English to look after his new chimpanzee research center at Lindi.[8] Daenens got the job, and soon started building his own three-bedroom house in a corner of the compound, where the basic structures of the camp, including the hangars, had already been installed.

At this point, Godelieve's son, Dirk, arrived and took up the story. He told me that he and his mother had flown out to Stanleyville in August 1957, at which point there were 175 chimps at the camp, the most they had ever had. Before their first visit to Lindi, they were injected with IPV by Courtois — which suggests either that there was no OPV left in Stanleyville at that time, or that this was still considered to afford the surest protection for whites. Although he and his mother lived in Stanleyville, Dirk was a frequent visitor to Lindi, and he was the first to confirm that the chimps' diet had been remarkably human. They were, he said, fed a lot of fruit, especially oranges and bananas, but they also got sugarcane, fresh bread, eggs, and milk powder. The biggest treat of all was cream, which was used to persuade the chimps to take their medication and which, together with the vaccines and drugs, was kept in a big petrol-driven fridge in the office. Dirk sketched me a very precise map of the Lindi compound.

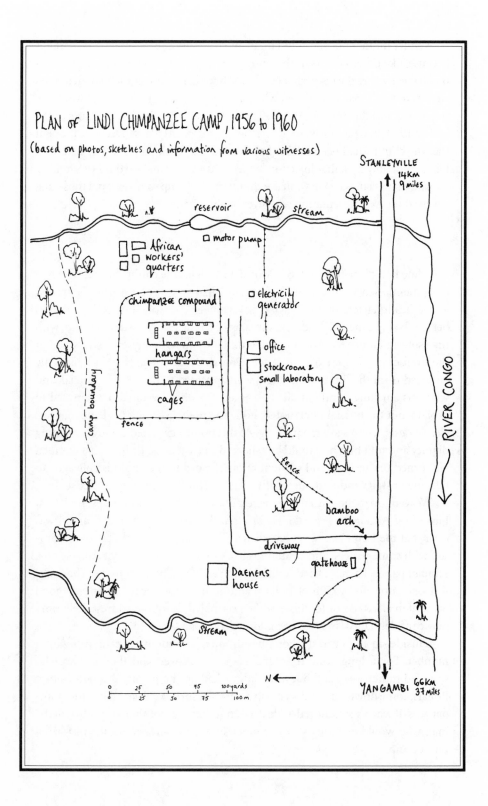

PLAN OF LINDI CHIMPANZEE CAMP, 1956 to 1960

(based on photos, sketches and information from various witnesses)

STANLEYVILLE
14 km
9 miles

reservoir
stream

motor pump

African
workers'
quarters

electricity
generator

chimpanzee compound

hangars

office

Stockroom &
small laboratory

cages

fence

camp boundary

RIVER CONGO

fence

bamboo
arch

driveway

gatehouse

Daenens
house

stream

0   25   50   75   100 yards
0   25   50   75   100 m

N ←

YANGAMBI  66 km
37 miles

Neither mother nor son could recall much about the experiments — perhaps because, like other visitors to the camp, they were never allowed inside the second hangar where the research took place. They did remember that blood samples were taken and that sometimes, when a chimp died, that the animal would be trepanned and the brain extracted. They eventually flew back to Belgium at the end of 1959, to be followed by Robert in June 1960. Madame Daenens thought that the chimps had been released at the end, but Dirk thought they had been killed, probably by lethal injection, which was the normal method of sacrifice. He said that as far as he knew, all the chimps in the camp were used up; those that survived the experimentation were eventually sacrificed.[9]

The time had come to search out Monsieur Rollais, the chimp-hunter who had been mentioned so often, and here again I had some good fortune. I arrived at the headquarters of the Belgian government pensions office five minutes before closing time one Friday, at the start of a long holiday weekend, and, with my esoteric French, was having some difficulty making myself understood at the front desk. We were deep in Anglo-French debate when two men suddenly emerged from the lift. One of them, who appeared to be a senior official, and who was smelling faintly of alcohol, asked me what I wanted. I attempted to explain, but the official interrupted, none too politely, with a fusillade that was clearly designed to send me packing. At this point I gathered up my remaining dignity and told him he should be ashamed to treat a visitor in such a manner. He turned on his heel, and without another word to me, told his colleague to take me upstairs and find out whether the person I was seeking still existed.

We went up to the sixth floor; the rest of the building was now deserted. First I asked for Alexandre Jezierski. He brought the name up on screen, and it was clear that the Gabu Nioka vet had died a few years previously. He busied himself with some papers, and behind his back I jotted down the last address on a scrap of paper. Then we tried Rollais; I didn't have a Christian name. There was just one entry, for a Gilbert Rollais, and he lived in France. Again, my good Samaritan affected not to notice while I scribbled down the address. Belgium's new confidentiality laws had been flouted, but I had the necessary.

Outside, in the nearest phone booth, directory inquiries came up with a number. For a long, long time, there was no answer, and then a man who sounded rather weak and out of breath picked up the phone. Yes, said Gilbert Rollais, come down on Sunday; it will be my pleasure to tell you about the chimpanzees. It was a six-hundred-mile drive, but that was nothing to speak with the man who would certainly know as much as anyone alive about the history of Lindi camp.

As I neared his hometown in Brittany, the terrain changed dramatically. The flatlands of Normandy were left behind, and now there were isolated flint cottages, and small hills topped with deciduous woodland, remnants of ancient forest. I stopped in one of these woods for breakfast, and strolled off down an earth track through a thick new growth of bracken and past tall bushes of broom, festooned in yellow. The air was sweet with springtime, and away in the valley a cock was crowing.

It took some time to find the home of Gilbert Rollais, which turned out to be a new bungalow on the edge of town, overlooking freshly plowed fields. I rang the bell, and a cleaning woman came to the door; she led me through to the living room, and there I found the famous chimp hunter seated in a reclining chair. He had a crumpled face and a sweet smile, but was clearly not well, for both of his legs appeared to be swollen. He explained that he had caught some strange virus out in Africa, which none of the tropical specialists in Paris or Antwerp could diagnose. He had been planning on traveling a lot in his retirement, but this wouldn't now be possible.

I had been half expecting an ogre, one of those colonials who have trophies on the wall and speak of their African assistants as "boys." But this man was gentle, and his eyes shone. His trophies were African gourds, statues, and musical instruments, and there were framed photographs of pygmies and the great sweep of the Congo River. Here was a man who still loved the continent.

We spoke only in French, and although I did not appreciate every nuance of our lengthy conversation at the time, a friend later translated the tape. Over the next five hours, with his photos and stories, Gilbert Rollais related the more intimate side of Lindi camp and its inhabitants.

He was, he told me, sixty-eight years old, and had spent nearly forty of those years in Africa. Between 1949 and 1953 he had managed the zoo at Brazzaville (across the river from Leo), where he became an expert in capturing gorillas, chimpanzees, and other animals. Some of the chimps were sold to a dealer who supplied the American space program, and Rollais later heard that one of "his" animals became the first American chimp in space.[10]

Later he moved to the Congo, where he first became manager of the zoo in Stanleyville, and was later appointed head of the chimpanzee capture program for Lindi. Officially he was employed by the Service of Water, Forests, Game and Fishing, but unofficially he was under the direction of Ghislain Courtois. The capture program was most intense between 1956 and 1958, and after that he joined another famous hunter, Jean de Medina, at the capture station at Epulu, in the Ituri forest — the same "Camp Putnam" that Koprowski and Norton visited in 1957. After the Belgians left, he returned to Kinshasa, and served as an adviser to the Congolese wildlife service from 1961 until his retirement and return to France in 1984.

He proudly showed me a medal he had been awarded by President Mitterrand, and another from President Mobutu of the Congo. He pointed out with some chagrin that the Belgians had never followed suit, even though his most important work had been for them.

I asked him to tell me about the chimps he had supplied to Lindi, and he explained that there had been three major phases to the collections. The first, between 1956 and 1958, was for the polio program under doctors Courtois and Koprowski, and was by far the most intensive. Later, in 1958, he collected for some Belgian doctors who were studying arteriosclerosis, and then in August 1959 he was asked to collect a third group of chimps for another research program (which seemed likely to have involved either cancer research or the export of live animals to the United States and Belgium). I asked how many chimps he had collected for polio and he told me that "it must have been around three hundred." He remembered nothing about Deinhardt's hepatitis work, but this was not surprising given that the program had employed chimps left over from the polio research.

We discussed the figures some more, but it was clear that he was uneasy on the subject, perhaps fearing that I would bring the animal rights lobby down on his head. Nonetheless, his total of "around 300" chimps for the polio research provided support for the figure of nearly 400 that my own research had produced. Together with the other collections, it seemed that the total number of chimps brought to Lindi camp between 1956 and 1960 was likely to have exceeded 500, most of them in the first twenty-one months of the camp's existence.

Next I wanted to know how he had set about capturing the animals. He told me that he was the only European involved, but that he had had between 150 and 200 African helpers. Many of them were pygmies, who would prepare their own hand-woven nets from lianas. An individual net was normally thirty to forty yards long, but during the hunting they would string many nets together into a single unit, perhaps 500 yards long, and six feet high. They allowed for a fair bit of slack, so that animals running into it would end up trapped within. The technique was for a trapper to follow a group of chimps to their night roost in a tree, and for the net to be strung out in the bush, around three sides of the tree, during the latter part of the night. At first light, beaters would advance forward from the open section, shouting and banging tin cans, and the chimps would drop to the ground and be driven into the long, low net and the hunting party hidden behind.

In the early days, the captured chimps would be trussed hand and foot and hung from wooden poles during the journey back to the temporary camp set up nearby. Soon, however, they found that too many of the chimps suffered badly as a result of restricted circulation, or heatstroke, so they began using makeshift wooden cages, constructed ad hoc at the place of capture. In the camp, the chimps would be moved into cages with iron bars, for the more lengthy transfer to Lindi on Rollais's five-ton truck. If a chimp died during transportation, the body would be handed over to the doctors.

Rollais told me that although chimps usually travel in groups of from twelve to twenty, they would rarely net more than four or five at one time. Sometimes the whole troop would escape through the branches of the trees, so they would catch nothing. He said that they concentrated on young animals, aged up to five or six years, and would allow older chimps to escape, since some could weigh up to eighty kilograms (180 pounds), at which weight they were highly danger-ous and far too large for the scientists to handle. I asked whether mothers did not fight to protect their young,[11] and he agreed that sometimes a chimp had to be killed, or else would die in a fall when they chopped down the tree in which it was hiding.[12] "If we could avoid killing them, we did so," he added.

Altogether, he estimated, they must have staged between 100 and 120 cap-ture operations over the four years of Lindi's existence, each lasting a day or two. He went to many different areas, he told me, starting with areas on the left bank, where *Pan paniscus* is found.[13] The pygmy chimps were easier to catch than the common chimps, but also harder to keep alive; like everyone else, Rollais spoke of the pygmy chimps refusing to eat because of the stress of captivity. He said that he tried lots of remedies, which included paying African women to put the chimps on their backs like babies, wrapped in *kitenges,* like babies, and to feed them milk from a bottle. He also spoke about caging the two species together, but said that although some *paniscus* learned new eating habits from the *troglodytes,* there had also been a lot of fights, which the pygmy chimps tended to lose. For this reason, they abandoned the *paniscus* capture program, although they would still buy the occasional animal if it was offered for sale, or found in a local market.

After that initial failure, he started collecting common chimps, *Pan troglodytes.* This species proved to be much sturdier and ate a lot of different foods — not only fruits, vegetables, and groundnuts, but also human foods like cooked rice, honey, jam, and biscuits. Rollais had even seen the Africans feed the chimps meat, spicy sauces, and alcoholic drinks, "which they took very well."

When these chimps fell ill, he said, it was normally with lung problems, sca-bies, or dysentery. Perhaps the extemporized diet had something to do with the latter, but he also mentioned the particular problem posed by *Klebsiella pneu-moniae.* He added that because they realized how sensitive the chimps were to human infections, they used to check the keepers' health once a week.

He recalled a few more interesting details. The hangars, he said, had been constructed specially in Stanleyville, and brought in pieces to Lindi by motor-ized barge. He told me that they had not caught other monkeys during the chimp hunts, mainly because this required a different capture technique — that

of cutting down the trees all around the tree where the monkeys were sheltering, to limit their means of escape, and then putting up nets before chopping
down the final tree. And although he recalled that the Stanleyville doctors had
kept a few monkeys in the animal house, he felt sure this had been of minor
importance compared to the chimp work.

He recalled little about the actual chimp research, since this was not his field.
Besides, by the time he delivered the apes to Lindi he was usually tired out and
only wanted to get back to Stanleyville for a shower and a whiskey. But he did
tell me that at the beginning, when foreign researchers visited, they used to go
back home with chimp blood and also with live chimpanzees to use in their own
laboratories. He said that he had been given some vaccine in a capsule right at
the start of the operation, and he knew that many parts of Province Oriental
had been vaccinated after they had tested the vaccine in the chimps. "I believe
that one of the conditions was that because the Belgian Congo had helped [with
the research], it should also be first to benefit," he explained.

As for Koprowski, he had only met him the once, when he visited one of his
small capture camps at Wanie Rukula. Koprowski had apparently taken a photo
of Rollais's longtime African girlfriend, Therese, feeding a baby chimpanzee
milk through a bottle. The polio researcher said that he would have to take
Therese and the chimp to America, to show the people there this wonder — a
line that clearly amused Therese rather more than Gilbert.

———————

Gilbert Rollais and I kept in touch regularly over the next two years, and he
wrote me several letters providing such details as the precise locations where he
had caught his chimpanzees.[14] He also sent me some of his powerful photos of
Lindi, and the often harrowing chimpanzee capture photos. These included
several of the cages inside the hangars, some of the chimps being caught and
carried — and one of Djamba, in chains, squatting atop the "Mission Courtois
Koprowski" sign at the entrance to Lindi.

Afterward, I thought back to his account of how the chimps had been captured, and realized that there had probably been a subtext. This really had been
a different era, one when there was a completely different mentality about the
rights of animals. Rollais told me that his first job in Stanleyville, in 1955, had
been to collect animals for Professor Vandebroek, an "evolutionary researcher"
from Leuven, who wanted chimpanzee skulls and skeletons. Initially Rollais told
me that he had been capturing live chimps for another program, but that any
that were killed in the course of the hunt would be put aside for Vandebroek.
They were later placed in large petrol drums, and then boiled to remove the flesh.
Toward the end of the afternoon, however, he made it clear that the purpose of

the mission had not been to collect live chimpanzees. "He wanted dead animals. I wasn't very pleased by it, but it was necessary. So I did my job."

The terrible testament to Vandebroek's research is still to be found in the basement of the Africa museum, at Tervuren, just outside Brussels. Here, among the dusty drawers and cupboards, are more than 100 skulls and 26 skeletons, mostly from *Pan paniscus*.

Then I realized that even when collecting for the Laboratoire Médical, Rollais must have experienced a conflict of interests. I wondered what would have happened to the larger chimps that became entangled in the net. Would they really have been released, as Rollais had claimed? Or were the hunters partly paid in kind, with chimpanzee meat? There were differing views about the acceptability of such a practice to the local people. Ghislain Courtois told a conference audience that "In Central Africa, the natives readily eat monkey meat, but generally they do not eat chimpanzees."[15] But when Rollais, who probably had more experience of such matters, was telling me about dressing the baby chimps in green pullovers to keep them warm, he added that the Africans thought him crazy, "because for them, the chimpanzee is for eating . . . it [was] like putting a green pullover on a cow."[16]

I was planning to see Gilbert Rollais again in October 1996 (this time with an assistant who spoke fluent French), but when I phoned to make arrangements, I learned that he had died two months earlier. The mystery virus had finally had its way with him.

Despite the terrible trade in which he was involved, Gilbert was (from a fifties perspective) merely supplying his scientific masters with the means to conduct crucial research, and I believe he tried to minimize the suffering of the animals in his charge. On a personal level, I shall always remember him for his kindness and sincerity, and in retrospect I am perhaps glad that there were certain questions I never got to ask him.

# 44

---

## THE BELGIAN VACCINE

---

At this stage, I clearly needed to find out more about the Belgian-made version of CHAT vaccine. Remarkably, the only official statement about where CHAT and Fox had been made came in Koprowski's article in the *British Medical Journal*, which applied to the vaccine used in the first trials in Province Oriental and Ruzizi. It stated that "the large pools representing each strain were prepared in the laboratories of the Wistar Institute."[1] The only clues in the literature that suggested that there might have been any Belgian-made pools featured in Plotkin's articles of 1961, which contained figures referring to CHAT pools named DS and De Somer.[2]

However, Gaston Ninane would have none of this. He insisted that apart from the early batches of CHAT and Fox fed in capsule form in 1957 (and perhaps the vaccine fed in response to the epidemics in Province Oriental), the rest of the OPV used in the Belgian Congo and Ruanda-Urundi had been made in Belgium. He said that live vaccine simply could not be transported from the United States to the Congo by plane — that unrefrigerated liquid vaccine would get too warm and deteriorate en route. With regard to the origin of the vaccine used in the Ruzizi Valley, at least, somebody had to be mistaken.

Apart from the timing, the other thing that was unclear about the change to the Belgian version of CHAT was how it had been effected. Had it involved one of the CHAT seed pools from the Wistar that had then been put into tissue culture in De Somer's lab, to make one or more production lots? If so, then who had provided the tissue culture material — Koprowski, or the Belgians themselves? Alternatively, did "pool DS" indicate that both the seed pool and the vaccine therefrom had been prepared separately in Belgium?

---

My first meeting on this subject was also one of the strangest in the course of this investigation. It was with Monique Lamy, who had worked with Pieter De Somer in the very early days, and who had later left his laboratory in order to graduate in medicine. Sadly, it seemed that the wonderful young woman recalled by Mortelmans had been marked emotionally, as well as physically, by a tragic tram accident that had cost her a leg. Whatever, she seemed angry and resentful from the very start of the interview.

Part of the problem might have been the fact that the French interpreter whom she had asked me to bring along had to cancel at the last minute, so we ended up speaking mainly in broken English. But whatever the reason, getting information from Dr. Lamy proved to be a thankless task.

What she did vouchsafe is as follows. She said that she had started working for Professor De Somer in 1955, and that she began doing vaccine production for him in 1956. For the first four years she and her colleagues produced what she called "Salk vaccine" (the Belgian version of IPV), but from 1960 onward they also produced the Sabin vaccine. This vaccine work started at the University of Leuven, but transferred soon afterward to a private company, RIT (Recherche et Industrie Thérapeutif), which was based at a castle in the small village of Rixensart. As substrate for both Salk and Sabin vaccines, she said, they had always used the kidneys of the cynomolgus macaque, from the Philippines.

At this point, I said that I believed that De Somer had also worked with a version of Koprowski's CHAT. She said that he had, but that they never produced it. I asked her to clarify, and she said they had only tested CHAT virus, but had never produced any vaccine. I told her that one pool of the vaccine had been called CHAT DS, or CHAT De Somer, and that I would show her the paper if she wished. She declined. She simply repeated that they had not produced vaccine for Koprowski, but that she personally had tested his strain intracerebrally in rhesus monkeys and found that it caused paralysis. "The virulence, for us, it is bad," she explained. When I asked which Koprowski strain, she told me both — the Type 1 and the Type 3, CHAT and Fox. I asked if Koprowski had been told about this, and she said that De Somer had doubtless informed him. She herself had not had direct contact with Koprowski.

This was extraordinary. Monique Lamy's claim that De Somer had never produced the Koprowski vaccines went against what I had been told by several other sources, including Koprowski himself. At the same time, she was claiming that both CHAT and Fox paralyzed monkeys, which contradicted what had been reported in the literature, for Koprowski had stated in a letter to the *British Medical Journal* that De Somer's lab (and four others) had tested CHAT vaccine intracerebrally in monkeys and had not detected a single case of paralysis.[3]

I said that if she liked, when I got back to England, I would fax her the Koprowski letter, but she answered, "For me, it is no more interesting." I said that if she was claiming that a vaccine that had been used widely around the world had caused paralysis in monkeys and was therefore not safe to use, then surely this was of considerable importance, and it was important to try to understand what had happened. "It is all history for me, all history," she replied. She added that Koprowski's vaccines, unlike Sabin's, had never been on the market, to which I replied that CHAT had been fed to some nine million people in Europe, Africa, and America. She asked me to prove it, and I gave her some details. Then she repeated: "We are not doing any production for Koprowski, that is sure." At this point, I got out Plotkin's paper, showing the DS pool, and she said, "That doesn't mean anything." I told her that there was another paper that showed the full name of the pool as De Somer, and she replied: "That is your problem, but not my problem."

And that was it. A few minutes later, she said that she had to go. I asked whether, if I brought the translator, I could come back again and ask some more questions, and she said "No, there is no more time." She repeated this twice more as I packed up my bag.

———————

One of the others mentioned by Jos Mortelmans was his former protégé in the Congo and Rwanda, Constant ("Stan") Huygelen. I went to see him at his palatial modern home on the edge of a village some miles outside Brussels, and he told me rather more of the background to the story.

He explained that RIT had started in 1945/6, when Pieter De Somer, at Leuven, had been approached by a young man who had inherited the family pharmacy and who wanted to expand. They founded the company together and by the late forties were producing large quantities of penicillin, then in short supply in Europe. The company prospered and moved to its present administrative headquarters at Genval. Then, in 1955, RIT arranged with Jonas Salk to begin large-scale production of inactivated polio vaccine. The first experimental lot was made in Leuven, at which stage the main workers had been De Somer, Monique Lamy, and another virologist named Abel Prinzie. In early 1957 RIT purchased the castle at Rixensart, not far from Genval, and began producing the vaccine on a huge scale. Because they were well ahead of vaccine houses in most other European countries, they exported a large amount of this IPV to the rest of Europe in the years 1957–1959.

In 1960, they began working on the Sabin OPV strains — first an experimental lot, and later mass production. In 1968 RIT was bought up by Smith Kline, which wanted to expand into vaccines, and it grew to become the leading vaccine manufacturer in the world, well ahead of the only other two big producers — Pasteur Mérieux and Lederle. Even today, with polio affecting fewer countries, it was still producing half a billion doses of polio vaccine a year.

Dr. Huygelen told me that he had once been based in central Africa — at Elisabethville in 1955–1957, and at Astrida (now Butare, the second city of Rwanda) from then until 1960. He had worked mainly on veterinary vaccines, but also on smallpox. He recalled that Stanley Plotkin had been with Courtois in Stanleyville for some time in 1959, "experimenting with the Koprowski live polio vaccine strains," but he recalled no vaccinations in Elisabethville, Astrida, or in Ruanda-Urundi, apart from the Ruzizi trial. After I inquired about vaccinations in Rwanda, he asked me: "You're not relating it to AIDS or anything, are you?"

In November 1960, Huygelen joined RIT, originally working with veterinary vaccines, but within a few months taking over the entire vaccine department.[4] By the time of his retirement in 1991, this department, which had started with eight people, was employing well over a thousand.

He told me that by 1960 Piet De Somer was loosening his ties with RIT, and though he continued on the payroll, visiting Rixensart once a month as a consultant, he spent most of his time at Leuven. Several years later he became rector of the university, and in the early seventies he resigned from RIT, after falling out with Smith Kline. Huygelen described De Somer as "a very intelligent person, [who] tried to do different things at the same time, and that's not always possible. . . . He was a very strong personality, so it shouldn't surprise you that there were some clashes. . . . I got on with him, but it [was] not always easy."

Before I had had the chance to ask about RIT's version of CHAT, Dr. Huygelen volunteered some interesting information. When he arrived at RIT, they were already working with both the Sabin strains and the Koprowski strains. They were never able to sell the latter, he told me, because at the 1960 Washington conference the Sabin strains were effectively given the nod — and were licensed in the United States soon afterward.

He went on to say that before his arrival RIT had made one batch of CHAT and another of Fox, each comprising about one hundred liters of concentrated vaccine. I asked him where these vaccines had been used, and he said that they were "given, I believe, free of charge to Poland." I asked him whether the CHAT batch produced at RIT had not been used in the Congo, and he answered that he thought not; he believed that the Congo vaccines had been produced at the Wistar Institute.

He also said that by the time of his arrival at RIT, only some fifty or sixty liters of these batches of CHAT and Fox remained. When I asked where they were now, he said he thought that both batches had been given to a virologist at Leuven in the early sixties, so that he could experiment with them in the lab. He could only recall that the man had an Italian name.

He told me that before his arrival, Monique Lamy had been in charge of vaccine production, manufacturing the vast batches of inactivated vaccine, as well as "the experimental batches of Koprowski and Sabin." He stressed that the company had "just produced the batches according to the recommendations which had been given by the developers of the strains."

When I asked him about Koprowski, Huygelen characterized him as "a difficult person . . . very outspoken and very few people would argue with him, except for Sabin and a few others." When I told him that Koprowski had been sweetness itself when I interviewed him, Huygelen said, "Oh, he can be very sweet, he can be very sweet!"

He stressed that the other important person working at RIT at that time was one Julian Peetermans, whose name had already cropped up perhaps a dozen times in the course of the conversation. He said that Peetermans would be the best person for me to speak with, since he had joined RIT straight from university in 1956, and had actually lived full-time in the castle in the early days, when vaccine production was just getting off the ground. He was now a vice president of the company. "I don't think there is anybody in the world who has that much experience of large-scale production of polio vaccine," he told me.

---

I went to see Julian Peetermans at his home that Sunday morning, and he turned out to be small and bookishly intense, with the air of someone who had poured his entire life's energy into a project. He made strong coffee, telling me that he drank two liters daily, and his intensity increased perceptibly during the morning, as we drank cup after cup. I could imagine him working to the limit, squeezing every last moment of time from the day — a tendency that I found rather admirable.

Over the course of the next four hours, Peetermans briefed me in minute detail about the processes involved in manufacturing and testing vaccines, the molecular biology of poliovirus, and the theory behind attenuation. And in the course of this extended tutorial, he told me a lot more about the history of RIT, and of its association with Koprowski.

Peetermans joined Piet De Somer, Monique Lamy, and Abel Prinzie at Leuven in December 1956, when they were still developing and testing their first batch of IPV.[5] In March 1957, Lamy and Peetermans transferred RIT's vaccine department to Rixensart — to what soon became known locally as the "Château des singes" — the "monkey castle." Meanwhile, De Somer and Prinzie remained at the university, running the virology department and its research arm — the Rega Institute, about which Peetermans was a little offhand, saying that it was involved with a lot of American and British research, and that "I don't know what they were really doing there." Dr. Lamy was in charge at Rixensart from 1957 until her departure from RIT in the early sixties, and Peetermans was production manager, a position he was to keep for the next two decades. His current title was head of the technical department, overseeing quality control.

His account of making vaccine for Koprowski was similar to that of Huygelen, though not exactly so. He said that De Somer had come to Rixensart one day and announced that Koprowski had asked them to make vaccine for him, "and we just did it." He said that this must have been in 1959 or 1960, before they started working with Sabin's strains.

Peetermans said that the seed viruses had come from Koprowski, and that they had grown them in tissue culture and tested them. Apparently they had employed their own substrate, the one that RIT already used for IPV, namely the kidneys of cynomolgus macaques. He did not remember how many doses of the vaccines they had made, save that it was "a very small number." He recalled that they had sent one batch to Poland, and that they might have sent some back to Koprowski. "It was just to help Koprowski or to collaborate with him, that was all. We did it for him as a contract manufacture, I think," he said, before adding that it had actually been more of a "gracious offer" to Koprowski, since, as far as he knew, they had not even been paid for it. Neither, he said, had Koprowski been paid for it. Because the vaccine had not been registered and was still an experimental product, it had no commercial value as such.

He added that since Koprowski's vaccines had never been registered in America, they did not have to adhere to the requirements published in Part 600 of the Code of Federal Regulations (unlike Salk's and Sabin's vaccines). These regulations applied to the source strain of attenuated poliovirus, the permissible number of passages from that strain, the substrate or substrates in which the vaccine could be grown, the temperature at which it had to be grown — even the quarantine requirements for monkey safety testing. The WHO published similar requirements, and the European Community had recently started doing likewise. Every producer had to follow these regulations and to fill in a protocol sheet to demonstrate that fact. "This is strictly, strictly, strictly regulated," Peetermans said. But such strict regulations had never applied to experimental vaccines like Koprowski's.

I asked Peetermans if he had received protocols from Koprowski, containing directions for how to grow his strains, and he said, "I don't think so. I don't know. . . . We multiplied and tested it [for safety], that's all."[6] In that case, I asked, did he still have any sample of the vaccine pools that RIT had made? "I don't think so, no," he answered. I told him what Huygelen had told me, about giving the remaining fifty or sixty liters of CHAT and Fox to someone at the virology department at Leuven, so that he could use them for lab experiments into polio RNA, and he said: "Then it went back to De Somer if this is true."

Two aspects of this struck me as remarkable. One was that they should have embarked on a first production of OPV so casually, as if it was merely another batch of the IPV they had been producing for years. The other was the fact that RIT had not been paid for the work. If the vaccine really was bound for Poland, behind the Iron Curtain, then this was indeed altruistic for a commercial vaccine

house.[7] However, manufacturing vaccine free of charge would have made a lot
more sense if the end product had actually been destined for the Belgian Congo
or Ruanda-Urundi.

When I told Peetermans that I had heard that the RIT strain of CHAT had
been used in Belgium's African colonies, he denied it. I explained that according to the *Bulletin of the WHO*, the CHAT and Fox vaccines used in Poland
had been supplied by Koprowski, and forwarded from the United States by the
Moore McCormack shipping line.[8] It seemed unlikely that RIT would have dispatched the finished vaccines to Koprowski, only for him to send them back to
Europe. He thought for a while and then said: "Well, it's just memory. And I was
not in charge of shipping them."

---

Later, Peetermans told me that the question of the final substrate was "important because it should give you high yields." I told him that Koprowski had frequently not made it clear which substrate he had used. Sometimes he had
reported that it was chick embryo when it was really monkey kidney. And
he had never specified the type of monkey from which the cells were taken.
Peetermans agreed that it was vital to record this accurately, as part of the passage history. "His passage history should be well documented. That's for scientific reasons. . . . You should be honest there, OK."

"On the other hand," he went on, "in the fifties [there] was probably much
less known about viruses growing and so on. And I think that it was done in laboratories, in university labs, in institutes . . . where people were . . . having ten
or twenty approaches all at the same time, which run in parallel. . . . That's what
you normally do if you want to go fast, and you don't know where you go. . . ."
This, clearly, was the process of trial and error that, as he had already explained,
was an intrinsic part of developing a successful vaccine.

But which animal had provided the cells for Koprowski's substrate? I asked,
and Peetermans told me he thought it had been made in monkey kidney. But
which monkey? I pressed. "I don't know," he said. "You mean if it was a macaque,
or a *Cercopithecus* [African green monkey], or a chimpanzee? I don't know what
it was. I don't know."

This was an important moment, for it was the first time that a vaccine-maker
had ever proposed the possibility that Koprowski's vaccines might have been
grown in chimpanzee cells. I asked him if he seriously thought that Koprowski
could have used chimpanzees. "Oh yes, but you never [used] chimpanzee kidneys," he replied. "They are not available; it's too expensive." I told him about
Lindi camp, and the large number of chimpanzees that were dying there, apparently from shock, from stress, or because they refused to eat. In these chimps, at
least, no pathogens had been found at postmortem. So, I asked, what could you

use that dead chimpanzee for? Peetermans got what I was driving at, and broke in. "Yes," he said, "but that's not a permanent source. You could use it once, but it's not a permanent source of tissue."

I said that some people believed that one of the reasons for the chimp colony was to provide a source of tissue culture material, one that was quite different to the cynomolgus monkeys that Sabin was using. "Why not?" responded Peetermans. "I don't know if it's true, but everything is possible. . . . There's only two possibilities . . . yes or no. I don't think that this is important unless you want to [investigate] the personalities of both these people, and their fight to become the Pope of live polio vaccine. . . . For a book that is fascinating, sure."

We talked some more about the personalities of Sabin and Koprowski, and Peetermans said: "People who are going to the top . . . are difficult people . . . at least for themselves, and probably also for the other people they affect. . . . If they are incorrect or . . . not honest . . . I cannot judge. . . . But I think to realize something [of great import], you should either be a very demanding person [or one] who's difficult."

We talked a great deal more. Peetermans agreed that lentiviruses such as HIV and SIV would not have been picked up by the testing procedures of the day, but equally, he said, they would not multiply in normal cells. But, I said, they *would* multiply in lymphocytes, which, surely, would always have been present in monkey kidney cultures in the fifties. Peetermans said that there would have been "practically none after trypsinization," the process of breaking down the kidneys into their constituent cells using the enzyme trypsin. This, I knew, was something I needed to look into.

Before I left, I asked once more whether he might not still have a sample of CHAT stored away somewhere in a freezer. Peetermans said he was sure that none of the vaccine remained at RIT, and added that they only kept vaccine strains with which they were working. There was always a risk of contamination, he said, and even if you kept experimental vaccines "in a freezer, or locked away somewhere," you might end up contaminating your working strains. "I think that there are research labs which still have that vaccine," he said, finally. "Koprowski must have something, I don't know."

Julian Peetermans had given me a fine perspective on the realities of vaccine-making in the fifties, even if he seemed uncertain about where Koprowski's strains had been used. But although I was a lot closer to the truth about the Belgian-made vaccine, I had still not quite got to the bottom of the barrel. There was more to come.

# 45

THE THREATS BEGIN

Before returning to England, I telephoned Stanley Plotkin's office in an attempt to arrange a second, briefer interview, since there were several questions that I had not had time to ask. I spoke to his secretary, and swiftly found that the mood had changed. She told me that Dr. Plotkin had asked for my full name and address, and copies of my most recent articles. When I got back home, I sent him the last three articles I had written — all dealing with AIDS in Africa — and said that I would get in touch again shortly in the hope of arranging an interview. I imagined that the subject of the articles might diminish Plotkin's willingness to talk about the Congo operation, but even if there was only a slim chance of completing the interview, it was worth trying.

His response was entirely unexpected. A fortnight later, a letter arrived from Richard Sprague, Koprowski's attorney. It reminded me that one of the conditions of my interviewing Koprowski in December was that I should provide him with taped copies of our meeting. Sprague added that he was now also representing Stanley Plotkin, who authorized him to request copies of the tapes made during my interview with him: one set for Plotkin, and another for Sprague. It seemed that the fact that I had previously written about AIDS had set alarm bells ringing. I could imagine Plotkin phoning Koprowski, and their comparing notes, and deciding that they had another Tom Curtis situation on their hands.

I was pleased that I had managed to get lengthy interviews with both Koprowski and Plotkin, even if both had been circumspect about questions relating to CHAT and the Congo research. But now, clearly, the doors were closing. Nonetheless, I did make one last attempt to get information direct from the two main protagonists.

Although I had copied the tapes of both Koprowski interviews months before, I had delayed sending them until I had enough spare time to make a full transcript, and prepare the follow-up questions, which he himself had invited me to send. This I now did.

I wrote back to Koprowski, apologizing for the lateness of my reply, and reminding him that the primary reason for my sending the tapes was to allow him the opportunity to correct any errors there might have been in what he said, and to fill in any gaps. I went on to request copies of some of the photos that Koprowski had told me he had, and lastly I submitted forty-three follow-up questions. The early ones were recaps, checking what he had meant on specific points, and then I asked all the other questions that seemed relevant. At this stage, there was no longer any point in holding back.[1]

I also wrote to Stanley Plotkin. I pointed out that I had gladly complied with his previous request for copies of my articles, but that I was less sanguine about this latest one. Because of the involvement of his lawyer, I would first need to transcribe the tapes, to check that I had said nothing that might be considered actionable. Second, this request was made retrospectively, whereas the agreement with Koprowski had been made before the interview.

In the end, I offered Plotkin a quid pro quo arrangement. During the interview, he too had invited me to send further questions by letter, and so I submitted fifteen follow-up questions and requested copies of three documents — the passage chart for CHAT, production details for one of the early feeding pools (or production lots) of CHAT, and the protocols signed with the Belgian, or Belgian Congo government about the Ruzizi and Leopoldville vaccinations. I promised to send him copies of the interview tapes once I had had positive responses to my questions and requests, and invited him to call me if he was able to comply with some, but not all. "Negotiation is always a civilised approach!" I ended. Then I wrote to Sprague, informing him of the action I had taken with both his clients.

---

Three weeks later, I got a reply from Stanley Plotkin. He wrote that my letter had confirmed the suspicion he had had toward the end of our interview: that my real interest was not in the history of OPV, but rather in the "spurious" OPV/AIDS theory. Consequently, he said that he refused to be quoted, and would not afford me a second interview.

In fairness, however, I must report his response to the hypothesis, which he appeared to have included as his definitive statement on the subject. He wrote:

> Conversations with Drs. Koprowski and Osterrieth also confirm that you believe that CHAT was made in chimpanzee kidney or African green monkey kidney contaminated with a putative relative of HIV. I can tell

you flat out that never happened. Chimpanzees then as now would have been a totally absurd substrate for a vaccine, considering the difficulty, the expense and the rarity of the species. African green monkey kidney cell culture was very new at the time and would have warranted comment and notice by myself. Thus, when my paper[2] says "Primary cultures of monkey kidney cells were used in all the work described here, except in the case of a single pool of CHAT virus which was prepared in a culture of human diploid cells as described elsewhere," it means rhesus monkey kidney, the only one which was used at that time for vaccine production. If there had been pools made in cells other than rhesus kidney it would have been worth mentioning as evidence to confirm or disconfirm that my method could identify CHAT no matter what its source.

As for the rest of my questions, he wrote that he had neither the time nor the photographic memory to answer them, and added that in any case, "there is no reason why I should do your work for you." It was certainly a well-written reply, and it pulled no punches. However, I was not bound by Plotkin's retrospective desire that I should not quote from the on-the-record interview that had taken place in March 1994, and I wrote back to inform him of that fact.

Plotkin's response had concentrated on one central question — that of the CHAT substrates. Even here, however, his claim was based on deduction, rather than personal experience or documentary evidence. And, as I already knew, the basic assumption underlying that deduction was wrong. I had already heard from Peetermans that RIT had used cynomolgus macaques to manufacture pools of CHAT — the same substrate Albert Sabin was using for his polio vaccines. Pierre Lépine was using baboon kidneys. And by 1961, when the paper Plotkin referred to in his letter was published, several vaccine-makers had already changed to African green monkeys to protect against the risk of SV40 contamination associated with the use of tissues from Asian monkeys.

Plotkin's claim that rhesus kidney was "the only one . . . used at that time for vaccine production" was based on thin air.

———————

A month later, I received a letter from Paul Osterrieth, who, as made clear by Plotkin's letter, had been in contact with Koprowski and Plotkin. It included copies of ten of the photos from his album, for which I had asked him during our first interview a year earlier.

This was a friendly gesture, but his letter was rather less amicable. Like Plotkin, Osterrieth no longer wanted to be quoted. In fairness, however, it is necessary that I report the most significant claims contained in his letter. First, he wrote, tissue cultures are never made from dead animals; "the organs have to be taken from animals which are killed for tissue culture purposes. That is one good reason not to have made tissue cultures from chimpanzees." Second, he added: "I did send minced kidneys from monkeys on some rare occasions but I think they were sent to Dr F. Deinhardt at W. Henle's lab at the Children's Hospital and not at the Wistar. I am 100% certain that I did not use chimpanzee organs for tissue culture."[3] This was a strange claim, for he had already told me that he had sent *chimp* kidneys (not merely monkey kidneys) to Deinhardt in Philadelphia, but it was good to have the statement that he himself had not tried to make tissue culture from chimp organs clearly on the record.

Last, he wrote, he would like to have, as soon as possible, copies of the tapes of our meetings, so as to be able to verify what he had said "in an unprepared and unformal conversation." Nonetheless, he closed the letter by stating that he respected my efforts and that his intention was "not to be mean."

I wrote back to Osterrieth in equally courteous tone, thanking him for the photos and the comments, but saying that — since I was now being asked for recordings of several of my interviews — that I had decided, after some thought, that I was not prepared to supply taped copies unless this had been agreed before the start of the interview. Neither was I prepared to be bound by a retrospective request not to quote or cite him, when I had briefed him about my book before the start of the conversation, and he had allowed me to tape the conversation in the full knowledge that he might be quoted. Despite these negative responses, I assured him that I would quote him accurately and in context, and that I would include his later comments, made in our second conversation and in his letter.

———

As for Koprowski, I sent him a brief reminder two months later, but from that side of the Atlantic there was only deafening silence. Until January 1995, that is, when I received another letter from Richard Sprague.

He informed me that he was now writing to me not only on behalf of Dr. Koprowski, but also on behalf of Dr. Plotkin and the Pasteur Mérieux, the vaccine house that he headed. With respect to the Plotkin interview of the previous spring, he wrote as follows: "As has been made, I believe, absolutely clear, Dr. Plotkin is entitled to a copy of his tape and, if you do not supply it promptly, appropriate action will be taken notwithstanding your residence in the United Kingdom." He objected to any connection between SIV, HIV, and the development of oral polio vaccine, and went on: "This letter is to put you on notice on behalf of all that I represent that any publication that is scientifically unsound and therefore obviously defamatory in nature will be promptly pursued in the appropriate courts against you and your publisher."

I was appalled by the letter. It demonstrated yet again that the response of Koprowski and colleagues to legitimate questioning about the development and experimental trials of CHAT in central Africa was first to avoid giving adequate or reliable answers, and second to attempt to use threats of litigation to silence the questioner.

For the first time, I took legal advice, which fully supported the letter that I sent back to Sprague three weeks later. I made several points. First, I observed that he had written me one previous letter on behalf of both his clients, not two letters, as he had claimed.[4] Second, he had stated in his letter that I had demanded information from Dr. Plotkin. In fact, I had *asked* Dr. Plotkin for information and *requested* some documents, in return for the tapes that he had requested from me. Third, he now said that it had been made absolutely clear that Dr. Plotkin was entitled to a copy of his tape. I responded that no such thing had been made clear, and that it was not Dr. Plotkin's tape of the interview, but mine. I added that I was no longer willing to supply a copy of the tape — not because of its content, but because of the way in which he and Plotkin had gone about trying to obtain a copy from me. "I don't, in short, take kindly to attempts to intimidate or bully me into compliance," I added.

If Koprowski and Plotkin thought that threats like these would silence me, they were wrong. My research had revealed compelling evidence to suggest that the OPV that they and their colleagues had fed in central Africa at the end of the fifties had somehow become contaminated with an SIV that was the forerunner of HIV-1, and I was willing to stand by that evidence. Furthermore, I had already enlisted the help of several scientists, each eminent in his or her own field, who had agreed to check my manuscript before publication (and I informed Sprague of this fact). My view (like that of Pascal, Alexander, Lecatsas, Elswood, Stricker, Curtis, Hamilton, and Martin before me) was that an event of such enormous import deserved open debate, rather than one that was terminated by legal threats. Fortunately, I signed soon afterward with a publishing house that was also not in the habit of being cowed into submission.

---

Appropriately enough, it was around this time that I gained some insight into how Koprowski had pursued his legal process against *Rolling Stone*, a process that, according to legal sources, had cost him about $300,000, and the rock magazine about half a million dollars.[5] I learned that he had provided no documentary evidence to counter Curtis's hypothesis that CHAT might be linked to the origin of AIDS, partly because relevant papers had been "lost in a move."[6] The main evidence he had submitted had consisted of two sworn affidavits that largely countered the OPV/AIDS hypothesis, one from the microbiologist Jonathan Allan, and the other from the retrovirus specialist Robert Gallo.

Allan pointed out, correctly, that the only SIV similar to HIV-1 was that of the chimpanzee, whereas Curtis's article had claimed the vaccine was grown in AGM or rhesus tissues (actually, he had suggested that nobody could be sure which tissues had been used). Thereafter, however, the affidavit was seriously flawed.

Allan's next two points were "Dr. Koprowski's protocol shows that he cultured his vaccine in monkey kidneys, which do not support the replication of SIV"; and "In order for monkey viruses to survive in lymphocytes, the T-cell growth factor is required and this was not present in Dr. Koprowski's vaccine." The first point, in which Allan appears to be maintaining that *clean* monkey kidneys, uncontaminated with lymphocytes, will not support SIV growth, is essentially irrelevant in that several commentators have pointed out that lymphocytes are ubiquitous in MKTCs, and were especially common in those made in the fifties.[7] (It also suggests that Allan has himself seen protocols for the pools of CHAT fed in Africa — 10A-11 and 13 — which, as it turned out, he had not.)[8] And the second point is an overstatement, for although T-cell growth factor facilitates the growth of viruses like SIV in lymphocytes, it is not a prerequisite.[9]

Robert Gallo's affidavit opens by stating that, in his opinion, Curtis's article "disparages Dr. Koprowski and is derogatory to his reputation"— a surprising claim, given his own positive comments about the viability of the hypothesis in the initial *Rolling Stone* article. Gallo goes on to state that "As I have been told, the Protocol for the preparation of Dr. Koprowski's vaccine called for the preparation of the vaccine in *monolayers* of monkey kidney cells. CD4+ T cells [lymphocytes] and macrophages are the target cells for HIV-1 infection. Monolayers of monkey kidney cells do not contain lymphocytes or macrophages as far as I know. Therefore, HIV-1 should not survive in such a culture."

Gallo continues: "I am advised that Dr. Koprowski used rhesus monkey kidneys in the preparation of his polio vaccine. It is widely known that rhesus monkeys *cannot* be infected with HIV-1.... Consequently, it is not possible that HIV-1 could be carried by rhesus monkeys and infect humans." Gallo's affidavit, it is becoming clear, is based on what he has been told by Koprowski or Koprowski's colleagues, but he has not himself seen any documentary evidence to support such claims. Given the wide range of claims that Koprowski had previously made about the manufacturing methods used for CHAT and Fox and the monkeys that provided cells for the substrate, these latest unsupported claims about substrate do not inspire confidence.

Gallo's final point reads as follows: "On page 108 of the article, under the heading 'It Could Happen,' Mr. Curtis implies that I agreed with him that Dr. Koprowski could have been responsible for the introduction of AIDS, although unintentionally, and I am quoted as stating 'It happens, sometimes, in medicine.' I was simply saying that honest workers sometimes make honest mistakes with adverse effects. I did not then, nor do I now, agree that Dr. Koprowski infected the human race with AIDS." All in all, Gallo's statement seems merely to reinforce Curtis's hypothesis that a medical accident could have occurred.

An immediate response to Allan's and Gallo's claims that SIV does not grow, or survive, in MKTC came from the eminent virologist Joseph Melnick, who submitted an affidavit in opposition to the Koprowski suit. In this, he stated: "In the late 1950s (as well as today) live attenuated polio vaccines were made in monkey kidney tissue cultures. These tissue cultures often contained small amounts of lymphocytes and macrophages. Such cells are now known to support the replication of SIV in culture."[10]

I later received a very helpful letter from Tom Curtis's brother, Michael Kent Curtis, who had just published a lengthy and impressive paper on the Koprowski/Curtis law case and the suppression of dissent in science.[11] He, too, had been concerned about Gallo's repeated stress on the fact that the vaccine had been made in monolayers, and had asked Professor Cecil Fox (a histologist who had been making MKTC since the fifties, when he also prepared time-lapse movies of these and other primary cell cultures) to explain exactly how a monolayer was prepared. Fox responded as follows:

> Initially, tissue which has been minced is placed in a culture flask with liquid cell culture medium. The flask is turned on its flat side and the cells are incubated on a horizontal surface. The epithelial cells spread out of the tiny bits of kidney and attach to the surface of the flask . . . [which] is covered by a single layer of cells like a flagstone floor. A casual observer might think this to be a pure culture, but when seen in time lapse movies it is apparent that other cell types are present such as macrophages, motile lymphocytes and fibroblasts. These are moving about on top of the monolayer and the macrophage component may persist for months.[12]

It appeared that monolayers, like other forms of MKTC, were liable to contain lymphocytes and macrophages.

Some years later, I spoke with Professor Fox myself, and he explained that in the fifties the preparation of tissue culture was very much an experimental procedure. He told me that lab technicians of that era used to say: "Well that worked pretty well; I'll throw a little bit of this in there."[13] One would imagine that at other times it was not the technicians, but those in charge, who might have taken such an initiative.

---

It was while reading Robert Gallo's affidavit that I suddenly recalled that it was a phone call from Gallo that had interrupted my second interview with Koprowski. Prompted by this, I did some research, and soon discovered that the two men were longtime associates. Gallo's book *Virus Hunting*, published in 1991, reveals that his early thinking about HIV vaccines had been influenced by contacts with Koprowski, Sabin, and Salk, but especially Koprowski.[14] And a 1985 paper proposing the theory (to date, unproven) that multiple sclerosis is caused by "a retrovirus that is related to, but distant from, the HTLV family" had Koprowski as first author and Gallo as last.[15]

Later I learned from several scientists that there was not merely a close professional relationship between Koprowski and Gallo, but also a close friendship, which apparently went back many years. For instance, back in December 1986, when Gallo was regarded by many as the leading figure in AIDS research, he had delivered the welcoming speech at "A Special Symposium in Honor of Hilary Koprowski," held at the Wistar Institute to celebrate the great man's seventieth birthday.[16]

One British virologist describes them as having "a father and son relationship. They're from different generations and they don't overlap in what they're interested in: they don't compete. Koprowski gets stuff in the National Academy of Sciences nominated by Gallo and vice versa. It's horribly close."[17]

---

There was another important development at the start of 1995 when, nearly a year after the meeting in Stockholm, Hans Wigzell and Carl-Rune Salenstedt wrote to Bill Hamilton with the results of the testing of the CHAT vaccine sample. They revealed that they had identified five different "lots" of CHAT 10A-11 vaccine, three of which had come direct from Koprowski, and two of which had been made at a later date at their own laboratories, SBL. They had arranged for all five to be tested for HIV and SIV by Jan Albert, one of the leading virologists at the newly created Swedish Institute for Infectious Disease Control (SIIDC). All five had produced consistently negative results.

They went on to state: "When it concerns protocols showing what monkey species have been used for the production of [the vaccine] virus we have not been able to find any. Consequently the origin of the Wistar lots is unknown to us." As for the Swedish-made lots, we could apparently "take it for granted that they were produced in *M. cynomolgus* tissue."[18]

The negative result was, admittedly, something of a blow to the theory, but on the other hand I had never really expected that we would receive a letter informing us of a positive result — that SIV or HIV had been found in CHAT vaccine.

Before long, however, I realized that there was far more to this brief communication than met the eye. First, there was the invaluable information about the origin of the different batches, which was contained on a separate sheet about testing procedures, written by Jan Albert. Two of the CHAT 10A-11 vaccine vials from Koprowski (marked merely "fl. 1" and "fl. 2") were dated February 10, 1958, while the other, which was marked "(501-510) P4" was dated the following day. This was just before the start of the Ruzizi campaign, in which the same pool,

10A-11, had apparently been used.[19] The two vials of Swedish 10A-11 were coded 2036 and 2330, and were dated April 5, 1963, and May 7, 1963.

What this immediately confirmed was that the terms "lot," "batch," and "pool" were, as I had long suspected, gloriously imprecise. All of these five batches (or "lots," as Wigzell called them) of vaccine were of pool 10A-11, and yet some had been prepared at different passage levels. There was certainly a difference between the Koprowski 10A-11 and the Swedish 10A-11, for the latter had been further passaged, apparently in cynomolgus kidney tissue, to enhance the titer.[20] And there might even have been a difference between the first two vials of Koprowski's vaccine and the third, for when I phoned Jan Albert, he told me that "P4" probably indicated that the third vial contained the fourth passage level of the virus.

In short, not all samples of CHAT vaccine, pool 10A-11, were identical. Different batches had been made in different laboratories, and had probably been prepared in tissue cultures originating from different monkey species. The seed pool of CHAT 10A-11 poliovirus *was* presumably homogeneous, but the production lots of vaccine could be further passaged in different substrates, with the end product still being referred to as the same pool.

The implications for the vaccine used in Ruzizi were wide-ranging. One possibility that now emerged was that in late 1957 or early 1958, Koprowski could have sent a sample of CHAT pool 10A-11 seed virus to De Somer, who could have passaged it further in another substrate, with the end product (still called CHAT pool 10A-11) being used in all, or part, of the Ruzizi Valley field trial.

What this demonstrated was that vaccine-makers like Koprowski apparently felt that their task was to attenuate poliovirus so that it was safe and immunogenic — and that if somebody then wished to passage it further to produce a final pool of vaccine in another substrate, that was their affair. Amazingly, the final substrate used for production lots was not seen as important enough to merit recording in the literature — or even, seemingly, in certain of the vaccine protocols. The bottom line was that experimental OPVs like Koprowski's could apparently be prepared in any substrate that successfully produced vaccine virus in large quantities. And the trusting consumer — the vaccinee — would be none the wiser.

There was no reference in the letter to Wigzell's previous promise to consider releasing some of the vaccine to a British lab to allow mitochondrial DNA testing for the host species. There was merely a bald statement from Jan Albert that "further analysis or additional testing of clinical samples from the vaccine trial cohorts is not warranted."

---

I had now made efforts to locate samples of CHAT vaccine on five different fronts. Officials from both the CDC[21] and the WHO[22] had told me that they had never received any CHAT samples for testing, a fact that was later confirmed by Koprowski's successor as director of the Wistar Institute, Giovanni Rovera.[23] Meanwhile, Meinrad Schar had written to inform me that "There are no samples of the CHAT oral polio vaccine in Switzerland available,"[24] and both Huygelen and Peetermans from RIT in Belgium had told me they believed that there was no vaccine remaining in their freezers.[25]

By contrast, the two establishments that did acknowledge that they held samples of CHAT vaccine — the Swedish Institute for Infectious Disease Control in Stockholm and the Wistar Institute itself — both refused to release any of the vaccine for independent testing. Bill Hamilton and I discussed this one evening, and speculated on why this should be. Were they afraid that some trace of an SIV contaminant might be found? Or were they, perhaps, concerned about what might be revealed about the substrate used to grow the vaccine?

---

My meeting with David Ho had taken place in December 1993, but by early 1995 he had still not published anything about the Manchester sailor sequence. Furthermore, he had not replied to my communications or sent me the promised documents from the Wistar committee.

But then in March 1995, I woke one morning to find that I had been well and truly scooped — for there on the front page of the *Independent* was the banner headline "World's First AIDS Case Was False," above a picture of David Carr in his Central Rovers football gear.[26] Despite the fact that I had been sitting on the information for fifteen months since the interview with Ho, and that it had been my decision not to break the story myself, it was hard not to feel a twinge of envy.

The article, which was followed by more detailed analysis on the next two pages, was written by the paper's science correspondent, Steve Connor, and was a first-rate piece of journalism. It told the story of the Manchester team's research, and Ho's follow-up investigation, which — it was now revealed — had failed to support the original findings. Connor wrote that, after taking advice from Gerry Myers (head of the HIV Sequence Database), Ho had concluded that the HIV-1 found in the tissues originally tested in Manchester must have come from a "modern" AIDS patient, one who had died in around 1990. But it was only when he tested the second set of tissues, finally sent by George Williams in February 1994,[27] that he discovered that they contained no HIV and, furthermore, that the DNA of the various samples proved that they came from at least two different individuals.

Connor did not beat about the bush. There were only two possibilities, he wrote: "[E]ither tissue samples were mixed up in a laboratory at Manchester University — something regarded as inconceivable — or the samples were deliberately switched."[28]

In one of the boxes accompanying the main article, Connor discussed how the new evidence would necessitate a rethinking of theories about how HIV-1 had originated. He had contacted Gerry Myers, who said that the elimination of the Manchester case had "bolstered his view that HIV came into being very recently . . . perhaps evolving from the monkey SIV just 35 years ago [1960]." Connor then analyzed the OPV/AIDS theory, which (he said) had several drawbacks, although the most significant one — that the Manchester sailor could not have been exposed to the Congo vaccine — had now been removed. However, he was rather more enthusiastic about Sergio Giunta's theory relating the origin of AIDS to the capturing of African monkeys for research purposes, and posited the introduction of reusable syringes and needles in Africa as a possible co-factor in the advent of the epidemic.

In traditional journalist style, Connor had phoned George Williams for his reaction to the story, and the pathologist responded: "I'm utterly, absolutely confident of the authenticity of that material. . . . We'll have to offer Ho further tissue. We should at least consider asking him to repeat it or get it done elsewhere. . . . I'd be quite happy to supply material to anyone who would take it on."

Since I had been trying to persuade Williams to provide some tissue samples from the case since 1991, and since he had given several different reasons for refusing, I felt that I should take him up on this offer. I phoned molecular biologist Mike Tristem, and we both wrote to Dr. Williams, formally requesting that he send Tristem a tissue sample. A few days later, I received a phone call from Dr. Williams's wife. She told me that her husband had handed over the legal side to the Medical Protection Society, and the medical side to the Central Manchester Health Care Trust (CMHCT), to whom she had forwarded our two letters. She added that she and her husband had been told not to discuss the matter further with anyone.

In the days that followed Connor's article, there was a frenzy of reaction. It emerged that the CMHCT had also taken over control of the remaining tissue samples — although nobody from the trust ever replied to the letters from Mike Tristem and myself. Gerald Corbitt, who had been in charge of the original testing, and who — since the end of 1992 — had declined to discuss the subject further with me, now told Steve Connor that since the recent revelations about the sequence he had wanted to write to the *Lancet* to retract his findings, but had been stopped from doing so by senior officials of the Trust.[29] However, the Trust's chairman wrote to the *Independent* to deny this,[30] and another Trust member, Professor James Burnie, told the *New York Times:* "There is no doubt the original findings as reported in *The Lancet* in July 1990 were correct. We have already carried out an informal inquiry which has validated this."[31] A few days later, the professor was rather less certain, when he revealed that the Trust had asked the United Kingdom's Forensic Science Service to retest the samples, and admitted that if they were shown to come from two patients, "we are then looking at a retraction in a big way."[32]

By this stage, David Ho's results had been rushed out in letter form in *Nature*,[33] and they revealed that the affair was even more complicated, since the various materials sent from Manchester appeared to contain the DNA of at least three different individuals. The letter also confirmed that Ho's lab had detected evidence of HIV quasispecies, which suggested that the source of contamination had been another clinical specimen from an HIV-1-infected person or an AIDS patient, rather than a cloned sequence used as a laboratory control.[34]

For my part, I was still feeling aggrieved with David Ho for breaking his word to me, and for sharing his findings with Connor instead. As it turned out, however, Ho was equally pissed off with Connor, who, he claimed, had got his scoop by breaking a verbal agreement to embargo the story until the publication of his own formal report in *Nature*.[35] (Steve Connor later denied this.)[36] Fortunately, all this worked to my favor, because a couple of months later Ho phoned to explain what had happened and to apologize. We ended up talking for almost an hour, during the course of which I once again asked if he could send a copy of the papers from the Wistar's expert committee on the CHAT hypothesis. He said that this time, without fail, he would get his secretary to photocopy and send them.

And as it turned out, the thirty-eight pages that arrived in the post a few days later were to have even greater implications for the case against CHAT than the formal announcement that David Carr, the Manchester sailor, had not had AIDS.

# 46

ALEXANDRE JEZIERSKI

One of the biggest disappointments of the Belgian research in 1994 was the discovery that the Polish vet, Alexandre Jezierski, was no longer alive. During 1993, I had come across several of his papers in the medical literature, and it was apparent that at his small laboratory at Gabu-Nioka in the eastern Congo, and without any of the resources of the huge labs in America, Britain, and France, he had conducted some highly individual research into oral polio vaccines.

The discovery that it was Jezierski who had escorted Hilary Koprowski and Tom Norton to Camp Putnam, or Epulu (situated some 150 miles from Gabu Nioka), was perhaps the most important revelation of my entire interview with Koprowski. For it confirmed that, at that crucial time in the development of CHAT, the American virologists had spent two or three days with a man who was already manufacturing his polio vaccines in the kidneys of local African primates, who had grown polioviruses in the kidney cells of chimpanzees, and who had conducted (or who was just about to conduct) small-scale vaccine trials in humans.

But it was not only with Koprowski that Jezierski had links. The more that I delved into the French and Belgian medical and veterinary literature of the period, the more I realized that this strange, angry figure served as a link, a common denominator, between many of the groups who were then making polio vaccine. As a Polish refugee, he was a stateless person, and seems to have affiliated himself to virologists of all nations: there was direct collaboration with Belgian and French teams, but he also had contacts with vaccine-makers from the United States, the

United Kingdom, and South Africa. Yet, as catholic as he was in his choice of col-laborators, he was just as ready — it seemed — to fall out with them.

I was never able to find Jezierski's curriculum vitae, but I did manage to piece together much of his career in the Belgian Congo from published articles and from others who had worked with him or visited his laboratory. Like many Polish Jews, he seems to have found his way to the Congo at around the time of the Second World War, when refugees with degrees were readily accepted by the understaffed colonial authorities.

By 1947, he was based at the veterinary laboratory in Elisabethville, and in 1950 he and his counterpart in the local medical laboratory, Jean Delville, co-authored three articles. One concerned a virus isolated from a child who appeared to be suffering from polio — the two men tried injecting the virus into a series of different mammals, including three *Cercopithecus* monkeys, a baboon, and a chimpanzee, to test their susceptibility to the virus.[1]

In 1953, Jezierski joined INEAC,* a farming and agronomy institute with headquarters at the small town of Yangambi, eighty miles downstream of Stanley-ville. He was appointed director of the veterinary lab at Gabu, which was attached to an animal husbandry research station and stock breeding farm at the town of Nioka, five miles distant. This fertile area had a high proportion of European set-tlers, and provided many of the vegetables for Stanleyville, five hundred miles to the west, which meant that the intervening road was well maintained. Although it was only an outlying station in the hills overlooking Lake Albert and Uganda, Gabu was important, for it produced animal vaccines for the entire colony.

In July 1953, a prominent member of Pierre Lépine's virology department at the Pasteur Institute in Paris, Georges Barski, visited the area in order to gather blood specimens for polio antibody studies. Barski took blood from five areas, including three different pygmy communities, and two villages near Gabu. In a related paper that he and Lépine wrote three years later, Barski expressed his particular gratitude to Dr. Jezierski, and thanked INEAC for its hospitality at the Gabu laboratory.[2] He also found a way to repay him, for by October 1953 Jezierski received samples of three strains of virulent poliovirus from the Pasteur Institute.

The four-page entry for Gabu in the INEAC annual report for 1953 indicates that Jezierski wasted no time in experimenting with the poliovirus strains. He continued the work begun with Delville by assessing the sensibility to polio-virus of the tissues of various different African monkeys — and other animals too. The entry ends, laconically: "Successive passages have brought about a marked attenuation of the strains, which are behaving like vaccine virus."

These few words indicate a quite astonishing fact — that in his small lab in the mountains of the eastern Congo, Alexandre Jezierski was already, in 1953,

* INEAC: Institut National Pour l'Étude Agronomique du Congo Belge.

## THIRTY SPECIES OF PRIMATES THAT HAVE BEEN USED TO MAKE MKTC FOR GROWING POLIOVIRUS, AND THEIR SIV STATUS

| | Monkey species — scientific name | Common name | SIV identified in 1990s | Reference |
|---|---|---|---|---|
| 1 | Cercopithecus ascanius ascanius | Black-cheeked white-nosed monkey | | Barski, Jezierski & Lépine, 1954 |
| 2 | Cercopithecus eucampyx | [Not identified] | | |
| 3 | Cercopithecus mitis | Blue monkey | * | " |
| 4 | Cercopithecus neglectus | De Brazza's monkey | Yes | " |
| 5 | Cercopithecus aethiops aethiops | Grivet (AGM) | Yes | " |
| 6 | Cercocebus aterrimus opdenboschi | Black mangabey | | " |
| 7 | Colobus badius | Western red colobus | | " |
| 8 | Colobus abyssinicus uellensis | Abyssinian black-&-white colobus | | " |
| 9 | Erythrocebus patas | Red monkey | Yes | " |
| 10 | Pan troglodytes | Common chimpanzee | Yes | Jezierski, 1955 |
| 11 | Colobus angolensis | Angolan black-&-white colobus | | " |
| 12 | Cercopithecus l'hoesti | L'Hoest's monkey | Yes | " |
| 13 | Cercocebus galeritus | Crested mangabey | | " |
| 14 | Cercopithecus hamlyni | Owl-faced monkey | Yes | " |
| 15 | Papio cynocephalus | Yellow baboon | Yes | " |
| 16 | Cebus capucina (South America) | Capuchin monkey | | Kaplan, 1955 |
| 17 | Papio sphinx | Mandrill | Yes | Lépine et al., 1955 |
| 18 | Cercopithecus aethiops sabaeus | Callitrix (AGM) | Yes | Hsiung & Melnick, 1957 |
| 19 | Cercopithecus aethiops pygerythrus | Vervet monkey (AGM) | Yes | " |
| 20 | Cercopithecus cephus | Mustached monkey | | " |
| 21 | Cercopithecus mona campbelli | Mona monkey (Campbell's) | | " |

| Monkey species — scientific name | Common name | SIV identified in 1990s | Reference |
|---|---|---|---|
| 22 *Cercopithecus petaurista buttikoferi* | Lesser white-nosed monkey | | Hsiung & Melnick, 1957 |
| 23 *Cercopithecus diana roloway* | Diana monkey | | " |
| 24 *Cercocebus torquatus atys* | Sooty mangabey | Yes | " |
| 25 *Cercocebus torquatus lunulatus* | White-crowned mangabey | Yes† | " |
| 26 *Macaca mulatta* (Asia) | Rhesus macaque | Yes† | " |
| 27 *Macaca cynomolgus* (Asia) | Cynomolgus macaque | Yes† | " |
| 28 *Perodicticus potto* | Bosman's potto | | " |
| 29 *Papio papio* | Guinea baboon | | " |
| 30 *Papio anubus* | Olive baboon | | " |

\* *C. mitis albogularis* (the Sykes' monkey) has been found to carry SIV, but is probably not the same *C. mitis* subspecies used by Barski et al.

† Only known to be SIV-infected in captivity.

AGM = African green monkey groups, which probably represent full species

Eleven of these species are known to carry SIV in the wild; three acquired SIV from other species in captivity.

attenuating poliovirus by successive passages in monkey tissue cultures. He was, in effect, running level with Albert Sabin, and was (in many respects) ahead of Hilary Koprowski, who would not begin to use MKTC until about a year later.

The lab's annual report for 1954 notes a leave of absence for Jezierski, who seems to have taken a busman's holiday, for he went straight to Paris to work with Barski and Lépine. Later that year a brief and remarkable paper by the three men explained that most workers who were growing poliovirus employed macaque tissues, while the Pasteur used tissues from baboons, but that this paper would explore the possibility of growing poliovirus in the tissues of other African monkeys originating from eastern Belgian Congo.

The paper described attempts to make tissue culture from the minced-up testicles of nine different monkeys (five *Cercopithecus* species, two *Colobus* species, one mangabey, and one red monkey), all of which had been captured or shot in the forests surrounding Gabu Nioka. The tissues of all these primates produced "good" or "very good" cell cultures, which proved sensitive to poliovirus. Also tested (both in Gabu and Paris) had been cell cultures originating from the tissues of seven other species of mammals, ranging from the bat to the cow, none of which supported the growth of poliovirus.

Clearly Jezierski was prodigiously active during 1954, for in the space of a single month at the start of 1955 he submitted three further articles on the subject, all published under his name alone, but describing him as working for the INEAC laboratory at Gabu and the virus department of the Pasteur Institute. This research involved seven new primates (including the chimpanzee and the yellow baboon), ten other mammals (ranging from the anteater to the elephant) and four reptiles (a tortoise, a turtle, a lizard, and a chameleon). Tissues were extracted in the field as soon as the animal was killed, and were minced up and made into cultures between two and twelve hours later. This time Jezierski used not only the testicles, but also spleens, lymph glands, kidneys, lungs, and muscle tissue.

The tissues of all the higher primates provided excellent cultures that were sensitive to poliovirus, and he was able to establish a correlation between the viral sensitivity of a species *in vivo* and *in vitro*.[3] In addition, he tested cells derived from the human placenta and from the muscle tissues of human and simian embryos, which also provided poliovirus-sensitive cultures. None of the non-primate cultures, however, were sensitive to poliovirus.

One of the other 1955 papers revealed that James Gear, from the South African Polio Research Foundation, was assisting Jezierski with some of the lab work, and that Lederle Laboratories (where Koprowski was then based) had provided Jezierski with some of his biomedical materials.[4]

The third paper constitutes the initial report of Jezierski's attempts to produce both a killed and a live polio vaccine. Although it was not spelled out, it appears that some of this work was conducted at Gabu, and some in Paris. Apparently Jezierski was still using cells from the monkeys' testicles, lymph glands, lungs, and spleen, but was beginning to favor the use of kidney cultures (prepared mechanically, rather than through trypsinization).

For his IPV, he employed tissues from the African green monkey and, like Jonas Salk, inactivated the poliovirus with formalin. For the OPV, he carried out twenty-one rapid passages (just as Sabin was doing in Cincinnati) of poliovirus Types 1, 2, and 3 in tissue cultures made from the kidneys of three different species of colobus monkey — *abyssinicus, badius,* and *angolensis.* Both his IPV and OPV produced antibodies in vaccinated monkeys, and protected them against challenge with virulent virus.[5]

These 1955 papers are quite remarkable. Some of the science is rather less sophisticated than the contemporary offerings of Salk, Sabin, and Koprowski, but all the important information is there — such as the source of the tissues used for viral culture, the method of producing the cultures, the number of poliovirus passages needed to produce an effective vaccine, the safety tests conducted, the quantities of virus used for vaccination and for challenge — and the length of time between the two. Given the difficulties that the great American and European vaccine-makers were experiencing, it seems extraordinary that merely by keeping up to date with the latest developments in the literature, and with very limited resources (a small vaccine lab and an abundant supply of monkeys), Jezierski should have been more than holding his own. Moreover, he was the only one of them to highlight the importance of the vaccine substrate. Not only did he clearly identify the species he himself used, but he also identified, in various of his publications, the species that other vaccine-makers were using: Sabin the cynomolgus macaque,[6] Lépine the baboon, Gear the African green monkey, and Salk the rhesus macaque.[7] He made no such claims for Koprowski, observing only that he had adapted his Type 1 virus to mice and cotton rats — which is what Koprowski was still reporting in his articles from that era.[8]

---

Perhaps members of the INEAC hierarchy were becoming restless about the extent of Jezierski's collaboration with the Pasteur, and the amount of time he was spending on human, rather than animal viruses. Whatever, his next contribution on the subject was not published until 1959, by which stage he had already been overtaken by his American rivals, and had left Gabu Nioka for good.

This 1959 article completes the extraordinary tale of Jezierski's oral polio vaccines.[9] He writes that tests carried out on African green monkeys and a chimpanzee confirmed that at an early stage of the passage in colobus tissue, the three polioviruses were already attenuated and conferred immunity. After sixty passages, Jezierski decided to adopt the more productive substrate of trypsinized kidneys — again from colobus monkeys. After ten passages in the new medium, viral titers had increased a hundredfold; after a further thirty passages, Jezierski plaque-purified the three strains and again proved their immunogenicity. At the 148th passage level, the viruses were titrated* in two different tissue cultures — made from colobus kidney and chimpanzee kidney — both of which showed that high titers had been attained. Sixty monkeys of different species were vaccinated with the new virus, and again it proved safe and effective.

At this point, Jezierski decided it was time to progress to the next level of testing and, basing his work on early experiments by Koprowski,[10] he fed the three attenuated polioviruses to a dozen chimpanzees. They were protected against challenge and suffered no ill effects, so Jezierski decided it was time to take the ultimate step. He decided to administer his vaccine to "human volunteers."

---

\* To titrate: To assess the concentration of a substance (in this case a virus) in solution.

He ended up feeding the three vaccine strains to twenty-one Africans, aged between twelve and twenty-one, at the mission hospital of Nyarembe, fifty miles north of Gabu up on the Ugandan border. Antibody response was good (save for those fed the vaccine cocktail, who developed decent antibody levels against only one of the three types), and there were no visible ill reactions. No dates are provided, but allowing three to four days for each MKTC passage, it seems likely that the chimp feeding would have taken place during 1956, and the human trial in either late 1956 or early 1957.

At the end of 1959, Jezierski's last communication about polio vaccines was published.[11] This reveals, among other things, that the three vaccine strains had reached the 210th passage level, and that he had carried out further studies on chimpanzees supplied by Jean de Medina, the head of the capture station at Epulu (formerly Camp Putnam). The article is followed by a discussion session in which Jezierski's paper is treated with skepticism by one speaker (Jos Mortelmans) and roundly rejected by the other — Paul Brutsaert, the senior Antwerp professor who delivered the opening address at the Stanleyville virus symposium in September 1957.[12]

Brutsaert ends his detailed critique: "The type of experimentation done by Jezierski cannot be done by one isolated man, however capable and hard working he is. One man just doesn't have the time for all the controls which are required, nor can he have a sufficient supply of animal material. Perhaps Dr Jezierski could interest a big European or American laboratory with research teams and unlimited materials." It seems likely that he was referring to labs like Koprowski's at the Wistar, or De Somer's at RIT.

Jezierski's reply is rather forlorn, concluding that "it is regrettable that . . . due to a combination of unforeseeable circumstances, this research had to be completely abandoned."

The INEAC annual reports reveal that Jezierski never returned from his tri-annual leave at the end of 1957. Perhaps he had finally trodden on too many toes, or perhaps senior members of INEAC were concerned about his apparently ad hoc experiments on human subjects. Certainly none of the papers ever mentions his seeking permission, or authority, to carry out the Nyarembe vaccinations.

---

By this time, several of his former collaborators had told me that Jezierski, despite his brilliance, was an extremely difficult man: arrogant, nervous, and quite unable to delegate or share responsibility. I wanted to find out more about his time at Gabu, and eventually I located Georges Lambelin, who had been Jezierski's deputy from 1953 to 1957, and who took over as director after his departure. Apparently he had not been involved with the polio program, which was purely Jezierski's research, for which he had had to obtain special permission from the directors of INEAC. Lambelin knew only that Jezierski had been trying to make tissue cultures from lots of different animals, and to attenuate poliovirus by consecutive passages. He recalled the many colobus monkeys, and also a group of chimps. "I have the impression that he was an excellent technician," he explained, "but his imagination was not exceptional. . . . He adapted various techniques, and worked very strictly with a high standard of scientific [accuracy]."

Eventually, after some prompting, Lambelin told me that he and Jezierski had not had a good relationship, and that Jezierski had got on even worse with the African staff. "He was very polite with the important people, and very disagreeable with the others. It was not pleasant to work with him." Furthermore, he apparently refused to train Lambelin, or to pass on any practical know-how about vaccine production. In the end, the problems became so evident to the INEAC hierarchy that in late 1957, when it was approaching the time for Jezierski's leave, they decided to fire him. Lambelin was instructed to abandon everything to do with polio, and to reorganize the lab purely on veterinary lines. There were a lot of monkeys there at the time, several of which were released, together with one chimpanzee, which was given to the polio researchers at Stanleyville.[13]

Jezierski apparently returned to Belgium, and was later reengaged at his old job, at the vet lab in Elisabethville. After independence, he joined the Food and Agriculture Organization in Rome, and after retirement he and his wife took an apartment in Brussels, where Jezierski died in 1991 (and she soon afterward).

I managed to locate one surviving relative by marriage, an antiques dealer from western Belgium, and it was he who apparently cleared out the Brussels flat after the couple died. In the process, he threw away most of Jezierski's papers. I got the clear impression that the antiques dealer had not especially liked his Polish in-law. He told me of Jezierski's lengthy collaboration with the Pasteur Institute, and of his links with South Africa. He also said that Jezierski had been very strange and mistrustful about money. He had holdings in banks all over the world, and in his later years used to drive across Europe in an old Citroën, leaving gold bars in this or that deposit box. He was also extremely cunning and good with his hands, and apparently used to spend hours at amusement arcades manipulating the miniature cranes, and winning wristwatches. At the end of his life he became rich, but the air of secrecy and mystery never left him, and after his death some two-thirds of a million dollars apparently went missing, inexplicably, from his estate.

---

I came across one other person who knew something about Jezierski's scientific achievements. In 1993, a Swedish veterinary virologist told me that Koprowski had been given the idea for his tissue culture techniques by a British vet, Gordon Scott, who had worked at Muguga in the fifties.[14] I located Dr. Scott, who told me that this was not the case — but yes, he had met Koprowski on several occasions, and knew of his polio work. He had also, it transpired, spent more than a month as the guest of Dr. Jezierski at Gabu in March and April 1954.

It turned out that shortly before this Tad Wiktor, who by then was director of the Stanleyville veterinary labs and already a fast-rising star in that service, was visiting Scott in Nairobi to learn about tissue culture techniques. (Perhaps my Swedish informant had got confused between the two Poles, Koprowski and Wiktor.) Suddenly the news came through that Jezierski had identified rinderpest (cattle plague) near Gabu. Wiktor flew there immediately, and Scott followed a few days later, bringing with him a supply of the latest rinderpest vaccine. Jezierski gave them the run of his lab, but because there were no freeze-drying facilities, Wiktor and Scott had to prepare fresh vaccine every day. For the next month, they rose at four each morning to kill rabbits and harvest their tissues for the vaccine substrate. The vaccination campaign managed to avert what could have been a serious outbreak of the cattle plague.[15]

Scott recalls that Wiktor — who, though much younger than Jezierski, was senior to him in the carefully delineated hierarchy — avoided wearing his uniform to work, so as not to embarrass his host with his copious epaulettes. He remembers the Pole as a martinet who had his African staff line up on parade at six each morning. He was, however, "staggered" by the fact that he was "pushing forwards the boundaries of science" in his little bush lab. Scott believes that at this stage Jezierski was working only on IPV, but had already begun to use kidneys in preference to other tissues; he recalls his mincing them up with fine scissors and placing the pieces in roller tubes. He accompanied Jezierski on some of his hunting expeditions, and observed him shooting colobus monkeys "with relish." Apparently this was a ritual that was repeated every week or so — and he always bagged two monkeys, in case one turned out to be diseased. Indeed, the one photo that Scott still has of Jezierski depicts him as a crew-cut, safari-suited professional hunter with rifle in hand and cigarette hanging from mouth. It gives no hint that this same man was a skilled virologist.

Though not a full participant, Scott was present at many of the sessions of the Muguga rabies workshop attended by Koprowski, Lépine, Wiktor, and Ninane in July 1955.[16] Apparently Alexandre Jezierski was not present, but given the nature of his three recently published polio articles, the fact that Wiktor and Scott had stayed with him the previous year, and that Lépine had been collaborating with him in Paris, it can be assumed that Koprowski heard all about him.

Scott was also present at the annual general meeting of the Kenyan branch of the British Medical Association at the end of January 1957, when Koprowski gave a formal address about OPV.[17] He told me that afterward a smaller group repaired to the house of Howard Binns, the Muguga director, for a sundowner, and that Koprowski played piano, showed them his boxes of vaccines, and then spoke for a while about his plans and ideas. Scott recalled only one specific detail of the discussion: "He posed the question [of] how many people had to be given the vaccine before the vaccine could be accredited — was it ten, a hundred, a thousand, ten thousand, a hundred thousand, a million?"[18] Apparently Koprowski told the vets that they were lucky — they could test their vaccines by challenging the definitive host with virulent virus, which makers of human vaccines could not.

Scott recalled that Jezierski's name came up during the course of that January 1957 soirée at Binns's house, and told me that Koprowski "almost certainly" visited his compatriot during the Congo trip that followed. He added that when he visited Gabu in 1954, he had first flown to Usumbura and then driven north to Jezierski's lab — a journey of more than five hundred miles, but one that had taken only a day — and surely the same route, I realized, as that taken by Koprowski and Norton three years later. Later, I was able to check the Sabena timetable for 1957, which confirmed that the weekly flight from Nairobi to Usumbura was on a Friday, which was the very day that the two Americans had left Nairobi.[19] The plane had had a forty-five-minute stopover at Entebbe, and another glance at Tom Norton's postcard to his daughters revealed that it had probably been written in transit, at Entebbe airport.

Tom Norton's photos had been taken as slides, and after Gail had them transferred to prints, they must have been inserted into the album in reverse order. Now, suddenly, the clues from Gail's photograph album, the Belgian newspaper clippings, and Hanka Wiktor's recollections were beginning to slot neatly into time and place. Now, at last, I was able to piece together the key events of Koprowski's *mensis mirabilis* of February 1957, which was so tragically to become, at the last, his *mensis horribilis.*

Hilary Koprowski and Tom Norton had clearly begun, not ended, their trip in Nairobi, and had flown from there to Usumbura on February 1, where they had spent the night with the Wiktors. My guess was that the Americans then dispatched their precious supplies of vaccine, CHAT plaque 20 and Fox, on the following day's flight to Stanleyville, so that they could be kept refrigerated at the Laboratoire Médical. They themselves must have set off north by road to see Alexandre Jezierski, and would probably have arrived at the Gabu lab on the evening of February 2. In all likelihood the three men would have visited nearby Lake Albert, and later proceeded to Camp Putnam, or Epulu, where they may well have met Jean de Medina, Jezierski's chimpanzee supplier. There at Epulu they must have parted, with Jezierski going back to Gabu, and the two Americans driving on to Stanleyville, arriving there on the fifth or the sixth.

This would have allowed the two Americans five or six days at Stanleyville and Lindi before Koprowski flew down to Leopoldville on the eleventh, to discuss his program of research with the medical authorities there. Norton was left behind to continue his work at the chimp station. Where Koprowski went next is not known for certain, though given his expressed intentions in Nairobi, he may have spent a week with Gear in South Africa.[20] His next documented

KOPROWSKI'S *MENSIS MIRABILIS* — FEBRUARY 1957

| | |
|---|---|
| Wed., Jan. 30 | Koprowski addresses the Annual General Meeting of the East African branch of the British Medical Association. |
| Thur., Jan. 31 | Koprowski has discussion with Kenyan medical officials. He spends the night at Muguga, near Nairobi (with Dr. Binns). |
| Fri., Feb. 1 | Koprowski and Norton fly to Usumbura via Entebbe. They spend the night with the Wiktors. Front-page article about Koprowski's vaccines appears in *East African Standard*. |
| Sat., Feb. 2? | Vaccines are forwarded by air from Usumbura to Stanleyville? |
| Sat., Feb. 2–Tues., Feb. 5 | Koprowski and Norton travel northward by road and visit Lake Albert (and possibly Gabu). Later they visit Epulu camp with Alexandre Jezierski, and then continue westward to Stanleyville. |
| Tues., Feb. 5 | First feeding of live poliovirus in cream to Lindi chimps. |
| Thur., Feb. 7 | Second feeding of live virus to Lindi chimps. That evening, Koprowski addresses a meeting in Stanleyville about the safety of his vaccines. |
| Fri., Feb. 8? | Koprowski and Courtois show two journalists around Lindi camp. |
| Mon., Feb. 11 | Koprowski flies to Leopoldville, possibly with Courtois, to discuss the Lindi polio research with the Congo's leading public health officials. Norton stays behind to continue the chimp work at Lindi. |
| Tues., Feb 12–Tues., Feb 19? | Koprowski goes to South Africa? (In Nairobi it was said that Koprowski intended to fly to Johannesburg for discussions with public health authorities there.) |
| Wed., Feb. 20 | Koprowski calls at the Medical Research Council in London to deliver a note about the safety of his vaccines. |
| Mon., Feb. 25 | Koprowski is in London with his father, who is recovering from prostate surgery. |
| Tues., Feb. 26? | Koprowski flies back to the United States. |
| Wed., Feb. 27 | Seventh anniversary of first feeding of OPV. Koprowski's new Type 1 vaccine, CHAT, is fed to six babies at Clinton State Farms. |
| Thur., Feb. 28 | Koprowski's father dies in Manchester. Koprowski flies to U.K. for the funeral. |

appearance is in London on February 20, when he left a note about his vaccines at the Medical Research Council. On the twenty-fifth, according to his own account, he was still in London with his father, who was recovering from surgery, and after that he flew back to America. It may well be that he was keen to be present at Clinton on February 27, his OPV anniversary, for the first formal feeding of CHAT to a group of six infants. The very next day, quite unexpectedly, his beloved father died. Koprowski immediately flew to Manchester for the funeral.

---

There was only one facet of this reconstruction that worried me. Although it seemed almost certain that the Americans had spent two or three days with Jezierski, there was no way of knowing whether or not he had briefed them on his polio research.

However, when I returned to America in June 1995, Tom Norton's daughter Ann showed me the folders of Tom's papers that Koprowski had borrowed from her mother, and which he had now finally returned. There was very little new material — much of it being multiple copies of papers I had already seen — but there was one page on which Tom Norton had sketched out some ideas for the Congo chapter in the book he and Koprowski had been planning to write. The penultimate entry read "Crocodile kidney TC = Jezairksi," which is clearly a reference to crocodile kidney tissue culture and to Jezierski.[21] It certainly sounded as if the three scientists had talked shop.

There were two areas of research where Jezierski was well ahead of Koprowski and Norton. First, he had been attenuating poliovirus in monkey tissue cultures for much longer than they had, and they would doubtless have relished the opportunity to pick his brains on the subject. And second, they would have wanted to know how easily other tissue cultures could be grown, and how effective they were as poliovirus substrates. In America, researchers were only using two species for tissue culture — rhesus and cynomolgus — but here was a man who had successfully grown poliovirus in the tissues of fifteen different African primates. These were seven guenons (*Cercopithecus* species), three colobus monkeys, two mangabeys, a red monkey, a baboon, and a chimpanzee. Every one of these species was locally abundant, and absurdly cheap to purchase.

Given the fact that they were about to work with chimps at Lindi, Koprowski and Norton would presumably have been especially interested in Jezierski's tissue cultures made from chimpanzee kidneys. His papers show that he used chimp kidney on at least two occasions. First he found that it made "very good" cultures, in which all three polioviruses produced visible cytopathic effect within three days. And second, at just around the time of the Koprowski visit, he used chimpanzee kidney tissue culture to do a comparative titration of his colobus-based vaccines.

Gordon Scott told me that Jezierski was "seeking fame and fortune through producing an attenuated polio vaccine," and that his wife seemed to endure the isolation in the hope that Alexandre's research would be recognized by a big organization, so that they could return in triumph from Africa to Europe. One suspects, therefore, that Jezierski would have done all he could to help — and impress — his compatriot-by-birth. After all, he might have reasoned, if he could win over this famous American virologist, who already carried a reputation for recognizing and exploiting genius in others, then fame and fortune would surely follow.

———————

One final question needs to be asked. Alexandre Jezierski fed experimental polio vaccines made from three types of colobus kidneys to twenty-one people in the Belgian Congo, probably in 1957. Although he injected these vaccines into egg yolks and tested them in monkeys, there were in reality no effective tests to weed out agents such as lentiviruses. In 1986, a group of Californian researchers found that individuals from one of his three species, the Abyssinian black-and-white colobus, also known as the guereza, showed evidence of infection with "HIV."[22] Does this not mean that we have another vaccine that conceivably could have transferred HIV-1 to *Homo sapiens*?

That question is easily answered — and in the negative. First, only a single colobus monkey was confirmed by the Californians as HIV-positive on both ELISA and Western blot, and this monkey was from the subspecies *Colobus abyssinicus kikuyensis,* found to the east of the Rift Valley, rather than *Colobus abyssinicus uellensis* (Matschie), from the western side, which Jezierski used for his vaccines. Furthermore, this report featured in a very early serosurvey of captive monkeys in American zoos (from the days when tests for HIV, rather than SIV, were still applied to monkeys), and SIV infection has not yet been confirmed in colobus monkeys in the wild.

In addition, although Jezierski's vaccine was fed at theoretically the right time (1957) and in the right country (the Congo) to be implicated, it was not fed in the right part of that country, for there are no indications of early HIV prevalence (or of an early eruption of AIDS) from the region around Nyarembe.[23]

It is certainly possible that Jezierski may have played a key role in the story of how AIDS began, but if he did it was because of the precedent he set. He may, it seems, have been a harbinger of doom, but he was not the central protagonist.

———————

One detail that is graphically illustrated by Jezierski's polio research is just how easy it was at the end of the fifties to set up ad hoc trials of vaccines in Africa. Furthermore, it is clear that not all such trials were properly recorded. In his case, the details of the experimental trial *were* written up in the literature — though in an article that could easily be overlooked, for very few other polio researchers have cited Jezierski's work in their papers.

Could there have been other polio vaccine trials, which were simply not recorded at all? The evidence suggests that there could have been, and that many of the colonial powers were quite cavalier about vaccinating their African "subjects" in the period before decolonization. The British Medical Research Council was already exploring the possibility of using the tissues of West African monkeys for polio vaccine production in 1955.[24] Afterward, the MRC proposed to send a team to West Africa, which could combine tissue culture research with virus studies in "what was likely to prove a hyperendemic area for poliovirus." There are no further reports of the mooted research, but it may be that these virus studies included an experimental vaccination in an area where natural resistance to polio was high.[25]

It is easier to follow the activities of the South Africans, for there are detailed reports that show that they field-tested their polio vaccine overseas before administering it at home. The OPV developed by Gear in African green monkey tissue was not tried out in South Africa until October 1960, a year after it had been used for the immunization of 200,000 in Mauritius, and more than a million in Kenya. One or two single-line references suggest that this vaccine was also fed to people in Kampala, Uganda (probably in late 1959).[26] The reasons why the vaccine was not used during the polio epidemic that swept part of Cape Province in October 1959 are not clear.[27]

For other experimental vaccines fed in Africa, the only remaining records lie in the archives of local newspapers or, more often, the memories of the participants. This is the case for many of the CHAT feedings in the Belgian Congo and Ruanda-Urundi, a summary of which will be presented later.

Some of the vaccine-makers liked to offer their vaccine informally and forty years later, one can learn of such episodes only through good fortune. It seems, for instance, that a certain amount of CHAT vaccine ended up in Kenya. While I was following up on Koprowski's visit there in January 1957, I talked with Geoffrey Timms, who had then been in charge of vaccine procurement for the colony — and who also happened to be George Dick's brother-in-law. He surprised me by volunteering that Koprowski had left behind about a thousand doses of the "no name" vaccine (presumably CHAT Plaque 20) in capsule form. Timms kept these in his freezer for a while, but "they were finally dismissed as either ineffective or dangerous or both, and I was told to destroy them" by someone in the colonial Ministry of Health.[28]

Dr. Timms gave me the address of another Kenyan doctor, Jimmy Harries, who had also had contact with Koprowski. I went to see Dr. Harries, and he told me that he had first met the Lederle man while on a WHO fellowship to America in 1956, when they had discussed the possibility of staging pilot vaccine schemes in Kenya. This idea was later vetoed by the Kenyan director of medical services, Dr. John Walker, who appeared to have read Dick and Dane's articles in the *British Medical Journal,* and was concerned that Koprowski's vaccines might revert to virulence and then spread among the Kenyan population. Nonetheless, when Koprowski visited in January 1957, he gave Jimmy Harries some doses of the new vaccine, which he later fed to his family over Sunday lunch. Harries was especially vulnerable to infection because he worked with polio patients in hospital.

The last variety of experimental trials are those that have been mentioned in the literature, but about which some doubt remains with regard to crucial details. An example would be the vaccination with one of Lépine's vaccines in and around Mitzic, Gabon, in late 1957. The title of the article in which this immunization was reported refers merely to a polio outbreak in the Gabonese bush — it is only in the last two paragraphs that the vaccination of more than two thousand people is quite casually revealed.[29] The man who carried out the vaccinations, Dr. L. J. André, who afterward rose to become director of the French Army Institute of Tropical Medicine, has since informed me that this was the first collective polio vaccination in the French territories of black Africa, and that all three vaccinations involved "injectable Lépine vaccine of the era," dispatched from Paris. Since sufficient vaccine was not immediately available, he wrote, they were sent a batch originally intended for another use. He could not say which substrate had been used, and added that no documents pertaining to the vaccination remained.[30]

Clearly Dr. André acted in good faith, but the work of Alexandre Jezierski prompts the question of whether the vaccine sent him was prepared in the Pasteur's normal substrate of *Papio papio.* In November 1954, at the WHO conference on polio vaccination held in Stockholm, Pierre Lépine revealed that the Pasteur had, in 1953, set up a specially equipped laboratory for vaccine production, and that both human cells and the kidneys of different African monkeys were being investigated.[31] (Jezierski, who seems to have spent the final six months of 1954 at the Pasteur, was clearly one of the major investigators.)[32] Lépine told the Stockholm audience that his lab was now producing one hundred liters of vaccine a week, and that some was being stockpiled for future use.

The possibility that the third dose of Lépine's vaccine administered at Mitzic might have been an injection of a live polio vaccine "booster" has already been discussed. But just as important as whether the vaccine was killed or live is the nature of the substrate employed. After the Geneva conference of July 1957, the floodgates seem to have opened for vaccine trials in Africa. The Mitzic immunization could have been a field trial of Lépine's strains made in one of Jezierski's fifteen monkey substrates, all of which — it would seem — he had brought to Paris. But if it was, which tissue was chosen?

If, for instance, the vaccine was prepared in the kidneys of one of the Epulu chimps supplied to Jezierski by Jean de Medina, this could theoretically explain why the HIV-1 Group O viruses found in Gabon and Cameroon are so different from the SIVcpz isolates found in the same area.[33] If a SIVcpz isolate genetically similar to HIV-1 Group O viruses is ever located from the region of eastern Congo around Epulu, this would strongly support such a hypothesis.

However, another intriguing clue is found in a paper from Lépine's department published in 1955. This details the finding of microscopic worms in tissue cultures made from the mandrill *(Papio sphinx),* and adds that these tissue cultures had been prepared in order to undertake vaccine therapy with "a non-inactivated vaccine."[34] In other words, this was research into a live vaccine and, given the year, probably a live vaccine against polio. There is no record of whether a live vaccine made in mandrill tissue culture was ever used in an experimental trial, but if it was, then the Mitzic vaccination must be a candidate. Mitzic lies at the heart of the mandrill's range, which includes Gabon, Equatorial Guinea, southern Cameroon, and southwestern Congo Brazzaville. Furthermore, the mandrill is host to a unique SIV, one of the five major lineages of primate immunodeficiency viruses — and some believe the oldest.[35]

---

Altogether, scattered through the literature of the fifties, there are reports of poliovirus being successfully grown in the tissues of 30 different nonhuman primates. These are the rhesus and cynomolgus macaques from Asia, one South American monkey (the capuchin), and 27 different species from Africa, including the chimpanzee (tested by Jezierski) and the sooty mangabey (tested by Hsiung and Melnick).[36]

Most of this work was purely for research purposes. But several of these substrates were later used to make experimental lots of polio vaccine, and it is certainly possible that some of these trial batches were then injected into, or fed to, humans — perhaps in Africa.

It is worth noting that during the 1980s and 1990s 11 of these 27 African primate species have been found to be naturally infected with SIV in the wild. Among these eleven, of course, are the chimp and the sooty mangabey, hosts to the SIVs thought to be the direct ancestors of HIV-1 and HIV-2.

# VII

---

CHARTING THE COURSE

---

*Ah! What avails the classic bent*
*And what the cultured word,*
*Against the undoctored incident*
*That actually occurred?*

— RUDYARD KIPLING, The Benefactors


*In solving a problem of this sort, the grand*
*thing is to be able to reason backwards. That is*
*a very useful accomplishment, and a very easy*
*one, but people do not practice it much.*

— HILARY KOPROWSKI, quoting Sherlock Holmes

THE HIV-2 ENIGMA

During a ten-week period in late 1994 and early 1995, I concentrated my research on a subject I had been studying on and off for the previous thirty months — the HIV-2 epidemic, and its likely sources.[1] Although I did not come up with a potential explanation for the epidemic as compelling as that for HIV-1, I did discover enough information to raise very serious doubts about the natural transfer theory, and to suggest that the hand of man might well have played a role here also.[2]

First, a brief recap. In 1985, a second human immunodeficiency virus was discovered,[3] and the following year this virus, which would later come to be known as HIV-2, was recognized among AIDS patients originating from Guinea-Bissau and Cape Verde.[4] In the years since then, virologists have realized that HIV-2 is less pathogenic and transmissible than HIV-1, that the viral load is lower (and it is therefore less often isolated from infectees), that perinatal transmission is rare, and that the incubation period is longer (with the best guess being some twenty years from infection to AIDS, as compared to roughly eleven years in the case of HIV-1). For all of these reasons, HIV-2 spreads less effectively than HIV-1, and is less equipped to break free from its region of origin to become a true pandemic.[5]

HIV-2 has been exhaustively studied, not least because of the widely held perception that the relationship with its simian precursor (which is generally thought to be SIVsm, the SIV of the sooty mangabey) is clearer than that of HIV-1. Many virologists feel that a better understanding of the natural history of HIV-2, in particular its methods of infecting cells and causing disease, might improve prospects for combating the more lethal HIV-1 epidemic.

The best review of early HIV-2 prevalence (and HIV-2-related AIDS) describes the epidemiological situation in 1989/90.[6] By that stage, it was already apparent that the virus had a distinctive distribution in the northwest of Africa, within a region bordered by Mauritania, Mali, and Niger in the north, and by Nigeria in the east. (See the map on page 339.) Outside this HIV-2 belt, prevalence fell away sharply, though several cases of HIV-2 infection had been identified in Portugal, France, and in Portugal's other former territories in Africa — Angola and Mozambique. By the early nineties, occasional cases of HIV-2 infection were being seen to the immediate east of the AIDS belt in Cameroon and Gabon, and on other continents in places like the United States, the Caribbean, Germany, India, and Brazil. In the latter two countries, historical links with Portugal seemed to be significant.

In 1989/90, the only country with high HIV-2 prevalence (of over 5 percent) in several urban and rural communities was Guinea-Bissau. The only other place where HIV-2 appeared to be well established throughout was Ivory Coast, where a medium prevalence (of about 2 percent) was encountered in many urban and rural areas. Among high-risk populations such as prostitutes and STD patients, HIV-2 prevalence of over 20 percent was encountered in Guinea-Bissau, Mali, Ivory Coast, Senegal, and Gambia — and in the latter two countries, Guinea-Bissan prostitutes were found to have significantly higher levels of HIV-2 infection than their indigenous coworkers. Geographically isolated states within the HIV-2 belt, or those that lacked international commercial links, such as Guinea Conakry (the former French colony to the immediate south of Guinea-Bissau), Sierra Leone, Liberia, and Togo, had strikingly low rates of HIV-2 infection.[7]

By 1990 HIV-2 prevalence still exceeded that of HIV-1 only in the extreme west of the HIV-2 belt (Mauritania, Senegal, Guinea-Bissau, Cape Verde, Gambia, Guinea Conakry, and Sierra Leone), mainly because HIV-1 was making rapid inroads throughout the eighties in countries in the center of the West African region. In Ivory Coast and Burkina Faso, roughly half of those who were testing positive for HIV-2 turned out to be "dually reactive," this being especially pronounced among high-risk groups and those sick with AIDS. Although it was initially assumed that these persons must be infected with both viruses, later research revealed that such antibody responses usually indicated that the subject had been exposed only to HIV-1.[8]

It is unfortunate that no attempt has been made to map AIDS incidence in West Africa by causative virus, but it is possible to make an informed estimate by adjusting national AIDS case totals according to the relative percentages of HIV-1 (including dual reactives) and HIV-2 infections detected serologically in suspected AIDS patients and, if data for these are unavailable, in hospitalized

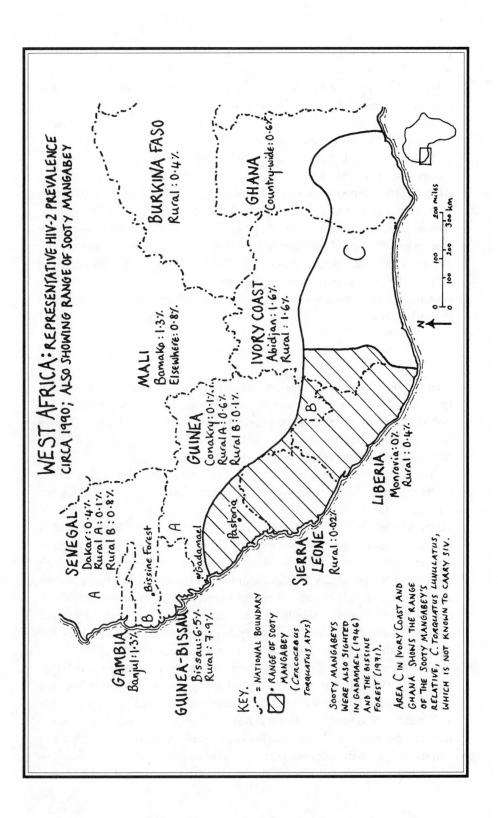

WEST AFRICA: REPRESENTATIVE HIV-2 PREVALENCE
CIRCA 1990; ALSO SHOWING RANGE OF SOOTY MANGABEY

GAMBIA
Banjul: 1·3%.

SENEGAL
Dakar: 0·4%.
Rural A: 0·1%.
Rural B: 0·8%.

GUINEA-BISSAU
Bissau: 6·5%.
Rural: 7·9%.

• Bissine Forest

• Gadamael

• Pastoria

GUINEA
Conakry: 0·1%.
Rural A: 0·6%.
Rural B: 0·1%.

MALI
Bamako: 1·3%.
Elsewhere: 0·8%.

BURKINA FASO
Rural: 0·4%.

SIERRA
LEONE
Rural: 0·02%.

LIBERIA
Monrovia: 0%.
Rural: 0·4%.

IVORY COAST
Abidjan: 1·6%.
Rural: 1·6%.

GHANA
(Country-wide: 0·6%.

KEY.
· — · = NATIONAL BOUNDARY
▨ = RANGE OF SOOTY
MANGABEY
(CERCOCEBUS
TORQUATUS ATYS)

SOOTY MANGABEYS
WERE ALSO SIGHTED
IN GADAMAEL (1946)
AND THE BISSINE
FOREST (1971).

AREA C IN IVORY COAST AND
GHANA SHOWS THE RANGE
OF THE SOOTY MANGABEY'S
RELATIVE, C. TORQUATUS LUNULATUS,
WHICH IS NOT KNOWN TO CARRY SIV.

N ←

0        100        200 miles
0    100    200    300 km

patients or those with TB.[9] In 1990, a total of 7,702 AIDS cases had been reported to the WHO from the West African region, of which I estimate that only some 1,447 (less than one in five) were attributable to HIV-2. More than a third of these HIV-2-related AIDS cases came from Ivory Coast, nearly 15 percent from Ghana, and almost 10 percent from Burkina Faso and Mali — meaning that 70 percent of all the cases in the region came from these four countries alone.

However, adjusting these figures for population produced a significant change, putting Guinea-Bissau in first place, with thirteen HIV-2-related cases of AIDS per 100,000 people, closely followed by Cape Verde with nine and Gambia with seven. Ivory Coast is now only fourth with four, and the remaining countries all have fewer than two cases per 100,000. It would therefore seem that, though by 1990 the bulk of the HIV-2 AIDS epidemic was centered on the more populous West African states in the middle of the region, the greatest density of HIV-2 AIDS, the epicenter, was located almost a thousand miles to the northwest, in the former Portuguese territories of Guinea-Bissau and Cape Verde, and in nearby Gambia.

There is considerably more evidence of archival HIV-2 infection than there is for archival HIV-1 infection, and this is partly due to the longer incubation period of the former, which means that by examining some of the HIV-2 AIDS cases from the seventies and early eighties, we can obtain a snapshot of a significantly earlier stage of the epidemic.

The earliest report pertains to an HIV-2-positive serum taken from a village in the Sassandra coastal region of western Ivory Coast in 1965. The researcher responsible for that test, Bernard Le Guenno, then of the Pasteur Institute in Dakar, Senegal, also identified another HIV-2-positive serum taken from a rural part of Abengourou region in eastern Ivory Coast in 1969.[10] Although the results appear reliable,[11] no portion of either of these archival sera remains, which means that the possibility of lab contamination cannot be ruled out. Neither are any further details available about the sample donors, or the precise villages from which they came. It should be noted that the part of western Ivory Coast, between Tai and Biankouma, where sooty mangabeys are found is fully 100 miles from Sassandra and some 250 miles from Abengourou.[12]

Le Guenno also identified retrospectively another HIV-2-positive sample dating from 1972. This had been taken from a fifty-two-year-old male from the coastal village of Kabrousse, in the Casamance region of southern Senegal.[13] By 1972 there were as many as 100,000 Guinea-Bissans taking refuge in Casamance from the liberation war.[14] Kabrousse lies just two miles north of the common border, and roughly sixty miles from the one part of Senegal — the Bissine Forest — where the sooty mangabey was still known to be present at the end of the 1960s.[15]

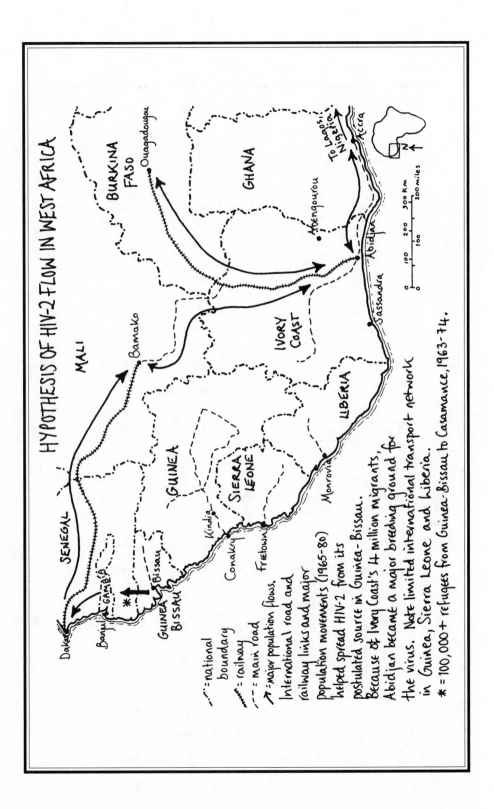

HYPOTHESIS OF HIV-2 FLOW IN WEST AFRICA

Dakar
SENEGAL
Banjul
GAMBIA
*
GUINEA
BISSAU
Bissau

MALI
Bamako
Ouagadougou
BURKINA
FASO

GUINEA
Kindia
Conakry
Freetown
SIERRA
LEONE

GHANA
Abengourou
Abidjan
Accra
To Lagos,
Nigeria

IVORY
COAST
Sassandra

LIBERIA
Monrovia

N

0   100   200   300 Km
0        100        200 miles

--- = national
        boundary
···· = railway
••••• = main road
↗ = major population flows.
International road and
railway links and major
population movements (1965-80)
helped spread HIV-2 from its
postulated source in Guinea-Bissau.
Because of Ivory Coast's 4 million migrants,
Abidjan became a major breeding ground for
the virus. Note limited international transport network
in Guinea, Sierra Leone and Liberia.
* = 100,000+ refugees from Guinea-Bissau to Casamance, 1963-74.

## RETROSPECTIVE EVIDENCE OF HIV-2 INFECTIONS CAUSED BY PROBABLE EXPOSURE BEFORE 1975

| No. | Year of birth/ Sex | Country of origin | Presumed place of infection | Probable date of exposure | Possible route of exposure | Reference |
|-----|------|------|------|------|------|------|
| 1 | 1935 M | Portugal | Guinea-Bissau | 1956–66 | Heterosexual contact | *Lancet,* 1988, 2(i), 221 |
| 2 | — | Ivory Coast | Sassandra, Ivory Coast | By August 1965 | (Blood sample) | *Trans. Roy. Soc. Trop. Med. Hyg.,* 1989, 83, 847 |
| 3 | — | Portugal | Angola | 1965–6 | Military service | 5th *Int. Conf. AIDS* (Montreal, 1989), MAP77 |
| 4 | 1933 M | Portugal | Angola, Guinea-Bissau | 1962–3 1964–7 | Prostitutes, transfusion (1966) | *Presse Méd.,* 1987, 16, 1981 |
| 5 | — | Portugal | Angola | 1966–8 | Military service | 5th *Int. Conf. AIDS* (Montreal, 1989), MAP77 |
| 6 | 1944 M | Portugal | Guinea-Bissau | 1966–9 | Military service, sexual contact | *Lancet,* 1987, 1(i), 688–689 |
| 7 to 21 | Fifteen males | North Portugal, France | West Africa | 1966–74 | Heterosexual activity | 9th *Int. Conf. AIDS* (Berlin, 1993), PO-CO9 |
| 22 | 1964 M | — | Portuguese Africa | 1968 | Transfusion | 5th *Int. Conf. AIDS* (Montreal, 1989), MAP77 |
| 23 | — | Portugal | Guinea-Bissau | 1968–9 | Military service | *Lancet,* 1987, 1(i), 688–689 |
| 24 | — | Portugal | Angola or Mozambique | 1968–74 | Navy service, Truck driver | *Lancet,* 1987, 1(i), 688 |
| 25 | — | Ivory Coast | Abengourou, Ivory Coast | By 1969 | (Blood sample) | *Trans. Roy. Soc. Trop. Med. Hyg.,* 1989, 83, 847 |
| 26 | 1937 F | Portugal | Portugal | 1969? | Wife of (6) | *Lancet,* 1987, 1(i) 688–689 |
| 27 | 1948 M | France | West Africa | 1970–5 | Bisexual sailor | *AIDS,* 1992, 6, 593 |
| 28 | — | Portugal | Guinea-Bissau | 1971–3 | Military service | 5th *Int. Conf. AIDS* (Montreal, 1989), MAP77 |
| 29 | — | Senegal | Casamance, Senegal | By 1972 | (Blood sample) | *Trans. Roy. Soc. Trop. Med. Hyg.,* 1992, 86, 301–302 |
| 30 | 1946 M | Mali | Kayes, Mali | By 1973 | Heterosexual activity? | *Lancet,* 1983, 2(ii), 1023 |

| No. | Year of birth/ Sex | Country of origin | Presumed place of infection | Probable date of exposure | Possible route of exposure | Reference |
|-----|------|------|------|------|------|------|
| 31 | 1926 F | France | France | 1974 | Transfusion from (6) | *Lancet*, 1988, 2(i), 510 |
| 32 | M (+wife) | — | Portugal | 1974 | Transfusion | *5th Int. Conf. AIDS* (Montreal, 1989), MAP77 |

A further 10 cases dating from 1966 to 1974 (2 from Ivory Coast, 2 from Nigeria, 2 from Gabon, 3 from Mali, and 1 from Senegal) were reported by Kawamura et al. (*Lancet*, 1989, 1(i), 385), but there is some uncertainty about the testing criteria used.

This was the only positive sample out of fourteen hundred sera taken from rural Casamance in 1972; when the same region was retested in 1990, HIV-2 prevalence was found to have increased tenfold, though it was still below 1 percent.

A further ten HIV-2-positive sera were reported in 1989 by a Japanese team that examined more than three thousand West African blood samples dating from 1966 to 1977.[16] Two positives originated from Ivory Coast and two from Nigeria in 1966, two from Gabon in 1967, and four from Mali and Senegal in 1973/4. These results were surprising, especially the early positive sera from Nigeria and Gabon, where HIV-2 was not otherwise recognized until the end of the eighties. However, there was a very high level of "uninterpretable" or "unidentified" readings, and the authors finished their letter: "The sera studied had been frozen for many years and/or had been thawed and frozen repeatedly, and this may have led to false positive screening tests."[17] Furthermore, it was unclear exactly which criteria had been used to establish HIV-2-positivity on Western blot,[18] which inevitably raised questions about the reliability of the results.

No pre-1980 sera from Guinea-Bissau (or Portuguese Guinea, as it was known until independence in 1974) appear to have ever been tested for HIV-2.[19] And yet of the 28 European cases of HIV-2 infection for which exposure can be linked to presence in Africa in the sixties or seventies,[20] 27 are connected to the former Portuguese territories of Guinea-Bissau and Angola.[21]

The earliest known case of HIV-2-related AIDS involved a man who lived in Guinea-Bissau between 1956 and 1966 (when he was aged twenty-one to thirty-one).[22] A formal report of his HIV-2 infection was published in 1988 by a team from the London Hospital for Tropical Diseases, who treated him for three months in the late stages of his illness.[23]

One of the doctors, Anthony Bryceson, has since provided some further details of the patient. Senhor José L. apparently ran a restaurant, and is therefore likely to have lived in the capital, Bissau, which is where the commercial life of the self-styled "overseas territory" was concentrated. He had sexual relations with many "local ladies" before getting married to a Portuguese woman (apparently in the early sixties). His first symptoms of fever, sweating, and weight loss began in 1974/5, and by the time he was referred to the London doctors in late 1978, he was "as sick a patient as we've ever had," with profuse watery diarrhea (caused by cryptosporidiosis) that led to a weight loss of some forty-five pounds. While in London, José also developed meningitis, oral and intestinal candidiasis, genital herpes, and a probable CMV infection. The doctors identified a T-cell defect and a shortage of lymphocytes, but the patient returned to Portugal just before Christmas, and is thought to have died there early in 1979. The man's HIV-2-positive widow and two children (born in 1964 and 1968, and of unknown HIV status) were apparently still in good health in 1993.

The next recorded case of HIV-2-related AIDS involved a Portuguese man who had worked in Angola between 1968 and 1974, first in the Portuguese navy, and later as a driver, taking trucks across the continent to Mozambique. He developed his first symptoms of AIDS in 1977, and died in 1980.[24] However, the second case according to the time of risk exposure involved an ex-member of the Portuguese navy who served in Angola between 1962 and 1964 and in Guinea-Bissau for the next three years; he is known to have had sex with prostitutes, but a blood transfusion in 1966 may represent his greatest risk factor. He emigrated to France in 1972, developed skin problems in 1979/80 and AIDS in 1986.[25] Another Portuguese man who served in Guinea-Bissau between 1966 and 1969, and who contracted a venereal disease there, also emigrated to France in 1972. In 1980 his wife developed her first symptoms of AIDS, as did he six years later.[26] Two French women who were transfused with this man's blood in 1974 and 1982 were both found to be positive for HIV-2 in 1988.[27]

The other traceable early European cases all feature ex-members of the military who served in Portugal's African wars between 1966 and 1974, or else partners of same, or persons transfused with their blood. The transfusion cases suggest that HIV-2 had entered the blood supply in Portuguese Africa by 1966, and that of France by 1974. Several of the infectees had apparently harbored the virus for more than twenty years without displaying any symptoms of AIDS.

Three of these early cases are known to have served not in Guinea-Bissau but in Angola.[28] However, since Guinea-Bissau is part of a contiguous zone of HIV-2 infection, and Angola is not, the former country is a far likelier source for their infections. Perhaps they stopped off for a few days in Guinea-Bissau en route to Angola — an especially plausible scenario if they were in the navy. Alternatively, it may be that they were infected in Angola by women who had previously had sex with veterans of the Guinea-Bissan conflict.[29]

HIV-2 also appears to have spread through most of Angola, especially among people displaced by the various wars that, tragically, have been waged there almost continuously over the last thirty years.[30] The virus has done the same in Portugal's other former African territory, Mozambique, where HIV-2 prevalence was between 1 percent and 3 percent in nine of the country's ten provinces by the late eighties.[31] Similarly, there is a high level of HIV-2 infection among female prostitutes in Portugal's former Indian holding of Goa.[32]

Portugal's fight to retain control in Angola, Mozambique, and Guinea-Bissau lasted from 1961 to 1975, and it is thought that at least 100,000 Portuguese fighters were present in the African theaters at all times from 1963 onward, with many thousands of African soldiers also involved. To protect the 3,000 whites in Guinea-Bissau, between 25,000 and 30,000 Portuguese soldiers were based there throughout the period 1963 to 1974, of whom 1,500 are thought to have lost their lives.[33] Others paid an equally high price — for the activities of the Portuguese military in Africa during this period clearly played a major role in the early dissemination of HIV-2.

---

Most of the foregoing information would seem to suggest that the hearth of HIV-2 is situated in Guinea-Bissau, and that young Portuguese conscripts were becoming infected during their period of military service in the sixties and seventies. The only apparently reliable information that suggests a different scenario (that HIV-2 was already quite widespread in West Africa during the sixties) consists of Le Guenno's two Ivorian samples from 1965 and 1969 that, sadly, are no longer available for confirmation by PCR.

This hypothesis of a Guinea-Bissan hearth is bolstered by the American virologist Patricia Fultz, who tested 440 Guinea-Bissan sera in 1980, and found that six (1.4 percent) tested positive for HIV-2 on three different assays. This is the earliest serosurvey to present convincing evidence of a low but significant level of HIV-2 infection in any community. In his 1991 thesis, Anders Naucler pointed out that the sera had actually come from "a rural area close to the capital."[34] For comparison, just over 7 percent of pregnant women from three "rural suburbs" of Bissau tested positive in 1987,[35] which might suggest that — in this area at least — the virus only achieved epidemic status and "took off" during the eighties. In retrospect, it seems that the first cases of AIDS in the country were probably seen in 1978 or 1979, at Bissau's main hospital.[36]

However, there are other features of the HIV-2 epidemic in Guinea-Bissau that are equally interesting. In 1987/8, a large epidemiological study conducted on pregnant women in the six major regional centers of Guinea-Bissau found HIV-2 prevalences of around 7 percent in two of them (Bissau and Bafata — the second largest town) and of between 2 percent and 4 percent in the other four.[37] Another study from 1991 reported HIV-2 prevalence of 8 percent in Caio — a rural rice-growing area on the coast.[38] Furthermore, in a large-scale survey conducted in 1986 on more than 2,700 Guinea-Bissans from all over the country, HIV-2 prevalence was found to be over 10 percent in urban areas and 7 percent in rural areas, with confirmation by at least two assays.[39] Individual results of over 5 percent prevalence were encountered at eleven sampling points in the west, north, and east of the country, and one in the south. Those tested apparently consisted of "general population and hospital patients,"[40] a vague description that reduces the epidemiological value of the study, and there is also uncertainty about the criteria required for the confirmatory tests.[41] Despite these caveats, the distribution of infections does suggest that HIV-2 was probably already widespread in most of the country by 1986.

Of course, what still needs to be explained is how HIV-2 could have spread so dramatically in a tiny state with a population of 800,000 — a backwater so remote that by 1989, when HIV-1 had swept through most of the rest of sub-Saharan Africa, only one out of a thousand hospitalized patients in Bissau would test positive for the latter virus, which causes 499 of every 500 cases of global AIDS. We shall look at this later in the chapter.

---

How did HIV-2 spread from its putative hearth? A glance at the epidemiology and regional geography allows one to trace the progress of HIV-2 outward from Guinea-Bissau and across the West African region. In 1990 the French geographer Amat-Roze published a compelling hypothesis, which proposed Guinea-Bissau and Burundi as the hearths of HIV-2 and HIV-1, respectively.[42] He pointed out that from an early stage of the two epidemics, the highest prevalences had generally been found in capital cities and truckstops — with two major exceptions being Ziguinchor, the capital of Casamance region in southern Senegal, and Bukoba, the capital of Kagera region in western Tanzania. Both were small regional centers in the heart of rural areas, but had very high HIV prevalence (43 percent and 50 percent, respectively) among their female prostitutes. According to Amat-Roze, these unexpectedly high levels of infection were the result of close links between these two small towns and the isolated hearths of Guinea-Bissau and Burundi. He described Ziguinchor and Bukoba as the "first foreign hubs" of the two epidemics.

For Guinea-Bissau, he pointed out that the years of fighting had prompted the flight of at least 100,000 refugees to Casamance region, where the people had close ethnic ties with northern Guinea-Bissau. (HIV-2 prevalence in the general urban and rural population of Casamance region was low relative to Guinea-Bissau, while prevalence among Guinea-Bissan prostitutes in Ziguinchor was far higher than among native Senegalese prostitutes. All this indicated that HIV-2 was traveling north from Guinea-Bissau, and not south from Casamance.)[43] From Ziguinchor, the prevalence of HIV-2 decreased the further north one traveled in Senegal, but the next highest infection levels of HIV-2 among prostitutes were to be found in Kaolack, 150 miles to the north, where the road from Ziguinchor intersected with the main east-west thoroughfare in the region, the railway from Dakar (the capital of Senegal) to Bamako (the capital of Mali). From the latter city, where 30 percent of prostitutes were infected by 1987, major macadamized roads lead east (to Ougadougou in Burkina Faso) and south (to Abidjan, in Ivory Coast). Abidjan, Amat-Roze maintained, had become the major "turntable" for HIV in the West African region — although the whole of the country, both rural and urban, had moderate HIV-2 prevalence. This was explained by the fact that by the nineties there were four million migrants from neighboring countries working in Ivory Coast — suggesting that some, when they returned home to plant their fields in the rainy season, took HIV-2 back with them.[44] According to the turntable scenario, the two HIV-2-positive sera from Sassandra in 1965 and Abengourou in 1969 might have come from immigrant workers rather than native Ivorians.

Amat-Roze supported this latter part of his hypothesis by citing the case of Nigeria, which brutally expelled about a million foreigners and closed its borders in 1983 (just as the two HIVs were beginning to spread across the region). By 1990, Nigeria had reported only 48 cases of AIDS from a population of some 88 million, of which just 20 were likely to be attributable to HIV-2.[45] Similarly isolated are the states of Liberia, Sierra Leone, and Guinea Conakry, which lie between Ivory Coast and Guinea-Bissau. Here, the natural geography of dense rain forest, intersected by deep valleys running down to the sea, means that there is no major thoroughfare linking them with the two countries that are the major centers of HIV-2 infection. Consequently, by 1990 they still had very few cases of HIV-2-related AIDS.[46]

———————

However, this epidemiological picture is not quite so simple because, as with HIV-1, there are different subtypes of HIV-2. The major subtype, A, is found throughout the West African region, but especially in the countries of the far west, such as Guinea-Bissau, Senegal, Gambia, and Cape Verde. Subtype B, by contrast, seems to be focused on Ivory Coast and Ghana, in the center of the region. These two types between them are apparently responsible for all the known cases of HIV-2-related AIDS, with the great majority being subtype A. There are three other subtypes, each represented by only a single known isolate, and none of these three grows in tissue culture. This fact, combined with the lack of AIDS-like disease in the three donors, and the apparent rarity of AIDS in the communities from which they originate, makes it tempting to surmise that they are nonpathogenic variants that are not well adapted to humans. Subtypes C and D are the Liberian isolates reported by Feng Gao and Beatrice Hahn in 1992; D clusters very closely with SIVsm, the SIV of the sooty mangabey, on the phylogenetic tree.[47] Subtype E is an isolate from a man originating from rural Sierra Leone, whose HIV-2 infection was only detected during medical inspection prior to a kidney transplant in the U.S.[48]

Molecular analysis indicates that there have been at least three introductions of sooty mangabey SIV to man, resulting in the HIV-2 subtypes E, D, and A/B/C — and perhaps as many as five, one for each subtype.[49] Significantly, it is not yet certain whether the two HIV-2 subtypes that definitely cause AIDS, A and B, represent two separate transfers from monkeys, or a single transfer in which two human variants diverged at an early stage (see figure on page 345).

It was around this point in my HIV-2 research that I stumbled across the great enigma. In articles on the subject of HIV-2, it is usually assumed that the natural range of the sooty mangabey, *Cercocebus torquatus atys*, embraces its apparent hearth in Guinea-Bissau. In fact, several articles (some illustrated by maps) claim that the range of the sooty extends from western Ghana, through the southern half of Ivory Coast, and then through Liberia, Sierra Leone, Guinea Conakry, and Guinea-Bissau, as far north as southern Senegal.[50]

In fact, such claims are wrong in two important respects. First, the mangabey found in Ghana and much of Ivory Coast is not the sooty mangabey, *C. t. atys*, but rather another subspecies, *Cercocebus torquatus lunulatus*, the white-collared mangabey. The official "border" between the two species is the Sassandra River, in western Ivory Coast.[51] SIV has never been found in the white-collared mangabey in the wild, although one individual living in a primate colony in Kenya, East Africa, became infected with SIVagm,[52] clearly acquired from one of the vervet monkeys (the east African subspecies of the AGM) that were also present in the colony.[53]

The second divergence from received wisdom about the range of the sooty is even more important to an understanding of the origins of HIV-2, and it pertains to the northern part of its range. During the late sixties, sooty mangabeys were twice identified in one small, protected area of southern Senegal — the Bissine Forest, some thirty miles east of Ziguinchor.[54] Another report claimed that the species was "probably" to be found in the even smaller national park of Basse-Casamance, in the extreme southwest of Senegal, down by the Guinea-Bissan border. A further report by the same author claimed, again without supporting evidence, that the monkey's rarity in Senegal was surprising, since it "was known in the two Guineas."[55] But in fact, despite several systematic searches, the sooty mangabey has not been seen in Guinea-Bissau in the last half century.

By good fortune, I managed to make contact with a man who had formerly worked on conservation projects in Guinea-Bissau, and he provided details of seven different surveys of the country's fauna, published in 1946, 1947, 1950, 1973, 1980, 1983, and 1989. The very first survey team had obtained a single sooty mangabey at Gadamael, a couple of miles from the southern border with Guinea Conakry.[56] However, all the surveys since 1946 had detected the presence of nine other monkey species, including four *Cercopithecus* species, two colobus, the red monkey *(Erythrocebus patas)*, and the local varieties of chimpanzee *(Pan troglodytes verus)* and baboon *(Papio papio)*. But there were no more sooty mangabeys, and the 1989 survey pointed out that without a new sighting, sooties ought to be considered extinct in the country. It recommended that a special investigation should be staged straightaway in the "last fragments of humid for-est in the south" — to establish once and for all whether any specimens were still present.[57] Significantly, the three surveys in the forties and fifties suggested that sooties had disappeared long before the start of the liberation war.

It began to appear that even if sooties had been present in the country back in the thirties and forties, they would have been restricted to a fairly specific forest habitat, which was apparently found only along the southern (and perhaps northern) borders. My informant explained that apart from chimps, the various monkeys were hunted widely for food and eaten by almost all ethnic groups save for the Moslems — who make up a third of the population and live mainly in the east. The preferred species for eating, he added, were Mona monkeys and Guinea baboons. Another wildlife report from 1989 stressed that monkey meat and bush-meat were generally only sold in towns that were close to hunting areas.[58]

What all this seemed to mean was that even if sooties had once been more widespread and a common source of food, few would have been consumed in the central and eastern parts of the country where HIV-2 was now so prevalent. Furthermore, the only part of the country where the presence of sooties had been confirmed was the south — the very part where there was least evidence of HIV-2 infection.

The very limited evidence of sooty mangabeys in Guinea-Bissau meant that there was a real problem for the theory of natural SIV transfer from that species to man. This was only underlined by the fact that not one of the twenty-eight archival HIV-2 cases mentioned above was known to have had links with an area where the sooty mangabey was present.

---

One can attempt to explain this apparent noncorrelation between the range of the sooty mangabey and the hearth of HIV-2 in a number of ways. One hypothesis is that HIV-2 may have been established in Guinea-Bissau for many generations, perhaps acquired in several places from a previously widespread population of sooty mangabeys, with some of those infections becoming well enough established to be passed on from human to human as HIV-2. With this scenario, the virus would have been present long before the 1960s, but it was only with the growing sexual activity in the war years that it began to spread exponentially.

However, there are several reasons for doubting this hypothesis. First, there is still no serological or historical evidence of HIV-2 infection prior to 1965. Furthermore, unlike another human retrovirus, HTLV-1, there is no evidence that HIV-2 was exported from West Africa to the New World with the slave ships.[59] Slaving from the mainland prospered from the early sixteenth century until the 1840s, with the Guinea-Bissan town of Cacheu serving as departure point for many of the Portuguese slave ships, most of which sailed to Brazil (where some 3.5 million slaves were landed at the port of Salvador).[60] Yet HIV-2 only emerged in Brazil, in high-risk groups in Rio and Santos, at the end of the 1980s, and there was still no evidence of HIV-2 infection in the vicinity of Salvador by the mid-nineties.[61]

Neither is there any evidence of early HIV-2 infection in the islands of Cape Verde, another former Portuguese "overseas territory," which lies some six hundred miles northwest of Guinea-Bissau. These islands were unpopulated until the fifteenth century, but over the next few hundred years they were settled by Portuguese seafarers and Guinean slaves, with the present population being descended from the intermixing of the two groups. By the early sixteenth century, the islands served as an entrepôt for Guinean slaves traveling out of Cacheu, a place where they could acclimatize for a few weeks or months before the long transatlantic voyage. Close links between the two former overseas territories of Portugal continue to this day, which encourages the view that if HIV-2 had been widespread in the former prior to the 1960s, then it would also have become established in the latter. However, three hundred sera collected from the Cape Verdean island of San Nicolao in 1963 all later proved to be HIV-2-negative. By contrast in 1990, a similar cohort from the same island showed an HIV-2 prevalence of 1.2 percent.[62] This suggests that HIV-2 arrived fairly recently not only on Cape Verde, but on the mainland also.

So, let us try a second hypothesis. The unusual C, D, and E subtypes seen in Liberia and Sierra Leone (especially subtype D, which is so similar to SIVsm) strongly suggest that individuals from this region may well have become infected with a form of HIV-2 through the preparation of sooty mangabey meat for the pot. Perhaps a hunter or monkey-meat seller from one of these places (or from Guinea Conakry or Ivory Coast, the other countries that make up the sooty's range) emigrated to Guinea-Bissau and brought the infection with him or her. There are three reasons for being skeptical about this theory. First, the C, D, and E variants do not grow in tissue culture, and their apparent rarity suggests that they may be equally unsuccessful at spreading between humans. Second, is it unlikely that many persons from these countries (where French and English are spoken) would be interested in emigrating to a country where Portuguese was the *lingua franca,* that was an economic backwater and that, from 1963 onward, was riven by war. And third, as already observed, there is only very limited evidence of HIV-2-related AIDS in Liberia and Sierra Leone — the countries where the sooty mangabey is abundant. By 1989, a total of 21 AIDS cases had been reported from Sierra Leone (including 16 cases likely to have been caused by HIV-2), and by 1990 just 5 had been reported from Liberia (including 3 likely HIV-2 cases). These were easily the lowest case totals per head of population for the entire HIV-2 belt.[63] If Liberian sooty mangabeys had failed to cause a significant level of AIDS among humans in Liberia, then were they really likely to have done so in Guinea-Bissau?

Another hypothesis is required. What if one of the nine monkey species found in Guinea-Bissau acquired SIV infection from the sooty mangabey, before that species became locally extinct? What if that species acquired a virus very similar to SIVsm, and then passed that variant on to man? The consumption of monkey meat is widespread in Guinea-Bissau, and it is served in restaurants in Bissau city to this day.[64] There are now several examples on record of cross-species transfer of SIVs from one monkey species to another.[65] The likeliest secondary hosts would be the chimpanzee and the baboon — the only two omnivorous monkey species. Indeed, two Swiss primatologists have observed a chimp killing and eating a sooty mangabey in the Tai forest of western Ivory Coast.[66] Furthermore, just as chimpanzees can be infected with HIV-1, and are therefore considered valuable in AIDS research,[67] baboons are the species of choice for the *in vivo* study of HIV-2.[68] If nothing else, this indicates that a baboon could theoretically have been infected with an HIV-2-like virus in the wild.

And yet nobody has yet discovered a wild baboon or chimp from West Africa that is infected by a virus similar to SIVsm or HIV-2. Also, since the mangabey locale in Guinea-Bissau in the forties (in the extreme south) is so different from the HIV-2-infected areas of today (in the north, west, and east), this hypothesis would require mangabeys to have been much more widespread a few generations ago, and (in all probability) for several cross-species transfers of SIV from mangabeys to chimps or baboons, and thence to humans, to have occurred in different localities. Even then, it would be necessary to explain why HIV-2 infection is common in eastern towns like Gabu, Sonaco, and Pirada, where the local Fula people are Moslems, and generally do not eat monkey meat.[69] Here again, it seems that too many details fail to correlate.

There is a further reason for doubting this hypothesis. Anne-Grethe Poulsen looked into the monkey-meat hypothesis during the course of a risk factor survey in persons aged fifty and more conducted in Bissau — and found that it was not borne out. Women aged fifty and more who had had experience of preparing monkey meat were almost twice as likely to be infected with HIV-2 as those who had not. Then, however, Poulsen learned that in Guinea-Bissan society, whereas women prepare most of the food, it is generally men who prepare the monkey-meat stew. And for men there was only a minimal correlation.[70]

Dr. Poulsen did, however, identify one correlation that might well be significant. She established that men who had served with the Portuguese army during the 1963–1974 liberation war were nearly five times more likely to be HIV-2-positive than those who had fought with Amilcar Cabral's PAIGC. And yet the guerrillas, living in the bush, would presumably have been far more likely to catch and eat monkeys. This intriguing correlation is bolstered by a further examination of those early centers of high seroprevalence. Between 1966 and 1974, more than half of the land area of Guinea-Bissau was effectively under the sway of the PAIGC — although the Portuguese military still controlled most of the towns.[71] Yet every single one of the seventeen towns and rural areas with high HIV-2 prevalence in the period 1986–1991 appears to have been controlled by the Portuguese rather than the guerrillas.[72]

We therefore need to look briefly at the history of the liberation war, and the risk factors that might be associated with the Portuguese side in particular.

---

In 1961, the Portuguese garrison in Guinea-Bissau totaled a thousand men. The guerrilla fighters mounted their first actions from the bush in 1962, and staged their first concerted attacks on Portuguese barracks in January 1963. Over the next sixteen months, as military reputations collapsed, the post of governor of the territory changed hands four times. Then, in May 1964, a new governor and military commander, a Nazi-trained "strongman," General Arnaldo Schultz,[73] arrived fresh from the conflict in Angola. He immediately initiated a "strategic hamlets" policy, whereby rural populations were pulled back into tightly controlled areas, allegedly for their own protection. This allowed the Portuguese military to bomb, napalm, and use defoliant spray upon presumed guerrilla strongholds in the bush.[74] But it is what went on within the restricted compounds that may be more relevant to the transmission of HIV-2. According to the veteran African historian Basil Davidson, every small Portuguese barracks had a brothel nearby, to bolster the morale of the fighting men (both Portuguese and indigenes).[75]

The failure of Schultz's approach is indicated by the volte-face embarked upon by his successor, Brigadier Antonio De Spinola, who was governor between the years of 1968 and 1973. In a belated effort to win back popular support, De Spinola adopted a "hearts and minds" policy, promising the local population, among other things, the best medical care in West Africa. This was quite a departure, because back in the fifties Portuguese Guinea had probably the poorest medical services in the region. In 1954, there was just one doctor for every 100,000 Guinea-Bissans.[76]

De Spinola changed all this. A white South African journalist who was visiting Guinea-Bissau in 1971 recorded that the clinic at Teixeiro Pinto (now Canchungo), catering for a regional population of eleven thousand, now boasted ten army-trained doctors, who had "launched a massive inoculation campaign against smallpox, yellow fever, cholera, diphtheria, tetanus and tuberculosis." This clinic would also have provided medical care for the people of the rice-growing zone at Caio, fifteen miles away (the same place where so many of the population would test HIV-2-positive twenty years later). In fact, the newfound altruism apparently even extended to other Africans in the region for, as the journalist records: "Tribesmen living in southern Senegal . . . made liberal use themselves of the free medical aid offered by Lisbon. Medical aid to potential enemies was regarded by the Portuguese as of good propaganda value and they helped where they could."[77]

---

This is not to insinuate that the Portuguese military might have deliberately introduced some dreadful disease into the Guinea-Bissan population. But it does highlight the attitude of the Portuguese to the native peoples living in their overseas territories during the dictatorship of Antonio Salazar, who ruled Portugal from 1932 to 1968. The fact that policy could shift so easily from bombing and napalming to providing the best medical care in the region suggests a ruthless and fickle pragmatism, a willingness to adopt any means that might sustain the hegemony.

Viewed from this perspective, the current high prevalence of HIV-2 within those parts of Guinea-Bissau, Angola, and Mozambique where the Portuguese once held sway is intriguing. What could have happened to cause this sudden eruption of the virus? One can postulate that one individual — a young Guinea-Bissan woman from near the border with Guinea Conakry, for instance, a woman who had recently skinned a sooty mangabey and become infected with SIVsm, and who later worked in a military brothel — may have infected soldiers with the virus. Perhaps the hectic sexual activity allowed the virus to mutate to a pathogenic variant — HIV-2. Perhaps the soldiers were then relocated, both to other barracks in Guinea-Bissau and to the other theaters in Angola and Mozambique — and prostitutes and soldiers in those places also became infected.

However, there are certain clues that argue against such a hypothesis, and they relate to the age-prevalence work of Anne-Grethe Poulsen and others. In Guinea-Bissau, HIV-2 seems to have infected an extraordinarily high proportion (over 15 percent) of persons aged over fifty, with the highest age-prevalence (22.6 percent) applying to persons aged fifty to fifty-five — those born between 1932 and 1937.[78] And although every comparative study finds that peak HIV-2 prevalence occurs later in life than peak HIV-1 prevalence (if only because viral load is lower, making HIV-2 less transmissible), it is noticeable that HIV-2 prevalence in Abidjan, Ivory Coast, seems to peak in persons ten to fifteen years younger than those in Guinea-Bissau.[79] One of the possible explanations is that older people in Guinea-Bissau seem to be infected with an HIV-2 strain of very low pathogenicity — in other words, they remain healthy and do not get AIDS. This, indeed, is what workers there have observed.

However, this still leaves the problem of how they might have become infected with the virus. Are we really to suppose that 15 percent of all the Guinea-Bissans born between 1910 and 1940 (aged between their twenties and fifties at the start of the high-risk period of the liberation war) contracted the virus through sexual contact during the hostilities? Or that they became infected by preparing the meat of the sooty mangabey — a species that appears to have disappeared from the country by around midcentury? Neither SIVsm nor HIV-2 are easily acquired viruses and the above scenarios fail to explain this quite extraordinary infection rate.[80]

I would tentatively float another scenario — partly, at least, on the basis of what we know about the likely origins of HIV-1 in central Africa. I would suggest that the present-day epidemiology of HIV-2 in Guinea-Bissau is more suggestive of a virus introduced accidentally by human hand — as, for instance, during a vaccination campaign. Here, an important clue is provided by the fact than in Poulsen's 1987 study, a mere 0.9 percent of Guinea-Bissans born between 1962 and 1967 were HIV-2-positive, but that this rose sharply to 7.5 percent for those born between 1957 and 1962, and 17.1 percent for those born from 1952 to 1957. To me, this suggests that some significant event may have occurred in Portuguese Guinea between the years of 1952 and 1962.

To date, I have been unable to obtain accurate records of vaccinations conducted in Guinea-Bissau during the fifties and early sixties, which is partly because — as an overseas territory rather than a colony[81] — the figures tend to be subsumed within the totals for Portugal itself.[82] But certain significant clues are revealed by a review of the contemporary Portuguese medical literature. There is a lot of concern about polio during this period, especially after the raging epidemic in Porto in 1958, and the relative merits of IPV and OPV are discussed extensively, with frequent references to both Koprowski and Lépine, and the latter's experiments into preparation techniques.[83] Several commentators during the fifties refer to OPV as the vaccine of the future,[84] although they also highlight the danger of contaminating viruses.[85] The only time during these years that a Portuguese speaker addressed the annual meeting of the European Association Against Poliomyelitis was in 1963, when Dr. de Castro Soares revealed that, since 1958, Portugal had been vaccinating with Salk's IPV (imported from the United States, Canada, and the United Kingdom), and that "oral live vaccines are not in use in Metropolitan Portugal yet."[86] His later repetition of this fact with respect to

"Metropolitan Portugal" (the mainland) suggested that OPV might already have been used in the overseas territories.

Another article from 1959 about polio in Angola seems to support this hunch. A Portuguese doctor from Luanda writes about the raging polio epidemic of 1951, and how the epidemiology of the disease seemed to "bracket" Angola with vaccination plans initiated in other African territories, especially on black children aged up to five years. (References elsewhere in the article to the significance of air connections with the French colonies and the Belgian Congo suggest which countries she means.) She ends rather vaguely by declaring: "In Angola, the campaign of vaccination against polio sketched out in 1957 has intensified somewhat in 1958, with the acquisition of about 26,000 doses of vaccine."[87] There is no reference to whether this vaccine was IPV or OPV, but her expression of hope that polio might cease to be a sanitary problem in Africa in the near future suggests that she is referring to the oral type used by the Belgians.

There are other clues that support this scenario. Portugal was always well represented at conferences on medical interventions in Africa. In September 1958, a huge conference on tropical medicine was held in Lisbon, at which three sessions were devoted to polio. Among the attendees were Albert Sabin, Pierre Lépine, Joseph Melnick, James Gear, Ghislain Courtois, and Hector Meyus. On the Portuguese side, there were dozens of senior officials from the ministry of health, and the chiefs of the health services of Guinea, Cape Verde, Angola, and Mozambique. One can imagine the clubbable Courtois in particular, fresh from the triumph of the Ruzizi/Lake Tanganyika vaccination, firing the imagination of Portuguese colleagues for the use of OPVs in Africa.

One of the most significant speeches at the conference was a brief address delivered by Joe Melnick's colleague, G. D. Hsiung, about the comparative susceptibilities of different monkey kidney cultures to enteric viruses like polio. Intriguingly, he reported that the tissues of two African monkeys, the baboon and the red monkey *(Erythrocebus patas)*, were more than twice as susceptible as rhesus monkey kidneys to polio. This also meant, of course, that they would give better yields.[88]

In fact, Hsiung and Melnick had already, in 1957, published a fascinating paper on this subject.[89] Concerned, like all scientists working with polio, by the temporary Indian ban on rhesus exports in 1955, the two Americans compared the effects of polio and other viruses on tissue cultures made from fifteen different African species and one Asian (the cynomolgus macaque) with the effects on rhesus macaque tissue cultures. They exposed the cultures to the same amounts of the various viruses, and counted the resulting plaques — and their results were fascinating.

Some species tested, like three different subspecies of African greens, were more susceptible than rhesus monkeys, not only to poliovirus, but also to other human enteric viruses such as the Echo and Coxsackie series. Several other species, like the red monkey, were also more susceptible than rhesus to polio-viruses, but were not at all susceptible to certain Coxsackie viruses. The four baboon species tested (including the Guinea baboon) were similarly susceptible to poliovirus, but had varying susceptibilities to the others. Members of a fourth group were very similar to rhesus in their responses to all the viruses tested. This latter group included the cynomolgus monkey, the Diana monkey — and two mangabeys — the white-collared mangabey *(Cercocebus torquatus lunulatus)* and the sooty mangabey *(C. t. atys)*.

Hsiung and Melnick's paper was mainly concerned with the suitability of different tissues for research purposes, but clearly several of these tissues (just like some of the fifteen African monkey tissues described in 1955 by Jezierski) would also be suitable for polio vaccine production. Probably the best tissues of all would be those from the fourth group, which closely resembled the well-characterized tissues of rhesus monkeys in their susceptibility to a wide range of human viruses.

If the Portuguese did decide to mount a polio vaccine trial, then where better to do it than Guinea-Bissau, which represented both a small and accessible population, and the overseas territory closest to Lisbon? And if they decided to manufacture their own vaccine for such a trial, then how better to minimize the chance of nasty viral surprises than by using a locally available substrate that behaved similarly to the extensively studied rhesus kidney?[90] Of the three African monkeys described by Hsiung and Melnick as responding like rhesus, the easiest for the Portuguese to procure would probably have been the sooty mangabey, which in the fifties was described as "abundant" or "present" in west-ern Guinea Conakry, Liberia, and Sierra Leone; in the latter it was even shot as a crop pest.[91]

As we have observed, the use of locally available monkeys to cultivate polio vaccine was, by this time, already a well-tried technique. The same approach had been used by Jezierski in the Congo from 1953, and by Gear in South Africa from 1954. Lépine's group at Paris had been using the kidneys of African mon-keys since 1954, while the British Medical Research Council team carried out experiments along similar lines at Fajara, in Gambia, in 1955. It is certainly pos-sible that others — like the Portuguese — also embraced the same idea, but that their experiments went unrecorded in the literature.

---

Lastly, I must reiterate that — so far, at least — there is no hard evidence to sup-port the hypothesis that a polio vaccine trial might have been staged in Guinea-Bissau in the late fifties or early sixties — let alone one that employed the kidneys of sooty mangabeys. This is merely one of several viable hypotheses that seek to explain how HIV-2 might have arrived in humans from monkeys, and why there is such a striking epidemiology of the virus in its apparent hearth.

However, what this scenario does demonstrate is that an "artificial" introduction of HIV-2 to *Homo sapiens* (one that involved human involvement) is by no means out of the question — even if the supporting evidence is not as strong as that for the HIV-1 groups, M and O.

# 48

INFECTION BY MOUTH

As I continued my researches into HIV-1 and HIV-2, the problems with the natural transfer theory only grew. Increasingly, it seemed a fallback hypothesis — one that offended nobody largely because it was noncontroversial (save to those Africans who were sensitive about the eating of monkeys), and all but impossible to disprove, or to prove.[1] Somewhere in the airy space between there floated the fact that — in many respects — natural transfer did not tie in at all well with the historical and geographical evidence on the ground.

I decided that perhaps a geneticist could offer some additional insights into how the HIVs might have come into being. For it was the geneticists and molecular biologists, with their sequence charts and computer programs, who had now been working for seven years or more reconstructing the prehistory of the primate immunodeficiency viruses (PIVs) from the study of contemporary SIV and HIV isolates. First they deduced the branching order of the viruses, which they depicted visually by drawing up a phylogenetic tree. Later, perhaps a little less confidently, they set the metronomes on their molecular clocks, in an attempt to calculate when the viruses depicted on the tree had first evolved.

In the years since his seminal article on the dating of the AIDS epidemic, Paul Sharp had precociously attained éminence grise status. Most of his recent articles on the molecular evolution of the PIVs had been collaborations with Beatrice Hahn, the young German-born molecular biologist resident in Birmingham, Alabama, who was also widely acknowledged to be at the cutting edge of AIDS research. Much like Philip Johnson and Vanessa Hirsch in the early nineties, Sharp and Hahn were slowly — branch by branch, tree by tree — mapping out the prehistoric forest of the PIVs on a molecular level.

I went to interview Paul Sharp at the genetics department of the University of Nottingham, which he had joined a year earlier. I had expected a man in his fifties, but he turned out to be two decades younger than that. He was aptly named and clearly knew the subject backward, but was nonetheless patient in his exposition of some of the less accessible aspects of molecular analysis. Despite the reddish tinge of his hair and his undisguised enthusiasm for the research, there was also something quite cool and detached about him.

My first question concerned his 1988 article about the "rates and dates of divergence" of the various HIV-1 Group M isolates.[2] Sharp told me that he and Wen-Hsiung Li still stood by all their findings. The branching order was almost certainly correct, and furthermore, they felt that they had set the molecular clock correctly too, with the African viral isolates diverging one from another (becoming separate viruses — as indicated by one branch splitting into two or more on the tree) in around 1960, and the American isolates (all of them subtype Bs) diverging in the mid-seventies. He was slightly less sure about the dating of the Haitian subtype B isolates — although the paper had suggested that they might have split from the African strains a few years before the American ones.

At that stage, in late 1994, there were seven recognized subtypes of Group M (A to G), but within three years there would be ten, delineated A to J. "All the evidence is that subtypes A to G are a starburst radiation," he went on, explaining that all the Group M subtypes seemed to emerge from the root of the tree — save for subtype B (the type that had infected people in the Caribbean, America, and Europe), which appeared to have branched from subtype D a little later than the others. He agreed that it could well be that a variant of D had "escaped" from Africa to one of these other places, where it had evolved separately into B.

Sharp told me that the first draft of the article had actually been written in 1986, and added: "I think we were very lucky. We came up with an answer which now looks very sensible." Other more recent articles had proposed very similar dates and evolutionary rates,[3] but none of them went so far as to propose a time for when HIV-1 had first appeared in humans. If Sharp's setting of the clock was correct, it had to be before 1960, but how long before remained unanswered.

---

At one stage, Sharp and Li had written a brief letter to *Nature* proposing that divergence between the HIV-1, HIV-2, and SIVagm arms of the tree had occurred 150 years ago,[4] but Sharp told me he now believed that it had happened "much, much earlier," and that the common ancestor of the two human viruses must have been found in monkeys. He added that the molecular clock appeared to be calibrated differently for the SIVs than for the HIVs, and that the divergence of the SIVs had quite possibly occurred several million years ago, when the different Old World monkey species started to evolve.

Sharp explained that sometimes the branches of the PIV phylogenetic tree represented viruses that had diverged with the speciation* of the hosts. Apparently this had happened with the SIVagm viruses, for different variants were found in the AGM subspecies that inhabited different parts of Africa.[5] However, the PIV tree and the primate family tree were not identical, which meant that some of the PIV branches had to represent cross-species transfers between hosts. For instance the SIV found in the Sykes' monkey (SIVsyk) was very different from the SIVagm range, and yet the host was a closely related *Cercopithecus* species.[6] Other examples of cross-species transfers included the transfers that had occurred in primate research centers from sooty mangabeys to macaques, and the recent discovery of an SIV that had crossed from an AGM to a baboon.

With respect to humans, there appeared to have been between three and five transfers from sooty mangabeys to produce the different "clades," or subgroups, of HIV-2,[7] while HIV-1 Group O and Group M also appeared to require at least two transfers from chimps.[8] The human species was thus far the only one to be infected with two very different PIVs — HIV-1 and HIV-2.

Sharp agreed that the most likely explanation for the origins of HIV-1 Group M and Group O was that two separate chimp SIVs had crossed to humans, but added that an alternative explanation might be that SIVcpz and HIV-1 had both originated independently from a common source. Both chimps and humans are omnivorous, and perhaps over the centuries both had eaten the same monkey species and got infected with a very similar strain. I said that this seemed far-fetched, but Sharp reminded me about the SIV-positive African green monkey from South Africa, the virus of which seemed to create some HIV-1-like bands on Western blot.[9] "Let's find the close simian relative to HIV-1," he said, indicating that he thought that there were even closer relatives than the existing isolates of SIVcpz. I asked whether it might be worth looking at *Pan paniscus* (pygmy chimps or bonobos) for an HIV-1-like virus, and he told me that just three days earlier he had mentioned in a fax to Beatrice Hahn that he wished someone would discover an SIV in a pygmy chimp.

It emerged that molecular biologists were still not certain whether the starburst of different HIV-1 clades, or subtypes, had occurred before or after the crossover to humans — whether there had been a single cross-species transmission to produce Group M, and another for Group O, or if there had been several transfers for each.

After we had talked the whole afternoon, and as the sky grew dark outside, I outlined the OPV/AIDS theory to Paul Sharp in more detail. His first reaction

---

* Speciation: When one species evolves (or branches) into two different species.

was that it would be difficult to correlate the HIV-1 trees with the evidence of spread. I pointed out that various pools of poliovirus, and various lots of those pools, had been produced, and then distributed as vaccine to different parts of central Africa. I further suggested that if one lot had become contaminated with different quasispecies of SIVcpz variants, as would be found in the kidneys of an infected chimpanzee, then this might represent the origin of the different subtypes. Alternatively, different vaccine lots could have been prepared from the kidneys of two or more SIV-infected chimps. Paul Sharp cautiously acknowledged that his papers on phylogeny contained nothing to oppose the theory — and also conceded that if the theory was correct, this could help explain the Group M starburst. But beyond that, he avoided making any response, saying merely that he would have to think about it further.

And this, indeed, is what he did. We exchanged several letters over the next year, and he sent me copies of his various articles, which, by this stage, were appearing thick and fast. One of his letters contained details of Beatrice Hahn's immediate response to the OPV/AIDS theory, delivered during a phone conversation — most of which centered on how the vaccine had been made and whether, in practice, it was feasible for it to have been contaminated. Some of these questions were readily answered; others could not be answered because the finer details of the manufacturing process had never been revealed. But by this stage, I knew that it was Dr. Hahn whom I needed to see next.

---

It was a numbingly hot day in the May of 1995 when I swung the car off Highway 59 North from New Orleans, and descended into Birmingham. During the sixties, this place was an infamous center of white supremacist intransigence, but thirty years later it had a different atmosphere entirely — that of a city reborn, full of optimism, energy, and ideals. One of the foci of that renaissance has been the University of Alabama, where two of the great names of AIDS research, Beatrice Hahn and Patricia Fultz, have set up base. Previous phone conversations with both had revealed that, though they spoke of each other with deference, they were not close collaborators. One got the sense of a tightly knit scientific community, of two confident, ambitious women, and of a burgeoning professional rivalry. I was looking forward to some academic passion, and I was not to be disappointed.

Hahn turned out to be by far the more informal of the two. Dressed in a silk shirt and jeans, she was very direct, both in her answers and her questions, and every bit as alert and impatient as I had been led to believe. She brought me up to date on her research, including the latest AGM work. Apparently they had tested members of both the eastern and southern African branches of the most geographically diverse subspecies of AGM, *Cercopithecus aethiops pygerythrus* (or vervet), and found that there was very little difference in the SIV sequences, even though the donor monkeys came from areas that were almost two thousand miles apart. All this gave further support to the hypothesis that the SIVagm strains had diverged with speciation, rather than through transcontinental migration of the host species. Furthermore, it supported the theory that AGMs might have served as the reservoir from which cross-species transmissions to other monkey species had occurred. An example was the SIVagm virus found in a Tanzanian baboon, which had probably acquired it by attacking and eating a green monkey from a nearby troop.[10]

Beatrice Hahn also provided further details on the two new subtypes of HIV-2 from Liberia.[11] She explained that according to her hypothesis, the two infectees had probably acquired their viruses as a result of hunting monkeys — or they might have had sex with someone who had been hunting monkeys two weeks previously. Hahn said she suspected that these were both dead-end infections that could not be passed on to other humans.[12]

When I asked why she thought there was so little AIDS in Liberia, in the areas from which the HIV-2 samples had been taken, she told me that AIDS probably came about through further passages in the human host, as might occur in bathhouses, or where a virus was passed from one person to another via an unsterilized needle. Perhaps such rapid passages had not occurred in Liberia. I told her that I had spoken to an Australian naturalist who had visited the mining area of Mount Nimba in northern Liberia, who had told me of widespread monkey-hunting by the miners, and of "Sodom and Gomorrah–like scenes" in the brothels of the nearby shantytown. OK, said Hahn, but perhaps nobody ever caught SIVsm from a monkey in the Mount Nimba area.

She added that they had tested thirty hunters, not one of whom had been HIV-2-positive, which suggested that transfer from monkey to monkey hunter was not a frequent event. Such transfers could have occurred in the past, she added, even leading to small flare-ups of AIDS, which would then die down again, leaving no trace. I said that there was certainly no evidence of such a flare-up in any part of Africa since medical papers on Africa started to appear, at about the beginning of the century. Nonetheless, I was impressed. This was almost the first time that I had met a proponent of the natural transfer school who had thought the arguments through to their logical conclusions.

––––––––––

We did not have time to talk about the OPV/AIDS theory that day, but agreed to meet again the following morning, so that I could expound the hypothesis. But the next day's meeting did not go well. Maybe Hahn felt that I had already taken too much of her time, or perhaps it was something to do with her forceful personality, but somehow my intended exposition never really got off the ground.

I started by pointing out the noncorrelation on a microcosmic scale between SIVsm and HIV-2 on the map of West Africa, and Hahn said that this was a moot point, but that there wasn't the systematic screening data available to prove it either way. She suggested that it might be that someone from Liberia had been infected with HIV-2 subtype A, and had then gone to Guinea-Bissau and started the epidemic there — that we just couldn't know such things. I pointed out that nobody had yet isolated a subtype A from Liberia — just a C and a D, which she was telling me were both dead-end infections. Furthermore, there appeared to be no HIV-2-related AIDS epidemic in Liberia. By contrast the epidemic in Guinea-Bissau (which seemed to be exclusively of subtype A) seemed far too deeply rooted and widespread to be started by just the one visitor, unless he or she was quite remarkably promiscuous, infectious, and widely traveled.

In her phone conversation with Paul Sharp about the OPV/AIDS theory, Hahn had suggested that SIV administered orally would be destroyed by the gastric juices in the digestive tract, but I reminded her that various articles had highlighted the importance of dendritic cells (such as those found in the tonsils) and Langerhans cells (found in the mouth) as receptor cells for HIV and SIV.[13] Furthermore, the fact that children had seroconverted after breast feeding, and gay men after having only oral sex, showed that acquiring HIV infection through the mucosa of mouth and throat was entirely viable. I pointed out that this could be exacerbated if somebody bit their tongue just before they were vaccinated, or if they had mouth ulcers or other oral lesions. In addition, several of the vaccinees were infants, and therefore had vulnerable immune systems.

But this was about as far as I got. Before I had a chance to go on, Hahn took over the floor, and proceeded to tell me why she thought that theories such as this one had no merit. I responded to her statements and inquiries as best I could, but nonetheless found being the questioned rather than the questioner an uncomfortable experience. Of course, I was not unaware that there might be some poetic justice here — the interviewer hoist with his own petard.

First she asked how this hypothesis would work physically — how could a polio vaccine transmit HIV? I told her that the key seemed to lie in the culture medium, the monkey kidney cells, in which the attenuated poliovirus had been grown. All right, she said, let's suppose that they didn't only use African greens, let's suppose that they also used chimps for some reason. The most important point, she went on, was that even if there were mononuclear cells (lymphocytes and macrophages) in the cell culture, how many could there be? Even if the lymphocytes contained SIV, would there really be a sufficient quantity to start an infection? She said that even in needlestick accidents involving persons who were jabbed with a needle that had just taken HIV-positive blood, only very few resulted in a new infection.

She carried on firing questions. What did they do with the culture super-natant* from the vaccine virus, before it ended up in a vial of vaccine? I said that it was filtered for bacteria, and then tested in monkeys and other animals to see if there were any obvious viral contaminants. Was it concentrated? By now I was getting somewhat flustered, but eventually I told her that it wasn't, but that it was usually diluted with saline solution before use. "The HIV particle [virion] is extremely labile [unstable], OK?" she responded. "And the idea that a single particle in a soup would give you an infection is simply naive. It doesn't."

I said I didn't think it was naive when one looked at the huge numbers vac-cinated. "You need to go over a certain threshold of infectious particles," she said. I asked her what kind of threshold, and she replied that nobody had tested this in humans. So, I asked, how did she know? Because, she said, people had carried out similar experiments to find out how many infectious SIV particles were required (either by intravenous injection or by mucosal infection) to establish infection in macaques. She said I should find out how many infectious particles were needed, and then work out whether it was remotely possible that contaminated tissue cultures could have contained a high enough titer of SIV to infect humans.

She told me that she knew the biology as well as the genetics, and that it was "far-fetched that you would have [high] enough titers on eight separate occa-sions to introduce eight separate subtypes, in such a way that [they] keep spreading in the population."[14] She explained that a virus would have to "evolve in a certain direction for some time in order to become a subtype," and that she had no idea "what type of geographical or social mechanism was required" to do that. My feeling was that several Lindi chimps infected with different vari-ants of SIV providing kidneys for a vaccine that was fed in many places was a scenario that could explain this — or even a single contaminated kidney being used to make vaccine that infected people with SIV at different vaccination sites, so that several human-adapted strains evolved separately (depending on the healthiness and genomes of the various hosts) and in isolation from each other. But by this stage the debate was hectic, and I never got to express this idea.

Beatrice Hahn added that if I was seriously pursuing this hypothesis, then I had to find out all the vaccine production steps, to see if it was viable that con-taminating cells could survive to the finished product. This was an excellent point, and almost the first time that anyone I had spoken with had addressed this focal question. She went on to explain that if the vaccine preparation had been left on a lab bench for three days to a week, then the chances were that all the virus would be dead. (This was not strictly correct, for HIV remains stable

---

* Supernatant: The liquid above a tissue culture preparation (e.g., oral attenuated poliovirus), which, after filtration, becomes the vaccine.

at room temperature for several days, and after a week there is only a "slight decrease" in living virus particles.[15] In any case, the vaccine should have been kept refrigerated at all times, so that the attenuated poliovirus would still be viable when fed to humans.) She said that if the tissue cultures had been centrifuged, then the chances were that the viral envelopes of any contaminating SIV would have fallen off. (However, there was no mention of centrifuging in the literature on CHAT.) I said that as far as I knew the only material hostile to SIV or HIV that might have been introduced to the tissue cultures would have been the trypsin, which, in the fifties, was commonly used to break up clumps of kidneys into constituent cells. Even then, it was simply not known whether trypsin had been used in the preparation of Koprowski's tissue cultures. "Find out — I mean get the facts," she admonished me.

I pointed out that it was extremely difficult to follow through the production steps, because the sole description of how CHAT had been prepared had been extremely skimpy, and because Koprowski now said that all the relevant details — even the species used to grow the vaccine — had been "lost in a move." Furthermore, even though the Wistar committee had found a single vaccine vial that might have been involved in the Congo trials, this had never been released for independent testing.

Hahn said that I didn't need the original vaccine, that I could do an experiment instead. She said all that was needed was to take the kidney from a SIV-infected macaque (perhaps even one that had simian AIDS, so that viral titer would be high), make the kidney cultures, and then infect them with attenuated poliovirus, in exactly the same way that it was done in the fifties. And then inject — or feed the vaccine to — an uninfected macaque. "If you can demonstrate that that rhesus macaque gets infected, then you'll have the ears of many people. If you can't, forget it," she told me.

I thought this clever and asked Hahn whether, if I could get hold of the original vaccine protocols, she would be willing to do such an experiment. She said that she would not — because she didn't believe that it was a valid hypothesis. "I have no stake one way or another," she went on. "I don't really give a damn. Except that to some extent . . . I'm curious." To me, this was taking world-weariness a step too far. I told her that I bloody well hoped that she was curious about what really happened, and asked just what it would require to persuade her that there might be some merit to the theory. To her credit, she hesitated for a few moments. Then she told me that the only thing that would persuade her as a virologist, as someone who grew viruses on a daily basis, was if I could produce documentary evidence to show that the tissue culture had enough infectious particles, and that the processing steps "didn't inactivate 99.9 percent of these viruses."

Much as I appreciated Beatrice Hahn's no-nonsense in-your-face frankness, I was also concerned by how little serious credence she was prepared to give to the hypothesis. She demanded documentary evidence to support the polio vaccine theory of AIDS origin, but was apparently prepared to accept the natural transfer theory without any such supporting documentary evidence.[16] At one point I mentioned epidemiology, and even before I had the chance to explain some of the correlations, she had already decried the science. On other occasions she described two fellow scientists as "a moron" and "dangerously stupid." I had interviewed both the men in question twice, and felt that although they were both misguided on one specific area of research, they were certainly brilliant in others. "Nobody is brilliant who says such bullshit," she snapped back. "There isn't such a thing as a person who is a total moron in one area, and very good in another." I felt that her own brilliance was perhaps colored by an unwillingness to suffer those less brilliant, or to appreciate those who had different areas of expertise.

Clearly she was now fretting to get back to work, and finally we agreed that she would examine my arguments in their totality, when they came out in the book. I asked her once more about minimum infectious doses, and she told me that I was about to see the right person. "Go and ask Pat Fultz," she said, chivvying me from her office. "That's what her life is about, that's what she does. Mucosally, intravenously, different strains . . . you name it, she's got it."

—————

Patricia Fultz turned out to be Beatrice Hahn's alter ego: perhaps a few years older, smartly and conservatively dressed, and considerably gentler in manner. I had sent her a couple of letters in the past, and she had replied in considerable detail about her work with the highly pathogenic SIVsmm(PBj14), an SIV strain from a sooty mangabey that was so virulent that pig-tailed macaques infected with it died within a couple of weeks, with their intestinal tissues simply melting away. This was a completely different disease presentation from normal simian AIDS.[17]

I asked Pat Fultz to tell me what was the minimum infectious dose for SIV in macaques and HIV-1 in chimps. She replied that in the case of retroviruses like SIV and HIV, which mutate so rapidly that they produce quasispecies of very similar variants, an infectious dose generally meant one (or perhaps two) infectious virions, plus perhaps a thousand or so noninfectious virions (variants that had developed mutations that did not allow them to propagate). The latter figure varied widely with every stock of virus, but it was always a large figure compared to the former. However, virions could only be seen and counted using an electron microscope, so the easier concept to deal with was the 50 percent animal infectious dose (AID50), which was calculated by diluting the virus stock until it would infect only half of the test monkeys. This was generally reckoned to equate with a 50 percent tissue culture infecting dose (TCID50); in other words, the same quantity of virus should infect the same cells *in vivo* and *in vitro*.

She told me that AID50 differed according to the route by which the virus was administered, be it intrarectally, intravaginally, orally, or intravenously. For both SIV in macaques and HIV-1 in chimpanzees, a lower dose was required for intravenous infection than infection through any of the three mucosal routes. Oral infection, she said, could require between ten and a thousand times more virus than injecting virus straight into the bloodstream. But then I asked whether, if there were breaks in the oral mucosa (like mouth ulcers or bleeding gums), this would render oral infection as effective as intravenous infection. "Yes; it's generally considered that that is so," Fultz answered.

She added that there did not seem to be a relationship between the amount of virus inoculated and progression to disease. Whether a macaque was injected with ten infectious particles or ten thousand, once infected, it would progress to simian AIDS at the same rate.

So, I said, recapping, theoretically one could take a single infectious virion and inoculate a macaque, causing simian AIDS. Fultz agreed, and told me that they had done something very similar with their acutely virulent strain, PBj14. They had taken a single infectious dose, injected it into a macaque, and caused lethal disease. This of course was a lab clone, which was already known to be infectious, in contrast to the normal population of infectious and noninfectious particles that would be found in the blood of an infected animal.

This was a significant moment in the investigation of the OPV/AIDS theory. For Patricia Fultz had confirmed that if a preparation (such as a dose of oral vaccine) contained even a single infectious virion of SIV, and if the vaccinee had lesions in the mouth, then that person could theoretically become infected as easily as if an SIV-contaminated IPV had been injected into that person's arm. Of course the quantity of infectious virions contaminating a vaccine would be a crucial factor, and could determine whether it caused a major disaster like the hepatitis-contaminated yellow fever vaccines of the thirties and forties,[18] or just a few infections. Nonetheless, just one infectious SIV virion in a cubic centimeter of oral polio vaccine could be enough to infect the human vaccinee with the simian virus.

———

Later, Pat Fultz went on to tell me about her vaccine development work. She said that she was no longer working with mangabeys, but only with chimps, developing and testing a vaccine against HIV-1. Most recently, her team had been evaluating the ability of HIV-1 isolates from different subtypes to infect and "superinfect" (i.e., doubly infect) chimpanzees, and they had discovered some very important information. They had infected some chimps with the

Euro-American strain, subtype B, but then had no difficulty superinfecting these chimps with subtype E viruses (commonly found in Africa and Thailand). Antibodies against one type were not effective against the other — which, said Fultz, "predicts that it would be extremely difficult to have an effective vaccine." Even worse, they had taken animals that had a very low level of subtype B infection (as might be caused by an attenuated vaccine) and had still managed to superinfect them with another strain of subtype B.[19] Not only had the "attenuated" HIV strain afforded no protection, but the superinfection also served to reactivate the original low-level infection.[20] This raised the possibility that an attenuated vaccine might combine with a wild-type virus to make a recombinant strain, which might be even more virulent or transmissible. From someone at the very forefront of AIDS vaccine research, these were alarming statements.

I asked Patricia Fultz about the implications for an attenuated vaccine against AIDS, and she answered that she didn't think it would ever happen, and that she herself would never get involved with such a vaccine. She said this was because HIV readily accumulates mutations with every replication cycle, which increased the possibility that new or recombinant strains of HIV would be created. She added that, since HIV is a retrovirus, there was another worrying possibility — that the vaccine virus might, with time, become integrated into the human genome, which could lead to oncogenesis and neoplastic disease (like cancer).

I wanted to know more about Ronald Desrosiers of the New England Regional Primate Research Center, who had appeared on network TV only a few nights earlier,[21] propounding the virtues of a live attenuated AIDS vaccine for humans — one in which the *nef* gene, which he felt conferred virulence, had been deleted by genetic engineering. In previous work, Desrosiers had reported injecting adult macaques with a *nef*-deleted vaccine, thus protecting them against challenge with virulent SIV.[22] Fultz told me that Desrosiers had been "vocal on the subject" for a couple of years now, but said that after her team had spoken at a meeting a couple of weeks earlier, and had given some preliminary results of their latest findings about reactivation, superinfection, and possible recombination, "my impression was he was not as enthusiastic anymore." I said that this was not the feeling I had got from the TV interview, in which he was still advocating an approach that, if it went wrong, could be absolutely disastrous. Fultz agreed. She also pointed out that in Desrosiers's own studies, the *nef*-deleted vaccine had protected the adult monkeys only after a period of eight or nine months.

Next I asked Pat Fultz to explain to me the mechanism whereby a virus like SIV could enter a new host and become pathogenic. She said that if the SIV used a receptor that was closely related to the receptor in the natural host, it could enter the cell of the new host, and if there were any spare proteins available that the virus needed, then it could replicate. As to whether or not it was pathogenic in the new host, this would depend on several factors. For instance the SIV from sooty mangabeys does not kill cells with CD4 receptors in the mangabey, but it does do so in macaques — hence the outbreaks of simian AIDS in primate research centers across America. There were many different ways, she said, in which the immune system of the new host could fail to mount an effective response to clear the virus. I asked if it was reasonable to suppose that SIVcpz — if introduced into humans — would replicate, and she said that it was, since the CD4 receptors and molecules in the two species were very closely related. As to whether or not it would be pathogenic, it was impossible to say, because nobody would deliberately stage such an experiment.

---

A few weeks before my meetings with Beatrice Hahn and Pat Fultz, a quite sensational paper had been published, which highlighted the whole question of the safety of live attenuated AIDS vaccines. Written by Ruth Ruprecht and colleagues from Harvard Medical School (where Ronald Desrosiers was also based), it reported an experiment in which three newborn macaques had been given SIVΔ3 (an attenuated multiply-deleted form of SIV almost identical to the one then being used by Desrosiers in his live vaccine research) — and all three had developed simian AIDS.[23] This was in stark contrast to the findings of the Desrosiers team with adult macaques.[24] Ruprecht concluded that because the virus had retained its pathogenic potential, such deleted variants should not be employed as live attenuated vaccines against human AIDS. Especially significant for my inquiry was the fact that these infant macaques had been given attenuated SIV orally, not intravenously.

I very much wanted to interview Desrosiers — and not just because of his advocacy of live attenuated AIDS vaccines. He had also been a member of the Wistar expert committee on the OPV/AIDS theory and, according to Brian Mahy at the CDC, had been the member delegated to arrange the testing of the Wistar's one sample of CHAT vaccine — something he had clearly not managed to achieve. Furthermore, according to Tom Curtis, it was Desrosiers who had written the final section of the committee's report dealing with the dangers of vaccines made in monkey kidneys, which he apparently considered "a ticking time bomb."[25]

Despite several requests by phone and fax, Ronald Desrosiers proved to be unavailable for interview throughout the period of my trip to the States, and he failed to contact me later as promised. Eventually I faxed him a letter containing five carefully worded and nonconfrontational questions.

A few days later, I received an envelope containing four articles, but no response to my questions. One of the articles was entitled "Asilomar: 20 Years

On" and concerned the international meeting held in 1975 at which scientists had examined the potential risks of the new science of genetic engineering. The article was written from the worldly-wise perspective of a commentator who felt that much of the concern about the potential dangers had been well intentioned, but misplaced, and it ended: "Those who would oppose freedom in the conduct of science are always with us, and we should ever be on our guard in defending the right to probe the unknown."[26] It seemed clear that Desrosiers was suggesting that those who opposed live AIDS vaccines in 1995 were similarly benighted.

Also included was a recently published response by Desrosiers to Ruprecht's paper, which strongly rejected the conclusion that his multiply-deleted strains were not suitable as candidate vaccines against AIDS.[27] It included the following paragraph:

> No live attenuated vaccine is 100% safe. The 10 vaccine-associated paralytic poliomyelitis cases that occur on average in the United States every year are the unfortunate price society must pay for the greater good of being protected on a larger scale. I do not expect, nor should anyone expect, a multiply-deleted HIV-1 vaccine to be 100% safe over the lifetime of tens of millions of individuals. What is important is the potential benefit versus the relative risk of the vaccine in the target population. This is not a vaccine approach for the general population, but is intended for high risk segments of world society. We need to remember how desperate the situation is in many parts of the world.

It seemed to me that Desrosiers was missing the point. If a live HIV vaccine should revert and spread, it would affect not only the vaccinee, but also the "general population." I was starkly reminded of the conclusion of Koprowski's address at the Geneva conference in July 1957, when he berated the audience with the need for large-scale clinical trials of OPVs with the following words: "Those of us who have worked in this field for years have to reach a point where we refuse to search indefinitely for strains which very often will fill imaginary criteria of attenuation."[28] Shortly after that, of course, Koprowski began his OPV trials in the Belgian Congo and Ruanda-Urundi.

The key question would be where one sought one's volunteers for such a vaccine trial — in which of those places where it was felt that the potential benefits by far outweighed the relative risks. Of course, the highest "high risk segments of world society" were to be found in sub-Saharan Africa, in exactly the same part of the world where the Koprowski trials had taken place forty years earlier, and where the clandestine trials of the Zagury-Gallo experimental AIDS vaccine had been staged in 1986.[29]

Ruth Ruprecht continues to be at the forefront of research into the amount of SIV (the "viral load") needed to infect, and cause disease in, macaques. In 1996 she published a paper showing that oral infection of macaques required 830 times more virus than intravenous infection, but 6,000 times less virus than intrarectal infection.[30] (This may surprise those who know that anal sex is more risky than oral sex in humans, but the discrepancy is presumably due to the traumatization of the anal mucosa that often occurs.) When asked on the phone whether a single virion of SIV could cause infection, even if given orally, Dr. Ruprecht confirmed the views of Pat Fultz by saying: "If that one virion is the infectious one, the answer is 'yes,'" but added that of course only one out of a thousand retroviral virions was actually infectious. What this illustrated was that there was not a threshold of infection as such, but that the chances of any one individual getting infected orally by an attenuated retrovirus were small. Of course, if one were talking about 200,000 individuals, the situation changed: one could then imagine that a tiny percentage of individuals — perhaps five, twenty, or fifty — might be unlucky.

In another fascinating paper published in 1996, Ruprecht and her team reported on retroviral infection studies conducted in mice and macaques, which had led her to develop the hypothesis of a viral threshold that, if exceeded, led to disease.[31] By contrast, animals with viral load below that threshold displayed a range of responses. Some cleared the virus altogether; some became infected subclinically (not getting disease); while others became immunocompromised by other factors, and thus progressed to disease at a later date. It was even possible (as Bill Hamilton had proposed back in 1993) that some members of high-risk groups like female prostitutes and gay men were effectively immunized against AIDS by early exposure to a low dose of virus.[32] The outcome depended largely on the host.

Ruprecht's work emphasizes the importance of the role played by individual host responses in determining the outcome of exposure to a low level of retrovirus (such as might be encountered in an SIV-contaminated polio vaccine, or a genetically deleted AIDS vaccine). So what, I asked her on the phone, did she think of the proposal to test live attenuated AIDS vaccines in humans? "It makes me shudder," she answered. She went on to explain that she was not against the concept of live AIDS vaccines per se, but she did feel that long-term safety studies were needed before such vaccines could be used in the open community.[33]

———————

Last, I must return to the microbiologist, Beatrice Hahn. On several points her comments to me turned out to be incorrect. An orally administered vaccine contaminated with SIV would not be destroyed by the gastric juices of the stomach — much of it would be absorbed by special receptors in the mouth or throat long before it entered the gastrointestinal tract. HIV or SIV can remain viable at room temperature for over fifteen days — considerably more than the three that she suggested.[34]

Most crucial of all was Hahn's claim that any viral contaminant in the vaccine would need to exceed a certain threshold dose before it caused infection. The work of Pat Fultz has shown that one infectious virion is enough for intravenous infection — and Ruth Ruprecht has demonstrated that primates can readily be infected by mouth. Fultz, meanwhile, has confirmed that the chances of oral infection are greatly increased if there are breaks in the oral mucosa. Such lesions would not only allow a portal of entry to the bloodstream, but they would be exactly the places where one would expect lymphocytes and macrophages — the sentinels of the body's defense system — to gather. It seemed that what Hahn had really been recalling in our interview was not a threshold of infection, but rather a threshold of disease like that proposed by Ruprecht — which is an entirely different concept.

However, Hahn did raise one very legitimate question about the OPV/AIDS theory — that of whether or not an SIV contaminant could have survived the vaccine-making process employed in the fifties. This, of course, is the most basic question of all — and one that both proponents and opponents of the theory need to confront. Unfortunately, we simply do not know precisely how CHAT vaccine was made.

Hahn had asked whether the tissue culture used to grow the vaccine virus had been centrifuged, suggesting that this would have irrevocably damaged any SIV, had it been present. Two virologists with extensive knowledge of tissue culture and virus cultivation told me that although centrifuging might have been used in the fifties to "throw down the cells" and separate them from cell-free fluids, this would have involved a "very low speed spin": not enough to destroy the envelopes of viruses like SIV, especially if those viruses were integrated into cells.[35]

One of the key questions is whether trypsin was used on the tissue cultures in which CHAT was grown and, if so, what impact that would have on the OPV/AIDS hypothesis. Trypsin is an enzyme that, since the mid-fifties, has been widely used in the early stages of tissue culture preparation. This is because of its ability to separate pea-sized lumps of kidney tissue into individual cells and small clumps of cells, thus guaranteeing that viruses such as polio, which are inoculated into the culture, have a greater surface area to infect, and therefore grow to a higher titer. By good fortune, trypsin also happens to be very effective at inactivating cell-free SIV or HIV. "Cell-free" refers to virions that are not integrated inside the tissue culture cells, but instead suspended in the supernatant — the fluids above those cells.

Before the use of trypsin became widespread, there were several alternative methods for making tissue culture.[36] These included stationary-tube cultures and roller-tube cultures (which David Kritchevsky recalled Tom Norton using at Lederle), but most significantly the suspended-cell or "Maitland technique."[37] Suspended-cell cultures were still deemed an acceptable substrate for OPV production by the WHO in 1960, even if it was concluded that "they do not lend themselves so well to subsequent observation for the presence of simian viruses and other agents [in comparison to trypsinized cultures]."[38]

The first key paper about trypsinizing monkey kidneys was published by Dulbecco and Vogt in 1954,[39] and by 1956, when Bodian, Rappaport, and Gear all published refinements to the technique,[40] Salk and Lépine were already using trypsinization to improve the viral yield of their IPVs. Later (after Koprowski left), Lederle did likewise for its OPVs.[41]

It is less clear what Koprowski himself did, especially for those first pools of CHAT produced in late 1956 and early 1957,[42] because not one of his papers relating to the CHAT and Fox strains makes any reference to trypsin or trypsinization before 1960.[43] There are, however, two clues that suggest he may have used trypsinized cultures — at least to develop the attenuated CHAT virus. The key article about the development of the CHAT strain of poliovirus states that "feces which contained virus were plated out in monkey kidney monolayer,"[44] and a later article also states that the single plaque passages had taken place in the same material.[45] The main method of producing monolayers (single sheets of epithelial cells) is through trypsinization, even if trypsin is not an "essential component" of the process, as some have claimed.

Back in 1993, an important letter about the OPV/AIDS theory, by Dr. John Garrett and colleagues from the National Institute for Biologic Standards and Control (NIBSC) in Potters Bar, United Kingdom, had been published in the *Lancet*.[46] They had carried out four experiments to investigate whether or not an SIV could have survived the vaccine manufacturing process and, in particular, trypsinization. Although such experiments could never prove whether or not OPV had introduced HIV to humans, this was probably the first time that anyone had taken the trouble to examine the viability of the hypothesis on a scientific basis.

First, Garrett examined fifteen OPV pools made by four different European and American manufacturers and released for use between 1975 and 1984, and found no evidence of HIV or SIV contamination. Second, he added HIV experimentally to MKTCs made from uninfected cynomolgus macaques, and found that the cultures did not support the growth of the virus. Third, he demonstrated that trypsin inhibited the infectivity of HIV. The results here were quite dramatic, for when he exposed cell-free HIV to standard strength 0.25 percent trypsin,[47] he found that after 30 minutes viral titer had been reduced 1,000-fold,[48] by 90 minutes it was reduced more than 10,000-fold, and after 23 hours of exposure, no detectable infectious virus remained.[49] His final experiment involved making tissue cultures from the kidneys of two SIV-positive cynomolgus macaques "under conditions used for the commercial production of polio vaccines." He found no evidence of detectable SIV in the cultures — either in the monolayers, or in the cell-free fluids above them.[50]

I eventually located John Garrett (by then retired) and interviewed him about the research he had carried out, which he acknowledged had been prompted by the controversy surrounding the OPV/AIDS theories of Curtis and Kyle.[51] It was clear that the first two experiments were more relevant to Kyle's hypothesis, which, as I have explained earlier, does not seem scientifically tenable.[52] But the last two findings were of direct relevance to the CHAT theory, and were therefore of real interest.

At first glance, Garrett's research appears to be a dramatic rebuff to that theory. However, if one looks a little more closely, things are not nearly so clear. Let us begin by looking at the experiment in which Garrett showed that trypsin rapidly inactivated cell-free virus.

First, we have no idea about how Koprowski and Norton prepared the substrate in which they passaged CHAT poliovirus in order to make up the large production lots of CHAT vaccine. It is on record that in America, "the major manufacturer and one other producer of inactivated poliovirus vaccine prepared vaccine exclusively in Maitland-type cultures."[53] Furthermore, Philip Minor, the principal virologist at the NIBSC, told me in interview that — like other vaccine producers — Albert Sabin used both the Maitland technique and trypsinization to prepare his early tissue cultures, and that it is certainly possible that Koprowski did likewise.[54] As has already been shown, Koprowski was far more preoccupied with the attenuation process than with the final substrate, so it could be that he used trypsinized monolayers to perfect his attenuated strains, and the cheaper Maitland technique to grow up the production lots of vaccine. Provided they were filtered and safety tested on monkeys and other animals, there was no innate reason not to use Maitland-prepared cells for the final substrate, for the serendipitous ability of trypsin to inactivate cell-free SIV was not yet appreciated. Of course, if Maitland cultures had been used for even part of that substrate, then the entire vaccine pool could have been contaminated with SIV.[55]

Second, even if Koprowski had used trypsin to make all his CHAT tissue cultures (those for CHAT virus attenuation and CHAT vaccine production), much still depended on the specific approach used. Garrett explained to me that in 1993 he and his colleagues had followed David Bodian's trypsinization technique published in 1956, which involved exposing the kidney fragments to trypsin for between eighteen and twenty-six hours — long enough to reduce cell-free SIV to a point where it was no longer detectable by PCR.[56] But in South Africa, Koprowski's friend James Gear advocated exposing the minced kidney to trypsin twice, for just ten minutes at a time.[57] Although this approach would have reduced cell-free SIV, it would certainly not have eradicated it.

Finally — and this is the crucial point — although trypsin would destroy most of the cell-free SIV, intracellular SIV (virus existing inside intact cells) would not be affected. It has been shown that fully mature virions of HIV or SIV can be present in many different types of cell, including macrophages[58] — and there is copious evidence that during the early days of vaccine production, macrophages would certainly have been present in most tissue cultures. The American histologist Cecil Fox has observed that monolayer cultures prepared in the fifties routinely contained both lymphocytes and macrophages, and that "the macrophage component [could] persist for months."[59] Another scientist of that era described watching "macrophages moving over the epithelial cells like vacuum cleaners."[60] Even as late as 1985 (at the beginning of the SIV scare), the British virologist Robin Weiss wrote that "in my experience, primary kidney epithelial cell cultures contain approximately 1% macrophages."[61] This is an important statement, for in the fifties (as today) the polio vaccines that are grown in MKTC employ *primary* monkey kidney cell cultures — in other words, cultures grown from the original cells extracted from the monkey, without further passage. (By contrast, secondary and tertiary cell cultures contain very few lymphocytes or macrophages.)

So, if macrophages are present in a monkey kidney monolayer, then after the trypsin is washed away, SIV can in practice bud from the outer surface of those macrophages and escape into the cell-free fluids (or supernatant) above. Indeed, it may even be that procedures such as the addition of poliovirus, freeze-thawing, and centrifuging (all of which can occur in vaccine-making) could facilitate the process whereby the cell walls of macrophages are destroyed, and fully mature SIV virions are released into the supernatant.[62] In vaccine-making, the primary supernatant is usually discarded but the secondary supernatant (once filtered and safety tested) is essentially the final vaccine, and any contaminating SIV therein could potentially infect the human vaccinee.

What all this means is that the experiments conducted by Garrett and others evaluated the possibility of SIV contamination of tissue culture prepared in the nineties, rather than the fifties. The key experiment by Garrett — in which he made monolayers from the kidneys of two SIV-positive macaques — was conducted on a very small scale, and therefore much depends on the precise techniques used. How carefully did he wash the kidneys, to remove any blood cells (including macrophages) that might have been present? (When I questioned him on this point, Garrett was able only to reiterate that he had used techniques employed in commercial vaccine production. But as an employee of the NIBSC, the body responsible for the control of British vaccines, one suspects that he would have been scrupulously careful about removing the types of cells in which SIV and HIV grow.) And what were the viral loads of the two macaques? Again, Garrett was unable to provide further details, but since the monkeys were asymptomatic, the amount of virus present in the blood may well have been low.[63] If other monkeys with a higher titer of virus had been employed (as might have been the case had he used African monkeys, which do not get visibly sick when infected), he might well have been able to detect SIV in the kidneys,[64] the kidney cell monolayers, and (after the trypsin had been washed away) in the cell-free fluids.

To his credit, John Garrett did concede that there were many ways in which his experiments might not, in practice, reflect what had actually gone on during the early days of OPV production. It was not easy, he explained, to reproduce tissue cultures like those of forty years earlier, when technology and knowledge of simian viruses had been comparatively primitive.

---

The fact is that with Tom Norton dead, Koprowski recalling nothing about the vaccine-making process, and all the relevant records apparently lost in a move between institutions, there is simply no way of knowing which precise techniques were used to prepare those early versions of CHAT poliovirus or, more importantly, those first batches of CHAT vaccine representing pools 4B-5 and 10A-11.[65]

Until such time as the detailed protocols for the first batches of CHAT vaccine do come to light, and we learn — perhaps — that trypsin *was* used, we can only say that the question of trypsinization does not impact on the OPV/AIDS theory, either for or against. And even if it does turn out that trypsin was used, this does not seriously damage the theory, because the enzyme would not destroy SIV inside cells such as macrophages, which would have been present.

But if the protocols relevant to early CHAT vaccine manufacture ever do resurface, then let us by all means stage Beatrice Hahn's experiment. Since we clearly cannot use the kidneys of SIV-infected chimpanzees to make an experimental lot of vaccine for humans, let us instead make a vaccine according to the CHAT protocols from the kidneys of SIV-infected macaques — including some with high viral load. If the vaccine that results contains SIV, then let it be fed to other macaques. Of course nobody would think of feeding vaccine experimentally to 215,000 animals, but let us bear in mind that this was the number of humans fed experimentally in the Ruzizi trial.

Alternatively, if the Mitzic trial is being simulated, then vaccine could be prepared by the Lépine method from a baboon that has been infected with SIV from a sooty mangabey. If a vaccine containing SIV is produced, then this could be injected three times into macaques, in the same way that two thousand people were thrice vaccinated at Mitzic.

However, two important experimental findings should be borne in mind. The chimpanzee is the only nonhuman primate that can readily be infected with HIV-1,[66] and this applies both *in vivo* and *in vitro*.[67] Similarly, both live baboons (of the *Papio papio* species used by Lépine) and baboon cells can be infected with HIV-2 (which, as we have seen, is equivalent to SIVsm).[68] In other words, the contamination hypotheses do seem to stand up in experimental terms.

# 49

PRESTON MARX AND

AN ALTERNATIVE HYPOTHESIS

A couple of days after my meetings with Hahn and Fultz, I had the opportunity to look round one of America's most famous primate research centers, that of Yerkes, situated a few miles outside Atlanta.

The center is located at the end of a long winding road through a wood, and is surrounded by a high wire fence to deter animal activists. Visitors stand in front of a video camera at the gate while their identities are checked, and are then admitted to the offices, which turn out to be a cluster of prefabricated huts. Behind these are several large enclosures for the various primate species.

I was shown round by the associate director, Tom Gordon, a soft-spoken man who had formerly been in charge of the sooty mangabey colony, which included the only breeding group of sooties in the United States. He told me that the Yerkes sooty mangabey group had been founded in the sixties, with a group of animals from a discrete area of Ivory Coast, though he thought that others had been acquired indirectly from Kansas City Zoo, and from a Department of Defense laboratory at Fort Knox, Kentucky.[1] The present colony comprised 150 sooties — all born at Yerkes — and included a breeding group of about eighty animals, most of which were SIV-positive. Only about 20 percent of the monkeys were antibody-positive at birth, but most of the remainder seroconverted within the first two years — which could, he said, be as a result of ingesting SIV through breast milk. There was another breeding group of some twenty SIV-negative sooties, housed in a separate area. A further fifty animals were involved in behavioral research and biomedical research, much of it relating to AIDS vaccine development.

As we walked around the facility, past the huge open-air enclosures for sooty mangabeys, white-collared mangabeys,[2] rhesus macaques, and pig-tailed macaques, and the smaller cages for other species like pygmy chimps and baboons, I noticed that the rhesus and SIV-positive sooties were separated only by a wire fence. It seemed to me that the fence was not substantial enough to prevent interspecies aggression — and possibly, therefore, cross-species transmission of SIV, though Tom Gordon assured me that it was. This led us conveniently to the subject of the likely origins of simian AIDS in primate research centers. I had already been talking about this with Pat Fultz, and now Tom Gordon further clarified the sequence of events.

It seemed that, starting in the sixties, American centers began to experience two different immunosuppressive conditions — one of which (first reported in 1983) turned out to be caused by a Type D retrovirus related to Mason-Pfizer monkey virus (MPMV),[3] while the other (first reported in 1985),[4] was caused by an SIV that had crossed species and become pathogenic in its new host. Most virologists distinguish the two by calling the Type D disease "SAIDS," and the SIV-related condition "simian AIDS," and I too shall use this terminology.

It was soon found that simian AIDS only occurred among Asian monkey species, and exhaustive surveys showed that Asian primates are not infected with SIV naturally in the wild.[5] The diseased animals had clearly acquired the infection somewhere in America — and from a species of African monkey that carries SIV asymptomatically. This was therefore a reverse of the situation that obtained in 1960, when SV40 came to the world's attention as a virus that was latent and harmless in Asian monkeys, but pathogenic in African species.

Eventually, retrospective analysis revealed that there had been at least five separate outbreaks of simian AIDS in the United States — four involving many animals, and the fifth just one. The first proven occurrence was a massive epidemic in a colony of stump-tailed macaques at the California Regional Primate Research Center at Davis. In the four years from 1976 to 1979, 49 of the 54 stump-tails died, and simian AIDS seems to have been responsible for at least three-quarters of the deaths. The earliest serological evidence of SIV in the Davis stump-tails is from 1974. However, opportunistic infections typical of simian AIDS had been occurring in stump-tailed, pig-tailed, and rhesus macaques at the facility since 1969, though these could not be proven to be SIV-related because no sera or tissues from that period remained. Once SIV had been introduced to the stump-tailed colony, it had clearly spread efficiently, with the key roles apparently being played by sexual transmission and vertical transmission through breast milk. Fighting appeared to be a less important transmission route.

Although the origin of the Davis simian AIDS outbreak in stump-tails could not be determined for certain, there were some powerful clues. Davis acquired about a dozen sooty mangabeys in the late sixties (some of which were later shown to be infected with SIVsm), and at least one of the early SIV-positive stump-tails is known to have been housed in close proximity to them.[6]

In 1978, the ill-fated stump-tail colony at Davis was broken up, with some of the survivors being sold on to other primate centers. Four of them ended up at Yerkes in 1981, and were incorporated into a new stump-tail colony there. All was well until 1988, but in the following two years 15 of the Yerkes stump-tails died from simian AIDS, including two of the animals transferred from Davis. Retrospective analysis of sera revealed that these two had been SIV-positive since at least 1980, meaning that they remained healthy for seven years or more after acquiring SIV. Of the 21 Yerkes stump-tails that were still alive, 20 tested SIV-positive.

A third episode was revealed by events at Delta Regional Primate Research Center at Tulane University in New Orleans, and here the agent of viral transfer was definitely human. In the seventies, the Delta leprosy researchers were encountering some difficulties because of the very few species that were susceptible to the disease. These included the sooty mangabey — and, strangely, the armadillo. To begin with, they conducted experiments on some two dozen sooties supplied by Yerkes, but the supply was limited. An attempt was therefore made to find a more readily available animal host by injecting lepromatous tissue from sooties into rhesus macaques. The macaques proceeded to get a lot sicker than expected; instead of leprosy, they developed simian AIDS.[7] The report of this episode, by Michael Murphey-Corb and Bobby Gormus, was the first to connect simian AIDS to sooty mangabeys.[8]

The first evidence of SIV, however, was reported by Ronald Desrosiers and his colleagues at the New England Regional Primate Research Center, just outside Boston.[9] In 1985/6 they screened some eight hundred of their primates, and isolated a lentivirus that would later be called SIV in one cynomolgus and five rhesus macaques, some of which were suffering visible symptoms of simian AIDS.[10] Two of the macaques had been involved in a serial passage experiment involving lymphoma tissue from a macaque born in the colony in 1972; another had clearly passed SIV to her offspring. The source of the remaining three infections was unknown, but it is worth noting that none of them sparked epidemics. Meanwhile, at Washington Regional Primate Research Center in 1986, an SIV was isolated from the tissue of a pig-tailed macaque that had died of lymphoma in 1982.[11]

SIV infection had thus been encountered in four different species of Asian macaques at five different regional primate centers in America. The phylogenetic tree showed that the rhesus and pig-tailed isolates (SIVmac and SIVmne) were the closest relations, while the stump-tailed isolates from Davis (SIVstm), the sooty mangabey isolates from Yerkes (SIVsm), and the HIV-2 isolates were roughly equidistant from each other on the same branch, indicating common ancestry. All this suggested two possibilities about the origins of the macaque SIVs. One was that the SIV clusters in macaque species at Davis/Yerkes, Delta, New England, and Washington could be traced back to separate transmission events from imported sooty mangabeys, with the genetic difference between the isolates representing the genetic variation of SIV in the various mangabeys imported from West Africa. The alternative explanation was that the macaque infections had a single source, perhaps back in the sixties, and that the different outbreaks since then were the result of macaque movements between different research centers, such as those of the Californian stump-tails, which took the infection to Yerkes.[12]

––––––––

As it happened, the following day in upstate New York I met someone who was able to put some more of the important pieces of the simian AIDS jigsaw in place. Preston Marx is the man who has probably done more than any other to disentangle the elements of the SIVsm/HIV-2 branch of the PIV family tree. He worked for more than a decade at the primate research centers at Davis and Holloman, and during the late eighties and early nineties made many visits to Liberia and Sierra Leone, the heart of the sooty mangabey's range, before both countries were torn apart by civil war. Marx and I had already talked several times on the phone, and he had invited me to visit him at LEMSIP (the Laboratory for Experimental Medicine and Surgery in Primates), the primate center in upstate New York where he was now permanently based as the representative of David Ho's organization, the Aaron Diamond AIDS Research Center.[13]

Marx told me that the famous virologist Carleton Gadjusek had very possibly played a crucial role in the simian AIDS story. Between the fifties and the seventies, he said, Gadjusek had done pioneering research into the rare brain disease called kuru,[14] which he concluded was caused by an atypical organism he termed a "slow virus" (though it later turned out to be a prion).[15] This research won him a Nobel Prize in 1976.

Much of Gadjusek's early work centered on inoculating pieces of brain infected by kuru (or other "slow virus" diseases) into the brains of chimpanzees, but Marx claimed that Gadjusek had also inoculated the material into sooty mangabeys at Davis. He established an infection, but then he ran out of mangabeys. So, according to Marx, "he did what any scientist would do" and tried to passage the infected mangabey brains into other animals — including, in this case, rhesus macaques and stump-tailed macaques.[16] Marx said that just as with the leprosy experiments at Delta twenty years later, he had also unknowingly transmitted SIV. The Davis macaques subsequently experienced outbreaks of lymphomas and opportunistic infections in both 1969 and 1974.

At that stage, of course, nobody knew what was responsible, and Marx told me that the disease had been "managed . . . out of the colony" by selling on the surviving animals from the stricken troops. Rhesus macaques were sent to New England, pig-tails (which had also become infected) to Washington, and much later stump-tails were dispatched to Yerkes. Marx said that the sequences of New England rhesus SIV and Washington pig-tail SIV were only 3 percent apart, indicating their common ancestry, and that Desrosiers' people at New England had recently found frozen tissues from the original Californian macaques that had been sent to NERPRC in 1970, and confirmed that they were SIV-positive.[17] This proved, Marx said, that the Davis outbreaks of 1969 and 1974 had involved simian AIDS.

According to Marx, therefore, all the simian AIDS found in American research centers could be traced to three separate experiments involving cross-species tissue transfers from sooty mangabeys: Gadjusek's inoculations into rhesus macaques, which caused the 1969 outbreak at Davis, together (indirectly) with the outbreaks at New England and Washington; Gadjusek's inoculations into stump-tails, which led to the 1974 outbreak at Davis, and the later one at Yerkes; and Bobby Gormus's inoculations into rhesus macaques at Delta, which led to the outbreak there.

This tidied up the mystery of simian AIDS in a satisfying way, but it raised some pertinent questions about the experimentation carried out at primate research centers. I was shocked by the cavalier way in which tissues and sera from one species had been introduced into other species, long after the risks of cross-species viral transfer had been highlighted by the SV40 debacle, and I was astonished that survivors from troops that had been stricken by mystery ill-nesses could have been casually sold to other centers, for use in experiments there. Furthermore, this apparent lack of monitoring and central control seemed to be echoed in other fields, like xenotransplantation (the transplanting of organs or cells from one species to another) — and here, of course, the impli-cations were even more frightening.

---

The subject of simian AIDS was fascinating for the perspective it afforded into how cross-species transfers of PIVs could occur, and I was intrigued that Marx believed that scientists were responsible — in this case through the inoculation of cells from one monkey species to another.

However, the main reason for my wanting to speak with Preston Marx was that he was the man who seemed to be doing the shoe-leather epidemiological research that might permit an explanation of the HIV-2 epidemic in West Africa. During our phone conversations, I had pointed out to him the noncor-relation between the sooty mangabey range and what appeared to be the epi-center of HIV-2 in Guinea-Bissau, and we had thrown around various ideas about the failure of HIV-2 to be carried across the Atlantic with the slave trade.

Marx began telling me something about his West African research. He said he had visited West Africa about a dozen times between 1988 and 1994, six times to Liberia and six to Sierra Leone. In the former, he had driven up and down the main road from Monrovia and Harbel to Zorzor in the north, collecting samples from the pet sooty mangabeys that he found along the way. It was near Zorzor that he took his "photo worth a thousand words," of a ten-year-old girl cradling a pet mangabey, which illustrated the close contact between human and monkey in this part of Africa. He told me many households kept pets, and of these more than half were sooty mangabeys, most of which were extremely tame. He had a photo of one mangabey sitting in the backseat of his jeep, for all the world like a four-year-old on a trip to the beach. I told him that this sort of contact seemed to have been going on for at least sixty years, as demonstrated by Graham Greene's account of a walking safari through Sierra Leone and Liberia in 1935, which twice mentions pet monkeys — and their propensity for biting.[18]

Marx also collected several live mangabeys, both from houses and restaurants (where he saved them from the pot), and these were kept at the Liberian Institute for Biomedical Research (LIBR), which had long supplied the United States with chimpanzees for hepatitis research. Later, he took two dozen sera from these mangabeys back to America, and found that two were SIV-positive, one of which provided a viral isolate. Marx added that no SIV research was conducted at LIBR, so there was no chance of contamination. In 1991 he and Ronald Desrosiers had published a paper on this first SIVsm sequence from Africa, which — just like the SIVsm sequences from sooties in American research labs — turned out to be closely related to HIV-2. Marx concluded the paper by proposing that there were ample opportunities for human exposure to SIVsm in Sierra Leone, Liberia, and Ivory Coast, either through the keeping of mangabeys as pets, or through their being killed for food.[19] Essentially, he was proposing a straightforward theory of natural transfer.

In 1990, the civil war in Liberia put a stop to Marx's research before he had had a chance to conduct an HIV survey of the human population. Instead, he transferred his investigations to Sierra Leone. He and C. J. Peters (the head of the Special Pathogens Unit at the CDC, who was researching Lassa Fever) decided to pool resources, and they collected 15,000 sera from villagers living in the northern quarter of the country, where (as elsewhere) sooty mangabeys were abundant. Marx tested some 9,300 of the sera and discovered, to his great surprise, that HIV was even rarer than Beatice Hahn had found in her Liberian survey. Remarkably, only nine of the sera tested HIV-positive: seven with HIV-1 and just two with HIV-2. Marx was discovering exactly the same paradox I had encountered in the country-by-country statistics in the HIV/AIDS Surveillance Database. HIV-2 was simply not present in rural Liberia and Sierra Leone on any appreciable level. Something didn't add up.

When they sequenced the two HIV-2 viruses, they found that one was a subtype A, while the other, code-named "Lua," was 28 percent divergent from all known HIV-2s, and therefore seemed to comprise a new clade, which would subsequently be characterized as subtype F.[20]

Marx also investigated a smaller area in the east of Sierra Leone, bounded by Bo, Kenema, and the diamond-mining town of Panguma, collecting samples from about a hundred pet mangabeys, of which only two proved to be SIV-positive. Intriguingly, they both clustered with HIV-2 subtype E, the only other member of which, "PA," was David Ho's Sierra Leonean dialysis patient from Los Angeles.[21] Later, it was discovered that PA had been born in a village just fifty miles from where one of the pet mangabeys was found.[22]

Marx concluded that the low SIV prevalence among the pet mangabeys was because they had mostly been captured as infants, and the majority of mangabeys in the wild seem to seroconvert through sexual contact. He thought that this might also be the reason why African green monkeys living on St. Kitts and other Caribbean islands had tested SIV-negative, even though SIVagm has probably been around for millions of years.[23] The sailors on the slave ships would in all probability have chosen young, immature monkeys to take on board, and perhaps none of these had been exposed to SIV before their trans-atlantic journey.

Marx also did the first-ever sequencing of SIV from wild sooty mangabeys, which involved a troop located some forty miles south of Kenema. Of the twenty-two in the troop, they managed to sample the blood of ten, four of which were SIV-positive — including more than half of the adults tested. Later, when they sequenced the four viral isolates, one proved to be a fairly typical SIVsm, but the other three were about 20 percent divergent, indicating the range of viruses to be found even within one group of mangabeys in the wild. Marx thought this was probably because young male mangabeys migrate from troop to troop to find mates.[24]

Preston Marx then tested thirty hunters and market women who sold monkey meat (which in Sierra Leone comes mainly from sooty mangabeys and Diana monkeys), and discovered that one of them, a market woman from Kenema, was apparently infected with HIV-2. He explained that she was not antibody-positive, but that he had found the *gag* gene, at the core of SIVsm, in her serum, and that it appeared to be close to the *gag* gene of SIVsmLib-1, a mangabey pet that had come from the Harbel plantation in Liberia.

All of this was starting, he felt, to make some sense. There was Beatrice Hahn's subtype D virus from Liberia, which was found to be closer to SIVsm isolates than to other HIV-2s, and which seemed to be a dead-end infection. There were the two pet mangabey isolates from Sierra Leone, and the closely related subtype E virus in the Sierra Leonean patient, PA, who died of kidney failure, with his HIV-2 infection not playing a part in the disease process. Then there was the seemingly healthy market woman from Kenema, and again there was the possibility of a closely related mangabey virus. Last, there was a confirming example from the United States — the technician who had developed antibodies to SIVsm after a needlestick accident at the Delta lab. Again, there was no sign of disease.

"All the clues are there," said Preston Marx, and at long last I got it. HIV-2 subtypes A and B were genuine HIV-2, the type that causes AIDS. But subtypes D and E — and probably C — were in reality instances of sooty mangabey SIV that had crossed to humans, but as dead-end infections that did not cause AIDS and that were not transmitted to others.[25] Marx called them "a very specific kind of infection which has been going on for eons."

My instant reaction to this scenario was that it was a beautiful piece of lateral thinking, and that Marx had, in all probability, unraveled the first half of the mystery of HIV-2. Of course, the second part of the enigma still remained. Why, in the seventies, did some of the SIVsm infections in humans become HIV-2s? Why did they become transmissible and pathogenic, and start causing AIDS?

Later that evening, I lay in bed thinking about the implications of Marx's remarkable theory of the difference between HIV-2 and SIVsm in humans. If he was right, then what it meant was that the natural transfer of SIV from monkey to human was not enough, on its own, to cause AIDS in the new host. Indeed, if Marx's sooty mangabey to macaque model was anything to go by, it needed a hell of a lot more. With the macaques, at least, it seemed that someone had to introduce SIV-infected cells artificially from another species before the virus "took" in its new host and caused disease. He seemed to have demonstrated that although natural transfer *could* occur, it was human-effected transfer that was required to complete the circle — and create AIDS. Indeed, I thought, some might go further and suggest that it was iatrogenic transfer — transfer effected by the physician or scientist.

---

The next day, we started off with a tour of the LEMSIP facility. We donned gowns, bootees, and gauze masks, and Marx showed me the macaques and tamarins, and finally the chimps. He explained that none of the experiments conducted on the chimps was lethal, that all the chimps had been bred in the United States (rather than brought from Africa), and that a "retirement facility" existed in Texas for those animals that were no longer required.

Back in his office, he got out a slide projector and launched into a formal presentation of his new hypothesis of how AIDS had come into being. He told me that this theory had already been delivered a few times to other interested parties. He began with a résumé of the various surveys we had discussed the night before. He followed by pointing out that his research had nailed down the link between SIVsm and HIV-2, but that nonetheless, the very low number of

HIV-2-positives in the northern survey had come as "a big shock." He realized that there must be a missing link between SIVsm and HIV-2.

Although there were now clear geographic correlations between HIV-2 subtypes D and E and SIVs from mangabeys living just fifty or a hundred miles away, and although his new SIVsm isolates from wild monkeys demonstrated that the virus had a much wider genetic diversity than previously thought, he had still not come up with a mangabey virus that was a convincingly close relative to the two main HIV-2 subtypes, A and B. It was then that he began thinking about the slave trade. He realized that if the standard explanation for the emergence of the HIVs was correct — that viruses present in isolated communities "broke out" as a result of the mass movements of people from countryside to cities in around 1960 — then the immunodeficiency viruses should certainly have emerged in the Americas at least a century before they did, as a result of this, the greatest of all mass population movements.

It was then that he realized that HIV-2 subtypes A and B probably did not have direct simian counterparts. For if SIVsm variants that were close relatives to A and B had existed in mangabeys and had been passed to humans anywhere in West Africa up to the mid-nineteenth century, then at least some of the eleven million slaves who had been carried across the Atlantic would surely have carried these HIV-2 infections with them. But HIV-2 had clearly not emerged in the Americas until it was imported in the 1980s.

The transient SIVsm infections in humans, however, were another matter. There was every possibility that some of the slaves had been infected with SIVsm, but because such infections would not have been passed to other humans, they would have died out after the first generation. There would be no detectable evidence of them today — unless PCR work on human bones ever became a viable means for recovering PIV.

Marx's conclusion was that there must have been another factor that caused a permanent genetic change in nontransmissible, transient SIVsm, turning it into the transmissible HIV-2 subtypes A and B, and that something similar had probably happened to turn SIVcpz into HIV-1. In a sense, he was back at the baseline paradox, though he had arrived there not just intellectually, but after proving the value of the various factors on each side of the equation. He had proved (at least for West Africa and HIV-2) that a culture had existed for hundreds of years that would allow SIVs to pass into humans, and yet the worldwide dissemination of HIV and the emergence of AIDS had not occurred until the 1970s.

The wild game handler in Liberia or Sierra Leone, be he a hunter or she a seller of monkey meat, could have been exposed to SIV-positive sooty mangabeys at any time over the previous several millennia. And yet there was clearly no HIV-2 at the time of the slave trade, or even, he argued, prior to the Second World War. Up to the forties or even later, he proposed, anyone who got SIVsm in the bloodstream probably got a transient infection for seven to twenty-one days, after which they might or might not seroconvert and present antibodies. In the case of the Kenema market woman, there had been no seroconversion, but merely traces of *gag* DNA left in the bloodstream. The same had been true of one of Beatrice Hahn's patients. But — and this was the key — there was no sexual spread. Whatever the recent change was, it was one that allowed the virus to pass from one person to another by the sexual route.

Finally it was time for Preston Marx to reveal his explanation for the emergence of AIDS. He slotted a new slide into the projector and there, on the screen, was the legend: "The Country Clinic Hypothesis." He gave the background by postulating a situation where a physician from an African hospital augmented his income by operating a small private surgery in a country clinic, where previously unknown invasive practices — like the injection of antibiotics and the reuse of needles — become commonplace. So, the monkey hunter or seller comes in to the clinic with an acute flu-like infection, a seroconversion illness caused by the entry of SIVsm into the bloodstream a week or two earlier, and wants an intramuscular injection of an antibiotic, which the doctor gives. The needle is not properly sterilized, and is used on the next patient. A couple of weeks later, that second patient gets an acute infection, and returns to the clinic for a further jab. And so it goes on. The new factor, he said, was the hypodermic needle — and in particular the reusable needle. It allowed rapid passage of the SIVsm virus from one arm to another arm, until it evolved into a new entity — HIV-2. Unlike SIVsm in humans, this new human virus persisted in the bloodstream, could be spread sexually, and caused disease.

Furthermore, he said, this was a testable hypothesis. He told me that when he had passaged SIVsm in macaques, they had got sick and then recovered. This, he thought, was similar to what happened when SIVsm was first introduced into humans: there was seroconversion, but infection was transient, and there was no fatal disease. However, if one transferred the resultant virus by rapid needle passage from one macaque to another, he proposed that there would be viral persistence in the genital tract, an increase in pathogenicity, and, finally, progression to disease. This seemed pretty reasonable to me, given Pat Fultz's work with the SIVsm PBj14 isolate, which, after passaging, had become so acutely lethal for macaques, but I had doubts that it represented an accurate simulation of what might or might not take place in the country clinic. But Marx was not to be diverted. With his experiment it would even be possible to go back to the various SIVsm/SIVmac isolates, he stressed, and then determine by PCR when the crucial genetic changes had occurred, when the virus started to cause immunosuppression, and when it became transmissible.

He pointed out that the combination of circumstances required to bring about AIDS cannot have occurred very often, and that this was focal to explaining why the AIDS epidemics had not occurred prior to now. It required a hunter to get infected with SIVsm (which his Sierra Leonean serosurvey had shown to be a very infrequent occurrence), and for the hunter to feel ill enough to go to the country clinic during the few crucial days of viremia;* it required the doctor to give an injection, and for him to reuse the same needle on his next patient or patients. "So if you multiply the probabilities, you may come up with something that's [so] rare that it hasn't yet happened in Sierra Leone," he pointed out.

"We used to talk in terms of lightning rods," Marx went on, well into his presentation mode by this point. "You know — lightning can't strike twice unless there's a lightning rod. The lightning rod's the needle. That's why it struck twice in the same place — HIV-1 in central Africa and HIV-2 in West Africa. . . . So my headline-grabbing statement is that the introduction of antibiotics in Africa [is] responsible for the HIV epidemics. That's a nasty thought."

The next slide was entitled "Loose Ends," and Marx pointed out that if invasive practices had occurred in the sooty mangabey zone prior to the Second World War, this would somewhat weaken the hypothesis. Had there been multiple tattooing on a single day? What about male and female circumcision ceremonies — were the knives cleaned between subjects? Or the smallpox immunization program in Africa — had needles been reused? On the last point, I told him that I had reliable reports about unsterilized needles being jabbed into arm after arm during smallpox campaigns in the Congo in the early sixties, which got Marx really hot. "Then this can substitute for the country clinic, if that's really true and if it happened in areas where [there are] sooty mangabeys," he said. "It has to be that," he went on, immediately postulating that intensive smallpox vaccination campaigns must have taken place in Ivory Coast and Guinea-Bissau, but not in Liberia and Sierra Leone. I told him that I had the figures at home, but that I was pretty sure that they would not support this part of his theory. I added my own belief — that the smallpox eradication program may have played some part in disseminating an existing virus, but not in the genesis of that virus.

We tossed the theory around some more. He told me that he had gone to Africa to investigate the natural-transfer hypothesis, but had come back convinced that something more was required. On this, I was entirely in agreement with him. And I was hugely impressed by his theory of transient SIVsm infections that were harmless and nontransmissible in humans, even if I had reservations about his Country Clinic hypothesis.

At this point I outlined the OPV/AIDS theory to him, and he told me his objections to it. What was the difference between this and the hunting and eating of chimpanzees, which must have been going on for eons, he asked? I said that chimp meat would usually be cooked, and besides, a vaccine was not like normal edible tissue (which is mostly muscle), but derived from a tissue culture

---

* Viremia: The period when virus is present in the bloodstream.

that had been produced under exactly the right conditions to encourage the growth of viruses. He acknowledged that if a vaccine made in chimp tissue had been fed to 100,000 people, then a rare event could have taken place, and said that the concept of a rare event was indeed important. But he said that even if chimp kidney had been used, it would be unlikely to have been SIV-positive, given the apparent rarity of SIVcpz. I pointed out that some 2 percent or 3 percent of chimp tissues tested thus far were SIV-positive, and that nobody had ever sampled chimps from the rain forest around Kisangani. There might be very high positivity in one local troop of apes (just as he had found widespread SIVsm infection in one wild troop of sooties, but zero seroprevalence in the other two troops he had tested).

———————

Preston Marx is a lovely, original thinker, and he has the energy and imagination to get out into the field to carry out the experiments that really need doing. He is exactly the sort of free-spirited scientist who will eventually crack the mystery of AIDS, through a combination of effort, spirit, and lateral thinking. However, as might be expected of someone who proposes so many original ideas, not all his theories hold up well under close scrutiny. An example of one that did not was his claim to have sequenced SIV from the skin of two red-capped mangabeys from Gabon, which he had procured from an American museum. The mangabeys dated from 1918, and he announced these findings at a conference as "the oldest known lentiviral sequences related to HIV."[26] However, by the time I met him two years later, he had to admit that the positive results had almost certainly represented lab contaminations.[27]

It is my belief that with his Country Clinic hypothesis of HIV-2 origin, Marx is also wide of the mark. First, by 1994 there were two accounts in the literature of lab workers who had seroconverted to SIV, and in neither case was there any mention of acute infection or flu-like illness.[28] Without an acute illness, it is much less likely that the hunter/market woman would go along to the clinic for an antibiotic injection during the stage of viremia. Second, HIV-2 is still happening in all the wrong places. Why did the human virus emerge in Guinea-Bissau, where there is no evidence that sooty mangabeys have been present since the 1940s (in other words, during the era of reusable needles)? And why do we see almost no HIV-2-related AIDS in Liberia and Sierra Leone, where sooties are common?

As regards the smallpox vaccination theory, the data once again fails to match the early prevalence of HIV-2. At the height of the smallpox eradication program, during the period from 1967 to 1971, vaccination was intense in three countries within the mangabey's range (Sierra Leone, Ivory Coast, and Guinea Conakry), but very low in Guinea-Bissau, where under 30 percent of the population appears to have been vaccinated.[29] This undermines Marx's proposal that smallpox vaccination may have replaced the country clinic in the genesis of HIV-2.

And lastly, if — as Marx claims — his Country Clinic hypothesis applies to HIV-1 as well, then we should have come across certain people in central Africa transiently infected with a virus that closely resembles SIVcpz. This we have not.

Preston Marx was halfway there. But still something more, I felt, was needed to explain why AIDS had erupted three times in the space of a few decades.

# 50

That classic 1975 book by Ivan Illich entitled *Medical Nemesis — The Expropriation of Health* explains it as follows: "The technical term for the new epidemic of doctor-made disease, Iatrogenesis, is composed of the Greek words for 'physician' *(iatros)* and for 'origins' *(genesis)*." Iatrogenic disease, he goes on, is illness that comes about as a direct result of the physician's intervention. It is very much a late-twentieth-century concept.

By this stage of my research, it seemed clear that there were really only two tenable hypotheses about how AIDS might have come into being. There was the theory of natural transfer — that a human acquired a monkey virus through that most "natural" of activities: hunting for food (and preparing it for the pot). And there was the theory of iatrogenic transfer — that the physician himself had unwittingly visited this disaster on the people he was seeking to protect.

Let us review the evidence. The work of Preston Marx has demonstrated that it *is* possible for a simian immunodeficiency virus to transfer to human beings (such as hunters, monkey meat sellers, and those who keep monkeys as pets). He has shown that this is a rare event, but that under exceptional circumstances the process of natural transfer works — at least in the case of the sooty mangabey. We simply do not know if this also applies in the case of the chimpanzee, but it is not unreasonable to suppose that it does.

But he has also demonstrated something that is even more important. He has shown that by itself, natural transfer of SIV to humans is not enough — *it does not result in AIDS*. His research suggests that a person who is casually infected with SIVsm will simply become a silent carrier of the virus, and will not pass it on or suffer as a result.

For this reason, he and several of his colleagues are now searching for the mystery factor that, they believe, when added to the equation, will transform a noninfectious, nonpathogenic dead-end SIV infection into a human-adapted HIV, which can spread and cause disease in its new host.

Whatever that factor is, it needs to be something that can prompt three outbreaks of AIDS (in point of fact: one pandemic, one epidemic, and one outbreak) to emerge in the second half of the twentieth century. It therefore needs to be something new, something that has come into play only recently — since the Second World War, let us say.

The traditional explanation, favored by so many of the great commentators on AIDS — including, it would seem, Robert Gallo and Luc Montagnier — is that at around the time that Africa came of age and grasped its independence, a combination of rapid urbanization, new travel opportunities, and new sexual minglings kicked the virus into overdrive, allowing HIV and AIDS to emerge from their rural hearth.

However, an increasing number of people believe that this explanation is wrong, and that the social phenomena described above are not nearly as "new" as they might at first glance seem. Let us examine the evidence that suggests that this vision of a pristine rural Africa, untouched by outside forces until the 1950s, is more myth than reality.

---

First, there is the slave trade. Approximately ten million people were forcibly shipped from the west coast of Africa, between present-day Senegal and Angola, across the Atlantic Ocean (mainly to Brazil, the Caribbean, and the southeastern United States) between the fifteenth century and 1865.[1] At least as many again died before they reached the New World.[2] At its height, in the 1840s, more than 100,000 slaves were exported each year.[3] The impact of this dreadful trade extended far into the interior of Africa, for the demand created by European and American slavers on the coasts was filled by African rulers in the hinterland, who waged war on each other in order to acquire new prisoners for sale.

In terms of the epidemiology of disease, the impact was massive, with African viruses and bacteria infecting many of those foreigners who visited the African shores and, of course, further pathogens being exported with the slaves.[4] Among those pathogens were retroviruses like HTLV-1, which passed from West Africa to the Caribbean and to the southeastern corner of the United States. And yet there is no evidence that either HIV-1 or HIV-2 arrived in the New World before the 1970s. This is significant, for slaves were taken from the whole of West Africa (including Guinea-Bissau, which was a center of slaving in the first four decades of the nineteenth century), from Cameroon, Gabon, and the interior of the Congo. This strongly suggests that transmissible and pathogenic variants of HIV-2 and HIV-1 groups O and M were not in existence prior to 1865 — otherwise such infections would have spread to the New World long before they did.[5]

Furthermore, although anti-slavery laws were eventually passed, slavery did not disappear from Africa overnight.[6] When the European and American slavers disappeared from the Congo, the vacuum was filled both by African slavers operating on the Lower Congo,[7] and by Arab slavers venturing in from the north and the east. The Arabs soon held sway over a large area of eastern Africa. By the late 1860s, almost 20,000 slaves a year were being exported from southern Sudan northward to Egypt, and about 30,000 a year from present-day Malawi to Kilwa on the Tanzanian coast, from where they were shipped to Zanzibar, Madagascar, the Comoros, and the Persian Gulf. By the 1880s, some 15,000 slaves a year were being brought down the long trail to Zanzibar from the eastern Congo, as witnessed by the explorer Henry Stanley and, later, by the writer Joseph Conrad, who arrived in 1890 at the falls that lie beside modern-day Kisangani, only to discover that the camp of the notorious Arab slaver Reshid was just ten miles upriver.[8] The last vestiges of the slave trade were not eradicated from German-held Tanganyika until 1900, and domestic slavery continued there for another four decades.[9] On the other side of the continent, the internal slave trade on the Lower Congo,[10] and the export of slaves from Angola to São Tomé continued until the First World War,[11] while slaves continued to be exported from Liberia to the Spanish island of Fernando Po up to the 1930s.[12]

The slave trade, therefore, caused massive population movements in many parts of sub-Saharan Africa until the end of the nineteenth century and, in some instances, well into the twentieth. Furthermore, the practice broke down traditional social structures, encouraging both sexual exploitation by the slave masters[13] and unprecedented sexual contact between slaves from different regions.[14] But although the areas providing the last shipments of slaves included those where chimpanzees are common[15] and where sooty mangabeys are abundant, there is no evidence that HIV-1 or HIV-2 emerged early in slave destinations like Zanzibar, Arabia, or Fernando Po.

Mass population movements in Africa did not end with the external and internal slave trade, for these were replaced in many parts of the continent by a system of forced labor, which was qualitatively little different. One example is the colony of Kamerun, established by the Germans in the southeastern corner of present-day Cameroon in 1884. The new colonial masters swiftly established plantations in the fertile lands between Mount Cameroun and the sea, and in the first few years, they imported workers from Liberia, Sierra Leone, Togo, Dahomey, Nigeria, and Congo. By the turn of the century this was proving too costly, but by establishing head and hut taxes, and by striking deals with chiefs in the agricultural lands around Foumban and Yaounde, they were able to pressurize Africans from these areas to work on the plantations. The new recruits (both volunteers and volunteered) were marched two hundred miles or more down to the coast, where they had to live in crowded barracks. They were unused to the hot, wet climate, and death rates were typically 7 percent to 14 percent per annum — yet until 1905, not one of the plantations had a physician. By 1913, just before the British takeover of Kamerun in the First World War, there were nearly 18,000 laborers, and apparently "a large proportion . . . died as a result of the migration experience."[16]

Meanwhile, in the so-called Congo Free State established as a personal fiefdom by the Belgian king, Leopold, in 1893, gangs of natives were rounded up to labor in the rubber plantations and to construct the Leopoldville-Matadi railway, which linked the new capital with the coast. African noncompliance was punished savagely — most infamously by the severing of hands. Word of atrocities leaked out, and eventually control of the Congo passed from the king to the Belgian government.

In 1911, the Union Minière de Haut Katanga was formed to exploit the huge copper deposits in the south, and new teams of labor recruiters were licensed. Their methods were still brutal and included launching manhunts, and taking village women hostage until their menfolk surrendered, to be roped together and led away. Naturally enough, this led to a recalcitrant workforce, so foreign recruiters were licensed, who cast their nets as far afield as Mozambique, Zambia, and Angola. Many of the foreigners recruited during the first decade of the mines had no medical examination at source, and death rates of 20 percent in the first year were not uncommon, with tick fever, dysentery, typhoid, and pneumonia the major killers.

The number of Katanga mines trebled to nine between 1922 and 1925, so an energetic recruiting campaign began in Ruanda-Urundi. To attract new workers, facilities were offered to wives who wished to accompany their menfolk; there are hints that the category of wives may have been broadly interpreted. This increased the success of the recruiting missions — so much so that by 1930, by which time the company was the world's largest producer of copper, nearly a third of the 13,000 Haut-Katanga miners were from Ruanda-Urundi. However, the twelve-day journey from Usumbura and the very different climatic conditions in Katanga made a serious impact on the immigrants' health, so that at the start of 1929, Banyaruanda women and children in the Katanga camps were dying at the appalling rates of 15 percent and 81 percent per annum, respectively. The company responded by establishing free medical facilities and vaccinating recruits against smallpox, typhoid, and meningitis, but eventually it was felt that the expense of such measures outweighed the cheapness of Ruanda-Urundian labor, and the recruitment center in Usumbura closed down in 1932.[17]

Meanwhile, an energetic program of road and railway construction got under way. During the twenties, paved roads in the Congo grew from 1,500 to 19,000 miles, and between 1920 and 1932 some 1,500 miles of track, including three new lines, were added to the railway network. These and other public works, such as the building of major ports on the rivers, involved further movement of migrant laborers across the land — and greatly facilitated further migrations. By 1927, one-quarter of the colony's adult male population was working for the government or private firms, and "the scale of labor migration was threatening the capacity of rural populations to sustain and reproduce themselves."[18]

The two world wars also caused massive demographic and social disruption — in Africa as elsewhere. During the First World War, there were two major African campaigns: one in German-held Kamerun, where 6,000 Germans eventually conceded defeat to a joint force of 19,000 French, British, and Belgians (with largely African troops), and the other in Germany's east coast colony of Tanganyika, where 15,000 German troops occupied 140,000 allies (nearly half of them African) for the entire four years of the war. Altogether, including porters and camp followers, over 750,000 East Africans took part in this campaign, and 100,000 died. Meanwhile, France's African colonies supplied 167,000 soldiers for the European theater, mostly from West Africa, but including 10,000 from French Equatorial Africa. The mass movement of peoples sparked a smallpox epidemic in Ivory Coast, and exacerbated a famine in Niger.[19]

During the Second World War, troops from French Equatorial Africa and French West Africa fought in France, the North African campaigns, and the Middle East. The British shipped men from their East African colonies to India and Burma. Altogether, about a million African troops (both volunteers and conscripts) and carriers were used in the Second World War, and they returned home with "very much widened horizons," thus fanning the winds of change that would eventually lead to the departure of the French and British colonizers. The second war also saw large numbers of working-class whites stationed in different African cities. Cultural and sexual exploration was very much a two-way process.[20]

To summarize, Africa did not lie quiescent between 1860 and 1960. In fact, the century following the end of the slave trade was characterized by a constant stream of peoples to and fro across the continent. As Leroy Vail from Harvard University put it: "[A]s early as the 1910s almost all of central Africa was connected by enduring webs of labor migrancy. By the 1930s, virtually no rural [population] in the region was . . . living in accordance with 'traditional village life.' . . . Thus, full-fledged urbanization . . . existed in the region for several decades before AIDS became evident." His letter was written in response to Kevin De Cock and Joe McCormick's paper about stable HIV prevalence in rural Yambuku,[21] and it ended: "In the light of this historical reality, one must seriously question the validity of the authors' explanation for the apparently uneven occurrence of AIDS in the rural and urban areas of contemporary central Africa as being the result of recent urbanization and social change."[22]

In other words, had any one of the three forms of HIV existed as a transmissible human virus during the first half of the twentieth century, and caused a low level of infection in a rural African community, it probably would not have remained sequestered for very long. In all likelihood it would have emerged in one of the large African mining centers or capital cities — and then on to the world stage. That it did not suggests that the different forms of HIV that we recognize today had not yet come into being as human viruses.

---

But what if, as some adherents of natural transfer have suggested, mass population movements and urbanization do not constitute the missing factor in the equation? What if the key factor was instead the introduction of the hypodermic needle, as Preston Marx and others have suggested? Or perhaps the new sexual freedoms enjoyed by migrant workers who were released from the traditional constraints of village life? Again, we need to look at the historical record.

There is a widespread misconception that injections were not widely practiced in Africa until after the Second World War. In fact, energetic vaccination programs and prophylactic treatments through injection were carried out throughout the interwar years, and not only in the mining areas. By 1930, a quarter of the population of French West Africa had been vaccinated against smallpox, and in 1936 a mobile vaccination team was introduced to continue the good work; yellow fever vaccinations also began during this pepiod.

A similarly interventionist approach was adopted against sleeping sickness. Between the two wars a Dr. Jamot introduced compulsory mass injections of atoxyl — first in what is now in the Central African Republic, then in Cameroon and the rest of French Equatorial Africa, and finally in French West Africa.[23] More than 140,000 were treated in the latter area alone. During the same period, the British initiated an effective anti-yaws campaign in southeastern Nigeria, next to the Cameroonian border. Medical officers injected arsenical and bismuth preparations in a process known as "bum punching." It is calculated that altogether half a million jabs may have been given yearly. The campaign lasted for much of the thirties and continued after the Second World War.[24]

Nowhere in any of the accounts of these campaigns is there any reference to needles being changed or sterilized between jabs, tasks that take extra time and manpower,[25] and that were not generally considered to be important until after the Second World War.[26] Instead, the emphasis is on jabbing arms or punching bums. Preston Marx was candid enough to admit that if there had been any major vaccination campaigns prior to the fifties and sixties in West Africa, it would tend to argue against his Country Clinic hypothesis, for such campaigns could have provided the "rapid passage factor" that he believes caused the recent emergence of AIDS. Of course, one cannot be sure that an SIV infection from a sooty mangabey (or chimp) would have transiently infected a local hunter or monkey meat seller prior to one of these mass vaccinations or mass injections. But the fact that so many such procedures were undertaken in the twenties and thirties in areas that included West Africa, Cameroon, and the Congo — areas widely felt to represent the hearths of the various outbreaks of AIDS — suggests that if the combination of occasional SIV transfers to man and multiple medical interventions involving needles was sufficient to launch an AIDS epidemic, then we would have seen AIDS many years before we actually did.

Another possible addendum to the natural transfer theory is the advent of new sexual freedoms. Let us therefore look at one specific community where the factors of monkey hunting and consumption and a high rate of exchange of sex partners were apparently combined. On Mount Nimba, which straddles Liberia's northern borders with Guinea Conakry and the Ivory Coast, lies a rich deposit of iron ore, and in the late fifties the Liberian American Swedish Minerals Company was set up to exploit this deposit.[27] As a result, the Liberian side of the mountain swiftly became a wasteland. By the time that the zoologist Malcolm Coe visited here in 1964 and 1966, he found that the miners had "killed virtually all the higher primates," for in Liberia all primates, including chimpanzees, are eaten.[28] He told me that sooty mangabeys had formerly been present in the area, but were now "very, very uncommon."[29] I was also told that the brothels of the Mount Nimba mines were some of the busiest in Africa, and that queues would start forming early on a Saturday evening, with some of the women servicing twenty or thirty miners in the course of the night.

The combination of sooty mangabey capture and consumption and a small number of women having sex with a large number of men could theoretically represent a situation in which an SIV could transfer to *Homo sapiens,* and then become a transmissible and pathogenic HIV-2 through rapid passage. And yet, even by the end of the 1980s, there had been no reports of AIDS or HIV infection from this community, and very few from Liberia as a whole. The same situation is found elsewhere in Africa. To the north of the Congo basin, where Stanley and the Arab slavers marched to and fro in the nineteenth century, and where labor recruiters wandered in the first three decades of the twentieth, venereal disease is now almost endemic, and is thought to be responsible for a localized belt of low fertility.[30] Again, we have a sexually wounded society, some of whose members have long been suffering from genital ulcers (which facilitate viral transfer), in an area where chimpanzees are quite frequently caught and eaten, and where an SIV transfer *could,* we presume, have taken root. And yet AIDS does not appear to have emerged in this region until the sixties or seventies. All of this suggests to me that chimp butchery and multi-partner sex, even when combined with high levels of VD, do not hold the key to the origin of HIV-1-related AIDS.

---

In fact, the most credible "mystery factor" to augment the natural transfer theory would probably be blood transfusions. These were already being used by Harvard scientists treating Allied casualties in Europe in 1916, but they began to be adopted more widely in countries around the world during the Second World War.[31] As far as I have been able to determine, their adoption in most of Africa came rather later — in the late forties or early fifties. The British physician Jack Davies recalls arriving in Kampala in 1945, and the fact that a government official was murdered in that year for trying to enlist blood donations from Africans. Apparently it continued to be difficult to procure African blood for transfusions until the 1950s. Hector Meyus, the Belgian hygiene official, arrived in Usumbura (now Bujumbura, Burundi) in 1952, and said that transfusions had been given for some years before that at Usumbura hospital. However, they were not, as far as he knows, administered at smaller hospitals, such as that at Rumange.[32]

Here is a technique that, in the early days, would have allowed unhindered transfer of blood — lymphocytes, viruses, and all — from one person to another, allowing not only infection, but perhaps also the rapid-passage factor that Marx and others are seeking. We can imagine that a hunter might have skinned a sooty mangabey (or a chimp), and then donated blood at the local mission hospital a month or so later, and that the unfortunate recipient of that blood might have acquired an SIVsm (or SIVcpz) that was all the more virulent and transmissible for its rapid progress through two humans.

It is certainly theoretically possible that the introduction of blood transfusions was the factor that converted transient, dead-end infections of SIV in humans into transmissible HIV and AIDS. Indeed, two Portuguese men who developed AIDS in the late eighties were apparently exposed through transfusions in Guinea-Bissau as early as 1966 and 1968.[33] However, it must be remembered that sooty mangabeys have apparently been extinct in Guinea-Bissau since the late forties, which makes it seem implausible that the Portuguese infectees might have received blood, on two separate occasions, from SIVsm-infected hunters. Furthermore, the earliest known cases of HIV-2-related and HIV-1-related AIDS (from the sixties and seventies) were apparently not linked to transfusions.[34]

It is also possible that the public availability of disposable needles and syringes, and their introduction to the African marketplace, played a role — as suggested by Jean Sonnet, Abraham Karpas, and others. The novelist V. S. Naipaul, traveling upriver on one of the famous Congo barges in 1975, observed large quantities of smoked monkey meat being sold on board, as well as hypodermic syringes, which he refers to as "new things."[35] Another writer, Helen Winternitz, traveling on the same river barge in 1983, again reported live monkeys, smoked monkey meat, and syringes being sold by the *commerçantes* on board.

On a broad level, hypotheses of origin like these — "natural transfer plus careless use of hypodermic needles," or "natural transfer plus transfusions" — provide some appealing correlations with the earliest known traces of HIV and AIDS. When looked at more closely, however, the fit is rather less attractive. Furthermore, such hypotheses, because of their nonspecific nature, are almost impossible to prove or disprove. But the key point is that they posit that natural transfers of SIVs from sooties and chimps have been happening for centuries, since man first hunted primates, but that other, far more recent factors caused the resulting dead-end SIV infections in man to transmogrify into infectious, transmissible HIV — and AIDS.

These theories, just like OPV/AIDS, propose that medical science played the crucial role in the advent of AIDS. But whereas I would propose an iatrogenic introduction of a simian virus to humans, proponents of these theories advocate a natural introduction to humans, but with modern medicine playing a significant role in onward spread.

---

Of course, such theories as these would be far more persuasive if we had some evidence that SIVs or HIV-like viruses were present in humans long before the first evidence of human AIDS. But we do not. Instead, the first instance we have of antibodies resembling HIV-1 in human blood remains the L70 sample obtained from Leopoldville in 1959, and the first reported cases of HIV-1-related AIDS are from the sixties and early seventies. Similarly, the first evidence of HIV-2 emerges in West Africa in 1965, and the earliest evidence of HIV-2-related AIDS (José L.) in 1974.

The apparent synchronicity of these dates suggests that primate immunodeficiency viruses are only recently arrived in humans, and that the process of their *introduction* was the crucial factor. It also suggests that although other factors such as transfusions and unsterilized injections are likely to have fueled the process of onward spread at a later stage, they were not essential to the process: AIDS would have emerged even without them.

Of course, it could be that nobody has yet systematically searched for large stored collections of blood samples from places like Guinea-Bissau and the Congo from the early fifties, the forties, or the thirties, to see if there is any evidence of early HIV-like viruses. But perhaps if Preston Marx and others from that school really want to put their theories to the test, they should start looking.[36]

If just one ancient human blood sample could be found containing a virus that branched very early on the HIV-1 phylogenetic tree (for instance, around the point of HIV-1/SIVcpz divergence), then this would enormously strengthen Marx's argument. And it needs hardly be added that if such a sample dated from 1956 or earlier, from before the time of the first polio vaccinations in Africa, then this would constitute a very serious (if not fatal) blow to the OPV/AIDS hypothesis. My own prediction is that no such sample exists.

---

Part of the reason for my skepticism is that so much of the available evidence from other sources — not only the geneticists with their phylogenetic trees, but also the epidemiologists and mathematicians — supports the idea that HIV-1 emerged in the mid-fifties, and from the Belgian Congo . . . in other words at the very time of the CHAT vaccinations, and from the very places where they occurred.

Various phylogenetic estimates for the emergence of the HIV-1 subtypes have been made by geneticists who have attempted to set the molecular clock, by estimating the time it takes for individual mutations in the HIV-1 genome to occur. Having made this calibration, they can then proceed to date the earliest nodes (divergence points between isolates) on the HIV-1 tree. The first published calculation, in 1988, was made by Li and Sharp. They estimated that HIV-1 "had existed in central Africa before 1960," and showed their first isolate branching off in 1958.[37] In 1989 Russell Doolittle proposed 1949–1969 for the advent of both HIV-1 and HIV-2.[38] In 1990, Querat and colleagues postulated 1961 or 1962 for the radiation of HIV-1 subtypes,[39] and Manfred Eigen proposed 1945–1960 for the divergence of the earliest African isolates, which, he suggested, were from the Congo.[40] In his classic article from 1994, Gerry Myers again proposed 1959 — this time for the star-like radiation of both HIV-1 groups, M and O,[41] and in the same year his colleague Bette Korber proposed 1960 for the beginning of the AIDS pandemic.[42] In 1995, Eddie Holmes and colleagues proposed 1947–1955,[43] and the following year Françoise Barré-Sinoussi proposed 1946–1966.[44]

There are other analysts who claim that the rate of PIV mutation is not constant — because substitutions (changes in the individual nucleotides in the genome) take place both forward and backward — and who therefore propose that the date of HIV-1 divergence from the SIVs was much earlier.[45] However, the preponderance of published reports that propose the very precise time period of the 1950s is quite striking.

Two other articles on this subject merit a mention. The first, a 1990 article by a group of French epidemiologists, proposed a date of 1952 plus or minus five years for the year in which more than ten persons were first infected with HIV, and suggested that this occurred in Leopoldville/Kinshasa.[46] The second, an article that described a method for assessing the global spread of HIV-1 based on an analysis of air travel between fifty-two major cities, concluded that 1965 was the first time that one hundred persons in one city were HIV-1-positive.[47] Again, the city in question was Kinshasa.

Thus several different methodological approaches point to the fifties as the time when humans first began to be infected with HIV-1, and to the city of Leopoldville/Kinshasa as the first to be infected. Once again the correlations with the CHAT campaigns in the Belgian colonies of central Africa between 1957 and 1960 are dramatic.

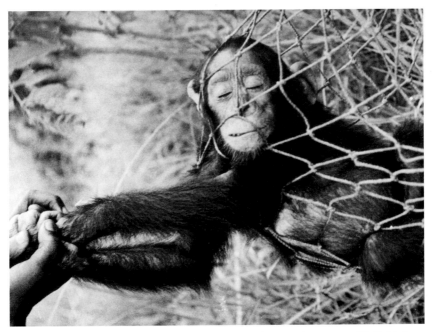

Chimp caught in a liana net by pygmies, at one of Rollais's base camps in the north of Province Oriental, 1958. *(Credit: G. Rollais)*

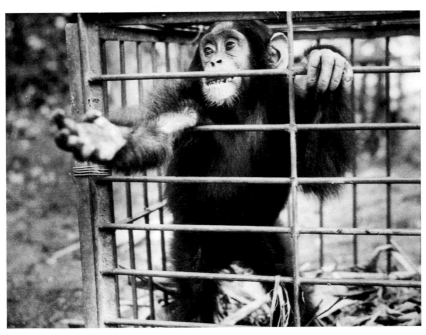

Chimp in a temporary cage at one of Rollais's base camps, before being transported to Lindi, circa 1957. *(Credit: G. Rollais)*

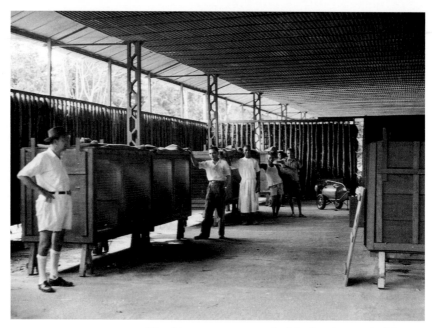

The chimp cages at one end of the first (quarantine) hangar at Camp Lindi, showing Robert Daenens and Gaston Ninane in the foreground. *(Credit: G. Rollais)*

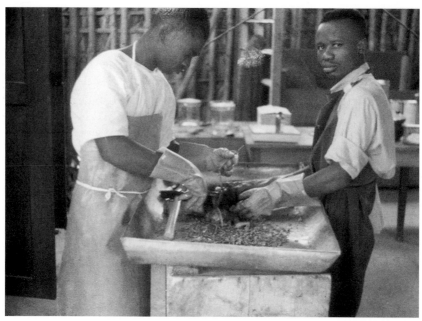

Two African assistants dismembering a dead chimp in the small "laboratory" at Camp Lindi, 1957. *(Credit: Gail N. R.)*

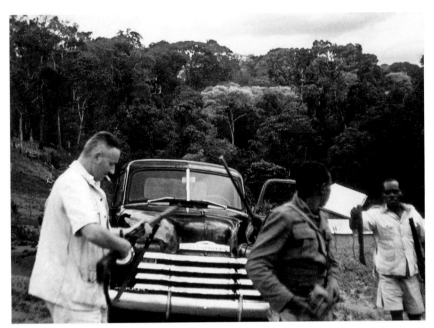

Alexandre Jezierski on a monkey-hunting expedition for the Gabu-Nioka laboratory, 1954. *(Credit: G. Scott)*

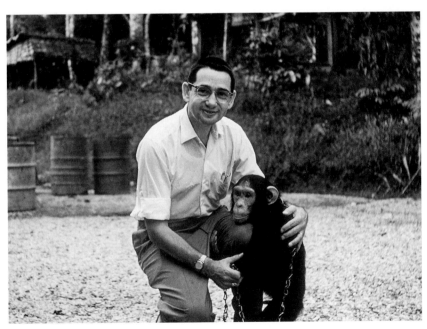

Henry Gelfand and chimpanzee friend, Camp Lindi, 1958. *(Credit: H. M. Gelfand)*

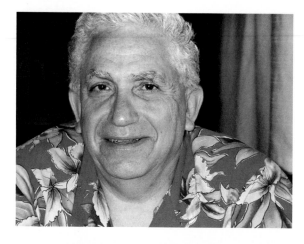

André Nahmias, 1995.
*(Credit: E. Hooper)*

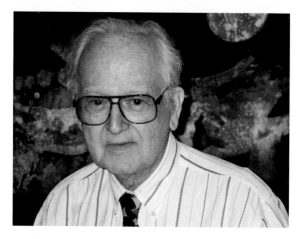

Joseph Melnick, 1995.
*(Credit: E. Hooper)*

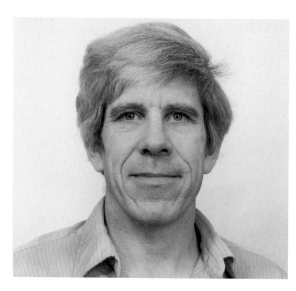

Bill Hamilton, circa 1981.
*(Credit: W. D. Hamilton)*

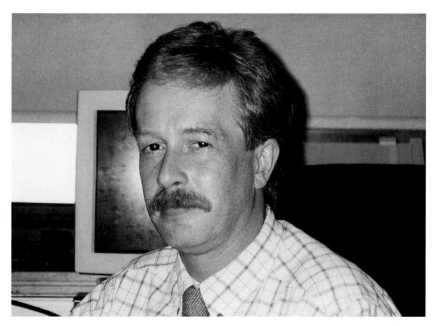

Paul Sharp, 1995. *(Credit: E. Hooper)*

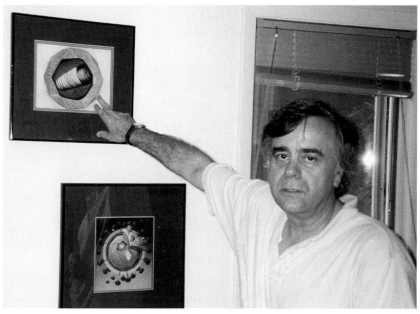

Preston Marx, and the human immunodeficiency virus, 1995.
*(Credit: E. Hooper)*

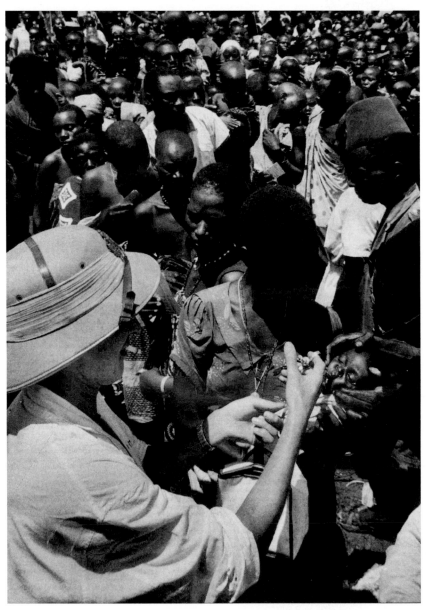

Agnes Flack vaccinating a "sea of Africans" with CHAT in the Ruzizi Valley, 1958. *(Credit: R. Phillips)*

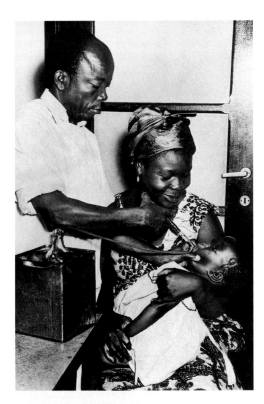

Child being vaccinated in Leopold-ville in 1959 with the "Koprowski live virus vaccine, which has been developed in the United States with the collaboration of the Stanleyville laboratories, and Lindi camp." *(Credit: H. Goldstein)*

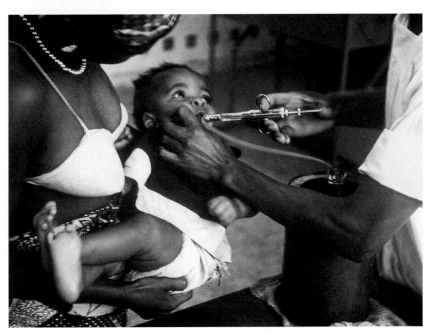

Another child vaccinated with chilled CHAT vaccine in Leopoldville, 1958. *(Credit: H. M. Gelfand)*

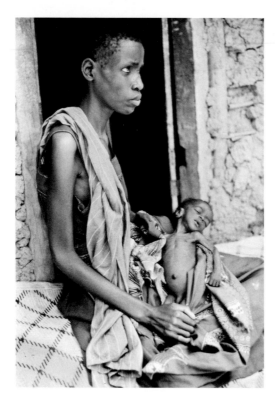

Florence and her baby son, Ssengabi, in Gwanda, near Kyebe, southern Uganda, 1986. Florence died one month after this photo was taken, and Ssengabi three months later. *(Credit: E. Hooper)*

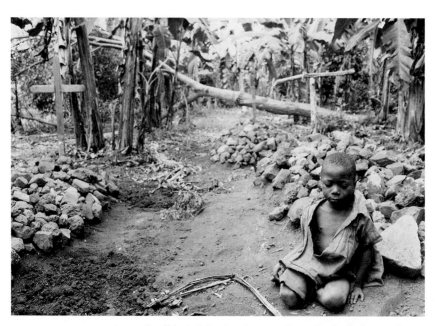

Small boy sitting in a banana plantation in Kyebe, southern Uganda. Surrounding him are the graves of family members, all of whom had, apparently, died of AIDS. *(Credit: E. Hooper)*

# 51

## WHAT HAPPENED

## AT LETCHWORTH AND CLINTON

In May 1995, as I was completing my American research, I had a lucky break. Finding myself with an unexpected spare couple of days, I phoned Tom Norton's seventy-nine-year-old widow, Priscilla, who was living six hundred miles away, to ask if I could visit for a brief interview. She made it clear that her memories of the period were limited (indeed, her daughters had already told me this), but said that I was welcome to give it a try.

We had an interesting chat, during which Mrs. Norton told me she thought she had posted fifteen or twenty of her husband's files to Dr. Koprowski — which, she estimated, had made a pile some three or four inches deep. (She held her hand above the table to indicate the depth.) This sounded like rather more than the amount of documentation that Koprowski had by then returned to her daughter Ann.[1] Unfortunately, of course, there was simply no way of checking whether Mrs. Norton's recollections on this point were accurate.

Later, she talked about the Africa trip her husband and Hilary Koprowski had made early in 1957. She confirmed my suspicion that they had first flown to Nairobi, and had gone on from there to Stanleyville. Tom had been out in Africa for some six weeks, she said, working on the polio vaccine at the chimp camp, but Dr. Koprowski had come back earlier. Although she appeared fairly well briefed on the issues, she recalled few details about the Lindi research, other than the fact that Tom was testing the vaccine on the chimps, either by feeding or by injection, she was not sure which.

Mrs. Norton's memories were rather sketchy, but she was not afraid of making it clear when she was not sure of something. Indeed, later in the interview I emphasized the importance of this. It was vital, I told her, that what she told me about were only the things about which she was certain; she confirmed that this was what she was doing.

Soon after this, I asked her whether she remembered anything about kidneys having been removed from the chimps. To my surprise, she said that she did. She said she thought that her husband had extracted kidneys from about four chimps, and had brought them back with him, presumably in four separate flasks. When I asked what made her think this, she said: "I wouldn't think they'd mix them up," which demonstrated that she was not unaware of the practical problems of lab technique and working with viruses.[2] She also said that Tom might have brought back some spinal cord material.

Later, when I asked whether her husband and the Stanleyville doctors had ever had to sacrifice any of the chimps, she answered: "What, to get out what they wanted? I guess so." I pointed out that sensibilities in the fifties must have been very different from those of today, and straightaway Priscilla Norton responded: "Well, they didn't broadcast it, that they killed them." The secrecy that had surrounded the activities at Lindi began at last to make some sense.

But what was even more interesting was the subject of Tom's return. Mrs. Norton agreed that this must have been around the middle of March 1957 (about a month and a half before he and Hilary formally moved from Lederle to the Wistar). She also agreed that Tom would probably have flown back to New York from Stanleyville by as direct a route as possible, because of the importance of getting the flasks of materials back swiftly. She said that there might have been about eight flasks in total, containing all the different materials, each of which would have been some twelve to fifteen inches high.

Then she added something really important. She told me that Tom had been picked up at the airport by Jim — who, she explained, was the driver at the Wistar Institute for many years in the fifties and sixties. Later, when I sought to confirm this, Priscilla Norton repeated that it was Jim who took the canisters her husband had brought back with him, and that he drove them down to the Wistar.[3]

So, according to Mrs. Norton, kidneys from the Lindi chimps were brought back from Stanleyville in March 1957, and were sent not to Lederle, where Koprowski and Norton were still working at the time, but to the Wistar. If she is correct, then the two scientists had access to chimpanzee kidneys from the time of their arrival in Philadelphia, where — to quote Koprowski — "this strain [CHAT] was again subjected to numerous laboratory procedures at the Wistar Institute for the selection of the least virulent particles."[4] Shortly afterward, the large pools of CHAT vaccine were manufactured for feeding in the Congo.

———

What I had learned from Priscilla Norton prompted me to a more vigorous questioning of some of my remaining American interviewees. Herald Cox had died back in 1986, but I spoke with his son, George Cox, himself a physician. He told me that his father had arrived at Lederle in 1941 and, when Hilary Koprowski joined the company a few years later, he had effectively put him in charge of the polio work, leaving him more or less to his own devices thereafter.

I asked Dr. Cox what had gone wrong between his father and Koprowski, and the whole tale came tumbling out. He cited several incidents, but was particularly outspoken about Koprowski and Norton's visit to the Congo, "I think it was totally without the approval or knowledge of my father. When he heard about it, he was very distraught and angry." He said that his father subsequently offered to resign, but instead the Lederle bosses supported him, which "led to Koprowski leaving under duress." George went on to say that "if Koprowski had really . . . done things aboveboard, it would have been a Lederle-Koprowski vaccine, not Sabin's, out there."

I asked George Cox how Koprowski had developed CHAT vaccine, and he told me that Koprowski had "collected it from somebody who'd received the Lederle vaccines, and simply renamed it. That's what my father said. . . . [The] powers-that-be knew that CHAT was a direct steal from Lederle, and . . . how it originated." He added: "You can't trust the man — what he says or what he writes."

Later that day, I went to see Stewart Aston, the former head of the virus production lab at Lederle, at his home a few miles from Lederle's headquarters at Pearl River. I had been impressed by his careful responses to questions on the two occasions when I had interviewed him in 1993, but was also aware that he was regarded as someone who could be relied upon to "toe the company line" in official interviews. Now I wanted to see whether, if approached at his own home, he would feel a little less constrained. He asked me to leave the tape recorder in my bag, which I did, but he spoke slowly enough for me to take accurate notes, and he responded to my questions with a degree of candor that was entirely unexpected.

The conversation turned to Koprowski's final two years at Lederle, from 1955 to 1957, and Aston told me: "He knowingly sent strains of virus outside the laboratory without permission. He was acting quite without proper authority." I pointed out that some of the strains he took out to the Congo in February 1957, three months before he moved to the Wistar, must have originated from Lederle. "It wouldn't surprise me," said Aston. "And that probably was the virus which some people think was the cause of HIV infection," he added.

At this point, I decided to tell him about my conversation with Priscilla Norton, and her recollection that chimp kidneys brought back by Tom Norton in March 1957 had been forwarded straight to the Wistar. In response, Aston became increasingly outspoken. "Hilary was not above under-the-table dealings," he said. "He was just acting very arrogantly, very independently, and not conducting himself in a straightforward manner."

I asked Aston what Koprowski and Norton might have used the chimp kidneys for, and he answered: "I can't think of any reason other than growing the virus. There's no point in using chimp tissue for safety tests. [For those], it's much cheaper and easier to use rhesus or African green monkey."

So what role, I asked, had Tom Norton played in all this? "Tom was a very excellent laboratory worker — very thorough, very meticulous. He was devoted to Hilary. It wouldn't surprise me at all if Hilary didn't use Tom. . . . I'd wager a guess that Tom, if he was reassured by Hilary: 'Oh this is perfectly safe — do this,' then [he] would do it without any question, in blind faith."

At the end, we talked some more about the possibility that the Congo episode may have given birth to AIDS, and Stewart Aston told me that he hoped that the book I was going to write would be "a warning against unauthorized, uncontrolled experimentation. I hope that your publishing this will . . . remind people that even though procedures [like vaccination] are very laudable and necessary, you do in fact have to make every possible effort to ensure that all safety procedures are satisfied."

---

By the end of 1995, I felt ready to take a final look at Koprowski's vaccines, and the history of their testing and feeding at different venues. New information that had come to light over the previous two years meant that many of the mysteries about his research could now be unraveled.

The first area of interest was the institute for handicapped children at Letchworth Village, in Thiells, New York, where Koprowski's friendship with the director of laboratories, George Jervis, had clearly been useful to him in several ways. The published record showed that Koprowski, Jervis, and Tom Norton had collaborated on feeding Koprowski's TN to twenty Letchworth children between February 1950 and March 1951, and on feeding TN and different strains of virulent virus to sixteen chimpanzees between September 1949 and October 1952. Later, of course, Jervis had participated in the vast Ruzizi field trial.

But I was beginning to realize that George Jervis had done much more than just feed Koprowski's vaccines to different subjects. He had in addition been in sole charge of a large and well-equipped laboratory. As the 1950 annual report for Letchworth Village expressed it: "Dr. Jervis is far too valuable to the department to be called on for routine clinical work."[5] The inference was that he should be left free to concentrate on research.

I visited Letchworth in the summer of 1995, just a few months before it was due to close. By this stage, the children had been moved elsewhere, but one of the remaining officials showed me round the handsome stone cottages, set amongst rolling parkland. We found a janitor who unlocked the building where

George Jervis used to work, and there in the basement was a spacious laboratory, now full of dusty glass and metalware.

That evening I visited Ruth Jervis, George's widow. She told me that her husband had worked at Letchworth from 1937 to 1968, and that Koprowski and Norton used to pay frequent visits to their house, with Koprowski usually playing piano after dinner. She added that her husband's major contribution to the polio research had been made in the laboratory, and confirmed that he had tested the vaccine on animals, including chimps.[6]

She astounded me by saying she had not known that the very first feeding of OPV in the world had involved one of the Letchworth children, and had taken place on her husband's authority.[7] However, she explained that George had been an eminent scientist in his own right, and had twice been nominated for the Nobel Prize, mainly for his work on the biochemical basis for retardation.

All that she recalled about his visit to Africa was that the flight from Idlewild had been postponed by a terrible snowstorm, but that she had seen her husband and Agnes Flack off the following day. I asked whether they had been carrying the vaccine with them, and Ruth Jervis told me she thought so, but wasn't sure. She added that her husband had returned from Africa before Flack, and that "he brought back the things he had to bring back with him." She could not say, however, what these were.

It was some time after this rather frustrating interview that I went back to the published records of the conference on "Biology of Poliomyelitis," which Koprowski had organized at the New York Academy of Sciences in January 1955. These reveal that several further trials of Koprowski's experimental polio vaccines, in addition to those formally reported in the mainstream literature, had been staged — almost certainly at Letchworth.[8] One of George Jervis's articles details the differing responses of various tissue cultures, experimental animals, and humans to administration of different poliovirus strains.[9] For example, the impact of six different variants of TN is compared in five different host systems: MKTC, monkeys, mice, rats — and humans. In this brief paper, Jervis also reported similar comparative studies of MEF-1 and SM, again adapted to MKTC.

Perhaps more than any other scientist at the conference, Jervis was showing the benefit of retaining a completely open mind about substrate. Try out every available material, he seemed to be saying, and see how it affects your vaccine virus for different hosts. Only by experimentation will you arrive at the perfect polio vaccine.

The discussion sessions at this conference reveal that Koprowski was coming to terms with the fact that, as demonstrated by both Sabin and Jervis, passage through monkeys and monkey tissues could be just as effective an attenuating factor as passage through obviously nonsusceptible hosts such as rodents and chickens.

It seems very likely that it was in the Letchworth lab that many of the collaborations between Jervis and Koprowski (the safety trials in macaques and chimpanzees, and the passage of various poliovirus strains in monkey kidney tissue culture) were conducted.[10] And yet there was a large animal house at Lederle, which apparently contained hundreds of cynomolgus and rhesus macaques and a small number of chimps — so why was Jervis needed? Perhaps this was a diplomatic way of avoiding conflict with Herald Cox, who was so vehemently opposed to the cultivation of polio vaccine strains in MKTC.[11] Whatever, it is clear that the collaboration between Jervis and Koprowski continued even after the latter's move to the Wistar, for the Moorestown paper reports that Jervis conducted CHAT vaccine safety tests on thirty-four rhesus and cynomolgus monkeys.[12] In short, throughout the crucial period this broadminded and innovative scientist appears to have played a key role in Koprowski's polio research.

---

However, within eight months of the 1955 conference in New York, Koprowski had shifted the venue for his polio vaccine trials to Clinton Farms, where most of the women prisoners who gave birth were happy to volunteer their infants, and often themselves, for vaccination.

During early 1995, I received two new documents that allowed a more complete unraveling of the research that took place at Clinton in the second half of the fifties. The first was a book that had just been published about Edna Mahan and the history of Clinton Farms, and this in turn led me to the boxed prison records, now held at the New Jersey State Archives in Trenton, where the minutes of the monthly meetings of the Clinton board of governors proved to be a veritable fount of information.[13]

The book, *Excellent Effect,* revealed that the Clinton penitentiary had been used for medical experiments for the better part of two decades, experiments not only involving polio, but also typhus, hepatitis, and other diseases.[14] This was in tune with Edna Mahan's belief that her charges should have the opportunity to do something positive for society, as reparation for their crimes. The only rewards offered to the volunteer participants were the end-of-experiment banquet, the possibility of a more sympathetic hearing before the parole board and, in the case of the OPV trials, the chance of spending additional time with their newborn children.

The initial discussions about the polio vaccine program took place between Joe Stokes and Edna Mahan on June 22, 1955,[15] and a research plan was presented to the board of governors by Andrew Hunt and Agnes Flack — and approved — in October 1955. Vaccinations began the following month, and the first progress report appeared in the December minutes. Apparently "the results are pleasing to the doctors — there have been no unusual developments of any kind," and already there were plans for *Life* magazine to do a photo story on the project. This article,[16] and another in the *Newark Evening News*,[17] were eventually published in October 1956, and apparently "except for a very few critical letters and telegrams, and one anonymous postal card, the reaction has been favorable."

A report by Flack and Hunt in February 1956 revealed that "inmates who are assisting (in the care of the babies) learn sterile techniques and receive $10 per month each from the Lederle Laboratories." Apparently one of the six original vaccinees (who had been fed TN) did not respond with antibodies, and had to be refed.[18] (For whatever reason this infant, who should have been designated No. 6, is omitted entirely from the published report of the first 25 cases.)[19] Over the ensuing months Stokes, Koprowski, and Norton visited frequently, and showed the project off to other scientists, including George Jervis and Dr. Anthony Payne (the Secretary to the Expert Committee on Poliomyelitis, at the WHO).

We now learn that the project is being conducted jointly by Lederle Laboratories and the "University of Pennsylvania Children's Hospital." This is clearly a reference to the Children's Hospital of Philadelphia, CHOP, which is situated on the university campus. However, all this changes early in 1957. On March 23, Stokes, Koprowski, Hunt, and Norton pay a visit to Clinton to discuss the polio research project, and it is announced that Koprowski and Norton "have left Lederle Laboratories, and are now associated with the Wistar Clinic of Philadelphia." They propose to close the project down at the end of April for about a month, by which time 46 babies would have been vaccinated and tested. By the time that the polio project reopens in May, the strict quarantine practices that had previously obtained are set aside, since they "are no longer necessary or even desirable." Dr. Stokes, we learn, is trying to find a foundation that will sponsor follow-up studies of the whole infant population of Clinton.[20] Some months later, Dr. Plotkin is also involved in discussions at Clinton on a similar project.

All this was fascinating, and placed in perspective the insistence by Paul Osterrieth that there was little or no collaboration between the Wistar and CHOP. For it was now apparent that these two institutions were collaborating on the Clinton polio vaccine study from May 1957 onward. A few months later, Fritz Deinhardt would be setting off to Africa for his hepatitis studies, which would involve his air-freighting chimp kidneys back to CHOP.

In the November 1957 minutes, we learn that Koprowski has invited Flack "to participate in the [polio vaccine] study currently underway in the Belgian Congo. Her assignment would be to serve as medical consultant under the U.S. Public Health Service, which is now responsible for the broadened program." Apparently she is due to leave on December 7 for six to eight weeks, and to immunize some 75,000 people. For whatever reason there is a delay, and by the time Flack finally leaves on February 17, 1958, there is an epidemic of a respiratory infection raging among the Clinton inmates. Several babies become so ill that they have to be transferred to the Hunterdon Medical Center, and Dr. Hunt is obliged to call at Clinton regularly to check on the infants in the polio study, and those in the measles and mumps vaccination program that Stokes and Koprowski had begun in January.[21]

From 1958 onward, there is less information in the minutes about the vaccine program, but *Excellent Effect* does reveal that the polio trials extended from the fall of 1955 right through until 1966. In March of that year, Tom Norton wrote Edna Mahan a charming letter thanking her for her cooperation, and for the very pleasant relationship they had enjoyed over eleven years. He continued: "[I]t is no exaggeration to say that the work at Clinton went far in its contribution to a live virus polio vaccine. The scientific data which came out of the Clinton studies were used not only by us, but by other people in the field. . . . They were not the sort of studies that make the headlines, but they were the sort of studies that must be made before the headline-making final results."[22]

---

Months after this, I spent another all-night session with the Clinton birth records, the published records of the vaccinations, and a perpetual calendar. By early morning, I had a pretty good idea of when most of the first ninety-odd infant vaccinees at Clinton had been vaccinated, and with which vaccines.

As already detailed, a total of 25 infants were fed either TN, SM N-90, or both vaccines between November 1955 and June 1956. In the next two months, a further seven infants were vaccinated, but only two of these immunizations were recorded in the literature. However, various clues suggest that all seven were fed with variants of SM N-90 as it was transmogrifying into CHAT.

After this, between October 1956 and January 1957 (while Koprowski was still at Lederle), there appear to have been seven feedings of the prototypes of the SM-45, CHAT, and Fox strains, which Koprowski would later announce at the Geneva conference just after his move to the Wistar.[23] Only the three Fox feedings in October and November 1956 are formally reported in the major article on the early Clinton trials,[24] but of the other four feedings, one must have involved SM-45,[25] and at least two must have involved an early version of CHAT. These two CHAT vaccinees were described as "BO" and "GA" in Koprowski's address to the Geneva conference. It turns out that these were the first two letters of the infants' surnames, which indicates that BO was fed on November 10, 1956, and GA on January 3, 1957. These appear to have been the first two CHAT feedings to humans, even before the feeding of CHAT to six Clinton infants on February 27, 1957.[26]

In his Geneva paper, Koprowski reported on the safety of the excreted viruses of BO, TA, and another vaccinee called GA.[27] The fecal virus from BO

## DATES OF POLIO VACCINATIONS AT CLINTON FARMS, NOVEMBER 1955 TO JUNE 1958

| Child Code No. | Type 1 vaccines | Type 2 vaccines | Type 3 vaccine |
|---|---|---|---|
| 1 | SM N-90: Nov. 8, 1955 | TN: Jan. 16, 1956 | — |
| 2 | SM N-90: (Nov. 10, 1955) | — | — |
| 3 | SM N-90: Nov. 15, 1955 | TN: Jan. 12, 1956 | — |
| 4 | SM N-90: Nov. 15, 1955 | TN: Jan 16, 1956 | — |
| 5 | SM N-90: Nov. 15, 1955 | TN: Jan. 16, 1956 | — |
| 6 | — | TN: Jan. 16, 1956 | — |
| 7 | SM N-90: Jan. 16, 1956 | — | — |
| 8 | SM N-90: Jan. 16, 1956 | — | — |
| 9 | SM N-90: Jan. 16, 1956; refed Mar. 2 & Apr. 13, 1956 | — | — |
| 10 | SM N-90: contact Jan. 16, 1956; refed Mar. 2, 1956 | — | |
| 11 | SM N-90: Jan 16, 1956; refed Mar. 2, 1956 | — | — |
| 12 | SM N-90: Jan. 16, 1956; refed Mar. 2, 1956 | — | — |
| 13 | SM N-90: Jan. 16, 1956 | — | — |
| 14 | SM N-90: contact Jan 16, 1956; refed June 13, 1956 | TN: Apr. 14, 1956; refed May 16, 1956 | — |
| 15 | SM N-90: Mar. 2, 1956 | TN: Jan. 16, 1956 | — |
| 16 | SM N-90: (Apr. 21, 1956) | — | — |
| 17 | SM N-90: May 16, 1956 | — | — |
| 18 | SM N-90: May 16, 1956 | — | — |
| 19 | — | TN: May 16, 1956 | — |
| 20 | — | TN: May 16, 1956 | — |
| 21 | SM N-90: May 16, 1956 | — | — |
| 22 | SM N-90: May 31, 1956 | — | — |

DATES OF POLIO VACCINATIONS AT CLINTON FARMS,
NOVEMBER 1955 TO JUNE 1958 (*continued*)

| Child Code No. | Type 1 vaccines | Type 2 vaccines | Type 3 vaccine |
|---|---|---|---|
| 23 | SM N-90: June 13, 1956 | — | — |
| 24 | SM N-90: June 13, 1956 | — | — |
| 25 | SM N-90: June 13, 1956 | — | — |
| 26 | SM N-90: (June 24, 1956) | — | — |
| 27 | No info available | | |
| 28 | No info available | | |
| 29 | No info available | | |
| 30 | No info available | | |
| 31 | No info available | | |
| 32 | SM N-90: (Aug. 27, 1956) | — | — |
| 33 | — | — | Fox: Oct. 20, 1956; Refed Nov. 10, 1956 |
| 34 | — | — | Fox: Oct. 18, 1956; refed Dec. 11, 1956 & July 15, 1958 |
| 35 | No info available | | |
| 36 | SM-45: (Nov. 7, 1956) | — | — |
| 37 | — | — | Fox: Nov. 9, 1956; Refed Dec. 11, 1956 |
| (38)=BO | CHAT: Nov. 10, 1956 | — | — |
| (39)=GA | CHAT: Jan. 3, 1957 | — | — |
| 40 | CHAT: Feb. 27, 1957 | — | — |
| 41 | CHAT: Feb. 27, 1957 | — | — |
| 42 | CHAT: Feb. 27, 1957 | — | — |
| (43) | CHAT: Feb. 27, 1957 | — | — |
| (44) | SM-45: Feb. 27, 1957 | — | — |
| 45 | CHAT: Feb. 27, 1957 | — | — |

| Child Code No. | Type 1 vaccines | Type 2 vaccines | Type 3 vaccine |
|---|---|---|---|
| 46=TA | CHAT: Feb. 27, 1957 | — | — |
| 47 | — | Jackson: Apr. 25, 1957 | — |
| 48 | Wistar: June 3, 1957 | — | — |
| 49 | CHAT: Dec. 4, 1957 | Jackson: June 26, 1957<br>P-712: Jan. 13, 1958 | Fox: Dec. 24, 1957 |
| 50 | Wistar: (Sep. 10, 1957) | — | — |
| 51 | No info available | | |
| 52 | No info available | | |
| 53 | CHAT: Dec. 4, 1957 | Jackson: Sep. 11, 1957 | Fox: Dec. 24, 1957 |
| 54 | Wistar: (Sep. 13, 1957) | — | — |
| 55 | Wistar: (Sep. 21, 1957) | — | Fox: (Dec. 21, 1957) |
| 56 | CHAT: Nov. 13, 1957 | Jackson: Sep. 11, 1957 | Fox: Dec. 24, 1957 |
| 57 | No info available | | |
| 58 | No info available | | |
| 59 | Wistar: (Oct. 3, 1957) | — | — |
| 60 | No info available | | |
| 61 | No info available | | |
| 62 | — | — | Fox: (Oct. 8, 1957) |
| 63 | No info available | | |
| 64 | Wistar: Oct. 8, 1957<br>CHAT: Dec. 4, 1957 | P-712: Jan. 12, 1958 | Fox: Dec. 24, 1957 |
| 65 | CHAT: Dec. 4, 1957 | P-712: Dec. 24, 1957 | Fox: Oct. 8, 1957 |
| 66 | CHAT: Nov. 13, 1957 | — | Fox: Dec. 24, 1957 |
| 67 | CHAT: Nov. 13, 1957 | — | — |
| 68 | CHAT: Nov. 13, 1957;<br>refed Dec. 4, 1957 | P-712: Jan. 13, 1958 | Fox: Dec. 24, 1957 |

DATES OF POLIO VACCINATIONS AT CLINTON FARMS,
NOVEMBER 1955 TO JUNE 1958 (*continued*)

| Child Code No. | Type 1 vaccines | Type 2 vaccines | Type 3 vaccine |
|---|---|---|---|
| 69 | CHAT: Nov. 13, 1957; refed Dec. 4, 1957 | P-712: Jan. 13, 1958 | Fox: Dec. 24, 1957 |
| 70 | CHAT: (Dec. 3, 1957) | — | Fox: (Oct. 23, 1957) |
| 71 | CHAT: Nov. 13, 1957; refed Dec. 4, 1957 | P-712: Jan. 13, 1958 | Fox: Dec. 24, 1957 |
| 72 | CHAT: (Nov. 13, 1957) | P-712: (Jan. 13, 1958) | Fox: (Dec. 11, 1957) |
| 73 | CHAT: (Dec. 4, 1957) | — | Fox: (Dec. 22, 1957) |
| 74 | CHAT: (Dec. 4, 1957; refed Dec. 24, 1957 & Jan. 13, 1958) | — | — |
| 75 | CHAT: (Jan. 13, 1958) | P-712: (Mar. 19, 1958) | — |
| 76 | CHAT: Dec. 24, 1957 | — | — |
| 77 | CHAT: (Jan. 9, 1958) | P-712: (Mar. 28, 1958) | Fox: (Jan. 9, 1958) |
| 78 | CHAT: (Jan. 12, 1958) | P-712: (Apr. 10, 1958) | Fox: (Feb. 14, 1958) |
| 79 | CHAT: Jan. 13, 1958 | P-712: Apr. 1, 1958 | Fox: Feb. 6, 1958 |
| 80 | CHAT: Jan. 13, 1958 | P-712: Apr. 1, 1958 | Fox: Feb. 6, 1958 |
| 81 | CHAT: Jan. 13, 1958 | P-712: Apr. 1, 1958 | Fox: Feb. 6, 1958 |
| 82 | CHAT: (Jan. 22, 1958) | P-712: (Mar. 19, 1958) | Fox: (Apr. 9, 1958) |
| 83 | Wistar: Apr. 1, 1958 | P-712: Apr. 23, 1958 | Fox: Feb. 6, 1958 |
| 84 | CHAT: Apr. 1, 1958 | P-712: Apr. 23, 1958 | Fox: Feb. 6, 1958 |
| 85 | Wistar: Mar. 4, 1958 | P-712: Apr. 30, 1958 | Fox: May 21, 1958 |
| 86 | CHAT: Mar. 4, 1958 | P-712: Apr. 1, 1958 | Fox: Feb. 6, 1958 |
| 87 | CHAT: Mar. 4, 1958 | P-712: Apr. 1, 1958 | Fox: Feb. 6, 1958 |
| 88 | Wistar: (Mar. 4, 1958) | P-712: (June 28, 1958) | Fox: (May 21, 1958) |

Details in parentheses indicate "best guesses."
Vaccines were refed after failed vaccinations, or — where indicated — contact experiments.

caused no adverse reactions, but when TA's excreted virus was processed and injected intraspinally into monkeys, three out of eight became slightly paralyzed. Once again, the virulence of the vaccine after intestinal passage was shown to vary greatly, depending on the vaccinee.[28]

By dating the vaccinations, it is revealed that the slight neurovirulence of TA's excreted virus could not have been known before the end of March 1957.[29] By this stage, Koprowski had already fed CHAT Plaque 20 to several people in Africa, including the Lindi chimp keepers and their families, and others in Stanleyville. In other words, the first African feedings had already begun even before a proper assessment had been made of the safety of the excreted CHAT vaccine virus.

Perhaps in response to the adverse TA results, Koprowski and Norton made a pool of excreted virus from GA, passaged five times in MKTC to increase titer, and found that this fecal virus caused no paralysis after injection into monkeys. And on this rather limited evidence of safety, Courtois was allowed to proceed, in May 1957, with the vaccination of nearly two thousand Aketi schoolchildren — apparently with the same CHAT Plaque 20 material in capsule form.[30]

Back at Clinton, at the end of April 1957, just a week before Koprowski formally took over at the Wistar, his experimental Type 2 strain, Jackson (which was Lederle's egg-adapted MEF-1 strain, readapted to MKTC) was fed for the first time to an infant of the same name. During the next five months — Koprowski's first months at the Wistar — just nine infants were fed, of which seven received Jackson or the experimental Type 1 strain, Wistar (which he mistakenly believed to be CHAT that had been adapted to a calf), in sequence with CHAT and Fox. It appears that Koprowski soon decided that Jackson and Wistar were not suitable strains, and that he should concentrate his research on the apparently more reliable CHAT and Fox. Between September 11 and October 8, 1957, there were another five unreported feedings, which probably involved tests of different variants of CHAT, as it transformed from Plaque 20 into pool 10A-11. It is possible that preparations based on different plaques were tried out, to see which gave the best antibody response; it is also possible that they experimented with different substrates.

Whatever, by November 13, 1957, a decision about the best variant seems to have been taken, because on that date five infants were fed CHAT — almost certainly pool 10A-11. From then until June 1958, twenty-six infants were fed, mostly with CHAT, Fox, and Sabin's Type 2 strain, P-712, in sequence. (The latter was introduced at the end of 1957, because of Koprowski's failure to develop a safe Type 2 strain.)

The suggestion that trial feedings of experimental polio vaccines continued at Clinton into the sixties is confirmed by later papers. One of Plotkin's articles from 1960 shows that the number of infant vaccinations had risen to 299, most of which presumably took place at the women's prison.[31] By 1962, 132 infants had been fed all three Koprowski strains (CHAT, WI-2, and WM-3) made in human diploid cells (HDCS), and although some of the trial vaccinees were premature babies fed at Philadelphia General Hospital, most would have been Clinton infants.[32] Other human feeding experiments with experimental polioviruses, (including versions of TN, which had been adapted to MKTC at different temperatures,[33] and variants of Fox that had been mutated by exposure to nitrous acid[34]) may also have taken place at the penitentiary.

It thus seems that for many years, Clinton served as the venue for Koprowski's initial human trials of experimental polio vaccines, not all of which were later fed on a wider scale. If any of those vaccines had been contaminated with SIV, then it would be among those who were born at Clinton Farms between 1956 and 1960, and whose mothers had volunteered them for the vaccine program, that one might expect to see the emergence of AIDS in the United States. To this end, I tried on several further occasions to find out more from James Oleske about the promiscuous drug-injecting sixteen-year-old from New Jersey who gave birth, in around 1973, to a baby who died of AIDS in 1979,[35] but he failed to respond to my calls or letters.

———————

David Ho was unable to see me during my trip to the States, but eventually, in June 1995, he phoned to explain what had happened about the Manchester sailor debacle. We ended up talking for nearly an hour, during which time he surprised me by agreeing with my proposal that medical science may well have been responsible for the onset of the AIDS epidemics. He seemed, however, to favor the theory proposed by his colleague Preston Marx — that the reuse of hypodermic needles in clinics and vaccination programs may have been responsible.

After his candor on the subject of iatrogenic transfer, I was surprised when Ho told me that, despite the disproving of the Manchester case, he would still "stand by most of the conclusion" of the Wistar committee's report. "This case [was] icing on the cake. . . . I don't think it was necessarily central," he added.

I pointed out to Ho how important it was for independent investigators, such as myself, to be given access to the materials that he and his colleagues had viewed while compiling the Wistar report. He agreed, and for the second time he promised that he would send me a batch of the relevant papers, and that this would include the protocol for CHAT. A few days later, a packet of thirty-eight pages arrived in the post.[36]

The first item to catch my eye was an undated single sheet of typescript entitled: "History of the use of CHAT strain 'Type 1' attenuated polio virus in humans." This, in fact, was the only document directly relating to the African trials in the whole packet. It revealed that at the time of writing, just two pools of CHAT had been used in humans. This was something I had been trying to find out for years.

The first of the two pools, which was not identified by number, had apparently been fed at a high titer to five children at Clinton Farms (which indicated that this referred to the official CHAT feedings on "Koprowski day" — February 27, 1957). The pool was also "put up in capsules," which were about one hundred times weaker, and fed to 80 people in Stanleyville and 1,978 children in the Aketi region.[37] The paper continued: "The second pool (Pool 10A-11), which is to be used in the 1958 Congo trials, has been given to 32 individuals at Clinton Farms, including 25 infants and 7 adults." The birthdates of the Clinton vaccinees allowed the paper to be dated between January 23 and January 27, 1958.

This was fascinating for two reasons. First, it was the only confirmation from a Wistar source that "the 1958 Congo trials" had involved feeding CHAT pool 10A-11.[38] This indicates that pool 10A-11 was used not only in the Ruzizi Valley trial between February and April 1958, but that it also may have been used for the twenty thousand vaccinations that were carried out in response to the epidemics in Gombari, Watsa, and Bambesa in the space of just six days, between January 27 and February 1, 1958. The dates suggest that a small pool of vaccine (not quite enough for the total number of vaccinees, for the vaccine ran out partway through the Bambesa vaccination)[39] must have been delivered to the Congo in late January 1958. The most obvious courier would have been Fritz Deinhardt, who flew from Philadelphia to Stanleyville for his hepatitis experiments at exactly that time, booking one seat for himself and one for his "box of shit."[40] It thus seems likely that this particular batch of vaccine would have been made in the United States, probably at the Wistar itself.

Intriguingly, the vaccinations in Moorestown began at exactly the same time,[41] and yet here it seems that the original unnamed pool (which is likely to have been 4B-5, which seems to have been Plaque 20, passaged once or twice in MKTC) was used instead of 10A-11.[42] Thus two trials staged simultaneously — one in the African bush and the other in a middle-class New Jersey suburb — used different pools of vaccine.

The documents from Ho included an analysis made by Bonnie Clause of the Wistar — at the request of the expert committee — about the sources of kidney for tissue culture used for vaccine production. She had searched the index of the *New York Times* from 1954 to 1961, and concluded that there had actually never been a total ban by India on monkey export, as Curtis had claimed in his article. (What Clause does not record is that the Indian curb on simian exports, though incomplete, did have a far-reaching impact on virus laboratories and vaccine houses around the world, for many began to make other arrangements.)

Neither could Clause find any evidence to support Curtis's contention that African monkeys might have been used for tissue culture purposes prior to the switch away from macaques in 1961. However, had she in addition perused the medical literature, she would have found that many different species of African monkey were examined for their tissue culture potential during the fifties, and that some were heavily used for vaccine production — for instance, the baboon by Lépine, and the African green monkey by Gear.

The packet also contained Koprowski's vaccine protocols, as referred to in the expert committee's report. However, it turned out that there were no protocols for any of the early pools of CHAT, such as those used in Africa. The three protocols enclosed all applied to vaccines made in the sixties. Two were for CHAT pool 23 and WM-3 pool 17 (the last Type 1 and Type 3 pools that Koprowski made in monkey kidney), and the other was for WM-3 pool 18 (made in human diploid cell strain). In fact, there was not even a complete protocol for CHAT pool 23, for only two of the five pages were included.[43]

However, the most important passage of the protocol was present, and this was the opening section of page 1. This reported that the strain was named CHAT — "an attenuated Type 1 polio virus strain" — and that the host cell was primary monkey kidney (MK). The next section, "Production of pool," is important, in that it offers us a better insight into Koprowski's polio vaccine production methods in MKTC (albeit those applying to 1960/61) than any other source. It is therefore worth quoting in full. It reads:

1. Origin of seed virus: A pool of CHAT virus was produced in monkey kidney cell monolayers at 37°C.
2. Cultivation of MK cells: Primary monkey cells were suspended in Eagle's Basal medium containing 10% Calf serum, plus 100 units of Penicillin and 100 g of Streptomycin per ml.[44] The above cell suspension was introduced into twenty 5 liter bottles: each bottle received 15 million cells suspended in 250 ml of medium. The bottles were incubated at 37°C. Complete monolayers developed in 7 days.
3. Cultivation of virus: The growth medium was removed and the monolayers (see above) were washed once with Hanks BSS. 25 ml of seed virus was added to each of the 20 bottles. Virus absorption proceeded at room temperature for 30 minutes. The bottles were rocked gently several times during the absorption period. Maintenance medium composed of Eagle's basal medium without serum was then added to each bottle to yield a fluid volume of 250 ml per bottle. The bottles were then incubated at 37°C for 48 hours at which time the cell sheets showed a marked cytopathogenic effect. The fluid and cell debris was then frozen in the culture bottle.

The section on "Post-production handling of pool" revealed that after harvesting, the virus fluids were passed through a Seitz St-1 filter, and then stored in glass bottles at minus 20°C.

The protocol reveals some interesting details. Although it is clear that both the attenuated poliovirus and the vaccine pool were prepared in MKTC monolayers, there is neither any specific mention of trypsin, nor of centrifuging.

Furthermore, it is clear that CHAT — like all polio vaccines made in MKTC — was produced in "primary monkey cells" (obtained straight from the animal's kidney, without further passage). As observed earlier, primary cells, in contrast to secondary and tertiary cells, are rich in lymphocytes and macrophages, the target cells for SIV and HIV.

In fact, the only process described in the protocol that would definitely have had some deleterious effect on a putative SIV contaminant was freezing to minus 20°C. Indeed, this was the one factor that the Wistar committee report had highlighted, stating that "the polio vaccine was subjected to at least two cycles of freezing and thawing . . . a procedure known to cause significant loss of SIV and HIV infectivity."[45] However, the committee's report provided no details of, or reference for, how much loss of titer freezing might cause, and several virologists who work with HIV and SIV, like Luc Montagnier, say that a significant amount of virus remains.[46]

Among the other items in the packet were two papers that shed some peripheral light on the issue.[47] There was a document entitled "Development of the Type 3, WM-3 strain," which comprised a detailed history, with complete passage chart, of the Type 3 vaccine that Koprowski was using in 1960. This only served to highlight the lack of a similar history or passage chart depicting the evolution of Koprowski's major vaccine, CHAT. And there was a more detailed document entitled "Requirements for the production of Koprowski strains of attenuated poliovirus vaccine," which had clearly been written in 1961 or later, again far too late to be relevant. However, this latter document was quite specific about the host cells, describing them as "either green monkey kidney tissue culture *(Cercopithecus aethiops)* or human diploid cell strain (WI-38)." These requirements, which had been published in different regions where Koprowski strains were used in the sixties, such as Croatia,[48] reinforced the total absence of precise information about the species of monkey kidney used to make the vaccine pools in the fifties.

But it was the last document in the packet that was potentially the most important. It was a Wistar Institute memo dated April 20, 1992, from Steven Holloway, the senior central services coordinator, and it contained a detailed list of the contents of a storage box, which, it was said, was now located in secured freezer number 178 in Room 369 of the institute. This storage box apparently contained seventy-three samples of polio vaccine and poliovirus from the late fifties and early sixties.

Most of the vials contained samples of four vaccines: CHAT, TN, Fox, and WM-III, and three of these vials had been "identified by Dr. Koprowski [as being] possibly related to the Congo trials." These were "CHAT pool 13," "Lederle Seed Type 1," and "WCh pool Wy 23 1:100 gel." The last appeared to be a sample of Wistar CHAT pool 23 as made by Wyeth, which, as far as I knew, had only been used in 1960/61, and never in the Congo. But the other two were interesting. CHAT pool 13 was the pool that had been fed in Leopoldville between August

1958 and April 1960. And although I doubted that "Lederle Seed Type 1" (which was probably SM N-90) had ever been fed in the Congo, it might have been revealing to compare it with its descendant, CHAT pool 13, to determine what differences there were between the two.

Of particular note was the presence of two Lederle Type 1 pools in the Wistar's freezers. These were not samples that had been extracted from the stool of a vaccinee, but the actual Lederle seed lots, and I wondered how Koprowski would explain this.

Despite the fact that there were two relatively early pools of Fox, pool 8 and pool 11, with the latter dating from June 1958, there were no samples of the early CHAT pools — 4B-5, 10A-11, and DS — which had apparently been fed in the Congo. I recalled Koprowski telling me that he personally had searched in the freezers for samples that might have been used in the Congo, and that nothing more had been found. Yet there was a real possibility that Fox pool 8 had been the one fed in Aketi in December 1957, or in Stanleyville in early 1958.[49]

In most cases, there was no indication whether the frozen vials in Room 369 contained seed-lots of attenuated poliovirus, or samples of the final vaccine production pools, passaged once or twice more in tissue culture and ready for administration to humans. But in his letter to *Science,* Koprowski had insisted that the samples stored at the Wistar "may represent seed lots used for production of vaccines," but were not vaccines as such.[50]

The Wistar had initially promised to test the poliovirus sample that might have been used in the Congo (presumably the sample of pool 13), and yet had never done so. One of the major reasons that had been given for not conducting such tests was that an inadequate quantity of the samples remained. But it so happened that Ho had sent me two versions of the first page of the freezer memorandum, on one of which the amounts of virus had been scribbled in the margin. The quantity of CHAT pool 13 was 5 milliliters, which, for testing purposes, represented a lot of virus, and certainly more than enough to provide several different laboratories with sufficient material to carry out exhaustive PCR analysis.

———————

There were two major revelations to come out of the Wistar committee material sent me by David Ho. One was that the expert committee had been provided with very little relevant data on which to base its findings, for most of the papers related to 1960 or 1961, two or three years too late to be relevant. The other was that a 5-milliliter vial of CHAT pool 13 was sitting in a sealed freezer at the Wistar Institute, still untested for SIV, HIV, and the mitochondrial DNA of the host cells.

To my mind, these papers also revealed something that I (and others) had long suspected. The final report of the Wistar's expert committee had preserved the status quo, but had failed to investigate properly the important issues raised by researchers like Tom Curtis and Louis Pascal.

---

Three years later, when this book was at the copyediting stage, I returned briefly to the United States, and was lucky enough to be able to speak with three of the women who had worked at Clinton in the late fifties, and who had been intimately involved with the vaccination program. They contributed a number of pertinent details about what had happened there. All three, despite advancing years, demonstrated that they were still articulate, sharp, and possessors of good memories.

The first of my interviewees was Mary Quarles Hawkes, the author of *Excellent Effect*, who had worked as classification officer at Clinton between the summer of 1956 and 1959. Her mother, Anita Quarles, was on the board of governors for almost thirty years, and Mary subsequently decided to write her doctoral dissertation about Clinton, beginning her archival research in 1963.

She was able to confirm a number of important details about the program. First, she said that although there had been no monetary benefits attached to having one's child vaccinated, mothers could earn a small stipend from working in the nursery as "medical aides," and babies who were in the polio vaccine program were allowed to stay at Clinton considerably longer than those who were not. Second, almost 40 percent of those who gave birth at Clinton were juveniles, below the age of eighteen. Third, although most of the infants who were released from Clinton were subsequently fostered, the majority were later returned to their own mothers when they were released. The exceptions, of course, were those infants whose mothers were serving life sentences. Last, she confirmed the important detail that "Aggie" Flack had carried the vaccines with her when she flew out to Africa. She added that Dr. Flack had subsequently been awarded an honorary degree, although she thought that this was probably not for her polio work, but rather for her research at Oak Ridge during the Second World War, where she had apparently developed a treatment for burns.

Mary Hawkes added that it was not unusual for infants born at Clinton to return, years later, as inmates. She cited one occasion when four generations of a family were incarcerated at the same time (a grandmother and mother who were involved in a numbers racket in Elizabeth, together with a delinquent daughter, who gave birth while she was inside). But she told me that the best person to see on this score was Dr. Julia Duane, a pediatric consultant who had attempted to organize a follow-up study on the Clinton mothers and babies.

Dr. Duane told me that she had taken over from Andrew Hunt as consultant at the Stevens Hospital nursery in August 1958, and that she had continued in that role until 1970. At the same time, she was employed under Dr. Hunt at the Hunterdon Medical Center, and as a volunteer who worked one day a week for Joe Stokes at CHOP. (She recalled the weekly conferences that Dr. Stokes had held there every Friday, and noted that Hilary Koprowski was often present.) Dr. Duane said that she assumed that Koprowski and Plotkin had been trying out their experimental vaccines on the Clinton infants, adding that "it bothered me that they were using these babies in this way." She claimed that all the infants at Clinton, without exception, were vaccinated (a point later echoed by Ruth Lorenzo), and that their mothers had first to sign an authorization form — a form that, she admitted, had not signified very much, in that "informed consent was not in existence in the fifties." If correct, however, this meant that there had actually been three types of infant vaccinees at Clinton: those who were numbered participants in the polio program, whose health and antibody status were followed up (normally for six months), and who were then included in the published scientific reports; those who were given numbers but who, for some reason, were not included in the reports; and those who — though vaccinated — were never given numbers (perhaps because they were "released" soon afterward).[51]

Julia Duane explained that, because of funding difficulties and procrastination by the decision-makers (such as members of the State Board of Child Welfare, and certain doctors and psychologists), she was never able to mount the follow-up study of Clinton babies. This was a great shame, she added, for so much valuable information might have been learned about the environments in which the children ended up. She confirmed, however, that most Clinton babies eventually ended up back with their natural mothers, adding that it was her impression that many of the children followed their mothers into crime, most especially crimes related to drug addiction.[52] For me, such details only reinforced the possibility that the promiscuous drug-injecting mother of James Oleske's pediatric AIDS patient born in 1973/4, might herself have been a Clinton baby born between 1956 and 1958.

Dr. Duane told me one more intriguing detail. She said that after I phoned to request an interview, she had phoned Stanley Plotkin, who had said that he recalled me, and would be interested to hear what I had to say. Dr. Duane did not, however, have a very good impression of Plotkin, saying that he had always seemed "protective and secretive" about the research he did at Clinton. "I don't think he ever took us into his confidence about what they were doing," she added.

My last interviewee was Ruth Lorenzo, who had worked as chief nurse at Stevens Hospital in Clinton for the entire duration of the polio vaccination program, from 1955 to 1966. Mrs. Lorenzo and I had spoken on the phone back in 1996, and although she had since suffered a stroke, which had affected her speech, she insisted on seeing me and did her best to answer my questions.

She was not the first person to intimate that Agnes Flack had not been universally liked by the Clinton staff. She said that Dr. Flack had herself asked to go to the Congo, adding "she didn't do anything unless there was publicity," and commenting that after delivering the babies in the hospital, Dr. Flack's interest in them ended. As for her own work, she told me: "We would keep getting new babies, and keep feeding them the vaccine. Over the course of time, we had three types of vaccine. I would draw the blood and take stool specimens. [They were] Dr. Koprowski's vaccines. At the beginning they were with Lederle, American Cyanamid. And then something happened, I don't know what, and then the study was for the Wistar Institute and the University of Pennsylvania."[53] She recalled that the Wistar had paid for her to hire five nurses, so that there should be someone in the nursery around the clock, and had also purchased a freezer for the specimens, and Pampers for the babies.

Ruth Lorenzo told me that the vaccine would come up from Lederle or the Wistar in test tubes, and they would then put it in formula and feed it to the babies. She said that some of the babies got ear infections, but that she did not know of any baby who had an adverse reaction after being immunized. "The vaccine was completely safe," she assured me.

Later, she got out her photo album of the Clinton years, and she was able to resolve some other important details. We were looking at a photograph of six infants, and she told me that this had been the very first group of vaccinees. Then she pointed to one of the babies, whom she named, and said that this boy had always been everyone's favorite, partly because he was deaf. Apparently his mother had contracted measles during her pregnancy. Later, I checked my files, and found that this confirmed something about which, until then, I had not been certain: that this boy had to have been "child No. 1" in the vaccine study at Clinton, and that he was the same child who was eventually transferred to the Crippled Children's Hospital, after a history of ill health.[54] Given Ruth Lorenzo's information, it certainly appeared as if his health problems might have resulted from his mother's getting of measles (especially if this was German measles, and it occurred during the first trimester), rather than any reversion to virulence of the vaccine virus.

During her reminiscences about the people at Clinton, Mrs. Lorenzo recalled a driver called Jim (whom she characterized as "a gofer, [but also] a gentleman"), who used to come up from the Wistar to collect the specimens. Jim's identity was further confirmed when we came across a photo in the album of a man who was clearly collecting a box of specimens from the nursery; the box had just been handed over by a much younger Ruth Lorenzo.[55] The former chief nurse immediately commented that the man in this photo wasn't Jim, but a driver from Lederle. This definite placing of Jim as the Wistar driver was important, for it also confirmed that the chimp kidneys that Priscilla Norton recalled her husband bringing back from the Congo in March 1957 had been delivered to the Wistar Institute, and not to his then employers at Lederle, in Pearl River.

# 52

WHAT HAPPENED AT LINDI

Back in the fifties, the promised report about the polio experiments on the Lindi chimpanzees by Ghislain Courtois, with Koprowski, Norton, Ninane, and Osterrieth as coauthors, which was frequently cited in other publications,[1] had never actually appeared.[2]

Four decades later, the mystery about the Lindi polio experiments had only deepened, for even those records of the work that must once have existed appeared to have been either lost, discarded, or destroyed. Koprowski said that those documents that he once held had been mislaid during a move between institutions. The accounts of the research in the annual reports of the Laboratoire Médical de Stanleyville contained minimal information. Ninane and Osterrieth, and others from the laboratory, explained that their papers had been left behind in the rush to depart the Congo. And representatives from the institutions where CHAT vaccine had been made, the Wistar Institute and RIT, claimed that the vaccine protocols and records of the safety and efficacy tests from the early period were no longer held. Of one thing I now felt certain: given the significance and scale of the Congo trials, such background documents should either have been permanently retained, or copies should have been lodged with a central body, such as the WHO.

So it was that after more than four years of research, I remained largely in the dark about the polio experiments conducted on the Lindi chimpanzees — from the numbers of animals involved to the types of experiments and research carried out. All I could do was to continue to investigate as many avenues as possible, in the hope that one of them might reveal more about what had actually happened. And then finally, late in 1996, as I was in the midst of writing this book, some important new details came to light — details that at long last allowed several aspects of the Lindi operation to fall into place.

---

But let us first review the information that is freely available in the medical literature — which amounts to just seven sentences. This represents the sum total of the published scientific information that came out of the polio research on the Lindi chimps — information relating to the safety and effectiveness of polio vaccines that were later fed to over nine million people.

In the *British Medical Journal* article, Courtois and Koprowski write of safety testing CHAT and Fox (confirming its lack of virulence) by injecting each vaccine into the spines of five Lindi chimpanzees. Apparently none of the chimps became paralyzed, although one (injected with Fox) developed mild lesions of the spinal cord, typical of polio. The authors also mention, in passing, that vaccination and challenge experiments were staged.[3]

The only other references come in brief contributions made by Koprowski and Courtois during the discussion sessions at the First International Conference on Live Poliovirus Vaccines, held in Washington, D.C., in June 1959.[4] At one point, in response to a paper by Joseph Melnick and his wife Matilda in which they report injecting Type 3 polio strains intraspinally in two chimpanzees, Koprowski says: "Dr. Courtois and I have injected 39 chimpanzees by the intraspinal route with different preparations and different variants of attenuated strains. Four chimpanzees out of 39 became paralyzed, and 10 out of 39 had lesions of CNS [central nervous system]. One of the strains used, the old SM virus, had a D+ character,[5] and out of five chimpanzees injected intraspinally, one was paralyzed with specific CNS lesions. These results prompt me to warn Dr. Melnick to use caution in his interpretation of his data obtained in two chimpanzees."

In response, Melnick pointed out that "if Dr. Courtois had not screened his [Koprowski's] strains for changes [indications of reversion to virulence] before testing in chimpanzees, then I am not surprised at the results which he obtained." Melnick also wondered whether the inoculum had been placed correctly in the spinal cord, adding that Sabin had injected his strains into a large number of chimpanzees without any signs of paralysis or spinal lesions.

Koprowski never revealed which "different preparations and different variants" of OPV he had tested with such dramatic results. We know only that five chimps were injected with CHAT Plaque 20 and five with Fox (pool unspecified),[6] and five with "the old SM virus" (SM N-90).[7] Presumably five other vaccine strains were tested on the twenty-four remaining chimps. These could have been trial vaccines like SM-45 or Wistar (Type 1), or Jackson (Type 2); different vaccine pools (e.g., 10A-11, 13, and 18 of CHAT); or pools prepared in different substrates.

The fact that three of these remaining twenty-four chimps became paralyzed, and that eight developed CNS lesions,[8] suggests that these vaccines were either incorrectly injected into the spine (as Melnick proposed) or that some, at least, were inadequately attenuated — and therefore too dangerous for human use.

At the next discussion session at the Washington conference, there was talk about the number of chimps that might become paralyzed if fed virulent virus at the same dosages, or titers, as normal polio vaccines, and Ghislain Courtois contributed the information that he had fed two sets of chimpanzees with large amounts of two virulent strains of poliovirus. Four of the twenty-five chimps fed "Mexican" (a Type 1 virus) had been paralyzed, as had five of those fed YSK (a wild Type 2 virus).[9]

These two brief statements suggested that by the middle of 1959 the intraspinal tests had involved thirty-nine of the Lindi chimpanzees, and the tests with virulent virus a further fifty.[10] How many others had been involved with vaccination and challenge, or with other research, was anybody's guess.

————

However, certain other details were revealed by Fritz Deinhardt's hepatitis work at Lindi in 1958, which was far better reported than the polio experiments. First there was the paper he published in the *American Journal of Hygiene* in 1962,[11] which gave details of three separate experiments involving a total of 47 chimps, 27 of which were identified by number, with the highest number being 416. However, the data was too sparse to allow any confident predictions about how many of these chimps had previously been involved in the polio research.

A further insight into the history of the chimp camp was afforded by the original reports about the hepatitis work made by the Henles and Deinhardt to the Armed Forces Epidemiological Board (AFEB).[12] The report for 1958/9, following Deinhardt's visit to Lindi between January and April 1958, features a fuller account of the hepatitis research carried out in Philadelphia in chimpanzee kidney tissue culture, as well as detailed medical charts for the 35 chimps involved in the first two hepatitis experiments at Lindi. It was apparent that nearly all the chimps involved had been infants or adolescents, aged from six months to six years; only two appeared to have reached the age of sexual maturity, between eight and ten.

The really important information, however, is not available in the published literature, even in internal reports like those for the AFEB. In late 1996, I drove down to southern Germany to visit Professor Jean Deinhardt, the English widow of the famous German virologist, who had written to me to say that she had come across her husband's databook for the chimp hepatitis experiments.

Much to my surprise, the databook revealed details not only of the hepatitis work, but also what may be the only documentation still in existence of the

Lindi polio research. It turned out that most of the 47 hepatitis chimps had also previously been involved in the polio program, which confirmed that the scientists were eager to make the maximum use of their experimental subjects.[13]

Somebody (almost certainly Paulette Dherte, the enterprising nurse who doubled as a lab assistant, or Paul Osterrieth)[14] had painstakingly listed the relevant polio research details for each animal, including precise dates of admission to the camp and of experimental procedures carried out — including blood samplings and, if appropriate, biopsy or autopsy. Furthermore, the book gave details of other long-stay chimps that had been used for the polio research, but were considered unsuitable for the hepatitis experiments.[15]

Each chimpanzee was identified not only by a number, but also by a name. Despite there being a few discrepancies, it was apparent that the chimps were probably numbered chronologically as they entered the camp. One of the earliest arrivals, number 4, Henriette, had apparently entered Lindi on June 22, 1956, which confirmed the memory of André Courtois that by the time of his holiday in Stanleyville starting in July 1956, the camp was already up and running.

Thereafter, it was now clear, the intake of chimps had been remarkable. By January 1957, 208 chimps had arrived in the camp; by May 1957, 321; by November, 396. But after that, as the hepatitis experiments started, the number of new chimps appears to have tailed off dramatically. By September 1958, only twenty further chimps had been brought to the camp in the course of ten months, and by February 1959 (the time of the third hepatitis experiment) there had been no new arrivals. Other sources indicate that there was a fresh influx of some 60 chimps in late 1959, probably for arteriosclerosis and cancer research, or perhaps for export to the United States and Belgium.[16]

It seemed that the most frenetic month at Lindi may well have been January 1957, the month before Koprowski and Norton arrived in Stanleyville to begin their polio experiments, for chimp number 143 joined the camp on January 11, and chimp number 208 on January 17.[17] However, by February 1958 and the start of the hepatitis work (which apparently "reused" those chimps that had survived the polio experiments), there are only three surviving chimps numbered between 100 and 300. This suggests that there must have been either a tremendously high natural death rate during 1957, or else a very heavy usage of the animals in research that involved their sacrifice.

The other period of high admissions appears to have been the late summer of 1957, just before Koprowski's second visit for the September symposium. This is confirmed by Dirk Daenens's recollection that when he first arrived in Stanleyville in August 1957, his father, Robert, the camp supervisor, told him that there were then 175 chimps present — the highest total there had ever been.[18] However, since the cumulative total had by then passed 370, we have to presume that by this date, more than half of all the chimps brought to Lindi had died — either naturally, or through euthanasia.

By February 1959, when the numbering had reached 416, there were apparently only 20 chimps available to be considered for inclusion in the third hepatitis experiment.[19] We know that twenty-seven of the thirty-five chimps used in the first two hepatitis experiments survived the experience,[20] but this still suggests that one way or another, at least 369 chimps had disappeared from Lindi in the space of thirty-two months.

The two polio experiments revealed by Deinhardt's databook are also interesting. The first involved the feeding of two types of virulent "wild virus" to the chimps: 20 were fed with YSK, the Type 2 poliovirus strain, 8 of them on February 7, 1957, the same date that Koprowski gave his speech at the nurses' school in Stanleyville, just after he and Norton arrived in town.[21] Nineteen chimps were fed with the Type 1 "Mexican" strain three months later.

This revealed that the feeding of virulent viruses, as reported by Courtois in 1959, had involved not two separate groups of 25, as I had assumed, but a maximum of 30 animals, of which 20 would probably have been fed both viruses.[22] There is no way of knowing how many of the 5 chimps paralyzed by YSK and the 4 chimps paralyzed by Mexican were severely or mildly affected, but we can assume that a maximum of 9 animals required euthanasia following this experiment.

The second polio experiment recorded in the databook took place on August 17, 1957, when 14 of the chimps later used for hepatitis work were fed with a Type 1 polio vaccine. Three months later, the same chimps were challenged with YSK, the virulent Type 2 strain. This, the only evidence in the databook of vaccination and challenge experiments, was a revelation, for it suggested that what really interested Koprowski was whether Type 1 vaccine could protect against wild Type 2 virus. This had been one of his pet theories for several years, and required an experiment that clearly could not be conducted in humans.[23] It seems possible that the research was conducted not just on 14 chimps, but on a total of 25 (to match the number earlier fed with YSK). We may presume that it was unsuccessful, and that Type 1 vaccine failed to provide protection to at least some of the experimental subjects, because Koprowski later had to resume his search for a Type 2 vaccine (always the problem in his set of three).[24]

The Type 1 polio vaccine fed to the chimps was identified in the databook as SM N-90, pool 14. I was surprised that the Belgian doctors were still experimenting with SM N-90, a strain that was — in August 1957 — clearly a Lederle rather than a Wistar vaccine. However, it occurred to me that this might have been the name that Koprowski had given the material produced from CHAT Plaque 20, when he first brought it to Stanleyville in February of that year. Since he was still officially a Lederle employee, he would perhaps, at that stage, not have wished to reveal the vaccine's new name.

No other details of polio experiments feature in the databook. However, I wondered whether other unreported experiments might have been carried out.

Dirk Daenens had mentioned that some chimps had been trepanned in order to remove the brains, but he might have been recalling routine autopsies rather than intracerebral safety testing, for by this stage injecting poliovirus or vaccine direct into the brain was known to be a far less sensitive safety test than doing so into the spine.[25] The 1958 Stanleyville lab report had stated that it was the intention, during 1959, "to complete with polio 3 the experiments finished with polio 1 and 2," but there is no further mention of this research in the following year's report. Then, of course, there was traditional vaccination and challenge (with the same poliovirus type). However, by this stage it was widely accepted that chimps, being far less easily infected by the oral route than man, were really not very good research animals in which to conduct this type of work.[26]

For the first time, I began to consider the possibility that perhaps no further polio research had been carried out on the Lindi chimps. Perhaps the three types of test referred to in the annual reports of the Stanleyville lab (which, in the most precise account, described them as "infection trials, tests of effectiveness, tests of intraspinal innocuity")[27] may actually have been those three experiments of which I already had details from the databook, and the report in the *British Medical Journal*.[28] It seemed possible that these three trials constituted the *whole* of the polio research conducted at Lindi, the research that was said to have allowed the perfection, the *"mise au point définitive,"* of the Koprowski strains.

If this was correct, then approximately 94 chimps would have been involved in the polio experiments conducted at Lindi between June 1956 and June 1959 (most of which would have taken place in the first year and a half, up to the end of 1957).[29] Of these 94 chimps, some 48 (the 9 animals known to have been paralyzed by virulent virus, and the 39 injected intraspinally — from which spinal cords had to be extracted) would presumably have been sacrificed.

---

The researchers themselves provided several different accounts of the number of chimps used in the polio work — both at the time, and when I interviewed them some thirty-five years later. André Courtois told me that his father had always said that 200 chimps had been involved, but when interviewed at Lindi in the spring of 1958 for a rather delightful article entitled "A Beer with Ghislain Courtois," the lab director informed his companion: "The station you see was created for Dr. Koprowski, vice-president of the NYAS, to help him in his research on an anti-polio vaccine," adding that he, Courtois, had "managed to obtain about 100 chimps for his service."[30] However, an article that appeared in the Usumbura paper *Centre Afrique* at the very same time, and which once again appears to have been based on information provided by Courtois, states that "some 400" captive chimpanzees in Province Oriental had "made a large and helpful contribution to the perfecting of the [vaccine] formula used today."[31]

Even the hunters who were responsible for providing the chimps offer differing versions. A retrospective article written in 1960 by Captain-Commander Lefebvre of the Department of Hunting and Fishing reported that Gilbert Rollais, the chimp-catcher, had been commissioned by the Stanleyville lab to provide one hundred chimps during 1956/7, and another 60 in August 1959.[32] However, when I interviewed him in 1994, Rollais told me that around 300 chimps had been brought to Lindi for the polio research. Interviewed in the same year, Gaston Ninane had eventually conceded that the figure could have been as high as 400.

But in the end, it would seem that the chimp numbering system is the most reliable guide to the number of chimps that arrived in the camp alive,[33] for the evidence suggests that no numbers were missed out, and that chimp 416 was indeed the 416th Lindi admission.

The databook had provided hard evidence that chimp number 346 ("Molotov"), which arrived at Lindi on July 12, 1957, was involved in polio research, and suggested that all the chimps up to number 403, "Madeleine," admitted on December 26, 1957, may have been so employed. The question this begs is — if only some 48 of the Lindi chimps had to be sacrificed as a direct result of the polio research, what happened to the other 300 to 350?

In order to answer this question, it is first necessary to try to establish how many Lindi arrivals died in the days following the trauma of their capture, caging, and transfer to the camp, or through being exposed to disease in the two crowded hangars. The head of the Stanleyville veterinary lab, Louis Bugyaki, recalls that there was initially a high death rate at Lindi, but that this fell to between 10 percent and 20 percent following his interventions. This was confirmed by Courtois in a conference address delivered in 1966. He reported many of the pygmy chimps died to begin with (he hints at 50 percent), but added that the death rate declined thereafter, dropping to 10 percent for common chimps "at the end of our captures."[34] Given these accounts, it seems reasonable to suggest that some 75 to 150 of the 350-odd chimps admitted to Lindi between June 1956 and July 1957 (and which we know to have been involved with the polio research) may have died of natural causes.[35]

If one adds the 48 chimps known to have been sacrificed following the polio research, this still leaves some 150 to 225, or roughly half the total, unaccounted for.

---

Let us look for a moment at the causes of death of those chimps that died "naturally." All sources, ranging from the recollections of Ninane, Osterrieth, and Rollais, to the retrospective articles Courtois wrote in 1966 and 1967, refer to two important processes being under way at Lindi. One was stress and loneliness following capture and incarceration, which often resulted in a chimp starving itself to death. The pygmy chimp, it will be recalled, was found to be especially prone to committing suicide in this way, and one of the countermeasures taken was to place a pygmy chimp in the same cage as a common chimp, so that the latter would teach the former how to adapt to the new food regime.

The other main cause of death in the camp was pneumonia, most often caused by strains of *Klebsiella* bacteria. Courtois writes: "It is surprising to see a germ which is usually an intestinal saprophyte in man cause such havoc in the chimpanzee."[36] Both he and Osterrieth proposed that the primary cause of these infections may have been an underlying viral infection, which allowed the *Klebsiella* organisms to proliferate and become pathogenic. Only the administration of the antibiotic Terramycin (a form of tetracycline) proved to be effective against *Klebsiella*, but some chimps continued to die, which is why other methods — such as clothing the chimps in children's shirts and pullovers — were also attempted.

In 1960, Pierre Doupagne prepared a conference address that included an analysis of 113 pathogenic isolates of different *Candida* species, which, he wrote, were becoming "more and more frequent" in the course of his laboratory analyses at Stanleyville.[37] Neither the organs that the isolates came from, nor whether they were human or primate in origin, is detailed in the paper, and nowadays, M. Doupagne cannot recall the details.[38]

One of the most characteristic AIDS infections in *Homo sapiens* is recurrent pneumonia caused by *Klebsiella pneumoniae*.[39] Another is candidiasis of esophagus, trachea, bronchi, or lungs caused by *Candida* species — those quintessentially opportunistic organisms. And one of the first articles about simian AIDS in rhesus macaques identified infections caused by *Klebsiella pneumoniae* and *Candida* species as shared features of simian AIDS and human AIDS.[40]

Even though we know that some patients at the Stanleyville hospital died as a result of their *Klebsiella* infections in the period up to July 1958,[41] we simply do not have enough evidence to propose that any of them had AIDS. By contrast, we know that many of the Lindi chimps were dying, and that an underlying viral infection was suspected. It therefore seems legitimate to consider whether any of them were suffering from simian AIDS. Of course, to advance such a hypothesis, one would first have to assume that one or more of the apes brought to Lindi arrived in the camp already infected with SIV.

On the basis of the current (somewhat limited) sampling, the SIV infection rate of common chimps would appear to be roughly 2 or 3 percent,[42] and we know that at least two of the three subspecies of common chimps (*Pan troglodytes troglodytes* from Cameroon and Gabon, and *Pan troglodytes schweinfurthi* from the Congo) can be infected with the virus in the wild. On this basis, one would expect between eight and twelve of the first 400 chimps at Lindi to have been SIV-positive on arrival. Perhaps more to the point, the fact that the chimps were procured in the course of about a hundred capture operations, carried out in diverse localities within a 120,000-square-mile portion of rain forest, makes it highly probable that at least one of the groups sampled was infected with SIV.[43]

It is clear that the policy of putting two or more chimps together in a cage could have allowed onward spread of the virus from animal to animal. Furthermore, we know that chimps of different species (*Pan troglodytes* — the common chimp, and *Pan paniscus* — the pygmy) were caged together, permitting a degree of interspecies contact unprecedented for tens of thousands of years, since they diverged genetically on the right and left banks of the Congo River. There could, therefore, have been a cross-species transfer of SIVcpz from *troglodytes* to *paniscus* (or even, perhaps, a hitherto undiscovered *paniscus* SIV could have passed the other way).

The examples provided by the transfer of sooty mangabey SIV into different macaque species show that the arrival of an immunodeficiency virus in a new host can cause simian AIDS, and in this instance it may be that the ravages caused by opportunistic organisms such as *Klebsiella pneumoniae* were the visible demonstrations of SIV cross-species transfer.

Preston Marx's research suggests that in the wild, most sooty mangabeys are SIV-negative until they attain the age of sexual maturity,[44] but this apparently does not apply to chimpanzees, for three of the four SIV-positive chimpanzees to have been identified to date are juveniles.[45] This suggests that, as with humans, positive mothers can infect their offspring — which is important, for virtually all the Lindi chimps were immature animals. But we know that another viable method of SIV transmission between individual animals, and between species, is through biting and scratching.[46] Rollais and Ninane both recalled the fights that used to take place between the chimps, and we know that many of the researchers were shocked by the way that the common chimps attacked their pygmy relatives. Another mode of viral transfer could have been through the touching and licking of other animals' genitals, for which *Pan paniscus* of all ages are well known.[47]

It would therefore seem perfectly possible that some of the Lindi chimps were already SIV-positive when they arrived at the camp, and plausible to suggest that further infections (including transfers of SIV between species) may have occurred during the animals' stay there.

––––––––––

Now for a brief look at the pygmy chimp. It is not certain what precise role *Pan paniscus* played in the polio research — but both Koprowski and Courtois have commented that it was initially decided to utilize *Pan paniscus* because of the similarity between the blood of that species and of *Homo sapiens*.

More of the relevant history was revealed in a syndicated newspaper article with a Brussels dateline that appeared in March 1959. This recorded that "between 70 and 80 chimpanzees of a species considered by scientists as 'blood relatives of man' were used for the experiments. They belonged to a rare thin-limbed species called *Pan paniscus,* not the more common *Pan satyrus* [*troglodytes*] species usually seen in zoos. The animals were caught in a region of the great rain forest on the southern side of the Congo river.... Unlike most chimpanzees, the *paniscus* is ... not easily acclimatised to captivity. A score or two of them died as soon as they were brought to the Lindi farm before Dr Courtois began to treat them with antibiotics."[48]

In his article about Lindi camp published in the sixties, Courtois writes that when, despite all their efforts, the pygmy chimps continued to die, they injected them with anabolic steroids and that finally a decision was taken to "utilize" the remainder of the captured *Pan paniscus.* This presumably means they were used up on the polio research, although no further specific details are provided.[49]

However, there are also different versions of the *Pan paniscus* story that come from two visitors to Stanleyville — one a science journalist, and the other a primatologist. During 1957, the great British travel writer John Hillaby (formerly the London science correspondent of the *New York Times* and a regular contributor to *New Scientist*), was making a grand tour of Belgium's African colonies, and on June 6 he visited Lindi camp. In his journal of the trip, he records that *Pan paniscus* were being used by Courtois and Koprowski for the polio experiments, that many were dying because they refused to eat anything but sugarcane, but that they were now being kept alive by Terramycin injections.[50] He describes the conditions at Lindi as "pathetic."

When interviewed about the episode in July 1996, just three months before his death, Mr. Hillaby told me that the Belgians had been loath to take him out to visit the camp, and "were unwilling to talk about what Koprowski was doing.... There was a reluctance everywhere to talk about the chimps. Of course, this whetted my appetite ... what were they using the chimps for?"

In February 1960, the Dutch chimp specialist Adriaan Kortlandt paid a visit to Stanleyville; by this time most — if not all — of the chimps appear to have been moved from Lindi to the laboratory itself. Kortlandt recorded in his journal that all eighty-six *Pan paniscus* captured by the Laboratoire Médical for use in the polio research program a year or two earlier had died within three weeks.[51] (When compared to the other accounts, this sounds like an apocryphal version of how they met their ends.) The primatologist was disgusted by the conditions at the lab, and he argued strongly against siting the mooted chimpanzee breeding colony in this area, writing: "This *Laboratoire Médical* is the most miserable scientific institution I have ever seen. About 50 or 60 chimpanzees are kept here for polio research in about 40 boxes measuring one cubic metre each, in a most filthy condition.... I must add that a well-informed man warned me not to touch the *Laboratoire Médical,* because when doing so I might cut my fingers."[52]

The only other use of the Lindi chimps recorded in the medical literature is as a source of kidneys to make tissue culture — as evidenced by the six shipments from Stanleyville to the Children's Hospital of Philadelphia for hepatitis research in 1958 and 1959.[53]

Chimpanzee kidney tissue culture, many observers agree, would also have constituted a very good substrate for vaccine production, provided one could be assured of two things. First, the kidneys would need to be proven free of the dangerous viruses virologists were encountering in growing numbers in simian tissues. Second, they would need to be cheap.[54] This was an important point, because by the end of the sixties *troglodytes* were costing $400 in the United States or Europe, or between $140 and $200 when purchased directly from sailors coming from Africa.[55] Sums like these represented a lot of money within the context of the times.

However, neither of these factors would have afforded insurmountable problems to the researchers at Lindi. One of the first things that Koprowski did at Lindi (presumably in February 1957) was to take sera from 111 of the chimps. He tested 100 of the sera (from animals that had spent up to three or four months at the camp) for the three types of poliovirus, and found that only four had antibodies, which indicated that the animals were well isolated and had not come into contact with many human pathogens. He then handed the other eleven sera over to Henle's people at Children's Hospital, who found them free of human viruses such as measles, mumps, influenza A, and Coxsackie B.[56] Courtois conducted other tests, and found that the Lindi chimps were not infected with tuberculosis.[57] In 1958, Fritz Deinhardt tested another 60 or 70, and found that none had antibodies to the infamous simian B virus, so often fatal for animal handlers and lab technicians.[58] The investigators may have also tested the animals or their sera for the presence of other simian viruses; there was certainly ample opportunity to do so. Whatever, it seems that the Lindi chimps were generally considered to be free of the more dangerous pathogens that might be communicated to humans.

The other factor — cost — was also clearly not a major obstacle. Once the project had been funded (and Courtois's budget sheet for October 1957 shows that the expenditure was relatively modest),[59] Courtois and Koprowski had an almost limitless supply of chimpanzees that was costing next to nothing. According to Jos Mortelmans, the cost of a chimp in Stanleyville at that time was only five to ten U.S. dollars.

We can therefore deduce that in the late fifties in Stanleyville, chimp tissues would have been a reasonable material in which to produce polio vaccines. Furthermore, as we have already seen, there are several other clues suggesting that either Koprowski or Courtois might have considered them to be a suitable substrate.

First, there is the meeting between Koprowski, Norton, and Alexandre Jezierski at the start of February 1957. By this stage, Jezierski had tried out all sorts of mammalian and reptilian tissues for making primary cultures, and had enjoyed remarkable success with the kidneys of African primates, especially the various colobus species. He had developed his own OPVs in these substrates, and had made at least two successful batches of chimpanzee kidney tissue culture.

The second piece of suggestive evidence is that in 1957, the question of substrate was still an open issue. There was a vigorous debate then under way about the best (i.e., safest, best characterized, most readily available) material for manufacturing a polio vaccine — and a logical approach to the question of the vaccine substrate might be to use cells which were as close as possible to those of the intended host — *Homo sapiens*.[60] The investigators themselves may have been thinking along these lines when they referred to *Pan paniscus* as "a blood relative of man."

The third pointer involves the widespread concern that the supply of monkeys might be interrupted, just as it had been in 1955, when the Indian government placed a temporary ban on the export of rhesus macaques.[61] That incident had initiated a flurry of activity among virologists, and several institutions had begun investigating potential new sources of monkeys for making tissue culture.

The fourth point is that by 1957 it was known that even chimps that had been fed virulent poliovirus and produced antibodies showed no trace of the virus *in their kidneys* — as demonstrated by David Bodian, in an important paper published the previous year.[62] This was further confirmed by the CHOP hepatitis researchers who, in 1959, revealed that the kidneys used for their tissue culture experiments in Philadelphia had originated from "several chimpanzees used for poliomyelitis studies at the Lindi camp [which] had to be sacrificed at intervals."[63] Since one of the experiments conducted on these cultures at CHOP was to inoculate them with stool suspensions from hepatitis patients, and then to investigate whether challenges with other viruses (including Type 1 polio) caused interference, this meant that the researchers must have been confident that the original cultures were devoid of poliovirus. By the same standard, tissue cultures made from the kidneys of chimps previously used in vaccine and challenge experiments would presumably have been considered a safe substrate in which to grow polio vaccine.

The fifth clue involves availability. If chimps were freely available at Lindi, then why not make use of their kidneys?[64] In fact, the question of whether other, unrecorded polio experiments (such as vaccination and challenge with the same poliovirus type) were conducted there is in some ways immaterial, since most such experiments would have left the researchers with a stock of healthy chimps that, from a scientific perspective, were still suitable for other uses. Furthermore, if a chimp "turned its face to the wall" and decided to die (as many apparently did), then its only possible use would have been to provide tissues (including kidneys for culture).

Sixth, there was no innate scientific reason not to use chimp kidneys. Already two other polio vaccines had been developed by techniques that included passaging the vaccine virus through a chimpanzee, and extracting virus from its stools. These two vaccines were Sabin's Type 2 OPV, P-712 Ch 2ab,[65] and an inactivated vaccine known variously as Brunden and Brunenders.[66]

Last, virologists know that tissue cultures are best made from the kidneys of immature animals, the cells of which have suffered less damage to their DNA, and therefore produce better cultures than those of adults. But even young chimps have generously sized kidneys, which would provide more usable tissue culture material than those of smaller primates like macaques and African greens.[67]

One other point should be added. If one feared that public and scientific reaction to the use of chimpanzee kidney tissue culture might be negative, one could, in all honesty, describe this material generically as monkey kidney tissue culture, MKTC. Although primatologists nearly always distinguish between "monkeys" and "great apes" like the chimpanzees, popular usage does not. Nonspecialist dictionaries define a monkey first and foremost as a nonhuman primate, which includes all animals from the apes to the marmosets.[68]

----

Whichever primate tissues were used to make CHAT, there appear to have been five main candidates for the laboratory in which the early Koprowski strains were manufactured. These are: Ghislain Courtois's lab in Stanleyville; Lise Thiry's lab (either at the Université Libre de Bruxelles, or at the Pasteur Institute of Brabant, on the edge of Brussels; Pieter De Somer's (either at RIT's castle at Rixensart, the virology department at Leuven, or the Rega Institute); George Jervis's at Letchworth Village; and that of Hilary Koprowski at the Wistar Institute in Philadelphia.

Gaston Ninane told me that during his leave of March to September 1957, he spent some weeks, apparently on his own initiative, at Lise Thiry's lab in Brussels, getting training in making tissue cultures. Two articles published by Thiry soon afterward reveal that she had been given samples of CHAT and Fox by Koprowski in July 1957, probably at the time of the Geneva conference, and that the viruses (among others) were then grown in different substrates, including human cell lines and "several batches of monkey kidney cultures."[69] It is even possible that Ninane helped with some of this work.

Paul Osterrieth began his leave in October 1957 — and was invited by Koprowski to spend some time at the Wistar, again to learn tissue culture techniques. Once again, CHAT would have been the natural virus to work with, and according to Priscilla Norton, four pairs of chimp kidney were already present in the lab, brought back by her husband in March. From about February 1958 onward, further chimp kidneys were arriving in Philadelphia, courtesy of Fritz

Deinhardt. It could be that some of these ended up at the Wistar, and some may have gone to Letchworth Village, where that hardworking scientist George Jervis is known to have helped Koprowski with tissue culture studies throughout the fifties. Whatever, there was certainly enough chimp kidney tissue from Stanleyville available in America during this period to carry out a great deal of research — and not only into hepatitis. There would, for instance, have been enough to conduct some fairly exhaustive tests for adventitious simian viruses, and then to produce enough tissue culture material to make a large pool of vaccine.

Paul Osterrieth returned to Stanleyville on February 23, 1958, the day before the start of the Ruzizi trial, and around this time began making "a little" tissue culture, possibly in the kidneys of locally available monkeys; he believes (but is not sure) that these were baboons. At that point, Fritz Deinhardt was still in Stanleyville — working on hepatitis and mincing up chimp kidneys. Throughout this period, routine autopsies were being carried out by Ninane on every chimp that died, and kidneys were among the organs extracted.

In the course of our final interview, Ninane admitted that he had tried to make a tissue culture from chimpanzee kidneys in Stanleyville, but had failed. Apparently he employed the Maitland technique, which does not require trypsinizing the cells — an action that would have helped inactivate cell-free SIV. It is clear that had he succeeded in making a chimp kidney tissue culture in this way, it could have been an extremely dangerous substrate.

Both the surviving scientists from Stanleyville, Ninane and Osterreith, deny that an experimental batch of CHAT was prepared in chimpanzee kidney tissue culture and fed to local people (even though there was no reason not to do this at the time). However, another possibility is raised by the 1959 Stanleyville lab report, written by Ninane (who had just then taken over as director). This states that during the year a large batch of polio vaccine was *"conditioné,"* or divided up, into 250,000 individual doses, and then dispatched to Usumbura. With chimp autopsies and attempts to make CKTC going on in the same lab, there is clearly a chance that accidental contamination of the vaccine could have occurred.

What of the other labs in Belgium? Here, the evidence is a little more circumstantial — but still intriguing. In December 1967, at a symposium on tissue cultures, Ghislain Courtois announced that "[m]ore than 10 years ago we sent kidneys from the Congo to Europe and they were quite satisfactory."

That "more than 10 years ago" indicates that Courtois was referring to 1957 or earlier. This was the very period when he personally dispatched skulls from seventy-nine chimpanzees[70] to the Museum of Central Africa at Tervuren, just outside Brussels. This suggests that the kidneys sent to Europe may have been chimp kidneys[71] — a proposition that, it may be recalled, was deemed plausible by Courtois's friend and colleague at that symposium, Joseph Mortelmans. Courtois's comment was made in the context of a discussion about the problems inherent in making monkey kidney tissue cultures, and the fact that the kidneys proved to be "quite satisfactory" almost certainly means that the Congo kidneys were made into culture on arrival.

As to who received those kidneys, the likeliest candidate has to be Pieter De Somer, who had been out in Stanleyville at the virus symposium in September and October 1957. Whether or not he had access to chimp kidneys, it seems very possible that he started manufacturing CHAT for use in Africa within weeks of his return.

By the summer of 1958, this possibility has become a certainty. In August 1958, when Henry Gelfand from Tulane University flew to Brussels to collect the CHAT vaccine that was to be used in part of the Leopoldville campaign, it was Courtois (then on leave from Stanleyville) who handed the vaccine over to him at the main public health laboratories. Gelfand recalls that Courtois had previously collected it from another lab outside Brussels[72] — which is presumably a reference to one of De Somer's labs. Apparently Piet De Somer and Ghislain Courtois were old friends.

All this information is independently confirmed by other sources. The Stanleyville vet, Louis Bugyaki, thought that chimp kidneys had been sent to the Koprowski team. Fritz Deinhardt's widow, Jean, was one of several virologists who told me that there was no intrinsic reason not to use chimp kidneys to make vaccine if they were available — in fact, she said, it was a logical thing to do. There is thus a lot of anecdotal evidence to support the scenario that chimp kidneys may have been used to produce a batch of polio vaccine, even if many of the protagonists (such as Koprowski, Plotkin, Ninane, and Osterrieth) deny that such a thing ever occurred.

Unfortunately, anecdotal evidence is all that is available. Koprowski, the Wistar Institute, and Julian Peetermans of RIT all insist that no records of this particular period remain — and both the Wistar and the Karolinska Institute have failed to release samples of CHAT vaccine for independent testing. Such testing might or might not detect the presence of an immunodeficiency virus. But it would have a good chance of shedding light on the question of which substrate was used to passage CHAT virus, and which was used to grow the vaccine.

---

There is a postscript to the Lindi story, and, like the rest of the tale, it is a sad one. In February 1961, Ghislain Courtois, now back in Belgium, wrote a letter to a Dr. Jan Stijns, the director of the medical laboratory at the tropical institute in Leopoldville, the same institute that Courtois had headed for his final year in the Belgian Congo.[73]

Toward the end of the letter, Courtois discussed what should be done with the chimpanzees remaining in Stanleyville. "The remainder of the animals could be released in the bush," he writes; "a portion — for instance a few couples — could be released on the Isle of Liculi. . . . They shouldn't *all* be released there, for there is not enough suitable habitat, but we could then consider recovering them in the future. The rest could be released in the big forest behind the zoo (as long as the zoo does not wish to make use of them)."[74]

This speaks volumes. Like so many of his colleagues, Courtois still retained hopes of returning, of playing a role, in the newly independent Congo. Clearly he still thought it might prove possible to continue the chimpanzee work. He had yet to come to terms with the fact that an era had come to an end.

The colonial interlude had, certainly, provided the country with schools and hospitals, railway lines and river steamers. But it had also been an era of benign paternalism: an era when 400-odd chimpanzees could be collected together and treated as "test-tubes containing human illnesses,"[75] an era when hundreds of thousands of Africans could be used to field-test different versions of an experimental vaccine — and nobody thought twice about it.

————————

In 1997, I received a very pleasant letter from the widow of Jean Brakel, who had been a "sanitary officer" at the Laboratoire Médical between 1956 and 1960, and who had helped Gaston Ninane with the vaccinations in response to epidemics in northern Province Oriental at the start of 1958. She explained that, apart from the pets, none of the Lindi chimpanzees had survived. She confirmed that there had been a high death rate on arrival at the camp, but then explained what had happened to the remainder.

"Apart from Jamba, born in captivity, all the others were sacrificed for experiments at Lindi," she wrote.[76]

# 53

The usage of chimpanzees at Lindi camp and by the Laboratoire Médical de Stanleyville between June 1956 and June 1960, most notably the death or sacrifice of 350 to 400 chimps involved in the polio experiments of 1956 and 1957, has probably, thankfully, never been equaled, either before or since. The fact that the chimps came from two different species that were frequently caged together, and that many died from relatively harmless pathogens, suggests that some, at least, of the animals were also infected with other, undetected viruses — including, perhaps, simian immunodeficiency virus. It is certainly possible that chimpanzee SIV spread further between animals (and perhaps between species) within the camp.

The fact that blood and tissues from the Lindi chimps, including kidneys, were flown from Stanleyville to Philadelphia (and in all likelihood to Belgium as well), and the fact that attempts to make chimpanzee kidney tissue culture took place in the first two (and very possibly all three) of those places, suggests in turn that one or more experimental batches of CHAT vaccine may have been produced in chimpanzee kidney tissue culture, some of which may have contained SIV. An additional possibility is that accidental contamination with chimpanzee SIV occurred in the Stanleyville laboratory, during the transfer of CHAT vaccine into vials.

Given the very real possibility, therefore, that batches of CHAT may have become contaminated with chimp SIV, it becomes vital to have as complete as possible a picture of where the vaccine was fed in the Congo and Ruanda-Urundi in the years before independence. What follows is a summary of the evidence, including important new details that came to light as this book was being written.

The very first CHAT vaccinations in central Africa involved feeding the vaccine in capsule form. These are the same capsules Koprowski and Norton offered to various doctors in Nairobi in January 1957, and which they then carried to Stanleyville. This vaccine was apparently first fed, in February, to the African "caretakers" living at Lindi camp and their families;[1] thereafter it was fed at weekly intervals to small groups of volunteers and children in Stanleyville.[2] Just over a thousand people seem to have been vaccinated, mainly at the laboratory, over the next twelve months.

In May 1957, 1,978 children attending two schools at Aketi, some 250 miles northwest of Stanleyville, were also fed these capsules, and the same pupils were given the Fox Type 3 vaccine in December of that year.[3] Although the Courtois article credits Michel Forro, the Vicicongo doctor, with "carefully monitoring" this vaccination, it seems that the vaccine was actually dispensed by missionaries, such as the Little Sisters of Turnhout.[4] Indeed, it seems likely that Dr. Forro may have already left Aketi by the month of December.[5] The casual nature in which this trial was conducted and the delegation of responsibility are remarkable, given that Aketi was probably the first time that OPVs made in monkey kidney had ever been fed on a large scale in an open community anywhere in the world.[6]

The next vaccinations, in chronological order, were those carried out by Gaston Ninane and Jean Brakel in January and February 1958 in response to the polio epidemics at Banalia, Gombari, Watsa, and Bambesa. Nearly 23,000 people of all ages were vaccinated, and it was here, apparently, that Ninane began feeding vaccine via a syringe attached to a vaccine flask — a method that would later be described as the "Koprowski system."[7] Supplies ran out partway through the final campaign in Bambesa, which suggests that a medium-sized batch was sent to the Congo shortly before the vaccinations began, and that this batch was quite separate from the larger batches used in the mass vaccination that began in Ruzizi at the end of February. The source of the vaccine used in Banalia in early January is uncertain — but vaccine for the last three campaigns, which were staged between January 27 and February 1,[8] may have been brought out from Philadelphia by Fritz Deinhardt, who arrived in Stanleyville in late January.

Between February 24 and April 10, 215,504 people were vaccinated in the Ruzizi Valley, and between Usumbura and Nyanza Lac, along the eastern shore of Lake Tanganyika.[9]

In the published accounts by doctors Koprowski and Courtois, there are few specific details about exactly where the vaccine was fed in this trial[10] but more information was provided in 1995 by Mr. George Flack, the ninety-two-year-old brother of Agnes Flack, from Clinton Farms. Dr. Flack died in 1989, but George was kind enough to send me not only a batch of news clippings, but also some of Agnes's photos, together with copies of her letters and appropriate sections of her diary.

According to these sources, Dr. Flack and George Jervis arrived in Stanleyville on February 20, where they met Ghislain Courtois for the first time, and then the three doctors boarded the onward flight to Usumbura. Four days later the feedings began, interspersed with lunches at local missions, dinners and cocktail parties in Bukavu and Usumbura, and sight-seeing excursions at the weekends.

During the first week, the vaccination teams were based at the small Congolese town of Kabunambo, the headquarters of the Mission Médicale de la Ruzizi, a service that provided medical care on both sides of the border and that (like Vicicongo at Aketi) enjoyed almost autonomous status.[11] To begin with, the feedings proceeded slowly, and Flack recorded the totals with precision. On the first day, 2,579 people were vaccinated; on the second, 704 were fed in the morning, and 1,037 in the afternoon.[12] These early feedings were fairly small scale, so that by the Friday the total had reached just 12,000. During the next fortnight, the doctors split into two teams, and another 50,000 vaccinations were carried out — presumably on both sides of the valley, in the Congo and Ruanda-Urundi.

In this first part of the campaign, the vaccine was spoon-fed, with each spoon being sterilized in a flame between vaccinees, but presently Ninane's syringe method was adopted, which speeded things up considerably.[13] On Monday, March 17, Dr. Flack wrote a letter in which she referred to vaccinating from 11,000 to 12,000 daily and likened her work to being on a production line, "competing with Ford and General Motors."[14] That same day George Jervis had to fly back home, and Flack reported that 72,500 vaccinations have been completed.

Although the diary forecasts that the teams "will probably finish polio about April 10," Flack herself stayed only another fortnight. She now moved into a hotel in Usumbura, and the momentum of vaccination grew. During this period, only two venues are mentioned by name: Bugarama, up at the northern end of the vaccination area, in the southern corner of Ruanda, where 8,000 are fed, and "Kulyande,"[15] where she recorded 12,413 vaccinees, which appears to have been a record. There may have been an incentive that day, because the team was accompanied by an American couple, Robert and Joan Phillips, who were filing reports from the area.[16] This is when Robert Phillips took his famous shots of Dr. Flack, in pith helmet, squirting vaccine into the mouth of an infant, as a sea of Africans stretches away into the distance — and it was these photos that, for many years up to 1992, were on display on the walls of the Wistar Institute, and that Koprowski provided to *Rolling Stone* for the Tom Curtis article.[17]

The running totals in the diary suggest that by the time that Gaston Ninane waved good-bye to Agnes Flack at Usumbura airport on the morning of March 30, about 150,000 people had been fed. This estimate is supported by an article that appeared in *Le Stanleyvillois* three weeks earlier, which revealed that Dr. Courtois was just beginning the vaccination of "some 150,000 natives" in the Ruzizi Valley.[18] It seems, therefore, that this represented the quantity of vaccine provided for the main part of the campaign, which had presumably been prepared at the Wistar Institute and brought out to Africa by Flack and Jervis. Courtois later reported that "in agreement with Dr. Jervis . . . the mother-solution" of vaccine was diluted about sixty times. Since each vaccinee received a squirt of one cubic centimeter, this means that just two and a half liters of concentrated vaccine would have been enough for the feeding of the 150,000 — an economy of scale rivaling that of the loaves and fishes.[19]

Dr. Flack, meanwhile, flew on to Johannesburg, where she enjoyed a week's vacation before returning to New York via Brussels, where she twice met with Lise Thiry, from the local branch of the Pasteur Institute. At the same time, Hector Meyus and Gaston Ninane were just completing their vaccination of a further 65,000 in Usumbura and alongside Lake Tanganyika.[20]

By this time, another vaccination had taken place in Stanleyville, with more than 3,000 men, women, and children from the military camps being vaccinated on that special Koprowski day — February 27, 1958. Fritz Deinhardt was apparently in attendance. Fox was fed to the same group in May.

A document submitted to the inspector general of hygiene in Brussels by his Congolese counterpart in September 1958 reveals that two further vaccinations took place in Province Oriental during the first half of 1958 — at the town of Rungu and at the gold mines of Kilo. Clearly there were also other vaccination campaigns. Gaston Ninane, for instance, recalls vaccinating along the eastern shore of Lake Kivu in Rwanda (probably in 1959), and at Lisala in Equateur province, at a date unknown.

The next major Congolese vaccination is the only one to be well documented — that of some 76,000 children in the capital, Leopoldville, between August 1958 and April 1960. Fox Type 3 vaccine was also fed, beginning in September 1959, and starting in the same month both vaccines were offered to European volunteers. André Lebrun, the effective director of hygiene for the city, says that he remembers helping to organize the vaccination of several thousand more in Leopoldville province, in the Bas-Congo region that lies between the capital and the Atlantic Ocean. He specifically recalled vaccinations at the ports of Matadi, Boma, and Muanda, and at the provincial capital of Thysville (now Mbanza-Ngungu).

In May 1959, Lebrun, Courtois, and Stanley Plotkin (visiting from the Wistar) held a press conference in Leopoldville to report on the continued success of the vaccinations, and the plans to extend them to children throughout the country. It was revealed that vaccinations had already taken place in several other towns, including Tshela in Leopoldville province, and Bukavu, Goma, Kalima, and Kindu in Kivu province. Furthermore, plans were announced to extend the vaccinations to 10,000 children in the region of Stanleyville,[21] 64,000 in the regions of Kabare-Lubudi,[22] and a million in Ruanda-Urundi.[23] Stanley Plotkin himself took part in the Leo and Stanleyville vaccinations, and in a further campaign in Kikwit, Kasai province, which had to be abandoned following local unrest.

Details of other small vaccination campaigns that took place ad hoc, dependent on collaboration with various individuals or groups, have been located more or less by chance. The small town of Bafwasende in Province Oriental was vaccinated during 1959, with the help of the local doctor.[24] Nurses working for the Baptist Missionary Society hospital at Yakusu vaccinated children attending mother-and-child clinics along a fifty-mile stretch of the Congo River, to the west of Stanleyville, in 1958 or 1959.[25] And at some time in late 1959 or early 1960, a campaign was staged at the large town of Coquilhatville ("Coq"), in Equateur province.[26]

The wide variety of sources for this information, which range from personal memories to newspaper articles, from internal reports to private correspondence, suggests that this is almost certainly not a complete list of all the CHAT vaccination campaigns conducted in the Belgian Congo in the years 1957–1960. The doctors who headed the colony's Hygiene Service during those years, and who might be expected to know the answers,[27] nowadays explain that no lists remain, or that they cannot recall any further localities.

However, the synopsis presented above probably includes most of the major CHAT campaigns conducted in the Congo during the final three years of colonial rule. It reveals that, in all probability, relatively few vaccinations occurred in the three central provinces of Equateur (two campaigns at Lisala and Coquilhatville), Kasai (no feedings), and Katanga (one planned vaccination at Lubudi).[28] By contrast, at least a dozen campaigns were staged in Province Oriental, five in Kivu province, and seven in Leopoldville province, including the carefully monitored campaign in the capital itself. In short, there does appear to be a clear geographical division between those areas of the Belgian Congo where CHAT was fed, and those where it was not.

—————

But what of Ruanda-Urundi, and the million vaccinations that were proposed there? I eventually managed to locate the former director of hygiene for the territory, Hector Meyus. He recalled that the vaccine had come from Stanleyville in special cool-boxes, and that he and Ninane had spent "four or five days together," vaccinating at the lakeside village of Rumonge, and possibly farther north as well — he mentioned Usumbura and the village of Kabezi. It was clear that he thought of the campaign as being quite distinct from that of Ruzizi, and it now seemed almost certain that there had been two separate trials. But at this point he suddenly downed a stein of good Belgian beer and said he could remember nothing more. His wife, however, later wrote me with the address of a sanitary officer who used to work for her husband, a man called Caubergh whom she thought would be able to help me.

I visited Hubert Caubergh at his home in late 1996, and he indeed turned out to be an invaluable source of information. This was partly because he had not been affected by the panic that obtained in the Congo in 1960. Ruanda-Urundi did not achieve independence until 1962, and Herr Caubergh left in late 1961, carrying copies of several important documents with him. Some of these had since been thrown out, but fortunately he had kept one vital paper in his personal file.

This paper contained details of the mass vaccination with CHAT of children in the southern half of the protectorate, Urundi, from 1959 to 1960 — and it listed exact totals of vaccinees for every vaccination point in every district or *territoire*. Even better, it also included full details of the Burundian children who had been fed in the two campaigns that made up the so-called Ruzizi Valley trial of February to April 1958. It was a superbly precise document, and provided exactly the type of detailed summary that was lacking for the Belgian Congo vaccinations.[29]

The Burundi campaign of early 1958, it was now revealed, had involved the vaccination of 58,787 children at twenty-seven different vaccination centers. (Caubergh had not recorded the feeding of adolescents and adults, but other evidence suggests there were about 82,000 of these.)[30] Most important, Caubergh's paper provided the first documentary confirmation from one of the vaccinators that CHAT feeding had occurred not only in the Ruzizi Valley (along the roads between Usumbura and both Bubanza and Bugarama), but also along the road running south from Usumbura, through Rumonge to Nyanza Lac.

Then there was the later campaign. Between December 20, 1959, and March 3, 1960, Caubergh and his colleagues vaccinated a total of 321,203 children, (some 83 percent of the target population of infants to five-year-olds) at 150 different vaccination centers in Urundi. They worked their way around the different *territoires*, starting in the east of the country, which had not featured in the 1958 campaign,[31] and ending up in two of the *territoires* that had already been vaccinated two years earlier: Usumbura and Bubanza (the latter containing the eastern side of the Ruzizi Valley).[32] The remaining two zones, these being Usumbura city center and the *territoire* of Bururi (containing the shoreline of Lake Tanganyika), were not revaccinated in 1959/60. By March 1960, therefore, most of the young children of Burundi (save for those from the inland areas of Bururi *territoire*, away from the lake) had been immunized with CHAT.[33]

After giving me a copy of this document, Hubert Caubergh added two important details. He told me that all the vaccine for the 1959/60 campaign had been made by RIT in Belgium, and forwarded through the Laboratoire Médical de Stanleyville, and that both Dr. Courtois and a representative from RIT were frequently present during the vaccinations.

He also recalled a mass vaccination in the northern part of the protectorate, Ruanda, which, he said, had taken place either shortly before or after that in Urundi. Although he had discarded the relevant paper, he recalled that only part of Ruanda had been vaccinated: the *territoire* of Cyangugu at the southern end of Lake Kivu, possibly followed by a part of Kibuye farther north on the lake and, in the east, the *territoire* of Astrida, followed by a small part of Nyanza, where the old Tutsi capital was sited. Later, I pointed out that the first Hutu uprising in Ruanda had begun in November 1959, and he agreed that 1959 was almost certainly the year when the Ruandan campaign had been staged, and that the uprising was very likely the reason why it had been abandoned. When I mentioned Gaston Ninane, and his memories of vaccinating along the eastern side of Lake Kivu within sight of the red-stained clouds above the volcanoes, Caubergh agreed that it was probably Ninane who had headed the Lake Kivu team, while he himself was in charge in Astrida and Nyanza. The 1959 report of the medical services of Ruanda-Urundi reports 137,390 polio vaccinations, and it seems likely that this was the total for the truncated campaign in Ruanda.

———————

Altogether, therefore, it seems that between February 1958 and March 1960, at least 660,000 vaccinations with CHAT were carried out in the Belgian protectorate of Ruanda-Urundi. This represents approximately 17 percent of the then 3.9 million population.[34] In all likelihood, more than 100,000 of the vaccinees were adults.[35]

The figures for the Belgian Congo are less precise, but it seems likely that about 330,000 were vaccinated with CHAT between February 1957 and June 1960,[36] which represented some 3 percent of the then population of 11 million. More than 60,000 of the vaccinees were adults,[37] and at least 6,000 persons were also fed Fox.

This makes a grand total of 990,000 CHAT vaccinees for Belgium's former African colonies in the years 1957–1960, and this figure does not include certain adult vaccinees, and those vaccinees who may have been fed in other campaigns that still await discovery. In all likelihood, therefore, the grand total is well over a million. This total is supported by Ghislain Courtois, who gave a speech at Lovanium in April 1960, and said that, with regard to Koprowski's OPV, "At this moment in the Congo and Ruanda-Urundi, the number of those vaccinated is not far from a million."[38]

———————

Which pools of CHAT vaccine were given in which places? Those fed in some of the individual African campaigns can be identified with certainty. The one relevant sheet of paper given to the Wistar expert committee investigating the OPV/AIDS theory reveals that the "first pool" of CHAT, which was fed to five Clinton infants (on February 27, 1957), was also produced in capsules that were fed in both Stanleyville and Aketi.[39] It seems that this first pool consisted of "material representing plaque 20"[40] (in other words CHAT Plaque 20, passaged one or more times in MKTC), and that it later came to be referred to as CHAT pool 4B, or 4B-5.

This same paper confirms that pool 10A-11 was "to be used in the 1958 Congo trials," and various clues suggest that this meant not only the intended vaccination in the Ruzizi Valley but also the four feedings in response to epidemics in Province Oriental.[41]

It is certain that the feeding of 215,000 people in the Ruzizi Valley and along Lake Tanganyika between February and April 1958 involved CHAT pool 10A-11.[42] Several sources make it clear that the 150,000-odd vaccinees fed in the valley itself by Flack and Jervis received vaccine prepared at the Wistar Institute. However, it seems likely that the final 65,000 doses, fed in Usumbura and along the lakeshore, were prepared elsewhere, possibly at one of De Somer's labs in Belgium.[43] It may even be that the researchers decided to compare the efficacy of American and Belgian batches of pool 10A-11 in different test areas, and that Koprowski reported only on the U.S. vaccine trial, while Courtois hinted at both in his article. (Koprowski did, however, include the total number of vaccinees from both trials. In those days, the number vaccinated without apparent mishap was crucial to the credibility of a vaccine manufacturer.)

A similar situation obtains with CHAT pool 13, which was used in the best-reported campaign of all, that conducted in Leopoldville. Henry Gelfand, from Tulane University in New Orleans, has a clear memory of collecting Belgian-made vaccine from Ghislain Courtois in Brussels in August 1958, and delivering it for use in the Leopoldville campaign.[44] However, comments by the Belgian and American vaccinators in Leopoldville in 1959 indicated that the vaccine had been made at the Wistar Institute.[45]

We have already discovered that vaccine pools are not necessarily homogeneous, and CHAT vaccine pools 10A-11 and 13, at least, would appear to have been made partly at the Wistar and partly in Belgium.[46]

As for the rest of the CHAT used in central Africa, we know from Caubergh that the vaccine fed to over 450,000 people in Ruanda and Urundi in 1959 and 1960 was made in Belgium by RIT and forwarded through Stanleyville. This would appear to have been pool DS, and it seems very possible that the other 1959/60 Congo vaccinations that are not formally documented in the literature involved the same Belgian-made pool.[47]

Very little is known about the Belgian-manufactured pools of CHAT and how they were prepared. It is possible that, as claimed at one stage by Ninane, the early Belgian pools — 10A-11 and 13 — employed both vaccine virus and tissue culture material from the Wistar, and that one was inoculated into the other in Belgium. However, the fact that pool DS was given a different name suggests that it may have employed CHAT from the Wistar that was given one extra passage at RIT in a Belgian-prepared tissue culture (perhaps one derived from the kidneys of cynomolgus macaques, as Dr. Peetermans recalls). All of this must remain conjecture, however, for apparently neither the records nor stocks of Belgian-made CHAT are still in existence.

———————

This issue of where and how the pools of CHAT vaccine were prepared is, of course, absolutely central to the story. One of the principal lines of defense offered against the OPV/AIDS theory (notably by Koprowski) has always been that the same vaccines were used in Africa and Europe, but that AIDS did not make an early appearance in those European venues where they were fed.[48] CHAT pool 13, it is pointed out, was fed to 76,000 children in Leopoldville — and was also given to children in Poland.[49]

However, in interviews, both Koprowski and Plotkin agreed that "pool" was an imprecise term. Plotkin explained that it could be taken either to mean a seed pool (the attenuated poliovirus in its pure form), or a production lot (a pool of vaccine used for feeding, which had been made from the seed pool by further passage or passages in a substrate like MKTC or HDCS).

Thus, whereas a seed pool of attenuated poliovirus would have been made at one place, at one time, in a single production run, production lots (or feeding pools) of polio vaccine could have been made at different times, at different places — and, most crucially, in different substrates. Both virus and vaccine, however, would bear the same generic name — such as "CHAT pool 13," or "pool DS."

One of the best illustrations of this is afforded by the five vials of CHAT pool 10A-11 tested in Stockholm, which were revealed to contain vaccine made in two different places, at three (or more) different times, and probably in at least two different substrates.[50]

Another example would be the field trial conducted by Drago Ikic in Croatia in 1963, when 11,000 children were fed Koprowski's improved Type 3 polio strain, WM-3. The blinded study was specifically designed to test the safety of the substrate, and on this occasion it was clearly reported in the literature that half of the vaccine had been prepared in MKTC, and half in human diploid cell strains.[51]

Perhaps the most important variable for a pool of vaccine is that of the substrate, and yet the substrate is the very issue about which Koprowski did not provide details — in particular regarding the species of monkey used — for the better part of a decade.[52]

Therefore, without proper records, there is absolutely no guarantee that the CHAT pool 13 fed in Leopoldville was the same as the CHAT pool 13 fed in Wyszkow, Poland, or that the pool 13 prepared at the Wistar was made in the same way as the pool 13 apparently prepared in Belgium. Equally, there is no way of knowing whether the CHAT pool 10A-11 fed to the population in the Ruzizi Valley in 1958 was prepared in the same way, made in the same substrate, as the 10A-11 fed along the east shore of Lake Tanganyika — or the 10A-11 sent by the Wistar to Sweden. It is apparent that different versions of the vaccine may have been prepared for different trials in Africa and Europe — or, alternatively, simply in order to increase the available quantity (or titer).

Unless one knows the exact history of how a vaccine is made — and can show, for instance, that only a single production lot was produced from a particular seed pool — one cannot point to a vaccine sample that is free from adventitious viruses, and use this as proof that other vaccine samples with the same numerical "title" are also free of viral surprises.

---

There are a few additional and important points to be made about the central African vaccinations with CHAT. The first concerns the way in which they were carried out — the question of whether vaccinees volunteered or were coerced. It will be remembered that Koprowski was heavily criticized, both in the United States and in Britain, for his description of the first children to be fed OPV (who were seriously handicapped) as "volunteers," but that by the mid-fifties he and his colleagues were taking care to obtain written consent — for instance, from the parents at Sonoma, and the mothers at Clinton. But how was this issue tackled with the one million vaccinees in central Africa?

The general approach appears to have been one of benevolent paternalism. The well-meaning vaccinators seem to have argued that since their African charges were uneducated and ignorant of the benefits of the procedure, they had to be persuaded to attend the *séances de vaccination* by whichever means were most effective.

What such an argument overlooks is the fact that the vaccines being used (at least in the early campaigns) were still experimental. CHAT, for instance, had been fed to only two Clinton infants (and tested intraspinally and intracerebrally in rhesus monkeys — though not, at that stage, in chimpanzees) when Koprowski began offering it freely to doctors in Kenya and the Congo in January and February 1957. In fact, all the African campaigns up to and including Leopoldville (which ended in April 1960) were described as "trials," and one suspects that many of the unreported feedings with Belgian-made vaccine had similar status. Not until September 1959, thirty-one months after the first Africans were fed CHAT, did the Belgian authorities consider the vaccine safe enough for white inhabitants of the Congo to be encouraged to seek immunization.

So how were the Africans encouraged to attend the early vaccination sessions? In Aketi, the first-ever mass trial, the schoolchildren were apparently informed that they would be receiving *bonbons*.[53] Ninane says that at Ruzizi people were told they would be getting "chocolate."[54] Agnes Flack's diary entry for the first day of the Ruzizi vaccination, February 24, 1958, notes: "Cooperation fantastic. Chief of village notified [that] everyone *had* to come and nobody said no."[55] Similarly, in Leopoldville, a decision was made to vaccinate all African children from infants to five-year-olds, which meant that "the population was called street by street by the administrative authorities the day before vaccination."[56] Once again, it would seem that refusing vaccination for one's child was not an option.

And how much benefit accrued to the participants in these trials? The *British Medical Journal* paper on the early African trials states that "Immunization of the total population of the community was decided upon only if 12% or more of the sera collected were found to have no antibodies against a given type of virus" (in other words, if at least 12 percent of the population lacked pre-existing immunity). Indeed, exactly 12 percent of the 84 pre-vaccination sera collected from the Ruzizi Valley were found to lack antibodies to Type 1 polio-virus.[57] On this basis, some 215,000 people were vaccinated. However, at a speech given at a conference in June 1958, just two months after the trial, Koprowski revealed that in actual fact only between 5 percent and 7 percent of the Ruzizi population lacked Type 1 antibodies, which meant that only between 11,000 and 15,000 of that vast number of vaccinees could potentially have benefited from the immunization campaign.[58] Later, in Leo, it was found that only some 60 percent of the CHAT vaccinations were actually effective in the African environment,[59] so it may be that just 3 percent of those fed CHAT in Ruzizi were actually immunized against polio as a result.

The Ruzizi paper also makes it clear that there was no *active* follow-up of the vaccinated population, even if medical authorities were asked to report "any occurrence of illness which could be attributed to vaccination." The fact that no such reports were made was later questioned by George Dick, who pointed out that even under normal circumstances, at least 150 of the 240,000-odd vaccinees reported in the *BMJ* paper should have died and many more fallen ill in the month following vaccination.

Even more alarming is the possibility that some of the vaccine batches may have reverted to virulence. All the early polio vaccines had a tendency to revert, as was frankly admitted by Stanley Plotkin, the managing director of the huge vaccine house Pasteur Mérieux, when he told me: "Even triple plaque purification would leave you with viruses that, in retrospect, were only mutated a few times, and so were capable of reversion. . . . Purification only leads to stability for a finite period."[60] He added that the vaccines most capable of reversion were the Type 3 vaccines, followed by Types 2 and 1, in that order.

Certainly Sabin had his problems,[61] as did Cox.[62] But Koprowski's strains seem to have had a particular problem with reversion and spread, as seen at Belfast.[63] Other worrying episodes include the four mysterious polio cases in the cottage next door to the TN trial at Sonoma[64] and the 120 polio cases which occurred in Province Oriental[65] (mostly close to vaccinated areas) in the first eight months of 1958.[66]

However, the potential of reversion was carefully investigated in Leopoldville, where a polio epidemic began in October 1958, in suburbs neighboring those where CHAT vaccination had started two months earlier. Over the next seventeen months 175 children developed polio in the city, of whom nearly 40 percent were vaccinees.[67] Stanley Plotkin ran quite exhaustive tests, concluding that the strains isolated from both vaccinated and unvaccinated cases of polio were genetically related to wild virus rather than vaccine virus.[68] But in an accompanying article, Sven Gard was far less sanguine. Having examined a number of isolates of excreted virus, not only from Leo, but also from the United States and Sweden, he concluded Koprowski's oral polio vaccines had the capacity to revert to virulence after human passage.[69] It is relevant to add that nowadays we know that after vaccination with OPV, poliovirus replicates for between several days and three months in immunocompetent people, and for much longer (a year or more) in persons who are immunodeficient.[70]

Subsequent developments, moreover, raised some real doubts about the efficacy of the Leopoldville vaccination campaign, for in 1961 the city saw the worst polio epidemic in its recorded history, with 296 cases (almost all in children) and 62 deaths. A Belgian doctor, Julian De Moor, who described this epidemic, admitted that "we don't know if this [the Type 1 poliovirus circulating in 1961] has the same characteristics as the wild virus circulating before the campaign of August 1958, or those of the attenuated CHAT vaccine strain."[71] A vaccination campaign initiated in 1961 failed, with only some 4,000 children being vaccinated. It was only in 1962, by which time the polio epidemic had alarmed most inhabitants, that the Service d'Hygiène was finally able to vaccinate 560,000 of the capital's population — this time with the Sabin vaccine.[72]

Even if there was a great population influx into Leo after independence,[73] it is remarkable that there should have been such a huge epidemic just one year after the mass vaccination of the under-fives (the age group that makes up over 95 percent of Africa's susceptible population)[74] with the Koprowski strains. It is also intriguing that by 1961 the residents of newly independent Leopoldville should have been so averse to vaccination, even when confronted with a raging polio epidemic. Perhaps for some, at least, the right to say "no" may have outweighed the perceived benefits of Western health care.

In fact, the African population was justified in its skepticism. The CHAT vaccine used in central Africa would seem to have achieved rather poor levels of immunization, and apart from the Leo campaign, it was not carefully monitored. Furthermore, as we have seen, there is evidence to suggest that this vaccine may have reverted to virulence and, even worse, may have been contaminated with one or more simian viruses. It is clear, from the perspective of the nineties, that instead of being ordered to attend the vaccination sessions by chiefs or colonial officials, or lured there with promises of *bonbons* and chocolate, the African "natives" of the fifties ought to have enjoyed the right to accept or refuse the vaccine, just like their American and European counterparts.

--------

The last intriguing question concerns which other organizations — apart from the Wistar Institute and RIT — were in any sense involved with the African CHAT trials. That the government of the Belgian Congo, and in particular the medical administration under Dr. Charles Dricot, had approved the entire process, from the setting up of the camp at Lindi to the mass vaccinations, has never been in question.[75] However, it is remarkable that so little documentation about the trials is available — and it would seem probable that somewhere in Belgian government records, perhaps among those closed Hygiène files in the Ministry of Foreign Affairs archives, a comprehensive account of the vaccinations *does* exist. The pronounced gap in the "Poliomyélite" correspondence file for the key period of October 1956 to July 1958, when there are copious entries before and after, is baffling.[76]

The degree of World Health Organization involvement in the CHAT trials has been a subject of some controversy, and requires clarification. In July 1957, after the Fourth International Poliomyelitis Conference at Geneva, the WHO's Expert Committee on Poliomyelitis, featuring Sabin, Lépine, Gard, Gear, Melnick, and eleven other eminent scientists (though not Koprowski) convened for a week-long session, at the end of which it issued a detailed report, which contained the statement that "the Committee strongly recommends that controlled field trials [of OPVs] be carried out for the purpose of testing further the value of these agents."[77] The committee recommended that several specific criteria should be met before such trials be allowed to proceed, among them that they should take place only under the most careful supervision, that participation be voluntary, and that ideally they be conducted in areas where poliovirus was endemic, and/or in the face of an impending epidemic. Another condition was that the vaccine strains used should meet certain criteria of safety.

This was a clear signal from these most eminent of scientists that properly conducted field trials of OPVs could now proceed in areas like Africa, where exposure to poliovirus occurred naturally at an early age. The committee's report prompted a front-page article in the *New York Times*,[78] and Koprowski referred to it in his *BMJ* article on the mass vaccinations in the Congo and Ruanda-Urundi, stating that it sanctioned his initiative.[79]

However, the CHAT trials in central Africa did not meet with the WHO approval Koprowski apparently expected. In December 1958, Dr. Payne, secretary to the WHO's expert committee, wrote to the *BMJ* in an attempt to clarify certain points. He confirmed that tests on "hundreds of thousands of people would be necessary" to confirm the safety of an OPV, but added that this was "a statement of fact and not a recommendation that such tests be carried out now." He went on:

> These large-scale tests should not be carried out until there is good presumptive evidence of safety and stability, based both on laboratory evidence and on small-scale human studies. The Expert Committee insisted most strongly on the need for a cautious extension of strictly controlled human trials under the most careful supervision. The criteria which should be fulfilled were specified in some detail. So far WHO has not given direct support to any trial of live poliovirus vaccine and, contrary to some reports, the "test" in the Belgian Congo was not supported by WHO.[80]

Although Dr. Payne does not spell out the reasons, it is quite clear that he and his colleagues felt that Koprowski's trials had failed to meet certain of the committee's criteria. With the evidence that we now have, we might suspect that the trials were deemed inadequate on several counts, including supervision, voluntary participation, a cautious increase in scale, and proven vaccine safety.[81]

This brings us to the final question — that of the degree to which the U.S. Public Health Service (and its various arms, like the CDC's Epidemiology Intelligence Service) may have been involved in Koprowski's research and vaccination trials in central Africa between 1957 and 1960. The official position is that it was not, and the major participants went to some lengths to confirm this. For instance, Stanley Plotkin, who was lead author of the second article about the Leopoldville vaccinations, is identified in that article both as a research associate of the Wistar Institute and a member of the Epidemiology Branch of the CDC of the PHS. A note carefully adds: "This work was done when Dr. Plotkin visited Leopoldville in May 1959 while on leave from the Public Health Service and the opinions expressed are those of the authors only."[82] During this period Plotkin apparently described himself as "only a scientific observer for the University of Philadelphia [sic] and the Wistar Institute."[83]

However, there were, of course, many sound reasons for the U.S. Public Health Service to be actively interested in the outcome of the trials in the Congo and Ruanda-Urundi. Certainly other participants in those trials — such as

Agnes Flack and Ghislain Courtois — were under the clear impression that the PHS *was* directly involved.[84] Furthermore, Hilary Koprowski received a PHS research project grant, number E-1799, for the "Study of attenuated strain of poliomyelitis virus"— a grant that was acknowledged in all his papers about central Africa, as well as in others, such as those on the Clinton investigations.[85]

But apart from this USPHS grant, there may have been certain less official contributions made. It is certainly possible that some informal financial contribution came from American sources to assist the construction of the large, new, and well-equipped laboratory and animal house that opened in Stanleyville in late 1957.[86] Otherwise this would have represented an extraordinary investment for the relatively impoverished Belgian colony to be making at that point in time, just as the African wind of change was beginning to blow. Perhaps the potential for chimpanzee research was viewed as a key factor, as suggested by the fact that construction work began at virtually the same time that Lindi camp opened, in June 1956.

The United States Public Health Service would not, of course, have been the only organization interested in the potential of an institution where chimpanzee research could be conducted. This is illustrated by the speech delivered in Lyon in 1966 by Ghislain Courtois, in which he gave the background to the attempts by the United States and Belgium to set up a chimpanzee breeding colony in the final year before independence. He first referred to the chimp camp at Lindi (established, he explained, in response to a proposal by Koprowski) and continued: "In the end we decided to move on to the second stage of our project, which involved trying to breed and raise the chimps. Contacts had been established with the American Public Health Service authorities, and a delegation led by Karl Meyer of the Hooper Foundation came to Leopoldville in 1960 to meet representatives of the Belgian Congo government."[87] Apart from Koprowski, the delegation represented a wide range of research interests, and was scheduled to include Willard Eyestone from the National Institutes of Health, Art Riopelle from Yerkes Primate Center, George Burch from Tulane University, and Cowles Andrus from Johns Hopkins.[88] However, the plans had to be abandoned due to the political unrest that followed.

At around the same time as the visit by Karl Meyer's delegation, one of the last CHAT vaccinations was taking place at the important town of Coquilhatville, northeast of Leo on the Congo River. Again, political events meant that the job of monitoring the vaccinations had to be abandoned, but a letter written by Courtois in February 1961 reveals that by then he had made arrangements for the CDC (rather than the Congolese or Belgian authorities) to analyze the stools and the pre- and post-vaccination blood samples.[89]

All this raises the question of whether the United States Public Health Service was to some extent using the Wistar (and, indirectly, the Laboratoire Médical) for the field-testing of American OPVs in Africa, a question that in turn leads us back to the roles played by Stanley Plotkin and Joseph Pagano. The two men were among the brightest stars of the Epidemiology Intelligence Service of the CDC (itself an arm of the Public Health Service), and both say that they volunteered to go on secondment to the Wistar soon after Koprowski took over, and that once there, they applied to work on the OPV program. A newspaper article from 1958 describes the Moorestown study as being carried out by Koprowski "in conjunction with a team of top epidemiologists representing the USPHS Communicable Disease Center field post that is located in Wistar,"[90] which suggests an official collaboration. Be that as it may, we do know that Plotkin and Pagano were central figures in the Wistar's OPV research throughout their periods of secondment, and did much of the organization of the field trials at Clinton, Moorestown, and Philadelphia in the United States, and in the Congo, Poland, and Croatia.[91]

One can only guess at the exact details of the understanding that appears to have existed between the PHS and the Wistar. Even if there were, at times, significant tensions between Koprowski and PHS officials,[92] it is apparent that the Wistar stood to benefit from the collaboration both materially and through association, while the PHS was eager to see the results of Koprowski's field trials in places like the Congo and Poland, especially when it was felt not to be safe or viable to conduct such large-scale OPV trials in the United States itself.

PHS officials would undoubtedly have been equally interested in, and supportive of, Sabin's trials in the Soviet Union. It seems possible that the reason why such trials were initiated and handled by independent researchers like Koprowski and Sabin, rather than at governmental level, was the fear of the worst-case scenario — and of the political fallout that would be generated should something go wrong with a mass vaccination in a foreign land.

Apparently there were no major mishaps in the Soviet trials — even if certain polio researchers suspect that the results may have been "cleaned up" for public consumption. Stanley Plotkin, for instance, told me: "In retrospect, I think some of those Russian data were, if not deliberately faked, then at least greatly exaggerated."[93]

However, given the absence of vital data, it is less easy to state categorically that nothing went wrong with the CHAT trials in the Congo.

# 54

CORRELATIONS WITH EARLY

## HIV AND AIDS

Gerry Myers, head of the HIV Sequence Database, has described the manner in which the different HIV-1 subtypes emerged in terms of "a star-like configuration suggestive of evolutionary radiation from a single ancestral virus."[1] To adapt his analogy, and to embrace the concept of several different subtypes emerging more or less simultaneously, I prefer the term "starburst," which was first coined, I believe, by Paul Sharp.[2] In fact, Myers postulated a twin starburst theory, whereby both groups of HIV-1, M and O, began diverging into different subtypes in or around the year 1959. The significance of that year, of course, is that this was when blood sample L70 was provided by a man from Leopoldville — which sample represents the earliest retrospective evidence of an HIV-1-like virus in humans.

This is confirmed by my own research, which has provided no persuasive evidence of HIV or AIDS existing *prior to* 1959. Those early cases that I investigated because they were clinically suggestive of AIDS — New York in 1924, Montreal in 1945, Memphis in 1952, Toronto in 1958, New York and Manchester in 1959 — now seem most unlikely to have been caused by HIV. Indeed, tissue samples from two of these cases have been tested by PCR, and no HIV was amplified.[3] We now know that in the one case where HIV-1 did seem to be a factor, that of David Carr, the result was probably caused by contamination.[4] The medical community now uses ICL (Idiopathic CD4+ Lymphocytopenia) as a catchall term for immunosuppression that is caused by factors other than HIV, and it is clear that several factors (including congenital immunodeficiency, unreported cancers and cancer treatments, and exposure to radiation and toxins) may cause a state of immunocompromise that mimics AIDS. There can be little doubt that since the dawn of humans, there have always been a small number of deaths from such unexplained failures of the immune system. Even today, medical science does not hold all the answers.

So what are the earliest traces of HIV and AIDS about which we can be either reasonably or absolutely confident?

Outside Africa, the earliest recognizable traces of AIDS are from North America, the Caribbean, and Europe. In the United States, apart from the questionable St. Louis case from 1968/9,[5] AIDS was first seen in the gay community in about 1978. In Haiti, we have one tentative case from 1978. And in Europe, there are the three Norwegians who developed first symptoms in the late sixties and who died of AIDS in 1976, together with other patients from France, Denmark, and Germany who developed their first symptoms in that same year. Of these six Europeans, only the German violinist lacked identifiable connections with Africa.

By contrast, within Africa, even though the recording of disease is far less systematic than in the West, we come across the first vestigial evidence of possible AIDS in the sixties, followed by a veritable flood of cases beginning in the early seventies, and continuing throughout that decade.

The most striking thing about these early cases is the very close correlation that exists — in both time and place — with the CHAT vaccinations that took place in central Africa between 1957 and 1960. It is time to pull all this data together, in order to show these correlations clearly.

———————

The first moderately persuasive case of AIDS in Africa is that of Jean Sonnet's patient Helene, who died in Leopoldville/Kinshasa in early 1962 from disseminated KS, pneumonia, fever, and bacterial infections of mouth and jaw. It will be recalled that Helene originated from Lisala, upstream on the river Congo, and that she first fell sick there with swelling of the lymph nodes some four years earlier. It will also be recalled that Dr. Ninane conducted a mass feeding of CHAT in Lisala,[6] on an unknown date between 1957 and 1960. It must be added, however, that despite the near certainty of both doctors Sonnet and Michaux that this was a case of AIDS, it has not been possible to confirm this by locating tissue or sera from the patient. I myself feel less than certain about this case, partly because of the very limited medical history prior to 1962, and partly because the main presenting symptom was KS, which quite often occurs in an aggressive form in Africa without the involvement of HIV.

The next African evidence is that provided by the Norwegian sailor, who first fell ill with AIDS-like symptoms in Norway in 1966, fully ten years before he and his wife and youngest daughter died of the syndrome. The stored blood of all three later tested positive for HIV-1. Arvid Noe's seroconversion seems likely to have taken place during one of his two visits to Africa. He went to West Africa in 1961/2, and to Mombasa, Kenya, in December 1964, and was clearly sexually

## CHAT VACCINATION CAMPAIGNS
## IN CENTRAL AFRICA, 1957–1960

| No. on map | Site of vaccination | Date of vaccination | Number vaccinated |
|---|---|---|---|
| 1 | Stanleyville[a] | Feb. 1957 to Jan. 1958; Feb. 1958; May 1959 | 18,883[d] |
| 2 | Aketi[a] | May 1957 | 1,978 |
| 3 | Gombari | Jan. 1958 | 2,925 |
| 4 | Watsa | Jan. 1958 | 14,569 |
| 5 | Banalia | Jan. 1958 | 3,798 |
| 6 | Kole | Jan. 1958 | 384 |
| 7 | Bambesa | Feb. 1958 | 2,350 |
| 8 | "Ruzizi Valley": Bugarama to Bujumbura to Nyanza Lac | Feb. to Apr. 1958 | 215,504 |
| 9 | Rungu | June 1958 | 4,000 |
| 10 | Kilo mines | July 1958 | 5,000 |
| 11 | Leopoldville[a] | Aug. 1958–Apr. 1960 | 76,000 |
| 12 | Lisala | 1958? | 1–5,000 |
| 13 | Bukavu | 1958 | 9,880 |
| 14 | Goma[b] | 1958/9 | 2,000 |
| 15 | Kindu | 1958/9 | 6,000 |
| 16 | Kalima | 1958/9 | 5,900 |
| 17 | Tshela | 1958/9 | 10,000 |
| 18 | Kikwit | May 1959 & Nov. 1959 | Unknown |
| 19 | Bafwasende | 1959 | 2,483 |
| 20 | Yaselia to Yakusu | 1959/60? | Unknown |
| 21 | Southern Ruanda: Astrida to Nyanza, and Cyangugu to Kibuye | 1959 | 137,390 |
| 22 | Lubudi[c] | 1959/60 | 64,000 |
| 23 | Boma | 1959/60 | Unknown |
| 24 | Thysville | 1959/60 | Unknown |
| 25 | Matadi | 1959/60 | Unknown |

| No. on map | Site of vaccination | Date of vaccination | Number vaccinated |
|---|---|---|---|
| 26 | Muanda | 1959/60 | Unknown |
| 27 | Rest of Urundi | Dec. 1959–Mar. 1960 | 321,203 |
| 28 | Coquilhatville | 1960? | Unknown |
| | | | TOTAL: More than 900,000 |

NOTES:

[a] Fox also fed in these places, between December 1957 and April 1960.

[b] This was reported as Boma in one newspaper article.

[c] This was reported as "Kabare-Lubudi" in one newspaper article.

[d] The individual vaccinations were 1,126, 3,102, and 14,655, respectively.

active on both occasions, as indicated by his twice contracting gonorrhea. In the next chapter, we shall look at the rather surprising resolution to his case.

After these two early cases, one of which is questionable, and for the other of which a degree of guesswork is involved in terms of the likely venue of infection, I have details of 24 other patients (either African, or visitors to Africa) who seem to have developed AIDS between 1973 and 1979, and a further 12 from the year 1980. Altogether, therefore, the list features 38 cases of postulated AIDS in Africa prior to the official recognition of the epidemic in the United States in 1981.[7] Fully 29 of these cases involve the Congo.[8]

The geographical spread is especially interesting. Thirteen cases relate to Kinshasa[9] and two to Kisangani. Four relate to Rwanda, Burundi (Bujumbura), or the adjoining area of eastern Zaire (Bukavu and Uvira), three to Equateur region (Lisala, Yambuku, and Abumonbazi), and two to Shaba region (Likasi and Lubumbashi). Another seven cases come from unspecified areas of the Congo. Of the remaining seven cases, four emanate from towns like Kalalushi (Zambia) or Kyotera (Uganda), which are close to the borders of the former Belgian colonies.

Of the 28 patients for whom a specific town is cited, 23 come from the Congo, Rwanda, or Burundi — and of these, fully 17 are linked to towns where CHAT was previously fed.[10] The other six are linked to places situated within 175 miles of towns where CHAT is known or believed to have been fed.[11]

Even if we include all 28 of the early AIDS patients who are linked to a named African town, 64 percent have connections to towns where CHAT was fed, and 82 percent to towns within 175 miles of places where CHAT was known

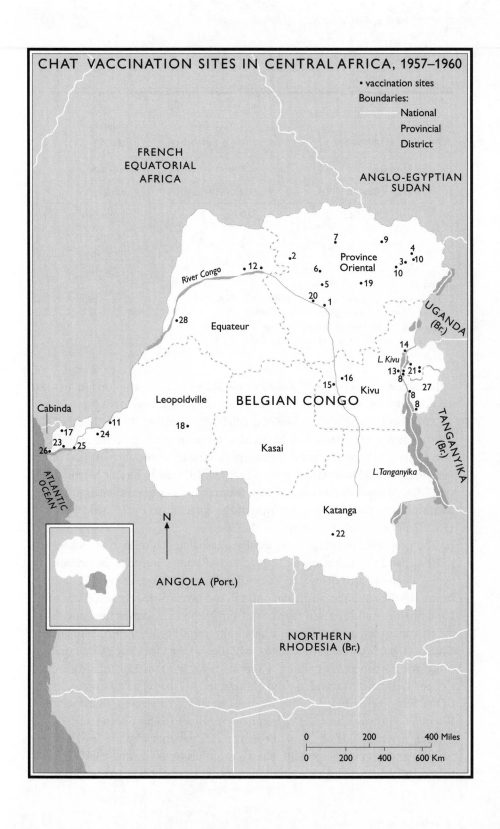

# CHAT VACCINATION SITES IN CENTRAL AFRICA, 1957–1960

- vaccination sites
Boundaries:
—— National
Provincial
District

FRENCH
EQUATORIAL
AFRICA

ANGLO-EGYPTIAN
SUDAN

Province
Oriental

- 7
- 9
- 4
- 10
- 2
- 3
- 10
- 6
- 5
- 19
- 12
River Congo

- 20
- 1

UGANDA
(Br.)

- 28
Equateur

- 14
L. Kivu
- 13
- 21
- 8

Cabinda

- 15
- 16
Kivu

- 27
- 8
- 8

Leopoldville

BELGIAN CONGO

TANGANYIKA
(Br.)

- 11
- 17
- 24
- 18

- 23
- 25
- 26

Kasai

ATLANTIC
OCEAN

L. Tanganyika

N

Katanga

- 22

ANGOLA (Port.)

NORTHERN
RHODESIA (Br.)

| 0 | 200 | 400 Miles |
| 0 | 200 | 400 | 600 Km |

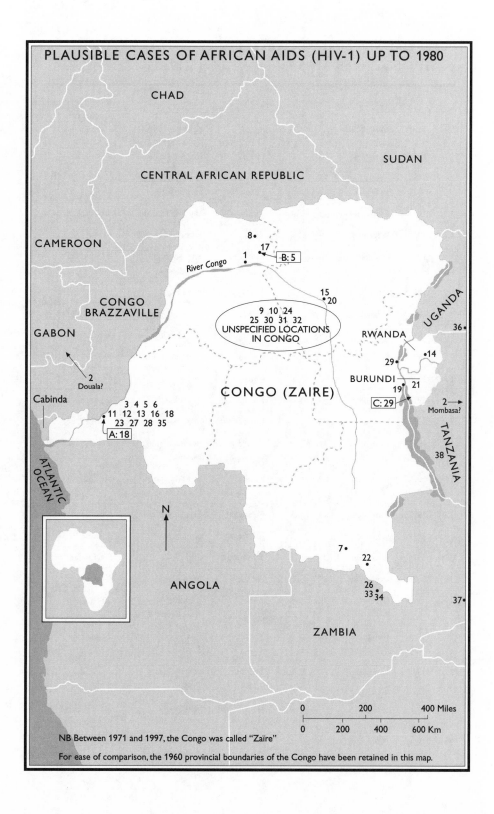

# PLAUSIBLE CASES OF AFRICAN AIDS (HIV-1) UP TO 1980

CHAD

CENTRAL AFRICAN REPUBLIC

SUDAN

CAMEROON

8●

17
1●     B: 5

River Congo

CONGO
BRAZZAVILLE

GABON

15
●20

9  10  24
25  30  31  32
UNSPECIFIED LOCATIONS
IN CONGO

UGANDA

36●

RWANDA

●14

2
Douala?

29●

BURUNDI

Cabinda

CONGO (ZAIRE)

19●  21

C: 29

2  →
Mombasa?

3  4  5  6
11  12  13  16  18
23  27  28  35

A: 18

TANZANIA

38

ATLANTIC
OCEAN

N
↑

7●

22
●

26
33 ●34

37●

ANGOLA

ZAMBIA

| 0 | | 200 | | 400 Miles |
|---|---|---|---|---|
| 0 | 200 | 400 | 600 Km | |

NB Between 1971 and 1997, the Congo was called "Zaïre"

For ease of comparison, the 1960 provincial boundaries of the Congo have been retained in this map.

## POTENTIAL AND CONFIRMED CASES
## OF HIV-1-RELATED AIDS IN AFRICA UP TO 1980

| No. | Year* | Nationality | Age* | Sex | Likely place of infection | Principal symptoms | Miles from known/ believed (#) vaccination site |
|---|---|---|---|---|---|---|---|
| 1 | 1962 | Congolese | 50 | F | Lisala | diss.KS, cachexia | 0 (same site) |
| 2† | 1966 | Norwegian | 20 | M | Cameroon/ Kenya | candid., dementia, resp. inf. | N/A |
| 3 | 1973 | Congolese | <1 | — | Kinshasa | candid., resp. inf. | 0 (same site) |
| 4 | 1974 | Belgian | 29 | M | Kinshasa | herpes, T. gondii | 0 (same site) |
| 5 | 1975 | Congolese | Young adults | | Kinshasa | diss. KS, Slim, lymph. | 0 (same site) |
| 6† | 1975 | Congolese | <1 | M | Kinshasa | pneumonia, candid. | 0 (same site) |
| 7 | 1976 | Belgian | 42 | M | Likasi | T. gondii, lymph. | 100 (#Lubudi) |
| 8† | 1976 | Danish | 46 | F | Abumonbazi | PCP, candid., diar. | 140 (Lisala) |
| 9 | 1976 | Congolese | 27 | F | Congo | salmonella, candid. | ? |
| 10 | 1976 | French | — | F | Congo | PCP | ? |
| 11 | 1976 | Congolese | <1 | — | Kinshasa | candid., septicemia | 0 (same site) |
| 12 | 1976 | Congolese | <1 | — | Kinshasa | diar., fever, resp. inf. | 0 (same site) |
| 13 | 1977 | Congolese | 34 | F | Kinshasa | herpes, crypto., candid. | 0 (same site) |
| 14† | 1977 | Rwandese | 29 | — | Kigali | candid., diar., lymph. | 50 (Butare) |
| 15† | 1977 | Canadian | 33 | M | Kisangani | herpes, septicemia | 0 (same site) |
| 16 | 1977 | Congolese | — | M | Kinshasa | Slim, fever | 0 (same site) |
| 17† | 1978 | Congolese | 26 | F | Yambuku | Slim, fever, ulcers | 90 (Lisala) |
| 18† | 1978 | Congolese | 29 | F | Kinshasa | herpes, diar. | 0 (same site) |
| 19† | 1978 | Greek | 30s | M | Uvira | multiple mycobacterial inf. | 10 (Ruzizi) |
| 20 | 1978 | Congolese | 39 | M | Kisangani | diss. KS, crypto., T. gondii | 0 (same site) |
| 21 | 1978 | Congolese | 24 | F | Burundi | crypto., CMV, PCP | ? |
| 22 | 1978 | Congolese | 40 | M | Lubumbashi | salmonella, agg. KS, Slim | 175 (#Lubudi) |
| 23 | 1978 | Congolese | — | — | Kinshasa | unknown | 0 (same site) |

| No. | Year* | Nationality | Age* | Sex | Likely place of infection | Principal symptoms | Miles from known/ believed (#) vaccination site |
|-----|-------|-------------|------|-----|---------------------------|--------------------|-------------------------------------------------|
| 24 | 1979 | Congolese | 24 | F | Congo | PCP, crypto. | ? |
| 25 | 1979 | Congolese | 30 | F | Congo | Slim, lymph. | ? |
| 26 | 1979 | Zambian | 25 | F | Kitwe | TB, candid., Slim | 290 (#Lubudi) |
| 27† | 1980 | Congolese | 33 | F | Kinshasa | Slim, candid., fever | 0 (same site) |
| 28 | 1980 | Congolese | 33 | F | Kinshasa | Slim, spontaneous abortions | 0 (same site) |
| 29 | 1980 | Congolese | 43 | M | Bukavu | PCP, candid., TB | 0 (same site) |
| 30 | 1980 | Congolese | 41 | M | Congo | crypto. | ? |
| 31 | 1980 | Congolese | 44 | M | Congo | EBV, CMV | ? |
| 33 | 1980 | Zambian | 22 | F | Kitwe | Slim, E. coli, fungal rash | 290 (#Lubudi) |
| 34 | 1980 | Zambian | 28 | M | Kitwe | Slim, T. gondii | 290 (#Lubudi) |
| 35 | 1980 | Congolese | — | F | Kinshasa | crypto. | 0 (same site) |
| 36 | 1980 | Ugandan | — | M | Rakai | agg. KS | 250 (Butare) |
| 37 | 1980 | Congolese | 55 | F | Chipata | agg. KS, splenomegaly | 680 (#Lubudi) |
| 38† | 1980 | Scottish | 45 | M | Tanzania | lymphoma, CMV, klebsiella | ? |

SYMPTOMS:
diss./agg. KS = disseminated/aggressive KS; candid. = candidiasis; resp. inf. = respiratory infection;
T. gondii = toxoplasmosis; lymph. = lymphadenopathy; diar. = diarrhea; crypto. = cryptococcal meningitis;
EBV = Epstein–Barr Virus.
\* = at onset of AIDS-like symptoms.
† denotes confirmed presence of HIV.

serapositive for HIV-1 antigens up to 1980/1
A: Kinshasa (1959:1; 1970:2; 1980:15)
B: Yambuku (1976:5)
C: Burundi (1980/1: Bujumbura 16; Rumonge 8; Kihanga 3; Muramvya/Ijenda 2)
(A and C are vaccination sites; B is 90 miles from a vaccination site.)

or believed to have been fed. Given the fact that there were such large areas of the Belgian Congo where no CHAT vaccinations occurred, the coincidence of place and time is quite striking — especially for a disease syndrome with such a long latency period.

But if one looks instead at known instances of HIV-1-positive blood samples taken in Africa in 1981 (Year Zero for AIDS) or earlier, the correlations with CHAT become even more remarkable. There are eighteen positive blood samples from Leopoldville/Kinshasa (one from 1959,[12] two from 1970, and fifteen from 1980).[13] There are five positive samples from 1976 from Yambuku, a place less than one hundred miles from the vaccination site of Lisala.[14] From Morvan's 1980/1 survey of Burundi, there are sixteen positive samples from Bujumbura, eight from Rumonge, and three from Kihanga — all of that were CHAT vaccination sites in 1958.[15] The two other HIV-positive sera identified by that survey were gathered from towns in the central mountains that were vaccination sites in 1959/60.[16] The only other proven HIV-1-positive bloods taken in Africa during this period are nine samples from prostitutes living in Nairobi, Kenya,[17] and one from Senegal.[18] In these instances, the blood samples were taken in the final year — 1981 — by which time HIV was traveling fast across national boundaries, often by air.[19]

These serological statistics are truly important, for they deal with proven samples of HIV-1-positive blood, some of which came from patients who are known to have progressed to AIDS. Again, the statistics tell their own story. Let us adjust to 1980, to match the AIDS statistics. Over 87 percent of all known samples of HIV-1 from Africa from 1980 or earlier come from towns where CHAT was fed.[20] And 100 percent come from places within one hundred miles of CHAT vaccination sites.

———

In Burundi, HIV-positivity clearly correlates far better with the 1958 than with the 1959/60 campaign. In the first campaign in Ruzizi and along Lake Tanganyika, some 141,000 Burundian adults and children were fed CHAT, and 27 positive samples were later detected in the vaccinated towns of Bujumbura, Rumonge, and Kihanga.[21] In the second campaign, some 320,000 Burundian children were fed, but only two HIV-positives were later detected from the vaccinated areas, both of which came from close to Bujumbura, and which may represent onward spread from there.

One is even tempted to point to the apparent correlation between HIV prevalence in 1980/1 and the areas where the second (possibly Belgian-made) batch of CHAT is believed to have been fed in 1958 (Bujumbura town and Rumonge), as against where the Wistar-made version is believed to have been fed (Kihanga).[22] However, caution is warranted, because the information about which batches were used where is only anecdotal.

However, there is one other epidemiological connection between CHAT and AIDS that needs to be mentioned, and although it does not relate to the earliest cases of AIDS, it provides perhaps the most telling positive evidence of all. It relates to the last three cases of AIDS of the seven described by Professor Jean Sonnet in 1987.[23]

Case 5 was a thirty-seven-year-old white Belgian male who had done voluntary service in the Congo between 1976 and 1978, and who had apparently had sex with many Congolese prostitutes during that period. He was found to be HIV-positive in 1985, and Sonnet informed me that he died of AIDS in 1989. Later, when I was given access to his medical records, I discovered where he had spent those two years in the seventies. It was in the small town of Lubudi, the one place in the whole of Shaba (formerly Katanga) province where CHAT had apparently been fed. At least, that was the intention, as announced by Courtois, Plotkin, and Lebrun at their press conference in May 1959.[24]

Cases 6 and 7 were a mixed-race couple, a Belgian cartographer and his Congolese wife, who were unusually old (seventy-one and fifty-four, respectively) when they were both found to be HIV-positive in Belgium in 1985. By 1988, both had died of AIDS. The intriguing thing about this particular story was that the couple left the Congo in 1968, and never returned. Both convincingly denied having had transfusions, abused drugs, or indulged in extramarital activity after their return to Belgium. The medical records did not, unfortunately, identify where the couple had lived in the Congo, but they did contain details of a hernia operation the husband had undergone in 1958 — in the town of Kikwit. He had also fallen ill with hepatitis in Kikwit at a time unspecified, which increases the likelihood that he had been living in the town for some time, rather than just passing through.

This was fascinating, for Kikwit was the place where Stanley Plotkin and a Belgian team carried out a CHAT vaccination in May 1959, one that apparently caused some problems among the local inhabitants. Two of these Belgian doctors, André Lebrun and Michel Vandeputte, later confirmed and enlarged upon the story Plotkin had told me. Apparently between a third and a half of the townspeople (including some whites) were vaccinated on the first day,[25] but on the second morning a group of Africans assembled, protesting that the white men who were taking pre-vaccination blood samples from some of the children were engaged in making *juju*, or witchcraft.[26] Stones were thrown, and the trial had to be abandoned. A further 600-odd Kikwit residents, equally divided between Europeans of all ages and African children, were vaccinated in November 1959.[27] Could the cartographer (and/or his wife) have been among those vaccinated in either May or November?

Once again, the coincidence of time and place was stunning. For in a strange echo of Lubudi in Shaba province, Kikwit was the only town in Bandundu province (formerly the eastern half of Leopoldville province) where CHAT vaccine had definitely been fed.

———————

Skeptics would argue that you can propose anything on the basis of epidemiological data — or press cuttings, or half-remembered stories from the past. Especially when they relate to the spread of a slow virus infection, one that allows years of opportunity for movement and maneuver. All those lists and maps and percentages may *look as if* they support the OPV/AIDS hypothesis, certainly, but what of the other possible explanations? What is to prove that the coming of independence and freedom from colonial travel restrictions did not allow a previously sequestered virus, recently crossed from simians to humans, to arrive in a big city such as Kinshasa, or perhaps in a town such as Stanleyville or Usumbura, and to begin its inexorable spread from person to person and from place to place?

Furthermore, in Leopoldville CHAT was fed only to whites, and to African children aged up to five years — in other words, those born in 1953 or later. And yet the individual who provided L70, the first HIV-positive blood sample, in 1959, was an adult African male.

But such objections can readily be answered — and partly by invoking the urbanization argument of the natural transfer school. In the late fifties, Leopoldville/Kinshasa became the biggest boom town in central Africa. Jean Sonnet informed me that, prior to 1958, Africans living in the Congo needed a travel pass to move from one district to another, and that these were only obtained after a medical checkup to exclude venereal disease.[28] It may be, therefore, that immigration to the capital suddenly increased in 1958, when the law was relaxed. This is backed up by population data: in 1958, Leo had 346,000 inhabitants;[29] in 1960 (the year of independence) 550,000;[30] and by 1984 it had officially grown to 2.5 million.[31] We can therefore assume that the influx to Leopoldville/Kinshasa would have included some adult vaccinees from other towns. Perhaps it included the mystery man who provided the first HIV-positive blood sample in 1959. Perhaps it even included Helene, who arrived from Lisala in 1962.

According to the OPV/AIDS hypothesis, therefore, the relatively slow emergence (or at least recognition) of AIDS in Kinshasa might be a result of two factors. It could result from the slow seeding of HIV in the capital by adult vaccinees arriving from other towns. Or it could represent the ten- to fifteen-year lag time before those Leopoldville children vaccinated in 1958–1960 achieved sexual maturity in the late sixties and seventies, and began to transmit the virus to others.

But in that case, skeptics might argue, why did no white colonial Belgians from Leopoldville get AIDS? Again, a relatively simple explanation. CHAT was only approved for use by the white population in August or September 1959, and by that time the vaccine-manufacturing process may well have been refined.[32] Since protocols and data about pools and batches and manufacturing methods apparently no longer exist, this can only be a guess. But there is some supporting evidence, based on other areas where CHAT was fed later rather than earlier. The vaccine fed to a third of a million children in Burundi beginning in December 1959 does not appear to correlate well with AIDS. Equally, we know that one of the last campaigns in the Congo, that at Coquilhatville (Mbandaka), the one Courtois later hoped to have monitored by the CDC, does not correlate with the early spread of HIV-1, for a retrospective test of 250 sera taken from Mbandaka in 1969 revealed no HIV-positives.[33] Intriguingly, one of the few whites in the Congo who may have been fed CHAT *prior to* August 1959 (the Belgian cartographer from Kikwit) did go on to get AIDS nearly two decades later.

But what about those adults who were vaccinated in 1957 and 1958 in places like Stanleyville, Lisala, the Ruzizi Valley, and Usumbura, or the four epidemic areas in Province Oriental? If this hypothesis is correct, why wasn't there an early emergence of AIDS among adults from those places?

The answer is that perhaps there was but that we have no proof. The available details are sketchy, but they include the fatal cases of *Klebsiella* pneumonia reported from Stanleyville in 1958 and the sudden rise of *Candida* infections in 1960. As we shall see later, there were cases of TB and generalized herpes in the early sixties among children born to mothers who had fled the violence in Rwanda.[34] In addition, it is possible that others died of strange diseases in the Congo, Rwanda, and Burundi in the sixties and early seventies, but that their deaths went unrecorded amid the general turmoil that obtained in large areas of central Africa at that time. For instance, within one week of independence at the end of June 1960, all but 100 of the Congo's 1,200 Belgian doctors had fled the country, "leaving all but six of the fledgling nation's 400 hospitals manned only by nurses and semi-trained 'medical assistants.'" A WHO doctor, one of 104 doctors and nurses flown in by the UN during the next four months, commented: "The Congo is just a few months short of returning to a medieval health pattern."[35] Rwanda suffered similar turmoil, and a more limited collapse of medical services, beginning in 1959, a process that was exacerbated after independence from Belgian trusteeship in 1962.[36]

The other crucial point is that it may well be that adults are far less vulnerable to orally administered SIV than infants, as demonstrated by the pioneering work of Ruth Ruprecht and colleagues from Harvard Medical School.[37]

Ruprecht's studies in macaques and mice led her to develop the disease threshold hypothesis, which proposed that humans infected with HIV would not develop AIDS if, during the early stage of retroviral infection, viral load remained low and did not rise above a certain threshold. She hypothesized that hosts infected with small amounts of virus could respond in several different ways. One

# UNROOTED PHYLOGENETIC TREE OF HIV-1 GROUP M

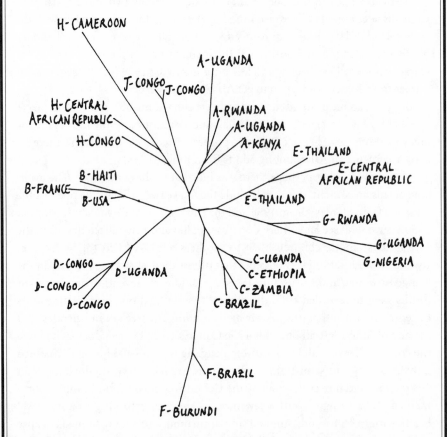

THE TREE, BASED ON SEQUENCES FROM THE V3 LOOP OF THE VIRAL ENVELOPE, WAS CALCULATED BY MAXIMUM LIKELIHOOD METHODS, AND IS BASED ON THAT FEATURED IN: T. LEITNER ET AL., "UPDATED PROPOSAL OF REFERENCE SEQUENCES OF HIV-1 GENETIC SUBTYPES"; HUM. RETRO. AIDS; 1997; III-1 to III-6.

way would be to eliminate all traces of viral infection, as appears to happen with some human infants who *serorevert* — testing HIV-positive at birth or during infancy, but HIV-negative some years later. Some victims of needlestick injury — inoculated with a tiny amount of HIV or SIV — respond rather differently, showing immune responses to HIV on a cellular level, but no visible signs of infection. A further response, perhaps occurring in the genetically fortunate, would be to develop latent infection or persistent smoldering infections, as appears to happen with long-term "nonprogressors" to AIDS, like some Nairobi prostitutes.[38] Such latent infections can sometimes become activated (in other words cross the viral threshold, and develop into full-blown AIDS) at a later stage — for instance, if the infectee becomes otherwise immunosuppressed.[39]

So, to extrapolate from this disease threshold hypothesis, if a large number of adults and children were exposed at the end of the fifties to tiny amounts of an HIV-1-like or SIVcpz-like virus through a contaminated oral vaccine, we would expect a very small number of adult vaccinees to become infected, and an even smaller number to cross the disease threshold and develop AIDS. By contrast, a larger proportion of infant vaccinees would be expected to develop latent infection after oral exposure to the virus. When some of these infants reached adulthood, they might become immunocompromised by other factors — such as the overall burden of disease in a tropical environment, contracting malaria or sexually transmitted disease, or simply getting pregnant — and begin the slow decline into AIDS.

Alternatively, these latently infected individuals could infect other less immunocompetent individuals, and these secondary contacts could go on to get AIDS. An example of this phenomenon is described by David Ho: a long-term survivor who seemed to be infected with a naturally attenuated form of HIV, but whose perinatally infected child died of AIDS.[40] Not only was the mother's latent HIV infection transmissible, but it was pathogenic in its new host. We would therefore expect to witness the secondary spread and increasing virulence of the virus from the mid-seventies onward, when the group exposed to HIV in infancy first entered the sexual network. This ties in nicely with the "Big Bang" of HIV-1-related AIDS, which Laurie Garrett and others identify as having occurred in central Africa in the mid-seventies.[41]

There is one additional clue that supports this hypothesis. In the Leopoldville campaign, some two thousand infants aged less than thirty days were fed fifteen times more vaccine virus than other CHAT vaccinees, in an attempt to ensure that they were immunized.[42] It is not known whether this also happened in other places where CHAT was fed in central Africa.

———

Let us for a moment assume that the OPV/AIDS theory has merit — and that one or more batches of CHAT vaccine was contaminated with a chimpanzee

SIV. How would this scenario square with the starburst of subtypes that Gerry Myers and other analysts believe to have occurred at around the time that HIV-1 arrived in humans?

In fact, the HIV-1 phylogenetic tree can very readily be explained by means of the OPV/AIDS hypothesis. First, it is clear that there may have been a strain of chimpanzee SIV circulating at Lindi camp. Alternatively, there may have been several divergent strains, originating from chimps captured in different parts of the rain forest (or even from chimps belonging to a single troop).[43] Furthermore, there may well have been further viral spread and divergence at the camp, between chimps of the same species, or of different species, which shared cages.

If one or more batches of vaccine became contaminated, then one or more variants of chimp SIV could have been introduced to humans at vaccination sites right across the Belgian colonies of central Africa.[44] However, because of the very small quantities of virus involved, only occasional individuals (predominantly infants or the already immunosuppressed) would become infected.

At this point, let us look at two different scenarios. First, let us imagine that a dozen unfortunate infants, located in different parts of the Congo and Ruanda-Urundi, became infected with a very small dose of SIVcpz originating from a single infected chimpanzee. Although all twelve babies would have been exposed to very similar quasispecies of SIV, each would react differently, depending on individual host factors such as genotype (genetic makeup) and general level of health. Furthermore, there might well be — in each case — a burst of mutation, as the simian virus struggled to adapt to the new human host. Now let us leave the babies to grow up, so that each relationship between virus and host is able to develop in complete isolation for fifteen or twenty years. Maybe three or four of the children might "cross the disease threshold," get disease and die. But by the mid-seventies, the remaining eight subjects could be hosting eight very different viruses, each of them human-adapted to a greater or lesser degree. What we now effectively have is eight different subtypes in various degrees of readiness for onward spread into the human population.

Now let us look at the second scenario, and imagine that several different isolates of chimpanzee SIV are introduced into Lindi camp, and that there is further viral spread within the camp. This time, let us imagine that many different batches of primary tissue culture are prepared from the kidneys of SIV-infected chimps, and used to produce vaccine, and that a dozen unfortunate infants in different parts of central Africa become infected with variants of SIVcpz that differ genetically by anything up to 25 percent. In time they grow up, and onward spread from these index cases allows at least some (let us once again say eight) of these variants to establish themselves in the new human host as different subtypes of HIV-1. For the first few years, these subtypes would develop in isolation from each other. However, as the years pass, and people

move about, these mini-epidemics would spread and begin to overlap geographically; before long, people would become dually infected, and new variants would begin to spring up through *in vivo* recombination.[45] (This, in fact,
is how the molecular biologists now reckon that subtype E, which is a recombinant, came into being.)

The polio vaccine/AIDS theory is probably the only hypothesis of origin
that can readily explain the starburst phenomenon. The starburst may represent a sudden explosive divergence of SIV isolates from a single chimp within
individual humans who live in geographical isolation from each other (scenario
1), or it may represent the virtually simultaneous introduction of several different chimp SIVs into humans (scenario 2).[46] Something very similar may have
happened with Group O if — as Gerry Myers believes — that too has a "star-
like configuration." It may be that fewer people were vaccinated in the "Group
O hearth," but the mode of introduction (injection) would have been that much
more efficient for introducing a viral contaminant, so a greater proportion of
vaccinees might have become infected.

One more clue about how the early stages of an AIDS epidemic may progress
is to be found in the work of the Belgian clinician Robert Colebunders, who
has spent much of the last decade looking at HIV-positive people who have
survived for long periods. In 1987, he reported on two HIV-positive Congolese
women from Kinshasa; these were possibly the first AIDS patients to be
described as "slow progressors," because of the gradual clinical course of their
illnesses. The women had survived seven and ten years respectively with typical symptoms of AIDS — although during that time both had suffered
repeated spontaneous abortions, and had lost children, and in one case a husband, to AIDS. The women were born in 1956 and 1957, and (when seen by
Colebunders) both had been living in Kinshasa for at least fifteen years.[47]
Nobody recorded whether they were actually born in Leopoldville/Kinshasa,
but if they were, they would presumably have been among those children vaccinated with CHAT.[48]

It may therefore be that these women represent primary infectees — people
who were infected with a tiny inoculum of SIVcpz in the fifties, and who
became slow progressors to AIDS, following an extremely gradual clinical
course. By contrast, their sexual partners or children seem to have suffered a
more rapid course of disease, which suggests that they might be secondary
infectees, who were exposed to a virus that by then had become human-adapted
and more pathogenic.[49] These examples may help explain why it took fifteen to
twenty years before the first wave of cases became apparent in places like
Kinshasa and Rwanda.[50]

Late in 1996, David Ho confirmed to me by phone that L70, the HIV-positive blood sample taken from Leopoldville in 1959, had produced a viral sequence, and that it was very close to the root of the HIV tree. This started me searching once more for further information about the donor of the L70 sample.

Unfortunately, the published information about the "Leo" series, which includes L70, is more limited than about any of the other eleven series described in Arno Motulsky's paper. We are told only that it consisted of 99 adults from Leopoldville, 78 males and 21 females, these being persons of mixed Bantu stock "originating from western and central Congo," of whom a few were hospital patients.[51] Jean Vandepitte thought that the Leo samples could have been taken at the hospital at Lovanium University, on the edge of the city.[52] Unfortunately, the specific data on L70, including his age and whether or not he was a patient, appear to have been discarded.[53]

It does seem remarkable that a blood sample taken at random so soon after the start of the CHAT vaccinations should have identified someone who was HIV-positive. And yet it may not be a coincidence — for there appear to be many links between the CHAT vaccinations and the Motulsky bleedings. We have already examined the possibility that L70 might have come from a man who emigrated from another town where CHAT had already been fed to adults, such as Stanleyville, Watsa, or Usumbura. But there is another possibility, too.

In his very first interview, Gaston Ninane mentioned that when Motulsky visited Stanleyville, he stayed for two or three weeks, during which time Motulsky accompanied him to some of the polio vaccination sessions. Ninane added that on at least one occasion they took blood at the same time, from the same persons. "When I took a sample of serum for antibodies, he took another sample for testing Glucose-6 [G6PD deficiency] and so on," he told me, though he was unable to recall which groups this had involved.[54]

Blood samples taken at the same time as polio vaccine feeding record prevaccination antibody status, and are useful only if one has post-vaccination samples with which to compare them. So is it possible that some other of Motulsky's sera might have been obtained at the same time as *post-vaccination* samples from persons previously fed CHAT? In fact, at least two of the groups that Motulsky studied do appear to have included persons who would have been fed CHAT six months to a year earlier, so it is possible that post-vaccination blood samples were taken at the same time.[55]

At another point in that first interview, Gaston Ninane volunteered that Motulsky's samples from Leopoldville had been taken "from people during the vaccinations." However, according to the published papers, only children aged up to five were being vaccinated in Leopoldville in early 1959.

But there is one possible explanation that might fit with the evidence. When supplies of CHAT were first delivered to Leopoldville in August 1958, perhaps Africans working at Lovanium University Hospital as medical, nursing, and support staff were checked for polio antibodies, and those lacking immunity against Type 1 were fed CHAT vaccine, to protect them in the course of their work. And perhaps a post-vaccination bleeding was arranged a few months later, to check whether they had been immunized — and some of these bloods, together with others from patients, were later offered to Motulsky, in whose hands they became the "Leo" series. The Belgian medical teams often shared resources in this manner (especially blood samples, which are time-consuming to obtain). For instance, when Michel Vandeputte described the polio antibody bleedings at Kikwit, he told me that part of each blood sample was kept in Leopoldville, and part was sent back to the Wistar.[56]

Furthermore, a contemporary article stresses that the taking of blood samples in Leopoldville became difficult after the unrest in January 1959, in which fifteen hundred Africans were arrested in a single suburb.[57] This makes it all the more likely that the Leo series was either derived from existing blood samples, or else was taken from a "safe" environment such as a university hospital.[58]

An examination of other papers written about blood sampling in the Congolese capital during the late fifties reveals that Motulsky's 99 Leo samples may have actually been taken by Jan Stijns, who conducted his own unpublished surveys of genetic markers in 1959.[59] Apart from being the director of the medical laboratory at the Institute of Tropical Medicine and a friend of Ghislain Courtois, Dr. Stijns apparently got to know Koprowski and Norton in Stanleyville in February 1957. He was a signatory of the "See you later alligator" postcard that the Stanleyville doctors sent to their American colleagues upon their return, and he also attended the virus conference in that city in September 1957. It is therefore at least possible that some of the bloods he took for genetic studies (and which he may have given to Motulsky) doubled as post-vaccination blood samples from CHAT vaccinees, provided as a favor to Koprowski.

All this is conjecture, supported only by some random anecdotal evidence from Ninane, Vandeputte, and others — and, once again, by the coincidence of time and place. Stijns is now dead, and nowadays neither Arno Motulsky nor Jean Vandepitte can remember any further details about the Leo series. However, Motulsky does accept the possibility that his samples from the Leo series could have come from Stijns, and that they "may well" have doubled as post-vaccination samples from polio vaccinees.[60]

All that can be stated with certainty, therefore, is that it is *possible* that L70, the earliest sample of HIV-positive blood, came from someone — or, indeed, from the sexual partner of someone — who had been fed CHAT some months earlier. If confirmed, this would clearly have enormous implications for the origins of AIDS, as well as for the provability of the OPV/AIDS hypothesis.[61]

STARBURST AND DISPERSAL

By 1997, it was possible to venture some informed guesses about how HIV-2 and the two HIV-1s might have emerged from their African hearths.

As already explained, HIV-2 is a virus of low virulence and infectivity, which has only barely emerged from its home ground in West Africa. The original zoonosis, that crucial transfer of a monkey virus to man, may have taken place in the countries of what used to be called French West Africa (such as Senegal, Guinea Conakry, or Ivory Coast), or in English-speaking west Africa (Liberia or Sierra Leone), or it may have occurred in Guinea-Bissau, but the sheer volume of early cases of HIV-2-related AIDS in the latter country suggests that this was the place where the human virus first began to cause disease.

From Guinea-Bissau, HIV-2 appears to have traveled northward with the refugee exodus to Casamance in Senegal, and then eastward and southward, along railways and arterial roads, down to its current epicenter in the human melting pot that is the Ivory Coast. Outside Africa, HIV-2 is almost entirely confined to the former colonial powers of Portugal and France, and to countries with Portuguese links, such as Brazil and India. There is a growing feeling that many of those infected with HIV-2 may not progress to AIDS,[1] and some have questioned whether HIV-2 would even have been recognized as a pathogenic agent, had it not been for the previous discovery of AIDS caused by HIV-1.

---

The outbreak of HIV-1 Group O has not spread far from its apparent hearth in Cameroon and Gabon. By the first part of 1997, occasional cases of Group

O–related AIDS had cropped up in neighboring countries (such as Equatorial Guinea, Nigeria, Chad, Niger, Benin, and Togo) and in other countries as far afield as Senegal, Kenya, France, Spain, Germany, and the United States — but the great majority were still found in Cameroon.

The virus is quite widespread there, having been found in all six provinces in which tests have been carried out. In some provinces, more than 5 percent of all HIV infections are caused by Group O. This variant has apparently not yet been isolated from the two provinces in the west, which were formerly colonies of the British, rather than the French.[2]

---

Now let us look at the main epidemic of AIDS, caused by HIV-1 Group M, with (at the time of writing) its ten well-defined subtypes, or clades, A to J. With one possible exception (B), it would appear that all the subtypes emerged from an African hearth, but at least seven of them have since spread to other parts of the world.

Subtype A is now found throughout Africa on a west-east axis, from Ivory Coast across to Kenya and Djibouti. Though common in Africa, it has barely spread to other continents.

Subtype B, the so-called Euro-American strain, will be discussed in more detail below.

Within Africa, subtype C is found mainly on the eastern side, but on a north-south axis, from Djibouti and Somalia down to Botswana and South Africa.[3] The ferry routes down the vertical slashes of Lake Tanganyika and Lake Malawi may have played an important role in its dispersal, as may the famously well-traveled Somali truck crews. Later, C "escaped" across the oceans to India and Brazil, and from these bases it began to spread vigorously in Asia and South America. By 1998, C had became the commonest subtype on the planet, and was reported to be causing half of all global HIV infections.[4]

Subtype D is almost exclusively found in the Congo, and in the east African countries of Ruanda-Burundi, Uganda, Tanzania, and Kenya. D is likely to have been involved in the Rakai/Kagera outbreak of the early eighties in which AIDS was first identified as a dangerous epidemic disease that affected the general population. Some believe that D may be an unusually aggressive subtype, causing more rapid disease and death.[5]

Most subtype E isolates come from the Central African Republic, along the border with the Congo, and there is one isolate from Cameroon. Otherwise, subtype E is found almost exclusively in Thailand, where it has virtually supplanted subtype B, which was the first clade to colonize the country in the mid-eighties. Research published in 1995 suggested that E is especially suited to heterosexual transmission, due to its propensity for infecting the vagina and the

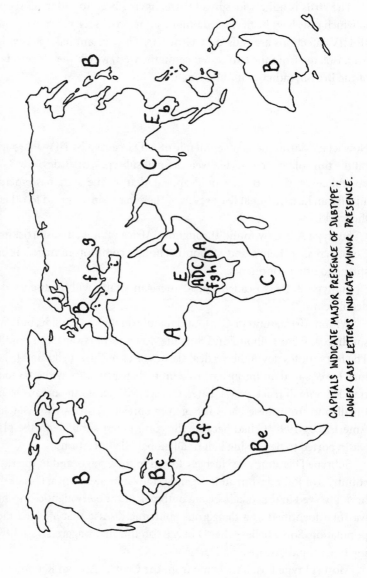

GLOBAL DISTRIBUTION OF HIV-1 GROUP M SUBTYPES IN 1997

CAPITALS INDICATE MAJOR PRESENCE OF SUBTYPE;
LOWER CASE LETTERS INDICATE MINOR PRESENCE.

tip of the penis. (By contrast, B, it was suggested, has adapted to being spread parenterally, as through needle-sharing, or abrasive anal intercourse.)[6] How E migrated from central Africa to Thailand is a mystery, but given the fame of Bangkok as a venue for sex tourism, it may have involved the vacation schedule of an international consultant. It has recently been confirmed that E is a recombinant virus featuring core proteins from subtype A, and envelope proteins from another clade that is perhaps now extinct.[7]

Subtype F is found in Congo and Cameroon,[8] but has also spread to Europe and South America. Several isolates have been located in Brazil, but by far the greatest number of subtype F sequences derive from children living in Romanian orphanages. Here HIV appears to have been spread by contaminated needles and by the unfortunate practice of "micro-transfusion," which was widely practiced in pediatric state institutions under Ceaușescu.[9] His regime gave many scholarships to African students, which may explain how the virus arrived in Romania in the first place.[10]

Subtype G is found in Congo and Gabon, but there has also been a nosocomial* outbreak at a pediatric hospital in Elista, southern Russia, where the source was traced to a blood transfusion given in Congo Brazzaville in 1981.[11]

Clades H, I, and J are less important, and seem quite rare. H is not known to have spread outside Congo and Gabon;[12] I has been found in Greeks living in Cyprus,[13] while J has been found in two Congolese living in Sweden.[14]

It seems significant that of the ten subtypes of HIV-1 Group M recognized by 1996, six (A, C, D, F, G, H) have been found in the Congo, one (J) in Congolese living abroad, one (E) in the south of the Central African Republic that borders the Congo, and one (I) in Cyprus, the Greek community of which has always had strong links with the Congo and, in particular, Stanleyville/Kisangani. (There were direct air connections between the two places in the fifties.)[15] In other words, nine of the ten subtypes have been isolated in the Congo, or from places which, or people who, had strong links therewith.[16] The odd one out is, of course, subtype B.

It would appear that the Congo has been home to a wide range of HIV-1 subtypes from an early stage of the epidemic, and it seems possible that all of the subtypes apart from B may have existed there, even if not all have yet been detected among the few hundred isolates sampled. This alone means that Congo is probably the best candidate venue for the Group M "starburst."[17]

---

At this point, it is worth looking back at two of the earliest epidemic outbreaks of AIDS — those in North America and Rakai/Kagera — in rather more detail, in

* Nosocomial: Hospital-based.

order to try to analyze some of the specific events involved in viral dispersal. The North American epidemic of AIDS in gay men and intravenous drug users was, of course, the first outbreak of the new condition to be recognized. This was in June 1981, but there is evidence of cases occurring as early as 1978. The epidemic was caused by the "Euro-American strain," subtype B, the only major clade to be found almost exclusively outside Africa. By contrast, in Rakai and Kagera, "Slim" was recognized as a new disease entity in about 1984, although the first cases may have occurred in the early eighties or late seventies. Because of the lack of isolates from this era, we cannot be sure which clade or clades sparked the epidemic, although the rapid course of some of the early cases suggests that the D clade, thought by some to be unusually virulent, may have been involved. This was the first outbreak of AIDS to be recognized in the general population of any region, for most of the early cases from places like Kinshasa, Kigali, and Lusaka involved only hospital patients.

However, as we have seen, the very earliest cases of AIDS and HIV infection emerged almost exclusively in the former Belgian colonies of the Congo, Rwanda, and Burundi where, at the time, they went unrecognized as a new disease entity. The major venue for these sporadic early cases was Kinshasa, but they also occurred in Equateur province (Lisala and Yambuku), Kisangani, Likasi, Uvira, Kigali, and Bujumbura.

This begs the question of whether there are identifiable routes along which HIV-1 might have passed in the sixties and seventies, which could have brought it from those former Belgian colonies to North American bathhouses and the Ugandan/Tanzanian border region in time to cause the epidemic explosions of the early eighties. And sure enough, if we turn to the history books, we shall find that there are.

―――――――――

On November 1, 1959, the first mass uprising by the Hutu majority against Tutsi rule took place in what is now Rwanda, and Hubert Caubergh says that it was probably this that cut short the intended countrywide immunization of children with CHAT, limiting that campaign to some 137,000 vaccinations.

In the weeks that followed, many of the tall Tutsi overlords were "cut down to size" by Hutus wielding *pangas,* and dozens of bodies, some dismembered, could be seen bobbing down the Kagera River toward Lake Victoria. The political climate had changed dramatically, and in September 1961, the Belgian administration bowed to pressure from the United Nations and the Catholic Church, and staged Rwanda's first countrywide elections, in which the main Hutu political party was swept to power. This prompted further fighting, and this time there was a massive exodus of Tutsis. By 1964, it was unofficially estimated that some 200,000 Tutsis, roughly half the total Tutsi population of Rwanda, had

# POSSIBLE GLOBAL SPREAD OF HIV-1 GROUPS M AND O

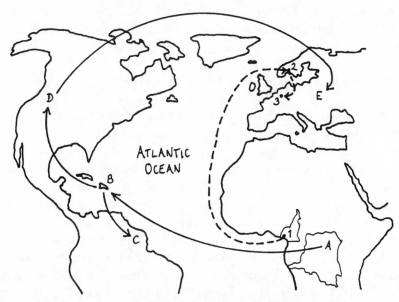

## HIV-1 GROUP M  ↗

KEY: A = CONGO
  B = HAITI
  C = FRENCH GUIANA
  D = NORTH AMERICA
  E = EUROPE

A→B : LATE '60s / EARLY '70s. THOUSANDS OF HAITIAN
  TECHNOCRATS RETURN FROM CONGO TO HAITI,
  A FEW CARRYING HIV.
B→C : 1974 ONWARDS. HAITIAN REFUGEES FLEE TO
  FRENCH GUIANA.
B→D : 1975 ONWARDS? HAITIAN TECHNOCRATS & REFUGEES
  (PLUS U.S. GAYS) TRAVEL TO NORTH AMERICA, ONE
  AT LEAST IS HIV-POSITIVE.
D→E : 1977 ONWARDS. U.S. GAYS CARRY HIV TO EUROPE.

## HIV-1 GROUP O  ↗

KEY: 1 = DOUALA
  2 = OSLO
  3 = KÖLN & THE RUHR

1 : 1961-62. ARVID NOE CONTRACTS HIV IN DOUALA, CAMEROON.
2 : 1962-67. ARVID RETURNS TO OSLO, AND INFECTS HIS
  WIFE AND, THROUGH HER, THEIR DAUGHTER.
3 : 1969-73. ARVID THE TRUCKDRIVER MAKES FREQUENT
  TRIPS TO THE RUHR. COULD THIS BE CONNECTED
  TO HEINRICH THE BISEXUAL VIOLINIST FROM KÖLN,
  WHO DEVELOPS AIDS IN 1976?

crossed to the Congo, Burundi, Tanganyika, and Uganda in the space of just over four years.[18]

This slice of history involves not just the mass movement of humans, but also that of human pathogens. The plight of the "regal" Tutsi aroused widespread sympathy and concern among the international community, and because this was the first major refugee crisis the post-colonial world had to handle, many of the diseases of the Tutsi refugees were recorded by the doctors who treated them. Looking back through the records now, more than thirty years later, one is struck by the fact that some of the diseases, especially those affecting young children, had clinical presentations typical of AIDS.

For instance, a group of Tutsi refugees who fled in 1962 from Cyangugu *territoire* in southwestern Rwanda to a mission station near Bukavu in the Congo displayed a very high incidence of tuberculosis. Of 21 refugee children who were treated for malnutrition in that year, 16 also had TB.[19] Cyangugu was one of the four Rwandan *territoires* where children were fed CHAT in 1959.

Similarly, in Kampala, Uganda, between 1962 and 1967, five cases of generalized *Herpes simplex,* which resisted all treatment, were recorded in apparently malnourished children, all of whom died. Two of the children were from Rwanda and one from Burundi. The two Rwandese children were especially interesting, for both had bronchopneumonia, and one was also diagnosed with TB and chicken pox. The text of Dr. A. C. Templeton's 1970 article about these children makes it clear that their families were "recent immigrants" to Kampala, suggesting that they were either Tutsi refugees from Rwanda, or else Hutu economic migrants.[20] The conclusion points out that *Herpes simplex* infections in Africa are normally transient rather than generalized, and that the virus is not normally a killer, but shrewdly adds that for those few who die from the infection, "it has been assumed that there is some form of deficient immunological response." Although it is doubtful whether any of the children were born before 1960, their mothers may have been among those vaccinated with CHAT.

In the course of following up on these cases, I came across the name of Jack Davies, who had headed the Pathology Department of Mulago Medical School in Kampala between the forties and sixties. I phoned him and, to my surprise, Dr. Davies promptly announced that he thought the first AIDS case in Uganda had appeared in 1960. I asked how he could be so precise, and he answered that he and his Mulago colleagues had been trying to establish a teaching collection of pathology slides, but after reviewing twenty thousand autopsies spread over seventeen years, had still not come across a case of *Pneumocystis carinii* pneumonia. Then, in 1960, an instantly recognizable case of PCP had cropped up. Dr. Davies recalled that the patient had been a man, and that in addition to the pneumonia he had had dysentery or some other form of wasting disease; but he could recall no other details, such as age or ethnic group.

By chance, Bill Hamilton was due to visit Uganda a few weeks later, and he spent an afternoon at the Mulago pathology labs, searching through the bound autopsy records for 1960 and 1961. Although he did not find Jack Davies's case of PCP, he did find three other interesting cases from 1960 and 1961. One, from 1960, ascribed death to "a heavy pure growth of *Klebsiella*";[21] the second case was of Kaposi's sarcoma with an unusual distribution, including the lymph nodes; the third was of KS plus several apparent opportunistic infections, including TB, pneumonia, and wasting. The entries under "tribe" indicated that all three patients were from Ruanda-Urundi.[22]

In summary, articles published in the mainstream medical literature and autopsy records from major hospitals like Mulago indicate that some of those who left Rwanda and Burundi in the late fifties and early sixties (and their off-spring) died from unusual diseases suggestive of immunodeficiency, or from common diseases with unusually virulent presentations.

There are, however, possible alternative explanations for the apparently low-ered immunity of these emigrants. Many of the refugees arrived in their coun-tries of asylum hungry, stressed, frightened, and therefore far more vulnerable to the impact of a variety of pathogens. The economic migrants, on the other hand, tended to be the poorest of the poor, living in quasi-slum conditions in urban areas where water supplies were inadequate and levels of hygiene mini-mal; women sometimes had to sell themselves in order to feed their children, and they suffered high levels of STDs. Without the opportunity to test by PCR some of the autopsy tissues from these apparently immunocompromised adults and children, there is no way of establishing the underlying cause.

Equally, however, it cannot be denied that something unusual may have been happening — and that some of these people *may* have been among the first to die of AIDS.

---

By 1995, I was becoming increasingly persuaded that the town of Butare (for-merly Astrida), in Rwanda — home to both the main army camp and the national university — could have played an important role in the genesis of the epidemic. For one thing, the prostitutes of Butare had tested 88 percent positive for HIV in 1984[23] — which suggested that the virus might have been seeded early in this community. For another, I had discovered that there were historical links between Butare and the area around Bukoba, in northwestern Tanzania, where the river Kagera propels its muddy waters out into Lake Victoria, and where the world's first outbreak of AIDS in the general population was seen.[24]

Hubert Caubergh had told me he thought that the CHAT vaccinations he conducted in the *territoires* of Astrida and Nyanza in 1959 had involved not only children, but also accompanying adults.[25] In fact, this important detail had already been established anecdotally by Bill Hamilton, who in August 1995 drove out into the villages around Butare (formerly Astrida), in two of which he came across people who would have been in their thirties in 1959, and who recalled having to walk into Astrida shortly before liberation, in order to receive an oral vaccination. This could only have been against polio.[26]

The first major outpouring of Tutsi refugees to Tanganyika (now Tanzania) occurred after the Ruanda elections in September 1961. Most were settled in camps just across the border, in Ngara district. Three-quarters of the first arrivals were from Gisaka, in Kibungu *territoire*, bordering Tanganyika, but about a fifth had fled from Astrida and Nyanza (the home of the old Tutsi court). Early in 1962, the new government of Tanganyika decided to move the refugees away from the reception camps in Ngara. However, there were ethnic and political differences between the different refugee groups. Those from Gisaka elected to move to the inland district of Karagwe (where they would eventually settle permanently), while the 3,000-odd refugees from Astrida and Nyanza were ordered to transfer to Bukoba district, along the lakeshore.[27] Between March and June, these latter refugees were settled at a camp at Nyakanyasi, on the north bank of the Kagera River, but in June the 2,000 refugees who remained were transferred into scatter settlements in two specific areas among the local Bahaya people. One was in Misenyi chiefdom, in the Kagera Salient, including the area around the Kagera Sugar Factory. The other was in Kiamtwara chiefdom, which embraces the area to the west of Bukoba town.[28]

These chiefdoms were areas where Bahutu migrant workers en route to Uganda had often, in the past, accepted temporary jobs as laborers on the Bahaya coffee plantations, and many had settled here among their employers. The Bahaya chiefs clearly hoped that the Batutsi refugees would integrate in similar fashion, but the aristocratic Astrida/Nyanza Tutsi had no intention of working as petty laborers, and the scatter settlement policy ended in disastrous failure. Many of the disgruntled refugees gravitated into Bukoba town, including some of the 12 percent who were defined as "non-viable family units," these being mainly old people with daughters, or widows with children. By year's end, these refugees were given the choice of remaining in Bukoba district or returning to Ngara, and apparently many of the refugees, especially unattached men and women, chose the former option.

The fact that the Tutsi refugees from Astrida and Nyanza, two *territoires* where CHAT was fed in 1959, spent much of 1962 in three specific parts of Bukoba district (the Kagera Salient, the area to the west of Bukoba, and Bukoba town itself), and that an unknown number settled there, is potentially significant. This is because, together with the border region around Lukunyu, these are the very parts of the district where AIDS would suddenly emerge with such devastating consequence twenty years later. By contrast, Karagwe, where the unvaccinated Gisaka Tutsi settled, witnessed hardly any AIDS in the early eighties.

There is an intriguing case of a two-year-old boy from Kagera district who died of aggressive KS at some time between 1964 and 1966. He had spent his whole life in the village of Ngando, which adjoins the Kagera Sugar Factory where the Tutsi refugees temporarily settled in 1962. Only the father was available to speak with a team of visiting British scientists, so it is possible that the mother was dead.[29] Apart from this pediatric case (which may well have been merely one of aggressive KS, rather than KS as a presentation of AIDS), I have come across no further reports of AIDS-like disease from the Bukoba/Kagera area in the sixties or seventies.

However, this is not difficult to explain, for we already have individual case reports of slow progressors to AIDS from elsewhere in Africa (like the women from Kinshasa studied by Colebunders, who may have been among those fed CHAT when they were children in 1958–1960).[30] It is therefore possible that an infant or young child who was immunized with the same vaccine in Astrida or Nyanza in 1959, and whose parents were among those who fled Rwanda and settled in Bukoba in 1962, could have been one of these slow progressors. By 1978 or 1979, when the Ugandan and Tanzanian armies began marching to and fro across this corner of Africa, such a child would have been around twenty years of age — and perhaps had sex with a soldier, or a partner of a soldier. Perhaps it required this further passage of HIV-1 in humans to render the virus more pathogenic and able to induce more rapid disease.

––––––––––

In March 1997, I interviewed Jack "Black Mamba" Walden, the former brigadier of the 207th Brigade of the Tanzanian People's Defense Forces (TPDF). He was then a major-general, and the Tanzanian military attaché in London — and he told me some fascinating things about the buildup to the Uganda/Tanzania war. He said that apart from the 208th (which was a regular army brigade), the other five TPDF brigades that invaded Uganda in 1979 were made up largely of volunteers from the people's militia — the semitrained fighting force that already provided security at village level in Tanzania. One of the reasons why the fighting was halted for three months after the Amin soldiers fled the Kagera Salient in October 1978 was that before pursuing them across into Uganda, these new TPDF recruits needed some further basic training. This took place in various military camps that were set up in the area to the south of the Kagera River — and it is these camps that played an important role in the seeding of HIV-1 in Uganda and Tanzania, and the emergence of the first population-wide epidemic of AIDS.

By November of that year, the 208th Brigade was based in a camp at Katoro, a village a few miles south of Kyaka bridge, with the 206th camped a short

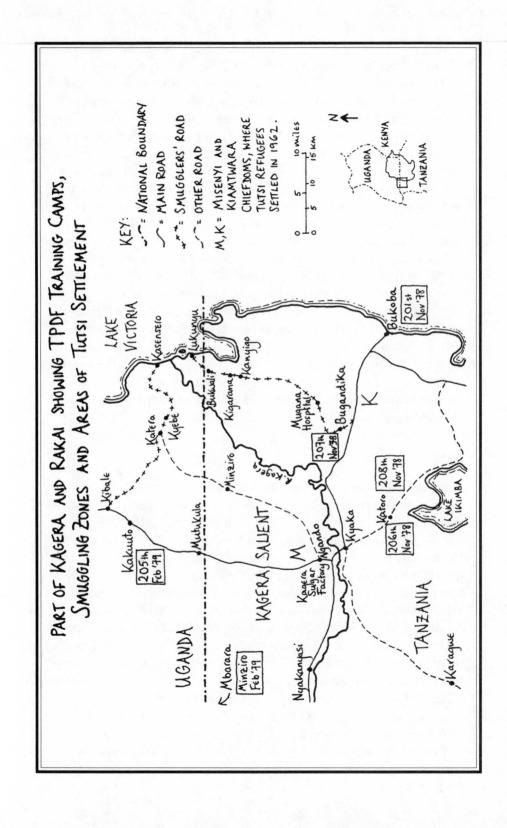

PART OF KAGERA AND RAKAI SHOWING TPDF TRAINING CAMPS,
SMUGGLING ZONES AND AREAS OF TUTSI SETTLEMENT

KEY:

.-'-.: = NATIONAL BOUNDARY

⌣ = MAIN ROAD

ᵡᵡᵡ = SMUGGLERS' ROAD

⌢ = OTHER ROAD

M,K = MISENYI AND KIAMTWARA CHIEFDOMS, WHERE TUTSI REFUGEES SETTLED IN 1962.

```
0        5        10 miles
|----|----|----|----|
0    5    10   15 km
```

N ↖

UGANDA
KENYA
TANZANIA

UGANDA

R. Mbarara

Minziro
Feb '79

Nyakanyasi

Kakuuto

205th
Feb '79

Kibale

Muhukula

Katera

Kyebe

KAGERA SALIENT

M

Kagera Sugar Factory Ngando

Kyaka

R. Kagera

Minziro

Bukwali

Kigarama

Kanyijao

LAKE VICTORIA

Kosensejo

Lukungu

207th
Nov '78

Muqana Hospital

Bugandika

K

Katoro

208th
Nov '78

206th
Nov '78

LAKE IKIMBA

TANZANIA

Karague

Bukoba

201st
Nov '78

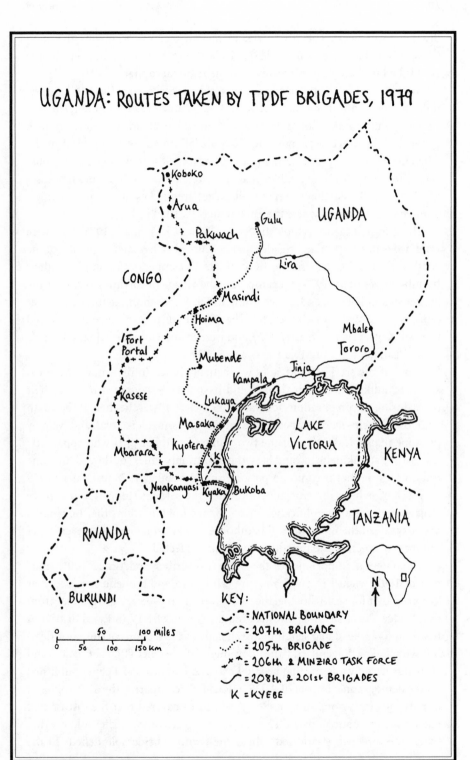

# UGANDA: ROUTES TAKEN BY TPDF BRIGADES, 1979

Koboko

Arua

Pakwach

Gulu

UGANDA

Lira

CONGO

Masindi

Hoima

Fort Portal

Mubende

Mbale

Tororo

Kampala

Jinja

Kasese

Lukaya

Masaka

LAKE VICTORIA

KENYA

Mbarara

Kyotera

K

Nyakanyasi

Kyaka

Bukoba

TANZANIA

RWANDA

BURUNDI

KEY:
⌐⌐⌐ : NATIONAL BOUNDARY
⌐⌐ : 207th BRIGADE
········ : 205th BRIGADE
×××× : 206th & MINZIRO TASK FORCE
⌐⌐ : 208th & 201st BRIGADES
K = KYEBE

N

0    50    100 MILES
0   50  100  150 KM

distance to the west. The 201st Brigade, meanwhile, was occupying the main town of Bukoba. It seems possible that by late 1978 HIV-1 had not yet become established in these three places, even in the regional capital.

By contrast, the 207th Brigade, under Walden, was based at Bugandika, a few miles to the north of the road between Bukoba and Kyaka. Although this is a rural area, it lies at the foot of the famous "Smugglers' Road," the murram track connecting Lukunyu, Kanyigo, and Bukwali (all noted for being hard hit by AIDS in the early eighties) to the rest of Tanzania. It was at Mugana Hospital, some three miles from Bugandika, that Margerete Bundschuh saw her first cases of AIDS in 1981. Furthermore, the village apparently lies in Kiamtwara chiefdom, one of the places where the Tutsi refugees settled in 1962.

These four brigades retook the Kagera Salient in January 1979, but there were two other Tanzanian brigades that assembled rather later. The men of the 205th arrived in Kagera region only in late December, and completed their training in February 1979 at a camp near the village of Kakuuto, just over the border in southern Uganda. (According to Dr. Bundschuh, Kakuuto was later especially badly affected by AIDS.) The last TPDF units to assemble passed through Kagera region in early 1979, and were formed into the Minziro brigade at the Ugandan town of Mbarara — again in February 1979.

None of the six TPDF brigades was actually based in the smuggling zone, and it is unlikely that the troops would have been encouraged to leave their bases during the preparations for war. Nonetheless, it was the men of the 207th who found themselves camped at the foot of the smugglers' road, and we may presume that at least some of the two hundred-odd bar-girls who apparently used to live at Lukunyu[31] would have traveled twenty miles southward for some fraternization. That two-month period from November 1978 to January 1979 may well have been the crucial period when the soldiers stopped in one place long enough for an amplification effect to take hold. It seems that Bugandika may have been the metaphorical bathhouse of Kagera region, with ever larger numbers of soldiers and prostitutes becoming infected.

The potential importance of the 207th was further underlined in the summer of 1997, when I received a phone call from Rand Stoneburner, a former WHO epidemiologist who, together with Daniel Low-Beer, a geographer from Cambridge University, was investigating the spread of HIV in Rakai district. A few months earlier, I had sent him a draft copy of the sections of this book dealing with Rakai, Kagera, and the movement of specific TPDF brigades, and Stoneburner now told me that he and Low-Beer had just had a paper published on the demographic impact of AIDS in Rakai. By comparing the age profiles of populations in various subparishes, they had discovered that the disease had had a truly dramatic impact on a microcosmic scale. Stoneburner told me that by far the three worst-affected subparishes, with considerable deficits in the normal populations of adults and younger children, were those at Kyebe, Katera, and Kibale. As I had learned from Walden, these were also the first three villages that the 207th occupied after crossing the border from Tanzania.[32] This suggested that members of this brigade were already HIV-positive by the time of the invasion, and that further sexual activity with local women in the course of the long route march north meant that an ever-increasing number of soldiers were infected by the time the brigade reached Masaka, Lukaya, and Kampala,[33] which themselves became known as centers of AIDS at an early stage of the epidemic.[34] Stoneburner was excited by the dramatic correlation of high HIV prevalence with the movements of the 207th, and was applying for a grant to study the relationship further, to see if the home villages of Tanzanian veterans from this brigade also became centers of infection in the eighties.

As for the other TPDF units, the 205th and Minziro brigades passed through Kagera region a couple of months after the 207th, by which time the virus may have spread further among local prostitutes. As with the 207th, the subsequent movements of these two brigades seem to correlate with areas of high HIV prevalence in Uganda, such as Mbarara, Kasese, and Fort Portal (for the Minziro) and Kakuuto, Hoima, and Gulu (for the 205th). By contrast eastern Uganda, which was liberated by the 201st and 208th brigades, did not experience a significant number of AIDS cases until several years later.

As hypothesized earlier, it seems that not only was there an epidemic explosion of HIV-1 at this point in time, but there may also have been a significant increase in virulence, perhaps caused by a virus entering a new host, or by the rapid passage of virus from person to person. Because the replication of HIV-1 is an error-strewn process, a sudden increase in infectees results in a huge increase in the number of viral mutants in circulation. Suddenly, the variants of low pathogenicity (which formerly favored host — and therefore viral — survival) no longer possess an evolutionary advantage. They tend to die out and, for a brief period at least, the viral strains that prosper are the more aggressive ones — like subtype D. Later in the epidemic, subtype D may have lost this advantage. Indeed, some have proposed that nowadays it may be too virulent for its own good, killing off its hosts before they have a chance to transmit infection to others, and that it is now being supplanted in this part of Africa by subtype A.[35]

This, therefore, is an instance in which well-documented historical events would seem to have played a crucial role in the early spread of HIV. It may be that elsewhere in central Africa one can trace the evolution of other subtypes to mass movements of people. But it is more likely that their early course would have been determined by less portentous events — a young man moving his place of work, perhaps, or a couple deciding to spend the night together.

At the start of 1997, I still suspected that one of the earliest infectees with a variant close to modern subtype B must have been the Norwegian sailor, Arvid Noe, who seemed likely to have been infected during his visit to Mombasa in December 1964. I even believed that his virus might represent the node on the tree at which Euro-American subtype B split from African subtype D.[36] Furthermore, I even had a hypothesis to explain how subtype D might have traveled down from Bukoba to Mombasa in time to meet Arvid Noe in 1964.

As stated above, apparently not all the Tutsi refugees returned from Bukoba to Ngara camp at the end of 1962. Some settled successfully in Bukoba, but apparently others again — those who had escaped with some money, or who were well educated and familiar with life at the royal court — decided to head toward the bright lights of Kampala, Nairobi, or Mombasa.[37] In the sixties, these cities were all part of the East African community, so passports were not required, and they were all accessible from Bukoba, thanks to the excellent ferry service operating on Lake Victoria. Ferries ran direct to Port Bell (near Kampala) and to Kisumu in Kenya, from where a daily train ran southward to Nairobi and Mombasa.

In fact, this link between Bukoba and Mombasa was already well established, since for at least fifty years a large proportion of the prostitutes working in Kenyan cities, especially Mombasa, have been Bahaya, the ethnic group indigenous to the Bukoba area.[38] In 1947, the British writer Elspeth Huxley visited Bukoba on her grand tour of east Africa and was told: "The main exports of Bukoba . . . are prostitutes and coffee, in that order."[39] It seemed eminently possible, therefore, that at some time between 1962 and 1964, one individual Tutsi or Muhaya woman might have transported HIV on this well-traveled route from Bukoba to Mombasa — and that one day in December 1964, she had met Arvid Noe as he disembarked from his ship.

However, as it turned out, my Rwanda-to-Norway subtype B hypothesis was entirely wrong.

---

Ever since my first contact with him in 1990, Stig Frøland had been diverting inquiries about the Norwegian sailor, while repeatedly promising that the sera would be analyzed by PCR, and the viruses sequenced. Finally, in 1997, he delivered. Rumors spread that the Norwegians had managed to obtain HIV-1 sequences from the autopsy tissues of both the sailor and his daughter. They did not, however, cluster with subtype D or subtype B. In fact, remarkably, they did not branch from the Group M bough at all, but from the Group O part of the tree.[40]

It was suddenly clear that Arvid Noe had not, after all, been infected in Mombasa in 1964.[41] He had clearly contracted his HIV infection more than two years earlier when, aged just fifteen, he had sailed from Norway for the first time on board the *Høegh Aronde,* a trip during which he was already sexually active, as evidenced by his having contracted gonorrhea. Between August 1961 and May 1962, the merchant ship sailed up and down the West African coastline, as far east as harbors in Nigeria and Cameroon, according to Karl Wefring.[42] The only significant Cameroonian port lies at Douala, which in turn lies close to the epicenter of the Group O epidemic that was first recognized in the nineties.[43]

This surprising discovery only reinforced the likelihood that it was during the sixties that viruses representing all three AIDS outbreaks first infected foreigners and escaped from Africa. Group O arrived in Norway with Arvid in 1962; HIV-2 arrived in Portugal with veterans of the Guinea-Bissau conflict in the mid-sixties; and Group M may well have traveled from the Congo to Belgium with the Kikwit cartographer in 1968.

Arvid's sequence also tied in with the tentative hypothesis that the Lépine vaccination in Mitzic in the final two months of 1957 might somehow have been connected to the outbreak of Group O viruses in humans. Both Mitzic and Douala were effectively administered as part of French Equatorial Africa until independence in 1960. The two lie less than five hundred miles apart, and are linked by a major road. Certainly it did not seem an unreasonable distance for a virus to travel in the space of four or five years. Perhaps, of course, the French polio vaccine had also been administered elsewhere in the region — including Douala itself.

And what of Herbert H. from Cologne and the chef from Gelsenkirchen: had these two early German AIDS cases also been infected with HIV-1 Group O? This seemed to be the most likely explanation — until, during the final edit of this book, another theory emerged that was even more persuasive than that of indirect contact with Arvid Noe during his truck-driving period. 1998 was a World Cup year, and there was an increasing volume of articles about tournaments of the past. One of these reminded me that in the 1974 finals, played in Germany, one of the competing nations had been the Congo or, as it was then known, Zaire: the only time that the country had qualified for the final stages. Hundreds of enthusiastic supporters accompanied the team, which was eliminated ten days later, after losing all three of its first-round games. I asked a friend to find out where these had been staged, and he discovered that the first had been in Dortmund (fifty miles from Cologne). The second and third had been played in Gelsenkirchen.[44] At long last, it seemed that the surprisingly early arrival of HIV and AIDS in Germany could be explained — and linked to the time that Zaire played away.

Of course, if correct, this meant that the two Germans were probably not infected with HIV-1 subtype B, or Group O, but with one of the African subtypes of HIV-1 Group M. As observed earlier, it would seem probable that, by good fortune, these early European infections did not spark an epidemic.

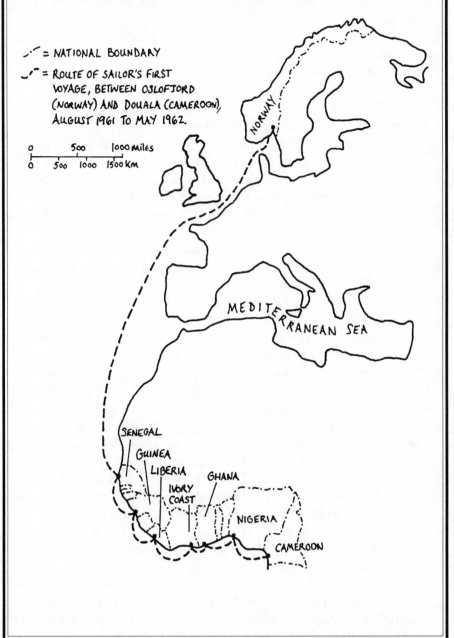

# THE TRAVELS OF THE NORWEGIAN SAILOR

--- = NATIONAL BOUNDARY

--- = ROUTE OF SAILOR'S FIRST
VOYAGE, BETWEEN OSLOFJORD
(NORWAY) AND DOUALA (CAMEROON),
AUGUST 1961 TO MAY 1962.

```
0        500      1000 MILES
0     500   1000  1500 KM
```

NORWAY

MEDITERRANEAN SEA

SENEGAL
GUINEA
LIBERIA
IVORY
COAST
GHANA
NIGERIA
CAMEROON

Soon after the announcement of the Norwegian sequence, there was an even more important development in terms of unraveling the prehistory of HIV-1, one that related to L70, the 1959 serum sample from Leopoldville. David Ho's group had obtained a sequence from the L70 sample, which they called ZR59, and they had found that it branched very near the root of the HIV-1 tree. The crucial question, of course, was how near. By the spring of 1997, the ZR59 sequence was being analyzed phylogenetically by Bette Korber from Gerry Myers's lab at Los Alamos, and by Paul Sharp in Nottingham, England. I sent David Ho some information on the provenance of the sample, and because of this — and the role I had played in helping to persuade André Nahmias to release the tiny remaining portion of serum for PCR analysis — it was decided that I too would be a coauthor on the ZR59 article.

In August 1997, David Ho sent me a first draft of the paper. It included the following passage:

> Collectively, these results show that ZR59 is extremely similar to the ancestral sequence for HIV-1 subtypes B, D and F. . . . The short but non-zero distance from ZR59 to the node for B/D/F suggests that the ancestral HIV-1 to these subtypes was introduced into Africans a few years before 1959. . . . Thus, it seems reasonable to speculate that the ancestor

PHYLOGENETIC TREE OF HIV-1, SHOWING SEVEN SUBTYPES OF GROUP M AND THE ZR59 ISOLATE, CALCULATED BY THE NEIGHBOR-JOINING METHOD

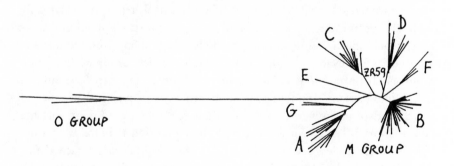

SOURCE:

T. Zhu, B.T. Korber, A.J. Nahmias, E. Hooper, P.M. Sharp & D.D. Ho; "An African HIV-1 sequence from 1959 and implications for the origin of the epidemic" (letter); *Nature;* 1998; 391; 594–597.

of the dominant form of HIV-1 was introduced into humans in the early part of the 1950s. . . . The factors that propelled the initial spread of HIV-1 in central Africa remain unknown, although the role of large-scale vaccination campaigns (perhaps with the use of non-sterilized needles) during that period should be carefully examined.

This was a remarkably frank statement about the likelihood that medical science had played the key role in initiating the major AIDS epidemic. It proposed that the first transfer to humans had occurred in the early fifties, and had initiated an immediate divergence (or "starburst") between subtypes A, C, D, and E. It proposed a secondary divergence between D and a branch representing B and F in about 1955 or 1956, and proposed that the ZR59 sequence from 1959 was a very early subtype D. Furthermore, it suggested that large-scale vaccination campaigns might have contributed to the primary spread of HIV-1.

My own opinion was that a much easier hypothesis to explain the starburst, one that did not require two stages — an introductory event and then needles — was that a vaccination campaign had *caused* the introduction from chimpanzees of several different SIV variants. However, this paper reporting the sequence was clearly not the venue to discuss such a hypothesis.

Even though the final published version of the paper was a little more cautious about dates, postulating that the ancestral Group M virus was introduced to humans "in the 1940s or the early part of the 1950s," this estimate was still remarkably close to the date of 1957–1959 required by the CHAT hypothesis.[45] And the difference was well within the margin of error, for the lack of SIVcpz samples and of other HIV-1 Group M samples from the fifties and sixties meant that there was considerable uncertainty about the early growth of this branch of the phylogenetic tree.

There are two significant possibilities that might affect the dating. One — as I have explained — is that the Group M subtypes actually represent the virtually simultaneous introduction of several divergent SIVcpz strains into humans — which would mean that the normal methods of dating nodes on the tree are, in this instance, invalidated. The other is that the earliest Group M divergence could have happened very rapidly, after one or more chimpanzee SIVs jumped species into humans, prompting viruses to evolve more quickly than usual, in order to adapt to the new host.[46] Both these scenarios would mean that the HIV-1 Group M/SIVcpz divergence could have occurred some years after the "forties or early fifties" date now postulated by Korber and Sharp.[47] Indeed, this was acknowledged by David Ho, who wrote the abstract that appeared at the head of the published article.[48] This ended with the crucial observation that all the Group M subtypes "may have evolved from a single introduction into the African population not long before 1959."

What this highlights is that the ZR59 sequence may in fact tie in very precisely with the OPV/AIDS hypothesis — and that it certainly does nothing to confound it. In other words, with regard to both time and place, the sequencing of the L70 sample provides further support for Louis Pascal's theory of origin.

---

The L70 sample — and its HIV-1 isolate, ZR59 — also demonstrated the flimsiness of a new theory about the way in which HIV-1 Group M had transferred to man, which had just been published by the Dutch retrovirologist Jaap Goudsmit, in his book *Viral Sex*.[49]

As explained above, only a handful of African subtype B isolates have been discovered — one each from Ivory Coast, Cameroon, Gabon, Uganda, and Rwanda. Remarkably, Goudsmit uses the Cameroonian isolate as the basis for his theory that a prototype form of subtype B from Cameroon was the ancestral HIV-1 Group M virus, from which all the other subtypes evolved. He proposes that "Proto-1B" must have migrated from Cameroon to Tanganyika (both German colonies from 1885 until the First World War) around the turn of the century, to reemerge in pathogenic form in Kagera in the early seventies — producing a starburst of African subtypes in the process. He also proposes that three hundred German settlers who returned to Germany in September 1939, at the start of the Second World War, were the source of the subtype B AIDS outbreak in Europe that, he claims, began in the port city of Danzig (now Gdansk) later that same year, and then spread through central Europe to Austria and Czechoslovakia — and eventually to North America.

There is a great deal of compelling evidence that argues against this hypothesis. First, the Danzig outbreak (of PCP, not AIDS) actually began in 1938, so the departure of the three hundred settlers from Cameroon in 1939 cannot be connected.[50] Second, Kamil Kucera has sent me six lung slides of pediatric PCP cases from Czechoslovakia in the fifties and sixties, two of which have been analyzed by PCR, showing no evidence of HIV.[51] Third, Goudsmit's theory runs entirely counter to the phylogenetic evidence, which clearly suggests that subtype B, far from being a prototype virus for HIV-1, actually branched from the tree slightly after the initial starburst of other Group M subtypes such as D. Fourth, he ignores the fact that the earliest black African B isolate, from Ivory Coast, dates from 1990/1, while the Cameroonian B was reported only in 1994. This is no basis for suggesting that subtype B originated in Cameroon. Instead it suggests that the African Bs were viruses that were reimported from America or Europe, after the advent of Euro-American AIDS in the late seventies. Last, there is the evidence provided by the 1959 sample, L70, that strongly suggests that the introduction of HIV-1 to man took place in the forties or fifties.

But recently there has been another twist to this story. After years of silence, Bob Garry, the man who found HIV-1 antibodies in tissues from Robert R., the St. Louis teenager who died in 1969, has announced that he has obtained HIV-1 sequences from these tissues, and that they represent "a typical subtype B virus."[52] On the phone, Garry told me that he still had checks to carry out, but that the data was "very strong." He said that this seemed to prove that Jaap Goudsmit was right and that HIV-1 was much older than most people thought. He added that he had received a grant from the NIH to carry out the study, and that this indicated their confidence that he was not sequencing a laboratory contaminant.

However, he went on to say that the Robert R. isolate appeared to be closest to two of the earliest HIV-1 isolates — LAI from France, and Gallo's HTLV-III-B. Apparently it diverged by 3 percent from these, rising as high as 4 percent or 5 percent in some regions. Despite Garry's confidence, this sounds far too close for comfort. Normally, when a sequence is that similar to a lab clone, virologists are immediately suspicious that there may have been inadvertent contamination. In this instance, contamination would seem a plausible scenario, in the course of the many attempts that have been made to isolate a retrovirus from the sample during the last ten years.[53]

———————

The ZR59 sequence indicates that Goudsmit and Garry are wrong, and that HIV is very likely to be a new human virus that has evolved rapidly in the last forty to fifty years. With this in mind, we should turn again to subtype B, which appears to have been the variant that escaped first from Africa, and that is responsible for the great majority of contemporary European and American HIV infections.

The likeliest candidate for the carrier of the ancestral B strain out of Africa is still the one suggested by Randy Shilts back in 1987 — one of the Haitian technocrats who worked in the Congo in the sixties and who later returned home, or re-emigrated to Europe or America.[54] Supporting this scenario is the fact that at least one AIDS patient examined in the Congo in 1983 was Haitian, and that at least one Haitian who developed AIDS in the United States in 1984 had formerly worked in central Africa.

However, there is another possible interpretation of the ZR59 sequence. If the CHAT hypothesis is correct, and if subtypes A, C, D, E, F, and so forth arose from separate introductions — through vaccination — of an SIVcpz contaminant to children and adults in central Africa in 1957–1960, then the unusual status of B could be explained if that subtype entered humans not in Africa but somewhere else — in Europe, perhaps, or America. According to this scenario, the first American infectee with subtype B could have been one of the infant vaccinees at Clinton Farms, from the group on which Koprowski tried out his experimental vaccine strains. Clinton, it would seem, was the only place in America where Koprowski fed the version of CHAT used in Africa — pool 10A-11.[55]

One candidate infectee, of course, would be James Oleske's patient — the promiscuous New Jersey drug injector who gave birth, at the age of sixteen, to a child who died of AIDS five years later, in 1979.[56] The woman in question would have been born some time between late 1956 and 1958 — just when the early versions of CHAT were being fed experimentally at the prison.

Dr. Oleske told me that the mother of this child was still alive in the nineties, when she appeared at another of his pediatric clinics. This suggests that she may have given birth to another HIV-infected child, but that she herself is still free of AIDS, even though she would (by that stage) have been infected with HIV for some thirty-five years. We know, however, that she experienced symptoms such as thrombocytopenia back at the time of her first pregnancy in 1973/4, which might be interpreted as one of the transient, smoldering infections that Ruth Ruprecht believes occur among persons with low viral load of HIV.[57] It appears possible that this mother may have been transiently infected with a small amount of immunodeficiency virus, but that she infected others — such as her daughter — with a more pathogenic variant, one that leads to AIDS.

It would also seem possible that the spread of the African HIV-1 subtypes and the Euro-American subtype, B, may have progressed at rather different rates. Certain of the major African subtypes (such as A, C, and D) may have first caused infection in adults, thereafter spreading slowly through the sixties — resulting, for instance, in the HIV-1 infection of one in 400 of Kinshasa women tested in 1970, and one in 120 of those tested in Yambuku in 1976. By contrast, if the B strain originated in an infant girl from Clinton (and if she was the only Clinton infectee), then it would have remained quiescent until the early seventies, when that girl (now a teenager) began having sex. If she infected her first daughter in 1973/4, she may also have infected some of her sex partners, or those with whom she shared needles. Certainly this scenario seems consistent with the first serological traces of HIV-1 in North America, detected among drug-injecting mothers (and one gay man) in 1977, presaging the explosion of the virus among gays and drug injectors between 1978 and 1982. During that period, the spread was even more rapid in the United States than in Africa.

---

Since the first reliable phylogenetic analysis of HIV-1 Group M isolates was published in 1988, much has been learned about the clustering of viruses into different clades, or subtypes, and the way in which recombination between subtypes can allow new variants to emerge. But relatively little has been learned about the early history of the epidemic. The sequencing of ZR59, however, changes all that.

Suddenly someone has twisted the focus knob on the microscope, and fascinating new details of that moment in time in 1959 have swung into view. Suddenly there is a new landscape, a new vantage point on the epidemic.

In the months and years to come, there will be further focus adjustments, and perhaps new slides to look at, too. Our understanding of the origins of AIDS will improve still further. But unless a totally convincing slide — from 1924 or 1945, for instance — reveals an ancestral human virus that lies at the very base of the HIV-1 tree, we should continue to bear in mind the very real possibility that humans have unwittingly unleashed this dreadful epidemic upon themselves.

# 56

## DEAD ENDS AND HIDDEN BENDS

In the final year of this research, ending in late 1997, I paid two further visits to Belgium, in an attempt to find out more about exactly who made the Belgian version of CHAT, and when.

As related earlier, Stan Huygelen and Julian Peetermans both thought that one pool of both CHAT and Fox vaccines had been prepared at RIT and sent — they said — to Poland. However, Monique Lamy, who had been the main vaccine-maker at RIT's Château des Singes when it opened in 1957, had told me that she had tested CHAT and found it too virulent for human use. She denied that any CHAT vaccine had been produced, and then declined to answer any more questions. The only thing that was clear from these interviews was that at least one person's memory was faulty.

I arranged to interview Lise Thiry, who for many years had headed the virology section at the Pasteur Institute in Brussels. She had been one of those who had attended the Stanleyville virus symposium in September 1957, with Piet De Somer and other luminaries from Belgium, and she had taken a keen interest in the Koprowski vaccines from then on. Since the fifties, Dr. Thiry has become more famous as a socialist senator in the Belgian parliament, and a champion of various issues, including vaccination and women's rights. André Courtois had told me that Koprowski would call on her first, whenever he came to Belgium.

Dr. Thiry was charming when I phoned her, inviting me to come to her house the following morning, but things were very different when I arrived. In the interim she had spoken with André Courtois, who had told her that he very much regretted speaking with me two years earlier. She now declined to discuss the vaccinations with me, adding that she strongly disagreed with what I was doing, and felt that I was wrongly impugning the safety of a vaccine. I tried to tell her some of the reasons why I had doubts about this particular vaccine, but she made it clear she was not interested. "You can write what you like in your book," she went on. "Say that I refused to answer your questions."

But within a few weeks I had discovered, quite by chance, that Dr. Thiry's connections with CHAT were more extensive than I had thought. I happened across two of her 1958 articles, which revealed that Koprowski had given her samples of CHAT and Fox in July 1957 — earlier than any other collaborator apart from Courtois in Stanleyville.[1] It seemed probable that Koprowski had had samples of the vaccines with him when he attended the Geneva conference that month. Gaston Ninane had told me that he too was present at the conference, and this might well have been the occasion when it was arranged for him to spend some weeks learning tissue culture techniques at Thiry's lab in Brussels — where, presumably, she already had possession of the Koprowski strains.[2]

Thiry's two papers reveal that she conducted experimental research into the behavior of CHAT, Fox, and other viruses in a total of twenty-three cell lines (including HeLa)[3] and five types of primary tissue cultures derived from "several animal species." Rabbit, guinea pig, and mouse are specifically mentioned, as are "several batches of monkey kidney cultures," which suggests that tissues from more than one monkey species may have been used.

These two articles were ascribed to Lise Quersin-Thiry, apparently her former married name. And this rang a faint bell. I already knew that Thiry had met Agnes Flack at Brussels airport when she returned from the Ruzizi trials, and had later shown her round the local branch of the Pasteur Institute. But now I went back to my copy of Agnes Flack's diary, and reviewed the entry for February 18, 1958, when Flack and Jervis were flying out from New York en route to Stanleyville and Ruzizi. It read: "Arr. Brussels 9:40 a.m. Met by Dr. Guerrsin- who took me shopping 1136 francs. Red carpet treatment at the airport. Chief of protocol met us and it was easy. Off again at 14:30 p.m." The shopping trip had involved buying replacement clothes after her luggage had been lost at Idlewild. But it was only now that I realized the identity of her guide, for "Dr. Guerssin-" was clearly Dr. Flack's version of Dr. Quersin-Thiry.[4]

The questions that must be asked are why the chief of protocol afforded Thiry and Flack "red carpet treatment" at Brussels airport, as Flack was about to board the plane for Stanleyville — and what it was that was rendered easy by his intervention. Presumably it was not merely the exportation of a pair of red slacks. And it was unlikely to have involved the American vaccine from the Wistar, for if flasks of that had already been on board the plane from New York,[5] they would presumably have been treated as transit goods, and transferred from one plane to the other as a matter of course. It occurred to me that this could have been the moment when some Belgian-made vaccine was loaded onto the plane, and it was this that required the helping hand of the chief of protocol.

The next year my research assistant, Sally Griffin, went back to Lise Thiry to ask her who had produced the oral polio vaccine used in the Congo. Thiry knew that Sally was my assistant, having met her the previous November, but this time she did at least answer one or two questions. She explained that no vaccine had been produced at her branch of the Pasteur Institute, and that Monique Lamy had done all the Belgian vaccine production at RIT, but she couldn't say which strains had been made. When Sally mentioned Agnes Flack, and the meeting at the airport, Dr. Thiry initially couldn't recall who that was. But when Sally talked about the lost luggage, and suggested that Thiry might have given some vaccine to Flack at the airport, Thiry replied that if she had handed over vaccine from Monique Lamy or someone, then she honestly couldn't remember it. Then she added that even if she had done this, she wouldn't feel ashamed about it.

At one point, just as in the first meeting, Dr. Thiry said that even if there was a one in a thousand chance of the OPV/AIDS hypothesis being right, then it was wrong to put such a hypothesis in a book, because it would "damage vaccinations and reputations." She said that already it was hard enough to convince people that vaccines were safe, and that such a book as mine could only do more harm than good. Sally Griffin tried to argue that the book was not questioning the safety of all vaccines, but rather one particular vaccine that had been made in the fifties, when tissue culture methods were not as advanced or safe as today — but to no avail. Soon afterward, Dr. Thiry made it clear that she would answer no more questions.

---

Clearly I needed to try to contact any others who might know something about the Belgian version of Koprowski's vaccine. Several such people were still living in the vicinity of Leuven, including members of Pieter De Somer's family, his former secretary, Janine Putzeys, and three other scientists who had worked at the Rega or RIT during this period. These were Michel Vandeputte, who had set up the first virology lab in Leopoldville in 1956 and carried out a polio antibody survey there the following year, before joining De Somer at the Rega Institute in 1960; Edward De Maeyer, a young Leuven graduate who started at the Rega in June 1957, before moving to America to work with John Enders at the end of 1958; and Abel Prinzie, who had worked with De Somer at RIT, and the Rega from 1955 onward.

The first thing to become clear from these meetings was that De Somer's trip to the Congo at the time of the 1957 virus congress had been a much grander affair than I had thought, and had probably lasted for the better part of two months. Michel Vandeputte recalled the excellent hospitality afforded the conference attendees by Courtois, and the visits made by De Somer, Koprowski,

Lise Thiry, and the others to Lindi camp and to the Wagenia fishermen at the Stanleyville rapids. He added that several of the visitors, including De Somer, had spent a day or two at the headquarters of the farming and agronomy organization INEAC, at Yangambi, fifty miles downstream from Lindi. This is intriguing, for this is the same organization for which Alexandre Jezierski was then working at Gabu, producing oral polio vaccine in the kidneys of African monkeys.

Professor De Somer's family contributed the information that he also spent a week with his brother, who worked as a judge in the town of Lusambo, in Kasai.[6] But this still left a month or so unaccounted for.

Michel Vandeputte told me that by the time of his 1957 Congo visit, De Somer was already interested in producing vaccine for Koprowski. But, like the others, Vandeputte was unable to tell me where else De Somer traveled in the Congo: whether he visited Jezierski, for instance, or had discussions with the colonial authorities in Leopoldville about the viability of a countrywide vaccination campaign, using Belgian vaccine.

De Somer must have returned to Leuven in October or November 1957 — and one is reminded of Courtois's comment in December 1967 that "more than ten years ago we sent kidneys from the Congo to Europe, and they were quite satisfactory." These might well have been chimp kidneys; but could this have been the occasion when they were sent? Certainly the polio program at Lindi was now coming to a close, to be supplanted by the smaller hepatitis program at the start of 1958. Perhaps this was viewed as an appropriate time for some of the chimps to make the ultimate sacrifice.

But surely no scientist would sacrifice a live chimpanzee just for its kidneys? Perhaps not, but David Bodian's work in 1956 had revealed that primates that had been exposed to poliovirus (even a virulent strain) retained no trace of that virus in their kidneys.[7] This meant that even those chimps that had been used in vaccination and challenge work could still safely provide kidneys to make tissue culture.[8] In other words, chimps could be used twice. In 1960, Ghislain Courtois had quoted extensively from Bodian's paper, showing that he was familiar with this research.[9]

I asked Edward De Maeyer whether it was possible that at the Rega Institute they had made vaccine from the kidneys of animals that had already been used for safety testing, and he said, "Maybe we did; I don't remember." Later, I asked whether chimp kidneys from the Congo could have been used, and he answered that they could have been, but that he recalled using only the kidneys of rhesus monkeys, which had been the sole species in the monkey house on the second floor of the Rega. He didn't know what had been used at RIT.

All this was tantalizing, but the breakthrough finally came when I interviewed Abel Prinzie, the other member of the Rega/RIT team in the early days. Prinzie told me that he had joined the Rega in 1955, a year after RIT had built the research institute as a gift to the University of Leuven. He was then a newly appointed associate professor of medicine, and part of his wages were paid by the university and part by RIT — "a foot in both camps," as he put it. At this stage, the virology department on the ground floor consisted of De Somer, Prinzie, and Monique Lamy (newly returned from Paris, where she had learned tissue culture techniques from Barski and Lépine). They had just one technician to help them, and when they began making tissue culture for the first time, they had to go to Antwerp to find a suitable monkey.

Early in 1955, De Somer and Prinzie approached the boss of RIT about making an IPV, and he gave them twelve months to get production on stream. By the end of that year, they had managed to produce a few vials of inactivated vaccine, and the two men vaccinated themselves, producing antibodies. They went back to their boss with the news that they had a vaccine, and he released more funds. Next they organized a trial vaccination of some eighty children of members of staff from the medical faculty; again, they appeared to be protected. By this time, at the end of 1956, they had fifteen technicians at the Rega working on IPV, and RIT purchased the castle at Rixensart, the Château des Singes, which was renovated and converted into a huge vaccine factory.

At the Geneva conference in July 1957, it was arranged that Prinzie would go to Pittsburgh to work with Jonas Salk, and he left in September of that year. During the next fifteen months, he frequently visited Koprowski and Plotkin at the Wistar at the other end of Pennsylvania; he recalls that, at this stage, "Koprowski and Sabin were fighting like dogs over a bone." Prinzie returned to Belgium in December 1958 to become head of the virus department at the Rega, and he formally transferred to RIT in 1965.

At first, when I asked him about the Koprowski strains, he replied that he and his colleagues had merely had discussions with Koprowski; they had never tested or used his strains. I said that I thought that they *had* produced some CHAT. Prinzie said that they had never produced it, but had just "sort of played around with [it] . . . just to get our fingers wet." I repeated that what I had heard from other RIT workers was that they had made one batch of CHAT and one of Fox on behalf of Koprowski. "You're right, you're right," he suddenly answered. "And this is in the days where Koprowski had contact with Courtois . . . and Plotkin. And they were going to go to the Congo, but they needed larger scale than they had produced by themselves. Because I believe that a large part of the vaccine that was used in the Congo was produced by our group. I was not personally involved, that's why my memory is hazy there."

This was a real breakthrough. Prinzie was the sixth scientist I had interviewed who had worked in the Rega Institute or RIT in the late fifties or early sixties, and yet he was the first actually to volunteer that they had produced much of the Congo vaccine. Prinzie went on to tell me that Courtois, whom he recalled as having created a "monkey-breeding station" in the Congo, had acted as go-between, linking the Koprowski group and De Somer. In those early days, he explained, everything was done by talking to friends. "One friend would say to another . . . 'Could you produce twenty liters of my strain, because it would help me?' It was more sort of give and take. . . . You get your good contacts. You never knew at that time — in '57 — Koprowski could have won the race. Therefore having Koprowski strains in hand could have been very useful. And working together with him in team was priceless, so why not?"

In a phone conversation a few months later, Dr. Prinzie provided some more specific details. Now he told me that as far as he knew, the Koprowski vaccine had first been produced in small batches at the Rega Institute, where Monique Lamy was in charge. The strains had arrived from America, and had been grown up in tissue culture to produce enough vaccine for the Ruzizi trial. He said that since this was only "a few hundred thousand doses," it was relatively small-scale production. He wasn't sure which monkey species had been used for tissue culture, but thought that it would probably have been rhesus or cynomolgus.

Prinzie recalled that later on, Stanley Plotkin had come to Belgium, to discuss with them what quantities of Koprowski's vaccines they could make, this time at RIT. "Plotkin was over here, and there was a plan for the large-scale exploration of the safety and efficacy of those strains. [De Somer] provided the possibility of making that vaccine that was not available in the U.S. In those days . . . regulations were not like now." These appeared to be the pools of CHAT and Fox that Peetermans had told me were made in 1959. So, according to Prinzie, Belgian production of CHAT and Fox had taken place in two stages: experimental small-scale production (possibly of a Belgian version of pool 10A-11) at the Rega in 1957/8, and larger scale manufacture (perhaps of pool DS) at RIT in 1959.

We talked more about those early days, and Prinzie said: "[It] really was an unknown territory, where you were stumbling into things you did not understand — and which sometimes (like SV40 or B virus) could be frightening. . . . [We were acting] in full innocence, not understanding what sort of Pandora's box we were opening. . . . We were at the dawn of oral vaccine, which of course was not killed. . . . There was nearly no control . . . it was minimal. . . . That is one of the major reasons why at some point people decided that to work with a dirty animal like the monkey was an impossible task."

Abel Prinzie also told me about a trip he made in 1955 to see Georges Barski and Pierre Lépine at the Pasteur Institute in Paris, where Monique Lamy had just been receiving her training. Over lunch in the cafeteria, Prinzie had started talking about tissue culture, but Barski swiftly interrupted, asking him to refrain from discussing such points at the table. When asked why, he explained that "you should never talk about what . . . we are doing together in cell culture outside the walls of my lab." This was a telling indication of the secrecy that surrounded the subject at the Pasteur — where, of course, they had just been collaborating with Jezierski, making experimental cultures from the kidneys of fifteen different African primates, including the chimpanzee.

When I asked Prinzie about the chimp camp at Lindi, he admitted that he did not know exactly what had been going on there, save that the researchers were checking the attenuation of the vaccine by feeding the chimps — and also by injecting them in neurovirulence tests that, he told me, later turned out to be "not very relevant." I asked whether they might not have also made use of the kidneys as a vaccine substrate. Prinzie replied promptly: "No, because it was recognized very early, of course, that the cohort population of chimps . . . could not produce enough kidneys." He pointed out that in the early days of making IPV at the Rega Institute, they had been using about 150 monkeys a month. The chimps, he said, were not available in those numbers.

---

At this stage it seemed vital to speak once more with Monique Lamy about the events of this period, especially the links between the Rega, RIT, and Lépine's lab at the Pasteur in Paris.[10] She confirmed that De Somer had sent her to the latter for a year in 1954/5 to learn tissue culture techniques, and said they had been using trypsinized cynomolgus kidneys to make their tissue cultures. Later, when it was pointed out to her that Lépine had reported using baboon kidneys at this time, she said: "It's possible, but I don't remember any more. It wasn't me who killed the monkeys. I just did culture." Intriguingly, she said she had not heard of Alexandre Jezierski, even though he had been at the Pasteur working with Barski and Lépine at the same time as herself.[11]

Lamy said that when she returned to Leuven, she had gone straight to the Rega Institute, where she started making tissue culture, and produced the initial pools of inactivated vaccine.[12] She claimed that only IPV had been made at the Rega, and that in 1957 she transferred to RIT's new facility in Rixensart to do industrial production of IPV (which, as before, she called Salk vaccine). She said that about twelve monkeys had been killed each day for their kidneys, and once again insisted that cynomolgus macaques were the only ones used. Lamy said that she was in charge, that Peetermans supervised production, and that altogether fifty people were employed making IPV, which was exported all over the world.

As for OPV, Lamy claimed that they started making Sabin vaccine in Belgium in 1962/3, after she had left RIT to study medicine. When asked specifically about the Koprowski strains, she said that she had received attenuated poliovirus strains from three different American manufacturers, and tested them intracerebrally in monkeys, and found that the two strains other than Sabin's were too virulent, especially Koprowski's. When told that Prinzie had said that they had produced vaccine for Koprowski, Lamy once again insisted that they had not done so — that the only OPV produced had been for Sabin.[13]

———

After thinking about all this some more, I realized that this latest evidence left two questions all but answered, but another one still wide open. It seemed almost certain that most of the CHAT and Fox used in 1959 in central Africa had been produced at RIT. This had been clearly stated by Prinzie, and independently confirmed by Ninane and Caubergh, both of whom had fed the vaccine in Ruanda-Urundi. (Even Huygelen and Peetermans, who said that the RIT-produced CHAT and Fox pools had been sent only to Poland, accepted that RIT *had* produced Koprowski's vaccines in 1959.) In all likelihood, at least some of the CHAT vaccine produced that year at RIT had been designated pool DS.

As regards the Leopoldville trial from August 1958 to April 1960, we have the primary evidence of Henry Gelfand from Tulane University, who recalls collecting vaccine from Courtois in Brussels in August 1958 and delivering it to the Congolese capital — this being vaccine that Courtois had previously collected from a lab just outside Brussels. Such a precise recollection indicates that at least part of the CHAT pool 13 used in Leo must also have been produced at one of De Somer's labs at Leuven University, the Rega, or RIT. (In interview, Koprowski suggested that RIT might have been involved.)

And yet, when one looks at the early epidemiology of HIV and AIDS, it is not pool DS that falls under the greatest suspicion of containing a contaminant SIV. And neither is it the pool 13 fed in Leopoldville. Certainly many of the early cases emerged there, but as discussed earlier, such was the population influx to Leopoldville from 1958 onward that the epidemic could have resulted from outsiders importing HIV to the Congolese capital.

It is rather the CHAT 10A-11 vaccine used in 1958 for the second (Lake Tanganyika) leg of the "Ruzizi Valley trial," vaccine that was fed in places like Usumbura and Rumonge, which coincides most precisely with the early appearance of HIV some years later. This is the correlation that is by far the hardest to explain away by any other hypothesis — or by coincidence. And it is for this batch, unfortunately, that we can be least certain about where the vaccine was made, and by whom.

In terms of documentary evidence, the paper in the *British Medical Journal* attests that the vaccines used in the early African trials, up to and including that at Ruzizi, were made at the Wistar. However, this paper only describes the first part of the Ruzizi trial, that staged in the valley itself. In terms of anecdotal evidence, we have reports from two sources that Flack and Jervis carried what was clearly American-made vaccine with them on the plane from New York in February 1958. There again, Flack's diary suggests that something else may have been loaded onto the plane at Brussels, perhaps bypassing normal procedures, as she and Jervis were in transit to Stanleyville and Usumbura. Lise Thiry says she has no recollection of such an event, though she does not deny that Belgian-made vaccine *could* have been put on the plane.

Ninane thought that from Ruzizi onward, all the CHAT fed in Africa had been made in Belgium. Prinzie, at the last, said that the "small-scale" production for the Ruzizi Valley trial had been carried out at the Rega Institute. But he also said that this was while Monique Lamy was in charge — which is quite clearly wrong, since both Lamy and Peetermans recall that Lamy left the Rega to take charge at RIT's castle when it opened in March 1957.

Clearly not everyone has clear memories of this period, and clearly not everyone has his or her facts straight. The vaccine fed in Usumbura and along Lake Tanganyika in April 1958 could have been made at the Wistar, or it could have been made in Belgium, at either the Rega Institute or RIT, either by Pieter De Somer or persons unknown. In addition, there would appear to be one other viable possibility.

----

Let us again review the sequence of events that begins in early 1958. Fritz Deinhardt, working principally on hepatitis, flies out to Stanleyville in late January. During the next three months he is, among other things, extracting kidneys from sacrificed chimpanzees, mincing them, and shipping them back to colleagues in Philadelphia to prepare tissue cultures for experimental research. "Vaccination[s] in face of . . . epidemic[s]"[14] take place in Gombari, Watsa, and Bambesa, between January 27 and February 1; at the final venue, Bambesa, only part of the village is fed, because of "insufficient vaccine." For a while, it seems, the stocks in Stanleyville are exhausted. On February 20, Agnes Flack and George Jervis fly to Stanleyville and then on to Usumbura; they are carrying supplies of CHAT for the Ruzizi Valley trial. On February 23, Paul Osterrieth returns to Stanleyville from six months' leave, during which time he has received training in tissue culture techniques at the Wistar Institute, at Koprowski's insistence. Flack, Jervis, and Ghislain Courtois begin the mass vaccination campaign in the Ruzizi Valley the following day. On February 25, they are visited by the bacteriologist Professor Welsch, from Liège, and by other senior public health officials, presumably Belgian. Shortly afterward, Gaston Ninane joins the vaccination team. Meanwhile, people from the Laboratoire Médical (probably Osterrieth and Paulette Dherte, perhaps with Deinhardt's assistance) vaccinate more than 3,000 soldiers at the military camp just outside Stanleyville on February 27.[15] On March 25, Jean Vandepitte arrives in Stanleyville to take over from Courtois, who departs on leave two days later. Osterrieth, for one, is not impressed with Vandepitte's modus operandi, and his rejection of the more laissez-faire regime established by Courtois over the course of many years; he decides that he will quietly disobey Vandepitte when he thinks fit.[16] Five days later, at the end of the Ruzizi Valley feeding, Gaston Ninane waves Flack off at Usumbura airport, and shortly afterward he flies back to Stanleyville. Within days, he returns to Usumbura with a new batch of vaccine, which he and Hector Meyus feed along the shores of Lake Tanganyika, finishing on April 10. Toward the end of April, Deinhardt returns to Philadelphia.

Ninane firmly believes that the second batch of CHAT vaccine that he brought back to Usumbura for the lakeside campaign was manufactured in Leuven, or at RIT. But he had been out in Ruzizi for the previous month, so it may well be that his belief is based purely on hearsay — on what he himself was told at the time. Perhaps one batch of the vaccine brought out from America or from Belgium by Flack and Jervis was stored in the freezer at the Stanleyville lab when they passed through in February, and then given to Ninane in April, so that he could conduct the feedings in Usumbura and along Lake Tanganyika. Or perhaps, while he was busy vaccinating in the Ruzizi Valley, someone else was busy preparing more vaccine in the Stanleyville lab.

We know that during this key period chimpanzee kidneys, ready-minced, were available in Stanleyville, courtesy of Deinhardt. We know that Ninane himself, at some stage, tried — unsuccessfully — to use chimp kidneys to make tissue culture there. We also know that during 1958 tissue culture from local primates (baboons, and possibly other species too) was successfully produced in the Stanleyville lab by Osterrieth. Between 1953 and 1957, Jezierski did exactly the same thing in the Gabu-Nioka lab, using tissue culture from fifteen different African primates, including chimps. We know, therefore, that making tissue culture from the kidneys of local simians was not hugely difficult; it was a viable procedure for an African laboratory at this time. This said, it must also be reiterated that both Ninane and Osterrieth deny that they themselves actually produced any chimp kidney tissue culture in Stanleyville.

This was at a moment when the Lindi polio research was coming to an end, and many of the apes were surplus to requirements. Yet the whole concept of the chimp camp had been to assist with medical and scientific investigations, and everyone involved wanted to make the best possible use of the research animals. At around this time, Ghislain Courtois sent the skulls of seventy-nine chimpanzees, roughly equally divided between *Pan troglodytes* and *Pan paniscus*, to the primate collection at the Africa Museum at Tervuren, halfway between Brussels and Leuven.[17] It seems very possible that some chimps may have provided skulls to the museum and kidneys to the laboratory. What is still uncertain is which laboratory.

Perhaps it was always the intention to mount trials of two different versions of the vaccine in early 1958. Or perhaps supplies ran out in Ruzizi, as they had earlier in Bambesa, and someone decided to produce another batch by passaging the vaccine virus (or the vaccine itself) once or twice more in a locally available substrate. Such an initiative could have been sanctioned by higher authorities, or it could even have been an off-the-cuff experiment by one individual doctor, perhaps with the discreet assistance of one of the sanitary agents, technicians, or nurses based at the *laboratoire*. As Jean Deinhardt, Fritz's widow, once told me with regard to growing poliovirus in chimp kidneys: "It would have been logical to try that.... [T]here would have been no contraindication to doing it." Although using such material as a human vaccine would have been a highly risky procedure, this was at the time when the lab director, Courtois, was spending most of his days out in Ruzizi, after which he left on vacation, and there was the uneasy interregnum under Vandepitte. It may be that for much of February and March 1958 the chain of command at the Laboratoire Médical was not entirely clear-cut.

If indeed a vaccine batch was produced in Stanleyville, then to whom would it have been fed? The answer, in all likelihood, involves the 65,000 souls vaccinated by Ninane and Meyus in Usumbura and along the shore of Lake Tanganyika at the start of April. In addition, the vaccine batch may have been given to the 3,000-odd soldiers fed at Stanleyville military camp on February 27. And conceivably it could have been fed to another 5,000 or so persons fed by Ninane (perhaps at around this time) in Lisala. These are the three most likely venues. The total comes to just under 75,000 vaccine doses. Even employing the less efficient Maitland suspended cell technique for making tissue culture, it would have required the kidneys of only about a dozen primates to make this quantity of vaccine. If trypsinization had been involved, just a single pair of kidneys would have been enough.

---

Forty years later, Courtois and Deinhardt are both dead. The American journalist Joan Phillips, who, with her late husband Robert, apparently met Deinhardt in Stanleyville during March 1958, is unwilling to talk about the meeting, or about what she recalls of the vaccine and the vaccinations. Osterrieth, after his original interview, now seems unwilling to talk further. Ninane *is* willing to talk, but we know that he was in Ruanda-Urundi, rather than Stanleyville, for much of the key period. We know that Professor Welsch was temporarily based at the Stanleyville lab at this time,[18] but he is now dead as well. The only other senior doctor employed by the Laboratoire Médical during early 1958, a medic from Luxembourg called E. Mangen (who, according to André Courtois, had frequent arguments with his father), is no longer traceable.

Until someone talks, or someone remembers more details, we will simply not know who prepared this particular batch of vaccine — a batch that may have become contaminated with the chimpanzee virus, SIVcpz, which is a close ancestor of HIV-1. But the crucial point is this. It could have happened this way. The apparatus was all in place that might very easily have allowed it to happen this way.

This may or may not be the solution to the mystery; the reader will come to his or her own conclusions. But whatever the finer details, it would seem possible that that February 1960 returnee from the Congo, the man who told the London *Times* reporter that "something untoward is brewing at Stanleyville," was correct in more ways than he knew.[19]

———————

So, let us get out the microscope, glance back through the box of slides — and review once again the accumulated evidence. The early AIDS cases, the early instances of HIV infection, and the wide range of different HIV-1 subtypes — all occur in the three central African countries where an experimental vaccine of unknown provenance, called CHAT, had been fed just a few years earlier. Now let us increase the magnification — to observe that it is not just the countries that coincide with the feeding of the vaccine, but the regions within those countries. Now zoom in further — down to town and village level. Look at Stanleyville, Lisala, Kikwit, Lubudi, Usumbura, Rumonge. The finer the resolution, the more precise the picture gets. The same precise parallels hold for the timings of the vaccinations and the emergence of the first traces of HIV.

We do not know exactly what happened at Lindi, but there is a huge and unexplained gap in the records of the experiments conducted there, and considerable secrecy surrounds the work carried out on the chimps — secrecy that continues to this day. What we do know is that two species of chimpanzee were housed in the camp, often in the same cages. We know that hundreds of the chimps that entered Lindi camp are unaccounted for, and that some of the chimps had symptoms of immunosuppression, suggesting they may have been infected with SIV. We know that at least six shipments of chimp kidneys were sent from Stanleyville to Philadelphia. Several of those who were indirectly involved in the research believe that many more pairs of kidneys were sent, both to the Wistar Institute, and to De Somer's labs in Belgium. Several of these contemporary observers believe that the only logical reason for sending those kidneys would have been to produce vaccine in them. Furthermore, it is clear that a pool of vaccine made in chimp kidney tissue culture could have been produced in Stanleyville itself.

The reader must make up his mind or her mind. I have made up mine. I believe that herein lies the truth. I believe that this is how the AIDS epidemic began.

# VIII

## HOW A RIVER IS BORN

*Everything flows and nothing stays.*

*You can't step twice into the same river.*

— HERACLITUS

# 57

## THE RECHANNELING OF HISTORY

Pathological liars are rare. The majority of people are, I believe, innately honest, if only because life teaches that the easiest way to live is with self-respect and a minimum of complication. However, for most people there seems to be a sliding scale — and a point at which lying does become an option. Many will lie when they feel their comfortable self-image to be threatened. Others will start to lie only when financial well-being is at stake. Only a few take it further, and would rather go to their graves than dissemble. There is no reason, of course, why scientists should be any different from the rest of the human race. They too have varying levels of integrity.

The process of lying is interesting too. One starts by swerving around the sharper and more dangerous corners of what is known to be true, to arrive at a position that is almost true, or that would definitely be true provided that some factor be realized, provided that $x$ equaled 6. This small refraction, and the realization that light can bend, allows one to maintain two parallel versions of truth — one for the heart, or perhaps for the best friend, or for the spouse in the dead of night. And the other, less precise version for the potential enemy, for the person who asks awkward questions and who might do one damage.

Time passes. Recollections become less sharp. The two parallel versions of truth fade in and out, and intertwine in the mists of memory. Finally, the process is completed. Two apples becomes three apples. A chimp changes to a giraffe, a zebra to a crocodile. And as far as one remembers, one was not even there at the time.

Hilary Koprowski is also, it would appear, aware of the problems of reporting facts and events accurately.

In August 1955, after Muguga, Dr. Koprowski was in the Transvaal, delivering a lecture about polio vaccines to the local branch of the South African Medical Association. He ended his speech as follows: "This lecture was purposely delivered neither in a euphoric nor in a discouraging tone. I would have liked my listeners to believe everything I said, but I did realize — particularly when I came to revise the talk — that verisimilitude falls short of truth, although the latter no man may ever know."[1]

His implication, it seems, is that God alone knows what the truth is.

———————

I still keep the ivory tortoise, that gift from Ann Courtois, on my computer table near the mouse. I like her idea of the African virtues of patience and perseverance, and I also like to view it as a symbol of my research — sometimes slow and plodding, sometimes jerky-necked with excitement when an especially juicy leaf hoves into view, but nonetheless lumbering forward, single-mindedly, toward its goal. It seems somehow appropriate that the tortoise is made of a substance that was far more acceptable back in the fifties than it is today — just like the monkey kidney tissue cultures around which this research has revolved.

One of my reasons for deciding to write this book in narrative fashion was that I felt it would enable not just the scientific information about the likely genesis of an epidemic to be detailed, but also something of the process of discovery. Furthermore, I hoped that this might help demonstrate how it was that so many of the original protagonists had developed memory loss about this particular period, and how it was that other members of the scientific establishment — including the great and the good — could have failed to spot (or to investigate) the evidence that lay beneath their noses.

In the six years after publication of the 1985 article by Phyllis Kanki and Max Essex, the article that demonstrated the presence of SIV in the African green monkey, a species that had previously provided kidneys to make polio vaccines,[2] it seems that only four people bothered to follow up the clues properly. One was the reclusive philosopher Louis Pascal, the true author of the OPV/AIDS hypothesis, and the man who first identified the risky vaccination campaign. The second was the brilliant but eccentric British venereologist John Seale, who submitted a 7,000-word paper on the subject to *Nature* in January 1990; it was never published.[3] The others were the two South African scientists Jennifer Alexander and Mike Lecatsas, who, without knowing of Pascal's or Seale's researches, proposed the polio vaccine hypothesis in letters to medical journals, and were then savagely criticized by their superiors.[4]

In 1991 the AIDS activist Blaine Elswood, his collaborator Raphael Stricker, and the journalist Tom Curtis took the research several steps further. Thereafter it was a disparate third wave, including science policy expert Brian Martin, evolutionary biologist Bill Hamilton, law professor Michael Kent Curtis, and journalist Julian Cribb,[5] who gave the theory further publicity and credibility.

And yet the clues were there to be found for any who cared to look. When I first learned of the OPV/AIDS theory in June 1992, I had been investigating theories of origin for more than two years. Suddenly, here was a more plausible explanation than any other I had come across, but I was still far from convinced. However, when further research consistently pointed to the same conclusion, I found, after several years, that I was starting to describe myself as "more than 90 percent persuaded" on the basis of the steadily accumulating stream of evidence. It was just as Louis Pascal had claimed in his broken boulder metaphor: as every new shard was uncovered, it fitted with the already hypothesized shape of the rock that must have plunged from the cliff above. As I write this today, there is still not a single significant fragment that conflicts with the theory.[6]

The hypothesis is supported not only by the richness and diversity of the fossil record — but also by the gaps in that fossil record, and the telling positions of those gaps. The events surrounding Lindi camp, the preparation of CHAT vaccine, and the field trials of that vaccine are characterized by missing records, faulty memories, obfuscation, and — on occasions — downright falsehoods. And yet of course, not every detail can be neatly excised from the archives. Like the debris from Pascal's smashed boulder, there will always be fragments of different sizes left behind for the geologist to examine.

But how is it that so many of those who should have been searching at the foot of the rockface — the virologists and vaccine-makers, the molecular and evolutionary biologists, even the epidemiologists — have failed to do their job?

There seem to have been several factors at play. First, most of them were not on the field trip: they were busy in their labs, peering into microscopes (or preparing grant applications). Second, there have been so many crackpot hypotheses of origin, so many silly and spurious conspiracy theories, that many observers became jaded and skeptical about iatrogenic theories per se. Third, many of those who had followed the controversy at a distance had read Koprowski's reply in *Science,* or heard about the Wistar expert committee's negative report, and had assumed that the matter had been laid to rest, that another theory had crumbled when subjected to the fierce light of scientific examination.[7]

But possibly there was a fourth reason too — one involving protection of the profession and fear of peer reaction. Because, if the OPV/AIDS theory was proved to be true, then the implications — and likely repercussions — were almost too awful to contemplate.

Some, the virologists and vaccine-makers, might feel that the theory could turn people against vaccines in general. Some, like primatologists, might be concerned that it would lead to awful retribution against African primates — especially chimpanzees. And some — those in certain institutions and pharmaceutical companies, or public health departments — would simply have dreaded the glare of unwanted publicity. Besides, they may have felt, why should they be held responsible for mistakes that occurred forty years earlier?

As for the protagonists, the men and women who were actively involved in the production and administration of polio vaccines used in central Africa in the fifties, one has to feel some sympathy. Their initial motive was essentially noble — to save lives — and nobody deliberately did anything to endanger humanity, or to create new and more serious medical problems. How were they to know that something could go wrong, that a new human virus could be introduced through the very vehicle with which they hoped to eradicate a deadly disease?

Whether or not any of these persons can be held directly culpable for the AIDS epidemic, what is unavoidable is that some of them bear a degree of responsibility. They were so preoccupied with winning the polio vaccine race that they failed to employ what, in retrospect, we can identify as sensible care and caution.

This can best be illustrated by one final quotation from Hilary Koprowski, from an article entitled "Tin Anniversary of the Development of Live Virus Vaccine." This was essentially the opening speech he delivered at the Second International Conference on Live Poliovirus Vaccines, in June 1960, to which he had added a few additional comments. One passage reads as follows:

> The poliomyelitis vaccine is administered orally, and many viruses find their way into the human body through the mouth. If one wishes to be a purist in this entire matter, then the licensing authorities should require all food items which are eaten uncooked to be tested for the presence of viral agents.
>
> Although it is permissible to be lighthearted about this whole matter of extraneous viruses, one should not at the same time be lightheaded. *If possible* [my emphasis], one should attempt to feed to millions of people throughout the whole world a preparation which would be free — so far as can be demonstrated within the limits of our present knowledge — from any virus other than polio.

From the perspective of the nineties, one can only say that when the stakes are as high as they were in this instance, one would have hoped for even more. Sometimes, doing one's best is just not enough.

And what of the response of the protagonists, nearly forty years after the events in question? The magnificent response to the OPV/AIDS theory would have involved a handing over of keys to filing cabinets and freezers, so that other scientists could independently examine the evidence. However, the impact of the AIDS epidemic has been so enormous, the human tragedy so great, that nobody should be surprised that the response has been rather less scientific, less noble.

Let us look, then, at what has actually happened since Pascal, Elswood, Curtis, and others first brought news of the broken boulder to public attention.

---

Most of the central figures who were involved with CHAT in the fifties strenuously maintain, at least in public, that there is no link between the vaccine and AIDS. They have been unable, however, to provide any physical or documentary evidence to support their position; indeed, there has been a discernable tendency for memories to prove inadequate, for records to become lost, and for samples of the vaccine to become unavailable. With respect to the latter, let us analyze the present state of play.

The proposal of the Wistar's expert committee that one of the CHAT samples, which "has been identified as possibly directly relevant to the Congo trials," should be tested by the CDC and the WHO seems to have died the death. Certainly the CDC was approached, and offered to help, but only if a second lab would also agree to test the sample — which apparently has never happened.[8]

This delicate situation was described in a letter from Giovanni Rovera, the director of the Wistar Institute, in November 1995. He wrote to inform me that the WHO had not responded to his approach "in an equivalent manner" to the CDC, and that the NIH had "likewise declined to test the sample because the limited quantity of virus stock available precluded comprehensive testing." He went on: "In consultation with my colleagues, I decided not to proceed in this matter since the results of any test on such a small sample of virus stock, no matter how competently performed, would not have been accepted in the scientific community as conclusive."[9] We now know from the freezer records that there are actually 5 milliliters of CHAT pool 13 available — more than enough to test at two labs (or even ten).[10] Remarkably, however, it is still not clear whether the CHAT vial at the Wistar contains a sample of the attenuated poliovirus seed pool, or the final production lot of vaccine. In its report, the Wistar committee referred to "vaccine stocks," whereas Rovera, in his letter, refers to "virus stock," which would seem to suggest that the sample is from a seed pool, just as Koprowski claimed in his letter to *Science*.[11] If this latter account is correct, and the sample is from the CHAT virus seed pool, then Rovera's letter embraces a strange logic, in that a seed pool is by its nature homogeneous, and it is therefore valid to test it. However, it is the vaccines (especially those fed in Africa) that are most important to test, since these were the materials fed to humans. Furthermore, there is more basis for concern about the vaccines, for we now know that much more care was taken about controlling the safety of the viral seed pools than that of the vaccine production lots.

Attempts to locate early samples of CHAT vaccine, like 10A-11 or 13, have not proved encouraging.[12] Meinrad Schar has informed me that there are no samples available in Switzerland.[13] In Belgium, Stan Huygelen and Julian Peetermans have made it clear that all the vaccine stocks have been given to others, or destroyed. Nobody seriously expects to find any remaining stocks in the Congo. This leaves only those few samples found in Stockholm, which were tested by Jan Albert, and found negative for HIV and SIV.[14]

However, there is an epilogue to that story, and a sad one to boot. After Hans Wigzell wrote to Bill Hamilton, in January 1995, with the results of the Stockholm testing of CHAT, Hamilton wrote back to Wigzell twice,[15] and phoned him five times, in the hope of persuading him to release a sample so that the mitochondrial DNA of the host (the species that provided the kidneys to make the vaccine) could be assessed. This was something that, during our meeting a year earlier, Wigzell had said that he might be willing to consider.[16] But not one of these communications elicited a reply.

Eventually, in July 1996, I wrote a letter to Wigzell,[17] who by now was *Rektor* (vice-chancellor) of the Karolinska Institute.[18] In this letter, I pointed out that Bill Hamilton had heard nothing more from him, and urged him once more to consider releasing a sample to test for the host species. I formally requested a reply from him, and added: "Clearly it would reflect much better [on you] . . . were you to release the samples now, rather than wait and risk being forced to respond in the context of the heated public debate which may well follow publication of my book." I showed the letter to Bill Hamilton before I sent it, and he approved its tone and content.

Just over a fortnight later, shortly before eight on a Sunday morning, I received a fax from Stockholm.[19] In it, Dr. Wigzell explained that he had only received Bill Hamilton's two letters; he had no record of his having phoned.[20] He went on to explain that he had "argued with relevant individuals within SIIDC" (the Swedish Institute and Infectious Disease Control) about whether the vaccine samples could be released, and had asked them to respond to Professor Hamilton; it seemed, he wrote, that they had not. He then went on to accuse me of using "black mail writings to achieve [my] ends." He continued: "This is the first time in my life that I have received a letter from some [one who] is using such deplorable methods."

I wrote back to assure him that no threat had been intended, and that I had rather been warning him about possible controversy in the future. I also asked him about the identity of the "relevant individuals within the SIIDC" who now held the CHAT vaccine samples.[21] Hans Wigzell never replied, and I decided not to pursue the matter further.

---

As for the documentary records about CHAT, and about the feedings in Africa, these too have proved hard to locate. Koprowski says that all the records about CHAT have been "lost in a move," even though his account of when this happened seems uncertain. Despite his statement, several pages of records about CHAT between 1958 and 1962 were provided by the Wistar Institute to the expert committee. However, only one page of these records was directly applicable to the CHAT vaccine of 1957/8, or to the 1958 vaccinations in Africa. David Ho has told me that he thinks that the Wistar provided the committee with just a "sample of what they had."[22] He was not implying subterfuge, but this does suggest that there may be further records that could usefully be examined.

Other sources have proved no better. In Sweden, the CHAT protocols, which were at one stage promised by Carl-Rune Salenstedt, never materialized. In Belgium, the relevant records about CHAT and Fox are unavailable at RIT and, it would seem, at the Rega Institute and the University of Leuven also. And the substantial file of poliomyelitis correspondence held at the Belgian Ministry of Foreign Affairs archives is completely devoid of entries for the months between November 1956 to July 1958. This equates precisely with the period one would most wish to view. Furthermore, the archives as a whole are surprisingly (though not completely) devoid of documentation about the vaccinations.

In the absence of written records, many people's memories are also proving inadequate. Gaston Ninane and Hubert Caubergh have revealed that much of the vaccine used in the Congo and Ruanda-Urundi was Belgian-made, but most of those involved at the Belgian end simply deny this. Peetermans and Huygelen say that the Koprowski vaccine RIT manufactured was not sent to the Congo, while Monique Lamy insists that no CHAT or Fox was ever produced in Belgium for human use. Of past employees at Rega and RIT, only Abel Prinzie has spoken out clearly on this key point.

Meanwhile Hilary Koprowski and Stanley Plotkin, the two men who effectively headed the vaccine program at the Wistar, have taken a different approach. When confronted with the possible links between CHAT and AIDS, they have threatened to sue. At the same time, they are suddenly keen to retell the story, but with a different spin, for they have published two new accounts of the vaccinations in recent years.

One constitutes a chapter in a 1996 book about the history of vaccination, which is coedited by Stanley Plotkin. Entitled "History of Koprowski Vaccine against Poliomyelitis," it was written by Koprowski in collaboration with his former assistant.[23] The second is a hitherto unpublished 1980 lecture by Koprowski about the development of OPVs that appears as an appendix in the fascinating autobiography by his wife, Irena Koprowska, published in 1997.[24]

Unfortunately, both of these recent versions of events contain errors. One involves the origin of the name of CHAT, which is still inaccurate.[25] Another is the claim that the increase of virulence of the viruses excreted by George Dick's vaccinees would nowadays "evoke no surprise, [but] Dick considered it the signal to campaign in the newspapers against attenuated virus vaccination." (In reality, the increase in virulence of TN that Dr. Dick reported in the medical literature [not in the press] was of an extremity that caused the WHO expert committee to conclude: "[A]ll are in agreement that this is an example of a strain which should not be used."[26]) A third example comprises Koprowski's two different accounts of the Ruzizi trial, which, he implies, was staged wholly or partly in response to a polio epidemic.[27] This simply is not so, and furthermore it does not tally with what Koprowski and Stanley Plotkin told me in interviews in 1993 and 1994, which was that the purpose of the Ruzizi trial was to assess the viability of mass vaccination with an OPV.[28] It seems strange that these errors have appeared *since* 1994, and in publications that, from Koprowski's and Plotkin's perspectives, were apparently designed to put the record straight.

Other themes in the chapter in Plotkin's book are interesting for other reasons, particularly with respect to Koprowski's relationship with his two great (and now posthumous) rivals for the OPV crown. Of Herald Cox, he writes: "I still regret the rupture . . . between us," while for Albert Sabin he claims that "if we fell out during the late 1950s and 1960s owing to the pressures of competition . . . the passage of time has removed all rancor." This is in marked contrast to the speech reprinted in his wife's book published the following year, in which Koprowski complains that Sabin questioned the safety of his original decision to feed OPV to children, saying that it could have started an epidemic, and later "graciously quoted" his [Koprowski's] pioneering work in only one of his own polio articles.

Koprowski's recycling of these more scathing remarks about Sabin after the latter's death is lent added piquancy by the fact that, in the final year of his life, after the OPV/AIDS controversy broke, Sabin was a better friend to Koprowski than any other of his erstwhile colleagues.

When Elswood and Stricker submitted their article about polio vaccines and AIDS to Luc Montagnier, coeditor of *Research in Virology,* Montagnier sent the text to Koprowski, inviting his reply — and Koprowski immediately forwarded a copy to Sabin.[29] The great man replied to Koprowski on March 3, 1992, a year to the day before he died, and was vigorous in defense of his former adversary. He described the Elswood/Stricker paper as "a most irresponsible communication by two ignorant people," and claimed that the cytopathic virus that he had identified back in 1959 in the large lot of CHAT used in the Congo trials "could not possibly have any relationship to SIV and certainly not to HIV." Besides, he added, "the large lot of vaccine prepared for the Congo field trials was made in *macacus rhesus* kidney cultures which are not known to harbor SIV."

Sabin provided no supporting evidence for these two important claims.[30]

He invited Koprowski to transmit his comments to Montagnier, adding that he could not understand why *Research in Virology* would consider publication of an article such as Elswood's. Sabin's letter was duly forwarded to Paris, together with a contribution from Koprowski that contained several mistakes, such as his assumption that HIV could not be transmitted orally.

A month later, as the controversy grew in the wake of Curtis's *Rolling Stone* piece, Koprowski again approached Sabin, this time asking him to sign a statement responding to the OPV/AIDS theory, which he planned to circulate to "a group of concerned scientists" and then submit to the press. Sabin advised Koprowski that "your proposed statement is unnecessary and will only give Tom Curtis the additional publicity which he seeks." He added that Curtis had been to see him "on a fishing expedition against you in which I refused to participate. I accused him of irresponsible journalism." He added that Curtis had been saying that if there was still any of the Congo vaccine in existence, it should be tested — but Sabin advised Koprowski against cooperating, on the grounds that "a test on 10 ml — even 100 ml — of a large lot proves nothing about what may have been present in the remainder of the lot."

Koprowski replied to say that he agreed "that sending the statement out will only increase the stature of Tom Curtis and the quicker he will be put in proper place the better it is for all of us." He seemed to be hinting that the OPV/AIDS hypothesis potentially placed all the fifties manufacturers of oral polio vaccine in the same boat.

According to several reports, it was shortly after this, at the start of May, that Stanley Plotkin met with Luc Montagnier in Paris to discuss the OPV/AIDS theory.[31] The fact that this much rumored meeting had involved just the two of them was confirmed by Tom Curtis who, it turned out, had interviewed Leonard Hayflick during the late spring of 1992. Curtis recalled Hayflick saying that he had recently met with Stanley Plotkin in Paris, "and that Plotkin . . . had spoken to Luc Montagnier, and reminded him that the French had done some experiments in Africa with baboons [giving polio vaccines made in baboon kidney], and that perhaps the French might have started the epidemic."[32] Curtis went on: "I don't know if there was a cause/effect relationship or not, but certainly it was after this that Luc Montagnier was far less interested in publishing the theory [of] Elswood and Stricker."

In June 1992, Montagnier decided to publish Elswood's article — but in a much shortened version as a letter, to which he now invited Koprowski and Sabin to respond. This time Sabin declined to help further, and when the letter was finally published in February 1993, it contained no rejoinder from either scientist. Montagnier did, however, add his own editorial comment, stating that since no polio vaccine had ever been made from the tissues of chimpanzees, host to the SIV closest to HIV-1, "it is difficult to imagine how massive contamination of polio vaccines . . . could have occurred."[33]

What is intriguing about all this is the manner in which Sabin leaped to Koprowski's defense. It seems very strange that Sabin should tell Koprowski, in a letter, which substrate he (Koprowski) had used for his own polio vaccines, as used in the Congo. Significantly, from then on Koprowski stuck to this line, claiming in his letter to *Science* that he had used only the kidneys of rhesus macaques for his vaccines, but then adding — inaccurately — that they had been captured either in India or the Philippines; (rhesus macaques are not found in the Philippines; Koprowski presumably meant cynomolgus macaques).[34] Two of Koprowski's other claims in that letter (that back in the fifties Sabin tested a sample of a seed-lot of CHAT virus rather than a sample of CHAT vaccine, and that the contaminant he found therein was a foamy virus) are not contained in any of Sabin's letters to him, and run counter to what is reported in the literature. Both, therefore, would appear to be questionable.

---

If a virus closely related to HIV-1 (and especially to an archival sample of HIV-1, such as L70) was ever found in chimpanzees from the rain forest of the eastern Congo, where the Lindi chimpanzees were collected, this would not, of course, provide final confirmation of the OPV/AIDS hypothesis, but it would render it mighty persuasive. The natural transfer school would then have to explain why AIDS had emerged in the very areas where CHAT vaccine was fed, rather than on the north bank of the Congo (if the ancestral virus had been found in the common chimpanzee, *Pan troglodytes schweinfurthi*), or the south bank (if the ancestral virus turned up in the pygmy chimp, *Pan paniscus*).

With respect to this issue, an interesting article was published in 1994 by a team from Robert Gallo's lab, who reported finding a new retrovirus (a Simian T-Cell Lymphotropic Virus or STLV) in the pygmy chimpanzee.[35] The authors claimed that the antibody pattern on Western blot was "identical" to the indeterminate HTLV-1 and HTLV-2 antibody-positivity that had been described in pygmy tribes such as the Bambuti and the Bakola. The discussion section claimed that these ancient tribes and the pygmy chimps had "lived in a common habitat for thousands of years," and proposed that the virus might have passed from pygmy chimps to pygmies through hunting practices. The claim was a strange one, for the Bambuti live in northeastern Zaire, and the Bakola in Cameroon, both of which are separated from the habitat of *Pan paniscus* by several hundred miles — and by the Congo River, which has been an effective barrier to nonhuman primates for at least eleven thousand years, but probably much longer. There is no evidence of pygmy peoples on the south bank of the river; pygmies and pygmy chimps can therefore hardly be said to share "a common habitat." At the end of the article, Hilary Koprowski is thanked "for helpful discussion."

In the conclusion of this paper, the proposition that the pygmy chimp virus might have transferred horizontally to humans through hunting and butchery was likened to the transfer of SIV to humans to produce HIV-2. What the authors did not mention, but what they may have been implying, was that their model would be all the more appropriate if it was ever discovered that pygmy chimps were carriers of an SIV that was closely related to HIV-1 in humans.

However, a later paper by a Belgian team about the same pygmy chimp retrovirus came to very different conclusions. Unlike Gallo's group, the authors had sequenced the virus, and discovered that it was "not closely related to the African pygmy virus."[36] Of course, this also served to undermine the Gallo group's theory of horizontal retroviral transfer occurring as a result of the hypothetical hunting of pygmy chimps by pygmies. The main difference between the PIVs and the PTLVs, the Belgian team highlighted, was the evolutionary time scale, for whereas HIV and SIV had diverged in the space of "centuries," the PTLVs had diverged over "tens of thousands of years."

No SIV has yet been found in the pygmy chimp, though as far as I know very few animals have been sampled. My own guess, however, is that when blood is sampled from the groups among which Gilbert Rollais conducted his captures (from common chimps living in the rain forest to the north and east of Kisangani, and from pygmy chimps inhabiting the forest to the south and west), a variant of SIV will be found that will group very closely with the early HIV-1 Group M viruses like ZR59. To my knowledge, no chimp from this area has yet been sampled for the presence of SIV.

———

When one asks scientists who were not directly involved with CHAT vaccine how they think it was made, most of those who have looked into the affair (at least the open-minded ones) admit that there is no hard evidence as to which kidneys were used. As detailed above, Albert Sabin claimed at the last that CHAT was prepared in rhesus kidneys, but without explaining how he knew that. By contrast, in the course of seven years of investigations into OPV/AIDS I have come across five specialists in virology, vaccine-making, or both — two Belgians, two Americans, and one Briton — who believe that the tissues of African primates, including chimpanzees, have been involved.

The first two such specialists are the former Stanleyville vets, Joseph Mortelmans and Louis Bugyaki. The latter specifically recalled being told by colleagues at the Stanleyville medical lab that chimp kidneys had been sent to both the United States and Belgium. The third specialist was Stewart Aston, the Lederle lab man, who, when he learned that Tom Norton's widow had said that Tom had brought back chimp kidneys that had been delivered to the Wistar, responded that in his opinion they must have been used for growing CHAT.[37]

The fourth and fifth men have to remain anonymous. One is a famous English scientist who was involved with the manufacture of polio vaccines from 1955 onward. The institution where he worked had used rhesus and cynomolgus macaques for both safety testing and tissue culture, and in the early days they were all kept in one big cage, which often contained as many as fifty monkeys at one time. He frankly admitted to me that the dangers of cross-species viral transfer had simply not been realized, but said that soon after his arrival the establishment in question changed to a policy of two to a cage and one month's quarantine before use.

We talked about the species that had been used by other polio manufacturers, and when I asked him about Koprowski, he told me that back in the fifties, "there was a question of using kidneys from Africa which came up." So, I asked, was he saying that Koprowski had used the kidneys of African monkeys to make his vaccines? "Oh, I think so, yes," he responded immediately. "I thought it was fairly well known that he was using African monkeys." He asked me whether it was not recorded anywhere, and I told him that nothing had been written in the literature, and that the relevant papers and protocols appeared to have been lost during a move. He roared with laughter. Later, he pointed out that Koprowski had had close links with Gear in South Africa, and that the South Africans had been using vervet monkeys at the time. "He might have [gone] there to get them," he offered. I pointed out that most of Koprowski's research had been conducted in central Africa, not South Africa, but he merely repeated that "the South African virologists would have known what was going on."

This, of course, was why I had written to James Gear in 1993. He, however, had sidestepped the question, suggesting: "Perhaps you should write to Dr Koprowski himself in regard to the answer of these questions," before forwarding a copy of my letter to Koprowski, almost scuppering my interview with him in the process. In reply to a further letter, Gear wrote: "Whether Koprowski's vaccines were contaminated . . . would only be confirmed when the virus is isolated or its presence shown in them."

My British informant was most insistent that his remarks about Koprowski's vaccines should not be attributed to him by name. So was the American virologist I spoke with, who in 1995 was a senior scientist at the CDC. He too was frank, not only about Koprowski, but about other contentious issues, such as the testing of live vaccines against HIV. He summarized the ethical issue as follows: "Is there a case for trying a live AIDS vaccine in a population in which 90 percent will die from it anyway?" He was also very gung-ho about the issue of xenotransplantation, for instance of baboon livers in AIDS patients. It was clear that here was a man who believed, like Ronald Desrosiers, that scientific advances required bold steps and an element of risk-taking.

When we turned to the OPV theory, he volunteered that the only way it would work was if chimp kidneys had been used to make the vaccine. At that moment, my tape recorder clicked off, and he expressed relief, even though I continued taking notes. "Maybe it is not so far-fetched — that the vaccine was made in chimp kidney," he went on. "They were certainly making the vaccine with [monkey] kidneys: no doubt about that. And if they found a chimp, I don't think they would be too discriminating about using that kind of kidney." I asked him if he was sure about that, that Koprowski's team had been making the vaccine from monkey kidneys out in Africa. "I think that's what they were doing over there," he replied. Later on, he added: "It was my understanding they were using African green monkey, not chimpanzee. On the other hand, the chimp kidney is a frightful theory."

We talked about the possibility of acquiring infection through the mouth. "If you take stock HIV-1 and gargle with it, you can get infected," he said, thus conceding that infection could take place through the oral mucosa. So, I asked, if chimp kidneys had been used, then the theory would be viable? "Is this off the record?" he checked. I told him it was. "If chimp kidneys were used, of course they [vaccinees] could get infected," he said.

At the end, we argued about whether or not it was important to write about the theory. I said that if this was actually what had happened, then surely it was vital to bring the full story out into the open, thereby lessening the risks of similar unintentional catastrophes in the future. He disagreed. "No. If the theory's correct, it would make the U.S. responsible for the AIDS epidemic, and [we would] possibly have to go and take care of those people over there with AIDS." He had got up to escort me out, but I was still scribbling his words down in my notebook. "You can keep this inflamed, and you can keep waving it, but I'm not sure that you're going to get anywhere with it," he went on. As we walked toward the door, he added that if I quoted him on any of this, he would simply deny he had said it.

When we shook hands, I pressed him one more time, saying that if the OPV/AIDS theory had merit, then surely it was vital that the truth came out. "I don't know if truth in itself has merit," he answered. "I think that truth which makes a contribution has merit."[38]

---

What I found stunning about this interview was that, for the first time, an eminent scientist was saying that he thought Koprowski had been making vaccine from the kidneys of African primates, and that if (as seemed possible) chimpanzees had been involved, then this could indeed have led to the birth of AIDS. And yet his response to this was — what good will it do to rock the boat?

Is he correct? Should embarrassing mistakes be buried underground and not brought to the public's attention, lest their revelation cause avoidable controversy and huge compensation claims? Does blowing the whistle only serve to inflame the situation?

On one level, what he says is right. Revelations about the events surrounding the CHAT trials in central Africa are almost bound to cause controversy and anger — especially among people with AIDS, among Africans, and, indeed, among all those who were used as experimental subjects back in the fifties. The latter category embraces not only colonial subjects, but also prisoners, handicapped children, and inner-city indigents.

And yet on most other levels, I think that the CDC professor is deeply wrong. And I believe that the majority of people, whether scientists or members of the general public, will — like me — feel horrified by the cynicism and self-interest inherent in his words.

One example of a man who believes that scientific controversy should not be brushed under the carpet is the venerable virologist Joseph Melnick, who remained above the fray during the fifties, and who continues to do so today. In interview, he makes it clear that he has many reservations about the OPV/AIDS theory; nonetheless, he vigorously defends the right of scientists (and others) to propound such hypotheses — and insists that the relevant vaccine samples should be tested for possible SIV contamination.[39]

In the affidavit that he submitted in opposition to the defamation suit brought by Koprowski against the publishers of *Rolling Stone,* Melnick wrote the following: "I am deeply concerned that the mere reporting on a scientific theory by Mr. Curtis . . . could become the subject of a libel suit. How AIDS originated is a presently unanswerable question, and there are many theories, all of which have strengths and weaknesses, all of which have supporters and detractors. The appropriate forum to debate and test those theories is the laboratory environs, not the courtroom. Indeed, I am troubled that if this libel suit were allowed to proceed, then any researcher or scientist could be subjected to litigation simply by setting forth a theory that was unpopular, or that might later be proven to be incorrect."[40]

Melnick has hit the nail fair and true. It is essential that the tradition of discussion and dissent in science — the right of free speech — should not be curtailed.

So let us look for a moment at what has happened to those who have dared to question the safety of Koprowski's vaccine. According to Blaine Elswood, some publishers were afraid to print Tom Curtis's articles because, after the court case, he was viewed as someone who attracted litigation.[41] Louis Pascal, after fighting valiantly to get his words and ideas into print for eight long years, has not been heard from since 1995. For myself, I have already been threatened with litigation by a lawyer representing Koprowski and Plotkin, even before this book is published.

I say shame on them, for trying to conduct their science through the courts. They have had several years now in which to produce some evidence to show that the OPV/AIDS hypothesis is misguided, or to demonstrate that the CHAT trials did not lead to the arrival of HIV-1 in humans. Instead, they say the documentary evidence has gone missing, and they have repeatedly shied away from testing any remaining sample of CHAT. As for the arguments they have advanced against the hypothesis, most of these have been either flimsy, or flawed, or misleading.

Let them come up with some material or documentary evidence that demonstrates that this theory is wrong, and I shall be happy to acknowledge that fact. Otherwise I, for one, will continue to believe that they are wrong, and I shall continue to feel free to write about the hypothesis.

# 58

WHEN THE LEVEE BREAKS

The band plays, and the river flows on. In the Western world, at least, there are signs that the flood is abating, that AIDS is on the retreat. The number of AIDS deaths in the United States fell for the first time in 1996, largely as a result of the new combination therapy championed by David Ho and others.[1] With this first glimmer of hope, there could surely be no more appropriate time to look seriously, once again, at the origins of this terrible disease.

However, physicians and epidemiologists emphasize that there are no grounds for complacency. The new therapies are available only to the wealthy. Furthermore, they do not constitute a cure, in that tiny amounts of dormant HIV remain in the bloodstream. If patients cannot tolerate, or remember to take, the precisely regulated regime of pills (and in practice many reject or forget them), then HIV swiftly reemerges in pathogenic form. Even worse, in early 1999 it was revealed that "up to 30 percent of Americans newly infected with HIV now carry a strain resistant to the new drug therapies."[2]

In the U.S., AIDS is now spreading faster among women than men, and new HIV infections continue apace, especially in the inner cities.[3] This suggests that in the industrialized world the virus is moving from its original target group, gay men, to the general population, especially its poor and disadvantaged members. However, a new complacency among some gay men who reject safe sex practices may presage a resurgence of the virus among that group.[4]

Elsewhere in the world, in some of the earliest infected countries like the Congo and Uganda, levels of HIV infection seem to have plateaued, and even to be falling, largely because so many of those at risk have already become infected.[5] The new amplification area of Africa is the south, where the highly transmissible subtype C has become established. In the late eighties, HIV was almost unknown in the Botswana conurbation of Francistown; by the late nineties, nearly half of its pregnant women were seropositive.[6] As the millennium ends, more than two-thirds of all those living with HIV and AIDS are still from sub-Saharan Africa.[7]

Yet it is in previously pristine regions like Asia, Latin America, and the old Soviet bloc that HIV and AIDS are nowadays making their most dramatic inroads, and where the worst of the epidemic will eventually be seen, if only because of the larger populations at risk. As early as 1994, India had more HIV-positive people than any other country on earth.[8]

By the end of 1998, an estimated 47.3 million people had become infected with HIV since the start of the epidemic, of whom 13.9 million had already died of AIDS.[9] By the millennium, the cumulative figures are likely to be approaching 55 million people infected with HIV, with over 16 million AIDS deaths. In the first day of the year 2000, roughly 15,000 people around the planet are expected to become infected with HIV.

Some point out that globally, more people die each year of other illnesses such as acute respiratory infections, malaria, and diarrheal diseases. For the moment, this is true, but whereas the worldwide death rates for those conditions remain fairly stable, those for AIDS keep on rising. Furthermore, AIDS is a slow disaster, and although its effects are less immediately dramatic, on a day-to-day scale, than the influenza epidemic of 1918, or the Black Death, its long-term impact will be far, far greater. This is because such a large proportion of those with AIDS are adults in the prime of life, in their reproductive years, while so many others are babies and young children. This results in a top-heavy population pyramid, where the only group minimally affected (at least for HIV-1-related AIDS) is the elderly. Even worse, for every person with AIDS in the developing world, another five to ten are effectively tied up tending to them. The overall impact on the health of the community is massive. The future social and economic impact of the AIDS pandemic is almost too huge to calculate.

The AIDS epidemic has undoubtedly been the major public health disaster of the twentieth century, and — some maintain — it is already the greatest of all time. As I write, in 1999, virtually 1 percent of humanity is infected with the virus. In years to come, that figure could rise to 5 percent. Julian Cribb, in *The White Death*, points out that some researchers claim that a billion people could be infected by the year 2050.[10]

Despite the advances being made with therapies for the already HIV-infected, there can be little doubt that a safe vaccine represents the ultimate solution to the problem of AIDS. But one of the greatest concerns is that new and more transmissible variants of HIV will evolve, leaving medical science forever chasing shadows, developing vaccines that will not prove effective against every version of the virus. There are also real doubts about the safety of some of the candidate strains, especially the live attenuated versions.

Vaccines are one of the greatest triumphs of medical science — some would say the greatest. Every year they save the lives of tens of millions of humans and hundreds of millions of animals. The vast majority of vaccines are safe, and have been proven so over the course of many years. And perhaps the brightest jewel in the crown is the polio vaccine.

The race to conquer poliomyelitis and develop a vaccine was a wonderful, imaginative, and heroic scientific enterprise. Those fumbling beginnings back in the dawn of virology led directly to the situation we have today, where the breaking of the chain of wild poliovirus transmission is a realistic goal for the near future. Already the virus has been eradicated from the Americas,[11] and only one case was reported from Europe in 1997.[12] Ironically, because the recent political upheavals have interrupted polio vaccination initiatives, the Congo is now one of the strongholds of the virus.[13] However, it is now almost certain that once "National Immunization Days" are staged there and in other vulnerable countries, poliomyelitis will become the second viral disease — after smallpox — to be eradicated from the human race through medical intervention.

This will be a magnificent achievement, for which the great pioneers of tissue culture development and polio research, such as John Enders, Renato Dulbecco, Joseph Melnick, David Bodian, Jonas Salk, Sven Gard, Albert Sabin, Herald Cox, and Hilary Koprowski deserve enormous credit.

On the other hand, it is important not to forget that one key aspect of the great leap forward in polio vaccine development was intrinsically flawed. It is now clear that some of the early tissue cultures used to develop vaccines were contaminated with simian viruses, and that virologists had little true idea of the potential magnitude of the risks they were taking in the name of medical progress.[14] Put simply, there were not enough checks and balances in place during the fifties to ensure that a live vaccine prepared from monkey kidneys was safe and free from viral surprises.

To look through some of the early reports about the standardization of polio vaccine manufacture is a truly sobering experience. In 1960, the WHO Expert Committee on Poliomyelitis, in its third report, observes that rhesus and cynomolgus macaques and African green monkeys are generally used for primary tissue culture, though "other species may also be found to be suitable." There are, in other words, no stipulations as to species in these recommendations.[15]

It is only in 1962 that an additional line enters the requirements for OPV. Now it is explained that "[m]onkeys of a suitable species, in good health, and which have not previously been used for experimental purposes of significance to the safety of the vaccine, shall be used as the source of kidney tissue for the production of seed virus and vaccine."[16] One wonders what prompted this new stipulation — and whether, prior to 1962, certain vaccine lots were prepared in the kidneys of monkeys that had previously been used for other experiments — ones that did not leave residual poliovirus in the kidney. An example would be polio vaccine safety tests, and vaccination and challenge tests, such as those conducted at Lindi.

The annual proceedings of the International Congress of Microbiological Standardization are also something of an eye-opener. In 1960, when recommendations for the manufacture of OPV are published for the first time, it is stipulated that "only monkey kidney tissue cultures may be used," but there is no reference to the species.[17] (These recommendations applied only to the Sabin strains, which were licensed for the first time that year. All the OPVs made before that, whether by Sabin, Cox, or Koprowski, were deemed to be experimental strains, and there were no legal requirements that applied to their manufacture.)

Another address at the same conference begins with a startling admission about the conditions under which the monkeys used for MKTC were housed and transported in the years before 1960. "In the early days of large scale vaccine production from monkey kidney tissue culture," comments Dr. C. L. Greening from the United Kingdom, "increasing world-wide demands for monkeys resulted in indiscriminate purchase from uninspected and often totally unsuitable animal centres. Minimum attention was given to transport conditions in aircraft or ships, and it was common practice to house stock monkeys at laboratories or animal farms . . . in large cages holding upwards of 150 animals."[18]

At the following year's conference, the president candidly admits in his opening address: "It seems astonishing in retrospect that the need for biological standardization was not earlier recognized. . . ."[19]

---

So what harm, if any, was done by this rather belated application of proper manufacturing standards to the process of polio vaccine production? For years it appeared that the SV40 slip-up was not going to prove serious for humans, but in 1994 we learned otherwise. Michele Carbone and colleagues demonstrated that this adventitious virus, which had been present in tens of millions of doses of the early generation IPVs and OPVs,[20] was being found in tumor tissue from people with pleural mesothelioma.[21] This is a pulmonary cancer that has now reached epidemic proportions among construction workers, and is expected to have killed 80,000 Americans by the year 2015.[22] The etiology is not yet proven, but it now seems very possible that many mesothelioma sufferers have experienced a two-stage process: SV40 exposure (presumably through polio vaccines between 1955 and 1961), and exposure to asbestos thereafter.

Sadly, of course, the SV40 story is not the only instance in which the inadequacy of past scientific knowledge can be linked to the later incidence of disease, or even the unintentional creation of a novel disease. One example from the animal kingdom is canine parvovirus (CPV), which suddenly emerged as a new disease of dogs in 1977, and within two years had spread across the six continents. Genetically, CPV is very close to a live vaccine that was developed in the seventies against feline panleukopenia virus (FPLV), which causes disease in cats.[23] Many virologists now believe that CPV evolved "in the course of deliberate or accidental adaptation of FPLV strains to replicate in canine cells," during the development of the live vaccine.[24]

Another example, even better known, was the deliberate introduction of the myxoma virus of the South American forest rabbit into the European rabbit population of Australia. In the forest rabbit, the virus causes minor illness, but in the European rabbit it proved lethal, killing 99.8 percent in the first wave after its introduction. The impact on the Australian ecosystem was far more dramatic than had been anticipated when government scientists approved the experiment in a bid to control soil erosion — and attempts were later made to reduce the pathogenicity of myxoma virus by genetic engineering.

Other examples of the accidental creation of new diseases involve zoonoses, the transfer of animal diseases to humans. The most notorious of recent years involves a double species jump — the inadvertent (some might say careless) transfer of scrapie from sheep to cows, creating "Mad Cow Disease" (bovine spongiform encephalopathy, or BSE),[25] and then the inadvertent transfer of BSE from cows to humans, creating new variant Creutzfeldt-Jakob disease (v-CJD) or "human BSE" as it is now being called.[26] The first step involved the feeding of ground-up body parts of scrapie-infected sheep to unsuspecting cattle, and the second the feeding of ground-up bits of cattle, in the form of hamburgers, meatballs, and pies, to unsuspecting humans. The latest alarming development in this story is the possibility that v-CJD may be capable of spreading from human to human through blood transfusion.[27] This is all the more worrying because not until the end of 1997 was a test developed to recognize the presence of the causative agent in asymptomatic infectees.[28]

Another candidate for an iatrogenic disaster, though not yet confirmed, is "Gulf War syndrome." Scientific opinion is presently divided as to whether this syndrome is the result of exposure to Iraqi biological and chemical weapons, a hyperimmune reaction to the cocktail of vaccines and antitoxins many Allied combatants were obliged to take, exposure to organophosphate insecticides, exposure to depleted uranium in artillery shells, or some combination of the above. However, increasing evidence is emerging that the Allied use of vaccines — including experimental ones — was excessive. One combatant claims to have had eighteen inoculations (some of which were unrecorded or secret) in the space of three days, and it has been revealed that an official warning about the risks of multiple vaccinations was ignored by the British Ministry of Defence.[29] The United States has belatedly called a presidential inquiry, but the British government has spent several years denying the existence of the syndrome.[30] These official responses, characterized by delay and denial, are further depressing reminders about the reluctance of those in authority to acknowledge responsibility for their own mistakes — especially the more dangerous and politically damaging ones.[31]

The examples above involve unintended scientific blunders — occasions when someone miscalculated and the effects were noticeable enough to be documented years later. But not all such episodes were the result of blunders. From the end of the Second World War until the late sixties, the general perception was that the scientist held the keys to the kingdom, and that the scientist's knowledge and wisdom could provide all the answers. If someone in a white coat decided that a test should go ahead, then go ahead it must.

This, therefore, was the era when anthrax bombs could be dropped over Scottish islands,[32] when U.S. army scientists could break lightbulbs filled with "harmless" bacteria on the New York subway,[33] when prisoners could be paid to have their testicles irradiated,[34] when unsuspecting hospital patients could be injected with plutonium,[35] and when more than two hundred underground nuclear tests could be staged secretly in the United States[36] — together with another 250 experiments in which radiation was deliberately released into the atmosphere.[37] The period between the forties and the early sixties was one of Cold War–driven paranoia, when government officials and scientific experts were considered the final arbiters of ethical as well as logistical conundrums. In times such as these, times of ordinary madness,[38] it was but a small matter to stage a vaccine trial in a faraway place, without the process having to be approved by any but the colonial government in charge, and without any checks and balances to ensure the safety of the participants.

---

The river glistens, and moves onward to the sea. Sometimes, in the throbbing heat, one cannot be sure what is real and what is not. Away on the northern shore, for instance, the light flashes on two shiny objects among the trees — perhaps the roofs of warehouses, perhaps some strange encampment in the bush. The place is full of mysteries such as these, but as one slides past in the haze they slip easily from the mind.

Because of the lack of documentation, many of the details of the research conducted at Lindi camp are not known, although sometimes glimpses are caught through the trees. We do know, however, that the second part of the project, that of opening a chimpanzee breeding farm in the Congo to provide animals for scientific research, was well into the planning stage before the political situation after independence caused its abandonment.[39] We can only guess at the experiments that might have been conducted on the chimp population, although we do have some clues, because the United States instead decided to set up a breeding colony on home soil — at Holloman Air Force Base in New Mexico.

By 1966 there were 160 chimpanzees in the Holloman colony — a population approaching that of Lindi at its height, in 1957. Many of the experiments conducted there were related to air force projects, including the training of chimpanzees Ham and Enos for the first space flights in 1961. Other research was conducted into pressurized environments (simulating deep sea diving), and retinal burns (presumably simulating exposure to atomic blasts).[40] Further work was conducted in collaboration with civilian scientists, and prominent among the experiments were attempts at transplanting chimpanzee kidneys into humans. This xenotransplantation research was pioneered by Keith Reemstma and Tom Starzl, who independently staged a total of nineteen experiments between 1963 and 1965.[41] The most successful kidney recipient survived for nine months after the transplant, and even briefly returned to her job as a teacher.

What is horrifying about this information is that we now know that at least one SIV-infected chimp arrived at Holloman in 1963 — this being Marilyn, from whom SIV was isolated and sequenced by Beatrice Hahn's team some thirty years later.[42] Since many of the chimps were allowed to play together in a thirty-acre "Consortium" across from the main laboratory, it is certainly possible that this SIV-positive chimp could have cross-infected others during the years that followed, including some of those providing kidneys for the human grafts.

As far as we know, all of the human recipients eventually died of kidney failure, but what if one of them had actually become infected with SIVcpz, and had gone on to infect his or her spouse with a human-adapted version of the virus? It is clear that this episode, just like Voronoff's chimp testicle grafts of the twenties,[43] and the injections of chimp blood by malaria researchers like Blacklock, Adler, and Rodhain between the thirties and fifties,[44] *could* have started the AIDS epidemic there and then. That they apparently did not must be judged "a close shave" — just as Hans Wigzell later described the OPV/AIDS theory.

However, the risks did not end in the sixties, for organ grafts from primates to humans have continued ever since. In 1964, the first attempt was made to transplant a chimpanzee heart into a human — an experiment extended by Christiaan Barnard in 1977, when he used hearts from a baboon and a chimp as temporary backups for patients whose human heart transplants had failed. The most famous recipient was Baby Fae, who survived just twenty days with a baboon heart in 1984.[45]

Later, in 1992, Tom Starzl resumed his research, this time transplanting baboon livers into humans.[46] His greatest success was a patient who survived for two months before succumbing to opportunistic infections brought on by the massive doses of immunosuppressive drugs administered to prevent organ rejection.[47]

Of course, such immunosuppressive drugs also served to minimize the resistance the transplant recipients mounted against the primate viruses that were undoubtedly present in the donated organs. Alarmingly, researchers at the Southwest Foundation for Biomedical Research, who supplied Starzl's baboon in 1992, were apparently not informed that the animal was to be used for xenotransplantation; the baboon is known to have been infected with three viruses, and may have been host to others not yet discovered. Starzl says he will do "whatever it takes to stop people dying," but Jonathan Allan, the Southwest microbiologist who testified for Koprowski in the *Rolling Stone* defamation case, is scared by the implications of such ventures across the species barrier. "Starzl may say that he sees no real ethical issues here. . . . But if you don't see them, then you're the wrong person to be making the decisions," he says.[48] Of particular concern is the fact that placing a primate organ inside an immunosuppressed human is probably the perfect way to encourage a monkey virus to jump species.

In 1995, there was a new departure when an AIDS patient from California, Jeff Getty, was given a bone marrow transplant from a baboon in a last-ditch attempt to save his life.[49] Although the transplant failed and though the baboon cells quickly died, Mr. Getty's health improved (as a result, he believes, of the radiation treatment he received at the time of the transplant), and he was soon able to resume his hobbies of sailing and weight training.[50] However happy one may feel for Jeff Getty, many believe that this story represents an alarming development within the context of zoonoses. For although Getty apparently signed a form pledging to refrain from sexual relationships or sharing eating utensils with others, there is still a very real possibility that he — or more likely another recipient of baboon cells — might unwittingly infect other persons with a human-adapted baboon virus. Such a virus might prove to be slow acting (like HIV), or highly virulent (like Ebola); it might be nontransmissible among humans, or it might prove to be highly infectious. As more and more xenotransplants from primates are attempted, the likelihood increases that undetected simian viruses or prions will be given a means to become established in the human species.

A 1995 discussion paper on xenotransplantation by CDC and FDA scientists concluded: "In this new field . . . what constitutes an acceptable risk in the balance between caution and progress is a matter of public concern, not merely a private matter for individual scientists, physicians and patients to decide." The same paper admits that it is hard to eliminate the risk of viral spread, and that "Once there is a problem in the general population, public health measures can decrease, but not eliminate that risk."[51] The calm, rational tone helps disguise the fact that fingers, once again, are running along the lid of a box of furies.

A new approach to the shortage of donor organs has involved breeding trans-genic pigs from embryonic cells into which human genes have been introduced. This reduces the risk of rejection when the pigs' livers are transplanted into humans. This was greeted by some as a welcome development, because pigs and humans are far removed on the evolutionary scale, making cross-species viral transfer less likely.[52] In 1997, however, it was discovered that pigs can carry at least two retroviruses, both capable of growing in human cells. The vice-president of research and development at one of the U.S. companies pioneering human clinical trials acknowledged that the pig livers were likely to contain these retroviruses, but commented: "If we stopped and worried about everything which could go wrong in medical experiments we'd never achieve anything."[53]

Xenotransplantation is clearly an issue of such momentous importance that it demands a great deal more open discussion and open research (conducted in a closed environment) before any further experiments are mounted in humans.[54] The potential benefits to those thousands of people awaiting transplants are huge — but so are the risks, and the risks may apply not just to donor recipients, but to the species as a whole. Lifetime monitoring of organ recipients is simply not enough — especially when nobody really knows what to monitor, or how to interpret the findings.[55]

Otherwise, if we allow xenotransplantation to become an established prac-tice by default, it may be our children and grandchildren who will be faced with the futile task of trying to shove the genie back in the bottle.

---

As that old sage Heraclitus pointed out, some 2,500 years ago: "You can't step twice into the same river." Every moment there are new points of contact between humans and the world around them, some of which hold immense hope for the future, some of which are fraught with the potential for disaster. And sometimes the light dims, and the boundaries between the two begin to blur.

In September 1997, a group of American scientists announced, amid con-siderable publicity, that they had pledged themselves as volunteers for human trials of Ronald Desrosiers's live AIDS vaccine. In all, fifty members of the International Association of Physicians in AIDS Care (IAPAC) offered them-selves as guinea pigs. The group's executive director, Gordon Nary, explained: "We cannot sit around for 16 years and continue to debate how quickly we can do trials." His deputy director, Jose Zuniga, added: "We are not calling for a trial tomorrow, or even the next day. [But] bold steps should be taken while observ-ing good science." Another group member admitted: "Of course I'm scared. I think that any volunteer would be scared."[56]

I was scared too. I phoned Ruth Ruprecht, who told me: "It's unsafe. These types of vaccine are unsafe." She added that her team had been testing one of

Desrosiers's strains, SIVΔ3 (a macaque SIV with three deletions, these being of the *nef* and *vpr* genes, and a sequence from the LTR, or long terminal repeat). Of the ten infant macaques to which they had given the multiply-deleted virus, nine had now become diseased, of which five had developed simian AIDS. Worse still, two adult macaques given SIVΔ3 had also developed disease, one of which had gotten full-blown AIDS. In Ruprecht's hands, neither the *nef*-deleted nor the triple-deleted SIVs developed by Desrosiers had proved to be properly attenuated either for infant or adult monkeys.[57]

That call by the IAPAC deputy director for the taking of "bold steps" reminded me of Desrosiers's response to my letter, in which he had avoided answering any of my questions, but had included a batch of articles, among them one that featured the following homily: "Those who would oppose freedom in the conduct of science are always with us, and we should ever be on our guard in defending the right to probe the unknown. . . ."[58]

To my mind, what was at stake here was not "the right to probe the unknown," but the question of acceptable and unacceptable risks. In October 1998, at the fourth time of asking (and as this book was in the final stages of editing), I finally got to interview Professor Ronald Desrosiers. He turned out to be mustachioed, energetic, and committed, and considerably less frightening than he sometimes appeared in his public relations forays on television.[59] I got the impression that he was now adopting more of a softly, softly approach; whether or not this was a conscious device I could not tell, but it was certainly very welcome.

To get it out of the way, I decided to ask Desrosiers about the Wistar CHAT sample at the start of the meeting. He had never been delegated to organize the testing, he said; he had merely made some phone calls to see whether anybody was prepared to carry it out. He commented that it "would be a pretty awesome responsibility" to test the sample, and added: "There may have been some difficulties identifying the particular lots in question . . . if Koprowski doesn't remember, how would we be expected to work it out?" Later, when I asked whether the CHAT sample could not usefully be tested to determine the mitochondrial DNA of the host, he refused to be drawn. He told me that Koprowski had never actually appeared before the Wistar committee, although he had spoken privately to Frank Lilly. The committee, he added, had only had a couple of meetings in New York. Later, he changed this to "two, three, four meetings . . . it wasn't a lot."

When we started talking about live attenuated AIDS vaccines, Desrosiers stressed, from the outset, that the key factor had to be safety. He told me that his group had now developed two new multiply-deleted variants of SIV, called Δ3X and Δ4. The latter had had three of the virus's nine genes deleted, together with a sequence from the LTR. Desrosiers said that he considered both mutants to be "highly attenuated," and added that — in his opinion — they struck an appropriate balance between safety and efficacy.[60] He believed that similar deletions could produce an attenuated version of HIV.[61]

All this sounded encouraging, but then Ruth Ruprecht's name was mentioned, and he became visibly upset and defensive.[62] He was openly skeptical about the fact that almost all of her monkeys that had received either the SIVΔnef and SIVΔ3 strains (strains that, he said, he himself had given her) seemed to have fallen sick or died from simian AIDS. These results, he stressed, were very different from those that his own team was encountering. However, when I pressed for details of his own results with these, his first two attenuated strains, he revealed that in his own Δnef trials, three out of seventeen macaques had developed high viral loads of SIV, and/or had developed simian AIDS within 5.1 years, and that the same had happened to five of sixty macaques given the Δ3 strain, and followed for 3.2 years. (In other words, he too had experienced reversions, and it appeared that the difference between his results and Ruprecht's was merely one of scale.)

He said that, by contrast, they had had no problem cases with either macaques given SIVΔ3X, and ten monkeys given SIVΔ4, and monitored for a mean of 2.8 years — which suggested that his new variants might be safer.

We moved on to the question of vaccine trials, and Desrosiers told me that within the next year or two he hoped to initiate large-scale safety trials of his latest attenuated vaccine in two hundred or three hundred rhesus macaques (he had just submitted the funding proposal earlier that week). If these were successful, he said, there might be a willingness in the scientific community to proceed to the first very limited trials in humans — perhaps in cancer patient volunteers with only a year or so to live. If there were no adverse indications, they could then move on to testing ten, twenty, or fifty people — perhaps physician volunteers, like those from IAPAC — and if that went well, they could eventually proceed to a large-scale field trial, involving 10,000 or so people living in a high-risk area. (He suggested Uganda or southern Africa as possible venues.) He emphasized that a realistic timescale for the latter trial would be after they had accumulated "ten, twelve, fifteen years" of data, but said that the sooner the large-scale monkey trial could be staged, the sooner they could move forward to a large-scale trial in humans.

He stressed that his live vaccine should be one that was kept in the wings, as a supporting act that would only need to be brought on if all the leading players fell out of contention. But it was clear that he felt that none of the other candidate AIDS vaccines had very much chance of success. The present situation, he said, was that "a complex set of social factors [is] going to influence what happens. . . . There is no company with enough money to back live attenuated [vaccines]; it's just too risky. . . . Part of what IAPAC is trying to do is champion the unchampioned approaches — which eventually may have an enormous impact for the developing world."

At this point, we started discussing what could happen if a field trial of a live AIDS vaccine were to go wrong. Desrosiers was quite frank about the risks, and admitted that the worst-case scenario would be if the vaccine began to revert to virulence (and therefore give people AIDS) after thirty or so years. But, he felt, if this was to happen, then the first cases would emerge much earlier (after ten or fifteen years, for instance), with the implication being that this would allow enough time for the large-scale field trials to be halted.

This sounded eminently reasonable, although there did seem to be an inconsistency in his proposed timetable. He had told me that he envisioned staging those human field trials in ten to fifteen years' time. However, by then his group would only have been able to monitor human vaccinees with normal life expectancy (such as the IAPAC volunteers) for between five and ten years. What if one of those volunteers suddenly suffered a decline in CD4 count, and developed AIDS, some twelve or fifteen years after being vaccinated? It seemed to me that by that time, several hundred thousand (and perhaps several million) people around the world might have received a live AIDS vaccine that was capable of reversion.

Near the end of our conversation, as he was giving me a lift back into Boston, I asked Desrosiers whether he was concerned that a government under huge political pressure from a large and vociferous HIV-positive lobby (perhaps an African or Asian government) might be tempted to take his live AIDS vaccine and release it early — before those slow, careful, step-by-step safety tests had been carried out, before scientists could be really confident that it was safe. After all, a live vaccine is just that, and can be harvested from the body of the vaccinee (as others had demonstrated with OPV). Desrosiers had to admit that he would not be able to prevent such a development, but he was still gung-ho, and confident that good sense would prevail. Besides, he said reassuringly, he could not see the vaccine being given to the whole world within his lifetime.

---

As we approach the end of the century, there are several much safer candidate vaccines against AIDS — such as inactivated vaccines and subunit vaccines — that are either already in human trials, or awaiting final clearance. Just as IPV was less efficacious than OPV (yet probably safer, once the early gremlins had been removed), so these other candidate vaccines may prove to be less efficacious than their live cousins, but also far less risky.

In the mid-nineties, Phase 1 safety trials of certain of these candidate vaccines began in Brazil, Thailand, and Uganda, involving volunteers from high-risk groups, such as gay men, intravenous drug users, and military recruits. Clearly participants could not be deliberately exposed to HIV, so now the scientists are waiting "to see what unfolds in the natural course of things — who becomes infected and who does not."[63] It will be several years before there are meaningful results to analyze.

Richard Marlink, executive director of the Harvard AIDS Institute, is one of the more prominent scientists who are calling for a start to be made on AIDS vaccine trials in the United States. In 1994, the National Institutes of Health halted planned trials of genetically engineered vaccines based on HIV's envelope gene, gp120 — an event linked to a preliminary vaccine trial in which five participants became HIV-positive, despite receiving the vaccine.[64] Vaccine initiatives worldwide promptly ground to a halt,[65] with one of these few institutions not to shelve its plans being Plotkin's Pasteur Mérieux.[66] Many scientists felt that the events of that year represented a disaster, in that vaccine development had been "set back a decade."[67] In 1997, Marlink commented: "Had the first generation of AIDS vaccines been approved, human trials could have begun in 1994, costing some $20 million annually over three years. And had the vaccines worked in people, the expense of the trials could have been recouped by the first 500 cases of AIDS prevented."[68]

He, too, likens the story of AIDS vaccines to that of polio vaccines back in the fifties. He points out that in 1955, when the Salk vaccine was licensed, it was far from being a perfect solution to the polio problem, but for all that the rate of paralysis was found to be 72 percent lower in vaccinated than in unvaccinated children. In the seven years following 1955, thousands of children who would otherwise have contracted polio were instead protected, and Salk's preparation thus provided an invaluable stopgap until a better vaccine, Sabin's OPV, was approved in 1962. The lesson, Marlink believes, is this: "Do not let a better vaccine of the future preclude a potentially life-saving one now."

This book is not a proper place for a discussion of the merits and demerits of the group of AIDS vaccines currently under trial in humans. Nonetheless, there is good evidence to suggest that several of the candidate strains (such as those based on protein subunits and synthetic peptides) are safe. The doubts surround whether they will be effective in protecting against HIV, and especially against different groups and clades of HIV. Professor Marlink believes that it is high time to begin trials of some of the candidates in the United States, while continuing to develop the live vaccine option — to be kept, as Desrosiers puts it, "in the wings."

---

The parallels between AIDS and polio are legion, and clearly the debate about trials of Desrosiers's live AIDS vaccine echoes the debate about the safety of live polio vaccines in the fifties. Then, as now, there was a fearsome disease causing worldwide concern, and tremendous public pressure for a cure. In 1959, as in 1999, there was a race among scientists to be first, a race fueled by the real and burning desire to do something worthwhile, to contribute something to humanity, but also fired by more selfish motives, such as the desire for prestige and potentially huge profits.

In 1963, soon after the SV40 scare had focused minds, that wonderful historian of the polio years, John Rowan Wilson, wrote the following: "You do not know what the full implications of discoveries are, until you have made them. Epidemic poliomyelitis is an example of this. It was, in effect, created by hygienic measures designed to deal with other diseases. The measures designed to protect the world from polio may, in their turn, for all we know, lead to some other quite unexpected consequence which may be to man's disadvantage."[69]

If Wilson was thinking about SV40, then it appears that he may have been right, given the increasing evidence of links with mesothelioma. But perhaps he was even more prescient in his warning, given the apparent links between another of those protective measures against polio, and the subsequent emergence of AIDS. Whether or not the OPV/AIDS theory is correct, a growing number of doctors and scientists are coming round to the view that AIDS is very likely to be an iatrogenic condition.

Is it possible that this story will come round full circle yet again? Are we once again in danger of introducing a new iatrogenic disease in an attempt to eradicate an existing one?

If what Desrosiers says is correct, then the main motivation behind the IAPAC vaccine initiative was to engender publicity, and to focus attention on the importance of proceeding with live HIV vaccine development and, when appropriate, trials. And it certainly seems that part of the thinking behind the fifty volunteer pledges was to provide some hope to the millions in the developing world, people who stand far too high a chance of becoming infected with HIV in the course of their lifetimes.

These are splendid, noble motives, and nobody would question the bravery and commitment of the volunteer physicians, all of whom must have been deeply touched by the tragedy of AIDS to have made such a selfless offer. Yet they have failed to address the central dilemma posed by live vaccines: the potential for eradication (and the supplanting of wild viral variants with harmless, domesticated ones) married nervously to the danger of reversion, recombination, and spread.[70] In this instance, the dilemma is rendered even more acute by the extreme mutability of the HIV genome.

Very few (if any) of the public statements by the human trial volunteers broach the most worrying aspect of all — that of the potential for spread of a reverted virus.[71] Of particular note is a two-page article written by Jose Zuniga, IAPAC's deputy director, at the time of the group's vaccine initiative in 1997.[72] Zuniga, who is also political editor of the glossy IAPAC journal, explains that the article contains "our association's official responses to some of the most commonly asked questions by the media and general public." There is no reference to the risk of spread. Instead, Zuniga reveals that if live HIV vaccine trials are forbidden in the United States, several of his volunteers "have expressed willingness to participate in trials of other potential live-attenuated vaccine candidates outside the U.S." He also says that: "The U.S. must not expect people in developing countries to take risks that people in the U.S. are not willing to take."

This is commendably democratic, but if it indicates a willingness to countenance more informal trials of an experimental vaccine, perhaps even clandestine trials in developing lands of the type that has gone wrong so often before, then this is a deeply worrying development. Even more disturbing is an account of the 1997 IAPAC press conference, which reveals that "the volunteers made clear that they intended to find a way of going ahead with the experiment irrespective of the outcome of the [FDA] talks."[73]

Such statements are doubtless colored by the despair many feel about the ravages that the epidemic has already brought — especially among groups such as gays and hemophiliacs. After nearly two decades, and still no vaccine in sight, it is understandable that many of those touched by the horror of AIDS should feel a temptation toward heroic gestures — a willingness, even, to risk their lives "for the greater good of the world."

The well-meaning physicians seem not to have considered that if something should go wrong with the vaccine, they have not simply volunteered themselves as guinea pigs: they have volunteered local communities where the trials are staged; they have volunteered the whole of humanity.[74] One hopes that they will reconsider the implications of their offer, will think again about the dangers of reversion and spread — especially when the immediate risks would, in effect, be imposed on a country far from home.

But what of potential guinea pigs from other parts of the world? It is not inconceivable that some individuals and governments from the developing world might be tempted toward participation in live AIDS vaccine trials, possibly by ethical motives, possibly by offers of cash. This is one of the dangerous situations that Jonathan Mann was trying to warn African governments about, back at the start of the nineties.[75] Sadly, Dr. Mann is no longer with us, but one hopes that there are other wise counselors on whom we can rely to help us distinguish between what is sensible and what is rash. One hopes, but one also worries. Do we, as a species, have sufficient safeguards in place, enough *independent* checks and balances, to ensure that when the men in white coats, or those in gray suits, get it wrong — as they surely sometimes do — that their mistakes will not be the end of us?

In one of my many conversations with the late David Dane, we got to talking about AIDS vaccine trials, and how they should be staged. David commented: "The problem is where to try out these AIDS vaccines. Should we use Rwandans and Ugandans as guinea pigs, when [we're] going to use [the vaccines] in the

West anyway? . . . The ghost of Koprowski's Ruzizi trial is hovering all around these discussions."[76]

The biotechnological advances of the last twenty-five years hold out tantalizing promises of human advancement and happiness, but they also confront us, potentially, with the greatest dangers that our species has ever faced. Are we mature enough to proceed cautiously, and sensibly, amid that understandable clamor from the optimistic, the egotistic, the foolhardy, and the desperate, amid those pressing demands to take bold steps before it is too late? Or are we about to make the same mistakes all over again?

---

The river flows onward. The square-sided riverboat, with its five great barges lashed behind, slides forward into the west, toward the great red disc on the horizon, toward a future suffused with red. Ahead, through the heat-haze, through the sizzle and glimmer, and a few hundred miles downstream, lies Kinshasa. Behind lies Kisangani and its medical laboratory and nearby, overgrown by jungle, the two concrete foundations — all that now remains of Lindi camp.

These same ancient barges may have carried the human immunodeficiency virus back in the fifties, in the very early days of spread. This great floating community, with its own doctors and traders and cooks and prostitutes, this body of crushed humanity, is one of the means whereby the virus may have been transported down to the capital, and onward to the world at large.

Dotted across the channel ahead are floating islands of water hyacinth, introduced from abroad to make the river more beautiful. Nowadays they are strangling the life from this, the main transport artery of central Africa — another well-intentioned and cavalier gesture gone wrong. The river narrows here, with sandbanks dividing the main course of the stream, and some of the passages have been overwhelmed by the floating carpets of tendrils and flowers. The captain gives them a wide berth, knowing what may happen if he passes too close.

The sun sets, and the tropical night falls quickly. Down below in the heart of the boat there are beery whoops and shouts, and clouds of *ganja;* sinuous Lingala rhythms slide away across the water. But here on the prow is a quiet man with an important job. He stares out along the line of the searchlights, and speaks carefully into his walkie-talkie, giving the right course to the captain up on the bridge. His knowledge of the reaches and shallows of the river, his educated reading of the rippling water and its ever-changing moods, protects the human cargo floating behind.

Apart from his sharp eye and sound judgment, the pilot is chosen for his sobriety and seriousness. Over the years he has proved these qualities many times. He has resisted the temptation to take shortcuts where none exists —

along channels that are too shallow, or through innocuous-looking pockets of floating vegetation — because he knows from experience that such bold initiatives are all too often disastrous, and result in the barges running aground on the sandbars, or trapped in the water hyacinth, sometimes for days at a time. He knows the places along the banks where the dead barges rest, unburied and rusting in the sun. He knows that the well-being and safe passage of the people on board are his responsibility, and he takes his job seriously.

As we float downstream into the west, are we also in the care of experienced pilots and sober captains? Can we sleep easy, confident in the knowledge that we are well protected from the harsher and less predictable elements of our great river of Science?

In 1990, when I started researching this book, the "Why now?" question involved just two viruses: HIV-1 and HIV-2. The existence of a third HIV, later called HIV-1 Group O, was revealed soon afterward.

But then in September 1998, during the final stages of editing, there was another significant development when François Simon and colleagues from Paris, Cameroon, and Gabon announced the discovery of a fourth human immunodeficiency virus,[1] which they christened "HIV-1 Group N."[2] The original isolation came from a forty-year-old Cameroonian woman with AIDS who was tested in June 1995, and rescreening of 700 stored sera from HIV-1-positive Cameroonians collected between 1988 and 1997 produced evidence of three further infections with the virus. One of these positive samples was taken in 1992, although it may be that earlier sera that caused atypical reactions on Western blot (such as those reported from Cameroon and Gabon in the eighties)[3] will also turn out to have been caused by Group N viruses. The original infectee subsequently died, confirming that the new variant was pathogenic for humans.

Sequence analysis showed that Group N was genetically different from the other two HIV-1s, suggesting that it was the result of a separate transfer from primates. On the phylogenetic tree, the Group N virus was positioned marginally closer to SIVcpz-gab-1, the SIV from the first Gabonese chimp, than to HIV-1 Group M or Group O, which suggested that the virus could have originated when a local chimp SIV was transferred into humans.

It was intriguing that both of the minor variants of HIV-1 (O and N) had a clearly identified hearth in the Cameroon/Gabon area of west central Africa.

We do not yet know how far — or how quickly — this fourth HIV will (or has) spread in humans, but a commentary piece accompanying the original report, written by the Pasteur Institute's Simon Wain-Hobson, predicted that the Group N viruses were unlikely to make much headway against the M Group "on a worldwide percentage basis."[4] He added that according to "Murphy's Law [Murphy; 4004 BC]," the N viruses would, however, doubtless make the business of antibody testing that much more difficult.

---

Then, on January 31, 1999, another sensational development. News services around the world began reporting that scientists had solved the twenty-year puzzle of how the AIDS epidemic began.

Beatrice Hahn, Feng Gao, and other members of the team from Birmingham, Alabama, had called a press conference to announce the findings of their research, which was due to be published three days later as a letter in *Nature*. As is necessary on these occasions, the scientific content had been somewhat dumbed down, and portioned into easy, bite-size lumps. In this instance, the dish had also been spiced up by such piquant ingredients as chimpanzee conservation, and the possible development of an AIDS vaccine. It was hardly surprising that one excited BBC interviewer described it as "probably the most exciting discovery about AIDS in the past couple of decades."

At the press conference it was announced that a team of American and British researchers had "discovered the origin of the AIDS virus"; apparently they had "tracked it down" to a virus, almost identical to HIV-1, which they had found in a certain type of chimpanzee. The epidemic, it was explained, had probably begun when hunters were exposed to infected blood while cutting up chimpanzees for meat. Apparently this particular variety of chimp had been virtually exterminated in recent years, because of the increasing levels of bush-meat consumption in this part of Africa. "It took us twenty years to find out where HIV-1 came from — just to realize that the very animal species which we have identified is at the brink of extinction," said Beatrice Hahn. Feng Gao made the dramatic plea: "Please don't kill the chimps." It was pointed out that eating chimp meat could be dangerous (in that one might become virally infected), and that if the chimps disappeared altogether, then so might the chance to make a vaccine against AIDS.

Paul Sharp was another key member of the scientific team, and he was interviewed in his lab at Nottingham University. He said that the virus had probably been in chimpanzees for "hundreds of thousands of years." When asked why it had not transferred to humans before now, he said: "It probably has. There have probably been many occasions when the virus has been transmitted to humans over thousands of years, but it's been changes in this century in Africa — population movements — that have allowed the virus to spread out from rural areas and start a pandemic."[5]

Beyond repeating that the puzzle of the origin of AIDS had now been solved, and that HIV-1 had come from chimpanzees, few of the reporters were very sure about how to interpret the latest findings. Some focused on Sharp's theorizing, and informed their readers unequivocally that the AIDS virus was "thousands of years old." Several (picking up on comments made at the press conference, and not realizing that this news was far from new) seemed fixated by the fact that chimps are apparently immune to the virus, whereas humans are not.[6] Others again vaguely suggested that knowing where HIV-1 came from must provide new hope for a vaccine, but were none too specific about the details. Many concentrated on the conservation aspect, pointing out that logging companies were opening up the previously pristine African rain forest, where they were quickly followed by hunters with guns, who were slaughtering apes on a massive scale in the interior.[7]

Only one or two of the journalists highlighted what was, in reality, the key detail — namely the researchers' conclusions that all three types of HIV-1 had originated from the SIV found in the *Pan troglodytes troglodytes* subspecies of chimpanzee, which is found only in west central Africa.

I obtained an advance copy of the *Nature* paper early on the Monday morning.[8] Stripped of the hype of the press conference, it revealed that what Hahn's team had done was complete the sequencing of the fourth chimpanzee SIV isolate, the one originating from Marilyn, the chimp from Holloman Air Force Base that had died in 1985. The viral sequence, SIVcpz-us, was the same one they had been working on when I had visited Birmingham four years earlier. More recently, they had done mitochondrial DNA analysis on the four chimp samples — and confirmed that three of them (SIVcpz-gab-1, SIVcpz-gab-2, and SIVcpz-us) came from *Pan troglodytes troglodytes,* while the fourth (SIVcpz-ant, isolated from Noah, the Congolese chimp reportedly seized by Belgian customs officials) came from *Pan troglodytes schweinfurthi.*[9] Then they did phylogenetic analysis on the four chimp viruses, together with representative HIV-1 isolates from Group O, Group M, and the new group, N.

When they came to produce their phylogenetic tree of HIV-1/SIVcpz, they found that the three SIVs from *Pan troglodytes troglodytes* clustered most closely with HIV-1 Group N. (They concluded that N was actually a recombinant strain, containing portions of both HIV-1 and the SIVcpz from *troglodytes.*) The next closest relationship was with HIV-1 Group M. HIV-1 Group O was rather more distantly related, while cpz-ant, the SIV from *Pan troglodytes schweinfurthi,* was the most divergent sample of all. On the basis of this, the scientists concluded that all three HIV-1 groups — M, N, and O — had evolved from the SIV found in *Pan troglodytes troglodytes.* What they were saying, in effect, was that all three versions of HIV-1-related AIDS (the outbreaks caused by Groups N and O, together with the major Group M pandemic) had originated from the Cameroon/Gabon/Congo Brazzaville region of west central Africa.

I was intrigued by these conclusions. Back in May 1995, when I first interviewed Beatrice Hahn and Feng Gao in Birmingham, Alabama, they explained that they had received large quantities of frozen tissue from Marilyn's brain, liver, lymph node, and spleen in August 1994 from Charles Arthur, a scientist based at the National Cancer Institute lab at Fort Detrick.[10] Gao told me that he had made his first attempt at sequencing in about March 1995, and had managed to tease out two short sequences from *gag* and *pol*, at the core of the virus. He added that it appeared that SIVcpz-us might be a recombinant: the *pol* sequence looked like a genuine chimp SIV, whereas the 520 nucleotides they had from *gag* suggested that it possessed elements from both SIVcpz and HIV-1 Group O. Hahn, however, told me that these sequences indicated that the isolate was another chimp lineage, and that it branched off before the HIV-1 Group O viruses from Cameroon. (She even sketched me a tree in which cpz-ant — from the Antwerp *schweinfurthi* chimp — branched off first, followed by cpz-us and then HIV-1 Group O. After that came the SIVcpz isolates from Gabon, and finally the bush of HIV-1 Group M isolates.) Two years later, in June 1997, Paul Sharp told me they had worked out part of the SIVcpz-us sequence, but not enough to resolve its position on the phylogenetic tree. In June 1998, he said that they had now sequenced the entire genome, but hadn't yet decided how to write it up. "The precise branching order depends on which side of the genome you look at," he explained.

Yet now, less than eight months later, they were announcing that the SIV isolates from the U.S. and Gabonese chimps clustered together, and that they all branched off the tree after Group O and before Group M. I was surprised by how much difference there was between their original positioning of cpz-us on the tree, and their final, published analysis. If nothing else, this revealed that incomplete viral sequences can be greatly misinterpreted.

There was another difference too. When we met in 1998, Paul Sharp had still been proposing that the origin of both of the major chimp SIV lineages (SIVcpz-gab and SIVcpz-ant) and both the HIV-1 groups (M and O) could be another small SIV-infected monkey (perhaps from the *Cercopithecus* genus), from which both chimps and humans had become infected twice. I thought this sounded far-fetched, and told him so. Yet now, in February 1999, he and Hahn were not only certain that all the groups of HIV-1 had come from chimps, but had apparently narrowed it down to a particular subspecies.[11]

It was clear that I needed to speak to Paul Sharp again. I waited a few days for the media excitement to die down, and then phoned him in Nottingham. He was just off to teach, but said he had a few minutes. I decided to ask the three key questions straightaway. Could he be certain that the SIVcpz from *Pan troglodytes troglodytes* was the source for all three known groups of HIV-1? "That's certainly what the trees look like," he answered. Did any members of his team have a new isolate of *Pan troglodytes schweinfurthi,* either extant or in the pipeline, on which they were basing their analysis? "Not that I know of," he replied. But what if other *schweinfurthi* SIV isolates were obtained that had sequences closer to Group M? "That would change the picture," he said. "All we can go on is the information that is available, and the information looked quite sound." This was a very different conclusion to that contained in the paper, where it was stated unequivocally that: "*P. t. troglodytes* is the primary reservoir for HIV-1 and has been the source of at least three independent introductions of SIVcpz into the human population."

A few days later, Sharp and I had a longer chat in which he was able to state his position more fully. He told me that Françoise Barré-Sinoussi, in Paris, had sampled another thirty or so *Pan troglodytes troglodytes,* and found three more that were SIV-positive. So far, they had sequence data for just one virus, and it appeared to sit happily near the other SIVcpz isolates from *troglodytes.* Later, in response to my mentioning that Jane Goodall in Tanzania might have information about *Pan troglodytes schweinfurthi,* Sharp told me that Beatrice Hahn had already made approaches to Goodall about possible noninvasive ways of procuring samples from some of the chimps at the Gombe Stream reserve.

I asked him why his views had changed so rapidly since the previous time we had spoken. Apparently, one factor had been the publication of the new sequence for HIV-1 Group N, and another had been their testing the mitochondrial DNA of Noah, the host animal to cpz-ant, and their confirmation that — alone among the four chimpanzee hosts — he was *Pan troglodytes schweinfurthi.* At that point, he said, the thing that had excited him was finding correspondence between the chimp phylogeny and the SIVcpz phylogeny: both appeared to have a cluster of three and one outlier, suggesting that there had been "host-dependent evolution of viruses."

"Looking at the trees of the viruses, the phylogeny of the three *troglodytes* viruses is absolutely convincing with the origin of Group N and Group M being just other viruses from the same branch of the tree," he said. In fact, he went on, "without the geographical origin evidence, the one we would be least confident about would be Group O."

The talk of evidence of geographical origin was timely. I asked him whether he had any evidence of early HIV-1 Group M infections in the *troglodytes* range, which embraced Cameroon, Gabon, Equatorial Guinea, and Congo Brazzaville. "You would know that better than I," he replied. He added that they believed that the arrival of HIV-1 Group M in man had occurred before the Second World War. I agreed that the Norwegian sailor case demonstrated persuasively that Group O had been present in Cameroon by the start of the sixties, but told him that I could find no evidence suggesting that the Group M virus had been present in any of the *troglodytes* countries prior to the eighties, quite late in the global epidemic.[12] "I'm surprised you're taking a lack of evidence as a positive" was Sharp's response.

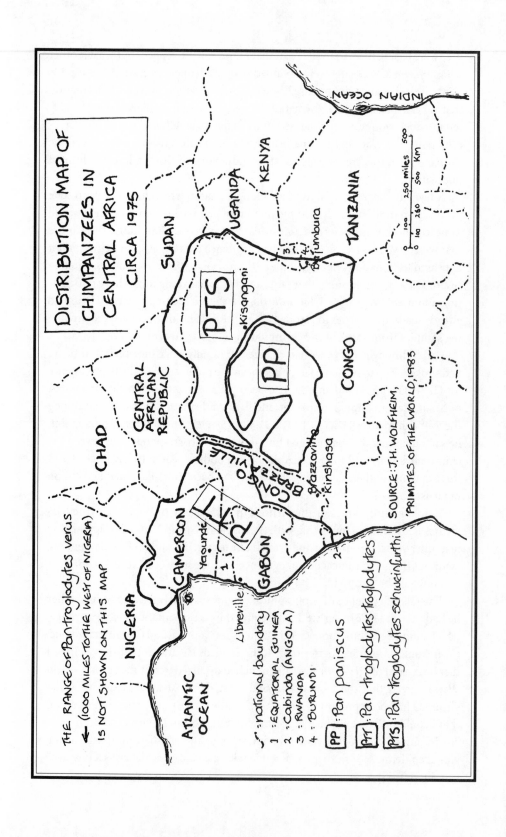

DISTRIBUTION MAP OF CHIMPANZEES IN CENTRAL AFRICA CIRCA 1975

THE RANGE OF *Pan troglodytes verus* ← (1000 MILES TO THE WEST OF NIGERIA) IS NOT SHOWN ON THIS MAP

: national boundary
1 : EQUATORIAL GUINEA
2 : CABINDA (ANGOLA)
3 : RWANDA
4 : BURUNDI

PP : *Pan paniscus*
PTT : *Pan troglodytes troglodytes*
PTS : *Pan troglodytes schweinfurthi*

SOURCE: J.H. WOLFHEIM, 'PRIMATES OF THE WORLD', 1983

ATLANTIC OCEAN

NIGERIA

CHAD

CENTRAL AFRICAN REPUBLIC

SUDAN

UGANDA

KENYA

TANZANIA

CONGO

CAMEROON
Yaounde

Libreville

GABON

CONGO BRAZZAVILLE
Brazzaville
Kinshasa

Kisangani

Bujumbura

INDIAN OCEAN

0  100  250 miles  500
0  100  250  500 Km

In any case, Paul Sharp had an alternative idea. "Where did the 1959 virus come from?" he asked. I agreed that Leopoldville, where the blood sample containing the 1959 Group M virus had been taken, lay only 150 miles or so from the southern extent of the *troglodytes* range, albeit on the other side of the Congo River. And I acknowledged that viruses, like humans, can easily travel 150 miles and cross rivers. However, I said, from an epidemiological perspective, it seemed a far-fetched scenario. It required the monkey-hunter to become infected in one of the *troglodytes* lands to the north of the River Congo, to leave no evidence of his infection in that area, to infect someone in Leopoldville, and for this event to start a chain of infection that progressed exclusively eastward, across more than a thousand miles of rain forest, through the Belgian-held territories of Congo, Rwanda, and Burundi, in time to start the explosion of AIDS in east Africa in the early eighties.

Sharp was not discomfited. He said that in the course of the AIDS epidemic, "we see an enormous impact of chance events and movements around the world." He cited the arrival of subtype B in the United States, and of subtypes B and E in Thailand; each introduction had probably been caused by the arrival of a single virus. I conceded that founder effect was clearly involved in these instances, but pointed out that the United States and Thailand are distant and separate from Africa, meaning that (in each instance) a single air passenger had almost certainly played the key role. By contrast, the shape of the epidemic within Africa, where viruses could move to and fro in all directions by land or river, would be subject to a completely different set of conditions.

By this stage, we were both becoming a little more animated. "There is only one Group M epidemic — [the transfer] happened just once — and you can't put a probability on the sort of events you're talking about," said Paul Sharp. How did he know? I asked. What indicated to him that there hadn't — for instance — been multiple introductions, perhaps by iatrogenic means, which gave birth to the different subtypes? "If you start to hypothesize about multiple introductions, the rules are all changed," he responded. He asked me how many introductions I wanted, and I said that my belief about how the Group M epidemic began was not dependent on multiple introductions — it could be many, several, or just one. I in turn asked him — three times — how multiple introductions would affect his mooted start date of 1940 or earlier. It would bring that date forward in time, would it not? "Of course it would, yes," he replied eventually. "But I don't think that at all plausible."

———

To get some better perspective on all these issues, I decided to phone Simon Wain-Hobson, the Pasteur geneticist who had obtained the first complete sequence of SIVcpz and published it back in 1990.[13] He mentioned the *Nature* article as soon as he picked up the phone, and he didn't sound happy. I asked what he felt about the paper. "It's bad taste," he said. "It's scientists trying to be politically correct." He pointed out that when he and his colleagues had written their 1990 paper, which had enlarged upon the initial report of chimp SIV published by Martine Peeters in 1989,[14] they had deliberately played down the chimpanzee ancestry of HIV-1, "precisely because we were frightened they would kill the [chimps]." He clearly felt that Hahn and her colleagues had overstated the conservation angle at the press conference. "Beatrice has sold it very, very efficiently," he added, somewhat ruefully.

He told me that he thought the paper technically sound, but that he differed from the authors when it came to interpreting the data. He said that the Marilyn isolate, SIVcpz-us, "seems to be closer to one of the N group [HIV-1 Group N] viruses." He was less certain that the *troglodytes* SIVs represented the source of HIV-1 Group O. So what about Group M? I asked. Did he think that the SIV isolates from *Pan troglodytes troglodytes* represented a convincing origin for HIV-1 Group M? The answer was emphatic: "No."

Why not? I asked. He said that there was only one SIV from *Pan troglodytes schweinfurthi* featured in the paper, and that nobody knew exactly where in the *schweinfurthi* range it had come from. He said that the rumor he had heard was that the infected animal, Noah, had previously been living in a zoo somewhere in the Congo, and that it had been "smuggled out." Certainly this one *schweinfurthi* isolate seemed to be more distantly related to the HIV-1s than the three *troglodytes* isolates, but this was insufficient evidence on which to base the theory that the *troglodytes* SIVs were the source of all three known HIV-1s. "What can you say?" he went on. "What if *schweinfurthi* viruses are very divergent, and one happens to be closer to [Group] M?"

"Chimps are reservoirs," he went on, "[but] the precise details are unclear. Beatrice is milking it too much. . . . We have one or two details — and people make these fantastic theories." He added that she had told him two years earlier that they were having "big problems amplifying the virus" from Marilyn, and that the fragments they had got were like HIV-1 Group O.

Despite being a geneticist, Simon Wain-Hobson has a good sense of the early history of HIV and AIDS, and he said that as far as he knew, the epicenter of the main AIDS epidemic had been on the other side of central Africa, in countries like Uganda, Rwanda, and Burundi, rather than in the *troglodytes* range in west central Africa. "The question is," he went on, "how did it get through to east Africa?"

So which animal did he think was the likely reservoir for HIV-1 Group M, the virus that causes 99 percent of the world's AIDS cases? "If I had to place my money, and you held a gun to my head, I would say go for schweinfurthi," he said. "All you need is three [more SIV isolates from] schweinfurthi, and you can demolish her [Beatrice Hahn's] theory."

---

Over the following days, I thought some more about Paul Sharp, and the fact that he is "no longer hedging his bets."[15] He believes that the Group M precursor virus arrived in man from *troglodytes* chimps in west central Africa in 1940 or earlier, and in response to my argument about there being no epidemiological evidence to support this, told me: "I don't have a feeling for a lack of evidence [of early Group M viruses] in Cameroon and Gabon."[16] He is, of course, a geneticist, and not an epidemiologist. And he is correct in that you can't put a *statistical* probability on how an epidemic will progress or develop. One can, however, develop an informed opinion, based on as much relevant data and information as possible. And if Sharp and his colleagues are going to report on a subject as important as the origin of AIDS — if they're going to tell the world that they have solved the puzzle — then they do, perhaps, have some sort of obligation to develop an informed opinion about other aspects of the debate before they make their announcement.

This, I believe, they have failed to do. Much of their presentation at the press conference seems to have been based on old, recycled opinions (natural transfer plus population movements and promiscuity equals AIDS) or on exaggerated titbits gleaned from the media (like Hahn's statement that *Pan troglodytes troglodytes* was "at the brink of extinction"). Apparently she and her team had first learned about the logging roads and the chimpanzee bush-meat trade just two months earlier.[17]

Put bluntly, do Sharp, Hahn, and Gao really have the broad picture? As far as I know, none of them has ever spent time in Africa. Neither do they appear to have spent much time looking at African history. Sharp believes that Group M has been in humans for at least six decades, and that "by the seventies, the Group M epidemic had been raging for some time." But his evidence for this is entirely theoretical. It is based on how he chooses to set the pendulum on his molecular clock, and on his dogged certainty that Group M has a single source.

But where is the evidence on the ground to support this conclusion? As I have tried to show in chapter 50, there have been massive population movements in the countries where the *troglodytes* chimpanzee lives (principally Cameroon, Gabon, and Congo Brazzaville)[18] for several centuries, from the time of the slave trade, through the forced-labor era of the early twentieth century, to the time of the First and Second World Wars. Of particular relevance is the fact that in the five years following 1940 (the latest date that Sharp favors for the transfer of the Group M precursor to humans), thousands of soldiers from French Equatorial Africa fought against fascism in North Africa and the Middle East.[19]

However, there is, to date, still no evidence that the Group M virus was present in any of the countries in the *troglodytes* range prior to the eighties.[20] As for the pygmies living in northern Congo Brazzaville and southern Cameroon (a group who might be expected to be exposed to chimpanzee viruses during hunting, and one living close to where the two geographically identified SIVcpz *troglodytes* viruses originated), HIV-1 infections were zero in the late seventies,[21] and still "very rare" by the early nineties.[22]

Let us look again, in more detail, at what Sharp's Group M hypothesis actually involves. Let us imagine a chimpanzee-hunter from French Equatorial Africa who becomes infected with SIVcpz in, let us say, present-day Congo Brazzaville in the 1930s. Ideally, this man should infect nobody in his local region, but needs to travel a considerable distance for an African at that time (at least 150 miles, but probably much more) and to cross the Congo River, in order to infect someone else in Leopoldville. The newly adapted human virus has to remain sequestered in Leopoldville for the next thirty to forty years, causing multiple infections according to Sharp, but with AIDS-like disease (such as the highly noticeable cryptococcal meningitis, or invasive KS in young adults) only being observed for the first time by local and foreign doctors from about 1975 onward.[23] According to this scenario, the virus would begin to break free from the confines of Leopoldville/Kinshasa in about 1970, in time to get seeded in eastern and southern Congo (in towns such as Kisangani, Lubumbashi, and Uvira, and — intriguingly — in rural areas such as Yambuku and Abumonbazi) by the second half of the seventies, in the Kagera region of Tanzania by 1978, and in Burundi (where there were multiple infectees in Bujumbura and rural Rumonge) by 1980/1.[24] Back in the west, in Congo Brazzaville, the home of the hunter, Group M makes its first recorded appearance in that same year, 1981.[25]

One has to compare this scenario with the OPV/AIDS theory, the multiple-introduction version of which postulates several separate viral transfers to infants, children, and adults between 1957 and 1960, the first detection of the virus in an adult in 1959, and the first reliable recognitions of AIDS in different parts of Congo, Rwanda, and Burundi between thirteen and twenty-three years later. As has been documented, nearly all of these sightings take place either in, or very close to, former vaccination sites — a fact that is not easily explained if HIV-1 Group M really has evolved from an SIV found only in *Pan troglodytes troglodytes* (unless a few *troglodytes* chimps were also present at Lindi).[26]

Paul Sharp uses the example of the explosion of subtype B viruses in North America to support his claim that chance events play an important role in viral spread. This is true for the Western world in the jet plane era, but it is not a compelling analogy for Africa in the 1930s. To my mind, a better analogy would be that of seed dispersal. Intercontinental spread is like the seed that is swallowed by a bird, and sown when the bird's stool falls to earth perhaps hundreds of miles away, while local spread is like the seed that is picked up by a gust of wind, and deposited just a few yards from where it started. In both cases, all that is necessary for regeneration is that the seed lands in fertile soil. However, one can see that in the former instance chance events (a forest fire, a tree-felling program) could conceivably remove the plant from its initial hearth, leaving only the dispersed seeds to survive, but in the latter instance an eradication of hearth (but species survival elsewhere) is far harder to postulate, except over a lengthy evolutionary timescale. The problem for Sharp with the seed dispersal analogy is that the "birds" (in this case, planes) had evolved only a few years before the 1930s, and were still rare in Africa before the Second World War. For that era, it is far less plausible to postulate the type of far-flung dispersal that would subsequently result in an ugly flowering in the Congo, Rwanda, Burundi, Tanzania, and Uganda, but without leaving any trace of the plant in what is claimed as the original seed bed of west central Africa.

There was no discussion of the early epidemiology of HIV-1 Group M, or its related disease, in Hahn and Sharp's paper; this was a detail that did not fit neatly with the hypothesis. Instead, there was merely the broad claim that *P. t. troglodytes* is "a primate whose range coincides precisely with areas of HIV-1 group M, N and O endemicity,"[27] which, given the relatively late emergence and low prevalence of HIV-1 Group M within most of that range, gives what I would maintain to be a misleading impression.[28] Of far more relevance than this claim is the fact that for Group O and Group N, there is a clearly definable viral hearth in the *Pan troglodytes troglodytes* area, whereas for Group M, this evidence of viral hearth is entirely lacking.

Of course, Sharp and Hahn's hypothesis, which involves repeated casual transfers of SIVcpz to humans (especially monkey-hunters), still requires a separate explanation for why the virus suddenly became pathogenic for humans on three occasions in recent years. Hahn has stated that "increasing urbanization, breakdown of traditional lifestyles, population movements, civil unrest and sexual promiscuity . . . likely triggered the AIDS epidemic,"[29] which brings us back to the views of the natural-transfer school, as propounded in the 1980s. Hahn does not take into account the more recent studies by Preston Marx, which strongly suggest that natural transfer and a late-twentieth-century lifestyle are not, by themselves, enough to create an outbreak of AIDS.

---

Hahn and Sharp's paper *is* valuable in many respects. In particular, it is important to have it clearly and unequivocally documented that the chimpanzee is the reservoir from which the HIV-1s have emerged. It is also commendable that they have called for more research into the relationship between SIVcpz and HIV-1, through further screening of the various chimpanzee species and subspecies, and of human populations living in the same locales. This research (especially into SIVcpz) has been sorely needed for many years now. As for the spin they have imparted to the SIV infection of chimps (enjoining people not to kill them, both for their own safety, and so that a vaccine against AIDS can be developed), this seems scientifically tenuous — even if it is an undeniably imaginative approach, and one that is targeted at a laudable goal. It remains to be seen, however, what the reaction will be when this news filters through to Africa. Will it deter people from buying chimpanzee bush-meat? Or will it encourage the perception of chimps as carriers of dangerous illnesses, and a new wave of carnage?

One can see why this noncontroversial hypothesis of how AIDS began possesses a great and natural attraction for the scientific community, especially those who may have carried out medical interventions in Africa during the fifties.

The problem with the Sharp/Hahn paper, as Simon Wain-Hobson so vividly pointed out, lies with its interpretation. He is not the only one to feel that the *Nature* paper contains an assumption too far, a massively important conclusion based on incomplete evidence.

Eric Delaporte is the director of the retrovirology lab at ORSTOM, at Montpellier in France, which has done a lot of important research into African SIVs during the nineties. Also working at ORSTOM is his wife, the Belgian virologist Martine Peeters, who was the first to report on the existence of SIV in the chimpanzee (and who was included as a coauthor on the *Nature* paper). Despite this, Delaporte says that the paper, and Hahn's presentation of it to the world, contained "not a lot of new things, but a lot of publicity." He clearly believes that the origin of HIV-1 Groups O and N is now settled, but when I expressed my doubts about whether Group M had also evolved from the SIV of *Pan troglodytes troglodytes,* he said: "We have the same feeling. . . . It is not excluded that there is another source for [Group M]. We are still looking for another nonhuman primate virus."[30]

So, let us once more review the genetic evidence. The Sharp/Hahn hypothesis is based on the difference between three *Pan troglodytes troglodytes* isolates, and a single isolate from *Pan troglodytes schweinfurthi.* Information about the provenance of the latter isolate is extremely patchy — save for Wain-Hobson's belief that Noah, the host, spent some time in a Congolese zoo. However, in February 1999 I was reliably informed by a Belgian primatologist, who wishes to remain anonymous, that Noah (together with a second chimp, Nico) was originally given by President Mobutu to the late king of Belgium (Baudouin) during the latter's visit to the Congo in 1986. My informant deduces that it was diplomatically unacceptable to decline the gift, and that the two chimps were therefore put on a plane out of Kinshasa, but that because their importation contravened CITES regulations about primates, they were apprehended by customs officials upon arrival in Belgium in June of that year. He believes that the chimps may originally have been gifts from local chiefs, or that they came from one of the city zoos (such as those at Kinshasa[31] or Lubumbashi), or from the animal center at Epulu, in eastern Congo.[32]

It is clear that before he left the Congo, Noah may well have been caged with other chimps, quite possibly with both *schweinfurthi* and *troglodytes*. There may, therefore, have been intraspecies or cross-subspecies transmission of SIV, and this alone could be relevant to the divergent nature of the Noah isolate, cpz-ant.

SIVcpz-ant may or may not be typical of the SIVs found in *Pan troglodytes schweinfurthi*. At this stage, we simply do not know. As pointed out earlier, chimps do not like to cross rivers, and groups can therefore become sequestered in different geographical locales in the rain forest. Furthermore, they are omnivorous, and eat other monkeys.[33] There may, therefore, be much wider divergence among SIV isolates found in a chimp subspecies such as *P. t. schweinfurthi* than among those found in herbivorous primates, like AGMs or sooty mangabeys.

There is also another factor that needs to be borne in mind. Back in 1961, Belgian researchers (including Paul Osterrieth and Gaston Ninane) reported "markedly variable" blood properties among 175 chimps (158 *schweinfurthi*, originating from six different locations in the eastern Congo rain forest, together with 17 pygmy chimps from south of the river). The researchers proposed that the geographically isolated *schweinfurthi* group from Mambasa should be considered as a "special group," different from the other *schweinfurthi*, on the basis of their highly divergent blood characteristics.[34] They went so far as to suggest that these Mambasa chimps might even be related to chimp subspecies found in other regions of Africa, such as those to the west.[35]

The 175 blood specimens were taken from chimps that were involved in the Lindi experiments (probably in 1957),[36] and the blood studies paper reveals that 21 of these chimps were from the Mambasa group.[37]

As far as I can determine from the literature, there is no record of *schweinfurthi* chimps — apart from Noah — having been sampled for the presence of SIV or HIV-1.[38] However, Noah's SIV sequence shows that *schweinfurthi* can be infected, and — as suggested above — it may transpire that both seroprevalence and viral divergence in the wild will turn out to be considerably greater than currently thought. On this point, therefore, Paul Sharp and I strongly agree: there needs to be more sampling of *schweinfurthi* from different parts of the rain forest.

Because we don't know from where in the Congo Noah originated, this sampling needs to take place in at least two geographically distinct parts of the *schweinfurthi* range. I personally would suggest sampling from the southeastern part of the range (such as Tanzania — near Jane Goodall's Gombe Stream reserve, perhaps), and from the northeast (such as Kibale Forest in Uganda). Both these places are presently accessible. I would also suggest, when the political

situation allows, sampling from at least two of the regions in the eastern Congo
rain forest that formerly served as collection points for Lindi — such as those
around Banalia and Mambasa.[39]

If SIVs from *schweinfurthi* chimps originating from Banalia, Mambasa,
Kibale Forest, and Gombe Stream turn out to be genetically close to the SIVcpz-
ant from Noah (and therefore more distantly related to the HIV-1 groups than
the *troglodytes* SIVs), then — and only then — will the geneticists be able to
propose persuasively that the SIV of *Pan troglodytes schweinfurthi* is not the
source of HIV-1 Group M in man, that it does not represent the origin of the
major AIDS pandemic.

There is also another avenue that needs to be investigated. Bill Hamilton
believes that the ancestral nonhuman primate host of the Group M virus may
well turn out to be the pygmy chimp, *Pan paniscus,* and that the human epidemic
may have started when an SIV from that species was transferred to man — either
directly, or via *schweinfurthi,* after cross-species transfer at Lindi camp. I agree
with him, though I am less certain that *paniscus* is a better bet than *schweinfurthi*
as the Group M precursor host. I have learned informally of four *Pan paniscus*
being sampled for SIV; all were negative.[40] However, it is clear that more pygmy
chimps need to be sampled, to discover whether this species also carries its own
version of the simian virus.

---

What follows (barring one or two minor changes — for instance to the next-
but-one paragraph) is the original postscript to this book. It was written in
October 1997, prior to the announcements about HIV-1 Group N and the *Pan
troglodytes troglodytes* hypothesis of source. It now features, in effect, as a postscript to the postscript — and even though it might appear to have been written with the benefit of hindsight, that is not the case.

During the latter half of 1997, after the first draft of this manuscript had
already been submitted to the publishers, I and my research assistant Sally
Griffin made a four-week trip to West Africa, to visit Guinea-Bissau, Guinea
Conakry, Gambia, and Senegal. What we discovered there came as a considerable surprise, for it revealed that the vaccine mentioned by Leonard Hayflick to
Chuck Cyberski and Tom Curtis in 1992 — into which I had by then carried
out some preliminary research — had actually been used far more extensively
than I had suspected.

This new information reinforced the possibility that another polio vaccine
(apart from Koprowski's) could have been involved with the onset of the HIV-2
and HIV-1 Group O epidemics. As it now transpires, it may also have been
involved with the genesis of HIV-1 Group N, and even — if Sharp and Hahn

turn out to be correct with their *Pan troglodytes troglodytes* theory — with that of HIV-1 Group M as well.

We learned that Lépine's polio vaccines had been administered to populations in different towns and rural areas throughout French West Africa (later Senegal, Guinea Conakry, Ivory Coast, Mali, Niger, Burkina Faso, Benin, and Mauritania) and French Equatorial Africa (later Cameroon, Gabon, Congo Brazzaville, and the Central African Republic). The vaccinations apparently took place between 1957 and 1964 — both before and after the independence of these countries. The very first inoculations were apparently staged in 1957 around Pastoria, near Kindia, in what is now Guinea Conakry. As far as is known, none of these African vaccinations has ever been formally reported in the medical literature — with the exception of the campaign in response to the polio epidemic around Mitzic, in Gabon.

There were apparently two sources for the monkeys that provided kidneys to make the vaccines. These were Pastoria (which, apart from being a well-equipped research lab, was also the Pasteur Institute's main primate collection center in Africa) and Brazzaville in Congo Brazzaville, where another arm of the Pasteur Institute is based. From Pastoria, thousands of Guinea baboons and African green monkeys, and a smaller number of patas monkeys, were shipped to France to provide tissue culture materials for both killed and live polio vaccines; hundreds of chimpanzees (*Pan troglodytes verus*) were also dispatched for use in safety testing and other experiments. According to reliable sources, both verbal and documentary, other locally available primates — including sooty mangabeys — were also captured during the early days (up to and including the late fifties), and were gang-caged with the other monkeys. This raises the possibility that some of the early batches of vaccine used in France's African colonies could have been made in the kidneys of baboons that had acquired SIV from sooty mangabeys. Baboons are known to attack and eat other monkeys, and they can be infected with HIV-2 *in vivo* and *in vitro*, so this is a viable scenario.

Although we could find no documentary evidence suggesting that Lépine's polio vaccines had also been given in Portuguese Guinea (now Guinea-Bissau), two of the other Pasteur Institute vaccines administered in French West Africa during this period (those against rabies and yellow fever) are known to have been shared with Portuguese Guinea, which is a contiguous territory. It is therefore quite possible that Lépine's IPV (and/or his attenuated polio vaccine) was also administered there. Intriguingly, Guinea-Bissans from Canchungo and Caio (the latter being the village with the highest known rural HIV-2 prevalence in the world) spoke of intensive vaccination campaigns with unknown vaccines during the early sixties — many of them organized by doctors from the Portuguese army. One man claimed that compliance had been compulsory.

The animals provided from Brazzaville appear to have included the mandrill (from the baboon family) and the chimpanzee.[41] The one article in the scientific literature about mandrill use at the Pasteur Institute in Paris during this period describes mandrill tissue cultures being used for the preparation of "non-inactivated" vaccines.[42] This would appear to be a reference to live polio vaccines, which may be relevant to Lépine's theories about injecting a live polio vaccine (to provide long-term immunity) after two previous injections with IPV. This raises the possibility that a mandrill used to make live or killed injected polio vaccine (such as that administered around Mitzic in northern Gabon in late 1957) might have acquired SIV from one of the Brazzaville chimps. It is also possible, of course, that there is a simpler explanation — and that the tissues of the local chimpanzees (*Pan troglodytes troglodytes*) were themselves used as experimental vaccine substrates.

---

Let me be quite clear about this. Though reliable, this information about Lépine's vaccines is still only preliminary, and it does nothing to weaken the powerful and extensive links reported in this book between the vaccines fed in Belgium's former African territories, and the first spluttering appearances of the major AIDS pandemic.

However, it is important to note that we now have four strains of HIV (HIV-1 Group M, N, and O, and HIV-2), and that all four have cropped up first in areas where vaccinations with polio vaccines made in monkey kidney tissue culture occurred in the fifties and sixties. We know that one of these vaccines was made in the tissues of an African primate, while details about the identity of the other primate host were never reported.

Further research into these issues — by scientists from several different fields — is continuing.[43] I, too, am still looking into the theory of iatrogenic transfer.

I believe that at this point there is a case for an official investigation to be launched — by a committee of independent scientists — into some of the issues raised in this book. Certain possible approaches are suggested in the appendices, and I would be happy to submit evidence if requested. Hopefully others who have knowledge of these events will decide to contribute what they know, allowing more and more of the details of the early course of the river, details that are presently "obscured by clouds," to be revealed.

E.H.

West Sussex and Somerset, England

May 1999

SOURCE:
Prepared specially for this book by Brian Foley,
Ph.D., HIV Database, Theoretical Biology and
Physics Group, Group T-10, Los Alamos National
Laboratory, Los Alamos, NM 87545, USA. The
alignment from which this tree was constructed is
available at http://hiv-web.lanl.gov/.

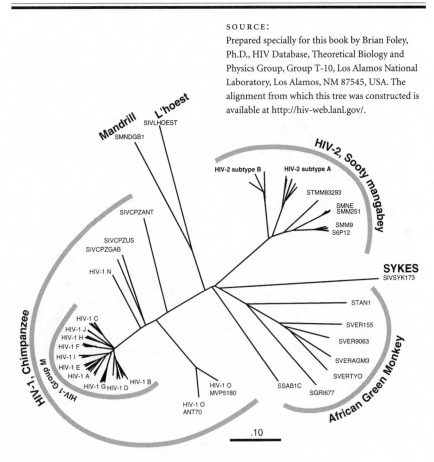

KEY:
SMM9 and SMM251: SIV sooty mangabey
STMM83293: SIV stump-tailed macaque
SMNE and S6P12: SIV pig-tailed macaque
STAN: SIVagm (tantalus)
SVER: SIVagm (vervet)
SGRI: SIVagm (grivet)
SSAB: SIVagm (sabaeus)
The other SIVs, and the HIV-2s, are self-explanatory, as are the HIV-1s, which are identified either by
Group (M, O, or N), or — in the case of Group M — by subtype (A to J).

Professor Foley comments: "It is readily apparent that the HIV-2 viruses are related to sooty mangabey
viruses . . . [but] we have yet to find the chimp group that gave birth to HIV-1 Group M." He was highlighting the fact that although we can now be confident that the HIV-1s evolved from chimpanzee viruses,
nobody has yet tested a chimp virus (from whichever species or subspecies) that clusters closely with
Group M, in the same way that SIVsm clusters closely with the HIV-2 viruses.

## Appendix A

### ARGUMENTS FOR AND AGAINST

### THE OPV/AIDS HYPOTHESIS

(What follows is a distillation of the arguments examined in this book. For a complete understanding of these arguments, we refer the reader to the text itself.)

#### FOR:

1. The extremely high correlation between the locations of African towns and rural areas where CHAT vaccine was fed between 1957 and 1960, and the locations of early instances of HIV-1 infection and AIDS.
2. The fact that the earliest known sample of HIV (L70, the Leopoldville blood sample taken in 1959) is coincident in time and place with a major trial of CHAT vaccine.
3. The fact that the L70 isolate branches near the root of the HIV-1 Group M tree, suggesting that the introduction of HIV-1 to humans took place only a few years earlier, and thus could have occurred in 1957/9, when the CHAT feedings were taking place in the Congo.
4. The fact that fourteen years after the discovery of the HIV-positive L70 sample, nobody has found a sample of HIV-1 from *before* 1959 or, more to the point, from before the time of the first CHAT feedings in 1957.
5. The fact that the only known close viral relative to HIV-1 is the SIV of the common chimpanzee, and that 350 to 400 chimps at Lindi camp were sacrificed in experiments to perfect CHAT vaccine. (Some eighty of these were pygmy chimpanzees; the rest were common chimps.) The deaths of less than half of these 350 or more chimps can be accounted for by "natural wastage," or by known experiments that required sacrifice.

6. The statistical likelihood (based on currently observed seroprevalence among sampled chimps) that between eight and twelve of the Lindi chimps would have been naturally infected with SIV upon arrival at the camp, and that SIV might have spread further through the practice of caging chimps (including chimps of different species) together. (Apparently it was common practice to house a common chimp and a pygmy chimp together in the same cage, but at one stage the researchers also housed several chimps together in a number of large cages.) The high incidence of opportunistic infections, especially *Klebsiella* pneumonia, among these chimps *suggests* that some may have been suffering from simian AIDS as a result of cross-species transfer of SIV within the camp.

7. The evidence from several sources that chimp kidneys from Lindi camp were sent from Stanleyville to Philadelphia (Children's Hospital and/or the Wistar Institute) and the evidence suggesting that they were also sent to Belgium.

8. The fact that Alexandre Jezierski, whom Koprowski and Norton met in the Congo in early 1957, had successfully used the kidneys of fifteen different African primates — including chimpanzees — to grow poliovirus, and later produced both killed and live polio vaccines in kidney tissue cultures from several of these primates. He is also known to have passaged an attenuated poliovirus (intended for use as a polio vaccine) in chimp kidney tissue culture.

9. The fact that Gaston Ninane attempted to make tissue culture from chimp kidney in the Stanleyville lab, though apparently without success.

10. The absence of documentation relating to the Lindi polio research in chimpanzees. There is virtually no published data about the research, and promised papers on the subject failed to appear.

11. The fact that the species of monkey used as the substrate for CHAT vaccine was, unusually, never reported in the literature of the day.

12. The fact that many of those directly involved with CHAT manufacture have apparently been unable to recall crucial details, such as the type of tissue culture used, and where the vaccines were administered.

13. That from a scientific and practical perspective, chimpanzee kidneys might have been viewed as the ideal substrate for a polio vaccine such as CHAT. Chimp kidneys were known to be able to grow poliovirus to a high titer. They were cheap and easily available at Lindi, and research carried out in Philadelphia and Stanleyville had proved them to be free of the more dangerous known human pathogens. Further clues include the fact that it would have been logical to have employed primate cells that were as close as possible to those of human cells, and the references by the Lindi researchers to the pygmy chimpanzee (their initial preferred research

animal) as the "blood relative of man"; the 1955 Indian ban on monkey export, which had raised concerns about kidney supply; the availability of a large stock of immature animals (the kidneys of which are ideal for making cultures); and the fact that some of the animals had already been used for other experiments, meaning that they were already destined for sacrifice. These considerations could have outweighed any concerns about the adverse public reaction that such a use of chimpanzees might have sparked — even in the 1950s.

14. The fact that in 1992, Hilary Koprowski was quoted as giving at least four different versions of which monkey species was used to manufacture CHAT. He finally decided that the monkey he had used was the rhesus macaque. The claim that he (Koprowski) had used rhesus to grow CHAT was made in a letter written to Koprowski by Albert Sabin in March 1992, shortly after the OPV/AIDS controversy broke. However, there appears to be no documentary evidence to support this claim.

15. The fact that Koprowski's papers relevant to CHAT have apparently been "lost in a move," and that Koprowski has given contradictory accounts about the circumstances of the loss.

16. The fact that there is a complete absence of records for the crucial period between November 1956 and July 1958 in the "polio correspondence" held at the Belgian foreign ministry archives — a period that coincides with the Lindi research and the early polio vaccine trials in the Congo.

17. The fact that Koprowski's 1992 letter to *Science* seeking to disprove the OPV/AIDS theory contained a high level of error and inaccuracy.

18. The fact that most of the findings of the Wistar Institute's expert committee, which concluded that the OPV/AIDS theory was highly unlikely, have since been invalidated. In particular, the claim that HIV was present in the tissues of the Manchester sailor is now thought to have been based on a lab contamination. Furthermore, the oral route is now known to be a means whereby SIV or HIV can enter the body and establish infection.

19. The fact that both the Wistar Institute and the Swedish Institute for Infectious Disease Control have failed to release samples of CHAT for independent analysis. In the former case, this reneges on a previous publicly declared offer to do so.

20. The fact that early polio vaccines are known to have contained several contaminating simian viruses (including SV40, to which tens of millions of IPV and OPV recipients were exposed).

21. The fact that in the 1950s, primary monkey kidney tissue cultures (such as those used for the manufacture of many polio vaccines, including CHAT) were routinely contaminated with lymphocytes and macrophages, which are the main target cells for SIV and HIV.

22. The fact that, according to Albert Sabin, the CHAT vaccine lot used in Ruanda-Urundi in 1958 was contaminated with an unidentified simian virus.

23. The fact that the CHAT vaccination trials in central Africa involved one million individuals. The huge number of vaccinees increases the possibility that a low-level SIV contaminant could have been transmitted to a few unfortunate individuals — and thence could have spread further between humans.

24. The fact that infant vaccinees in the Congo and Ruanda-Urundi received fifteen times the standard dose of CHAT vaccine.

25. The fact that on one occasion, Dr. Koprowski is known to have misreported in the medical literature the final substrate used for manufacture of a polio vaccine.

26. The fact that the natural transfer theory for the origin of AIDS contains several inherent difficulties. In particular, it cannot easily explain the recent and almost simultaneous emergence of the four outbreaks of AIDS, and the fact that pygmy groups (who appear to have hunted and eaten chimpanzees since time immemorial) were not found to be infected with HIV-1 when tested in the early stages of the epidemic.

27. The fact that there is evidence to suggest that, apart from the pandemic of HIV-1-related AIDS, the outbreaks of HIV-2, and HIV-1 Groups O and N may also have been started through vaccine-related accidents.

### AGAINST:

1. The fact that — as far as is known — no sample of CHAT virus or vaccine has ever been tested and found to contain SIV or HIV.

2. The fact that despite much circumstantial evidence, there is no hard proof that chimpanzee tissues were ever used for CHAT vaccine manufacture.

3. The fact that other iatrogenic theories, such as those involving the introduction of blood transfusions or reusable hypodermic syringes in Africa, *could* explain how transient SIV infections in humans became transmissible and pathogenic for humans.

4. The fact that, thus far, the SIVcpz isolates most closely related to HIV-1 have been found in the *Pan troglodytes troglodytes* subspecies of common chimpanzee from west central Africa, and that the only example of SIV found in *Pan troglodytes schweinfurthi* (the common chimp found near Lindi camp and Kisangani, in the Congo) is more distantly related to HIV-1. However, it must be added that thus far only two *Pan troglodytes schweinfurthi* chimps and four *Pan paniscus* chimps appear to have been sampled (these are the two chimp species known to have been present at Lindi and Stanleyville).

# EXPERIMENTS AND INVESTIGATIONS THAT

# COULD BE CONDUCTED TO SHED FURTHER LIGHT

# ON THE OPV/AIDS HYPOTHESIS

1. The samples of early Koprowski polioviruses held by the Wistar Institute (especially CHAT pool 13 and Fox pool 8) could be tested in independent labs for the presence of SIV/HIV, and to establish which monkey species provided kidneys for tissue culture.

2. The samples of CHAT 10A-11 held by the Swedish Institute for Infectious Disease Control could be tested independently to establish which primate substrate was used to produce the vaccine.

3. A further search could be made at both the above institutions for post-vaccination serum samples taken in the fifties from CHAT vaccinees. Any found could be tested for SIV/HIV.

4. A further search could be made at both the above institutions for CHAT vaccine protocols, or other documents relevant to the vaccine. David Ho is of the opinion that more papers about the early polio vaccines may exist at the Wistar Institute.

5. A search could be made for archival sera from central Africa from before 1957, to see if there is any evidence of "ancient" HIV-1. Any authentic positive sample from before 1957 would provide a strong challenge to the polio vaccine hypothesis.

6. Further attempts could be made to establish the exact provenance of blood sample L70, taken from an unidentified male in Leopoldville in 1959, and later found to contain HIV-1. Jean Vandepitte is one person who might still have original data.

7. The stored skeletons (and, in some cases, formalinized bodies) of common and pygmy chimpanzees sent from the Congo to Tervuren could be examined for the presence of SIV. Many of these were collected from areas close

to those where Gilbert Rollais collected chimps for Lindi. In particular long bones, which might still contain dried marrow, are worth testing for SIVcpz DNA; if any is found, it could be sequenced, to see if it is more closely related to HIV-1 than other SIVcpz isolates. (Unfortunately the seventy-nine skulls from Lindi chimps sent to Tervuren by Ghislain Courtois in the late fifties are less promising candidates, although it might be worth testing one or two, to see whether there is any recoverable viral DNA around the jawbone.)

8. A scientific expedition could be mounted to those areas in the Congo rain forest where Gilbert Rollais collected common and pygmy chimps; I have details of the locations. To launch extensive capture operations might prove to be disruptive and establish an unfortunate precedent, but another option would be to test young chimps being sold at local marketplaces. Blood and/or stool samples could be taken, and tested for the presence of SIV; any positive samples could be sequenced.

9. Blood samples could be taken from longtime residents of Kisangani, the Ruzizi Valley, and Lake Tanganyika towns such as Rumonge — especially from those persons who are likely to have been fed with one of the early batches of CHAT vaccine. (Here, Hubert Caubergh's lists of vaccinated villages should be helpful.) Any HIV-positive samples could be sequenced, to see if they bear any unusual characteristics.

10. Similarly, attempts could be made to trace infants who were fed CHAT at Clinton State Farms in the late fifties. (I have the names of early vaccinees, and information about which vaccines — and sometimes which pools — were fed. If any persons have died of AIDS, stored tissues could be tested for the presence of HIV, and any detectable virus could be sequenced. In addition, bloods from those Clinton vaccinees who are willing to donate samples could be assessed for HIV-positivity.)

11. Attempts could be made to find out whether the teenager who gave birth to an HIV-positive baby in New Jersey in 1973/4 was originally a Clinton vaccinee. James Oleske might be able to help here.

12. Further attempts could be made (for instance among ex-workers at Lindi, Stanleyville, the Wistar Institute, the Rega Institute, and RIT) to establish whether chimpanzee kidneys were ever used to make tissue culture for producing CHAT vaccine.

13. Persons directly involved with CHAT manufacture and research, such as Hilary Koprowski, Stanley Plotkin, Monique Lamy, and Julian Peetermans, could be invited to answer questions about the exact details of manufacture.

14. Further tests could be conducted to investigate the viability of a contaminant SIV surviving the vaccine-making process. Since there is no evidence as to how Koprowski prepared his MKTC monolayers, the kidneys of a

rhesus macaque bearing a high titer of SIV could be prepared for tissue culture by four different methods: the Maitland technique, versenation, trypsinization by the Bodian method, and trypsinization according to Gear. The tissues could then be inoculated with an attenuated poliovirus, to simulate vaccine production, and the supernatant tested for presence of SIV. If the virus is present, a typical dose of "vaccine" could be fed to and injected into other macaques, to see whether they become infected by the SIV contaminant in the "OPV" or "IPV."

15. Similar vaccines could be prepared from baboon kidney tissue culture, to simulate those prepared in Pierre Lépine's laboratory.

16. Kidneys from SIV-infected chimpanzees are in short supply, but experimental polio vaccine lots (made as above, according to the methods of the 1950s) could perhaps be made from the kidneys of an AIDS patient who had donated organs for medical research. This would allow researchers to see whether HIV survived through to the final "vaccine."

17. As a test of the extent to which trypsin is able to inactivate SIV, a culture of SIV-infected macrophages could be prepared, trypsinized, and then the trypsin could be washed away, to see whether the cells produce further SIV in the days following.

*Acknowledgments*

By far the most striking and heartwarming thing for me about researching and writing this book has been the remarkable number of people who have provided quite remarkably generous assistance. Many gave interviews, few of which were less than an hour in length — and several of which lasted much longer. In the great majority of cases, my questions were answered with candor and good humor. Others responded to inquiries by letter, fax, or phone. Others again provided support and sustenance of more subtle varieties.

All those in the following list have helped in one or other of these ways. Regrettably, it is not an exhaustive list, and to those whose contributions have not been mentioned, I must apologize in advance. You know who you are. Many others have been omitted deliberately, either at their own request, or because there is reason to doubt that they would welcome their names being published here.

In addition to the unnamed ones, therefore, my sincere thanks go to the following persons:

Peter Aaby, Caroline Akehurst, George Alexander, Jennifer Alexander, Fred Allingham, Lawrence K. Altman, Michael Anders, Arnaud André, Frank Andrew, Roy Ansell, Isolde Antonio, Koya Ariyoshi, Wilbur Armand, Mick Askew, Stewart Aston, Pascu Atanasiu, Boko Atkinson, Andrew Bailey, E. H. Barker, Tony Barnett, John Barrie, Arthur Bartley, Ann Bayley, Rebecca Bell, Valerie Beral, John Berry, Wilfred Bervoets, Gunnil Biberfeld, Peter Bird, Mrs. Blackwell, Bill Blattner, Rev. John Blease, Thomas Bøhmer, Marie-Antoinette Bossut, Margerete Böttiger, Jean Brakel, Jean-Mark Brakel, Hans-Dieter Brede, Moya Briggs, Billie Broadus, Anthony Bryceson, Susan Buchbinder, Alan Buckley, Louis Bugyaki, Harold Burger, Donald Burgess, Fritz Buser, Ib Bygbjerg, Kekoura Camara, Lois Camp, Margaret Carswell, Richard Carver, Hubert Caubergh, Jacques Cerf,

David Chadwick, Martin Chandler, Francis Charlton, Susan Chesters, Hanne Christensen, Pat Christie, Ivor Citron, Brian Clapham, John Clayton, Andrew Cliff, Nathan Clumeck, Malcolm Coe, Lady B. Cole, William Cole, Robert Colebunders, Ilsa Colman, John Connolly, John Cook, Jim Cooper, Gerald Corbitt, André Courtois, George Cox, Donna Cragle, Geraldine Crane, John Crewdson, Jeff Crisp, J. W. Crofton, Anne Cullen, James Curran, Michael Kent Curtis, Tom Curtis, James Cutler, Chuck Cyberski, Dirk Daenens, Ed Dahl, Patricia Daley, Angus Dalglish, Bill Darrow, Colin Daverage, Glyn Davies, Jack Davies, Anton De Bont, Etienne De Cock, Kevin De Cock, Jeanne and Bruno De Medina, Jean Deinhardt, Jean Delville, Godelieve Desmedt, Jan Desmyter, Ronald Desrosiers, Elliot C. Dick, Andrew Dickson, Karen Dorn-Steele, Larry Douglas, Pierre Doupagne, William Drake, Selma Dritz, Peter Drotman, Julia Duane, Renato Dulbecco, Marjorie Dunbar, John Durbin, Graham Eagland, Blaine Elswood, Memory Elwin-Lewis, Milton Evans, Johan Evensson, Paul Ewald, Peter Fallon, O. D. Fisher, Ginny Fitzgerald, David Fitzsimons, George Flack, Alan Fleming, Pete Fletcher, Tom Folks, Alex Forro, Cecil Fox, Caroline Franklin, Alvin Friedman-Kien, Patricia Fultz, Lars Gurtler, Feng Gao, Sheree Garbutt, Martin Gardner, Keith Garfield, John Garrett, Bob Garry, Dorothy Garside, Eldene Gatlin, Derek Gay, Henry Gelfand, John Gerrell, Paul Gigase, Charles Gilks, Bernard Gingell, Tom Gordon, Jay Gould, Manfred Grunwald, Frederich J. Graboske, Victor P. Grachev, Charles E. Graham, Rick Graves, Frank and Sheila Gray, Val Green, Nancy Griffiths, Michael Grosse, Jackie H., Bjorn Hagmar, Beatrice Hahn, Peter Hanaway, Jimmy Harries, Mary Quarles Hawkes, Alistair Hay, Leonard Hayflick, Charles L. Heaton, Hermann Heimpel, Joe Held, Mr. Helsby, Gertrude Henle, Gordon Hennigar, Nancy Hessol, Arlene Hetherington, David Heymann, Cliff Heyworth, R. Hicks, Sister Hieronyma, John and Katy Hillaby, Max Hilleman, Vanessa Hirsch, David Ho, Eddie Holmes, Harvey Holmes, Marilyn Hornbuckle, Michael Hooten, Colin Houston, Rev. Andrew Huckett, Anders Hugo-Perrson, Klaus Hummeler, Andrew Hunt, Michael Hutt, Constant Huygelen, Danny Irvine, Harold Jaffe, Marilyn Janczewski, P. G. Janssens, Hermann Jervell, Ruth Jervis, John Jewell, Martin Johnson, Philip Johnson, Serge Jothy, Dr. Juel-Jensen, Judy Jurgi, Elise K., Daniel Kanyerezi, Abraham Karpas, John C. Kelliher, Gerry Kendall, Olen Kew, Dr. Kim-Farley, Dr. Kissane, M. Kivits, Lars Kjellen, Pat Klinke, Jack Kneeland, John Knowelden, Michael Koch, Bob N. Kohmescher, Hilary Koprowski, Lillian Kornitsky, Adriaan Kortlandt, David Kritshevsky, Jack Kutti, Walter Kyle, Ann and Al L., Richard Lacey, Georges Lambelin, Monique Lamy, Rowland Lansdell, Ahmed Latif, André Lebrun, Gerasmos "Mike" Lecatsas, Melvyn Legg, Andrew Leigh-Brown, John Leonard, Bettina Lerner, Jay Levy, Rod Lomas, Ruth Lorenzo, Francis Lothe, Daniel Low-Beer, Sebastian Lucas, Ray Luff, Erik Lycke, Gardner Macmillan, Brian Mahy, F. F. Main, Bob Manor, Philippe Marechal, Richard Marlink, Preston Marx, Brendan and Josephine Mason, Michael Mason, Myra

McClure, Joe McCormick, Angus McCrae, Elizabeth McGee, Ken McGinley, Michael McGuiness, Joan McKenna, Joseph Melnick, Thomas Mertens, Hector Meyus, Jean Michaux, Donna Mildvan, Olive Miles, Clarence Mills, Julie Milstein, Philip Minor, Jan Moass, Luc Montagnier, James D. Moore, Jolyn Wells Moran, Bror Morein, Karl Morgan, Joseph Mortelmans, Jacques Morvan, Arno Motulsky, E. E. Muirhead, Gerry Myers, André Nahmias, Lily Namba, Janice Neary, Thomas Nelson, Anton Nemeth, Roland Neveu, Berit Nilsen, Gaston Ninane, Baxter Nisbet, John Noble, Stan Norris, Priscilla Norton, Jack Nowlan, Carmel O'Doherty, Tobin John O'Hare, Terry O'Keefe, Paul O'Malley, James Oleske, Paul and Odette Osterrieth, Russell Ozanne, Keith P., Joseph Pagano, Elaine Page, Betty Papageorge, Tim Parsons, Stefan Pattyn, Phillips Pearson, Roger Pearson, Julian Peetermans, Martine Peeters, Arthur Perrin, Tom Peterman, Martha Phan, Ian and Maureen Phillips, Joan Phillips, M. C. Pike, Anthony Pinching, Arthur Pitchenik, Margaret Pitt, Sheila Plank, Stanley Plotkin, Walter Plowright, James Porterfield, Anne-Grethe Poulsen, Brian Powers, Carol Preston, Edmund Preston, Abel Prinzie, Mary Quarles, Renee Quintine-Grey, Gail R., G. W. Rainsbury, Herbert Ratner, Robert Redfield, Hubert Renson, Rothenberg Richard, Howard Richardson, Fr. Michael Ricquet, Carole Riddich, Julian Perry Robinson, Gilbert Rollais, Willem Roodenburg, Robert Root-Bernstein, Eric Roper, Joseph Rotblat, Jane Rowley, Ruth Ruprecht, Jean Rutsaert, Walter Rydz, Albert Sabin, Heloisa Sabin, Carl-Rune Salenstedt, Martin Salwen, Don Schollar, Gordon Scott, Thomas F. McNair Scott, John Seale, Sister Severia, Paul Sharp, Connie Sharpe, Don Shenton, H. R. Shepherd, Randy Shilts, Roger Short, Alex Shoumatoff, Roger Signor, Mervyn Silverman, L. Robert Smith, Eva Lee Snead, John Sninsky, Bill Snyder, Jean Sonnet, Tom Sorohan, John Spalding, Michael Spencer, Wallace Stark, Michael Steel, Larry and Ruby Steele, Graham Stephens, Ernest Sternglass, Wolfram Sterry, Alice Stewart, Roy Still, Rand Stoneburner, Trevor Stretton, Raphael Stricker, A. E. Stuart, Charles Stuart-Harris, Peter Stumbke, John Taylor, Richard Tedder, Lise Thiry, Jim Thomas, Pauline Thomas, Jo Thompson, Helge Timmerman, Geoffrey Timms, Jeanette Todrick, Tom Todrick, Ronald Tovey, Mike Tristem, Tom Unwin, Dirk Thys Van Der Audenaede, Bernard Vandercam, Rachel Van Der Meeren, Win Van Hoef, Jean Vandepitte, Boris Velimirovic, Paul Volberding, Per Wahlen, Jonas Wahlstrom, Simon Wain-Hobson, John B. Walden, Terry Washington, James Watanabe, Maria Wawer, Arthur Weatherill, Constance Webb, Jonathan Weber, Nick Wedd, Carolyn Weeks-Levy, Karl Wefring, Robin Weiss, Claude Weitz, Lorna Wells, Albert White, Roger Whitehouse, Hans Wigzell, Anna Wiktor, John Wilkinson, George Williams, Sidney Wilmer, Tom Wilson, Peter Woodham, Ann Woods, Chris Woods, Ray Wraxall, Pearce Wright, and Zofia Wroblewska.

Certain other individuals and organizations merit a special mention. First and foremost are the primary publishers (Little, Brown and Penguin), both of whom deserve enormous credit for the courage and meticulous attention to detail that they have demonstrated in the course of bringing this book to print. Next are the librarians and archivists who have helped in my research, most of which relates to the period before 1960, which is not covered by computerized databases like Medline. I have used nearly twenty libraries and archives in all, but seven have been particularly helpful. First and foremost is the wonderful library at the London School of Hygiene and Tropical Medicine at Keppel Street in London, which has provided most of the medical references. Next come two other libraries in Britain and the United States — the Royal Society of Medicine library in Wimpole Street, London, and the National Library of Medicine at Bethesda, on the NIH campus. These may well be the best medical libraries in the world, and between them they have provided virtually all the missing articles in my reference lists — and some more besides. Next come three archive sections — those at the Medical Research Council in Park Crescent, London, the Public Record Office at Kew, London, and the Ministry of Foreign Affairs in Brussels, all of which have provided some remarkable material. Last but not least is the library at Worthing in West Sussex, which has been my local facility for eight of the nine years it has taken to write this book. The staff have been unfailingly kind and helpful, going out of their way to track down books and articles, even those which were not immediately locatable through the inter-library loans service. To these and all the other librarians who have offered such intelligent and enthusiastic assistance, I doff my cap and say thank you.

I would also like to express gratitude to three organizations that have generously mailed me background data on a regular basis. These are the Centers for Disease Control (for the *Morbidity and Mortality Weekly Report*), the Health Studies Branch of the U.S. Bureau of the Census (for the *HIV/AIDS Surveillance Database,* the bible of HIV seroepidemiological research), and Group T-10 at the Los Alamos National Laboratory (for the annual editions of *Human Retroviruses and AIDS,* the PIV sequence database).

Next are those who have helped finance the project. These include Eric Stern, who made a generous contribution to research funds; Professor Bill Hamilton, who responded to my request for a loan by instead providing a grant (albeit one that was eventually repaid); and most significantly my parents, who supported me throughout a two-year period when there was no other cash coming in.

There are many people who have provided significant intellectual input to this book, some of whom deserve to be singled out. They include the eight people who were kind enough to read the manuscript and supply detailed comments and criticism: evolutionary biologist Bill Hamilton; AIDS expert Professor M.; virologist David Dane; molecular biologist Fergal Hill; surgeon Wilson Carswell, with his vast experience of African medicine; science policy expert Brian Martin; and legal experts Liz McNamara and Ruth Collard. All eight have, in addition, provided an exceptional amount of encouragement, help, and advice, sometimes over a period of several years. I am especially indebted to Bill, who suggested the title of the book (later further refined at the prompting of the Little, Brown publisher, Sarah Crichton), together with many of the ideas that feature in the prologue. Special thanks also go to Brian, who has, for some time, served as an informal clearinghouse for information about the OPV/AIDS theory, and has set up a useful web site at: http://www.uow.edu.au/arts/sts/bmartin/dissent/documents/AIDS/.

A debt of gratitude is also owed to those who have investigated the central hypothesis in detail, and who have shared discoveries and insights with me — notably Tom Curtis, Blaine Elswood, Raphael Stricker, Jennifer Alexander, Mike Lecatsas, and Michael Kent Curtis. Four others deserve special praise for their particular intellectual generosity — Louis Pascal, the effective founder of the OPV/AIDS theory, who provided many helpful letters, together with large bundles of invaluable commentary and source articles; the late George Dick, who gave me his entire polio archives of books and conference abstracts; Kamil Kucera, who sent me hundreds of pages of handwritten notes — in English — about his research into *Pneumocystis carinii;* and Jean Sonnet who, in the last months of his life, provided important material about suspected early AIDS cases in the Congo, and who arranged for me to have access to the rest of his papers after his untimely death. Much of the inspiration for this book has come from those mentioned in the last two paragraphs, though any mistakes — if mistakes there be — are mine and mine alone.

My thanks go also to those friends and colleagues who, by their actions and support, have helped me get through a period of my life that has variously been intense, stimulating, obsessive, lonely, and surprisingly joyful. These include my wonderful New York agent, Carl Brandt, whose sound advice and constant encouragement have been invaluable; his London counterpart, Bill Hamilton (not the scientist); my editor at Little, Brown, Roger Donald, who believed in the project from the start; my editor at Penguin, Stefan McGrath, who has provided much sensitive advice during the final months; copy editor Mike Mattil, whose keen eye and ready wit have been constantly in evidence, as has his ability to perform casual miracles; Sarah Drayton, who assisted during the final stage of the editing, most notably with technical terms; Pete Raffell, who helped with many of the photographs; and all those friends and extended family members who put me up and put up with me in the course of my many research trips. The latter include Sue Raffell, Peter Bird, Eric Stern and family, Jonathan and Jeanette Purdey, Kate Todrick, Mark Lockwood, Michael and Grace Anders, Mina Howe, Frank and Judy Hooper, Lennox Roosen, Jane Nantale, and Hilda and Gert Vervaecke.

These acknowledgments cannot be complete without a special mention for Sally Griffin, who started out as a temporary research assistant in mid-1996, and who ended up helping in every conceivable way over a period of eighteen months: translating papers, transcribing interviews, drawing maps and charts (including those that feature in the text), researching, interviewing, analyzing, and editing. I am extremely pleased that at the end of that period, Sally took up a post in Africa, working with children affected by HIV and AIDS. By that time she had become a good friend, as had her mother, Pat, and together they did much to help me cope with the long and difficult illnesses suffered by my parents, Eileen and Eric Hooper.

And it is to them, my mother and my father, that the final accolade must go. They supported and encouraged me — and provided love, enthusiasm, and good counsel in equal measure. It is they, finally, who allowed me the room to produce this book. And although neither of them lived to see it appear in print, at least both knew that it would do so, and read much of the manuscript before they died.

ED HOOPER
West Sussex and Somerset, England
January 1999

# Notes

I have been somewhat selective about the authorship of group-written articles, but generally the first-named author and at least one other (such as the second or last-named author) are credited. *Index Medicus* abbreviations have been employed.

The four most commonly cited references have been abbreviated in the endnotes as follows:

*BMJ* 58 — G. Courtois, A. Flack, G. Jervis, H. Koprowski, and G. Ninane, "Preliminary Report on Mass Vaccination of Man with Live Poliomyelitis Virus in the Belgian Congo and Ruanda-Urundi," *British Medical Journal*, 1958, 2(i), 187–190.

*NYAS* 57 — T. M. Rivers (ed.), "Cellular Biology, Nucleic Acids and Viruses," *Special Publications of the New York Academy of Sciences*, 1957, 5, 1–414.

*PAHO1* — "First International Conference on Live Poliomyelitis Vaccines: Papers Presented and Discussions Held (Washington, D.C., June 22–26, 1959)," *Pan American Sanitary Bureau*, 1959, Scientific Publication No. 44.

*PAHO2* — "Second International Conference on Live Poliomyelitis Vaccines: Papers Presented and Discussions Held (Washington, D.C., June 6–10, 1960)," *Pan American Sanitary Bureau*, 1960, Scientific Publication No. 50. [Both of the latter conferences were sponsored by the Pan American Health Organization (of which the Sanitary Bureau is a part); hence the *PAHO* abbreviation.]

## INTRODUCTION: *John Snow and the Water Pump*

1. M. S. Gottlieb et al., "*Pneumocystis* Pneumonia — Los Angeles," *MMWR*, 1981, 30, 250–252.
2. See L. Kramer, *Reports from the Holocaust: The Story of an AIDS Activist* (London: Cassell, 1995), p. 13. In fact, since — as we now know — AIDS was already occurring in several continents by 1981, it is already legitimate to call it a pandemic, as well as an epidemic.

3. A. Friedman-Kien et al., "Kaposi's Sarcoma and *Pneumocystis* Pneumonia among Homosexual Men — New York City and California," *MMWR*, 1981, 30, 305–308.

4. H. Masur et al., "An Outbreak of Community-Acquired *Pneumocystis* Pneumonia," *N. Engl. J. Med.*, 1981, 305(24), 1431–1438.

5. G. T. Hensley et al., "Opportunistic Infections and Kaposi's Sarcoma Among Haitians in the United States," *MMWR*, 1982, 31, 353–361.

6. N. J. Ehrenkranz et al., "*Pneumocystis carinii* Pneumonia among Persons with Hemophilia A," *MMWR*, 1982, 31, 365–367.

7. A. Ammann et al., "Possible Transfusion-Associated Acquired Immune Deficiency Syndrome (AIDS) — California," *MMWR*, 1982, 31, 652–654.

8. R. O'Reilly et al., "Unexplained Immunodeficiency and Opportunistic Infections in Infants — New York, New Jersey, California," *MMWR*, 1982, 31, 665–667.

9. M. A. Gonda, "The Natural History of AIDS," *Natural History*, 1986, 95, 78–81.

10. J. Crewdson, "The Great AIDS Quest: Science Under the Microscope," *Chicago Tribune*, November 19, 1989, section 5, pp. 1–16.

11. J. Maddox, "More on Gallo and Popovic," *Nature*, 1992, 357, 107–109. S. Connor, "US Aids Pioneer 'Lied over Research Finds,'" *Independent on Sunday* (U.K.), January 3, 1993, p. 1. However, after Gallo moved to appeal, the U.S. government withdrew its findings of scientific misconduct. See D. S. Greenberg, "Resounding Echoes of Gallo Case," *Lancet*, 1995, 345, 639.

12. R. Shilts, *And the Band Played On* (New York: St. Martin's Press, 1987), p. 439.

13. C.-E. Winslow, *The Conquest of Epidemic Disease: a Chapter in the History of Ideas* (Madison: University of Wisconsin Press, 1980), pp. 271–279.

14. Until 1996, it was widely thought that all those infected with HIV-1 would, sooner or later, progress to AIDS (unless they died of something else first). (The course of HIV-2 infection is less certain: some observers believe that certain strains of the virus are non-pathogenic, and do not cause disease.) In 1999 we know that a very small proportion of HIV-1-positive people are infected with strains of low pathogenicity, or else have a genetic makeup that provides some resistance to the effects of the virus. Also, there is triple therapy — see below.

15. Following the emergence of triple (or combination) therapy in 1996, we now believe that many of those who get infected with HIV (at least in the West) will survive. (See Anon, "Update: Trends in AIDS Incidence — United States, 1996," *MMWR*, 1997, 46(37), 861–867; Anon., "A New Lease of Life," *Guardian* (U.K.), May 12, 1997, section 2, p. 2.) However, becoming HIV-positive does still have dreadful consequences, for it means that either one can expect to become very sick (and possibly die), or else one will stay alive only through taking an onerous course of drugs every day for the rest of one's life. We now (in 1999) know that the bodies of some HIV-positive people will reject the therapies, while others will experience dangerous side effects. Other infectees again will fail to maintain the drug regime, and for these, HIV often reemerges at a viral load even higher than before. Furthermore, such drug regimes are extremely expensive (typically costing over $10,000 U.S. per person per year), and therefore provide no answer for most of those who live outside the industrialized sector of the world.

16. Anon., "AIDS in Africa," *AIDS-Forschung*, 1987, 1, 6–24. This first article was written anonymously, but was followed by a sequel that was not: A. Fleming, "AIDS in Africa — An Update," *AIDS-Forschung*, 1988, 3, 116–138. See also "Seroepidemiology of Human Immunodeficiency Viruses in Africa," *Biomed. & Pharmacother.*, 1988, 42, 309–320; and "AIDS in Africa," *Baill. Clin. Haem.*, 1990, 3(1), 171–205, both by the same author.

17. F. Barin, S. Mboup, M. Essex et al., "Serological Evidence for Virus Related to Simian T-Lymphotropic Retrovirus III in Residents of West Africa," *Lancet*, 1985, 2(ii), 1387–1389.

18. In 1992, it was announced that a third human immunodeficiency virus had been detected in patients from Cameroon, Gabon, and France, and this virus was later designated as HIV-1 (Group O), with the "original" virus now redesignated as HIV-1 (Group M). Thus, in the space of approximately a decade, three AIDS viruses — and three related AIDS outbreaks — had been recognized. And, as it turned out, there was even more bad news to come (see Postscript).

19. W. A. Blattner, R. C. Gallo et al., "The Human Type C Retrovirus, HTLV, in Blacks from the Caribbean Region, and Relationship to Adult T-Cell Leukemia/Lymphoma," *Intl. J. Cancer*, 1982, 30, 257–264, and W. A. Blattner, R. C. Gallo et al., "Human T-Cell Leukemia/Lymphoma Virus-Associated Lymphoreticular Neoplasia in Jamaica," *Lancet*, 1983, 2(i), 61–64.

## CHAPTER 1: *Frozen in Time: 1959*

1. Anon., "Nationalism's Rapid Growth in the Congo: Arrests Continue," *Times* (U.K.), February 2, 1959, p. 6.

2. The name changes of these countries can be somewhat confusing. The Belgian Congo became the Democratic Republic of Congo (sometimes Congo-Kinshasa) at independence in 1960, and was renamed the Republic of Zaire in 1971. It reverted to its original name, the Democratic Republic of Congo, just as the first draft of this book was being completed, in May 1997. The country that lies on the north bank of the river, directly opposite the Congolese capital, Kinshasa, was formerly known as the "Middle-Congo," one of the four territories of French Equatorial Africa; it became Congo Brazzaville in 1960, and was renamed the Republic of Congo in 1991. To minimize confusion, this latter country will be referred to throughout this book as "Congo-Brazzaville," and the former Belgian Congo will be referred to as "the Congo" or "Congo." It is mainly in the latter country that the events described in this book take place. Where interviewees refer to "Zaire" instead of "Congo," it is because their original usage has been retained.

3. A. G. Motulsky, J. Vandepitte, and G. R. Fraser, "Population Genetic Studies in the Congo. I. Glucose-6-Phosphate Dehydrogenase Deficiency, Hemoglobin S and Malaria," *Am. J. Hum. Gen.*, 1966, 18(6),514–537; and E. R. Giblett, A. G. Motulsky, and G. R. Fraser, "Population Genetic Studies in the Congo. IV. Haptoglobin and Transferrin Serum Groups in the Congo and in Other African Populations," *Am. J. Hum. Gen.*, 1966, 18(6), 553–558.

4. Enzyme-linked immunosorbent assay (ELISA), Western blot (WB), immunofluorescence assay (IFA), and radioimmunoprecipitation assay (RIPA).

5. A. J. Nahmias, M. Schanfield, A. Motulsky, P. Kanki, M. Essex et al., "Evidence for Human Infection with an HTLV III/LAV-like virus in Central Africa" (letter), *Lancet*, 1986, 1(ii), 1279–1280.

6. A. G. Motulsky, "A University of Washington Historical Connection: The Detection of HIV in Central Africa in 1959," *U. Wash. Med.*, 1987, 13, 64.

7. The blood from eight groups was frozen and flown back to Seattle; four groups provided finger-prick specimens that were studied only in the Congo. See Motulsky et al., "Population Genetic Studies in the Congo. I."

8. A. G. Motulsky, personal communications, November 1990 and February 1991.

9. J. Vandepitte, personal communication, May 1993.

10. The historical account in this chapter is based on articles that appeared in the *Times* (U.K.) during the weeks of David Carr's engagement (January 31, 1959) and death (August 31, 1959). J. A. Condon, *Reddish Remembered* (Metropolitan Borough of Stockport, 1983) was also useful for the local history.

11. The clinical information in this chapter is based on David Carr's medical notes (viewed with permission of the next of kin), held at the royal infirmaries of Manchester and Stockport, and on conversations with David's physicians, John Leonard, Trevor Stretton, and Rowland Lansdell, one of his nurses (Carole Riddick), his GP (Jack Nowlan), the pathologist (George Williams), his fiancée ("Elsie"), the surviving members of his family, and with nearly two dozen of his friends and workmates. The medical notes made available to me included the gross pathological findings at autopsy, and many of the microscopic postmortem findings feature in G. Williams, T. B. Stretton, and J. C. Leonard, "Cytomegalic Inclusion Disease and *Pneumocystis carinii* Infection in an Adult," *Lancet;* 1960, 2(ii), 951–955.

12. A granulomatous disease of unknown origin, which may resemble TB.

13. C. D. Anderson and H. J. Barrie, "Fatal *Pneumocystis* Pneumonia in an Adult," *Am. J. Clin. Pathol.,* 1960, 34(4), 365–370.

14. Further information comes from Dr. Hennigar and Dr. Martin Salwen, (head of pathology at Kings County Hospital, Brooklyn in the nineties) and from the autopsy report. Also helpful were two of Ardouin's relatives, members of the Haitian-American community in New York, and John Crewdson of the *Chicago Tribune,* who was kind enough to share his background notes on the case.

15. G. R. Hennigar, H. A. Lyons et al., "*Pneumocystis carinii* Pneumonia in an Adult, Report of a Case," *Am. J. Clin. Pathol.,* 1961, 35(4), 353–364; and H. A. Lyons, K. Vinijchaikul, and G. R. Hennigar, "*Pneumocystis Carinii* Pneumonia Unassociated with Other Disease," *Arch. Intern. Med.,* 1961, 108, 929–936.

16. E. W. Walton, "Giant-Cell Granuloma of the Respiratory Tract," *BMJ,* 1958, 2, 265–270.

17. P. W. Nichols, letter to the editor, *N. Engl. J. Med.,* 1982, 306(15), 934–935. D. Huminer, J. B. Rosenfeld, and S. D. Pitlik, "AIDS in the Pre-AIDS Era," *Rev. Infect. Dis.,* 1987, 9(6), 1102–1107. R. Sabatier, *Blaming Others. Prejudice, Race and Worldwide AIDS* (London: Panos Institute, 1988), p. 35.

18. The "Cutter incident," at the start of the U.S. vaccination campaign in 1955, resulted in 260 cases of paralysis and eleven deaths.

19. Nowadays, with the ability to study viruses genetically, we know that the different approaches to viral attenuation in 1959 were effectively rather primitive, hit-and-miss versions of genetic engineering.

20. *PAHO1;* see discussion on pages 577–579. Further information was provided in interview by attendees at that conference, including doctors Cabasso, Dick, Gard, Lebrun, Koprowski, Melnick, and Plotkin.

21. A. B. Sabin, "Present Position of Immunization against Poliomyelitis with Live Virus Vaccine," *BMJ,* 1959, 1(i), 663–682. (See especially pages 677–678.)

22. *PAHO1,* p. 579.

23. Sabin was responsible for the development of several viral vaccines, including those against dengue fever and Japanese B encephalitis. Later he spent years investigating a possible viral etiology for cancer.

24. Tim Radford, "Year 2000 Date to Wipe Out Polio," *Guardian* (U.K.), July 3, 1993.

25. The first viral disease to be conquered by man was smallpox, in October 1977.

26. A. B. Sabin, "Acute Ascending Myelitis Following a Monkey Bite, with Isolation of a Virus Capable of Reproducing the Disease," *J. Exp. Med.*, 1934, 59, 115–135.

27. A. B. Sabin, "HIV Vaccination Dilemma" (letter), *Nature*, 1993, 362, 212. See also A. B. Sabin, "Improbability of Effective Vaccination against Human Immunodeficiency Virus Because of Its Intracellular Transmission and Rectal Portal of Entry," *Proc. Natl. Acad. Sci.*, 1992, 89, 8852–8855.

28. H. Koprowski, "Albert B. Sabin (1906–1993)" (obituary), *Nature*, 1993, 362, 499.

29. This paper was eventually published as B. F. Elswood and R. B. Stricker, "Polio Vaccines and the Origin of AIDS" (letter), *Res. Virol.*, 1993, 144, 175–177.

30. Joseph Pagano, personal communication, November 1993.

31. Gaston Ninane, personal communication, August 1992.

32. David Kritchevsky, personal communication, November 1993.

33. Abel Prinzie, personal communication, November 1996.

CHAPTER 2: *Frozen in Space: A Rural Epicenter in Africa*

1. This account mainly consists of events that occurred during the author's first visit to Kasensero in August 1986, but the interview with John took place during a second visit in February 1987. See E. Hooper, *Slim* (London: Bodley Head, 1990), chapters 4 and 13.

2. See R. Mugerwa, N. Sewankambo, J. W. Carswell et al., "AIDS in Uganda," *Symposium on AIDS in Africa* (Brussels, 1985), poster P10, which begins with two crucial observations: that there is a new disease in Rakai district, and that it has been named "Slim" by the people of that district.

3. Examples include E. Hooper, "An African Village Staggers under the Assault of AIDS," *New York Times*, September 30, 1986, pp. C1–C3; E. Hooper, "AIDS in Uganda," *Swiss Rev. World Affairs*, 1987, 37(4), 24–27; E. Hooper, "AIDS Hits Villages," *Development Forum*, November–December 1986, 14(9), 1–5. Perhaps the finest of Roland Neveu's fine series of photographs appeared in the *Times* (U.K.), October 27, 1986, p. 14 (but with an inaccurate and inappropriate caption).

4. D. Serwadda, N. K. Sewankambo, A. Lwegaba, J. W. Carswell et al., "Slim Disease: A New Disease in Uganda and Its Association with HTLV-III Infection," *Lancet*, 1985, 2(ii), 849–852; and J. W. Carswell (editor), "AIDS in Uganda — A Review," *Health Information Quarterly*, Ministry of Health, Uganda, 1986, 2(4), 22–43. See also E. Hooper, *Slim*, pp. 38, 58, and 256.

5. Examples: R. Nordland, R. Wilkinson et al., "Africa in the Plague Years," *Newsweek*, December 1, 1986, pp. 44–46; P. Murtagh, "Death Is Simply a Fact of Life," *Guardian* (U.K.), February 4, 1987; M. S. Serrill, "In the Grip of the Scourge," *Time*, February 16, 1987, pp. 34–35; R. Bazell, "The Plague," *New Republic*, June 1, 1987, pp. 14–15; B. Walker, "Whole Villages Ravaged by the 'Slim Disease,'" *Sacramento Bee*, December 13, 1987, pp. A1, A14; Anon., "Uganda — Land beyond Sorrow," *National Geographic*, April 1988, 173(4), 468–491; J. Kierans, "The Land of the Living Dead," *Daily Star* (U.K.), January 30, 1990, pp. 18–19.

6. For example: H. Timmerberg, "Das Dorf, aus dem Aids kommt," *TEMPO* (Germany); April 4, 1987, pp. 54–65; E. Hale, "AIDS Hits Africa; Infection Ripples throughout Continent," *Gannett News Service* feature dated October 11, 1987; A. Shoumatoff, "In Search of the Source of AIDS," *Vanity Fair*, July 1988, pp. 94–117.

7. "The Epidemiology of AIDS in Uganda," talk delivered by Samuel Okware to National Seminar on AIDS, Kampala, Uganda, August 28, 1987.

8. R. Bazell, "The Plague"; see also R. Henderson, "Truth about AIDS Reaching Those Who Least Need It — Disease Particularly Fierce in Africa," *Baltimore Sun*, November 29, 1987, 87(47), 1A and 20A.

9. B. Walker, "Whole Villages Ravaged by the 'Slim Disease.'"

10. A. Shoumatoff, "In Search of the Source of AIDS."

11. This diagnosis is controversial, in that the deaths were officially ascribed to typhoid fever and TB. At the time, Carswell suspected that the prisoners were perhaps being selectively starved to death. It was only years later that he suspected that they might have died of Slim. If so, this must have been Slim with a very short latency period. Otherwise, the epidemiology is more suggestive of a pathogen like typhoid circulating in the prison, or even of a warder or warders deliberately contaminating the food or water of these most hated of prisoners.

12. M. Arseneault, *Un rêve pour la vie* (Montreal: Libre Expression, 1997). Also, Dr. Teasdale Corti, personal communication (February 1996) and Michel Arseneault, personal communication (March 1997).

13. M. Essex, S. Mboup, and P. J. Kanki (editors), *AIDS in Africa* (New York: Raven Press, 1994), p. 678.

14. L. Garrett, "The Fatal Curse of Juliana's Cloth," *Newsday* (New York); December 26, 1988, 3, 26–29 (part of her powerful "AIDS in Africa" series, which appeared between December 26 and 28, 1988).

15. F. Mhalu, G. Biberfeld et al., "Prevalence of HIV Infection in Healthy Subjects and Groups of Patients in Tanzania," *AIDS*, 1987, 1, 217–221. See also: J. Z. J. Killewo, G. Biberfeld et al., "Incidence of HIV-1 Infection among Adults in the Kagera Region of Tanzania," *Int. J. Epidem.*, 1993, 22, 528–536.

16. L. Garrett, "The Fatal Curse of Juliana's Cloth," see pp. 3 and 28.

17. J. Killewo et al., "Prevalence of HIV-1 Infection in the Kagera Region of Tanzania: A Population-Based Study," *AIDS*, 1990, 4, 1081–1085. These high prevalences subsequently got even worse. In 1992, all 842 inhabitants of Bukwali, a village between Kanyigo and Lukunyu in the border region, were serotested by two different assays, and 13.35 percent were found HIV-positive. Since this included all age groups, it suggested that over a quarter of all adults in the village were infected. (Philippe Krynen, "Partage Tanzania," Bukoba, Tanzania; personal communication, June 1993.) Unfortunately, the well-meaning M. Krynen was later picked up by the Peter Duesberg school (which then included Joan Shenton of *Meditel* and Neville Hodgkinson of the *Sunday Times* [U.K.]), which claims that there is no AIDS epidemic in Africa. Krynen claimed that the results showed that HIV prevalence in Bukwali was much lower than had been reported elsewhere, although how anyone could suggest that the infection of a quarter of a village's adult population was "low" beggars belief. Even the fact that, of the 87 confirmed HIV-positives who were examined clinically, a quarter (23) displayed serious AIDS symptoms, while a further quarter (20) demonstrated AIDS-Related Complex (ARC) or nonspecific symptoms, failed to lead him to the obvious conclusion — that Bukwali was suffering a catastrophic epidemic of AIDS, and that HIV was the cause. See "The Plague That Never Was," *Sunday Times* (U.K.), October 3, 1993, pp. 10–11, for Neville Hodgkinson's dubious interpretation of Krynen's data. For further discussion of these contentious issues, see E. Hooper, "Empty Bottles; Empty Vessels," *AIDS Newsletter* (U.K.),1993, 8(9), 2–7.

18. Dr. Bundschuh did, however, witness several cases of Kaposi's sarcoma during the 1960s and '70s which, she writes, were "very different [from] Kaposi growing in Aids," which she first witnessed in 1983.

19. Margerete Bundschuh, personal communication, July 1995.

20. "Observer bias" should also be taken into account: in any epidemic the first recognized cases are likely to involve those with the fastest progression of disease.

21. Also known as "prodromal AIDS," ARC embraces a wide range of early symptoms, including lymphadenopathy, splenomegaly, and wasting (as in this instance). Other typical early presentations of AIDS include oral thrush and chicken pox (*Herpes zoster*).

22. A. D. Burt, C. R. Shiach, C. G. Isles et al., "Acquired Immunodeficiency Syndrome in a Patient with No Known Risk Factors: A Pathological Study," *J. Clin. Pathol.*, 1984, 37, 471–474. Also see: C. R. Shiach, C. G. Isles, S. G. Ball et al., "Pyrexia of Undetermined Origin, Diarrhoea, and Primary Cerebral Lymphoma Associated with Acquired Immunodeficiency," *BMJ*, 1984, 288, 449–450; and L. Morfeldt-Manson and L. Lindquist, "Blood Brotherhood; A Risk Factor for AIDS?" (letter), *Lancet*, 1984, 2(ii), 1346. Also personal communications from doctors Shiach, Ball, and Isles, 1996 and 1997.

23. W. M. H. Behan et al., "HTLV-III-Seropositivity in AIDS" (letter), *Lancet*, 1984, 1(ii), 1292.

24. The couple first met in December 1979, and it is believed that prior to this the girlfriend (who frequented a large hotel in Dar) may have had sexual relations with TPDF soldiers returning from the Ugandan war.

25. In March 1997, Major-General Jack "Black Mamba" Walden confirmed that it was the Soviet-made B-21 multiple rocket launcher (known sardonically as the "Stalin organ") that had made such an impact before the Tanzanian assault on Katera camp.

26. E. Hooper, *Slim*, pp. 59–60. See also T. Barnett and P. Blaikie, *AIDS in Africa — Its Present and Future Impact* (London: Belhaven Press, 1992), p. 43.

27. T. Barnett and P. Blaikie, *AIDS in Africa*, p. 44, and E. Hooper, *Slim*, p. 28.

28. Other notable early press reports from Rakai include E. Kitaka, "Disease Fear in Central Africa," *Compass News Features*, October 11, 1985 (the first by several months); Anon., "AIDS Kills 100 Monthly in Rakai," *Weekly Topic* (Uganda), March 20, 1986, pp. 1 and 16; C. Bond, "AIDS Epidemic Ravages Uganda," *Guardian* (U.K.), May 16, 1986; C. Bond, "AIDS Lays Waste to Uganda," *New African* (U.K.), July 1986, pp. 29–31; and C. Watson, "Aids-Hit Uganda Learns to Love Carefully," *Independent* (U.K.); December 4, 1986.

29. See A. Shoumatoff, "In Search of the Source of AIDS," pp. 94–117. Shoumatoff's journey took him to Guinea-Bissau (where HIV-2 is the dominant virus), Congo, Kenya, and finally Uganda, and his account is a fine amalgam of whimsical travelogue and incisive science. A lengthier version appears in his book *African Madness* (New York: Knopf, 1988).

30. See R. Hayes et al., "A Community Trial of the Impact of Improved Sexually Transmitted Disease Treatment on the HIV Epidemic in Rural Tanzania; 1. Design," *AIDS*, 1995, 9, 919–926, and its sequel by H. Grosskurth et al., "2. Baseline survey results," *AIDS*, 1995, 9, 927–934.

31. E. Hooper, *Slim*, pp. 59–60.

32. *Chambers's World Gazetteer and Geographical Dictionary* (London: Chambers, 1957), p. 717.

33. L. Garrett, "The Fatal Curse of Juliana's Cloth," see pp. 3 and 26. A fuller version is given later in Laurie Garrett's book *The Coming Plague — Newly Emerging Diseases in a World out of Balance* (New York: Farrar, Straus and Giroux, 1994), pp. 334–335.

34. Margerete Bundschuh, personal communication, 1995.

35.  This same phrase was also used by a nurse who had tended to many of the early AIDS patients in Rakai district.

36.  Rand Stoneburner, of the WHO Global Programme on AIDS, and Daniel Low-Beer, of Cambridge University Department of Geography, personal communications, 1995 and 1996.

37.  T. Barnett and P. Blaikie, *AIDS in Africa,* pp. 74–75.

38.  Margerete Bundschuh and Bill Hamilton, personal communications, 1995, citing information from Tanzanian and Ugandan locals, respectively.

39.  Full title: President for Life Field Marshal Al Hadj Dr Idi Amin Dada, VC, DSO, MC, Lord of All the Beasts of the Earth and Fishes of the Sea, Last King of Scotland, Conqueror of the British Empire in Africa in General and Uganda in Particular. Source: G. Foden, "Who Else Was Out to Get Amin?," *Guardian* (U.K.), September 21, 1996.

40.  See T. Avirgan and M. Honey, *War in Uganda — The Legacy of Idi Amin* (Dar es Salaam: Tanzania Publishing House, 1982). This is an outstanding eyewitness account of the 1978/9 war, and, as far as I know, the only such detailed account to appear in print. Most of the background information about the war has been drawn from this excellent source.

41.  A few hundred Ugandan liberation fighters also assembled in Kagera and later joined the invasion force.

42.  L. Garrett, "The Fatal Curse of Juliana's Cloth," see pp. 3 and 26.

43.  Jack Walden says he left 100 to 200 men behind at Katera to cover the brigade's rear, and that this unit was moved back to Kyaka bridge sometime during 1979. (Personal communication, March 1997.) However, local residents recall a much larger number of TPDF soldiers, and say that most of them moved down to a new camp beside Kyebe trading center. (Bill Hamilton, personal communication, August 1995.)

44.  N. Miller and R. Yeager, "By Virtue of Their Occupation, Soldiers and Sailors Are at Greater Risk," *AIDS Analysis Asia,* 1995, 1(6), 8–9.

45.  M. Musagara, S. Okware et al., "Sero-prevalence of HIV-1 in Rakai District, Uganda," *4th International Conference on AIDS and Associated Cancers in Africa* (Marseilles), 1989, poster 010, p. 117 of abstracts. See also T. Barnett and P. Blaikie, *AIDS in Africa,* p. 36.

46.  A. Dunn, S. Hunter et al., "Enumeration and Needs Assessment of Orphans in Uganda — Survey Report, April 1991," Save the Children Fund (social work department), Kampala, Uganda, 1991, pp. iv and 49.

47.  V. Asedri, "790,522 Ugandans Are HIV Positive," *New Vision* (Uganda), December 1, 1989, 4(271), 1, quoted in part in *Slim,* by E. Hooper, pp. 380–381. Also see HIV/AIDS Surveillance Database, available from Health Studies Branch, International Programs Center, Population Division, U.S. Bureau of the Census, Washington, D.C. 20233-8860. Phone: (301) 457-1406. Fax: (301) 457-3034. Updated at regular intervals.

48.  J. W. Carswell, "HIV Infection in Healthy Persons in Uganda," *AIDS,* 1987, 1, 223–227; and E. Hale, "Uganda in the Front Line in Battle against AIDS," *Reporter-Dispatch* (White Plains, N.Y.), October 11, 1987. This latter article apparently includes some of the early results of Uganda's national serosurvey, for Masaka and Tororo districts. By 1992, there were indications that these early regional variations might already have disappeared, which only reinforces the importance of early serological data for tracking the initial footprints of HIV within a community. One can only imagine what insights a national survey of blood conducted in 1982 might have provided.

49.  D. Serwadda et al., "Slim Disease: A New Disease in Uganda and Its Association with HTLV-III Infection."

50.  E. Hooper, *Slim,* pp. 98–107, 250, 278–286.

51. For instance, in December 1990 Uganda announced a total of 21,719 AIDS cases, and Tanzania announced 21,208 cases three months later. The national totals have stayed comparable ever since. Tanzania's population is, however, almost half as large again as Uganda's.

52. T. Avirgan and M. Honey, *War in Uganda*, p. 72.

53. In this instance, orphans were defined as children below the age of eighteen who had lost at least one parent.

54. T. Barnett and P. Blaikie, *AIDS in Africa*, pp. 30–31. The survey report by Dunn and Hunter ("Enumeration and Needs Assessment of Orphans in Uganda") incorporates the twenty-one new subcounties of Rakai district, whereas this reference relates to the thirteen subcounties under the old system, but the basic trends remain the same. In this book, only seven representative subcounties have been detailed.

55. M. J. Wawer, N. K. Sewankambo et al., "Dynamics of Spread of HIV Infection in a Rural District of Uganda," *BMJ*, 1991, 303, 1303–1306.

56. W. B. Wood, "AIDS North and South: Diffusion Patterns of a Global Epidemic and a Research Agenda for Geographers," *Professional Geographer*, 1988, 40, 266–269.

57. This is an appropriate place to puncture an important fallacy about HIV epidemiology in Africa — that high HIV prevalence coincides with a trans-African highway running from Mombasa through Nairobi and Kampala and right across to Kinshasa in Congo. This mythical highway was first reported by Sharon Kingman and Steve Connor in their otherwise excellent book *The Search for the Virus* (London: Penguin, 1989, second edition), see figure 19 on p. 213, and their account has since been repeated elsewhere (e.g., G. Myers, "Phylogenetic Moments in the AIDS Epidemic," in S. S. Morse [editor], *Emerging Viruses* [Oxford University Press, 1993], pp. 120–137). This road certainly exists between Mombasa and eastern Congo, and is an important factor in HIV spread, but to the west of this, no very effective highway exists. In actuality, road transport across the great basin of the Congo is nowadays extremely limited, especially in the rainy season, and most human traffic occurs instead on the river ferries.

58. W. Namaara, and F. Plummer et al., "Cross Sectional Study of HIV Infection in South Western Uganda," *Second International Symposium on AIDS and Associated Cancers in Africa* (Naples), 1987, abstract TH-37, p. 91 of abstracts.

59. J. W. Carswell, "HIV Infection in Healthy Persons in Uganda," and E. Hale, "Uganda in the Front Line in Battle Against AIDS."

60. E. Hooper, *Slim*, p. 303.

61. J. W. Carswell et al., "Prevalence of HIV-1 in East African Lorry Drivers," *AIDS*, 1989, 3, 759–761.

62. M. J. Wawer, N. K. Sewankambo et al., "Dynamics of Spread of HIV Infection in a Rural District of Uganda," *BMJ*, 1991, 303, 1303–1306; see map on p. 1304. The same report detailed 50 percent prevalence among adults in Kyotera and 36 percent in Kalisizo adults.

63. Two other hypotheses of spread have also been reported in the literature. One of them, which sought to link reported AIDS cases in Uganda to former patterns of migrant labor, was unpersuasive, since even its author admitted that it was based on an inadequate data base. See C. W. Hunt, "Migrant Labour and Sexually Transmitted Disease: Aids in Africa," *J. Health. Soc. Behav.*, 1989, 30, 353–373. The other was published in 1990 by a team from Cambridge University, who reported that a "highly significant positive correlation" existed between Uganda's 1989 district-by-district totals of reported AIDS cases and recruitment patterns from the early eighties for the former Uganda National Liberation Army (the name of the Ugandan army from the end of the liberation war in 1979 until

1985, when Milton Obote was toppled). The hypothesis was afforded some support by 1987 prevalence data, which revealed high levels of HIV infection around Gulu and Kitgum, the two main towns of Acholi, and in Ankole region, which were the main areas of UNLA recruitment. However, its impact was substantially weakened by the fact that its published version featured a map indicating that its authors had wrongly included Masaka and Rakai — two districts of very high HIV prevalence — in Ankole region. See M. R. Smallman-Raynor and A. D. Cliff, "Civil War and the Spread of AIDS in Central Africa," *Epidemiol. Infect.*, 1991, 107, 69–80.

64.  The Ugandan sex researcher Christine Obbo provides some further support for the above scenario. In an unpublished paper, she analyzes the interplay between cross-border coffee smuggling, fishing, small-time *magendo* (black market trading), and sexual activity, which increasingly obtained in lakeside and border villages from 1975 onward, and has this to say with respect to the 1978/9 war: "During the war, as defeat was [imminent], Amin claimed that his soldiers had reported a strange wasting disease among the Tanzanians across the border. As usual people dismissed this as one of Amin's fantastic claims, but it seems that he was referring to what people now know to be AIDS." This information is unsourced, so it is hard to know whether it is based on historical fact. C. Obbo, "Sexual Relations before AIDS," paper presented at the Seminar on Anthropological Studies Relevant to the Sexual Transmission of HIV (Sonderborg, Denmark, November 19–22, 1990), and available on request from the International Union for the Scientific Study of Population, Rue des Augustins 34, B-4000 Liège, Belgium.

65.  See J. Levy, "HIV Pathogenesis and Long Term Survival," *AIDS*, 1993, 7, 1401–1410, especially figure 2.

66.  R. Shilts, *And the Band Played On*, p. 197 is the source for this rather vivid image.

67.  A. Anzala, F. A. Plummer et al., "Incubation Time to Symptomatic Disease and AIDS in Women with Known Duration of Infection," 7th International Conference on AIDS (Florence, 1991), abstract TUC103. This paper reported that the median interval from seroconversion to AIDS among female prostitutes in Nairobi was forty-five months.

68.  G. W. Rutherford, N. A. Hessol, P. M. O'Malley et al., "Course of HIV Infection in a Cohort of Homosexual and Bisexual Men: An 11 Year Follow Up Study," *BMJ*, 1990, 301, 1183–1188.

69.  Bill Hamilton, personal communication, 1995.

CHAPTER 3: *"A Mysterious Microbe":*
*Early Evidence of AIDS in North America*

1.  R. Shilts, *And the Band Played On: Politics, People and the AIDS Epidemic* (New York: St. Martin's Press, 1987). For all its naming of names and tendency to factionalize, this is an evenhanded and levelheaded Grand Tour through the early years of the recognized epidemic. The book represents the fruit of many years of conscientious research and, despite its several small errors, on the important stuff Shilts almost invariably gets it right. Also worthy of honorable mention is chapter 11 of L. Garrett, *The Coming Plague: Newly Emerging Diseases in a World out of Balance* (New York: Farrar, Straus and Giroux, 1994). This provides a fine, updated overview but, because of its theme, is rather too ready to bracket AIDS conveniently with other emerging viral diseases and, despite its considerable scholarship, is sometimes inaccurate on specifics. Also see L. Kramer, *Reports from the Holocaust: The Story of an AIDS Activist* (New York: St. Martin's Press, 1994); A. G. Fettner

and W. A. Check, *The Truth about AIDS — Evolution of an Epidemic* (New York: Holt, Rinehart and Winston, 1984); and F. and M. Siegal, *AIDS: The Medical Mystery* (New York: Grove Press, 1983). One other noteworthy book is J. Leibowitch, *A Strange Virus of Unknown Origin: A True Medical Detective Story* (New York: Available Press, 1985), which contains many original nuggets of thinking, but an equally large number of factual errors and an extraordinarily flowery writing style, which the translator has done little to improve.

2. M. S. Gottlieb et al., "*Pneumocystis* Pneumonia — Los Angeles," *MMWR,* 1981 (June 5), 30, 250–252. The first published report on AIDS.

3. A. Friedman-Kien, L. Laubenstein, K. Hymes, F. P. Siegal, S. Dritz, M. S. Gottlieb et al., "Kaposi's Sarcoma and *Pneumocystis* Pneumonia Among Homosexual Men — New York City and California," *MMWR,* 1981, 30, 305–308.

4. R. M. Selik, H. W. Haverkos, and J. W. Curran, "Acquired Immune Deficiency (AIDS) Trends in the United States, 1978–1982," *Am. J. Med.,* 1984, 76, 493–500.

5. H. W. Haverkos and J. W. Curran, "The Current Outbreak of Kaposi's Sarcoma and Opportunistic Infections," *CA — a Cancer Journal for Physicians,* 1982, 32(6), 330–339; H. Masur et al., "An Outbreak of Community-Acquired *Pneumocystis Carinii* Pneumonia," *N. Engl. J. Med.,* 1981, 305, 1431–1438.

6. Two patients, for instance, had KS that apparently went into clinical remission after chemotherapy — one was Jewish, and the other an Italian with a history of KS in his family. See K. B. Hymes, L. J. Laubenstein et al., "Kaposi's Sarcoma in Homosexual Men — A Report of Eight Cases," *Lancet,* 1981, 2(i), 598–600. See also H. W. Jaffe, D. J. Bergman, and R. M. Selik, "Acquired Immune Deficiency Syndrome in the United States: The First 1,000 Cases," *J. Infect. Dis.,* 1983, 148(2), 339–345, in which Jaffe comments that some of the sixty-one AIDS patients without apparent risk factors may represent the expected "background" level of KS.

7. See M. S. Weinberg and C. J. Williams, "Gay Baths and the Social Organization of Impersonal Sex," in M. P. Levine (editor), *Gay Men — The Sociology of Male Homosexuality* (New York: Harper and Row, 1979).

8. See R. Shilts, *And the Band Played On,* pp. 19 and 39, where he claims that the average bathhouse patron at this time had a 33 percent chance of leaving the baths infected with either syphilis or gonorrhea.

9. This figure should be viewed in the context of Michael Callen — the singer and long-term AIDS survivor — and Gaetan Dugas, the Canadian air steward, each of whom is reported to have had between 2,500 and 3,000 lifetime partners — or one of the CDC AIDS interviewees of 1982, who had had 2,000 sexual contacts in the previous year alone. See L. Garrett, *The Coming Plague,* p. 271; and M. Callen, *Surviving AIDS* (New York: HarperCollins, 1990). Also see R. Shilts, *And the Band Played On,* pp. 83 and 132.

10. F. P. Siegal, D. Armstrong et al., "Severe Acquired Immunodeficiency in Male Homosexuals, Manifested by Chronic Perianal Ulcerative Herpes Simplex Lesions," *N. Engl. J. Med.,* 1981, 305(24), 1439–1444. Also see F. Siegal and M. Siegal, *AIDS: The Medical Mystery,* pp. 1–12.

11. The 1993 case definition for AIDS issued by the CDC involves essentially the same opportunistic infections (or else a single CD4+ lymphocyte count below 200) in an HIV-positive person. CD4 count and HIV status are now officially enshrined within the case definition of AIDS. See S. B. Harris, "The AIDS Heresies," *Skeptic,* 1995, 3(2), 42–79, especially Figure 1.

12. H. W. Jaffe, W. W. Darrow, J. W. Curran et al. "National Case-Control Study of Kaposi's Sarcoma and *Pneumocystis Carinii* Pneumonia in Homosexual Men: Part 1,

Epidemiological Results," *Ann. Intern. Med.,* 1983, 99(2), 145–151, Table 1 of which features one of the earliest AIDS case definitions published by a member of the CDC AIDS task force. For an updated case definition, including CD4+ T-lymphocyte categories, see *MMWR,* 1992, 41, RR–17, 1–19.

13. For this useful term I am indebted to Alex Shoumatoff's "In Search of the Source of AIDS," in *African Madness* (New York: Knopf, 1988).

14. See H. W. Jaffe et al., "AIDS in the United States."

15. H. H. Neumann, "Use of Steroid Creams as a Possible Cause of Immunosuppression in Homosexuals" (letter), *N. Engl. J. Med.,* 1982, 306(15), 935.

16. W. W. Darrow, "Time-Space Clustering of KS Cases in the City of New York: Evidence for Horizontal Transmission of Some Mysterious Microbe," CDC memorandum to Chairman, Task Force on Kaposi's Sarcoma and Opportunistic Infections, March 3, 1982.

17. Descriptions of these and other gay establishments mentioned in this chapter are contained in *Bob Damron's Address Book #80,* published in 1980 by Bob Damron Enterprises Inc., P.O. Box 14-077, San Francisco, CA 94114.

18. D. M. Auerbach, W. W. Darrow, H. W. Jaffe, and J. W. Curran, "Cluster of Cases of the Acquired Immune Deficiency Syndrome — Patients Linked by Sexual Contact," *Am. J. Med.,* 1984, 76, 487–492.

19. See W. W. Darrow, "AIDS: Socioepidemiological Responses to an Epidemic," which is chapter 6 in W. F. Skinner (editor), *AIDS and the Social Sciences: Common Threads* (Lexington: University Press of Kentucky, 1991).

20. See p. 101 of W. W. Darrow et al., "The Social Origins of AIDS: Social Change, Sexual Behavior, and Disease Trends," which is chapter 5 in D. A. Feldman and T. M. Johnson (editors), *The Social Dimensions of AIDS: Method and Theory* (New York: Praeger, 1986).

21. See the various figures on pp. 88 and 89 of Darrow, "AIDS: Socioepidemiological Responses to an Epidemic."

22. These are numbered chronologically, NY1 to NY22, according to date of onset of symptoms, in the accompanying diagram.

23. The hairdresser Michael Maletta, who — apart from Dugas — is the only individual in the cluster to link patients from Los Angeles and New York.

24. For instance, W. W. Darrow, "Trip Report to New York City July 12–16 and August 3–6, 1982," CDC memorandum to Coordinator, CDC Task Force on AIDS, September 3, 1982. In the course of three interviews and a lengthy correspondence, Bill Darrow has also provided a great deal of very helpful background information, while taking care not to identify individual patients.

25. R. Shilts, *And the Band Played On,* pp. 438–439.

26. One of the best studies, from the researchers at the San Francisco City Clinic, concluded that 51 percent of HIV-positive men progress to AIDS within ten years of infection. See G. W. Rutherford, N. A. Hessol, P. M. O'Malley et al., "Course of HIV-1 Infection in a Cohort of Homosexual and Bisexual Men: An 11 Year Follow Up Study," *BMJ,* 1990, 301, 1183–1187.

27. See P. Ewald, *Evolution of Infectious Diseases* (Oxford: Oxford University Press, 1994), especially pp. 125–127 and 135–136.

28. These are NY1 (the black air steward who frequently visited Haiti), NY5 (Nick Rock, a frequent visitor to the Caribbean in the seventies, when he was employed on all-gay cruises), NY9 (the French ballet instructor), NY11 ("Cosmic Energy," as he was nicknamed, whose myriad sexual partners included NY17 and probably Michael Maletta, Nick, and Enno, between 1976 and 1977), NY14 (the link between the "heavy sex group"

and the "trend setters"), NY17 (the Pleasure Chest employee), NY18 (an Italian who was a member of FFA between 1976 and 1978), and NJ1 (about whom little documentation is available, but who may conceivably have been a drug injector — as were many of the early New Jersey cases — and who apparently contracted AIDS in 1978).

29. Criteria for inclusion in the cluster were, Darrow says, "very rigid." There had to be "reciprocity in the naming process," or, if one partner was dead, the contact had to be confirmed by a close friend. Dugas was himself suspected of having had at least two other direct contacts within the cluster.

30. In reality (as detailed in chapter 1) this man was Jamaican, but moved to Haiti in childhood.

31. G. N. Stemmermann et al., "Cryptosporidiosis — Report of a Fatal Case Complicated by Disseminated Toxoplasmosis," *Am. J. Med.,* 1980, 69, 637–642.

32. L. R. Smith and C. L. Heaton, "Actinomycosis Presenting as Wegener's Granulomatosis," *JAMA,* 1978, 240(3), 247–248.

33. M. Elwin-Lewis et al., "Systemic Chlamydial Infection Associated with Generalized Lymphedema and Lymphangiosarcoma," *Lymphology,* 1973, 6(3), 113–121.

34. L. Weinstein et al., "Intestinal Cryptosporidiosis Complicated by Disseminated Cytomegalovirus Infection," *Gastroenterology,* 1981, 81, 584–591.

35. Even earlier American AIDS cases from the mid-seventies have been mooted by interested observers who are not themselves physicians (such as writers and journalists), but seem to be anecdotal and unreliable. Such reports include that of a baby with PCP born in 1976 to a drug-injecting mother in San Francisco (J. Adams, *AIDS: The HIV Myth* [London: Macmillan, 1989], p. 184), or AIDS in 1976 in an intravenous drug user (A. Shoumatoff, *African Madness* [New York: Knopf, 1988], p. 163). The normally reliable John Crewdson refers to a suspected 1975 case of AIDS presenting as PCP in a previously healthy black infant of seven months living in New York City ("How Long Has Virus Been Stalking Victims?," *Chicago Tribune,* October 25, 1987, p. 20), but the original report of the case makes it clear that the infant enjoyed a full recovery after treatment (M. Rao et al., "*Pneumocystis Carinii* Pneumonia: Occurrence in a Healthy American Infant," *JAMA,* 1977, 238, 2301).

36. B. L. Evatt et al., "Coincidental Appearance of LAV/ HTLV-III Antibodies in Hemophiliacs and the Onset of the AIDS Epidemic," *N. Engl. J. Med.,* 1985, 312(8), 483–486.

37. J. W. Curran, B. L. Evatt et al., "AIDS Associated with Transfusions," *N. Engl. J. Med.,* 1984, 310(2), 69–75.

38. A direct ELISA antibody test; see chapter 7.

39. H. W. Jaffe, W. W. Darrow et al., "The Acquired Immunodeficiency Syndrome in a Cohort of Homosexual Men: A Six-Year Follow-Up Study," *Ann. Intern. Med.,* 1985, 103, 210–214.

40. IFA and Western blot; see chapter 7.

41. Paul O'Malley, personal communication, 1995. See also G. W. Rutherford, P. M. O'Malley et al., "Course of HIV-1 Infection in a Cohort of Homosexual and Bisexual Men: An 11 Year Follow Up Study."

42. C. E. Stevens et al., "Human T-Cell Lymphotropic Type III Infection in a Cohort of Homosexual Men in New York City," *JAMA,* 1986, 255(16), 2167–2172.

43. Cladd Stevens, personal communication, 1995.

44. J. D. Moore, E. J. Cone, and S. S. Alexander, "HTLV-III Seropositivity in 1971–1972 Parenteral Drug Abusers — a Case of False Positives or Viral Exposure?" (letter), *N. Engl. J. Med.,* 1986, 314, 1387–1388; also James Moore and Steve Alexander, personal communications, 1991.

45. W. R. Lange et al., "Followup Study of Possible HIV Seropositivity among Abusers of Parenteral Drugs in 1971–72," *Public Health Reports* (Washington), 1991, 106(4), 451–455.

46. One hopes that additional sera from the seventies will be tested in future — including some of the samples taken from thirteen thousand gay New York men from 1974 to 1978, as part of the hepatitis B vaccine baseline studies. See W. Szmuness, C. E. Stevens et al., "A Controlled Clinical Trial of the Efficacy of the Hepatitis B Vaccine (Heptavax B): A Final Report," *Hepatology*, 1981, 1(5), 377–385.

47. Pauline Thomas and Renée Quintine-Grey (New York City Department of Health), personal communications, 1995. See also P. Thomas et al., "HIV Infection in Heterosexual Female Intravenous Drug Users in New York City, 1977–1980" (letter), *N. Engl. J. Med.*, 1988, 319(6), 374.

48. L. Garrett, *The Coming Plague*, p. 310.

49. Art Ammann, Selma Dritz, and Jay Levy, personal communications, 1995.

50. H. Burger et al., "Long HIV-1 Incubation Periods and Dynamics of Transmission Within a Family," *Lancet*, 1990, 336, 134–136; and Harold Burger, personal communication, 1993. This, the only early pediatric case to be written up in detail, involves a child who was born in December 1977 and who was found to be HIV-positive (but symptom-free) in 1990. Her brother, born in 1973, is HIV-negative. Her mother was an intravenous drug user in New York City between 1975 and 1977, and was married to a fellow drug injector, whom she left when she became pregnant with her daughter. The mother is HIV-positive and in 1990 developed PCP. Her live-in lover from 1978 to 1988, whose only discernible risk factor was heterosexual contact with the woman, was also found to be HIV-positive in 1988, shortly before he died of AIDS.

51. For instance, 10 percent of the original fifty GRID cases assessed in the national case-control study had used heroin on at least one occasion. See H. W. Jaffe, W. W. Darrow, J. W. Curran et al., "National Case-Control Study of Kaposi's Sarcoma and *Pneumocystis Carinii* Pneumonia in Homosexual Men: Part 1, Epidemiological Results," *Ann. Intern. Med.*, 1983, 99(2), 145–151; see Table 4.

52. See M. Bulterys et al., "HIV-1 Seroconversion after 20 Months of Age in a Cohort of Breastfed Children Born to HIV-1-Infected Women in Rwanda" (letter), *AIDS*, 1995, 9(1), 93–94.

53. P. Thomas et al., "HIV Infection in Heterosexual Female Intravenous Drug Users in New York City, 1977–1980."

54. See, however, R. F. Garry et al., "Documentation of an AIDS Virus Infection in the United States in 1968," *JAMA*, 1988, 260(14), 2085–2087. But, as revealed later in the book, there is some uncertainty about the validity of the results.

55. See J. Leibowitch, *A Strange Virus of Unknown Origin*, pp. 62–64; and S. Garfield, *The End of Innocence: Britain in the Time of AIDS* (London: Faber and Faber, 1994), pp. 60–69.

CHAPTER 4: *High Days and Holidays — The Haitian Interchange*

1. J. D. Stamford (editor), *Spartacus International Gay Guide*, 11th edition (Amsterdam: Spartacus, 1981).

2. P. Farmer, *AIDS and Accusation: Haiti and the Geography of Blame* (University of California Press, 1992), see especially pp. 145–147.

3. Surgeon Ralph Greco, who visited the island annually from 1976, claimed in 1983 that it had become "a very popular holiday resort for Americans [gays] . . . during the last

five years." See R. Greco, "Haiti and the Stigma of AIDS" (letter), *Lancet,* 1983, 2(ii), 515–516.

4. This was certainly the case in 1980, for in that year one of Bill Darrow's New York interviewees took a Caribbean cruise on board the newly relaunched luxury liner S.S. *Norway,* and stopped off for several nights in Port-au-Prince, where he had sex with four or five different men. The man developed KS two years later, though whether he was infected before or after his visit to Haiti is, of course, a moot point. W. W. Darrow, personal communication, 1995.

5. See A.-C. d'Adesky, "Silence + Death = AIDS in Haiti," *Advocate,* 1991, 507, 30–36. Also see P. Farmer, *AIDS and Accusation,* p. 147.

6. There had been even earlier warnings. In February 1981 a bodyguard to President Jean-Claude Duvalier flew to New York from Port-au-Prince, to be treated for disseminated candidiasis and tuberculosis that proved to be refractive to treatment. R. Shilts, *And the Band Played On* (New York: St Martin's Press, 1987), p. 56.

7. A. E. Pitchenik et al., "Opportunistic Infections and Kaposi's Sarcoma among Haitians: Evidence of a New Acquired Immunodeficiency State," *Ann. Intern. Med.,* 1983, 98(3), 277–284. J. Vieira, S. H. Landesman et al., "Acquired Immune Deficiency in Haitains — Opportunistic Infections in Previously Healthy Haitian Immigrants," *N. Engl. J. Med.,* 1983, 308(3), 125–129. G. T. Hensley et al., "Opportunistic Infections and Kaposi's Sarcoma among Haitians in the United States," *MMWR,* 1982, 31, 353–361.

8. R. Shilts, *And the Band Played On,* p. 135; and W. W. Darrow, personal comunication.

9. Letter from A. Friedman-Kien to J. Curran and W. Darrow, July 9, 1982.

10. P. Farmer, *AIDS and Accusation,* p. 146.

11. Anon., "Acquired Immunodeficiency Syndrome (AIDS) Update — United States," *MMWR,* 1983, 32, 309–311.

12. A. DeLand and A. Campbell, *Fielding Travel Guides: Worldwide Cruises 1994* (Fielding Worldwide Inc., 1994), pp. 178–179.

13. Anon., "If It's Tuesday, This Can't Be Haiti," *Sunday Punch* (San Francisco), March 31, 1991.

14. Examples: P. Moses and J. Moses, "Haiti and the Acquired Immunodeficiency Syndrome" (letter), *Ann. Intern. Med.,* 1983, 99(4), 565; and J.-L. Leonidas et al., "Haiti and the Acquired Immunodeficiency Syndrome" (letter), *Ann. Intern. Med.,* 1983, 98, 1020–1021. The most detailed of such theories appears as: A. Moore and R. D. Le Baron, "The Case for a Haitian Origin of the AIDS Epidemic," in D. A. Feldman and T. M. Johnson (editors), *The Social Dimensions of AIDS: Method and Theory* (New York: Praeger, 1986), pp. 77–94. G. W. Shannon et al., *The Geography of AIDS — Origins and Course of an Epidemic* (Guildford Press, 1990) is also worth a look; in chapter 3, the Moore/Le Baron hypothesis — involving the use of animal blood in voodoo ceremonies, homosexuality among voodoo priests, increasing levels of gay tourism from North America, and Haitian migration to (not from) central Africa — is summarized and then refuted (see pp. 40–45).

15. Letter from W. R. Greenfield, *JAMA,* 1986, 256(16), 2199–2200.

16. L. K. Altman, "The Confusing Haitian Connection to AIDS," *New York Times,* August 16, 1983, p. C2; see also R. Greco, "Haiti and the Stigma of AIDS."

17. Anon., "Update: Acquired Immunodeficiency Syndrome — United States," *MMWR,* 1985, 34, 245–248.

18. R. Sabatier, *Blaming Others: Prejudice, Race and Worldwide AIDS* (London: Panos Publications Ltd., 1988), p. 43.

19. J. W. Pape et al., "Risk Factors Associated With AIDS in Haiti," *Am. J. Med. Sci.,* 1986, 29(1), 4–7. For sound analysis on why many Haitian men denied homosexuality or

bisexuality, see V. Casper, "AIDS: A Psycho-Social Perspective," chapter 11 of D. A. Feldman & T. M. Johnson, *The Social Dimensions of AIDS,* especially pp. 198–201.

20.  A. G. Fettner and W. A. Check, *The Truth About AIDS — Evolution of an Epidemic* (New York: Holt, Rinehart and Winston, 1984), pp. 115–117. See also R. Bazell, "The History of an Epidemic," *New Republic,* August 1, 1983, pp. 14–18.

21.  J. W. Pape et al., "Characteristics of the Acquired Immunodeficiency Syndrome (AIDS) in Haiti," *N. Engl. J. Med.,* 1983, 309(16), 945–950.

22.  G. E. Noel, "Another Case of AIDS in the Pre-AIDS Era," *Rev. Infect. Dis.,* 1988, 10(3), 688–689; M. Laverdiere et al., "AIDS in Haitian Immigrants and in a Caucasian Woman Closely Associated with Haitians," *Can. Med. Assoc. J.,* 1983, 129, 1209–1212. See also A. E. Pitchenik et al., "Opportunistic Infections and Kaposi's Sarcoma among Haitians," Table 1, patient 12.

23.  J. W. Pape and T. M. Johnson, "Epidemiology of AIDS in the Caribbean," quoted in P. Farmer, *AIDS and Accusation,* p. 131.

24.  The Collaborative Study Group of AIDS in Haitian-Americans, "Risk Factors for AIDS among Haitians Residing in the United States — Evidence for Heterosexual Transmission," *JAMA,* 1987, 257(5), 635–639.

25.  J. B. Schorr et al., "Prevalence of HTLV-III Antibody in American Blood Donors" (letter), *N. Engl. J. Med.,* 1985, 313(6), 384–385.

26.  See V. Casper, "AIDS: A Psycho-Social Perspective," in D. A. Feldman and T. M. Johnson, *The Social Dimensions of AIDS,* p. 199.

27.  He is said to have previously been a virgin (F. P. Siegal and M. Siegal, *AIDS: The Medical Mystery* [New York: Grove Press, 1983], p. 85), and he denied homosexual activity or other risk factors. See also J. Andreani et al., "Acquired Immunodeficiency with Intestinal Cryptosporidiosis: Possible Transmission by Haitian Whole Blood," *Lancet,* 1983, 1(ii), 1187–1191; and J. Leibowitch, *A Strange Virus of Unknown Origin* (New York: Available Press, 1985), pp. 30–31.

28.  Both these cases are mentioned in B. Somaini, "Acquired Immunodeficiency Syndrome in Switzerland," *Eur. J. Clin. Microbiol.,* 1984, 3(1), 67; see Table 1.

29.  D. B. Rose and J. S. Keystone, "AIDS in a Canadian Woman Who Had Helped Prostitutes in Port-au-Prince" (letter), *Lancet,* 1983, 2(i), 680–681. See also J. Leibowitch, *A Strange Virus of Unknown Origin,* p. 28.

30.  J. Leibowitch, *A Strange Virus of Unknown Origin,* pp. 63–64.

31.  P. Hagen, *Blood: Gift or Merchandise — Towards an International Blood Policy* (New York: Alan R. Liss, 1982), pp. 166–168.

32.  See, for instance, R. Severo, "Impoverished Haitians Sell Plasma for Use in the U.S.," *New York Times,* January 28, 1972, p. 2. This reveals that some 350 Haitians a day had, since May 1971, been selling their plasma to Hemo-Caribbean for four to five dollars a liter, that between five thousand and six thousand liters a month were exported to the United States and another four thousand liters to Germany and Sweden. Those selling their plasma were "among the nation's poorest and most backward citizens," among whom TB, tetanus, gastrointestinal diseases, and malnutrition were prevailing conditions, but the company's technical director assured the writer that "few, if any, diseased persons slip through."

33.  B. L. Evatt et al., "Coincidental Appearance of LAV/HTLV-III Antibodies in Hemophiliacs and the Onset of the AIDS Epidemic," *N. Engl. J. Med.,* 1985, 312(8), 483–486.

34.  A. Stepick, "Haitian Refugees in the U.S.," Minority Rights Group (London), Report No. 52, 1982, pp. 9–12.

35.  Arthur Pitchenik, personal communication, 1995.

36. S. Landesman, "The Haitian Connection," chapter 3 of K. M. Cahill, *The AIDS Epidemic* (London: Hutchinson, 1984).

37. M. Laverdiere, "AIDS in Haitian Immigrants and in a Caucasian Woman."

38. L. Gazzolo et al., "Antibodies to HTLV-III in Haitian Immigrants in French Guiana" (letter), *N. Engl. J. Med.,* 1984, 311(19), 1252–1253.

39. Analysis of data from Pape ("Characteristics of AIDS in Haiti") on early cases of AIDS seen in Haiti. In addition, F. P. Siegal and M. Siegal, *AIDS: the Medical Mystery,* p. 70, relates the story of a woman from Haiti's neighbor, the Dominican Republic, who developed AIDS-like symptoms in New York in 1979. Dr. Siegal tells me that the woman's stored blood proved to be HIV-positive when tested five years later.

40. For further discussion of this hypothesis see Pape, "Characteristics of AIDS in Haiti" and P. Farmer, *AIDS and Accusation,* pp. 130–140.

41. *Vodun* helped millions of slaves cope with the dreadful tortures and oppression of plantation life, and eventually provided the political framework that enabled these slaves to organize and overthrow their despotic masters — to become the first independent black state in the New World. See the excellent R. I. Rotberg, "Vodun and the Politics of Haiti," in M. L. Kilson and R. I. Rotberg (editors), *The African Diaspora* (Cambridge: Harvard University Press, 1986), pp. 342–365.

42. See J. W. Pape and T. M. Johnson, "Epidemiology of AIDS in the Caribbean," p. 39.

43. How many Haitians actually worked in the Congo during the sixties and seventies is a moot point. I have been unable to procure any official figures, and the estimates in different books vary wildly. Jacques Leibowitch and Robert Gallo appear to have been the first to receive credit for the theory in print (see J. Seligmann et al., "Tracing the Origins of AIDS," *Newsweek,* May 7, 1984, pp. 62–63), but they do not specify a figure. In "Acquired Immunodeficiency Syndrome in a Heterosexual Population in Zaire," *Lancet,* 1984, 2(i), 68, Peter Piot writes of "several thousand professional people [going] from Haiti to Congo between the early 1960s and the mid-1970s," and this is probably the best estimate.

44. Boris Velimirovic, personal communication, 1993.

45. See The Collaborative Study Group of AIDS in Haitian-Americans, "Risk Factors for AIDS among Haitians Residing in the United States," especially Table 5 on page 638.

46. According to Harold Jaffe, the consultant on the project, "we no longer have the raw data." Harold Jaffe, personal communication, 1995.

47. R. Shilts, *And the Band Played On,* p. 50; and D. Mildvan, "Opportunistic Infections and Immune Deficiency in Homosexual Men," *Ann. Intern. Med.,* 1982, 96(1), 700–704; (see Patient 2, p. 701).

48. Donna Mildvan, personal communications, 1995.

CHAPTER 5: *Early Traces in Europe*

1. R. M. Du Bois et al., "Primary *Pneumocystis carinii* and Cytomegalovirus Infections" (letter), *Lancet,* 1981, 2(ii), 1339.

2. David S., personal communication, 1994.

3. Ib Bygbjerg, personal communication, and R. Shilts, *And the Band Played On* (New York: St. Martin's Press, 1987), pp. 34–35. Of course, it may be that an early American visitor (such as Gaetan Dugas in 1977) had already seeded the virus in Denmark.

4. J. Gerstoft, I. Bygbjerg et al., "Severe Acquired Immunodeficiency in European Homosexual Men," *BMJ,* 1982, 285, 17–19.

5. R. J. Biggar et al., "Low T-Lymphocyte Ratios in Homosexual Men — Epidemiologic Evidence for a Transmissible Agent," *JAMA,* 1984, 251(11), 1441–1446.

6. B. D. Bultmann, K. Kratzsch, H. Heimpel et al., "Disseminated Mycobacterial Histiocytosis Due to M. Fortuitum Associated with Helper T-Lymphocyte Immune Deficiency," *Virchows Arch. (Pathol. Anat.),* 1982, 395, 217–225; plus Hermann Heimpel, personal communications, 1995.

7. W. Sterry et al., "Kaposi-Sarkom und aplastische Panzytopenie — Gleichzeitiges Auftreten bei einem Patienten," *Der Hautarzt,* 1979, 30, 540–543.

8. W. Sterry et al., "Kaposi's Sarcoma, Aplastic Pancytopenia, and Multiple Infections in a Homosexual (Cologne, 1976)," *Lancet,* 1983, 1(ii), 924–925.

9. Wolfram Sterry, personal communication, 1993.

10. Indeed, one of the earliest papers on the European epidemic, Anon., "The Epidemiology of AIDS in Europe," *Eur. J. Cancer Clin. Oncol.,* 1984, 20(2), 157–167, remarks on the early evidence of AIDS in Europe (especially Germany and France) and adds that, by contrast, "[i]t is peculiar that very early cases have not been reported among US citizens."

11. Donna Mildvan, personal communication, 1995.

12. J. L'age-Stehr, "Acquired Immune Deficiency Syndrome in the Federal Republic of Germany," *Eur. J. Clin. Microbiol.,* 1984, 3(1), 61.

13. M. P. Glauser and P. Francioli, "Clinical and Epidemiological Survey of Acquired Immune Deficiency Syndrome in Europe," *Eur. J. Clin. Microbiol.,* 1984, 3(1), 55–58.

14. J. B. Brunet, "Acquired Immune Deficiency Syndrome in France," *Eur. J. Clin. Microbiol.,* 1984, 3(1), 66.

15. A good demonstration of the fact that KS in a gay man is not always a reliable marker of AIDS can be found in the early papers by the Brunet group. They feature the case of a widely traveled gay Frenchman who developed AIDS-like opportunistic infections in 1982, but who had been diagnosed with KS a full decade earlier, in 1972. Although it is possible that he already had AIDS in 1972, it is in retrospect much more likely that he was first exposed to the KS agent (perhaps in the late sixties) and only later on to HIV. See J. Brunet et al., "AIDS in France: The African Hypothesis," chapter 42 of A. Friedman-Kien (editor), *The Epidemiology of Kaposi's Sarcoma and Opportunistic Infections* (Chicago: Year Book Medical Publishers, 1984).

16. J. B. Brunet, J. Leibowitch et al., "Acquired Immunodeficiency Syndrome in France," *Lancet,* 1983, 1(i), 700–701; J. Leibowitch, *A Strange Virus of Unknown Origin* (New York: Available Press, 1984), p. 23; and D. Brenky and O. Zemor, *La Route du SIDA: enquête sur une grande peur* (Paris: Londreys, 1985), p. 30.

17. A. G. Saimot, J. Leibowitch et al., "HIV-2/LAV-2 in Portuguese Man with AIDS (Paris, 1978) Who Served in Angola in 1968–74" (letter), *Lancet,* 1987, 1(i), 688.

18. J. B. Brunet et al., "AIDS in France: The African Hypothesis."

19. N. Clumeck et al., "Acquired Immune Deficiency Syndrome in Black Africans" (letter), *Lancet,* 1983, 1(i), 642.

20. I. C. Bygbjerg, "AIDS in a Danish Surgeon (Zaire, 1976)" (letter), *Lancet,* 1983, 1(ii), 925.

21. J. Vandepitte et al., "AIDS and Cryptococcosis (Zaire, 1977)" (letter), *Lancet,* 1983, 1(ii), 925–926.

22. N. Clumeck, J. Sonnet et al., "Acquired Immunodeficiency Syndrome in African Patients," *N. Engl. J. Med.,* 1984, 310(8), 492–497; see p. 493.

23. N. Clumeck, "Acquired Immune Deficiency Syndrome in Belgium," *Eur. J. Clin. Microbiol.,* 1984, 3(1), 59–60.

24. N. Clumeck et al., "Acquired Immune Deficiency Syndrome in Black Africans."

25. J. B. Brunet, "Acquired Immune Deficiency Syndrome in France."

26. M. McEvoy, "Acquired Immune Deficiency Syndrome in the United Kingdom," *Eur. J. Clin. Microbiol.*, 1984, 3(1), 63–64. However, the U.K. figure was not entirely accurate. In 1984, various letters and articles were published about the first British patient to have been diagnosed with AIDS, a Scott who appears to have been infected in Tanzania in 1979 or 1980.

27. S. S. Frøland, K. W. Wefring, T. Bøhmer et al., "HIV-1 Infection in Norwegian Family before 1970" (letter), *Lancet*, 1988, 1(ii), 1344–1345.

CHAPTER 6: *HIV and AIDS in Central Africa*

1. A. C. Bayley, "Aggressive Kaposi's Sarcoma in Zambia," *Lancet*, 1984, 1(ii), 1318–1320. See also A. C. Bayley, R. G. Downing et al., "HTLV-III Serology Distinguishes Typical and Endemic Kaposi's Sarcoma in Africa," *Lancet*, 1985, 1(i), 359–361; and L. K. Altman, "New Form of Cancer Seen in African AIDS Patients," *New York Times*, December 9, 1985, pp. A1 and B10.

2. Anne Bayley, personal communication, 1996.

3. Michael Rolfe, personal communication, 1989.

4. E. Hooper, "AIDS Epidemic Moves South through Africa," *New Scientist*, July 7, 1990, p. 22.

5. P. Piot, F. A. Plummer et al., "Retrospective Seroepidemiology of AIDS Virus Infection in Nairobi Populations," *J. Infect. Dis.*, 1987, 155(6), 1108–1112.

6. A. O. K. Obel et al., "Acquired Immunodeficiency Syndrome in an African," *E. Af. Med. J.*, 1984, 61(9), 724–727.

7. D. Serwadda, N. K. Sewankambo, A. Lwegaba, J. W. Carswell et al., "Slim Disease: A New Disease in Uganda and Its Association with HTLV-III Infection," *Lancet*, 1985, 2(ii), 849–852.

8. T. Jonkheer et al., "Cluster of HTLV-III Infection in an African Family," *Lancet*, 1985, 1(i), 400–401.

9. A somewhat inaccurate version of this case appears in J. Leibowitch, *A Strange Virus of Unknown Origin* (New York: Available Press, 1985), p. 24. This fuller account represents a personal communication from Ib Bygbjerg, 1993.

10. P. Riley, "AIDS Epidemic Threatens to Sweep Central Africa," *Sunday Times* (U.K.), October 13, 1985.

11. P. Van de Perre, N. Clumeck et al., "Female Prostitutes: A Risk Group for Infection with Human T-Cell Lymphotropic Virus Type III," *Lancet*, 1985, 2(i), 524–527.

12. M. Bulterys, P. Van de Perre et al., "Long-term Survival among HIV-1-Infected Prostitutes" (letter), *AIDS*, 1993, 7, 1269. Unfortunately, no further information on T-cell count or HIV status was provided for the survivors.

13. Rwandan HIV Seroprevalence Study Group, "Nationwide Community-Based Serological Survey of HIV-1 and Other Human Retrovirus Infections in a Central African Country," *Lancet*, 1989, 1(ii), 941–943.

14. G. Bugingo et al., "Etude sur la seropositivité liée a l'infection au Virus de l'Immuno-deficiencé Humaine au Rwanda," *Rev. Méd. Rwanda*, 1988, 20(54), 37–42.

15. For a dramatic example of urban-to-rural spread, see P. Van de Perre et al., "HIV Antibodies in a Remote Rural Area in Rwanda: An Analysis of Potential Risk Factors for HIV Seropositivity," *AIDS*, 1987, 1, 213–215.

16. N. Clumeck et al., "AIDS in Black Africans," *Lancet*, 1983, 1(i), 642; and J. B. Brunet et al., "Acquired Immunodeficiency Syndrome in France," *Lancet*, 1983, 1(i), 700–701.

17. T. C. Quinn, J. M. Mann, J. W. Curran, and P. Piot, "AIDS in Africa: An Epidemiological Paradigm," *Science*, 1986, 234, 955–963.

18. The location of this one rural case could be significant in the light of information revealed later in the book.

19. P. Van de Perre, P. Lepage, N. Clumeck et al., "Acquired Immunodeficiency Syndrome in Rwanda," *Lancet*, 1984, 2(i), 62–65.

20. P. Piot, J. B. McCormick et al., "Acquired Immunodeficiency Syndrome in a Heterosexual Population in Zaire," *Lancet*, 1984, 2(i), 65–69.

21. B. Lamey and N. Melameka, "Aspects cliniques et épidémiologiques de la cryptococcose à Kinshasa — à propos de 15 cas personnels," *Méd. Trop.*, 1982, 42(5), 507–511. The eighteen-month period during which the fifteen patients were observed is not specified, but Vandepitte's 1985 presentation (see n. 22) records a sudden increase in cryptococcal meningitis cases in Kinshasa in 1978, which suggests that the Lamey study may well have started then.

22. Additional information is provided by J. Vandepitte et al., "Cryptococcal Meningitis and AIDS in Kinshasa, Zaire," [First] International Symposium on African AIDS (Brussels, 1985), presentation O4/II, which reports that cases of cryptococcal meningitis (without immunodeficiency) were seen in Kinshasa at the rate of one per year from 1952 to 1977, whereas forty-four cases (all fatal) were diagnosed at the Kinshasa University Hospital alone between 1978 and 1984.

23. Collaborative Study Group of AIDS in Haitian-Americans, "Risk Factors for AIDS among Haitians Residing in the United States," *JAMA*, 1987, 257(5), 635–639.

24. Indeed, even before Piot's team was seeing its first cases of AIDS in Kinshasa hospitals, there is independent evidence that suggests that the syndrome was also being witnessed, unrecognized, elsewhere in the country. In September 1983 the American writer Helen Winternitz traveled from Kinshasa to Kisangani by riverboat, and en route she saw the funeral of a young boy, the son of a "prostitute who worked in the claustrophobic corners of the barges for ten cents a trick." Apparently the boy died of prolonged malnutrition, having "been thin for too long" — a picture that nowadays sounds suspiciously like pediatric AIDS. H. Winternitz, *East along the Equator — A Congo Journey* (London: The Bodley Head, 1987), pp. 56–57.

25. Jean Vandepitte, personal communication, 1993.

26. J. Vandepitte et al., "AIDS and Cryptococcosis (Zaire, 1977)" (letter), *Lancet*, 1983, 1(ii), 925–926.

27. D. Vittecoq, J. C. Chermann et al., "Acquired Immunodeficiency Syndrome after Travelling in Africa: An Epidemiological Study in Seventeen Caucasian Patients," *Lancet*, 1987, 1(i), 612–615. Also See D. Brenky and O. Zemor, *La route du SIDA: enquête sur une grande peur* (Paris: Londreys, 1985), p. 30. N. Clumeck, J. Sonnet et al., "Acquired Immunodeficiency in African Patients," *N. Engl. J. Med.*, 1984, 310, 492–497; see p. 493.

28. J. Sonnet et al., "Opportunistic *Rhodococcus Equi* Infection in an African AIDS Case (1976–1981)" (letter), *Acta Clin. Belg.*, 1987, 42(3), 215–216. Although the letter states that the Belgian patient had lived in both the Congo and Burundi before 1976, the man's widow denies this, saying that he first came to Burundi in 1977, and met her shortly afterward. If correct, this means that he infected her, not vice versa.

29. I. Bygbjerg, "AIDS in a Danish Surgeon (Zaire, 1976)" (letter), *Lancet*, 1983, 1(ii), 925.

30. In fact, according to Randy Shilts, she was a lesbian who had never hidden her sexuality. See R. Shilts, *And the Band Played On: Politics, People and the AIDS Epidemic* (New York: St. Martin's Press, 1987), p. 117.

31. Ib Bygbjerg, personal communication, 1993.

32. In May 1986, a serum sample from Grethe Rask was sent to Donald Hicks, then working in the CDC laboratories in Atlanta. Hicks has since told me that the sample tested positive on ELISA and a gel-based Western blot developed by his boss, Jane Getchell.

33. N. Nzilambi, K. M. De Cock, J. B. McCormick et al., "The Prevalence of Infection with Human Immunodeficiency Virus over a 10-Year Period in Rural Zaire," *N. Engl. J. Med.,* 1988, 318, 276–279. Joe McCormick claims that a similar proportion of samples from the Sudanese Ebola epidemics of 1976 and 1979 tested HIV positive, (J. McCormick and S. Fisher-Hoch, *The Virus Hunters — Dispatches from the Frontline* [London: Bloomsbury, 1996], pp. 190 and 195), but this claim is not substantiated by Françoise Brun-Vezinet, whom he cites as its source.

34. J. Getchell, D. Hicks et al., "Human Immunodeficiency Virus Isolated from a Serum Sample Collected in 1976 in Central Africa," *J. Infect. Dis.,* 1987, 156(5), 833–837.

35. This was thirty-two HIV-positives out of 283 prostitutes tested, breaking down into 4 of 47 (8.5 percent) in Lisala, 21 of 181 (11.6 percent) in Bumba, and 7 of 55 (12.7 percent) in Yandongi, a strikingly even distribution between the two towns on the Congo River and the rural area of Yandongi. This in turn suggests that the latter was not an "isolated village."

36. T. Campbell, "Air Crash Survivor Tries to Remember," *Edmonton Journal,* December 4, 1976. Further information supplied by attending physician Arnold Voth, Peter Lema of Pacific Western Airlines, and Andrew Geider, archivist at Canadian Airlines International Ltd.

37. E. Rogan Jr., L. D. Jewell, A. Voth et al., "A Case of Acquired Immune Deficiency Syndrome before 1980," *Can. Med. Assoc. J.,* 1987, 137, 637–638.

38. There is in fact one earlier case that is apparently serologically proven, as will be detailed later, but it is for a number of reasons controversial.

39. Arnold Voth, personal communications, 1993 and 1995.

40. A. Nemeth, G. Biberfeld et al., "Early Case of Acquired Immunodeficiency Syndrome in a Child from Zaire," *Sex. Transm. Dis.,* 1986, 13(2), 111–113. Further information supplied by Antal Nemeth and Gunnel Biberfeld.

41. Jean Vandepitte, personal communication, 1993, including information from Dr. L. Corbeel.

42. The tests were IFA (immunofluorescence assay), RIPA (radioimmunoprecipitation assay), and competitive ELISA.

43. Actually twelve-fold.

44. J. Desmyter, P. Goubau et al., "Anti-LAV/HTLV-III in Kinshasa Mothers in 1970 and 1980," 2nd International Conference on AIDS (Paris, June 1986), communication 110: S17g.

45. A. Nahmias, A. Motulsky, M. Schanfield et al., "Antibody to HTLV-III/LAV in Serum from Central Africa in 1959," [First] International Conference on AIDS and Associated Cancers in Africa (Brussels, 1985), presentation PO3; also A. Nahmias, A. Motulsky, M. Essex et al., "Evidence for Human Infection with an HTLV-III/LAV-like Virus in Central Africa, 1959," *Lancet,* 1986, 1(ii), 1279–1280.

46. A. O. Pela and J. J. Platt, "AIDS in Africa: Emerging Trends," *Soc. Sci. Med.,* 1989, 28(1), 1–8.

47. "In Search of the Source of AIDS," in A. Shoumatoff, *African Madness* (New York: Knopf, 1988), pp. 163–164 and 135.
48. K. B. Noble, "Political Chaos in Zaire Disrupts Attempts to Control AIDS Epidemic," *New York Times,* March 22, 1994, pp. A1 and A8.
49. After addressing the 3rd International Conference on AIDS in 1987, Zagury declined to answer further questions about his work from reporters. (R. Cooke, "Tests Foster Hope for AIDS Vaccine," *Newsday* (N.Y.), June 4, 1987, pp. 4 and 15.)
50. M. Roddy, "Aids Research Developing in Zaire," *Straits Times,* November 12, 1988.
51. See D. Zagury, B. Goussard et al., "Immunization against AIDS in Humans" (letter), *Nature,* 1987, 326, 249–250; and D. Zagury, R. Gallo et al., "A Group Specific Anamnestic Immune Reaction against HIV-1 Induced by a Candidate Vaccine against AIDS," *Nature,* 1988, 332, 728–731.
52. "Investigation of Non-Compliance with DHSS Regulations for the Protection of Human Research Subjects Involving the National Institutes of Health Intramural Research Programme, Final Report," Office for Protection from Research Risks (OPRR), Division of Human Subject Protections, March 26, 1993. For commentary, see C. Grady, *The Search for an AIDS Vaccine: Ethical Issues in the Development and Testing of a Preventive HIV Vaccine* (Bloomington: Indiana University Press, 1995), pp. 101–102.
53. C. Levine, "Children in HIV/AIDS Trials: Still Vulnerable after All These Years," *Law, Medicine and Health Care,* 1991, 19(3–4), 231–237.
54. P. M. Sharp, B. H. Hahn et al., "Cross-species Transmission and Recombination of 'AIDS' Viruses," *Philos. Trans. R. Soc. Lond. (Biol.),* 1995, 349, 41–47. See also W.-S. Hu and H. M. Temin, "Retroviral Recombination and Reverse Transcription," *Science,* 1990, 250, 1227–1233.


CHAPTER 7: *False Positives, and the Specter of Contamination*

1. Before June 5, 1981.
2. Since 1993, the CDC's expanded adult case surveillance definition of AIDS has included all HIV-infected persons with a CD4+ T-lymphocyte count of less than 200 per milli-liter, even if they have no symptoms. HIV has thus been officially enshrined as an inte-gral part of the definition of AIDS; indeed, some argue that AIDS should now be called "HIV disease." See Division of HIV/AIDS, CDC, "1993 Revised Classification System for HIV Infection and Expanded Surveillance Case Definition for AIDS among Adolescents and Adults," *MMWR,* 1993, 41(RR-17), 1–19. (This does not, however, affect the status of ancient cases of AIDS, for clinically plausible symptoms may still be officially diag-nosed as AIDS, even if HIV-positivity is — or was — never confirmed.)
3. There are many other factors that can cause immune disorders, especially in infants and children. To gain an unbiased perspective on the subject, the interested reader is advised to take a look at a good immunological textbook from shortly before the AIDS era, such as E. R. Stiehm and E. A. Fulginiti (editors), *Immunologic Disorders in Infants and Children* (Philadelphia: W. B. Saunders and Co., 1980), particularly the chapter by Art Ammann and Richard Hong entitled "Disorders of the T-Cell System" (pp. 286–348).
4. For HIV-1, the identifiable proteins include gp120 and gp41 from *env* — which encodes the envelope portion of the virus; p55, p28, p24, and p18 from *gag,* which encodes the core of the virus; and p65 from *pol,* which encodes the reverse transcriptase enzyme common to all retroviruses. In this nomenclature, "gp" stands for glycoprotein (found

in *env*), "p" for protein (found in *gag* and *pol*), and the numbers denote the molecular weights of the proteins. Nowadays the presence of at least one *env* and one *gag* antibody typical of HIV is necessary before an assay is deemed HIV-positive, but early tests were often so defined if a single protein — usually p24 — was found to be present.

5.  For an excellent and readable account of the problems inherent in HIV testing in the eighties, see S. Connor and S. Kingman, *The Search for the Virus* (London: Penguin, 1989), pp. 63–93.

6.  Michael Koch, *AIDS: Vom Molekul zur Pandemie* (Heidelberg: Spektrum, 1989), p. 3. This episode is requoted by Mirko Grmek in his *History of AIDS — Emergence and Origin of a Modern Pandemic* (Princeton: Princeton University Press, 1990), pp. 172–173; Grmek affords Brede's testimony real significance by referring to it as "the beginning of the present flare-up . . . of AIDS in epidemic form."

7.  Hans-Dieter Brede, personal communications during 1995.

8.  A review of three decades of the *South African Medical Journal*, between the mid-forties and mid-seventies, revealed only these three fatal cases of KS. (See L. W. Duchen et al., "A Fatal Case of Sarcoma Idiopathicum Haemorrhagicum of Kaposi," *S. Af. Med. J.*, 1953, 27, 1078–1083; and C. J. Uys et al., "Kaposi's Sarcoma Occurring in a Coloured Male," *S. Af. Med. J.*, 1958, 32, 577–580.) Two of these cases involved disseminated KS involving both lymph glands and viscera, but no other infections are mentioned that might lend support to a diagnosis of AIDS. The only miner with KS was a Malawian gold miner who "made an uncomplicated recovery" from the condition after removal of an intestinal blockage (T. Coetzee et al., "Kaposi Sarcoma — Presentation with Intestinal Obstruction," *S. Af. Med. J.*, 1967, 41, 442–445). All of these cases sound suspiciously like "classical" African KS.

9.  R. Sher et al., "Seroepidemiology of Human Immunodeficiency Virus in Africa from 1970 to 1974" (letter), *N. Engl. J. Med.*, 1987, 317(7), 450–451. Further sera taken from more than twenty-nine thousand workers in South Africa's gold and platinum mines in 1986 still showed a very low seroprevalence in Malawian immigrants (0.18 percent), and zero HIV prevalence in Botswanans, Mozambicans, Lesothans, Swazilanders, and South Africans (G. M. Dusheiko, B. A. Brink, R. Sher et al., "Regional Prevalence of Hepatitis B, Delta, and Human Immunodeficiency Virus Infection in Southern Africa: A Large Population Survey," *Am. J. Epidem.*, 1989, 129[1], 138–145). This evidence of extremely low HIV prevalence vis-à-vis central Africa is supported by the fact that the first recognized cases of AIDS in South Africa occurred in 1982 in white homosexuals (most of whom had visited the United States), but only in 1987 in black heterosexuals (B. D. Schoub et al., "Considerations on the Further Expansion of the AIDS Epidemic in Southern Africa," *S. Af. Med. J.*, 1990, 77, 613–618). See also the *HIV/AIDS Surveillance Database*, published at regular intervals by the Health Studies Branch, International Programs Center, Population Division, U.S. Bureau of the Census, Washington, D.C. 20233-8860 — an invaluable resource that summarizes HIV epidemiological data from all known sources.

10.  The cohort of 144 children appears to feature in H. M. Meyer, "Field Experience with Combined Live Measles, Smallpox and Yellow Fever Vaccines," *Arch. Ges. Virusforsch.*, 1965, 16, 365–366.

11.  J. S. Epstein, H. M. Meyer et al., "Antibodies Reactive with HTLV-III Found in Freezer-Banked Sera from Children in West Africa," 25th Interscience Conference on Antimicrobial Agents and Chemotherapy (Minneapolis, 1985), abstract 217.

12.  For instance: G. Hancock and E. Carim, *AIDS — The Deadly Epidemic* (London: Gollancz, 1986), p. 119; M. D. Grmek, *History of AIDS*, p. 136; and T. C. Quinn,

J. M. Mann, J. W. Curran, and P. Piot, "AIDS in Africa: An Epidemiologic Paradigm," *Science,* 1986, 234, 955–963; 956.

13. S. Z. Wiktor, T. C. Quinn et al., "Human T Cell Lymphotropic Virus Type 1 (HTLV-1) among Female Prostitutes in Kinshasa, Zaire," *J. Infect. Dis.,* 1990, 161, 1073–1077, features excellent sample Western blots of sera containing HTLV-1, showing the main protein bands of that virus to be p19, p24, p28, p36, gp46, and p53. (The protein bands reported in Epstein's paper, above, were p19, p28, gp46, and p65.)

14. A similarly dubious report of allegedly positive archival West African sera involved two samples taken in 1971 from the Mano people of northern Liberia, which tested repeatedly positive on ELISA, positive on RIPA (although one of the samples failed to react when retested), though minimally reactive by Western blot. The two alleged positives were an eighty-five-year-old woman and a sixty-year-old man, and there was no reactivity to HIV-2, the virus that was more likely to be present in West Africa prior to the late eighties. One of the coauthors later conceded to the author that the positive RIPA results were "dubious." F. Chiodi, G. Biberfeld et al., "Screening of African Sera Stored for More Than 17 Years for HIV Antibodies by Site-Directed Serology," *Eur. J. Epidem.,* 1989, 5, 42–46.

15. M. Kawamura, M. Hayami et al., "HIV-2 in West Africa in 1966" (letter), *Lancet,* 1989, 1(i), 385.

16. W. C. Saxinger, R. C. Gallo et al., "Evidence for Exposure to HTLV-III in Uganda before 1973," *Science,* 1985, 227, 1036–1038.

17. C. Saxinger, R. Gallo et al., "Unique Pattern of HTLV-III (AIDS-Related) Antigen Recognition by Sera from African Children in Uganda (1972)," *Cancer Res.,* 1985, 45 (Supp.), 4624s–4626s.

18. R. J. Biggar, R. C. Gallo, P. L. Gigase et al., "Kaposi's Sarcoma in Zaire Is Not Associated with HTLV-III Infection" (letter), *N. Engl. J. Med.,* 1984, 371(16), 1051–1052.

19. R. J. Biggar, W. A. Blattner et al., "Seroepidemiology of HTLV-III Antibodies in a Remote Population of Eastern Zaire," *BMJ,* 1985, 290, 808–810.

20. R. J. Biggar, S. Alexander, R. C. Gallo, W. A. Blattner et al., "Regional Variation in Prevalence of Antibody against Human T-Lymphotropic Virus Types I and III in Kenya, East Africa," *Int. J. Cancer,* 1985, 35, 763–767. In 1987, one of Biggar's several coauthors told me privately that he had been worried about the lack of correlation between their findings and those of others, and by the lack of apparent AIDS cases in Kenya (let alone Turkana region) before 1984. He said he wished he had withdrawn his name from the paper.

21. See W. R. Lange et al., "Followup Study of Possible HIV Seropositivity among Abusers of Parenteral Drugs in 1971–72," *Public Health Rep.* (Washington), 1991, 106(4), 451–455.

22. R. J. Biggar, P. L. Gigase, W. A. Blattner et al., "ELISA HTLV Retrovirus Antibody Reactivity Associated with Malaria and Immune Complexes in Healthy Africans," *Lancet,* 1985, 2(i), 520–523. See also R. J. Biggar, "The AIDS Problem in Africa," *Lancet,* 1986, 1(i), 79–82.

23. R. J. Biggar, "Possible Non-specific Associations between Malaria and HTLV-III/LAV" (letter), *N. Engl. J. Med.,* 1986, 315(7), 457. Members of the Gallo laboratory were not alone in making such errors, though others were possibly franker about reporting their problems. At around the same period Guy de Thé reported that, using ELISA, 40 percent of sera collected during the early seventies in Uganda, Kenya, Tanzania, and Ivory Coast were HIV-positive, but that only a few were reactive on Western blot, normally against p24 only, but "exceptionally against the whole spectrum of *gag* and *env* products." It

would be interesting to have these sera retested today, but without such a retest, one must assume that even the exceptional sera represented false positives.

24. J. A. Levy, G. Henle, W. Henle, G. Giraldo et al., "Absence of Antibodies to the Human Immunodeficiency Virus in Sera from Africa prior to 1975," *Proc. Natl. Acad. Sci.,* 1986, 83, 7935–7937.

25. J. W. Carswell, N. Sewankambo et al., "How Long Has the AIDS Virus Been in Uganda?" (letter), *Lancet,* 1986, 1(ii), 1217. See also J. W. Carswell, "HIV Infection in Healthy Persons in Uganda," *AIDS,* 1987, 1, 223–227, in which the author states that Biggar's and Saxinger's papers contain "confusing results."

26. P. J. Kanki, M. Essex et al., "Antibodies to Simian T-Lymphotropic Retrovirus Type III in African Green Monkeys and Recognition of STLV-III Viral Proteins by AIDS and Related Sera" (letter), *Lancet,* 1985, 1(ii), 1230–1232.

27. F. Barin, S. M'Boup et al., "Serological Evidence for Virus Related to Simian T-Lymphotropic Retrovirus III in Residents of West Africa," *Lancet,* 1985, 2(ii), 1387–1389; and F. Clavel, L. Montagnier et al., "Isolation of a New Human Retrovirus from West African Patients with AIDS," *Science,* 1986, 233, 343–346.

28. P. J. Kanki, M. Essex et al., "New Human T-Lymphotropic Retrovirus Related to Simian T-Lymphotropic Virus Type III (STLV-IIIagm)," *Science,* 1986, 232, 238–243.

29. P. J. Kanki, M. Essex et al., "Serologic Identification and Characterisation of a Macaque T-Lymphotropic Retrovirus Closely Related to HTLV-III," *Science,* 1985, 228, 1199–1201, which refers to "antibody-positive sera taken from Mm251–79" (i.e., macaque monkey 251, bled in 1979).

30. H. W. Kestler, R. C. Desrosiers et al., "Comparison of Simian Immunodeficiency Virus Isolates," *Nature,* 1988, 331, 619–622, which includes Essex and Kanki's reply on pp. 661–662. See also S. Connor, "Laboratory Mix-up Solves AIDS Mystery," *New Scientist,* February 25, 1988, p. 32.

31. Carol Mulder, "A Case of Mistaken Non-identity," *Nature,* 1988, 331, 562–563.

32. J. Brooke, "In Cradle of AIDS Theory, a Defensive Africa Sees a Disguise for Racism," *New York Times,* November 19, 1987, B2. See also D. Dickson, "AIDS: Racist Myths, Hard Facts," *AfricAsia,* May 1987, No. 41; 49–53.

33. M. Fukosawa, M. Hayami et al., "Sequence of Simian Immunodeficiency Virus from African Green Monkey, a New Member of the HIV/SIV Group" (letter), *Nature,* 1988, 333, 457–461.

34. C. Mulder, "Human AIDS Virus Not from Monkeys," *Nature,* 1988, 333, 396. See also R. Steinbrook, "Research Refutes Idea That Human AIDS Virus Originated in Monkeys," *Los Angeles Times,* June 2, 1988, Part 1; pp. 3 and 22.

35. There are countless articles on the subject of the HTLV-III contamination, but by far the best and most comprehensive is Crewdson's magnum opus (deserving — in many people's view — of a Pulitzer Prize), entitled "The Great AIDS Quest: Science under the Microscope," *Chicago Tribune,* November 19, 1989, Section 5 (Special Report), pp. 1–16. See also M. Gladwell, "At NIH, an Unprecedented Ethics Investigation," *Washington Post,* August 17, 1990, pp. A8–A9.

36. Dr. Gallo provided no evidence to support this characterization.

37. R. C. Chirimuuta and R. J. Chirimuuta, *AIDS, Africa and Racism* (privately published and available from R. Chirimuuta, Bretby House, Stanhope, Bretby, Derbyshire; DE15 0PT, U.K.; ISBN 0-951280-4-1-4, 1987), p. 1.

38. R. C. Chirimuuta, *AIDS, Africa and Racism,* pp. 142–143. The figures are those for July 1987.

39. For instance: R. Sabatier, *Blaming Others — Prejudice, Race and Worldwide AIDS* (London: Panos, 1988), especially pp. 47 and 57.

40. Herbert Schmitz, personal communication, 1995.

41. I. Wendler, A. F. Fleming, F. Hunsmann, H. Schmitz et al., "Seroepidemiology of Human Immunodeficiency Virus in Africa," *BMJ*, 1986, 293, 782–785.

42. Anon., "Evidence for Origin Is Weak," *New Scientist*, October 15, 1987, p. 27. Also see C. Rouzioux et al., "Absence of Antibodies to LAV/HTLV-III and STLV-III(mac) in Pygmies," 2nd International Conference on AIDS (Paris, 1986), poster 378.

43. It is probable that present-day pygmies have relatively little contact with the various subspecies of African green monkey, *Cercopithecus aethiops*, because they all inhabit the savanna regions, rather than the rain forests where the pygmies have resided, apparently for the last two thousand years — since being driven there by expanding Bantu populations at around the time of Christ. (See C. McEvedy, *The Penguin Atlas of African History* [London: Penguin, 1980], pp. 20 and 34.) Nonetheless, pygmies do hunt and eat a wide variety of forest primates.

44. A. Nahmias et al., "Evidence for Human Infection with an HTLV-III/LAV-like Virus in Central Africa, 1959," *Lancet*, 1986, 1(ii), 1279–1280.

45. See, for instance, A. Fleming, "AIDS in Africa — An Update," *AIDS-Forschung*, 1988, 3, 116–138.

46. E. Hooper, *Slim* (London: The Bodley Head, 1990), pp. 161–165.

47. Alex Shoumatoff, *African Madness* (New York: Knopf, 1988), p. 166. There is, of course, endless fun to be had with acronyms. In 1987, according to Shoumatoff, Russians were in the habit of interpreting AIDS as *"Amerikanskii Imperialisticheskii Dozhobnii Siphilis,"* or Imperialistic American Rear-End Syphilis (p. 184).

48. See K. B. Mullis, "The Unusual Origin of the Polymerase Chain Reaction," *Scientific American*, April 1990, pp. 36–43 for a fascinating (and very Californian) description of how Mullis's night drive along Highway 101, with female friend in attendance, led to the birth of the PCR concept.

49. Normally, exposure to heat like this would destroy enzymes, but the PCR process utilizes a variety of the DNA polymerase enzyme that was discovered in bacteria living in the geysers of Yellowstone National Park. (Richard Marlink, personal communication, 1998.)

50. S. Kwok, K. B. Mullis, J. Sninsky et al., "Identification of Human Immunodeficiency Virus Sequences by Using In Vitro Enzymatic Amplification and Oligomer Cleavage Detection," *J. Virol.*, 1987, 61(5), 1690–1694.

CHAPTER 8: *The Manchester Sailor*

1. This section constitutes part of a personal communication by cassette tape, from Dave's former fiancée in 1992.

2. Cytomegalovirus (CMV) would only be so named in 1960, the year after David Carr's death. See T. H. Weller et al., "Serologic Differentiation of Viruses Responsible for Cytomegalic Inclusion Disease," *Virol.*, 1960, 12, 130.

3. In 1956, the German microbiologist Herwig Hamperl reviewed several cases of fatal adult cytomegalic inclusion disease, and proposed that in three North American cases, death had actually been caused by a *Pneumocystis carinii* pneumonia coinfection. He also proposed that the two conditions seemed predisposed to occur in conjunction. (H. Hamperl,

"Pneumocystis Infection and Cytomegaly of the Lungs in Newborn and Adult," *Am. J. Pathol.*, 1956, 32, 1–13.) Three other fatal cases of cytomegaly and PCP had just cropped up in British cancer patients, so their opportunistic nature and tendency to "hunt as a pair" were now recognized on both sides of the Atlantic. (W. St. C. Symmers, "Generalised Cytomegalic Inclusion-Body Disease Associated with *Pneumocystis* Pneumonia in Adults," *J. Clin. Pathol.*, 1960, 13, 1–21.)

4. G. Williams, T. B. Stretton, and J. C. Leonard, "Cytomegalic Inclusion Disease and *Pneumocystis Carinii* Infection in an Adult," *Lancet*, 1960, 2(ii), 951–955.

5. G. Williams, T. B. Stretton, and J. C. Leonard, "AIDS in 1959?" (letter), *Lancet*, 1983, 2(ii), 1136.

6. K. B. Mullis, "The Unusual Origin of the Polymerase Chain Reaction," *Scientific American*, April 1990, pp. 36–43.

7. G. Corbitt, A. S. Bailey, and G. Williams, "HIV Infection in Manchester, 1959" (letter), *Lancet*, 1990, 336, 51.

8. C. Mihill, "Manchester Man had HIV 31 Years Ago," *Guardian* (U.K.), July 6, 1990. P. Wright, "Royal Navy Sailor Died of Aids 31 Years Ago," *Times* (U.K.), July 6, 1990.

9. Anon., "Aids Traced to Death in 1959," *Daily Telegraph* (U.K.), July 6, 1990.

10. For instance: P. Davison and S. Kingman, "How the First Aids Case Was Unravelled," *Independent on Sunday* (U.K.), July 8, 1990.

11. G. Bell, "Revealed: David Carr, the West's First Aids Victim," *Sunday Express* (U.K.), July 29, 1990.

12. The brain and liver samples from Carr tested negative.

13. J. Getchell, D. Hicks et al., "Human Immunodeficiency Virus Isolated from a Serum Sample Collected in 1976 in Central Africa," *J. Infect. Dis.*, 1987, 156(5), 833–837.

14. Williams et al., "Cytomegalic Inclusion Disease and *Pneumocystis Carinii* Infection in an Adult."

15. It was not until November 1992, at the third time of asking, that the Royal Navy finally revealed the dates on which he joined each ship. Even then, as will emerge later, the records provided were incorrect for two of the five vessels listed.

16. Anon., "Game of Hide and Seek with 'Subs' off Ulster Coast," *Belfast Telegraph*, July 9, 1956, p. 8.

17. I am especially grateful to the ship's official photographer on that voyage, John Noble, who went through his diary of the trip and recorded his account on cassette tape, just months before his death from cancer of the stomach in July 1992.

18. Anon., "H.M.S. Warrior in the Pacific," *Navy News*, June 1957.

19. N. Dombey and E. Grove, "Britain's Thermonuclear Bluff," *London Review of Books*, October 22, 1992, pp. 8–10.

20. E. Hooper and S. Griffin, "Blast from the Past," *New Statesman* (U.K.), May 16, 1997, pp. 32–33. Other evidence suggested that not just paternalistic cynicism, but also carelessness and ignorance, may have played a role here. In 1994 it was revealed that, as an economy, some of the radioactive debris that was needed for further research had been flown back to England not on a specially prepared RAF flight, but inside a diplomatic bag on a scheduled passenger plane. Anthony Bevine, "How FO Sent H-Bomb Fallout to Blighty by Passenger Plane," *Observer* (U.K.), February 6, 1994.

21. There had apparently been at least one hundred national servicemen in the thousand-strong crew.

22. Anon., "Another Atom Test Man Dies," *Daily Express* (U.K.), August 30, 1958, p. 7. Anon., "Did Death Rays Strike H-Ship Officer?," *Daily Herald*, August 30, 1958, p. 1. The

latter article says that a navy spokesman admitted that a security curtain had been drawn around the matter in the twenty-four hours after Lt. Franklin's death. Nowadays, Lt. Franklin's widow admits that she was manipulated by naval officers, who persuaded her to go along with their blanket pronouncement that there was no link to the bomb tests.

23. "Atomic Weapon Trials," Report by the Defence Research Policy Committee; dated May 20, 1953; C.O.S. (53)239; D.R.P./P(53)257 (available at the Public Records Office).

24. M. Ichimaru et al., "T Cell Malignant Lymphoma in Nagasaki District and Its Problems," *Japan J. Clin. Oncol.*, 1979, 9, 337–346. See also R. C. Gallo et al., "Origin of Human T-Cell Leukaemia-Lymphoma Virus" (letter), *Lancet*, 1983, 2(ii), 962–963.

25. E. J. Sternglass and J. Scheer, "Radiation Exposure of Bone Marrow Cells to Strontium-90 during Early Development as a Possible Cofactor in the Etiology of AIDS," *Annual Meeting of the American Association for the Advancement of Science* (AAAS), Philadelphia, Pennsylvania, May 18, 1986. See also J. M. Gould and B. A. Goldman, *Deadly Deceit: Low-level Radiation, High-level Cover-up* (New York: Four Walls Eight Windows, 1991), pp. 135–144.


CHAPTER 9: *AIDS in the Pre-AIDS Era?*

1. A. J. Nahmias, A. Motulsky, P. Kanki, M. Essex et al., "Evidence for Human Infection with an HTLV III/LAV-like Virus in Central Africa, 1959," *Lancet*, 1986, 1(ii), 1279–1280.

2. As, for instance, stated by Gerry Myers in "HIV: Between Past and Future," *AIDS Res. Hum. Retro.*, 1994, 10(11), 1317–1324.

3. D. Huminer, J. B. Rosenfeld, and S. D. Pitlik, "AIDS in the Pre-AIDS Era," *Rev. Infect. Dis.*, 1987, 9(6), 1102–1108.

4. Centers for Disease Control, "Revision of the Case Definition of Acquired Immuno-deficiency Syndrome for National Reporting — United States," *Ann. Intern. Med.*, 1985, 103, 402–403.

5. G. Corbitt, A. S. Bailey, and G. Williams, "HIV Infection in Manchester, 1959," *Lancet*, 1990, 336, 51.

6. R. F. Garry, M. H. Witte, M. Elvin-Lewis, C. L. Witte, S. S. Alexander, W. L. Drake et al., "Documentation of an AIDS Virus Infection in the United States in 1968," *JAMA*, 1988, 260(14), 2085–2087.

7. J. Desmyter and L. Montagnier, "Anti-LAV/HTLV-III in Kinshasa Mothers, 1970 vs. 1980," First International Conference on AIDS and Associated Cancers in Africa (Brussels, 1985), p. 12.

8. J. Leonard et al., "AIDS in 1959?" (letter), *Lancet*, 1983, 2(ii), 1136.

9. J. P. Vandenbroucke, "Tracking AIDS Epidemic in Libraries" (letter), *Lancet*, 1990, 336, 318–319.

10. Of these four cases, one involved a twelve-year-old Scottish girl who had suffered from disseminated and fatal *Mycobacterium avium* infection beginning in 1961. However, other family members, including her twin sister, had since contracted the same disease, which strongly suggested that congenital immunodeficiency was involved. (Dr. John Crofton, personal communications, 1991 and 1994. Original article: M. E. Schonell, J. W. Crofton et al., "Disseminated Infection with Mycobacterium Avium. 1. Clinical Features, Treatment and Pathology," *Tubercle*, 1968, 49, 12–30; see also the second part

of the article on p. 31–41.) Another case involved a twenty-three-year-old woman from Goteborg, Sweden, who died of an atypical mycobacterial infection in 1967, both of her doctors whom I contacted were "firmly convinced that the young woman was not suffering from an HIV infection," and indeed her personal and clinical history did not seem to support an AIDS diagnosis. (B. Hagmar, J. Kutti, P. Wahlen et al., "Disseminated Infection Caused by *Mycobacterium kansasii*," *Acta Med. Scand.*, 1969, 186, 93–99. Personal communications: Per Wahlen [February 1993] and Jack Kutti [May 1993 and February 1994].) The third case was discounted by Dr. Huminer himself, who confirmed my suspicion that his report of disseminated KS and T-cell immunodeficiency in a fifty-nine-year-old Jewish male was doubtful as an AIDS diagnosis, being more typical of the "classical KS" to which elderly Jewish males appear to be predisposed. (E. Flatau et al., "Malignant Evolution of Kaposi's Sarcoma with Impaired Cellular Immunity," *Harefuah*, 1977, 93, 242–244; and D. Huminer, "Was a Case of AIDS Reported in *Harefuah* before the First Publication on the Syndrome in the USA?" [letter], *Harefuah*, 1985, 109, 424–425.) The fourth of these cases, involving a fifty-two-year-old Japanese-American woman from Hawaii in 1978, was subsequently discounted as AIDS by its lead author, who retrospectively found that the patient's stored tissues tested HIV-negative, and identified a T-cell lymphoma that had probably caused the other infections. Interestingly, however, the patient was also negative on PCR for HTLV-I, which often causes T-cell lymphomas, especially among those of Japanese ancestry. (See also G. M. Stemmermann et al., "Cryptosporidiosis: Report of a Fatal Case Complicated by Disseminated Toxoplasmosis," *Am. J. Med.*, 1980, 69, 637–642. Grant Stemmermann, personal communication, April 1995.)

11. Dr. Heimpel's vague recollection that the soldier had been gay was never confirmed.

12. R. Owor, W. M. Wamukota, "A Fatal Case of Strongyloidiasis, with *Strongyloides* Larvae in the Meninges," *Trans. R. Soc. Trop. Med. Hyg.*, 1976, 70, 497–499. I was unable to gather any further information, despite writing several letters to the doctors involved.

13. P. W. Nichols, "Opportunistic Infections and Kaposi's Sarcoma in Homosexual Men" (letter), *N. Engl. J. Med.*, 1982, 306, 934–935. G. Williams, T. B. Stretton, and J. C. Leonard, "AIDS in 1959?" (letter), *Lancet*, 1983, 2, 1136. M. H. Witte et al., "AIDS in 1968" (letter), *JAMA*, 1984, 251, 2657.

14. M. Elvin-Lewis et al., "Systemic Chlamydial Infection Associated with Generalized Lymphedema and Lymphangiosarcoma," *Lymphology*, 1973, 6, 113–121.

15. J. M. Watanabe et al., "*Pneumocystis carinii* Pneumonia in a Family," *JAMA*, 1965, 193(8), 685–686.

16. H. A. Lyons, K. Vinijchaikul, and G. R. Hennigar, "*Pneumocystis carinii* Pneumonia Unassociated with Other Disease," *Arch. Intern. Med.*, 1961, 108, 929–936; G. R. Hennigar et al., "*Pneumocystis carinii* Pneumonia in an Adult: Report of a Case," *Am. J. Clin. Pathol.*, 1961, 35, 353–364.

17. C. D. Anderson and H. J. Barrie, "Fatal *Pneumocystis* Pneumonia in an Adult: Report of a Case," *Am. J. Clin. Pathol.*, 1960, 34, 365–370.

18. J. P. Wyatt et al., "Cytomegalic Inclusion Pneumonitis in an Adult," *Am. J. Clin. Pathol.*, 1953, 23, 353–362.

19. G. C. McMillan, "Fatal Inclusion-Disease Pneumonitis in an Adult," *Am. J. Pathol.*, 1947, 23, 995–1003.

20. The case histories that follow feature information obtained from local newspapers and archives, family doctors, clinicians, pathologists, workmates, relatives, and friends. In most

cases I was also given permission by the next of kin to view the original medical records. My thanks go to all of those who helped, many of whom asked not to be cited by name.

21. M. Elvin-Lewis et al., "Systemic Chlamydial Infection Associated with Generalized Lymphedema and Lymphangiosarcoma."

22. M. H. Witte, C. L. Witte et al., "AIDS in 1968" (letter), *JAMA*, 1984, 251, 2657.

23. R. F. Garry et al., "Documentation of an AIDS Virus Infection in the United States in 1968," *JAMA*, 1988, 260(14), 2085–2087.

24. John Crewdson, "Case Shakes Theories of AIDS Origin," *Chicago Tribune*, October 25, 1987, pp. 1 and 20. Barbara Jones, "18-Year Secret of AIDS Is Revealed," *Mail on Sunday* (U.K.), November 8, 1987.

25. My thanks to Bob Manor and Roger Signor of the *St. Louis Post-Dispatch* for their generous help on this case.

26. Drake (presumably at Witte's request) had reviewed the blocks in 1984, at the time of their joint letter to *JAMA* in which they first tentatively proposed a diagnosis of AIDS. It may be that they were not refiled properly when he returned them.

27. Steve Alexander, who was director of immunology at the Biotech company that manufactured the test, implied in a phone conversation in 1991 that the same assay had been used. See J. D. Moore, S. S. Alexander et al., "HTLV-III Seropositivity in 1971–1972 Parenteral Drug Abusers — A Case of False Positives or Evidence of Viral Exposure?," *N. Engl. J. Med.*, 1986, 314(21), 1387–1388.

28. An article appeared in *Science* soon afterward describing a similar break-in that had taken place at Robert Gallo's home, on August 11, 1990. B. J. Culliton, "Gallo Reports Mystery Break-in," *Science*, 1990, 250, 502.

29. An example of the growing skepticism is found in G. Myers et al., "Phylogenetic Moments in the AIDS Epidemic," in S. Morse (editor), *Emerging Viruses* (Oxford: Oxford University Press, 1993), pp. 120–137. For further developments on this case in 1997, see later in this book.

30. C. Szechenyi, "Army Documents Reveal Chemical Warfare Tests in St. Louis," *Kansas City Times*, June 4, 1980, pp. A1–A4. See also "Behavior of Aerosol Clouds Within Cities," *Joint Q. Rep.*, Chemical Corps, U.S. Army, July–September 1953, no. 5; p. 8ff.

31. J. Sawyer and W. Allen, "Army Duped City Officials in '53 Experiment," *St. Louis Post-Dispatch*, July 13, 1994, p. 1A. Also see Anon., "Smoke Screen to Bar Air Raid on City under Study," *St. Louis Post-Dispatch*, June 26, 1953, p. 1. This three-paragraph article was all the information the citizens of St. Louis were given to explain the strange happenings in the city; the first two words of the title were apt, at least.

32. James Coates, "CIA's Manhattan 'Tests': Experiments on New Yorkers?," *Chicago Tribune*, December 10, 1979. The biological, chemical, and mind-control experiments went under several code names, including MKNAOMI, MKULTRA, MKDELTA, and MKSEARCH. Records of the test programs were later ordered destroyed by the CIA doctor in charge, Sidney Gottlieb, but expense vouchers and other materials were left untouched, and subsequently produced in response to the Church of Scientology's requests under the Freedom of Information Act. The Coates article mentions 180 such tests being staged in the United States, but by 1980 the Scientologists had apparently discovered "well over 300." (Written statement for press distribution by Church spokesman Brian Anderson, August 14, 1980.)

33. The How test site comprised a 25-square-block area to the east of Grand Boulevard and north of Olive. The other test site, Item, was downtown (west of Memorial and north of Spruce).

34. Furthermore, of the three known and documented releases, one took place just five hundred yards south of Robert's house, with the aerosol clouds traveling toward it on the wind. J. Sawyer and W. Allen, "Army Duped City Officials in '53 Experiment." The graphic accompanying the article reveals that a dual-point release was staged at two points along Olive (east of Compton and west of University) at 11:40 P.M. on the night of June 19, 1953, and that the clouds traveled north. Robert's house on Delmar lay four blocks to the north.

35. E. L. Cook, "No Local Record of Army Sprayings," *St. Louis Globe-Democrat*, June 5, 1980, p. B1.

36. A. Tucker, *The Toxic Metals* (London: Pan Ballantine, 1972), pp. 174–205.

37. L. A. Spomer, "Fluorescent Particle Atmospheric Tracer: Toxicity Hazard," *Atmospheric Environment*, 1973, 7, 353–355.

38. The most vulnerable time is between one and three months, this being the period when infants lose maternal antibodies acquired in the womb, but are still in the process of building their own protection. See I. P. Roitt, *Essential Immunology* (Oxford: Blackwell, 1982), p. 114.

39. Army tests conducted in 1953 in Virginia and Minnesota employed a version of FP that was combined with spores of *lycopodium*, a drying agent derived from mosses. A Canadian pharmacologist commented that this variant could be dangerous if inhaled by babies, asthma patients, or the elderly. (Anon., "Germ Warfare Tests Cited," *Detroit Free Press*, June 9, 1980, p. 9A.) One of the army reports on these trials stated that "some human respiratory exposures are reported. . . . The assumption that dry biological materials will behave like the FPs (fluorescent particles) insofar as stability . . . [is] concerned needs to be proven in additional field tests involving both materials." (Anon., "US Germ War Tests Disclosed," *San Diego Union*, June 9, 1980.) It should be noted that many versions of luminous paint comprise zinc sulfide to which a tiny quantity of radium has been added, and that the manufacture of zinc cadmium sulfide FP passed at some stage before 1964 from the New Jersey Zinc Company to the U.S. Radium Corporation. It is known that some versions of FP incorporated radioactive materials such as Xenon 133. (See P. A. Leighton et al., "The Fluorescent Particle Atmospheric Tracer," *J. Appl. Meteor.*, 1965, 4, 334–348.) There is nothing to indicate that a form of FP including either radioactive or biological materials was ever used in St. Louis, though since accurate and detailed records of the individual tests have still not been released, one cannot be *certain* that only zinc cadmium sulfide was employed.

40. Huminer et al., "AIDS in the Pre-AIDS Era."

41. J. M. Watanabe et al., "*Pneumocystis carinii* Pneumonia in a Family."

42. The family's health problems need to be viewed in the light of the remarkable revelations about radiation releases from the Hanford reactors between 1944 and the mid-sixties (releases that included the deliberate venting of more than seven thousand curies of Iodine-131 on the night of December 2, 1949, in the infamous "Green Run"), and the greatly elevated incidence of leukemias and immune disorders (notably hypothyroidism) in the "Downwinders" area. These revelations came about largely through the efforts of the Hanford Downwinders Coalition, the Hanford Education Action League, and various campaigning journalists, most notably Karen Dorn-Steele, whose article "'Downwinders' — Living with Fear," *Spokesman Review* (Spokane), July 28, 1985, pp. 1–3, led the way. Other good examples of the genre: S. Gilmore, "Hanford's Nuclear Families," *Seattle Times/Seattle Post-Intelligencer*, July 29, 1990, pp. A1–A7; E. Schumacher, "First Denial, Then Anger," *Seattle Times/Seattle Post-Intelligencer* (Pacific supplement), January 27, 1991, pp. 7–11; and

T. Paulson, "Radiation Guessing Game," *Seattle Times/Seattle Post-Intelligencer,* February 19, 1991, pp. B1–B4; also see Anon., "Thyroid Study a Sham, Some Say," pp. A1 and A8. Moscow lies some 120 miles due east of Hanford, but is directly downwind. In 1991, it was reported that residents of nearby Pullman "were exposed in the fifties to higher levels of cancer-causing radioactive particles than people living immediately around the Hanford nuclear reservation." See L. Nelson, "Inherit the Wind. Hanford: The Downwind Legacy; Day 1," *Lewiston Tribune,* March 30, 1991, pp. 1A and 5A.

43. V. A. Pilon, "Dissemination of *Pneumocystis*," *N.Y. St. J. Med.,* 1990, 121–122.

44. Such as J. Ruskin and J. S. Remington, "*Pneumocystis Carinii* Infection in the Immunosuppressed Host," in *Antimicrobial Agents and Chemotherapy — 1967* (American Society for Microbiology, 1968), pp. 70–76; J. H. Brazinsky et al., "*Pneumocystis* Pneumonia Transmission between Patients with Lymphoma" (letter), *JAMA,* 1969, 209(10), 1527; and T. R. Goersch et al., "Possible Transfer of *Pneumocystis carinii* between Immunodeficient Patients" (letter), *Lancet,* 1990, 336, 627. Nosocomial transmission has also happened frequently between elderly patients (see J. L. Jacobs et al., "A Cluster of *Pneumocystis carinii* Pneumonia in Adults without Predisposing Illness," *N. Engl. J. Med.,* 1991, 324(4), 246–250) and among infants, especially in nurseries (see L. O. Gentry and J. S. Remington, "*Pneumocystis carinii* Pneumonia in Siblings," *J. Pediatr.,* 1970, 76(5), 769–772).

45. J. L. Jacobs et al., "A Cluster of PCP in Adults without Predisposing Illness," see p. 249.

46. Anon., "Illness Report Denied," *Idahonian,* September 25, 1964, p. 3. This includes Larry's brother's statement that "the community is a beehive of unfounded rumour."

47. J. A. Kovacs et al., "*Pneumocystis carinii* Pneumonia: A Comparison between Patients with the Acquired Immunodeficiency Syndrome and Patients with Other Immunodeficiencies," *Ann. Intern. Med.,* 1984, 100, 663–671.

48. During World War II, all was suborned to the race to make the A-bomb, so corners were cut and safety compromised in order to save time. Once established, this precedent was hard to break, especially as the Soviet Union replaced Germany and Japan as the bête noire, and a new race — this time for nuclear supremacy — began. By the time it was realized just how much damage had been done to the local environment by the venting of radioactive particles into the air and the dumping of radioactive waste into underground pits or the Columbia River, it was too late to reverse the process. The response of the authorities was an all-too-human one — that of secrecy and denial, of pretending (even in the face of evidence to the contrary) that nothing was amiss.

49. See K. Dorn-Steele, "'Downwinders' — Living with Fear." In the six days that followed, I-131 levels in milk at Ringold, the small farming community that faces Hanford across the Columbia River, rose fifteen times over. During this same period, Hanford scientists were also concerned about the levels of zinc-65 in the milk of Ringold cows; Zn-65 is a potent emitter of gamma rays, and concentrates in the prostate gland. Larry was found at autopsy to be suffering from hyperplasia of the prostate.

50. *Final Report of the Advisory Committee on Human Radiation Experiments* (New York: Oxford University Press, 1996), pp. 334–335. The "volunteers" are said to have been members of Hanford's health physics staff (Idaho National Engineering Laboratory), and the report adds: "No evidence is available bearing on what these subjects knew or were told about the experiments or the conditions under which they agreed to participate." However, the main impact of 1–131 is on the thyroid, and it is not usually very immunosuppressive — which renders this scenario unlikely.

51. In the early days of atom bomb production, the scientists believed that releasing radioactive waste into the river was safe, given the dilution that would occur in such a vast

volume of water, but it is now known that fish concentrate radioactive isotopes in certain tissues, and that fish from the Columbia used to contain radioactive phosphorus,
P-32, at levels more than a million times higher than the river water. P-32, which also
emits gamma rays, is a potent element that lodges in bone and bone marrow, and is "an
initiator leading to cancer."

52.  Fred's father, a marine, died of leukemia in 1948, after participating in the clean-up
operations at Nagasaki at the end of the war.

53.  He claimed that this test was part of a much larger "pentomic" program, which had also
involved other trials elsewhere in the States. We know that between 1951 and 1958, at
the official Nevada Test Site, at least fifty-five thousand members of the U.S. military
were exposed, sometimes repeatedly, to battlefield nuclear weapons as part of the training of a "Pentomic army," which would be emotionally and physically equipped to fight
in the event of a nuclear war. The military personnel, mainly army and marines, were
involved in eight series of troop exercises (Desert Rock I–VIII), "designed to explore the
conditions and tactics of the atomic battlefield." For a vivid account of the training of
the pentomic (believed to derive from Pentagon and atomic) army, including being
marched to within a few yards of Ground Zero just an hour after "Smoky," a forty-four-
kiloton nuclear explosion on August 31, 1957, see H. L. Rosenberg, *Atomic Soldiers —
American Victims of Nuclear Experiments* (Boston: Beacon Press, 1980), pp. 114–124. In
R. Bertell, *No Immediate Danger — Prognosis for a Radioactive Earth* (London: Women's
Press, 1985), p. 70, the author states that altogether over a quarter of a million troops
and an unknown number of civilians "took part in military manoeuvres to prepare for
combat in a nuclear war," if one includes similar tests conducted by Canada and the
United Kingdom.

54.  In December 1993, Secretary of Energy Hazel O'Leary revealed details of 204 previously
secret underground tests conducted between the sixties and nineties, only 111 of which
had previously been detected by seismic devices. Many had been detonated simultaneously with announced tests. No information was provided about secret tests that may
have been conducted before 1963. Technically, therefore, it is possible that a subkiloton
nuclear explosion could have been staged in a remote part of eastern Washington in
1958, when seismic detection was not so sophisticated. See R. Norrish and T. Cochran,
*United States Nuclear Tests, July 1945 to 31 December 1992* (Washington, D.C.: Natural
Resources Defense Council, 1994), pp. 18–20. Also see "Nuclear Secrets" and "Testing on
Human Guinea Pigs," *Newsweek,* January 3, 1994, pp. 22–27, which refer to thirty-one
experiments conducted since 1945 in which American citizens were deliberately
exposed to radioactive materials (including plutonium, administered by injection),
sometimes without their knowledge.

55.  *Washington Atlas and Gazetteer,* first edition (Freeport, Maine: De Lorme Mapping
Company, 1988), pp. 7, 43, and 57.

56.  Two other examples of "synchronicity" must be pointed out, even though they may well
have no relevance to Alice's illness. The fluorescent particles used in the Army Chemical
Corps atmospheric tests of the fifties and sixties were developed by Stanford University,
in conjunction with a company called Metronics Associates — both of which are situated in Palo Alto. A 1965 paper about these experiments written by Philip Leighton
(who seems to have headed the program at both establishments) mentions that at least
one FP release took place in Palo Alto itself, although the year is not specified. (P. A.
Leighton et al., "The Fluorescent Particle Atmospheric Tracer," *J. Appl. Meteor.,* 1965, 4,
334–348, see p. 344.) Furthermore, there was a very high incidence of PCP among

patients at Stanford University Hospital during the sixties (including one case that coincided with Alice's job-searching in Palo Alto in May and June 1963). See J. Ruskin and J. S. Remington, "*Pneumocystis carinii* Infection in the Immunosuppressed Host"; L. O. Gentry and J. S. Remington, "*Pneumocystis carinii* Pneumonia in Siblings"; and J. Ruskin and J. S. Remington, "The Compromised Host and Infection. 1. *Pneumocystis carinii* Pneumonia," *JAMA*, 1967, 202(12), 1070–1074. Doctors Joel Ruskin and Jack Remington of the Palo Alto Medical Research Foundation, who reported these cases, were immunologists who specialized in studies of compromised hosts and the impact of opportunistic organisms such as *Pneumocystis carinii* and *Toxoplasmosis gondii*. Could these illnesses have been linked to the atmospheric test in the town, and could there be a connection to Alice's death the following year? This is not as absurd as it may sound, because a previous Chemical Corps germ warfare test, staged in the Bay Area in 1950, involving FP mixed with the bacterium *Serratia marcescens*, was linked to an outbreak of pneumonia at Stanford University Hospital, and the death of one man, in whose lungs the bacterium was later found. (R. P. Wheat et al., "Infection Due to Chromobacteria: Report of 11 Cases," *Arch. Intern. Med.*, 1951, 88, 461–466. Also see Anon., "Bay Area Blitzed in 1950 by Army Germ War Tests," *Washington Star*, September 17, 1979. Anon., "Trial Starts in Army Death Suit," *Stars and Stripes*, March 26, 1981.)

57.   However, the relationship between radiation exposure and immune dysfunction is becoming more and more apparent as the years pass. In 1998, a report presented to the U.N. General Assembly revealed that 90 percent of villagers who had lived near the Soviet nuclear test site at Semipalatinsk (now in Kazakhstan) in the fifties and sixties were now suffering from "immune deficiency syndrome." See D. Harrison, "A Secret Nuclear Tragedy," *Observer* (U.K.), October 4, 1998, p. 11. Furthermore, acute exposure to radiation can result in *rapid* development of breathing problems, as among the islanders of Rongelap, who were irradiated by fallout from the Bikini nuclear test in 1954; over half of those exposed developed upper respiratory diseases within the next two months (R. Bertell, *No Immediate Danger*, p. 70).

58.   Interestingly, this possibility, suggested to me by Tony Pinching in 1998, reflected a previous comment by the lead author on the case, James Watanabe, when I first contacted him in 1990. He pointed out that at the time of the deaths in 1964, Legionnaire's disease, like AIDS, wasn't known.

59.   See J. A. Kovacs et al., "*Pneumocystis carinii* Pneumonia: A Comparison between Patients with the Acquired Immunodeficiency Syndrome and Patients with Other Immuno-deficiencies," *Ann. Intern. Med.*, 1984, 100, 663–671, which points out that PCP "presents as a more insidious disease process" in patients with AIDS than those with other immunosuppressive diseases.

60.   G. R. Hennigar, H. A. Lyons et al., "*Pneumocystis carinii* Pneumonia in an Adult," *Am. J. Clin. Pathol.*, 1961, 35(4), 353–364.

61.   My sincere thanks to the *Chicago Tribune* journalist John Crewdson, who was kind enough to share with me his notes and contacts on this case. He too was skeptical that it was a genuine case of AIDS, mainly because Ardouin's wife had survived for so long after his death (she was still alive in 1991).

62.   J. L. Stoeckle, H. L. Hardy et al., "Chronic Beryllium Disease — Long Term Follow-Up of Sixty Cases and Selective Review of the Literature," *Am. J. Med.*, 1969, 46, 545–561.

63.   Nonetheless, it was still a high reading. It contained 9.1 micrograms of beryllium per liter; a toxic amount is deemed to be 20 micrograms.

64. From a handbook on clinical tests referred to by Martin Salwen, head pathologist at Kings County Hospital, Brooklyn, during our second interview in 1991.

65. Letter from Dr. Salwen to Dr. Hill, June 20, 1991. Reply from Hill to Salwen, July 29, 1992.

66. R. Rhodes, *The Making of the Atomic Bomb* (London: Simon and Schuster, 1986), p. 549.

67. R. A. Simpson, "Uranium in Canada — 1957," *Can. Mining J.,* 1958 (February), pp. 146–147. Also: "Rayrock Mines," *Can. Mining J.,* 1958 (March), p. 110; and "Rayrock Mines," *Can. Mining J.,* 1958 (September), p. 156; T. A. Mansell, "Northwest Territories — 1958," *Can. Mining J.,* 1959 (February), pp. 105–106; R. A. Simpson, "Uranium in Canada — 1958," *Can. Mining J.,* 1959 (February), pp. 144–146; and F. R. Joubin, "Development of the Uranium Industry in Canada," *Can. Mining J.,* 1959 (October), pp. 110–114.

68. R. Bertell, *No Immediate Danger,* p. 70.

69. See K. Adachi, *The Enemy That Never Was* (Toronto: McClelland and Stewart, 1991) for background to anti-Japanese feeling in mining and lumbering industries.

70. Information and background history were kindly provided by various public officials from Yellowknife and Hay River (NWT), and Uranium City (Alberta). Different branches of the Workers' Compensation Board and Rio Algom Ltd. also initiated unsuccessful searches.

71. There was no apparent damage to either thyroid or spleen at autopsy, which works against the radiation exposure hypothesis. However, Dr. Barrie acknowledged that both were examined rather perfunctorily, because he concentrated his attentions on the lungs.

72. R. C. Gallo et al., "Origin of T-Cell Leukemia-Lymphoma Virus," *Lancet,* 1983, 2(ii), 962–963.

73. M. S. Cappell and J. Chow, "HTLV-I-Associated Lymphoma Involving the Entire Alimentary Tract and Presenting with an Acquired Immune Deficiency," *Am. J. Med.,* 1987, 82, 649–654.

74. J. P. Wyatt, M. L. Trumbull, M. Evans et al., "Cytomegalic Inclusion Pneumonitis in the Adult," *Am. J. Clin. Pathol.,* 1953, 23, 353–362.

75. H. Hamperl, "Pneumocystis Infection and Cytomegaly of the Lungs in the Newborn and Adult," *Am. J. Pathol.,* 1956, 32, 1–13.

76. Peter Nichols, letter to editor, untitled, *N. Engl. J. Med.,* 1982, 306(15), 934–935.

77. Apart from the fact that Wyatt himself failed to spot the presence of PCP (which was little known outside Europe at the start of the fifties), there were at least two significant errors in his article on the case (J. P. Wyatt et al., "Cytomegalic Inclusion Pneumonitis in the Adult"). One involved the patient history — which was inaccurate in several respects, and ended up adding a month to Dick's life. The other involved the microphotographs, of which there were nine — four from Dick and five from the other patient featured in the article. However, one of the photographs — allegedly from Patient 1 — was actually a mirror image of one of the photos from Patient 2, at a different magnification. (Compare photographs 4 [p. 355] and 6 [p. 357]. My thanks to Dr. Gerald Corbitt for spotting this error.) Such errors raised questions about Wyatt's findings, and highlighted the fact that he had merely examined tissue sections from the two patients. He had neither had direct contact with them when alive, nor had he been present at the autopsies.

78. J. L. Ziegler, P. A. Volberding et al., "Non-Hodgkin's Lymphoma in 90 Homosexual Men," *N. Engl. J. Med.,* 1984, 311(9), 565–570.

79. *AIDS and the Third World,* Panos dossier (London: The Panos Institute, 1988), pp. 174–175.

80. Both women are photographed bare-breasted and one, pictured smiling as she emerges from a stream, is wearing military fatigue trousers.

81. HTLV-I infection ranges from 2 percent to 10 percent among the islanders from widely separated parts of the Solomons. (A. Gessain, R. C. Gallo, D. C. Gadjusek et al., "Highly Divergent Molecular Variants of Human T-Lymphotropic Virus Type I from Isolated Populations in Papua New Guinea and the Solomon Islands," *Proc. Natl. Acad. Sci.,* 1991, 88, 7964–7968.)

82. M. S. Cappell and J. Chow, "HTLV-I-Associated Lymphoma Involving the Entire Alimentary Tract and Presenting with an Acquired Immune Deficiency."

83. This conclusion was reinforced when Dick's former wife was found to be negative for HIV, but had a low titer of CMV — suggesting that she had been exposed in the past but that, like most people, had suffered no infection. Unfortunately, the lab did not test for HTLV-I, but it would certainly be interesting to learn if she had also been exposed to that virus.

84. H. Hamperl, "Variants of *Pneumocystis* Pneumonia," *J. Bacteriol.,* 1957, 74, 353–356.

85. Letter from Serge Jothy to Fergal Hill of June 4, 1991; letter from Dr. Hill to Dr. Jothy of July 29, 1992. As Dr. Jothy pointed out, HTLV-1 was another possibility, given the patient's Japanese background, but the slides were never tested for this virus.

86. In addition to these potential archival cases from the literature, there were also some rather more anecdotal accounts of apparent AIDS or HIV infection from the forties and fifties, which I investigated. They included "Shoga's disease" (literally "queer's disease," characterized by "diarrhea, weight loss and certain death") in Mombasa in the forties; a 1952 outbreak of pneumonia at RAF Melksham, a military camp close to Porton Down, England, in which three National Servicemen apparently tested positive for "HVI" (sic); and a report that the U.S. Army had found the sera of a few soldiers who had served in Africa in the last war to be HIV-positive. I checked these reports out in some detail and found them to be based on dubious information and, in all likelihood, barroom tales.

87. Primary CMV infections, leading to secondary colonization by *Pneumocystis carinii,* may also have been involved in the cases of Dick G. and Mrs. Sadayo. (Tony Pinching, personal communication, 1998.)

88. Similar tests were also carried out by the Soviet and French governments.

89. However, two of Laurence's five patients apparently showed evidence of reverse transcriptase activity, suggesting that they might be infected with a retrovirus of some sort. This has never, as far as I know, been confirmed.

90. Anon., "AIDS Minus HIV?," *Lancet,* 1992, 340, 280; Anon., "AIDS without HIV," *BMJ,* 1992, 305, 271.

91. S. Harris, "The AIDS Heresies — A Case Study in Skepticism Taken Too Far," *Skeptic,* 1995, 3(2), 42–79.

92. See epigram on p. 42 of previous reference.


CHAPTER 10: *Theories of Origin, Propounded and Refuted*

1. In several instances, additional reasons why theories can be disproved have been omitted because of lack of space.

2. For example, a pamphlet entitled *Voice of Revival* (unsourced, undated) remonstrates against a "society which tolerates adultery, homosexuality, incest, paedophilia, sale of addictive drugs, corruption in high places etc. . . . God warned Israel of the consequences of flouting His instructions, 'Then the Lord will make your plagues remarkable, and the plagues of your children shall be great and persistent plagues, with evil and long-lasting sicknesses. He shall also bring on you all the diseases of Egypt (Africa) of which you were afraid; and they will cling to you'. (Deuteronomy; 28; v59–60, Interlinear Bible — Baker)." The pamphlet concludes: "AIDS is one of the several signs heralding the end of this age; Armageddon is at hand!"

3. F. Hoyle and C. Wickramasinghe, *Lifecloud* (1978), *Evolution from Space* (1978), and *Diseases from Space* (1979) (London: Dent and Sons). Since all these books were published before 1981, there is, of course, no mention of AIDS.

4. P. Newmark, "AIDS in an African Context," *Nature*, 1986, 324, 611.

5. M. O. McClure and T. F. Schulz, "Origin of AIDS," *BMJ*, 1989, 298, 1267–1268.

6. R. Jackson, "Hitler's Labs Created AIDS Virus," *Sun* (U.S.), January 3, 1989.

7. The history of the Soviet allegations is taken mainly from "The U.S.S.R.'s AIDS Disinformation Campaign" (Foreign Affairs Note), U.S. Department of State (Washington, D.C.), July 1987. See also A. Veitch, "Germ of Doubt," *Guardian* (U.K.), December 20, 1985, p. 16. The history of the American allegations has been reconstructed from published articles and commentaries.

8. V. Zapevalov, "Panic in the West, or What Is Hidden behind the Sensation about AIDS" (translated title), *Literaturnaya Gazeta,* October 30, 1985. The article sourced the information to "the well-respected Indian newspaper *Patriot,*" but neglected to mention that it emanated from an anonymous letter, and that this letter had apparently been published more than a year earlier. It also featured a three-paragraph postscript about the allegations in Seale's interview in *Executive Intelligence Review* published twelve days earlier. This was such a speedy and dramatic response that it would seem likely that it was sanctioned — if not planted — by the KGB.

9. "AIDS, Its Nature and Origin," by Jakob and Lilli Segal of Humboldt University, East Berlin, GDR, no publication details, no date, but clearly written in April 1986 or earlier. The article was later revamped and published as J. Segal, L. Segal, and R. Dehmlow, "Das AIDS — seine Natur und sein Ursprung," *Streitbarer Materialismus,* July 1988, 11, 7–68.

10. The Segals theorized that after a year during which the prisoners showed no symptoms, the scientists probably declared the new pathogen too innocuous for military purposes, and released their test subjects; "and it would have been logical for these former convicts to head for a nearby big city, not the nearest, Washington, because the climate of the capital would hardly be favourable for them, but more probably New York."

11. "AIDS and the Security of the Western World" (interview: Dr. John Seale), *Executive Intelligence Review,* October 18, 1985, pp. 54–57. *EIR* is published by Lyndon LaRouche, the right-wing politician from California, who apparently believed that the true extent and nature of the AIDS epidemic was being concealed, and that HIV could be spread casually from person to person by bodily contact, or through the air, by aerosol transmission, or the bites of insects. During 1986, LaRouche and *EIR* set up a "Biological Holocaust Task Force" that published a 150-page report entitled "An Emergency War Plan to Fight AIDS," at $250 a copy. They were also behind a group calling itself PANIC (the Prevent AIDS Now Initiative Committee) that advocated mandatory HIV testing, and the quarantining of HIV positives and those with AIDS, and which was instrumental

in putting Proposition 64, which argued for such measures, on the California ballot sheet. Seale apparently testified in favor of Proposition 64 at preliminary hearings before the California legislature in September 1986, and campaigned in its favor in the weeks that followed. (C. Gregg, "Unclean, Unclean: The Plague Mentality," *New Internationalist,* March 1987, pp. 12–14.) Although the proposition was defeated in November 1986 by a margin of 70 percent to 30 percent, the initiative achieved some of PANIC's aims, in that it served, to an extent, to legitimize the debate. The whole germ warfare origin controversy needs to be viewed within the context of Proposition 64, with which it appears to be inextricably linked. Although during 1985 and 1986, Seale and LaRouche apparently agreed on many aspects of the AIDS debate, Seale seems to have started to alter his views during the summer of 1986. By August he was merely claiming that the AIDS virus *might* have been man-made, and that either Soviet or American laboratories could have been responsible, since "any determined person, with access to the Aids virus in any laboratory, could start an epidemic in any country which thereafter would inevitably spread to every country" ("AIDS Virus Infection: A Soviet View of Its Origin" [letter by Z. A. Medvedev, reply by J. Seale]; *J. Roy. Soc. Med.,* 1986, 79, 495). Dr. Seale has right-wing political views, and some of his conference speeches reveal him to be a homophobe. Nonetheless, I believe that his often highly controversial contributions to the AIDS debate, especially during 1985 and 1986, were prompted more by genuine alarm about what he considered to be the scientific world's casual attitude toward an impending global disaster than by any conscious desire to sensationalize or misinform. Many aspects of his theorizing about AIDS were clear-sighted, and it is perhaps not his fault that his ideas were embraced by a whole range of others — many of whom (like LaRouche, the Streckers, and certain Soviet journals) had their own fish to fry. Between 1987, when he ceased to campaign for mandatory testing, and 1990, when he stopped working on AIDS altogether, John Seale produced some excellent analysis of the epidemic, emphasizing that AIDS has to be viewed in the context of a zoonosis, a disease that had crossed species from animal to man, and examining the various ways (all of them more plausible than biowarfare experiments, and some of which will be examined later in this book) in which such a transfer might have occurred. I am grateful to Dr. Seale for his detailed discussions of these issues, and for lending me, for a period of several months, his apparently uncensored files and papers from this period.

12.   Theodore Strecker, "This Is a Bio-Attack Alert," typed manuscript dated March 28, 1986. Robert's name was omitted from the title page. To some extent the manuscript was inspired by an interview that had appeared a few days earlier in the men's magazine *Omni,* in which virologist Carlton Gadjusek maintained that Communist scientists had their own passkeys at Fort Detrick, and outnumbered their American counterparts in some laboratories. In fact, the Streckers took this information entirely out of context, for Gadjusek continued: "With . . . U.S. citizens and foreign Communist investigators here, obviously there is no 'secret' bacterial warfare activity going on." (Interview with D. Carlton Gadjusek, *Omni,* March 1986, 34, p. 106.)

13.   Their major piece of "evidence" consisted of two lengthy memoranda about viruses and immunity published by the WHO in 1972. A. C. Allison, H. Koprowski et al., "Virus-Associated Immunopathology: Animal Models and Implications for Human Disease. 1. Effects of Viruses on the Immune System, Immune-Complex Diseases and Antibody-Mediated Immunologic Injury" and "2. Cell-Mediated Immunity, Auto-Immune Diseases, Genetics, and Implications for Clinical Research," *Bull. WHO,* 1972, 47, 257–264 and 265–274.

14. The "Bio-Attack Alert" ended with a list of "correct responses," including the retaking of the virus labs ("by force if necessary"), the mobilizing of the National Guard, the arrest and trial of those responsible, the seizure of records, and the necessity of warning the American people "that the enemy is ashore and advancing. Inform all scientists concerning the true nature of the disease and its origin. Someone may have a cure." This paper was posted to the U.S. president and vice-president, state governors, members of cabinet, and the heads of various government agencies including the NSA, CIA, and FBI. President Reagan was given three weeks in which to respond, and it seems that he failed to meet the Streckers' deadline. Also see R. Strecker, "AIDS Virus Infection" (letter), *J. Roy. Soc. Med.,* 1986, 79, 559–560.

15. W. C. Douglass, "WHO Murdered Africa," *Health Freedom News,* published by the National Health Federation, PO Box 688, Monrovia, California 91016, September 1987, reprinted as separate pamphlet (*WHO Murdered Africa — Just As We Said*) by the NHF in 1992. Such claims were later enlarged by another Strecker acolyte, Alan Cantwell Jr., who published them in rather less strident form in a book stridently entitled *AIDS and the Doctors of Death.* Theodore Strecker was found shot dead, his rifle beside him, in August 1988 . . . "perhaps not so unexpectedly, considering his views about the nature of AIDS," according to his brother, who hinted at foul play, even though the official verdict was suicide. Robert fought on alone, claiming to have "absolute theoretical proof that the cure for AIDS lies in the development of time reversed nonlinear conjugate wave pulsed electro-magnetic radiation." (Letter from Robert Strecker to John Seale, dated March 15, 1989.) In another letter to the evolutionary biologist Dr. David Penny, who had written an article for *Nature* proposing a theory of AIDS origin that differed from his own, he asked whether the journal "has been reduced to being authored, reviewed and read by anencephalic morons." The "true nature of AIDS," he told Dr. Penny, was revealed in his own "AIDS virus infection" letter.

16. A. J. Nahmias et al., "Evidence for Human Infection with an HTLV III/LAV-Like Virus in Central Africa, 1959" (letter), *Lancet,* 1986, 1(ii), 1279–1280. S. S. Frøland et al., "HIV-1 Infection in Norwegian Family before 1970" (letter), *Lancet,* 1988, 1(ii), 1344–1345.

17. N. Nuttall, "Old Soviet Aids Myth Exposed," *Times* (U.K.), March 19, 1992, p. 18.

18. For a particularly paranoid example, see G. Glum, *Full Disclosure — The Truth about the AIDS Epidemic* (Los Angeles: Silent Walker Publishing, 1994). For a well-balanced repudiation of Strecker's theories, see D. Gilbert, "Tracking the Real Genocide," *Covert Action Quarterly,* Fall 1996, 58, 55–64.

19. It seems likely, for instance, that at least one chimpanzee SIV was present in an American primate colony as early as 1963. See R. V. Gilden, L. O. Arthur et al., "HTLV-III Antibody in a Breeding Chimpanzee Not Experimentally Exposed to the Virus," *Lancet,* 1986, 1(i), 678–679.

20. J. Marks, *The Search for the Manchurian Candidate — The CIA and Mind Control* (London: Allen Lane, 1979) contains good background on Dr. Sid Gottlieb and the CIA and Chemical Corps drug testing and chemical and biological warfare testing programs that went under a variety of different code names, including MKSEARCH, MKNAOMI, and MKULTRA.

21. See J. Kwitny, *Endless Enemies — The Making of an Unfriendly World* (New York: Congdon and Weed, 1984), pp. 65, 67, and 71. For the original testimony, see "Alleged Assassination Plots Involving Foreign Leaders — An Interim Report of the Select Committee to Study Governmental Operations with Respect to Intelligence Activities," Report No. 94–465, U.S. Government Printing Office (Washington, D.C.), 1975, pp. 20–21 and 29–30. The

latter report comprises hearings before Senator Frank Church, and features Gottlieb's testimony, given under the alias "Joseph Scheider," and Devlin's, given as "Victor Hedgman," as well as intriguing hints that the lethal agent was intended to be incorporated into a vaccine, either injected or oral. Gottlieb gave "rubber gloves, a gauze mask and a syringe" to Devlin, so that the lethal material could be injected into "some substance that Lumumba would ingest" (pp. 24–25). Another senior CIA officer, "Michael Mulroney," was told by Devlin in October 1960 that he had "a virus in the safe," and later testified "I knew it wasn't for someone to get his polio shot up to date" (p. 41). In December 1960, a European forger and former bank robber, code-named WI/ROGUE, appeared on the scene; he had apparently been trained by European CIA agents in "medical immunization," though it is unclear whether or not he was intended to be used as the hired assassin (pp. 45–48).

22. R. Lederer, "Chemical-Biological Warfare, Medical Experiments and Population Control," *CovertAction Information Bulletin,* Summer 1987, 28, 33–42; see notes 36 and 43.

23. "Testimony before a Subcommittee of the House Committee on Appropriations," Department of Defense Appropriations for 1970 (Washington, D.C.: U.S. Government Printing Office, 1969), quoted in R. Harris and J. Paxman, *A Higher Form of Killing* (London: Chatto and Windus, 1982), p. 241. Another (apparently fuller) version, quoted on pp. 5–6 of L. G. Horowitz, *Emerging Viruses: AIDS and Ebola, Accident or Intentional?* (Rockport, MA: Tetrahedron, 1996), claims that further testimony revealed that "a research program to explore the feasibility of this could be completed in approximately 5 years at a total cost of $10 million," and that "tentative plans [had been] made to initiate the program," although they had then been postponed for the two years previous to 1969. The source of this additional material was allegedly Theodore Strecker, through an FOIA application. The Horowitz book is a particularly entertaining attempt to tie in biological weapon scenarios (including the birth of the Ebola and AIDS viruses) with the WHO, the CIA, the OTRAG rocket base in the east of the Congo, and even Richard Preston, author of *The Hot Zone.* It is best taken with a pinch of salt.

24. See W. Szmuness, C. E. Stevens et al., "A Controlled Clinical Trial of the Efficacy of the Hepatitis B Vaccine (Heptavax B): A Final Report," *Hepatology,* 1981, 1(5), 377–385; and D. P. Francis, J. W. Curran et al., "The Prevention of Hepatitis B with Vaccine: Report of the Centers for Disease Control Multi-Center Efficacy Trial among Homosexual Men," *Ann. Intern. Med.,* 1982, 97, 362–366. Also A. M. Schwartz and T. L. Chorba, "Hepatitis Vaccine and the Acquired Immunodeficiency Syndrome" (letter), *Ann. Intern. Med.,* 1983, 99(4), 567–568; and M. I. McDonald, D. T. Durack et al., "Hepatitis B Surface Antigen Could Harbour the Infective Agent of AIDS," *Lancet,* 1983, 2(ii), 882–884.

25. Some groups were especially suspicious about Wolf Szmuness, the Polish émigré who had been in charge of the hepatitis B vaccine trials, and whose past history included seven years spent in exile in Siberia during World War II, from where he defected to the United States. (A. Kellner, "Reflections on Wolf Szmuness," *Prog. Clin. Biomed. Res.,* 1985, 182, 3–10.) His background, combined with the suspicions that AIDS had arisen through contamination of the hepatitis B vaccine, encouraged the view in some quarters that he was either a Soviet spy or else a double-agent, advancing the interests of white heterosexual supremacists. (See, for instance, A. Cantwell Jr., *AIDS and the Doctors of Death — An Inquiry into the Origins of the AIDS Epidemic* [Los Angeles: Aries Rising Press, 1988], pp. 101–105.)

26. See M. R. Hilleman et al., "Clinical and Laboratory Studies of HBsAg Vaccine," in G. M. Byas (editor), *Viral Hepatitis* (Philadelphia: Franklin Institute Press, 1978), pp. 525–537. Mentally handicapped children at Willowbrook State School, Staten Island, New York,

had been used in various hepatitis experiments (including exposure trials) since the late fifties by Dr. Saul Krugman. The "school" was apparently closed down in 1976, in the wake of controversy about the treatment of its child patients, and Hilleman's study documents nine months of follow-up, suggesting that the inoculations probably began in 1975 at latest. This date of 1975 for the first U.S. vaccinations is confirmed by R. T. Ravenholt, "Role of Hepatitis B Virus in Acquired Immunodeficiency Syndrome," *Lancet*, 1983, 2(ii), 885–886. Hilleman gives no information about the identity of the second set of trial subjects, who were HB-positive, but they may have been gay men. A total of 666 New York gays had already been enrolled in baseline surveys in preparation for HB vaccine studies in 1974/5 (see W. Szmuness et al., "Hepatitis B Vaccine," *N. Engl. J. Med.*, 1980, 303(15), 833–841).

27. One early article frankly tackled the problem of potential slow virus contamination of HB vaccines, concluding that it "would not be expected." See R. H. Purcell et al., "Hepatitis B Vaccines — On the Threshold," *Am. J. Clin. Pathol.*, 1978, 70, 159–169.

28. J. A. Golden; C. E. Stevens, "No Increased Incidence of AIDS in Recipients of Hepatitis B Vaccine" (letter and reply), *N. Engl. J. Med.*, 1983, 308(19), 1163–1164.

29. F. B. Hollinger, "Hepatitis B Vaccines — to Switch or Not to Switch" (editorial), *JAMA*, 1987, 257(19), 2634–2636.

30. H. Ratner, "Monkey Viruses, AIDS and the Salk Vaccine, Parts 1 and 2," *Child & Family*, 1988, 20, 134–138.

31. J. A. Morris, "Long-term Follow-up after SV40 Inoculation" (letter), *N. Engl. J. Med.*, 1982, 306(19), 1176–1177. See also L. P. Weiner et al., "Isolation of Virus Related to SV40 from Patients with Progressive Multifocal Leukoencephalopathy," *N. Engl. J. Med.*, 1972, 286(8), 385–390. For recent confirmation of an association between a cancer and SV40 exposure, see L. Carbone et al., "Simian Virus 40–Like DNA Sequences in Human Pleural Mesothelioma," *Oncogene*, 1994, 9, 1781–1790; P. Brown, "Mystery Virus Linked to Asbestos Cancer," *New Scientist*, May 21, 1994, p. 4; and Anon., "A Shot in the Dark," *New York*, November 11, 1996, pp. 38–43 and 85.

32. E. L. Snead, "AIDS — Immunization Related Syndrome," *Health Freedom News*, 1987, 6(6), 14–45.

33. For example, see J. Teas, "Could AIDS Be a New Variant of African Swine Fever Virus?" (letter), *Lancet*, 1983, 1(ii), 923; and J. Beldekas, J. Teas et al., "African Swine Fever and AIDS" (letter), *Lancet*, 1986, 1(i), 564–565. (This theory also had conspiratorial undertones, since it had previously been reported that the CIA was responsible for introducing ASF to Cuban pigs in 1971, in a bid to destroy the country's economy and bring down the Castro regime. See D. Fetherston and J. Cummings, "Cuban Outbreak of Swine Fever Linked to CIA," *Newsday* [New York], January 9, 1977, p. 5.)

34. Later, they allegedly found that some pigs tested positive for HIV antibodies, while some AIDS patients tested positive for ASF virus — results that were roundly rejected as false positives by the CDC. See "Pigs, AIDS and Belle Glade" (editorial), *New York Times*, June 3, 1986, p. A26.

35. See A. Moore and R. D. Le Baron, "The Case for a Haitian Origin of the AIDS Epidemic," in D. A. Feldman and T. M. Johnson (editors), *The Social Dimensions of AIDS: Method and Theory* (New York: Praeger, 1986), pp. 77–94. This theory is also well summarized in G. W. Shannon, G. F. Pyle, and R. L. Bashshur, *The Geography of AIDS — Origins and Course of an Epidemic* (New York: Guilford Press, 1990), pp. 40–45. See also P. Moses and J. Moses, "Haiti and the Acquired Immunodeficiency Syndrome" (letter), *Ann. Intern. Med.*, 1983, 99(4), 565–566.

36. A. Cantwell, *AIDS and the Doctors of Death*, p. 131.

37. P. K. Lewin, "Possible Origin of Human AIDS" (letter), *Can. Med. Assoc. J.*, 1985, 132, 1110.

38. H. P. Katner, "Origin of AIDS" (letter), *J. Natl. Med. Assoc.*, 1988, 80(3), 262.

39. See M. A. Gonda, "Bovine Immunodeficiency Virus," *AIDS*, 1992, 6, 759–776. Further-more, those humans exposed to BIV accidentally (e.g., by needle-stick accidents) have not become infected. See K. Schneider, "AIDS-Like Virus Is Found at High Rate in U.S. Cattle," *New York Times*, June 1, 1991.

40. A. Karpas, "Origin of the AIDS Virus Explained?," *New Scientist*, July 16, 1987, p. 67; and A. Karpas, "Origin and Spread of AIDS" (letter), *Nature*, 1990, 348, 578. The theory was based on a previous exposition: F. Noireau, "HIV Transmission from Monkey to Man" (letter), *Lancet*, 1987, 1(ii), 1498–1499.

41. A. Kashamura, *Famille, sexualité et culture: essai sur les moeurs sexuelles et les cultures des peuples des Grands Lacs africains* (Paris: Payot, 1973).

42. U. Rahm and A. Christiaensen, "Les mammifères de l'île Idjwi (Lac Kivu, Congo)," Musée Royale de L'Afrique Centrale, Tervuren, Belgique, *Annales Serie IN-8, Sciences Zoologiques*, 1966, 149, 1–35.

43. By contrast, an SIV has been isolated from the other subgroup of this species, *C. mitis albogularis*, the Sykes' monkey, which is found only to the east of the Rift Valley, in Kenya, Tanzania, Mozambique, and South Africa. However, this particular SIV, now termed SIVsyk, is but a very distant relation to HIV-1. See P. Emau, H. M. McClure, P. N. Hirsch et al., "Isolation from African Sykes' Monkeys (*Cercopithecus mitis*) of a Lentivirus Related to Human and Simian Immunodeficiency Viruses," *J. Virol.*, 1991, 65(4), 2135–2140.

44. P. Wright, "Smallpox Vaccine 'Triggered AIDS Virus,'" *Times* (U.K.), May 11, 1987, pp. 1 and 18.

45. R. R. Redfield et al., "Disseminated Vaccinia in a Military Recruit with Human Immunodeficiency Virus (HIV) Disease," *N. Engl. J. Med.*, 1987, 316(11), 673–676; see also N. A. Halsey and D. A. Henderson, "HIV Infection and Immunization against Other Agents," *N. Engl. J. Med.*, 1987, 316(11), 683–685. Although the last case of smallpox occurred in 1977, and the eradication of the disease was officially announced in 1980, the soldiers of many countries are still vaccinated against smallpox in case it is ever employed as an agent of biological warfare.

46. The WHO responded promptly to quash the *Times* article, with a press release (WHA/5, "WHO Says Concentrate on Action to Prevent AIDS," May 11, 1987) that came out the same day.

47. Copy of six-page discussion paper apparently written by the consultant (unsourced, untitled, undated), made available by Pearce Wright. It contains a number of provable factual errors.

48. In fact, even lower levels of smallpox vaccine quality control are revealed by "The Global Eradication of Smallpox: Final Report of the Global Commission for the Certification of Smallpox Eradication, Geneva, December 1979," WHO (Geneva), 1980, especially pp. 27–29; and F. Fenner, "Lessons from the Smallpox Eradication Campaign," in R. A. Lerner et al. (editors), *Vaccines '85* (Cold Spring Harbor, NY: Cold Spring Harbor Labor-atory, 1985), pp. 143–146.

49. The two papers referenced above make it clear that smallpox vaccine is generally pre-pared in animal skin. However, before 1967 "methods for manufacturing biologically sterile vaccine in eggs or cell cultures were . . . in use in a few places . . . [but] there were problems with the heat stability of such vaccines" (Fenner). I have checked the literature

fairly exhaustively, and it appears that the only cell cultures used for human trials of smallpox vaccine were based on chick embryo and rabbit kidney — and there is no reason to suspect that either of these could have become accidentally contaminated with HIV or SIV.

50. E. Sternglass, *Secret Fallout, Low-Level Radiation from Hiroshima to Three Mile Island* (New York: McGraw-Hill, 1981).

51. The Nuclear Test Ban Treaty was signed by the United States, the Soviet Union, and the United Kingdom on August 4, 1963, and prohibited the testing of nuclear weapons in space, above ground, and under water. However, France and China have staged atmospheric tests after this date, while South Africa and Israel are suspected of having done so.

52. E. J. Sternglass and J. Scheer, "Radiation Exposure of Bone Marrow Cells to Strontium-90 during Early Development as a Possible Co-factor in the Etiology of AIDS," paper presented at the AGM of the American Association for the Advancement of Science, May 18, 1986, Philadelphia.

53. V. M. Hirsch, P. R. Johnson et al., "An African Primate Lentivirus (SIVsm) Closely Related to HIV-2," *Nature,* 1989, 339, 389–392. T. Huet, S. Wain-Hobson et al., "Genetic Organization of a Chimpanzee Lentivirus Related to HIV-1" (letter), *Nature,* 1990, 345, 356–359.

54. Indeed, it was clear by 1988 that the African green monkey theory of origin had been based upon a laboratory error. See chapter 7.

55. These outbreaks of simian disease were first reported as being possibly related to the human AIDS epidemic in 1983. (R. V. Henrickson, M. B. Gardner et al., "Epidemic of Acquired Immunodeficiency in Rhesus Monkeys," *Lancet,* 1983, 1(i), 358–360.)

56. See, for instance, R. Sabatier, *Blaming Others: Prejudice, Race and Worldwide AIDS* (London: Panos Institute, 1988), p. 50.

57. For example, Anon., "Monkey Eaters' Lives at Risk," *Daily Telegraph* (U.K.), February 18, 1987.

58. E. O. A. Asibey, "Wildlife as a Source of Protein in Africa South of the Sahara," *Biological Conservation,* 1974, 6(1), 32–39. See also S. Connor, "Great Apes Face Extinction as Food Trade Grows," *Independent* (U.K.), October 26, 1994, p. 7.

59. L. Thompson, "AIDS Virus: From Monkey to Man," *Albuquerque Journal,* October 14, 1985, p. B1.

60. L. Montagnier, "Origin and Evolution of HIVs and Their Role in AIDS Pathogenesis," *J. AIDS,* 1988, 1(6), 517–520; R. C. Gallo, "HIV — The Cause of AIDS: An Overview of Its Biology, Mechanisms of Disease Induction, and Our Attempts to Control It," *J. AIDS,* 1988, 1(6), 521–535; Anon., "HIV Infection 'Almost Certainly' Came from Animals," *Pharmaceutical J.,* September 14, 1991, p. 355; Anon., "Luc Montagnier Interview," *Omni,* December 1988, pp. 102–134.

61. J. Desmyter, J. Vandepitte et al., "Origin of AIDS" (letter), *BMJ,* 1986, 293, 1308.

62. K. M. De Cock, "AIDS: An Old Disease from Africa?," *BMJ,* 1984, 289, 306–308.

63. This "new roads, urbanization and new sexual freedoms following independence in Africa" hypothesis has been repeated in countless texts. One of the best written is P. Gould, *The Slow Plague — A Geography of the AIDS Pandemic* (London: Blackwell, 1993).

64. F. Brun-Vezinet, L. Montagnier et al., "Lack of Evidence for Human or Simian T-Lymphotropic Viruses Type III Infection in Pygmies" (letter), *Lancet,* 1986, 1(ii), 854.

65. R. Colebunders, H. Taelman, and P. Piot, "AIDS: An Old Disease from Africa?" (letter), *BMJ,* 1984, 289, 765.

66. P. W. Ewald, "The Evolution of Virulence," *Sci. Am.,* April 1993, pp. 86–93.

67. R. C. Gallo, "HIV — The Cause of AIDS."

68. N. Nzilambi, K. M. De Cock, J. B. McCormick et al., "The Prevalence of Infection with Human Immunodeficiency Virus over a 10-Year Period in Rural Zaire," *N. Engl. J. Med.*, 1988, 318, 276–279.

69. One of the three subjects, for instance, was already infected by the age of seven — presumably either perinatally or parenterally.

70. G. Jean-Aubry, *Joseph Conrad in the Congo* (New York: Haskell House Publishers, Ltd., 1973).

71. J. Cribb, *The White Death* (Sydney: Angus and Robertson, 1996), pp. 102–107.

72. A. Karpas, "Origin and Spread of AIDS" (letter), *Nature*, 1990, 348, 578; J. Seale and Z. Medvedev, "Origin and Transmission of AIDS. Multi-Use Hypodermics and the Threat to the Soviet Union: Discussion Paper," *J. Roy. Soc. Med.*, 1987, 80, 301–304. Here, Seale and his Soviet coauthor give a range of examples from Africa, the United States, and the Soviet Union of HIV (and such other viral diseases as hepatitis B and Ebola hemorrhagic fever) being spread through the use of improperly sterilized hypodermic needles.

73. S. Giunta and G. Groppa, "The Primate Trade and the Origin of AIDS Viruses" (letter), *Nature*, 1987, 329, 22.

74. J. Creamer (editor), *Biohazard: The Silent Threat from Biomedical Research and the Creation of AIDS* (London: National Anti-Vivisection Society, 1987), see especially pp. 2–3 and 25–32.

75. C. Gilks, "AIDS, Monkeys and Malaria," *Nature*, 1991, 354, 262. For further background, see R. S. Desowitz, *The Malaria Capers — More Tales of Parasites and People, Research and Reality* (New York: Norton, 1991), pp. 123–142.

76. G. Kolata, "Theory Links AIDS to Malaria Experiments," *New York Times*, November 28, 1991, p. B14.

77. The only known chimp experiments that occurred in Africa involved the inoculation of two European men in Freetown, Sierra Leone, West Africa with blood taken from a malaria-infected chimpanzee (*Pan troglodytes verus*) in 1922, the animal subsequently died. B. Blacklock and S. Adler, "A Parasite Resembling *Plasmodium Falciparum* in a Chimpanzee," *Ann. Trop. Med. Parasit.*, 1922, 16, 99–107. However, there is no evidence that this subspecies of chimp is (or has ever been) infected with an SIV. By contrast, there is no evidence to suggest that any malarial research involving human injections with chimp blood has ever occurred in *central* Africa, where we know that some chimps, at least, of the subspecies *Pan troglodytes troglodytes* and *Pan troglodytes schweinfurthi* are infected with an SIV that is close to HIV-1. A similar theory cited the erstwhile practice of attempting to boost the dwindling sex drives of elderly men by giving them testicular grafts from monkeys, especially chimpanzees and baboons. This research was pioneered by the Russian scientist Serge Voronoff in the twenties, but was discontinued a few years later when shown to be both ineffective and dangerous. (R. G. Gosden, "AIDS and Malaria Experiments" [letter], *Nature*, 1992, 355, 305. See also D. W. Hamilton, *The Monkey Gland Affair* [London: Chatto and Windus, 1986], and R. G. Hoskins, "Studies on Vigor. IV. The Effect of Testicle Grafts on Spontaneous Activity," *Endocrinology*, 1925, 9, 277–296.) Again, these experiments involved the West African chimp, and almost certainly took place too long ago to have been relevant.

78. Charles Gilks told me that the two experiments he identified in which sooty mangabey blood was allegedly injected directly into man were reported in German medical jour-

nals in 1909 and 1910. (H. von Berenberg-Gossler, "Beitrage zur Naturgeschichte der Malariaplasmodin," *Arch. Protistenk.*, 1909, 16, 245–280; also see R. Gonder et al., "Experimentelle Untersuchungen über Affenmalaria," *Centralbl. Bakteriol. Parasitol., 1 Abt. Orig.*, 1910, 54(3), 236–240. Also see commentary in J. Rodhain and L. Van den Berghe, "Contribution à l'étude des plasmodiums des singes africains," *Ann. Soc. Belge Méd. Trop.*, 1936, 16, 521–531.) Although these articles indicate that the monkeys involved were *Cercocebus fuliginosus* (an alternative early name for the sooty mangabey), the only German colonies in West Africa during this period were Togoland and Kamerun (now Togo and Cameroon), in which the white-collared mangabey (*Cercocebus torquatus torquatus*) is found, but not the sooty. The white-collared mangabey has a predominantly fuliginous (smoky gray) body, but is not host to the "correct" SIV.

79. Charles Gilks, personal communication, 1996.

80. R. Root-Bernstein, *Rethinking AIDS — The Tragic Cost of Premature Consensus* (New York: The Free Press/Macmillan, 1993). H. P. Katner, "Origin of AIDS" (letter), *J. Natl. Med. Assoc.*, 1988, 80(3), 262.

81. R. J. Ablin et al., "AIDS: A Disease of Ancient Egypt?" (letter), *N.Y. St. J. Med.*, 1985, 85, 200–201.

82. L. André, "Le S.I.D.A. a-t-il déjà existé?," *J. Méd. Trop.*, 1987, 47(3), 229–230. Syphilis was first seen in the Old World among soldiers at the siege of Naples in 1495, and the disease spread across Europe in epidemic fashion in the remaining years of that century. The source of the outbreak is generally ascribed to the opening up of the New World by Christopher Columbus, whose first two voyages of exploration — in 1492 and 1493 — featured visits to the Isle of Hispaniola — which, of course, includes Haiti, that land of pigs and scapegoats.

83. T. Appelboom et al., "The Historical Autopsy of Erasmus Roterodamus (c. 1466–1536)," in T. Appelboom et al., *Art, History and Antiquity of Rheumatic Diseases* (Brussels: Elsevier, 1987), pp. 76–77. My original source for the last three paragraphs was M. D. Grmek, *History of AIDS — Emergence and Origin of a Modern Pandemic* (Princeton: Princeton University Press, 1990), pp. 110–111.

84. See R. B. Mitchell, *Syphilis as AIDS* (Austin, Texas: Banned Books, 1990), and Harris L. Coulter, *AIDS and Syphilis — The Hidden Link* (Berkeley: North Atlantic Books, 1987), including an interview with Joan McKenna on pp. 77–92.

85. R. Root-Bernstein, *Rethinking AIDS — The Tragic Cost of Premature Consensus.*

86. J. A. Sonnabend and S. Saadoun, "The Acquired Immunodeficiency Syndrome: A Discussion of Etiologic Hypotheses," *AIDS Res.*, 1984, 1(2), 107–120.

87. R. Lederer, "The Origin and Spread of AIDS," *CovertAction Information Bulletin*, Summer 1987, 28, 48–54; especially p. 48.

88. See, for instance, S.-C. Lo, "Isolation and Identification of a Novel Virus from Patients with AIDS," *Am. J. Trop. Med. Hyg.*, 1986, 35(4), 675–676; and K. Wright, "Mycoplasmas in the AIDS Spotlight," *Science*, 1990, 248, 682–683. Luc Montagnier continues to believe that a mycoplasmal cofactor is involved, as will be discussed later. Nowadays, the standard response of most virologists to co-factorial theories is that it is hardly surprising that HIV should have different pathogenic potential depending on whether or not other pathogens are present.

89. Robert Root-Bernstein, personal communication, 1995. In the same phone conversation, Root-Bernstein told me that he was still looking at three other possibilities: that HIV was "necessary, but not sufficient [on its own]" to cause AIDS; that HIV "synergized" with

something else like alcohol or barbiturates to cause AIDS; or that AIDS was really an autoimmune disease — a possibility that he was then investigating by experiment. He promised to contact me further if he had interesting results, but I did not hear from him again.

90. See, for instance, P. H. Duesberg, "AIDS Epidemiology: Inconsistencies with Human Immunodeficiency Virus and with Infectious Disease" (advertisement), *Proc. Natl. Acad. Sci.,* 1991, 88, 1575–1579; and P. Duesberg, "AIDS Acquired by Drug Consumption and Other Noncontagious Risk Factors," *Pharmac. Ther.,* 1993, 55, 201–277.

91. A few examples. I asked why, when an HIV-positive and an HIV-negative child were born to an HIV-positive mother, only the first child went on to get AIDS. Such anecdotal stories, he replied, are worthless unless reproduced in large numbers. (This is a valid point, but one that he tended to use *ad infinitum.*) I asked him about Patricia Fultz's work: How could a pure clone of a highly virulent form of SIVsm cause simian AIDS when introduced into macaques and SIV-negative (but not SIV-positive) sooty mangabeys? He said that we could not be sure that the clone was uncontaminated with other organisms. When I asked why rural people in Africa had themselves recognized AIDS, or Slim, as a new condition, he insisted that he saw nothing new, but only old diseases under new names. I urged him to go to Africa and find out for himself. As far as I know, he never did.

92. J. Cohen, "Duesberg and Critics Agree: Hemophilia Is the Best Test," *Science,* 1994, 266, 1645–1646.

93. Research published in 1995 revealed that in an HIV-positive individual, between 100 million and a billion HIV virions are produced daily, and there is a proportionate level of production and destruction of CD4 lymphocytes. In other words HIV does, after all, behave like a typical virus — and it is the proliferation of slightly mutated versions ("quasispecies") of HIV within the body that eventually overloads the immune system and causes the decline into full-blown AIDS. See D. D. Ho et al., "Rapid Turnover of Plasma Virions and CD4 Lymphocytes in HIV Infection," *Nature,* 1995, 373, 123–126; and X. Wei, B. H. Hahn, G. M. Shaw et al., "Viral Dynamics in Human Immunodeficiency Virus Type 1 Infection," *Nature,* 1995, 373, 117–122. See also S. Wain-Hobson, "Virological Mayhem," *Nature,* 1995, 373, 102 for excellent analysis.

94. For a riposte to the position of Duesberg and his journalist supporters like Celia Farber, Joan Shenton, and Neville Hodgkinson that there is no AIDS epidemic in Africa, see E. Hooper, "Empty Bottles, Empty Vessels," *AIDS Newsletter,* 1993, 8(9), 2–7.

95. J. Cohen, "The Epidemic in Thailand," *Science,* 1994, 266, 1647.

96. J. Cohen, "Could Drugs, Rather Than a Virus, Be the Cause of AIDS?," *Science,* 1994, 266, 1648.

97. J. Cohen "Could Drugs, Rather Than a Virus, Be the Cause of AIDS?" An independent panel from Duesberg's own university, Berkeley, later found his assertions groundless.

98. P. H. Duesberg, *Inventing the AIDS Virus* (Washington, D.C.: Regnery, 1996).

99. If he does so, his chances are not good. Three lab workers who, in separate incidents, were inadvertently injected with pure clones of HIV have all since demonstrated a severe loss in CD4 cells, and one developed PCP just under six years after his probable HIV exposure. See J. Cohen, "Fulfilling Koch's Postulates," *Science,* 1994, 266, 1647. Those readers who are still unpersuaded should take the trouble to read and evaluate some of the Duesberg camp's literature, especially *Reappraising AIDS,* the monthly magazine published by the Group for Scientific Reappraisal of the HIV/AIDS Hypothesis, 7514 Girard Avenue, #1–331, La Jolla, CA 92037, USA; fax: (619) 272-1621. They should also

refer to perhaps the best of the ripostes to Duesberg's arguments: S. B. Harris; "The AIDS Heresies — A Case Study in Skepticism Taken Too Far," *Skeptic,* 1995, 3(2), 42–79. On p. 72, Harris proposes a practical (and useful) way in which Duesberg, if sincere, could self-inject HIV.

CHAPTER 11: *Gerry Myers and the Monkey Puzzle Tree*

1. Richard Rhodes, *The Making of the Atomic Bomb* (New York: Simon and Schuster, 1986), p. 676.
2. G. Myers, K. MacInnes, and L. Myers, "Phylogenetic Moments in the AIDS Epidemic," in S. S. Morse (editor), *Emerging Viruses* (Oxford: Oxford University Press, 1993), pp. 120–137.
3. HIV Sequence Database, edited by Gerry Myers and Bette Korber, Los Alamos National Laboratory, T-10, MS K710, Los Alamos, New Mexico 87545. (Updated annually.)
4. R. C. Gallo et al., "Origin of T-Cell Leukemia-Lymphoma Virus," *Lancet,* 1983, 2(ii), 962–963. Also: A. Fleming, "HTLV from Africa to Japan" (letter), *Lancet,* 1984, 1(i), 279; and S. Hino et al., "HTLV and the Propagation of Christianity in Nagasaki" (letter), *Lancet,* 1984, 2(i), 572–573. There were apparently many contacts between Japanese locals and Portuguese/African crews during this period, including sexual ones.
5. F. Fenner, "Lessons from the Smallpox Eradication Campaign," in R. A. Lerner et al. (editors), *Vaccines '85* (Cold Spring Harbor, N.Y.: Cold Spring Harbor, 1985), pp. 143–146.
6. Gerry Myers may have been wrong about these two specific examples, although batches of Hilary Koprowski's polio vaccines were certainly made in Croatia, then part of Yugoslavia. His mention of Poland, where *American-made* Koprowski strains were fed to many millions, also suggests that he may have been thinking of these vaccines.
7. K. Shah and N. Nathanson, "Human Exposure to SV40: Review and Comment," *Am. J. Epidemiol.,* 1976, 103(1), 1–12.
8. Later, this lack of an association between SV40 and cancer would be disputed. See M. Carbone et al., "Simian Virus 40–Like DNA Sequences in Human Pleural Mesothelioma," *Oncogene,* 1994, 9, 1781–1790.
9. As revealed later, this was clearly Preston Marx.
10. M. Grmek, *History of AIDS: Emergence and Origin of a Modern Pandemic* (Princeton: Princeton University Press, 1990).
11. Part of the reason for Myers's skepticism was that he believed that André Nahmias had used up all of the L70 sample on his various antibody tests, and that none remained for PCR work.
12. This was an interesting comment, as I later realized, since baboon kidneys were used to prepare a French inactivated polio vaccine in the fifties and sixties.
13. This virus was later reported in R. De Leys, M. Van den Haesevelde et al., "Isolation and Partial Characterization of an Unusual Human Immunodeficiency Retrovirus from Two Persons of West-Central African Origin," *J. Virol.,* 1990, 64, 1207–1216.
14. P. Charneau, L. Montagnier, F. Clavel et al., "Isolation and Envelope Sequence of a Highly Divergent HIV-1 Isolate: Definition of a New HIV-1 Group," *Virol.,* 1994, 205, 247–253.
15. H. Tsujimoto et al., "Isolation and Characterization of Simian Immunodeficiency Virus from Mandrills in Africa and Its Relationship to Other Human and Simian Retroviruses," *J. Virol.,* 1988, 62, 4044–4050.

16.  P. R. Johnson, V. M. Hirsch et al., "Simian Immunodeficiency Viruses from African Green Monkeys Display Unusual Genetic Diversity," *J. Virol.,* 1990, 64(3), 1086–1092.

17.  The callitrix, or *Cercopithecus aethiops sabaeus.*

18.  The grivet, or *Cercopithecus aethiops aethiops.*

19.  At this point, the fifth PIV group was still privileged information, but Myers encouraged me to go and interview Vanessa Hirsch, who briefed me about the unusual Sykes' monkey SIV. See P. Emau, H. M. McClure, V. M. Hirsch et al., "Isolation from African Sykes' Monkeys (*Cercopithecus mitis*) of a Lentivirus Related to Human and Simian Immunodeficiency Viruses," *J. Virol.,* 1991, 65(4), 2135–2140. The full sequence was eventually published in V. M. Hirsch, H. M. McClure et al., "A Distinct African Lentivirus from Sykes' Monkeys," *J. Virol.,* 1993, 67, 1517–1528.

20.  This interesting hypothesis about the African green monkey was later investigated by a team of French researchers in West Africa. See G. Galat, J.-L. Rey et al., "Des singes et des retrovirus," *Dossier ORSTOM Actualités,* no. 40, pp. 1–8. (This pamphlet is undated, but was apparently published in 1993 or 1994.) ORSTOM's research method is sensitive enough to detect a reduction of life expectancy of as little as 5 percent in SIV-positive AGMs, but it will be eight years before they have any definite results.

21.  P. N. Fultz, H. M. McClure et al., "Identification and Biologic Characterization of an Acutely Lethal Variant of Simian Immunodeficiency Virus from Sooty Mangabeys (SIV/SMM)," *AIDS Res. Hum. Retro.,* 1989, 5(4), 397–409.

22.  These were later reported in V. Courgnaud, P. N. Fultz, L. Montagnier et al., "Genetic Differences Accounting for Evolution and Pathogenicity of Simian Immunodeficiency Virus from a Sooty Mangabey Monkey after Cross-species Transmission to a Pig-tailed Macaque," *J. Virol.,* 1992, 66, 414–419.

23.  P. R. Johnson, G. Myers, and V. M. Hirsch, "Genetic Diversity and Phylogeny of Non-human Primate Lentiviruses," in W. C. Koff et al. (editors), *Annual Review of AIDS Research,* vol. 1 (New York: J. Marcel Dekker, 1991), pp. 47–62.

24.  This assumes that the rate of divergence is the same in the United States and Africa — an assumption that Myers said was "probably true."

25.  An updated version was eventually published almost three years later, as Myers et al., "Phylogenetic Moments in the AIDS Epidemic."

26.  See Myers et al., "Phylogenetic Moments in the AIDS Epidemic," p. 127. However, in her book *The Coming Plague* (New York: Farrar, Straus and Giroux, 1995), Laurie Garrett claims on pages 378–379 and footnote 200, page 665, that Myers uses the term "Big Bang" for the later "phylogenetic moment" — the start of the AIDS pandemic in the mid-seventies. I think that this is incorrect.

27.  T. F. Smith, G. Myers et al., "The Phylogenetic History of Immunodeficiency Viruses," *Nature,* 1988, 333, 573–575.

28.  In fact, Z321 *was* atypical in that it later turned out to be a recombinant virus, comprising a subtype G core and a subtype A envelope. D. J. Choi et al., "Sequence Note: HIV Type 1 Isolate Z321, the Strain Used to Make a Therapeutic HIV Type 1 Immunogen, Is Intersubtype Recombinant," *AIDS Res. Hum. Retro.,* 1997, 13(4), 357–361. Perhaps for this reason, Myers's estimate of the HIV-1/HIV-2 node was far too recent.

29.  The researchers had studied the divergence of two sheep lentiviruses, visna (from Iceland) and South African ovine maedi visna (SA-OMVV), which according to the historical evidence could be dated to the Icelandic importation of Karakul sheep from Germany in 1933, and concluded that mammalian lentiviral radiation (when the PIVs had separated from ungulate lentiviruses, like visna) had occurred in around A.D. 1560 and HIV-1/

HIV-2/SIVagm divergence in around A.D. 1790. See G. Querat et al., "Nucleotide Sequence Analysis of SA-OMVV, a Visna-Related Ovine Lentivirus: Phylogenetic History of Lentiviruses," *Virol.*, 1990, 175, 434–447.

30. P. M. Sharp and W.-H. Li, "Understanding the History of AIDS Viruses" (letter), *Nature*, 1988, 336, 315; and S. L. Yokoyama et al., "Molecular evolution of the Human Immuno-deficiency and Related Viruses," *Mol. Biol. Evol.*, 1988, 5, 237–251.

31. W. W. Denham, "History of Green Monkeys in the West Indies, Part 1. Migration from Africa," *J. Barbados Mus. Hist. Soc.*, 1981, 36, 221–229.

32. R. M. Hendry et al., "Antibodies to Simian Immunodeficiency Virus in African Green Monkeys in Africa in 1957–62" (letter), *Lancet*, 1986, 2(i), 455. L. J. Lowenstine et al., "Seroepidemiologic Survey of Captive Old-World Primates for Antibodies to Human and Simian Retroviruses, and Isolation of a Lentivirus from Sooty Mangabeys (*Cercoce-bus atys*)," *Intl. J. Cancer*, 1986, 38, 563–574. Apparently two hundred AGMs from the islands of St. Kitts, St. Lucia, Barbados, and Nevis were tested, and all found negative for SIV. (See Anon., "Status Report on Simian Retroviruses," WHO document BLG/POLIO/ 87.2, 1987, p. 2.)

33. J. S. Allan, V. M. Hirsch, P. R. Johnson, G. M. Shaw, B. H. Hahn et al., "Species Specific Diversity among Simian Immunodeficiency Viruses from African Green Monkeys," *J. Virol.*, 1991, 65(6), 2816–2828.

34. Later, it emerged unexpectedly that SIVagm is only very rarely passed from mother to baby in the wild, bites and sex being the normal modes of transmission. It might there-fore have been that the exported West African monkeys were too young to be infected. See J. E. Phillips-Conroy, R. C. Desrosiers et al., "Sexual Transmission of SIVagm in Wild Grivet Monkeys," *J. Med. Primatol.*, 1994, 23, 1–7.

35. R. F. Khabbaz, T. M. Folks et al., "Simian Immunodeficiency Virus Needlestick Accident in a Laboratory Worker," *Lancet*, 1992, 340, 271–273; Anon., "Seroconversion to Simian Immunodeficiency Virus in Two Laboratory Workers," *MMWR*, 1992, 41(36), 679–681.

CHAPTER 12: *AIDS and Polio Vaccines*

1. The first proposition of a version of the OPV/AIDS theory in a medical journal had occurred in 1989. See G. Lecatsas and J. J. Alexander, "Safe Testing of Poliovirus Vaccine and the Origin of HIV Infection in Man" (letter), *S. Af. Med. J.*, 1989, 76, 451.

2. The virologist was Dr. Myra McClure, whom I first interviewed in December 1990. It was Louis Pascal who correctly deduced that Ratner had been her informant.

3. W. S. Kyle, "Simian Retroviruses, Poliovaccine, and Origin of AIDS," *Lancet*, 1992, 339, 600–601. Further information was kindly supplied by Mr. Kyle.

4. C. Lincoln and R. Nordstrom, "Sabin Polio Vaccine for Herpes Simplex," *Schoch Letter*, 1976, 26(10), 17. A. Tager, "Preliminary Report on the Treatment of Recurrent Herpes Simplex with Poliomyelitis Vaccine (Sabin's)," *Dermatologica*, 1974, 149, 253–255.

5. Walter Kyle, personal communication, May 1996.

6. Chadd Stevens, personal communication, 1995.

7. "Oral Polio Vaccines and HIV" (informal document prepared by CDC and FDA), November 1994.

8. T. Curtis, "The Origin of AIDS: A Startling New Theory Attempts to Answer the Question 'Was It an Act of God or an Act of Man?,'" *Rolling Stone*, March 19, 1992, issue 626; pp. 54–60, 106, and 108.

9.  S. A. Plotkin, A. Lebrun, G. Courtois, and H. Koprowski, "Vaccination with the CHAT Strain of Type 1 Attenuated Poliomyelitis Virus in Leopoldville, Congo. 3. Safety and Efficacy during the First 21 Months of Study," *Bull. WHO,* 1961, 24, 785–792.

10. *BMJ* 58.

11. R. J. Biggar, C. Saxinger et al., "Seroepidemiology of HTLV-III Antibodies in a Remote Population of Eastern Zaire," *BMJ,* 1985, 290, 808–810.

12. R. J. Biggar, "Possible Nonspecific Associations between Malaria and HTLV-III/LAV" (letter), *N. Eng. J. Med.,* 1986, 315(7), 457–458.

13. D. S. Dane, G. W. A. Dick et al. "Vaccination against Poliomyelitis with Live Virus Vaccines: 1. A Trial of TN Type II Vaccine," *BMJ,* 1957, 1(i), 59–65. G. W. A. Dick, D. S. Dane et al., "Vaccination against Poliomyelitis with Live Virus Vaccines: 2. A Trial of SM Type I Attenuated Poliomyelitis Virus Vaccine," *BMJ,* 1957, 1(i), 65–70. G. W. A. Dick and D. S. Dane, "Vaccination against Poliomyelitis with Live Virus Vaccines: 3. The Evaluation of TN and SM Virus Vaccines," *BMJ,* 1957, 1(i), 70–74. My thanks to Gerry O'Kane for his help with preliminary research in Belfast.

CHAPTER 13: *The Race to Conquer Polio:*
*Early Research and Inactivated Polio Vaccines*

1.  This brief history of vaccination and IPV development is largely derived from histories written and published soon after the acceptance of the Sabin vaccine, among them: J. R. Wilson, *Margin of Safety* (London: Collins, 1963); R. Carter, *Breakthrough — The Saga of Jonas Salk* (New York: Trident Press, 1966); P. J. Fisher, *The Polio Story* (London: Heinemann, 1967); and A. Klein, *Trial by Fury — The Polio Vaccine Controversy* (New York: Scribner's, 1972). The J. R. Wilson book is by far the finest of these accounts, containing a shrewd and well-informed overview of the polio saga by a doctor who was deputy editor of the *British Medical Journal* for much of the fifties. Wilson manages to be commendably evenhanded, but it should be borne in mind that his account was apparently commissioned by Lederle Laboratories in order to "put the record straight." Also see A. Chase, *Magic Shots* (New York: William Morrow, 1982).

2.  From *vacca,* Latin for "cow."

3.  One exception might be the vaccine cocktails administered to some combatants in modern wars. There are growing indications that Gulf War syndrome may be linked to immunizations with multiple agents, some unlicensed. See R. Norton-Taylor, "MoD Ignored Warning on Gulf Drugs," *Guardian* (U.K.), October 29, 1997.

4.  T. M. Rivers, "Immunity in Virus Diseases with Particular Reference to Poliomyelitis," *Am. J. Public Health,* 1936, 26, 136–148. See particularly the discussion by James P. Leake, p. 148.

5.  In both cases, the official diagnosis was a heart attack.

6.  J. F. Enders et al., "Cultivation of the Lansing Strain of Poliomyelitis Virus in Cultures of Various Human Embryonic Tissues," *Science,* 1949, 109, 85–87.

7.  "Section of Epidemiology and Preventive Medicine: Discussion on Poliomyelitis Vaccination in 1956," *Proc. Roy. Soc. Med.,* 1957, 50, 1067–1073, featuring J. Knowelden on pp. 1072–1073.

8.  J. R. Wilson, *Margin of Safety,* p. 146.

CHAPTER 14: *The Race to Conquer Polio: Oral Polio Vaccines*

1.  This is often referred to as the first time that a human was immunized by OPV — but strictly speaking this is inaccurate because, in 1950, there were no reliable antibody tests to establish whether a vaccinee was lacking immunity to a poliovirus type prior to vaccination, and had acquired immunity after vaccination. Victor Cabasso, personal communication, 1993.

2.  An inhabitant of Indiana and, by inference, a matter-of-fact, unassuming midwesterner.

3.  David Dane, personal communication, April 1996. See also R. Carter, *Breakthrough: The Saga of Jonas Salk* (New York: Trident Press, 1966), pp. 110–111.

4.  H. Koprowski, *Proceedings of a Round Table Conference on Immunization of Poliomyelitis* (Hershey, PA: National Foundation for Infantile Paralysis, March 1951).

5.  R. Carter, *Breakthrough*, pp. 109–110.

6.  R. Carter, *Breakthrough*, p. 110. Almost three decades later, Koprowski would claim in a speech (later reprinted in a book by his wife) that he knew he "would never get official permission from the State of New York" for this first trial, but went ahead nonetheless after obtaining permission from the parents. (Irena Koprowska, *A Woman Wanders through Life and Science* [Albany: State University of New York Press, 1997], appendix, p. 298.)

7.  H. Koprowski, G. A. Jervis, and T. W. Norton, "Immune Responses in Human Volunteers upon Oral Administration of a Rodent-Adapted Strain of Poliomyelitis Virus," *Am. J. Hyg.*, 1952, 55, 108–126.

8.  Anon., "Poliomyelitis: A New Approach," *Lancet*, 1952, 1(i), p. 552.

9.  This was so named because the donor of the original sample was a member of the British Middle East Forces in the Second World War.

10. H. Koprowski et al., "Adaptation of Type 1 Strain of Poliomyelitis Virus to Mice and Cotton Rats," *Proc. Soc. Exp. Biol. Med.*, 1954, 86, 238–244; H. Koprowski et al., "Administration of an Attenuated Type 1 Poliomyelitis Virus to Human Subjects," *Proc. Soc. Exp. Biol. Med.*, 1954, 86, 244–247.

11. H. Koprowski, "Practical Application of Living Virus Vaccines," in *The Dynamics of Virus and Rickettsial Infections* (New York: Blakiston Company, 1954), pp. 270–291. The speech was given at a symposium held in Detroit, Michigan, October 21–23, 1953.

12. A. B. Sabin, discussion at the end of Koprowski's paper in *The Dynamics of Virus and Rickettsial Infections*, pp. 289–290.

13. H. Koprowski et al., "Immunization of Children by the Feeding of Living Attenuated Type I and Type II Poliomyelitis Virus and the Intramuscular Injection of Immune Serum Globulin," *Am. J. Med. Sci.*, 1956, 232(4), 378–388.

14. H. R. Cox, "Trial Vaccines and Human Welfare," *Lancet*, 1953, 2(i), 1–5.

15. A. B. Sabin, "Present Status of Attenuated Live-virus Poliomyelitis Vaccine," *JAMA*, 1956, 162(18), 1589–1596.

16. R. Dulbecco and M. Vogt, "Plaque Formation and Isolation of Pure Lines with Poliomyelitis Viruses," *J. Exp. Med.*, 1954, 99, 167–182.

17. A. B. Sabin, "Present Status of Attenuated Live-virus Poliomyelitis Vaccine."

18. A report by Albert Sabin, featuring in Annex B in WHO/Polio/17; WHO meeting on Poliomyelitis Vaccination, Stockholm, November 21–25, 1955. This work is summarized in A. B. Sabin, "Oral Poliovirus Vaccine," *JAMA*, 1965, 194(8), 872–876; see especially p. 874.

19. "India Cuts Export of Some Monkeys," *New York Times*, March 11, 1955, p. 27.

20. Conference on "Biology of Poliomyelitis," *Ann. N.Y. Acad. Sci.*, 1955, 61(4), 737–1064. See particularly "Part II. Susceptibility of Cells and Organisms to Poliomyelitis," pp. 806–894. See also "Committee on Laboratory Investigations of Poliomyelitis," minutes of the First Meeting held on July 14, 1955, [U.K.] Medical Research Council; MRC.55/658.

21. G. W. A. Dick and D. S. Dane, "The Evaluation of TN and SM Virus Vaccines," *BMJ*, 1957, 1(i), 70–74.

22. *NYAS* 57.

23. V. J. Cabasso, H. R. Cox et al., "Cumulative Testing Experience with Consecutive Lots of Oral Poliomyelitis Vaccine," *BMJ*, 1960, 1(i), 373–387.

24. "Expert Committee on Poliomyelitis: Second Report," *WHO Technical Report Series* No. 145, WHO (Geneva), 1958, with particular reference to pp. 25–27.

25. A.M.-M. Payne, "Poliomyelitis Vaccine" (letter), *BMJ*, 1958, 2(ii), 1472–1473.

26. S. Plotkin, A. Lebrun, G. Courtois, and H. Koprowski, "Vaccination with the CHAT Strain of Type 1 Attenuated Poliomyelitis Virus in Leopoldville, Belgian Congo. III. Safety and Efficacy during the First Twenty-one Months of Study," *PAHO2*, 466–473.

27. F. Przesmycki et al., "Vaccination against Poliomyelitis in Poland with Koprowski's Live Attenuated Strains," *PAHO2*, 522–532.

28. Da Silva et al., "Studies of Orally Administrated Attenuated Live Virus Poliomyelitis Vaccine in Newborns and Infants under Six Months" (staff meeting report), *U. Minn. Med. Bull.*, 1957, 29, 133–150.

29. V. J. Cabasso, H. R. Cox et al., "Cumulative Testing Experience with Consecutive Lots of Oral Poliomyelitis Vaccine." See also J. R. Wilson, *Margin of Safety* (London: Collins, 1963), p.187.

30. *PAHO1*.

31. G. W. A. Dick and D. S. Dane, "The Evaluation of Live Poliovirus Vaccines," *PAHO1*, 6–13. Further comments about the lack of follow-up of the Ruzizi vaccinees, and the paucity of useful information gained from the trial, appear in G. W. A. Dick and D. S. Dane, "Vaccination Against Poliomyelitis in the United Kingdom," *Brit. Med. Bull.*, 1959, 15(3), 205–209; see especially p. 208.

32. See A. Lebrun, G. Courtois, H. Koprowski et al., "Preliminary Report on Mass Vaccination with Live Attenuated Poliomyelitis Virus in Leopoldville, Belgian Congo," *PAHO1*, 410–418; and S. A. Plotkin and H. Koprowski, "Epidemiological Studies of the Safety and Efficacy of Vaccination with the CHAT Strain of Attenuated Poliovirus in Leopoldville, Belgian Congo," *PAHO1*, 419–436.

33. An example of Koprowski's barbed wit: "Sabin's excellent presentation reminds me of [a description of John Donne by C. S. Lewis]: 'These diverse excellencies are usually held together by Donne's adoption of the role of pleader — by his argument. The argument may be on different levels . . . fanciful . . . or serious.' Since most of Sabin's arguments were, I hope, in the serious category . . ." (NYAS 57, p. 128). It appears that many scientists (apart from Sabin) felt attacked by such flourishes. At a 1955 conference, Thomas Francis spoke as following in his summarizing speech: "Doctor Koprowski has fortunately provided a fine text with his references to Bertrand Russell and Aristotle. It happens that I recall, too, that in one of his *Unpopular Essays,* Russell pointed out that we frequently remember a man for the brilliant sayings ascribed to him and forget many of his absurdities." T. Francis Jr., "Summary and Review of Poliomyelitis Immunization," *Ann. N.Y. Acad. Sci.*, 1955, 61(4), 1057–1058. For comment on Koprowski's tendency to

harangue in speeches and articles, see J. R. Wilson, *Margin of Safety,* pp. 141–142 (and pages following for examples).

34. *PAHO1,* discussion by J. Melnick and A. B. Sabin, p. 577.

35. A. B. Sabin, "Present Position of Immunization against Poliomyelitis with Live Virus Vaccines," *BMJ,* 1959, 1(i), 663–682; see especially 677–678.

36. H. Koprowski, "Live Poliomyelitis Vaccine" (letter), *BMJ,* 1959, 1(ii), 1349–1350.

37. Anon., "Too Many Polio Vaccines?" *Time,* May 2, 1960, pp. 68–70. It is unclear whether or not this was a reference to Sabin's claim that CHAT and Fox reverted to virulence.

38. "Preliminary Data on Viremia in Man after Oral Administration of Live, Attenuated Poliovirus Vaccine," including information from R. Murray; WHO report WHO/BS/Int/19, November 3, 1960.

39. J. L. Melnick, "Problems Associated with the Use of Live Poliovirus Vaccine," *Am. J. Public Health,* 1960, 50(7), 1013–1031.

40. M. E. Flipse et al., "A Preliminary Report on a Large-Scale Field Trial with the Oral Cox-Lederle Attenuated Poliomyelitis Vaccine in Dade County (Miami), Florida," *PAHO2,* 435–444.

41. J. R. Wilson, *Margin of Safety,* pp. 216–218.

42. For instance: V. M. Zhdanov, "Large-Scale Practical Trials and Use of Live Poliovirus Vaccine in the USSR," *PAHO2,* 576–588.

43. H. R. Cox, "Trial Vaccines and Human Welfare."

44. R. Rustigian et al., "Infection of Monkey Kidney Tissue Cultures with Virus-Like Agents," *Proc. Soc. Exp. Biol. Med.,* 1955, 88, 8–16.

45. R. Hull et al., "New Viral Agents Recovered from Tissue Cultures of Monkey Kidney Cells," *Am. J. Hyg.,* 1956, 63, 204–215. This vitally important paper detailed the finding of eight simian viruses (plus another two possibles) in monkey kidney tissue cultures prepared by two different methods — the Maitland technique and trypsinization. It also detailed the finding of simian viruses in eight other North American labs, concluding: "The greatest significance of these viruses has been their appearance in tissue cultures used to produce and to test poliomyelitis vaccine." Hull added that only rarely had such viruses proved capable of surviving the formaldehyde treatment involved in making Salk vaccine, but made no comment about live, untreated vaccines like the OPVs.

46. H. Malherbe and R. Harwin, "Seven Viruses Isolated from the Vervet Monkey," *Br. J. Exp. Pathol.,* 1957, 38(5), 539–541.

47. B. H. Sweet and M. R. Hilleman, "Detection of a 'Non-Detectable' Simian Virus (Vacuolating Agent) Present in Rhesus and Cynomolgus Monkey-Kidney Cell Culture Material. A Preliminary Report," *PAHO2,* 79–85.

48. B. E. Eddy et al., "Tumors Induced in Hamsters by Injection of Rhesus Monkey Kidney Cell Extracts," *Proc. Soc. Exp. Biol. Med.,* 1961, 107, 191–197.

49. Expert Committee on Poliomyelitis, Third Report, *WHO Tech. Rep. Ser.,* 1960, 203, 1–53.

50. L. E. Burney, "Live Poliomyelitis Vaccine Status," *Public Health Rep.* (Washington), 1959, 74(11), 983–984.

51. H. Koprowski, "Live Virus Vaccines against Poliomyelitis" (letter to the surgeon general of the United States of America, August 25, 1960), WHO document WHO/BS/Int./16, October 27, 1960. H. Koprowski, "Live Virus Vaccines against Poliomyelitis" (letter to the editor of the *British Medical Journal,* September 7, 1960), WHO document WHO/BS/Int./15, October 27, 1960. H. Koprowski and S. Plotkin, "Notes on Acceptance Criteria and Requirements for Live Poliovirus Vaccines," WHO document WHO/BS/IR/85,

submitted to the WHO Study Group on Requirements for Poliomyelitis Vaccine, November 1, 1960.

52.  H. Koprowski and S. Plotkin, "Notes on Acceptance Criteria and Requirements for Live Poliovirus Vaccines."

53.  L. Hayflick and P. S. Moorhead, "The Serial Cultivation of Human Diploid Cell Strains," *Exp. Cell Res.*, 1961, 25, 585–621. L. Hayflick, S. A. Plotkin, T. W. Norton, and H. Koprowski, "Preparation of Poliovirus Vaccines in a Human Fetal Diploid Cell Strain," *Am. J. Hyg.*, 1962, 75, 240–258.

54.  Anon., "Live Poliovirus Vaccine Approved; Worldwide Trials Reported," *Science*, 1960, 132, 606–607.

55.  F. Buser et al., "Immunization with Live Attenuated Polio Virus Prepared in Human Diploid Cell Strains, with Special Reference to the WM-3 Strain," *Proceedings of the Symposium on the Characterization and Uses of Human Diploid Cell Strains*, (Opatija, Yugoslavia, 1963), 381–387. J. S. Pagano, M. Böttiger, S. Gard et al., "The Response and the Lack of Spread in Swedish Schoolchildren Given an Attenuated Polio-Virus Vaccine Prepared in a Human Diploid Cell Strain," *Am. J. Hyg.*, 1964, 79, 74–85.

56.  D. Ikic, "Poliovaccines Prepared in Human Diploid Cells," *First International Conference on Vaccines Against Viral and Rickettsial Diseases of Man*, Pan American Health Organization Scientific Publication No. 147; May 1967, 185–189.

57.  L. Hayflick, "The Coming of Age of WI-38," *Adv. Cell Culture*, 1984, 3, 303–316; S. Plotkin, L. Hayflick, D. Ikic, H. Koprowski, and F. Perkins, "Serially Cultured Animal Cells for Preparation of Viral Vaccines," *Science*, 1969, 165, 1278–1283.

58.  H. R. Cox, V. J. Cabasso et al., "Immunological Response to Trivalent Oral Poliomyelitis Vaccine," *BMJ*, 1959, 2(ii), 591–597.

59.  H. M. Gelfand, "Oral Vaccine: Associated Paralytic Poliomyelitis, 1962," *JAMA*, 1963, 184(12), 948–956; A. B. Sabin, "Oral Poliovirus Vaccine: History of Its Development and Use and Current Challenge to Eliminate Poliomyelitis from the World," *J. Infect. Dis.*, 1985, 151(3), 420–436.

60.  V. P. Grachev, "World Health Organization Attitude Concerning the Use of Continuous Cell Lines as Substrates for Production of Human Virus Vaccines," in A. Mizrahi (editor), *Viral Vaccines* (New York: Wiley-Liss, 1990), pp. 37–67.

61.  A. M. Lewis, "Experience with SV40 and Adenovirus-SV40 Hybrids," in *Biohazards in Biological Research*, Proceedings of a Conference held at the Asilomar Conference Center, California; January 22–24, 1973 (California: CSH, 1973), pp. 96–113; K. Shah and N. Nathanson, "Human Exposure to SV40: Review and Comment," *Am. J. Epid.*, 1976, 103, 1–12.

62.  M. Carbone et al., "Simian Virus 40–Like DNA Sequences in Human Pleural Mesothelioma," *Oncogene*, 1994, 9, 1781–1790; P. Brown, "Mystery Virus Linked to Asbestos Cancer," *New Scientist*, May 21, 1994, p. 4; P. Wechsler, "A Shot in the Dark," *New York*, November 11, 1996, 39–43, 85.

63.  Y. Ohta, M. Hayami et al., "Isolation of Simian Immunodeficiency Virus from African Green Monkeys and Seroepidemiologic Survey of the Virus in Various Non-Human Primates," *Int. J. Cancer*, 1988, 41, 115–122.

64.  R. Carter, *Breakthrough*, p. 354.

CHAPTER 15: *Dr. Dick and Dr. Dane*

1. Sadly, George Dick died in 1997 and David Dane in 1998. I owe both men a great debt of gratitude for the wonderful long-term assistance they provided to my researches. Both doctors checked the text of this chapter and confirmed its accuracy; since it was written long before their deaths, I have decided to retain the original tenses.

2. George Dick, personal communication, August 1992.

3. A. M. McFarlan, G. W. A. Dick, and H. J. Seddon, "The Epidemiology of the 1945 Outbreak of Poliomyelitis in Mauritius," *Q. J. Med.*, 1946, 59, 183–208.

4. D. S. Dane, G. W. A. Dick et al., "Poliovirus Antibody in Children in Northern Ireland," *Lancet*, 1956, 1(ii), 481–483.

5. Examples include H. Koprowski, T. W. Norton, G. A. Jervis et al., "Clinical Investigations on Attenuated Strains of Poliomyelitis Virus: Use as a Method of Immunization of Children with Living Virus," *JAMA*, 1956, 160, 954–966; H. Koprowski, T. W. Norton, G. A. Jervis et al., "Immunization of Children by the Feeding of Living Attenuated Type 1 and Type 2 Poliomyelitis Virus and the Intramuscular Injection of Immune Serum Gobulin," *Am. J. Med. Sci.*, 1956, 232(4), 378–388; H. Koprowski, T. W. Norton, K. Hummeler et al., "Immunization of Infants with Living Attenuated Poliomyelitis Virus: Laboratory Investigations of Alimentary Infection and Antibody Response in Infants under Six Months of Age with Congenitally Acquired Antibodies," *JAMA*, 1956, 162, 1281–1288.

6. Whereas IPV immunizes only the vaccinee, OPV (as a live virus) tends to spread to non-vaccinees, eventually — in theory — conferring "herd immunity" on entire pockets of population. Thus an OPV trial could interfere with the ability of scientists to monitor antibody responses in an IPV trial.

7. G. W. A. Dick, "Proposed Trials of Live Attenuated Type 1 Poliomyelitis Virus Vaccine," Report to the Committee on Clinical Trials of Poliomyelitis Vaccines, 1955, Medical Research Council document MRC.55/702.

8. Most of the islanders lacked polio antibodies, and would therefore have been vulnerable to a disastrous "virgin soil epidemic" had the dangerous Type 1 poliovirus been imported on a ship from the Cape, where it was endemic. The motives were not, of course, solely altruistic, for this also represented an opportunity to conduct a "sealed" experiment on the isolated island community of 292 persons. Potentially, such a trial would allow for long-term studies of antibody response, and the fact that everyone would be vaccinated simultaneously effectively eliminated the potential problem of reversion to virulence of the vaccine virus among nonvaccinees. J. H. S. Gear, "Live Virus Vaccine Studies in Southern Africa," *PAHO2*, 474–481; see especially p. 475. George Dick, personal communication, 1994.

9. Anon., "Polio Vaccine in Northern Ireland," *BMJ*, 1956, 1(i), 697. *Report on Health and Local Government Administration in Northern Ireland* (H.M.S.O. Belfast, 1956), p. 2 of the introduction by F. F. Main, the chief medical officer.

10. Meanwhile, a field test of Brunenders (a slightly less virulent, but correspondingly less immunogenic, version of Salk's IPV) was being conducted on nearly 180,000 children on the British mainland. Brunenders was not brought to Ulster, so if Dick's trials were successful, a larger scale field trial of Koprowski's strains could still be staged in an area where IPV had never been used.

11. "Committee on Clinical Trials of Poliomyelitis Vaccines: Minutes of the Ninth Meeting," 1956, Medical Research Council document MRC.56/377.

12. Anon., "Minister Tells of Plan to Defeat Polio," *Belfast News-letter,* February 22, 1956, p. 3. By this stage George Dick had already announced that he would be looking for ten volunteers from the general public before the end of 1956, and suggested that — if all went well — the trial would be extended to involve a hundred or more volunteers in 1957, and "some thousands of people" in 1958. (Anon., "1,000 in Big Polio Test," *Belfast Telegraph,* February 9, 1956, p. 1.)

13. Koprowski et al., "Clinical Investigations on Attenuated Strains of Poliomyelitis Virus," see especially p. 959.

14. It appears that no records remain of the 190 persons fed TN in the United Kingdom, but Dick, Dane, and other doctors from the era recall that the adult vaccinees were faculty members from Queens University in Belfast, and doctors working under Ritchie Russell, an enthusiastic proponent of live virus vaccination who headed the polio treatment programs at two hospitals near Oxford. The children and infants appear to have included the offspring of the adult volunteers, together with some who were vaccinated by their own GPs in Northern Ireland (in Belfast and other provincial towns), or by Ritchie Russell or Roy Vollum in Oxford.

15. George Dick, personal communication, 1994.

16. Anon., "Poliomyelitis Vaccination: Live Attenuated Vaccines Given by Mouth," Report of the Medical Research Council for the year 1955–1956 (London: H.M.S.O., 1956), p. 17.

17. J. R. Wilson, *Margin of Safety* (London: Collins, 1963), p. 166.

18. D. S. Dane, G. W. A. Dick et al., "Vaccination against Poliomyelitis with Live Virus Vaccines: 1. A Trial of TN Type II Vaccine," *BMJ,* 1957, 1(i), 59–65; G. W. A. Dick, D. S. Dane et al., "Vaccination against Poliomyelitis with Live Virus Vaccines: 2. A Trial of SM Type I Attenuated Poliomyelitis Virus Vaccine," *BMJ,* 1957, 1(i), 65–70; G. W. A. Dick and D. S. Dane, "Vaccination against Poliomyelitis with Live Virus Vaccines: 3. The Evaluation of TN and SM Virus Vaccines," *BMJ,* 1957, 1(i), 70–74.

19. H. Koprowski et al., "Clinical Investigations on Attenuated Strains of Poliomyelitis Virus," see p. 966.

20. The SM vaccine used by Lederle after Koprowski's departure in 1957 was triple plaque purified by the Dulbecco method, and was therefore a very different vaccine strain.

21. "Expert Committee on Poliomyelitis: Second Report," *WHO Tech. Rep. Ser.,* 1958, no. 145, pp. 1–83; see p. 24.

22. Not all of the Belfast team were so comfortable with the SM results. A pediatrician with the team sent me a speech he had written about the vaccinations, in which he reported that "minor illnesses or symptoms were recorded in nine of the sixteen persons successfully vaccinated [with SM] or infected by contact." (See O. D. Fisher, "Clinical Surveillance of Poliomyelitis Virus Vaccination, with Follow Up of Subsequent Immunity," speech read at 9th International Pediatric Congress (Toronto, 1958). It is worth noting that there was a serious polio epidemic in Belfast and adjoining areas, starting in June 1957, with 225 cases of paralysis; all 174 isolations from patients revealed Type 1 poliovirus. (See Anon., *Report on Health and Local Government Administration in Northern Ireland During the Year Ended 31st December 1957* (Belfast: H.M.S.O., 1958), pp. 2–3. None of the Belfast doctors, however, believed that this could have been linked to the SM vaccinations in 1956.

23. *NYAS* 57.

24. In his published address to the New York meeting, Koprowski claimed with regard to SM that "[i]ts contagiousness remains quite low." Later, he presented results of his own safety tests of excreted SM, carried out during 1956, which, he said, represented "evidence . . . definitely at variance with the results obtained . . . by Dick et al." *NYAS* 57, 128–133.

25. One year later, in December 1958, Koprowski was introduced as the New York Academy of Sciences president, succeeding Boris Pregel, a physicist who was also president of the Canadian Radium and Uranium Corporation. See Anon., "The 20-Hour Week Is Predicted Soon," *New York Times,* December 5, 1958, p. 19.

26. Address given by G. W. A. Dick, *NYAS 57,* pp. 134–137.

27. J. R. Wilson, *Margin of Safety,* pp. 167–169.

28. See note from George Godber to chief medical officer, dated May 18, 1956, in file MH55 2459 at Public Record Office, Kew, London. See also memorandum 24/Gen/3507 (AMD 5) from director general of Army Medical Services to deputy directors and assistant directors of (army) medical services dated May 16, 1956, in file MH55 2459.

29. "Committee on Clinical Trials of Poliomyelitis Vaccines," minutes of the Ninth Meeting held on March 7, 1956, Medical Research Council document MRC.56/377. Interestingly, this was the only MRC meeting on clinical trials of polio vaccines during this hectic period that was attended by army personnel.

30. "Committee on the Clinical Trials of Poliomyelitis Vaccines," minutes of the Seventh Meeting held on December 9, 1955, MRC Document MRC.56/63.

31. In addition, John Connolly, who had helped cowrite the damning papers on SM and TN, and who (in 1993) was head of virology at Queen's University in Belfast, initiated a freezer search for SM and TN, but reported back that there were no samples to be found. None of the members of H.M.S. *Whitby*'s crew whom I interviewed recalled oral vaccinations while in Derry, but oral vaccines tend to be less memorable than injected ones.

32. S. Gard, "Field and Laboratory Experiences with the CHAT Strain Type 1 Poliovirus," *PAHO2,* 187–190.

## CHAPTER 16: *"What Happens When Science Goes Bad"*

1. T. Curtis, "The Origin of AIDS," *Rolling Stone,* March 19, 1992, pp. 54–61, 106–108.

2. In his article, Curtis explained how Elswood, with whom he had worked on previous stories about alternative therapies for AIDS, had written him in August 1991 enclosing photocopies of various pertinent articles, and a note reading: "Here's a bombshell story just waiting for an investigative reporter."

3. R. B. Stricker and B. F. Elswood, letter to the editor, *Lancet,* 1992, 339, 867.

4. T. Curtis, "Did a Polio Vaccine Experiment Unleash AIDS in Africa?" *Washington Post,* April 5, 1992, p. C-4. See also the response by Malcolm Gladwell: "It's Possible, but Not Likely," which follows on p. C-5.

5. Louis Pascal's "What Happens When Science Goes Bad. The Corruption of Science and the Origin of AIDS: A Study in Spontaneous Generation" is published as Working Paper No. 9 by the University of Wollongong Science and Technology Analysis Research Program. It is available free from Science and Technology Studies, University of Wollongong, NSW 2522, Australia; fax: +61-2-4221 3452; e-mail: brianmartin@uow. edu.au. The same piece, together with much related material about the theory, is also published on the web at: http://www.uow.edu.au/arts/sts/bmartin/dissent/documents/AIDS/.

6. B. F. Elswood and R. B. Stricker, "Polio Vaccines and the Origin of AIDS," draft copy dated May 11, 1992. This article was eventually published in *Medical Hypotheses,* 1994, 42, 347–354.

7. L. B. Seeff et al., "A Serological Follow-up of the 1942 Epidemic of Post-Vaccination Hepatitis in the United States Army," *N. Engl. J. Med.,* 1987, 316(16), 965–970.

8.  Examples of Curtis's articles in the *Houston Post* include "Vaccines Not Tested for HIV?" March 18, 1992, pp. A-1, A-12; "Expert Says Test Vaccine," March 22, 1992, pp. A-1, A-21; "Polio Experts Support Vaccine Tests for HIV," March 26, 1992, pp. A-1, A-18; "Discovery Too Grave to Imagine," April 5, 1992, pp. A-1, A-32; "Do Cold, Hard AIDS Facts Lie in Freezer?" May 8, 1992, pp. A-1, A-15; "Scientists Urge Screening of Polio Vaccine for HIV," July 17, 1992, pp. A-1, A-18; "Doctor Wants Houston Researcher to Test Polio Vaccines for AIDS Link," July 18, 1992, p. A-9; "Scientists Urge Major Changes in How Polio Vaccines Made," October 23, 1992, p. A-16.

9.  J. Cohen, "Debate on AIDS Origin: Rolling Stone Weighs In," *Science,* March 20, 1992, 255, 1505.

10. T. F. Schulz, "Origin of AIDS" (letter to the editor), *Lancet,* 1992, 339, 867; also the following letters by R. B. Stricker and B. F. Elswood, and H. Ratner, pp. 867–868.

11. Elswood later told me that this information came from Chuck Cyberski, a TV producer with AIDS, who had questioned Hayflick privately at the end of a gerontology conference.

12. P. Singer (editor), *Applied Ethics* (Oxford: Oxford University Press, 1986).

13. Interview with Eva Lee Snead, broadcast on *Natural Living with Gary Null,* WABC (New York), May 31, 1987.

14. Eva Lee Snead later published her theories in a book, beguilingly entitled *Some Call It "AIDS" — I Call It Murder!* and subtitled: *The Connection between Cancer, AIDS, Immunizations and Genocide* (San Antonio, TX: AUM Publications, 1992). The book was dedicated "to God; maybe together we can save mankind," and ended its acknowledgments with "A heartfelt THANK-YOU to the Texan State Board of Medical Examiners, who by revoking my medical license enabled me to have the time to research and write this book." On the back was a photo of a glamorous woman with big hair and teeth, who turned out not to be Ms. Snead, but rather someone who had enjoyed her book. The text itself — all 529 closely-printed pages — had clearly involved a huge amount of research, but possessed very little direction or ability to sort wheat from chaff.

15. P. J. Kanki, J. Alroy, and M. Essex, "Isolation of T-Lymphotropic Retrovirus Related to HTLV-III/LAV from Wild-Caught African Green Monkeys," *Science,* 1985, 230, 951–954.

16. *BMJ* 58.

17. H. Koprowski, "The Tin Anniversary of the Development of Live Poliovirus Vaccine," *PAHO2,* 5–11.

18. P. M. Sharp and W.-H. Li, "Understanding the Origins of AIDS Viruses," *Nature,* 1988, 336, 315.

19. Adenovirus vaccines were the only other common vaccines made in MKTC, and were injected into more than 100,000 U.S. military personnel between 1958 and 1961. Source: K. Shah and N. Nathanson, "Human Exposure to SV40: Review and Comment," *Am. J. Epidem.,* 1976, 103(1), 1–12.

20. G. Myers, "HIV: Between Past and Future," *AIDS Res. Hum. Retro.,* 1994, 10(11), 1317–1324.

21. This rarely calculated figure represents cumulative risk, whereas HIV prevalence data provides only a snapshot of the percentage of a population infected at one moment in time. Pascal concluded that the total number of persons alive (in 1991) who would get AIDS had to include at least five million homosexuals, over a hundred million Africans, and further hundreds of millions from elsewhere in the Third World, most notably South America and Asia.

22. This is no longer true, because a partially effective inactivated vaccine has now been developed against an animal lentivirus — feline immunodeficiency virus. M. J. Hosie

and J. M. Flynn, "Feline Immunodeficiency Virus Vaccination: Characterization of the Immune Correlates of Protection," *J. Virol.*, 1996, 70(11), 7561–7568.

23. L. Pascal, "Modern Medicine Started AIDS: How the AIDS Virus Was Transferred from Monkeys to Humans via Contaminated Polio Vaccine," unpublished paper, dated November 20, 1987.

24. Shortly after this the journal ran an editorial defending its decision not to publish Pascal's lengthy article. R. Gillon, "A Startling 19,000 Word Thesis on the Origin of AIDS: Should the JME Have Published It?" (editorial), *J. Med. Ethics*, 1992, 18, 3–4.

25. This is unfair, if only for the reason that Pascal himself has already conceded that a "postal mix-up" had delayed the process for eighteen of those months.

CHAPTER 17: *Louis Pascal*

1. H. Ratner, "Monkey Viruses, AIDS and the Salk Vaccine" (Parts I and II), *Child & Family*, 1988, 20, 134–138. Ratner sent copies of this and other articles to various virologists, including Myra McClure.

2. H. Ratner, "An Untold Vaccine Story," *Child & Family*, 1980, 19, 191–194, continued in *Child & Family*, 1988, 20, 50–59; *Child & Family*, 1988, 20, 139; *Child & Family*, 1988, 20, 322–327; *Child & Family*, 1990, 21, 109. H. Ratner, H. R. Cox et al., "The Present Status of Polio Vaccines, 1960," *Child & Family*, 1980, 19, 195–213, continued in *Child & Family*, 1980, 19, 259–280. H. Ratner, "The Devil's Advocate and the Salk Vaccine Program: 1955: A Contribution Toward an Objective Evaluation," *Child & Family*, 1988, 20, 61–69, continued in *Child & Family*, 1988, 20, 140–157.

3. I prefer to describe the "monkey bite theory" as the "natural transfer theory," and to refer to "isolated" rather than "lost" tribes. The title of "natural transfer" is meant to highlight the fact that the hunting and butchery of monkeys has been a natural part of life in sub-Saharan Africa for millennia; since it is not a new process, it cannot — by itself — explain the recent emergence of AIDS.

4. Anon., "Hope or Horror? Primate-to-Human Organ Transplants," *J.N.I.H. Res.*, 1992, 4, 37; Lorraine Fraser, "AIDS Secret of Ape Liver Trial Patient," *Mail on Sunday* (U.K.), September 13, 1992, p. 15.

5. Some four hundred copies of "What Happens . . ." had been distributed by the end of 1992. Brian Martin, personal communication, June 1996.

6. In fact, retroviruses called foamy viruses are regular contaminants of MKTC. On average, they take nearly eight weeks to produce any cytopathic effect in tissue culture. See E. F. Baker, "Latent Simian Foamy Viruses," *S. Af. Med. J.*, 1989, 76, 451–452.

7. R. F. Khabbaz et al., "Simian Immunodeficiency Virus Needlestick Accident in a Laboratory Worker," *Lancet*, 1992, 340, 271–273.

8. This version of the first Apollo moon missions is not universally accepted. An international space conference held in July 1996 heard from John Rummel, formerly in charge of the planetary protection program at NASA, that insufficient time had been allowed to design quarantine systems against an "Andromeda strain." He told the conference that "they spent $24 million on something that, in the end, satisfied almost nobody." See C. Arthur, "Bugs from Space a Threat to Earth," *Independent* (U.K.), July 16, 1996. Although this account rather spoils Pascal's metaphor, it only adds to the impact of his overall argument about scientific irresponsibility.

9.  The potential danger of contaminating viruses in vaccines made in MKTC had been highlighted by Koprowski's boss, Herald Cox, as early as 1953. (H. R. Cox, "Viral Vaccines and Human Welfare," *Lancet*, 1953, 2[i], 1–5.) These dangers should, of course, have been taken into account by all those who were making human vaccines in monkey kidney substrates.

CHAPTER 18: *The Counterattack Begins*

1.  T. Curtis, "Did a Polio Vaccine Experiment Unleash AIDS in Africa?," *Washington Post*, April 5, 1992, p. C-4.
2.  T. Curtis, "The Origin of AIDS. A Startling New Theory Attempts to Answer the Question 'Was it an Act of God or an Act of Man?'" *Rolling Stone*, March 19, 1992, pp. 54–61, 106–108.
3.  Like many topical magazines, *Rolling Stone* postdates each issue to ensure maximum sales.
4.  J. Cohen, "Debate on AIDS Origin: *Rolling Stone* Weighs In," *Science*, 1992, 255, 1505.
5.  "Possible Origins of AIDS," letter by C. H. Fox, pp. 1259–1260; letter by T. Curtis, p. 1260; letter by J. Cohen, pp. 1260–1261; all found in *Science*, 1992, 256.
6.  See, for instance, G. Ruckle, "Studies with the Monkey-Intra-Nuclear-Inclusion-Agent (MINIA) and Foamy-Agent Derived from Spontaneously Degenerating Monkey Kidney Cultures. I. and II.," *Arch. Virusforsch.*, 1958, 8(2), 139–166 and 167–182; G. E. Stiles, J. L. Bittle, and V. J. Cabasso, "Comparison of Simian Foamy Virus Strains Including a New Serological Type," *Nature*, 1964, 201, 1350–1351. For a review, see J. J. Hooks and C. J. Gibbs, "The Foamy Viruses," *Bact. Rev.*, 1975, 39(3), 169–185.
7.  H. Koprowski, "Live Poliomyelitis Virus Vaccines: Present Status and Problems for the Future," *JAMA*, 1961, 178(12), 1151–1155; see particularly pp. 1153–1155.
8.  A. B. Sabin, "Properties and Behavior of Orally Administered Attenuated Poliovirus Vaccine," *JAMA*, 1957, 164(11), 1216–1223; see especially table 8.
9.  J. Gear, "The South African Poliomyelitis Vaccine," *S. Af. Med. J.*, 1956, 30, 587–594.
10. S. Spencer, "Oral Polio Vaccine: The Best Yet?" *Saturday Evening Post*, July 23, 1960, pp. 20–21 and 87–90. M. M. da Silva et al., "Studies of Orally Administered Attenuated Live Virus Poliomyelitis Vaccine in Newborns and Infants under Six Months," *U. Minn. Med. Bull.*, 1957, 29, 133–150. The latter article is especially interesting, for it reports the first small-scale OPV trials carried out (in Minnesota) by the Cox-Cabasso group at Lederle, after it took over the reins from Koprowski and Norton. The article mentions specifically that the material used for the Fox Type 3 feeding "was grown in monkey kidney tissue (cynomolgus) in Povitsky bottles." (By contrast, the Type 1 vaccine used, SM-45, represented a final passage in CETC of a vaccine virus previously passaged in MKTC; here the species of monkey is not specified.) The article states that the vaccines were made available to the Minnesota team by Lederle in January 1957, so we know that Lederle scientists were using cynomolgus kidneys — at least to grow Fox vaccine — prior to that date. January 1957 was also the month in which Koprowski and Norton set off for the Belgian Congo; they officially left Lederle in April 1957.
11. P. Lépine and M. Paccaud, "Contribution a l'étude du virus spumeux (foamy virus)," *Ann. Inst. Past.*, 1957, 92(3), 288–300.
12. See, for instance, P. Lépine, "La problème des vaccinations antipoliomyélitiques et l'appréciation du niveau d'immunité des populations," 3rd Symposium of the European

Association against Poliomyelitis (Zurich, September 1955), in which Lépine states that Salk's vaccine is made in the kidney cells of rhesus monkeys (*Macaca mulatta*).

13. Anon., ["Requirements for the Production of the Koprowski Strains of Attenuated Poliovirus Vaccine"], *Immunolski. Zavod. Radovi* (Yugoslavia), 1964, 2, 124–125. The original text is in a Slavonic language.

14. H. Koprowski, "AIDS and the Polio Vaccine" (letter), *Science*, 1992, 257, 1024–1026.

15. R. J. Biggar et al., "ELISA HTLV Retrovirus Antibody Reactivity Associated with Malaria and Immune Complexes in Healthy Africans," *Lancet*, 1985, 2(i), 520–523; R. J. Biggar, "Possible Nonspecific Associations between Malaria and HTLV-III/LAV" (letter), *N. Engl. J. Med.*, 1986, 315(7), 457.

16. The Fox isolate came from an asymptomatic polio infectee in 1950 or 1951 (T. Lownes, "How the New Polio Vaccine Is Made," *Miami Herald*, January 17, 1960), but the strain was not successfully attenuated by Koprowski (as his first Type 3 strain) until 1956. Evidence: in May 1956, Joe Stokes commented: "work on attenuation of Type 3 is being carried out by Dr. Koprowski and his colleagues. They seem to be successful in isolating apathogenic substrains through the use of plaque technique." (See J. Stokes Jr., "Discussion," [*Am. Med. Assoc.*] *J. Dis. Child.*, December 1956, p. 453, which pertains to the sixty-sixth annual meeting of the American Pediatric Society, held May 9–11, 1956.) We know that Koprowski's first exploration of the plaque technique came when Renato Dulbecco, its originator, plaque-purified SM for him in August 1955 (see *NYAS* 57, table 1, p. 128). Koprowski's Fox strain was first fed experimentally to humans in June 1956, and to babies at Clinton in October 1956. (B. W. Hotchkiss, "Babies Being Fed Live Polio Virus," *Newark Evening News*, October 24, 1956, pp. 1 and 2.)

17. J. Morvan et al., "Enquête séro-épidémiologique sur les infections à HIV au Burundi entre 1980 et 1981," *Bull. Soc. Path. Exot.*, 1989, 82, 130–140.

18. B. Godefroid et al., "Etude sur la séropositivité liée à l'infection au Virus de l'Immuno-deficiencé Humaine au Rwanda," *Rev. Méd. Rwanda*, 1988, 20(54), 37–42.

19. B. Standaert et al., "Acquired Immunodeficiency Syndrome and Human Immuno-deficiency Virus Infection in Bujumbura, Burundi," *Trans. R. Soc. Trop. Med. Hyg.*, 1988, 82, 902–904.

20. *PAHO1*, see pages 416 and 497.

21. F. Przesmycki et al., "Vaccination against Poliomyelitis in Poland with Koprowski's Live Attenuated Strains," *PAHO2*, pp. 522–532.

22. HIV/AIDS Surveillance Data Base; U.S. Department of Commerce: Bureau of the Census, Washington D. C. 20233–0001, December 1993 edition.

23. J. Sonnet et al., "Early AIDS Cases Originating from Zaire and Burundi (1962–1976)," *Scand. J. Infect. Dis.*, 1987, 19, 511–517.

24. J. H. Wolfheim, *Primates of the World: Distribution, Abundance, and Conservation*, (Seattle and London: University of Washington Press, 1983), pp. 490–501 and 475–483.

25. *PAHO1*, pp. 577–579.

26. H. Koprowski, "Live Poliomyelitis Vaccine," *BMJ*, 1959, 1(ii), 1349–1350.

27. H. Koprowski, "Live Poliomyelitis Virus Vaccines: Present Status and Problems for the Future," *JAMA*, 1961, 178(12), 1151–1155; see particularly p. 1154.

28. Louis Pascal's analysis revealed that eleven of the textual entries were numbered two figures too low, two were numbered one figure too low, while two footnotes were not marked in the text at all.

29. Both Tom Curtis and the British evolutionary biologist Bill Hamilton responded in detail to Koprowski's *Science* letter, though *Science* never published their replies. For the

full texts of both, see J. Cribb, *The White Death* (Sydney: Angus and Robertson, 1996), pp. 254–262.

30. P. Manson, "Theories Tying AIDS to Contaminated Vaccines Date Back to 1988," *Houston Post,* August 19, 1992, p. A-14.

31. T. Curtis and P. Manson, "Scientists Urge Screening of Polio Vaccine for HIV," *Houston Post,* July 17, 1992, p. A-1.

32. T. Curtis and P. Manson, "Doctor Wants Houston Researcher to Test Polio Vaccines for AIDS Link," *Houston Post,* July 18, 1992, p. A-1.

33. T. Curtis, "Officials Continue to Ignore Signs of AIDS-Vaccine Link," *Houston Post,* August 19, 1992, p. A-1.

34. C. Basilico, C. Buck, R. Desrosiers, D. Ho, F. Lilly, and E. Wimmer, "Report from the AIDS/ Poliovirus Advisory Committee," September 18, 1992, released at a press conference in New York on October 22, 1992, available from Brian Martin, Department of Science and Technology Studies, University of Wollongong, NSW 2522, Australia; fax: +61-2-4221 3452; e-mail: brianmartin@uow.edu.au.

35. Presumably the committee meant 1957 to 1960, the dates of the Koprowski vaccination campaigns in the Congo.

36. For discussion on this point, see T. Curtis, "AIDS Theories" (letter), *Science,* 1993, 259, 14. However, as I later discovered, the dates were not, after all, of relevance.

37. J. Cribb, *The White Death,* pp. 178–180.

38. "The Wistar Institute of Anatomy and Biology Responds to Advisory Committee's Report on the Origin of AIDS," Wistar Institute press release, dated October 22, 1992.

39. G. Kolata, "Theory Tying AIDS to Polio Vaccine Is Discounted," *New York Times,* October 23, 1992, p. A16.

40. For instance, Anon., "Panel Nixes Congo Trials as AIDS Source," *Science,* 1992, 258, 738–739. This brief article, which proposed that the Manchester sailor case had administered "the putative coup de grâce" to the OPV/AIDS theory, only added to the impression that the coverage *Science* had afforded the theory during 1992 was less than evenhanded. See J. Cribb, *The White Death,* pp. 168–170 and 180.

41. T. Curtis and P. Manson, "Scientists Urge Major Changes in How Polio Vaccines Made," *Houston Post,* October 23, 1992, p. A16.

42. B. Rule, "Institute Will Investigate Possible Link between AIDS and Polio Vaccine," Associated Press wire story, March 6, 1992; Anon., "AIDS Story Prompts Libel Suit," *Science,* 1992, 258, 1567.

43. For the resolution of the Koprowski vs. AP case, see later in the book.

44. M. K. Curtis, "Monkey Trials: Science, Defamation, and the Suppression of Dissent," *William & Mary Bill of Rights J.,* 1995, 4(2), 507–593, with particular reference to pp. 526–529.

45. See M. K. Curtis, "Monkey Trials: Science, Defamation, and the Suppression of Dissent"; this lengthy article by Tom Curtis's brother is the key reference on this subject. See also B. Martin, "Stifling the Media" (letter), *Nature,* 1993, 363, 202; B. Martin, "Sticking a Needle into Science: The Case of Polio Vaccines and the Origin of AIDS," *Soc. Stud. Sci.,* 1996, 26, 245–276; B. Martin, "Political Refutation of a Scientific Theory: The Case of Polio Vaccines and the Origin of AIDS," *Health Care Analysis,* 1998, 6, 175–179; W. D. Hamilton, "AIDS Theory vs. Lawsuit" (unpublished letter to *Science*), in J. Cribb, *The White Death,* pp. 254–257.

CHAPTER 19: *An Untimely Passing*

1.  J. Sonnet et al., "Early AIDS Cases Originating from Zaire and Burundi (1962–1976)," *Scand. J. Infect. Dis.,* 1987, 19, 511–517.
2.  J. J. Sonnet, J. L. Michaux, and M. De Bruyere, "An Early AIDS Case in a Zairian Woman Presenting with an Aggressive Variant of Kaposi's Sarcoma in 1962," 1984, draft paper. Compare with Q. Chess et al., "Serum Immunoglobulin Elevations in the Acquired Immunodeficiency Syndrome (AIDS): IgG, IgA, IgM and IgD," *Diagnostic Immunol.,* 1984, 2, 148–153, which reveals that Helene's IgA and IgM levels were even higher than those of the typical AIDS patient (in whom such levels are usually elevated) and that her IgG level, at 1365, was identical to that of the average AIDS patient.
3.  R. L. Colebunders and A. S. Latif, "Natural History of HIV Infection in Adults," *AIDS,* 1991, 5 (suppl. 1), S103–S112 — a classic article on the presentations of AIDS in Africa.
4.  C.-K. Yeh et al., "Oral Defence Mechanisms Are Impaired Early in HIV-1 Infected Patients," *J. AIDS,* 1988, 1(4), 361–366.
5.  By contrast, in 1960 Sonnet and Michaux had witnessed another fatal case of KS in Leopoldville, but one in which the disease had taken fully ten years to run its course. Both doctors felt confident that this first fatal but indolent KS case was not HIV associated. J. Sonnet, J. L. Michaux, and J. De Cort, "Angiosarcomatose de Kaposi à localisations cutanées ganglionnaires viscerales et osseuses avec hyperprotidemie et anomalies des globulins du système gamma," *Acta Clin. Belg.,* 1961, 16(3), 313–331.
6.  N. Nzilambi, K. M. De Cock, J. B. McCormick et al., "The Prevalence of Infection with Human Immunodeficiency Virus over a 10-Year Period in Rural Zaire," *N. Engl. J. Med.,* 1988, 318(5), 276–279.
7.  N. Nzilambi et al., "The Prevalence of Infection with HIV over a 10-Year Period in Rural Zaire." See also K. M. De Cock, "AIDS: An Old Disease from Africa?" *BMJ,* 1984, 289, 306–308.
8.  In Professor Sonnet's article, it is recorded that Maria met and married Daniel in Bujumbura in 1973, and that they had their first child in 1974. In fact, Daniel did not arrive in Burundi until 1977, and Maria's first child was by another man.
9.  Other examples of unpublished papers by Jean Sonnet: "AIDS in African Patients" (1983); "Le tableau clinique du syndrome de déficit immunitaire acquis chez 13 Africains de race noir" (1984); "Syndrome d'immunodépression acquise aux infections opportunistes mortelles chez 6 Zairois," with J. M. Brucher et al. (1984).

CHAPTER 20: *The Congo Trials*

1.  *BMJ* 58.
2.  However, see G. Blanc and L.-A. Martin, "Premiers essais de prophylaxie de la poliomyélite par virus vivant fixé au lapin. Innocuité de la méthode," *Bull. Acad. Natl. Méd.,* 1953, 137, 230–234, which describes the administration of a live polio vaccine virus (made in rabbit tissue) to several thousand Moroccans at the start of the fifties. See also the authors' previous article about the preparation of the vaccine in *Bull. Acad. Natl. Méd.,* 1952, 136, 655–662.
3.  G. Courtois, "Vaccinations antipoliomyéletique par virus vivant au Congo Belge," *Ann. Soc. Belg. Méd. Trop.,* 1958, 38, 805–816.

4. T. F. Schulz, "Origin of AIDS" (letter), *Lancet,* 1992, 339, 867.
5. *NYAS* 57.
6. These are the references to the missing article on the chimpanzee research that feature, respectively, in notes 1 and 3, above.
7. J. Morvan, B. Carteron et al., "Enquête séro-épidémiologique sur les infections à HIV au Burundi entre 1980 et 1981," *Bull. Soc. Pathol. Exot.,* 1989, 82, 130–140.
8. F. Rodhain, "Arboviruses humaines au Burundi: Résultats d'une enquête séroépidémiologique, 1980–1982," *Bull. Soc. Pathol. Exot.,* 1987, 80, 155–161.
9. Rwandan HIV seroprevalence study group, "Nationwide Community-Based Serological Survey of HIV-1 and Other Human Retrovirus Infections in a Central African Country," *Lancet,* 1989, 1(ii), 941–943.
10. These were ELAVIA and LAV-1, French versions of ELISA and Western blot.

CHAPTER 21: *Primate Immunodeficiency Viruses*

1. M. Peeters, T. Huet et al., "Isolation and Partial Characterization of an HIV-Related Virus Occurring Naturally in Chimpanzees from Gabon," *AIDS,* 1989, 3, 625–630.
2. M. Peeters, M. Van den Haesevelde, L. Kestens, P. Piot et al., "Isolation and Characterization of a New Chimpanzee Lentivirus (Simian Immunodeficiency Virus Isolate cpz-ant) from a Wild-Captured Chimpanzee," *AIDS,* 1992, 6, 447–451. See also Anon., "A New Chimp Virus?" *New Sci.,* October 27, 1990.
3. Luc Kestens, personal letter, September 1994.
4. F. Gao, P. M. Sharp, G. M. Shaw, B. H. Hahn et al., "Human Infection by Genetically Diverse SIVsm-Related HIV-2 in West Africa," *Nature,* 1992, 358, 495–499.
5. A. André, G. Courtois, G. Lennes, G. Ninane, and P. M. Osterreith, "Mise en évidence d'antigènes de groupes sanguins A, B, O et Rh chez les singes chimpanzés," *Ann. Inst. Past.,* 1961, 101, 82–95.
6. J. Desmyter et al., "Anti-LAV/HTLV-III in Kinshasa Mothers in 1970 and 1980," 2nd International Conference on AIDS (Paris, June 23–25, 1986), Communication 110, abstract S17g, 106.
7. A. J. Nahmias et al., "Evidence for Human Infection with an HTLV-III/LAV-Like Virus in Central Africa, 1959" (letter), *Lancet,* 1986, 1(ii), 1279–1280.
8. This was not just coincidence, for I learned later that Desmyter had advised Nahmias about which assays to use. According to Desmyter's letter to Nahmias dated October 29, 1985, he (Desmyter) used five different assays on the 1970 and 1980 samples.
9. N. Nzilambi et al., "Perinatal HIV Transmission in Two African Hospitals," 3rd International Conference on AIDS (Washington, D.C., June 1987), abstract TH.7.6.
10. See the Zaire (Congo) section of the HIV/AIDS Surveillance Database; U.S. Department of Commerce: Bureau of the Census, Washington, DC 20233–0001; 1993 edition.
11. G. Lecatsas and J. J. Alexander, "Safe Testing of Poliovirus Vaccine and the Origin of HIV Infection in Man" (letter), *S. Af. Med. J.,* 1989, 76, 451.
12. S. F. Lyons, C. J. Dommann, and B. D. Schoub, "Safe Testing of Live Oral Poliovirus Vaccine" (editorial), *S. Af. Med. J.,* 1988, 74, 381.
13. E. F. Baker, "Latent Simian Foamy Virus" (letter), *S. Af. Med. J.,* 1989, 76, 451–452.
14. B. D. Schoub, C. J. Dommann, and S. F. Lyons, "Safety of Live Oral Poliovirus Vaccine and the Origin of HIV Infection in Man" (letter), *S. Af. Med. J.,* 1990, 77, 51–52.

15. Vero cells are a continuous cell line (but one that originates from the same species — the African green monkey).

16. Reply to the Schoub letter by G. Lecatsas and J. J. Alexander, *S. Af. Med. J.,* 1990, 77, 52.

17. G. Lecatsas and J. J. Alexander, "Origins of HIV" (letter), *Lancet,* 1992, 339, 1427.

18. By this stage, Tom Curtis had reported that Warren Cheston, a vice-president of the Wistar Institute, had said that they had found "a number of samples of polio vaccines that were put in our freezer back in the 1950s," and that Claudio Basilico, cochair of the Wistar expert committee, had acknowledged that some of the samples "were very likely to have been used" in Africa. See T. Curtis and P. Manson, "Doctor Wants Houston Researcher to Test Polio Vaccines for AIDS Link," *Houston Post,* July 18, 1992, pp. A-1 and A-9.

19. *NYAS* 57.

20. R. V. Gilden, L. O. Arthur, C. E. Graham et al., "HTLV-III Antibody in a Breeding Chimpanzee Not Experimentally Exposed to the Virus" (letter), *Lancet,* 1986, 1(i), 678–679.

21. Later, I discovered that this had involved research into hepatitis — Feng Gao, personal communication, May 1995.

22. W. D. Hillis, "An Outbreak of Infectious Hepatitis among Chimpanzee Handlers at a United States Air Force Base," *Am. J. Hyg.,* 1961, 73, 316–328. This article also includes the information that between 1958 and 1960, almost all of the chimps brought to Holloman AFB were purchased from vendors in Yaounde, Cameroon, so Cameroon may well be the source of the SIV-positive Holloman chimp imported in 1963.

23. W. Janssens, P. Piot et al., "Phylogenetic Analysis of a New Chimpanzee Lentivirus SIVcpz-gab-2 from a Wild-Captured Chimpanzee from Gabon," *AIDS Res. Hum. Retro.,* 1994, 10(9), 1191–1192.

24. In interview in 1995, Hahn sketched me a phylogenetic tree, in which SIVcpz-us branched on the side of SIVcpz-ant, the smuggled chimp from Antwerp, but on the opposite side of the HIV-1 Group O cluster from the two chimp SIV isolates from Gabon. Further developments are reported later in this book.

CHAPTER 22: *Pierre Lépine and the Pasteur Institute*

1. L. J. André and E. André-Gadras, "Cas de poliomyélite observés dans un district de brousse du Gabon," *Méd. Trop.,* 1958, 18, 638–641.

2. P. Lépine and V. Sautter, "Sur l'absence dans le vaccin français de l'agent vacuolant (virus SV40)," *Acad. Nat. Med.,* 1962, 146, 112–115; A. Nicolas, D. Cherby, and B. Montagnon, "Absence du virus simien SV 40 (agent vacuolant) dans le vaccin antipoliomyélitique preparé selon la technique Lépine," *Acad. Natl. Méd.,* 1962, 146, 116–119.

3. Joint CCTA/WHO Training Course on Rabies, July 11–28, 1955, held in Muguga, near Nairobi, Kenya. List of course attendees and further details kindly provided by Gordon Scott and Roy Ansell.

4. P. Lépine, "Prophylaxie de la poliomyélite: Présent et avenir," *Bull. WHO,* 1955, 13, 447–472; see p. 469.

5. Discussion by Pierre Lépine, *NYAS* 57, 148–149.

6. At the end of the published speech, Lépine promised that a detailed report of the chimp work would appear later in the *Annales de L'Institut Pasteur* (his house journal), though it would seem that it never appeared.

7. Anon., "Le vaccin du professeur Lépine sera vendu par une firme pharmaceutique américaine," *L'Echo de Stan* (Stanleyville, Belgian Congo), June 24, 1957. The story is sourced to Agence France Presse.

8. Discussion by Pierre Lépine, in *Papers and Discussions Presented at the Fourth International Poliomyelitis Conference; International Poliomyelitis Congress, July 8–12, 1957* (Philadelphia: J.B. Lippincott, 1958), pp. 154–155.

9. Expert Committee on Poliomyelitis: Second Report, *WHO Technical Report Series*, 1958, see 1–83; especially 25–57.

10. Dr. André later wrote a letter in which he stated that this was the first collective vaccination in France's black African territories, and claimed that all three injections had been identical, and had employed the "well-known inactivated Lépine vaccine made at the Institut Pasteur of Paris." Interestingly, however, he added that the vaccine "wasn't available straight away. The level of production was not enough, so we were sent a lot intended for another use." L. J. André, personal communication, August 1997.

11. H. Koprowski, "Etat actuel de l'immunisation contre la poliomyélite avec des virus vivants atténués," *Rev. Lyon. Méd.*, 1959, 8, 39–40. This was part of the report of the Symposium International de Virologie held at Lyon in June 1958.

12. Lépine in discussion following Koprowski's address, *Rev. Lyon Méd.*, 1959, 8, pp. 45–46.

13. D. Gouere, "Epidémiologie de la poliomyélite et vaccinations antipoliomyélitiqes en France," Eleventh Symposium of European Association of Poliomyelitis and Allied Diseases (Rome, October 1966), pp. 84–85; M. R. Radovanic, "Present Epidemiological Situation of Poliomyelitis in Europe (1964–1968)," Twelfth Symposium of European Association of Poliomyelitis and Allied Diseases (Bucharest, May 4–7, 1969), 15–28; see Annex II on p. 21.

14. G. Blanc and L.-A. Martin, "Innocuité pour l'homme du virus poliomyélitique fixé au lapin. Hypothèses sur le pouvoir protecteur d'un tel virus," *Bull. Acad. Natl. Méd.*, 1952, 136, 655–663.

15. G. Blanc and L.-A. Martin, "Premiers essais de prophylaxie de la poliomyélite par virus vivant fixé au lapin. Innocuité de la méthode," *Bull. Acad. Natl. Med.*, 1953, 137, 230–234.

16. P. Lépine, "Prophylaxie de la poliomyélite: Présent et avenir"; see p. 465.

17. P. Lépine and M. Paccaud, "Contribution a l'étude du virus spumeux (foamy virus). 1. Etude des souches FV I, FV II, FV III isolées de cultures de cellules renales de cynocephales," *Ann. Inst. Past.*, 1957, 92(3), 289–300.

18. In fact, as I later learned, Pastoria continued to supply primates to Paris even after independence. See the postscript.

19. A. Nicolas et al., "Absence du virus simien SV 40 (agent vacuolant) dans le vaccin antipoliomyélitique preparé selon la technique Lépine."

20. P. J. Kanki, J. Alroy, and M. Essex, "Isolation of T-Lymphotropic Retrovirus Related to HTLV-III/LAV from Wild-Caught African Green Monkeys," *Science*, 1985, 230, 951–954.

21. P. M. Sharp, K. L. Robertson, F. Gao, and B. H. Hahn, "Origins and Diversity of Human Immunodeficiency Viruses," *AIDS*, 1994, 8 (suppl. 1), S27–S42; see S38–S39.

22. The only confirmed SIV sampling of Guinea baboons I have managed to trace was done by Anders Naucler, who tested four baboons, twelve African green monkeys, and ten mona monkeys from Guinea-Bissau, and found them all SIV-negative. Anders Naucler, personal communication, March 1998.

23. T. Kodama et al., "Prevalence of Antibodies to SIV in Baboons in Their Native Habitat," *AIDS Res. Hum. Retro.*, 1989, 5(3), 337–343.

24. M. J. Jin, P. M. Sharp, B. H. Hahn et al., "Infection of a Yellow Baboon with Simian Immunodeficiency Virus from African Green Monkeys: Evidence for Cross-Species Transmission in the Wild," *J. Virol.*, 1994, 68(12), 8454–8460.

25. "Too Close for Comfort?" (*Wildlife on One,* BBC1 TV broadcast [U.K.], 1991), film about the chimpanzees of the Tai National Park, Ivory Coast, assisted by scientific adviser Christophe Boesch. See also G. Teleki, "The Omnivorous Chimpanzee," *Sci. Am.*, 1973, 228(1), 32–43.

26. H. J. A. Fleury et al., "Virus Related to but Not Identical with LAV/HTLV-III in Cameroon" (letter), *Lancet,* 1986, 1(ii), 854; E. Delaporte et al., "HIV-Related Virus in Gabon," 3rd Conference on AIDS in Africa (Naples, 1987), TH-28.

27. R. De Leys, M. Van den Haesevelde et al., "Isolation and Partial Characterization of an Unusual Human Immunodeficiency Retrovirus from Two Persons of West-Central African Origin," *J. Virol.*, 1990, 64, 1207–1216; M. Van den Haesevelde et al., "Molecular Cloning and Complete Sequence Analysis of a Highly Divergent African HIV Isolate," 7th International Conference on AIDS (Florence, 1991), MA1157.

28. P. Charneau, L. Montagnier, F. Clavel et al., "Isolation and Envelope Sequence of a Highly Divergent HIV-1 Isolate: Definition of a New HIV-1 Group," *Virol.*, 1994, 205, 247–253; see pp. 252–253.

29. G. Myers, "HIV: Between Past and Future," *AIDS Res. Hum. Retro.*, 1994, 10(11), 1317–1324; see p. 1318.

30. J. N. Nkengasong et al., "Antigenic Evidence of the Presence of the Aberrant HIV-1$_{ant70}$ Virus in Cameroon and Gabon" (letter), *AIDS*, 1993, 7(11), 1536–1537.

31. S. Connor, "New Strain of HIV Beats Blood Tests," *Independent on Sunday* (U.K.), April 3, 1994, p. 1.

32. H. Agut, L. Montagnier et al., "Isolation of Atypical HIV-1-Related Retrovirus from AIDS Patient" (letter), *Lancet,* 1992, 340, 681–682.

33. S. Saragosti, "Variability of HIV Type 1 Group O Strains Isolated from Cameroonian Patients Living in France," (9th) Colloque des Cent Gardes, 1994, pp. 109–112.

34. F. Honoré, "Les 'singeries' de l'Institut Pasteur à Kindia et à Paris," *L'Illustration* (Paris), April 23, 1927, no. 4390, pp. 407–409.

35. G. Lefrou and V. Michard, "Etude sur les causes de mortalité des chimpanzés en captivité à l'Institut Pasteur de Kindia (1950–1956)," *Ann. Inst. Past.*, 1957, 93, 502–516; see especially p. 504.

36. Blaine Elswood, personal communication, February 1993.

37. *Research in Virology* is one of three titles that have emerged from the ashes of the venerable *Annales de l'Institut Pasteur.*

38. This was partly because Chuck Cyberski died of AIDS shortly afterward, and partly because, during my time-pressured interviews with Hayflick and Plotkin, there were more important questions to ask. Many years later, I learned that in May 1995, Louis Pascal wrote a letter to Bill Hamilton in which he quoted from a letter dated May 17, 1992, which he had received from Chuck Cyberski. The Cyberski letter included the following passage: "Two weeks ago I interviewed Leonard Hayflick. . . . The conversation made me wonder what is going on. He was well aware of the storm of controversy raised by the *Rolling Stone* article and vehemently denied using African green monkeys. However, he never refuted the underlying premise of contamination; instead he went on to tell an interesting story about a vaccine the French were experimenting with at the same time — in French Equatorial Africa — using baboon kidney cultures! Perhaps one of the most striking revelations was his admission that he was in Paris two weeks earlier, meeting with Luc

Montagnier, Hilary Koprowski and Stanley Plotkin. . . . One can only wonder what was discussed!" This is yet another version of the meeting, and this time Montagnier is said to have taken part, as well as Koprowski. By the time I read Pascal's letter to Hamilton, I had come across slightly different versions of this alleged meeting from Jennifer Alexander, Blaine Elswood, and Pascal, but the primary source for all three was the late Chuck Cyberski. As will be revealed later in the book, this primary account by Cyberski was also inaccurate, although a similar meeting to the one he described did in fact take place in Paris. In his letter to Hamilton, Pascal stressed that by the time of the Paris meeting, the existence of highly divergent strains of HIV-1 from Gabon and Cameroon (some of which would later come to be called HIV-1 Group O viruses) had been recognized for some years. (See notes 26 and 27, above.)

39. B. F. Elswood and R. B. Stricker, "Polio Vaccines and the Origin of AIDS" (letter), *Res. Virol.*, 1993, 144, 175–177.

40. This raised the question of whether baboon kidney might have been used as the substrate for the Sabin strains of OPV, when they were adopted and manufactured in France. This is a possibility that by the end of my research in May 1999, I had still not managed to investigate properly.


CHAPTER 23: *The Norwegian Sailor*

1. H. L. Vis et al., "Aspects cliniques et biochimiques de la malnutrition proteique au Kivu Central," *Ann. Soc. Belg. Méd. Trop.*, 1965, 45(6), 607–628.

2. R. Root-Bernstein, *Rethinking AIDS — The Tragic Cost of Premature Consensus* (New York: Free Press, Macmillan, 1993).

3. W. C. Von Glahn and A. M. Pappenheimer, "Intranuclear Inclusions in Visceral Disease," *Am. J. Pathol.*, 1925, 1(5), 445–466, and patient autopsy, kindly supplied by Michael Shelansky, Chairman of Pathology, College of Physicians and Surgeons of Columbia University, New York City.

4. O. Busse, "Uber Saccharomycosis hominis," *Virchows. Arch.*, 1895, 140, 23–46.

5. J. Vandepitte et al., "Cryptococcal Meningitis and AIDS in Kinshasa, Zaire," [First] International Symposium on AIDS and Associated Cancers in Africa (Brussels, 1985), abstract 04/II.

6. Jean-Louis Michaux, personal communication, November 1992.

7. The first case in the Congo: J. Stijns and P. Royer, "Un cas de méningite à torulosis au Congo Belge," *Ann. Soc. Belg. Méd. Trop.*, 1953, 33, 483–486. The third case: P. Royer, J. P. Delville et al., "Observation d'un cas de torulose méningée et pulmonaire," *Ann. Soc. Belg. Méd. Trop.*, 1954, 34, 229–232.

8. See, for instance, H. P. Katner and G. A. Pankey, "Evidence for a Euro-American Origin of Human Immunodeficiency Virus (HIV)," *J. Natl. Med. Assoc.*, 1987, 79(10), 1068–1072.

9. M. Kaposi, "Idiopathisches Multiples Pigmentsarkom der Haut," *Arch. Dermatol. Syphilis*, 1872, 4, 265–273. Reprinted in English as M. Kaposi, "Classics in Oncology. Idiopathic Multiple Pigmented Sarcoma of the Skin," *CA — Cancer J. Clin.*, 1982, 32(6), 342–347 (see also introduction on Moriz Kaposi, 340–341).

10. L. H. Breimer, "Did Moriz Kaposi Describe AIDS in 1872?" *Clio Medica*, 1984, 19, 156–159.

11. Confidentiality concerns were not paramount in the nineteenth century.

12. By contrast, Moriz Kaposi's second such patient, a distiller from Krakow seen the following year, died in hospital as a result of diarrhea, fever, and continuous bleeding —

and at autopsy it was discovered that the mysterious sarcoma was disseminated through-out his internal organs. However, like Leonhard Kopf, he was in his late sixties, an age group that is susceptible to classic KS.

13. The first recorded use of the name "Brodtes" [sic] had been in 1708. Anon., *"Prottes unser Heimatort"* (Vienna: R. Spies, 1979), pp. 22 and 156–157.

14. Manfred Grunwald, personal communication, June 1992.

15. It should be pointed out that, as the local blacksmith, Leonhard Kopf would also have served as the "animal doctor," and would therefore presumably have been required to tend to the horses of the Prussian cavalry. This might have put him at greater risk of exposure to a viral agent not found locally.

16. Gigase worked for FOMULAC — the Fondation Médicale de l'Université de Louvain au Congo — which also ran Lovanium University in Leopoldville.

17. See A. Thijs, "L'angiosarcomatose de Kaposi au Congo Belge et au Ruanda-Urundi," *Ann. Soc. Belg. Méd. Trop.,* 1957, 37, 295–307; M. S. R. Hutt and D. P. Burkitt, *The Geography of Non-Infectious Disease* (Oxford: Oxford University Press, 1986), pp. 134–137.

18. F. Lothe, "Multiple Idiopathic Haemorrhagic Sarcoma of Kaposi in Uganda," *Acta Uniona Contra Cancrum,* 1962, 16, 1447–1451; H. Schmid, "Kaposi's Sarcoma in Tanzania: A Statistical Study of 220 Cases," *Trop. Geogr. Med.,* 1973, 25, 266–276.

19. R. J. Biggar et al., "Seroepidemiology of HTLV-III Antibodies in a Remote Population of Eastern Zaire," *BMJ,* 1985, 290, 808–810.

20. R. J. Biggar, "The AIDS Problem in Africa," *Lancet,* 1986, 1(i), 79–83; see p. 80. R. J. Biggar, "Possible Nonspecific Associations between Malaria and HTLV-III/LAV" (letter), *N. Engl. J. Med.,* 1986, 315(7), 457.

21. Michael Hutt, John Cook, Jack Davies, John Taylor, and Francis Lothe.

22. Symposium on Kaposi's Sarcoma, May 1961, the papers of which were published as: "Unio Internationalis Contra Cancrum Acta," *UICC,* 1962, 18, 1–511.

23. Second Kaposi's Sarcoma Symposium, January 8–11, 1980, the papers of which were published as "Kaposi's Sarcoma," *Antibiotics and Chemotherapy,* 1981, 29, 1–103.

24. Y. Chang et al., "Identification of Herpesvirus-Like DNA Sequences in AIDS-Associated Kaposi's Sarcoma," *Science,* 1994, 266, 1865–1869; Y. Chang et al., "Human Herpesvirus-Like Nucleic Acid in Various Forms of Kaposi's Sarcoma," *Lancet,* 1995, 345, 759–761; N. Dupin et al., "Herpesvirus-Like DNA Sequences in Patients with Mediterranean Kaposi's Sarcoma," *Lancet,* 1995, 345, 761–762; D. Whitby et al., "Detection of Kaposi Sarcoma Associated Herpesvirus in Peripheral Blood of HIV-Infected Individuals and Progression to Kaposi's Sarcoma," *Lancet,* 1995, 346, 799–802.

25. A. E. Friedman-Kien, T. A. Peterman et al., "Kaposi's Sarcoma in HIV-Negative Homo-sexual Men" (letter), *Lancet,* 1990, 335, 168–169.

26. K. Kucera, "Exact Correlation in Epidemics of *Pneumocystis* Pneumonia," *Folia Parasitol.,* 1966, 13, 343–360.

27. L. L. Pifer et al., *"Pneumocystis carinii* Infection: Evidence for High Prevalence in Normal and Immunocompromised Children," *Pediatrics,* 1978, 61, 35.

28. Articles by C. Chagas in *Mem. Inst. Cruz* (Rio), 1911, 3, 219 and in *Bull. Soc. Pathol. Exot.,* 1911, 4, 467.

29. G. van der Meer and S. L. Brug, "Infection à *Pneumocystis* chez l'homme et chez les ani-maux," *Ann. Soc. Belg. Méd. Trop.,* 1942, 22, 301–309.

30. Occasional cases of PCP occur in children (i.e., those aged more than six months, who are no longer definable as infants), but are usually prompted by a lack of gamma globulin in

the blood, which results in an inability to fight infection. See Table 1 and pages 164–166 in A. Thijs and P. G. Janssens, "Pneumocystosis in Congolese Infants," *Trop. Geogr. Med.*, 1963, 15, 158–172.

31. R. Root-Bernstein, *Rethinking AIDS — The Tragic Cost of Premature Consensus*, pp. 14–16. J. P. Vandenbroucke, "Tracking AIDS Epidemics in Libraries" (letter), *Lancet*, 1990, 336, 318–319. David Ho, personal communication, December 1993.

32. A. Thijs and P. G. Janssens, "Pneumocystosis in Congolese Infants."

33. R. C. Ringholz, *Uranium Frenzy — Boom and Bust on the Colorado Plateau* (New York: W. W. Norton, 1989), p. 26.

34. During the forties, by far the richest uranium-bearing ores in the world, used for all of the early U.S. atomic bombs, were found at Shinkolobwe — also in the Belgian Congo, albeit some nine hundred miles to the south of Kilo.

35. The two blasts were code-named Mosaic G1 and G2, and took place off Monte Bello Island, Western Australia, on May 16 and June 16, 1956. See B. Wigmore and A. Rimmer, "Did YOU Sail on This Ship of Doom?," *The People* (U.K.), April 21, 1991; and D. Robinson, *Just Testing* (London: Collins Harvil, 1985). My sincere thanks to Ken McGinley of the BNTVA, Boko Atkinson of the Diana Association, and the dozens of other British nuclear test veterans who cooperated so generously with my research in 1991 and 1992.

36. This is relevant, because H.M.S. *Diana* called at various African ports, including Freetown, Luanda, and Mombasa (twice) on her way home from Australia.

37. Jachymov, formerly St. Joachimsthaler, is the home of the silver Joachimsthaler, or "thaler," which later gave its name to the U.S. dollar. The two coins have the same weight and silver content.

38. A. Pirchan and H. Sikl, "Cancer of the Lung in the Miners of Jachymov (Joachimstal)," *Am. J. Cancer;* 1932, 16(4), 681–722.

39. Most of the mining in these early days was carried out on the surface, and not in the deeper uranium-bearing lodes, and it may well be that many of these early illnesses were the result of inhaling sulfur dioxide fumes from the smelting of the sulfur-rich silver ores that are found in the area.

40. This remarkable history of mining in the Jachymov region from medieval times to the present was provided by the kindness of Dr. Vladimir Horak, who in 1992 sent me two lengthy letters with many relevant articles enclosed. My thanks to Tom Unwin for his painstaking translations from the Czech. See also J. Brabec, "Co nas stal uran" ["What Price Uranium?"], *Respekt* (Prague), August 12–18, 1991, pp. 7–8.

41. Information from a *Fine Cut* documentary on the postwar Czech political prisoners, broadcast February 22, 1992, BBC2 (U.K.).

42. Annotated map of Jachymov closed zone provided by Dr. Vladimir Horak.

43. Michael Rowbotham, "Mountains of Death," *Mail on Sunday* (U.K.), November 17, 1991, pp. 48–49.

44. However, the very first retrospectively confirmable cases of PCP (with convincing micro-photographs of *Pneumocystis* cysts) were reported from Rostock, Griefswald, and Berlin (Germany) in 1938, and Danzig (Poland) in 1939. It is possible that during this period, uranium ore from Shinkolobwe in the Belgian Congo was being imported through the Nazi-controlled Baltic ports to the German capital in preparation for the atom-bomb program. But another unfortunate possibility — mentioned by Kamil Kucera among others — is that eugenics-related medical experiments were already under way in certain Nazi-controlled nurseries in the mid-thirties.

45. J. Vanek, O. Jirovec et al., "Interstitial Plasma Cell Pneumonia in Infants," *Ann. Ped.,* 1953, 180, 1–21.

46. Article by J. Vanek and O. Jirovec; *Zbl. Bakt.,* 1952, 158, 120.

47. Gottwaldov (or Zlin), Olomouc, and Novy Jicin are all close to the town of Vsetin, a noted center of weapons manufacture.

48. Another possible correlation is with sulfur dioxide emissions from the burning of poor-quality "brown coal," especially in the region surrounding Most, just to the south of the Erzgebirge. This is part of a "Bermuda Triangle of pollution" at this mountainous corner of Poland, and the former states of East Germany and Czechoslovakia. However, the prevailing winds from the Most region are easterly, which is reflected by the sulfur dioxide measurements across the country. The brown coal theory thus fits less well with the epidemiology of PCP than the uranium mining and transport theory. It may well be, of course, that both factors have played a significant role since the last war.

49. Later, I came across a very strange book entitled *AIDS: Origin, Spread and Healing* by a German writer, Wolff Geisler (Koln: Bipawo Verlag, 1994). On pages 89–94, Geisler comments on these early clusters of PCP in Czechoslovakia, Germany, the Belgian Congo, and elsewhere, and in note A88 (p. 209) he draws attention to the correlation with uranium mining and its immunosuppressive potential. Geisler is, however, a committed conspiracy theorist who believes that AIDS is the result of a series of biological warfare experiments, beginning with the transfer to humans of EIAV (equine infectious anemia virus) in Germany before the First World War. One of the many shortcomings of his book (which does contain the occasional worthwhile nugget) is that he routinely interprets medical studies of infectious disease as representing evidence that the doctors involved have previously introduced the pathogenic agents to their patients. In the case of PCP, there is a potential kernel of truth in that widespread Nazi eugenics experiments did take place. But he extrapolates from this possibility to claim (without proof) that German scientists (including Herwig Hamperl) deliberately infected children in orphanages and hospitals in Germany, Poland, Czechoslovakia, Iran, and Korea with *Pneumocystis* before, during, and after the war, and that the practice was continued in the United States in the fifties and sixties. By making such blanket assertions, he ends up drawing attention away from the Nazi medical research, and a sensible appraisal of same.

50. Slides tested by PCR by Dr. Mike Tristem of Imperial College, Silwood Park, U.K., in April 1995; he found no evidence that HIV was present.

51. C. F. Lindboe, S. S. Frøland, K. W. Wefring et al., "Autopsy Findings in Three Family Members with a Presumably Acquired Immunodeficiency Syndrome of Unknown Origin," *Acta Path. Microbiol. Immunol. Scand.* (Sect. A), 1986, 94, 117–123.

52. S. S. Frøland, K. W. Wefring, T. Bøhmer et al., "HIV-1 Infection in Norwegian Family before 1970" (letter), *Lancet,* 1988, 1(i), 1344–1345.

53. At the request of doctors and family members, I have used a pseudonym for the Norwegian sailor.

54. The analysis had involved an early assay, perhaps one of poor sensitivity. However, there is another possible explanation for the error, which is revealed later in the book.

55. J. P. Getchell, D. R. Hicks, J. B. McCormick et al., "Human Immunodeficiency Virus Isolated from a Serum Sample Collected in 1976 in Central Africa," *J. Infect. Dis.,* 1987, 156(5), 833–837, which, for ten years after publication, constituted the oldest isolate of HIV-1.

56. Details of Arvid's naval career were obtained by Dr. Wefring from the Norwegian government Direktoratet for Sjomenn, and further particulars from the individual shipping

companies. The confidentiality laws in Norway have since been changed, rendering the procuring of further information difficult.

57. At the time of our meeting, HIV-1 Group O had not yet been identified and named, but there had been a report in 1990 of an unusual retrovirus resembling HIV-1 being found in two patients from Cameroon. R. De Leys et al., "Isolation and Partial Characterization of an Unusual Human Immunodeficiency Retrovirus from Two Persons of West-Central African Origin," *J. Virol.,* 1990, 64, 1207–1216.

58. D. W. Cameron, P. Piot, F. A. Plummer et al., "Female to Male Transmission of Human Immunodeficiency Virus Type 1: Risk Factors for Seroconversion in Men," *Lancet,* 1989, 2(i), 403–407.

59. J. N. Nkengasong, G. van den Groen et al., "Antigenic Evidence of the Presence of the Aberrant HIV-1 ANT70 Virus in Cameroon and Gabon" (letter), *AIDS,* 1993, 7(11), 1536–1537. P. Charneau, F. Clavel et al., "Isolation and Envelope Sequence of a Highly Divergent HIV-1 Isolate: Definition of a New HIV-1 Group," *Virol.,* 1994, 205, 247–253.

CHAPTER 24: *Switzerland and Sweden*

1. In the middle of 1990, Mann resigned after a series of clashes with the new WHO director-general, Hiroshi Nakajima, who did not share his conviction that AIDS was a human rights issue, and that the international community had to guarantee that any future therapies or vaccines would also be made available, free, to the Third World countries where they were most needed. Many feel that his departure coincided with the GPA's beginning to play a less dynamic role in coordinating the response to the pandemic. See R. M. Bhatt, "The Limits of Cooperation: The World Health Organization and the International Response to AIDS, 1981–1994," paper prepared for the annual conference of the International Studies Association (ISA), San Diego, April 1996, pp. 15–18. Jonathan Mann and his wife were among the tragic victims of the Swiss Air crash off Nova Scotia in September 1998.

2. "The Wistar Institute of Anatomy and Biology Responds to Advisory Committee's Report on the Origin of AIDS," Wistar Institute press release, October 22, 1992.

3. WHO internal memorandum on "Safety of Poliovaccines," prepared by M. H. Merson, R. J. Kim-Farley, and D. I. Magrath, marked 18/446/7VAC, dated May 8, 1992.

4. For the second claim, see T. Huet, S. Wain-Hobson et al., "Genetic Organization of a Chimpanzee Lentivirus Related to HIV-1" (letter), *Nature,* 1990, 345, 356–359. For the fourth claim, see Anon., "Seroconversion to Simian Immunodeficiency Virus in Two Laboratory Workers," *MMWR,* 1992, 41(36), 678–681; and R. F. Khabbaz, "Brief Report: Infection of a Laboratory Worker with Simian Immunodeficeincy Virus," *N. Engl. J. Med.,* 1994, 330(3), 172–177.

5. G. Lecatsas and J. J. Alexander, "Safe Testing of Poliovirus Vaccine and the Origin of HIV Infection in Man" (letter), *S. Af. Med. J.,* 1989, 76, 451.

6. See Simon Wain-Hobson interview later in this book.

7. Opinions expressed by Jennifer Alexander in interview, 1992.

8. B. Stone, "No AIDS Risk from Polio Vaccine," Food and Drug Administration Talk Paper, T92–29, April 6, 1992.

9. "T-Lymphotropic Retroviruses of Non-Human Primates," *Weekly Epidem. Rec.,* 1985, 60, 269–270.

10. "Acceptability of Cell Substrates for Production of Biologicals," report of a WHO Study Group, *WHO Tech. Rep. Ser.*, 1978, 747.

11. L. Hayflick, S. A. Plotkin, T. W. Norton, and H. Koprowski, "Preparation of Polio-virus Vaccines in a Human Fetal Diploid Cell Strain," *Am. J. Hyg.*, 1962, 75, 240–258; L. Hayflick, "The Coming of Age of WI-38," *Advances in Cell Culture*, 1984, 3, 303–316; L. Hayflick and P. S. Moorhead, "The Serial Cultivation of Human Diploid Cell Strains," *Exp. Cell. Res.*, 1961, 25, 585–621; see p. 587, Figure 1 for an explanation of the differ-ence between a cell strain (such as WI-38) and a cell line.

12. 1984 publication by WHO Department of Biologicals, BLG/84.2 Rev. 1, pp. 1–24.

13. G. Courtois, "Vaccination antipoliomyélitique par virus vivant au Congo belge," *Ann. Soc. Belge Méd. Trop.*, 1958, 38, 805–816.

14. "Poliomyelitis Vaccine. Salk. Use of Monkeys," note to (U.K.) Chief Medical Officer from "W. D.," dated April 21, 1955, Public Record Office reference: MH 55 2458.

15. R. Preston, *The Hot Zone* (New York: Random House, 1994).

16. Diagnostic tests for HIV and SIV have been available since 1984 and 1985, but those for prion diseases have proved more problematical. It was only after this chapter was writ-ten (1997) that diagnostic tests for "human BSE" were proposed for the first time. See A. F. Hill, J. Collinge et al., "Diagnosis of New Variant Creutzfeldt-Jakob Disease by Tonsil Biopsy" (letter), *Lancet*, 1997, 349, 99–100.

17. G. Courtois, "Vaccination antipoliomyélitique par virus vivant au Congo belge."

18. F. Buser et al., "Bestimmung der neutralisierenden Antikorper gegen Poliomyelitis vor und nach der Salk-Impfung bei Sauglingen un Kleinkindern," *Schweiz. Med. Wochenschr.*, 1958, 21, 530–532.

19. H. Koprowski, "Historical Aspects of the Development of Live Virus Vaccine in Polio-myelitis," *BMJ*, 1960, 2(i), 85–91; see p. 88.

20. The Fox pool was designated WFX, pool Wy 3–3, which indicates that it had apparently been made at the Wyeth laboratories — which later made the pools of CHAT and Fox for the huge Polish campaign.

21. F. Buser and M. Schar, "Poliomyelitis Vaccination with Live Poliovirus," *Am. J. Dis. Child.*, 1961, 101, 60–66.

22. S. A. Plotkin, "Recent Results of Mass Immunization against Poliomyelitis with Koprowski Strains of Attenuated Live Poliovirus," *Am. J. Public Health*, 1962, 52(6), 946–960; see p. 959.

23. F. Buser et al., "Immunization with Live Attenuated Polio Virus Prepared in Human Diploid Cell Strains, with Special Reference to the WM-3 Strain," *Proceedings — Symposium on the Characterization and Uses of Human Diploid Cell Strains* (Opatija, Yugoslavia, 1963), pp. 381–387.

24. M. Schar, "La vaccination antipoliomyélitique et l'épidémiologie en Suisse," *Proceedings of the 8th Symposium of the European Association of Poliomyelitis and Allied Diseases*, (Prague, September 23–26, 1962), pp. 82–84.

25. S. S. Kalter et al., "A Survey of Primate Sera for Antibodies to Viruses of Human and Simian Origin," *Am. J. Epidem.*, 1967, 86(1), 552–568. See Table 6 on p. 561.

26. N. G. Rogers, M. Basnight, C. J. Gibbs Jr., and D. C. Gadjusek, "Latent Viruses in Chimpanzees with Experimental Kuru," *Nature*, 1967, 216, 446–449.

27. One of Hull's many articles on this subject was R. Hull et al., "New Viral Agents Recovered from Tissue Cultures of Monkey Kidney Cells," *Am. J. Hyg.*, 1956, 63, 204–215.

28. J. Strom (editor), *The Poliomyelitis Epidemic in Stockholm 1953 — Epidemiological, Clinical and Laboratory Investigations* (Stockholm: Tryckeri AB Thule, 1956).

29.  S. Gard, M. Böttiger, and R. Lagercrantz, "Vaccination with Attenuated Poliovirus Type 1, the CHAT Strain," *PAHO1*, 350–354; M. Böttiger, S. Gard, and R. Lagercrantz, "Vaccination with Attenuated Type 1 Poliovirus, the Chat Strain. I. A Study of 20 Families," *Acta Paediatr. Scand.*, 1966, 55, 405–415.

30.  M. Böttiger, S. Gard, and B. Zetterberg, "Vaccination with Attenuated Type 1 Poliovirus, the Chat Strain. II. Transmission of Virus in Relation to Age," *Acta Paediatr. Scand.*, 1966, 55, 416–421.

31.  M. Böttiger, E. Böttiger, and B. Zetterberg, "Vaccination with Attenuated Type 1 Poliovirus, the Chat Strain. III. Antibody Response and Spread of Virus in Schoolchildren," *Acta Paediatr. Scand.*, 1966, 55, 422–431.

32.  S. Gard, "Poliovirus Vaccination in Sweden," *Proceedings of the 8th Symposium of the European Association of Poliomyelitis and Allied Diseases* (Prague, September 23–26, 1962), pp. 140–144. One further small trial of CHAT pool 26 (made in WI-26, an early form of Hayflick's human diploid cell strain, WI-38) followed, involving 135 children in an Uppsala school in 1962, but this was apparently the last time that any of Koprowski's strains were fed in Sweden. (J. S. Pagano, M. Böttiger, J. O. Bonnevier, and S. Gard, "The Response and the Lack of Spread in Swedish School Children Given an Attenuated Poliovirus Vaccine Prepared in a Human Diploid Cell Strain," *Am. J. Hyg.*, 1964, 79(1), 74–85; J. S. Pagano, M. Böttiger, and S. Gard, "Chat Type 1 Attenuated Poliovirus Vaccine Prepared on Human Diploid Cells: A Study in 135 Swedish Children. 1. Epidemiology and Results of a Trial," *Proceedings of the 8th Symposium of the European Association of Poliomyelitis and Allied Diseases* [Prague, September 23–26, 1962], pp. 498–507.)

33.  A. Lebrun, G. Courtois, H. Koprowski et al., "Preliminary Report on Mass Vaccination with Live Attenuated Poliomyelitis Virus in Leopoldville, Belgian Congo," *PAHO1*, 410–436; see p. 416; F. Przesmycki, "Vaccination against Poliomyelitis in Poland with Koprowski's Live Attenuated Strains," *PAHO2*, 522–532. These CHAT pools were also different from the experimental pool that Gard apparently worked with at the Wistar in 1959 — pool 19. (S. Gard, "Immunological Strain Specificity within Type 1 Poliovirus," *Bull. WHO*, 1960, 22, 235–242.)

34.  A. Nemeth et al., "Early Case of Acquired Immunodeficiency Syndrome in a Child from Zaire," *Sex. Transm. Dis.*, 1986, 13(2), 111–113.

35.  Margerete Böttiger's thesis appeared in 1966, and includes the following articles: M. Böttiger et al., "The Immune Response to Vaccination with Inactivated Poliovirus Vaccine in Sweden," *Acta Pathol. Microbiol. Scand.*, 1966, 66, 239–256; M. Böttiger, "Studies on Characteristics of Poliovirus" (parts I, II and III), *Arch. Ges. Virusforsch.*, 1966, 18(2), 119–154; M. Böttiger et al., "Vaccination with Attenuated Type 1 Poliovirus, the Chat Strain" (parts I, II and III), see notes 29, 30, and 31 above.

36.  Anon., "British Guests in Malmo," *Sydsvenska Dagbladet*, June 3, 1957.

37.  The only evidence I could find of any small-scale OPV trials having taken place on the west coast of Sweden involved a study conducted by Eric Lycke, who fed CHAT to thirty infants at a children's home just outside Sweden's second city of Gothenburg, some two hundred miles north of Malmo. N. Faxen et al., "Excretion Period of Attenuated Poliovaccine Virus in Infants," *Arch. Ges. Virusforsch.*, 1962, 12(1), 1–6.

38.  D. Huminer et al., "AIDS in the Pre-AIDS Era," *Rev. Infect. Dis.*, 1987, 9(6), 1102–1108; B. Hagmar, J. Kutti et al., "Disseminated Infection Caused by *Mycobacterium Kansasii*," *Acta Med. Scand.*, 1969, 186, 93–99.

39.  D. K. Smith et al., "Unexplained Opportunistic Infections and CD4+ T-Lymphocytopenia without HIV Infection — An Investigation of Cases in the United States," *N. Engl. J. Med.*,

1993, 328(6), 373–379. This paper includes details of three HIV-negative patients (all women) who suffered a disseminated mycobacterial infection similar to that of the Gothenburg patient.

CHAPTER 25: *An Introduction to HIV-2*

1.  B. Davidson, "Portuguese-speaking Africa," in M. Crowder (editor), *Cambridge History of Africa from about 1940 to about 1975* (Cambridge: Cambridge University Press, 1984), vol. 8, chapter 15, pp. 755–806.
2.  F. Barin, F. Denis, and J. S. Allan, "Serological Evidence for Virus Related to Simian T-Lymphotropic Retrovirus III in Residents of West Africa," *Lancet,* 1985, 2(ii), 1387–1389; F. Clavel et al., "Isolation of a New Human Retrovirus from West African Patients with AIDS," *Science,* 1986, 233, 343–346; F. Clavel, "HIV-2, the West African AIDS Virus" (editorial review), *AIDS,* 1987, 1, 135–140.
3.  J. M. Amat-Roze et al., "La géographie de l'infection par les virus de l'immunodéficiencé humaine (VIH) en Afrique noire: Mise en evidence de facteurs d'épidémisation et de régionalisation," *Bull. Soc. Pathol. Exot.,* 1990, 83, 137–148; M. Smallman-Raynor, A. Cliff, and P. Haggett (editors), *Atlas of AIDS* (Oxford: Blackwell Reference, 1992), pp. 126–127, 135, 174, 306–314. (Amat-Roze and Table 8.3(e) of the *Atlas* (p. 311) are also the main sources for the population movement map that appears in chapter 47.)
4.  M. Guydayer, L. Montagnier et al., "Genome Organization and Transactivation of the Human Immunodeficiency Virus Type 2," *Nature,* 1987, 326, 662–669; V. M. Hirsch et. al., "SIV from Sooty Mangabey Monkeys: An African Primate Lentivirus Closely Related to HIV-2," 5th International Conference on AIDS (Montreal, June 4–9, 1989), Abstract T.C.O.43; V. M. Hirsch et al., "An African Primate Lentivirus (SIVsm) Closely Related to HIV-2," *Nature,* 1989, 339, 389–391.
5.  M. Smallman-Raynor et al., *Atlas of AIDS,* technical appendix to chapter 8.3, pp. 313–314.
6.  HIV-1: A. R. Moss and P. Bacchetti, "Natural History of HIV Infection," *AIDS,* 1989, 3, 55–61. HIV-2 (anecdotal reports): R. Ancelle et al., "Long Incubation Period for HIV-2 Infection," *Lancet,* 1987, 1(i), 688–689; G. Dufoort et al., "No Clinical Signs 14 Years after HIV-2 Transmission by Blood Transfusion," *Lancet,* 1988, 2(i), 510. For a more detailed study of HIV-2 disease progression, see R. Marlink, P. Kanki et al., "Reduced Rate of Disease Development after HIV-2 Infection as Compared to HIV-1," *Science,* 1994, 265, 1587–1590.
7.  P. J. Kanki, M. Essex et al., "New Human T-Lymphotropic Retrovirus Related to Simian T-Lymphotropic Virus Type III (STLV IIIagm)," *Science,* 1986, 232, 238–243.
8.  H. W. Kestler III et al., "Comparison of Simian Immunodeficiency Virus Isolates," *Nature,* 1988, 331, 619–621; followed by reply from M. Essex and P. J. Kanki, pp. 621–622. S. Connor and S. Kingman, *The Search for the Virus — The Scientific Discovery of AIDS and the Quest for a Cure* (London: Penguin, 1989), pp. 227–229.
9.  J. M. Amat-Roze et al., "La géographie de l'infection par les virus de l'immunodéficiencé humaine (VIH) en Afrique noire."
10. P. J. Kanki and K. M. De Cock, "Epidemiology and Natural History of HIV-2," *AIDS,* 1994, 8 (suppl. 1), S85-S93.
11. P. N. Fultz et al., "Seroprevalence of HIV-1 and HIV-2 in Guinea Bissau in 1980," *AIDS,* 1988, 2, 129–132.
12. A. Naucler, "HIV-2 Infection and AIDS in Guinea-Bissau, West Africa" (thesis), Lund, 1991.

13. R. G. Marlink, P. Kanki, M. Essex et al., "Clinical, Hematological and Immunological Cross-Sectional Evaluation of Individuals Exposed to HIV-2," *AIDS Res. Hum. Retro.*, 1988, 4, 137–148.

14. A. Wilkins et al., "The Epidemiology of HIV Infection in a Rural Area of Guinea-Bissau," *AIDS*, 1993, 7, 1119–1122.

15. A book from 1973 claims the opposite: that Manjaco women only very rarely slept with Portuguese soldiers, that they married at the very young age of twelve or thirteen, and that after marriage they were "known for their fidelity." A. J. Venter, *Portugal's Guerrilla War: The Campaign for Africa* (Cape Town: John Malherbe Pty, 1973), pp. 131–132.

16. HIV/AIDS Surveillance Database, U.S. Department of Commerce, Bureau of the Census, Washington, D.C., December 1993.

17. A.-G. Poulsen et al, "HIV-2 in People over 50 Years in Bissau, Prevalence and Risk Factors," 8th International Conference on AIDS (Amsterdam, 1992), Abstract PoC 4132.

18. A.-G. Poulsen et al., "Prevalence of and Mortality from Human Immunodeficiency Virus Type 2 in Bissau, West Africa," *Lancet*, 1989, 1(ii), 827–830.

19. A. Shoumatoff, "In Search of the Source of AIDS," in *African Madness* (New York: Knopf, 1988), p. 142.

CHAPTER 26: *Paul Osterrieth and Fritz Deinhardt*

1. *BMJ* 58 was authored by Courtois, Jervis, Flack, Koprowski, and Ninane.

2. P. M. Osterrieth and P. Deleplanque-Liegeois, "Présence d'anticorps vis-à-vis des virus transmis par arthropodes chez le chimpanzé (*Pan troglodites*). Comparaison de leur état immunitaire à celui de l'homme," *Ann. Soc. Belg. Méd. Trop.*, 1961, 41, 63–72; A. André, G. Courtois, G. Lennes, G. Ninane, and P. M. Osterrieth, "Mise en évidence d'antigènes de groupes sanguins A, B, O et Rh chez les singes chimpanzés," *Ann. Inst. Past.*, 1961, 101, 82–95; F. Deinhardt, G. Courtois, P. Dherte, P. Osterrieth, G. Ninane, G. Henle, and W. Henle, "Studies of Liver Function Tests in Chimpanzees after Inoculation with Human Infectious Hepatitis Virus," *Am. J. Hyg.*, 1962, 75, 311–321; R. Delcourt, G. Ninane, P. Osterrieth, and M. Vastesaeger, "Le metabolisme lipidique du chimpanzé (*Pan satyrus schweinfurthii*)," *Acta Cardiol.*, 1964, 19, 531–545. The fifth article is the unpublished paper on polio research in chimps.

3. F. Deinhardt et al., "Studies of Liver Function Tests in Chimpanzees after Inoculation with Human Infectious Hepatitis Virus."

4. F. Przesmycki et al., "Report on Field Trials with Live Attenuated Poliomyelitis Vaccine of Koprowski in Poland," *Am. J. Hyg.*, 1960, 71(3), 275–284.

5. P. Osterrieth, "Proprietés biochimiques des Klebsiella," *Ann. Soc. Belg. Méd. Trop.*, 1958, 18, 721–730.

6. A. André et al., "Mise en évidence d'antigènes de groupes sanguins A, B, O et Rh chez les singes chimpanzés"; see p. 83.

7. G. Lefrou and V. Michard, "Etude sur les causes de mortalité des chimpanzés en captivité à l'Institut Pasteur de Kindia (1950–1956)," *Ann. Institut. Pasteur*, 1957, 93(4), 502–516.

8. J. A. Gagnon, *The Chimpanzee* (Basel/New York: Karger, 1970), pp. 69–99.

9. H. Koprowski, T. W. Norton, J. Stokes et al., "Immunization of Infants with Living Attenuated Poliomyelitis Virus: Laboratory Investigations of Alimentary Infections and Antibody Response in Infants under Six Months of Age with Congenitally Acquired

Antibodies," *JAMA*, 1956, 162(14), 1282–1288 (Clinton). H. Koprowski, T. W. Norton, J. Stokes et al., "Immunization of Children by the Feeding of Living Attenuated Type I and Type II Poliomyelitis Virus and the Intramuscular Injection of Immune Serum Globulin," *Am. J. Med. Sci.*, 1956, 232, 378–388 (Woodbine). S. A. Plotkin, H. Koprowski, S. N. Richardson, and J. Stokes, "Vaccination of Families against Poliomyelitis by Feeding and by Contact Spread of Living Attenuated Virus: Including Studies of Virus Properties after Human Intestinal Passage," *Acta Paediatr.*, 1960, 49, 551–571 (Moorestown).

10. H. Koprowski et al., "Immunization of Infants with Living Attenuated Poliomyelitis Virus." S. A. Plotkin, H. Koprowski, and J. Stokes, "Clinical Trials in Infants of Orally Administered Attenuated Poliomyelitis Viruses," *Pediatrics*, 1959, 23, 1041–1060. Also *BMJ* 58.

11. J. Stokes, H. Koprowski, K. Hummeler et al., "Passive-Active Immunization of Infants with Attenuated Poliomyelitis Viruses Administered Orally," Society Transactions, American Pediatric Society, 66th Annual Meeting (Buck Hill Falls, Pa.; May 9–11, 1956), published in (*Am. Med. Assoc.*) *J. Dis. Child.*, 1956, pp. 452–454.

12. F. Deinhardt et al., "Studies of Liver Function Tests in Chimpanzees after Inoculation with Human Infectious Hepatitis Virus."

13. Anon., "Monkey business," *Thermometer* (Children's Hospital of Philadelphia), 1958, 9(2), 3–6.

14. This was confirmed just a few years later by Bill Hillis, in his research on the chimps at Holloman Air Force Base. See W. D. Hillis, "The Outbreak of Infectious Hepatitis among Chimpanzee Handlers at a United States Air Force Base," *Am. J. Hyg.*, 1961, 73; 316–328.

15. W. Henle, "Studies on Viral Hepatitis," part of the *Annual Report to the Commission on Viral Infections of the Armed Forces Epidemiological Board*, covering the period March 1, 1958, to February 28, 1959; see p. 5, which shows that only four of the six shipments had been received by the latter date.

16. *BMJ* 58; see p. 188.

17. The most southerly volcano, Karisimbi, is 10,000 feet above the surface of Lake Kivu and roughly forty miles north of Kibuye. Clouds passing directly over the volcano would easily be seen at that distance, providing visibility was good.

18. A. J. Nahmias, A. Motulsky et al., "Evidence for Human Infection with an HTLV-III/LAV-Like Virus in Central Africa, 1959," *Lancet*, 1986, 1(ii), 1279–1280.

19. J. Vandepitte et al., "AIDS and Cryptococcosis (Zaire 1977)" (letter), *Lancet*, 1983, 1(ii), 925–926.

20. Professor Vandepitte added that there would have been sporadic early cases of AIDS before 1975, and later he wrote to inform me that the fourth child of the Zairean airline secretary (who herself died of AIDS in 1978) had died of a respiratory infection (probably pneumonia) and thrush in 1973. By contrast, the secretary's three previous children, born to a different father in the years up to and including 1970, remained healthy.

21. L. Montagnier, "Origin and Evolution of HIVs and Their Role in AIDS Pathogenesis," *J. AIDS*, 1988, 1, 517–520.

22. The Wistar expert committee had commented that this procedure was "known to cause significant loss of SIV and HIV infectivity, while reducing poliovirus titers only marginally."

23. T. Huet, S. Wain-Hobson et al., "Genetic Organization of a Chimpanzee Lentivirus Related to HIV-1," *Nature*, 1990, 345, 356–359.

24. It was now May 1993, almost three years since the appearance of the *Lancet* article about amplifying HIV from the Manchester sailor sample, and still nothing had been published

about the sequence. During 1992, I phoned Corbitt's lab frequently to check on progress. One time, Corbitt announced that Bailey had amplified about 800 nucleotides from the envelope gene, but when I phoned again three months later, he told me that, when sequenced, this had turned out to be "rogue DNA" — a lab contamination. Sources: phone conversations with Corbitt in February and May 1992, and with Bailey in May and August 1992.

25. H. Koprowski, C. W. Saxinger, R. C. Gallo et al., "Multiple Sclerosis and Human T-Cell Lymphotropic Retroviruses," *Nature,* 1958, 318, 354–360.

CHAPTER 27: *The Quieting of Louis Pascal*

1. In this Pascal was in good company, for when Albert Sabin said he had found a contaminant in CHAT in 1959, he had referenced the Ruzizi campaign, but then added that the same material had apparently been fed in Poland without mishap; he, too, clearly thought that just the one pool of CHAT had been used throughout the Congo. In fact, as I now knew, pool 10A-11 had been used in Ruzizi, pool 13 in Leopoldville (Congo) and in the small trial at Wyszkow (Poland), while pool 18 had been used in the Polish mass trial.

2. This account again differed from the story he had given me about having "definitely" established a *naval* link between Carr and Belfast.

3. The first part of his chapter in *Applied Ethics* was ascribed to one "Walter Bradford Ellis — a little-known pioneer in the field of over-population"; only later in the piece was it revealed that this was a clever device to manipulate the reader, and that Ellis and Pascal were actually one and the same. L. Pascal, "Judgement Day," in P. Singer (editor), *Applied Ethics* (Oxford: Oxford University Press, 1986), pp. 105–123.

4. He provided two pieces of supporting evidence. The first was an article that demonstrated that a superinfection with another retrovirus allowed HIV-1 to grow in HeLa cultures (P. Lusso, R. C. Gallo et al., "Expanded HIV-1 Cellular Tropism by Phenotypic Mixing with Murine Endogenous Retroviruses," *Science,* 1990, 247, 848–852. [The superinfection, in this instance, was with endogenous murine leukemia virus — MuLV — a mouse retrovirus.]) The second was a book, which reported that Microbiological Associates (the company that — in the early 1960s — had supplied Koprowski with monkey kidneys for certain of his tissue culture work, and which — Pascal surmised — could also possibly have supplied some of the kidneys for vaccine production) had, for thirteen years, been marketing a "prostate, benign, human adult" culture called MA160, when in reality the culture had been a HeLa contamination. See M. Gold, *A Conspiracy of Cells — One Woman's Immortal Legacy and the Medical Scandal It Caused* (Albany, NY: State University of New York Press, 1986), pp. 97–98 and 148.

5. C. Bernstein and B. Woodward, *All the President's Men* (New York: Simon and Schuster, 1974), pp. 71–73.

6. Y. Ohta et al., "No Evidence for the Contamination of Live Oral Poliomyelitis Vaccines with Simian Immunodeficiency Virus" (letter), *AIDS,* 1989, 3(3), 183–184. Pascal's initial refutation came in the form of a document entitled "Preliminary Notes Concerning Shortcomings of a Correspondence by Y. Ohta et al. . . . ," dated May 8, 1993.

7. C. Basilico, D. Ho et al., "Report from the AIDS/Poliovirus Advisory Committee" (released at a press conference held in New York City on October 22, 1992, and available from Brian Martin, Science and Technology Studies, University of Wollongong, NSW 2522, Australia; fax: +61-2-4221 3452; e-mail: brianmartin@uow.edu.au).

8. Y. Cao et al., "Identification and Quantitation of HIV-1 in the Liver of Patients with AIDS," *AIDS*, 1992, 6, 65–70, deals with humans and HIV rather than monkeys and SIV, but it makes the point nonetheless.

9. I am indebted to Bill Hamilton for suggesting this image.

## CHAPTER 28: *A Man of Many Ideas*

1. Item 30 in this list features the two final trials conducted by the Swedes in 1960/1 and 1961/2, involving some 4,212 children. These involved a vaccine prepared in Stockholm, which was based on CHAT 10A-11, but then passaged one further time in monkey kidney — using tissue culture prepared from the cynomolgus macaque. M. Böttiger, E. Böttiger, and B. Zetterberg, "Vaccinations with Attenuated Type 1 Poliovirus, the Chat Strain: III. Antibody Response and Spread of Virus in Schoolchildren," *Acta Paediatr. Scand.*, 1966, 55, 1–10.

2. For an analysis of phase 1, 2, and 3 trials with respect to AIDS vaccine testing, see J. P. Porter et al., "Ethical Considerations in AIDS Vaccine Testing," *IRB: A Review of Human Subjects Research*, 1989, 11(3), 1–4.

3. H. Koprowski, "Hybrids and Viruses: Reflections on Golden Past and Less Certain Future," in K. Maramorosch (editor), *Advances in Cell Culture* (New York: Academic Press, 1981), volume 1, pp. 1–13.

4. H. Koprowski, T. W. Norton, and W. McDermott, "Isolation of Poliomyelitis Virus from Human Serum by Direct Inoculation into a Laboratory Mouse," *Public Health Rep.*, 1947, 62(41), 1467–1476; see acknowledgments at the end.

5. H. Koprowski, G. A. Jervis, and T. W. Norton, "Oral Administration of Poliomyelitis Virus to Man and Ape — A Comparative Study," *Proc. Natl. Acad. Sci.*, 1954, 40, 36–39.

6. H. Koprowski, G. A. Jervis, and T. W. Norton, "Immune Responses in Human Volunteers upon Oral Administration of a Rodent-Adapted Strain of Poliomyelitis Virus," *Am. J. Hyg.*, 1952, 55, 108–126.

7. Koprowski appears to mean lacking antibodies to poliovirus Type 2, though Victor Cabasso later told me that in 1950 there were still no effective polio antibody tests available.

8. As far as I have been able to determine, only one of Koprowski's fellow polio researchers ever commented publicly on the virulence to monkeys of the TN strain used in those first trials — and that was four years after Koprowski's paper was published. See H. A. Wenner, "Vaccination against Poliomyelitis — The Current Status of 'Inactivated' and 'Attenuated' Virus Vaccines," *Pediatrics*, 1956, 17(2), 287–296; see p. 295.

9. H. Koprowski, G. A. Jervis, and T. W. Norton, "Oral Administration of a Rodent-Adapted Strain of Poliomyelitis Virus to Chimpanzees," *Arch. Ges. Virusforsch.*, 1954, 5, 413–424.

10. However, there is some confusion about the origin of TN. In their 1952 article in the *American Journal of Hygiene*, the authors rather disconcertingly claim that TN — a Type 2 strain — was originally isolated during attempts to adapt the Brockman strain of polio (a virulent Type 1 virus) to mice, concluding: "Since laboratory contamination cannot be excluded altogether, no discussion will be offered as to the exact origin." This is intriguing in the light of George Theiler's belief that the TN strain was very similar to one developed in his laboratory at the Rockefeller Institute (George Dick, personal communications, 1992 and 1993; Victor Cabasso, personal communication, 1993).

11. H. Koprowski, T. W. Norton, and G. A. Jervis, "Studies on Rodent Adapted Polio-myelitis Virus. I. Cerebral Resistance Induced in the Rhesus Monkey," *Bact. Proc.,* 1951, 51, 92.

12. M. Roca-Garcia and G. A. Jervis, "Experimentally Produced Poliomyelitis Variant in Chick Embryo," *Ann. N.Y. Acad. Sci.,* 1955, 61, 911–923; see Koprowski's *"Discussion,"* pp. 922–923.

13. G. A. Jervis, "Comparative Susceptibility of Tissue Culture Cells in Experimental Animals and Man," *Ann. N.Y. Acad. Sci,* 1955, 61, 848–851.

14. H. Koprowski, "Immunization against Poliomyelitis with Living Attenuated Virus," *Am. J. Trop. Med.,* 1956, 5, 440–452.

15. See *NYAS* 57.

16. The first passage history ends up in a chick embryo tissue culture (CETC) substrate. In the second scheme, however, if one makes thirteen passages in CETC plus one extra CETC passage (to equal the fourteen CETC passages in the first scheme), one is left with six monkey kidney tissue culture (MKTC) passages and five CETC passages; the final substrate now becomes MKTC.

17. V. J. Cabasso, G. A. Jervis, H. R. Cox et al., "Cumulative Testing Experience with Consecutive Lots of Oral Poliomyelitis Vaccine," *PAHO1,* pp. 102–134.

18. H. Koprowski, "Immunization against Poliomyelitis with Living Attenuated Virus."

19. Anon., "India Will Permit the Export of Monkeys to Be Used in Genuine Medical Research," *New York Times,* April 14, 1955, p. 21.

20. Copy of a letter to Dr. Fulton from Dr. A. M.-M. Payne, Section of Endemo-epidemic Diseases, WHO, dated June 20, 1955, Medical Research Council document MRC.55/558, LIP.2.

21. R. Dulbecco and M. Vogt, "Plaque Formation and Isolation of Pure Lines with Poliomyelitis Viruses," *J. Exp. Med.;* 1954, 99, 167–182.

22. MRC Committee on Laboratory Investigations of Poliomyelitis, Minutes of First Meeting, held on July 14, 1955. Medical Research Council document MRC.55/658.

23. A *British Medical Journal* editorial in 1958 indicates that British interest in African monkeys continued. It states: "It might in time be possible to obtain large numbers of monkeys from West, Central and East Africa. The African species are different [from Asian], but probably would serve well enough for the purpose of vaccine production, though more experience with them is needed to confirm this. Their collection in vari-ous parts of Africa is not yet properly organized, nor are there such good air services for transport, but there is little doubt that these difficulties could be overcome." Anon., "Monkeys for Poliomyelitis Vaccine" (editorial), *BMJ,* 1958, 1(ii), 1168–1169.

24. "Poliomyelitis Vaccination — A Review of the Present Position at a Meeting of Experts Convened by WHO" (Stockholm, November 21–25, 1955), Medical Research Council document MRC.55/1013; LIP.55/11, pp. 6 and 7. Also published as WHO document WHO/Polio/17, dated November 29, 1955.

25. *NYAS* 57. *Papers and Discussions Presented at the Fourth International Poliomyelitis Conference (Geneva, 1957)* (Philadelphia: J. B. Lippincott, 1958).

26. R. Dulbecco and M. Vogt, "Plaque Formation and Isolation of Pure Lines with Polio-myelitis Viruses."

27. Just over two years later, in his Alvarenga Prize Lecture of October 1959, Koprowski would describe CHAT in different terms. He said that it "represents a different strain from that used . . . in the initial vaccinations in 1953–6" (i.e., SM), and that it had been "subjected to numerous laboratory procedures at the Wistar Institute for selection of

the least virulent particles." H. Koprowski, "Historical Aspects of the Development of Live Virus Vaccines in Poliomyelitis," *Am. J. Dis. Child.*, 1960, 100, 428–439.

28. When different plaques are selected from the same petri dish, and each is inoculated into a new MKTC, these parallel plaques are said to represent a plaque line. In principle, the least virulent plaque of the plaque line, as evidenced by injecting material grown from that plaque into the brains and spines of monkeys (the monkey safety test), will be selected for the next stage of propagation, though in practice this is not always the case.

29. *NYAS* 57. There appear not to be any remaining records of the original spoken version of the New York speech (January 1957), but it was clearly quite different from the final published version (December 1957). There are various pieces of evidence. Koprowski refers to articles that were published only after the conference was staged; he describes himself as being a member of the Wistar Institute (even though he moved there only in May 1957); and he refers to the NYAS conference of January 1955 as having occurred "three years ago." Koprowski's prominent position in the New York Academy of Sciences (by the end of 1957 he was president-elect) apparently allowed him to adapt the text.

30. *BMJ* 58.

31. H. Koprowski, "Importance of Genetics of Viruses in Medical Research," *J. Hum. Gen.*, 1959, 34(4), 335–351; see p. 341.

32. F. Przesmycki et al., "Vaccination against Poliomyelitis in Poland with Types 1 and 3 Attenuated Viruses of Koprowski, 1. Virological Studies of the Vaccine Strains and Serological Studies of the Vaccinated Population," *Bull. WHO*, 1962, 26, 733–743.

33. The correct figure of vaccinations for the Congo is discussed later in the book.

34. L. Hayflick, S. A. Plotkin, T. W. Norton, and H. Koprowski, "Preparation of Poliovirus Vaccines in a Human Fetal Diploid Cell Strain," *Am. J. Hyg.*, 1962, 75, 240–258.

35. J. S. Pagano, M. Böttiger, J. O. Bonnevier, and S. Gard, "The Response and the Lack of Spread in Swedish School Children Given an Attenuated Poliovirus Vaccine Prepared in a Human Diploid Cell Strain," *Am. J. Hyg.*, 1964, 79, 74–85. F. Buser et al., "Immunization with Live Attenuated Polio Virus Prepared in Human Diploid Cell Strains, with Special Reference to the WM-3 Strain," *Proceedings — Symposium on the Characterization and Uses of Human Diploid Cell Strains* (Opatija, 1963), pp. 381–387. D. Ikic, "Polio Vaccines Prepared in Human Diploid Cells," *First International Conference on Vaccines Against Viral and Rickettsial Diseases of Man, Papers Presented and Discussions Held* (Washington, D.C., November 7–11, 1966), Pan American Health Organization Scientific Publication No. 147, May 1967, 185–189.

36. S. A. Plotkin, B. J. Cohen, and H. Koprowski, "Intratypic Serodifferentiation of Polioviruses," *Virol.*, 1961, 15, 473–485. The only other CHAT pool I had come across in the literature, "WI seed lot, pool 19," had featured in a paper written by Sven Gard during his sabbatical at the Wistar, and appeared to have been used only experimentally in the lab. There is also evidence of a pool 16 in the Wistar freezers (see later).

37. The reference to 4B occurred in a table in a paper (H. Koprowski, "The Role of Markers of Poliovirus in Attempts to Identify Strains Isolated from Man during a Mass Vaccination Program," *PAHO1*, 135–139; see Table 5, p.138) that described the trials in Leopoldville (where pool 13 was fed) and Moorestown, New Jersey. It therefore seems likely that 4B, or 4B-5, was fed in the latter place. In table 6 of an internal WHO document ("Factors Influencing a Successful Vaccination with Live Poliovirus," WHO/BS/IR/84, submitted by S. A. Plotkin on October 27, 1960, to the Study Group on Requirements on Polio-myelitis Vaccine), there was a comparison of the CHAT vaccines fed (and excreted) at different Koprowski vaccine trials, such as Leopoldville (13), Poland (18G-11), Switzerland

(10A-11) and "New Jersey–Philadelphia." This suggested that the same pool (4B-5) may have been used in both of the limited open trials of CHAT staged in the United States, conducted in Moorestown (New Jersey) and Philadelphia. The timing suggests that it was probably the first CHAT pool used for feeding, and that it was produced even before Koprowski joined the Wistar.

38.   S. A. Plotkin, "Factors Influencing a Successful Vaccination with Live Poliovirus." This was later formally published in the *Proceedings of the Sixth International Congress of Microbiological Standardization*, Wiesbaden, Germany, September 1960 (Berlin: Hoffman Verlag, 1961), pp. 48–73.

39.   Tom Curtis, personal communication, 1992.

## CHAPTER 29: *Hilary Koprowski — Opening Moves*

1.   H. Koprowski and H. Uninski, "Ammonia Content of Canine Blood after Oral Administration of Ammonium Salts and Ammonia," *Biochem. J.*, 1939, 33, 747–753.

2.   I. Koprowska, *A Woman Wanders through Life and Science* (Albany: State University of New York Press, 1997).

3.   E. H. Lennette and H. Koprowski, "Human Infection with Venezuelan Equine Encephalomyelitis Virus. A Report of Eight Cases of Infection Acquired in the Laboratory," *JAMA*, 1943, 123, 1088–1095.

4.   VEEV's qualities as an "incapacitating agent" meant that it fast became one of the major weapons in the U.S. biological arsenal. (See "The Problem of Chemical and Biological Warfare," Volume II of *CB Weapons Today*, by the Stockholm International Peace Research Institute [London: Paul Elek, 1973], pp. 70–71.) The preparation, during the fifties, of VEEV of varying strengths by the Special Operations Division of the Army Chemical Corps, based at Fort Detrick, is discussed in John Marks, *The Search for the Manchurian Candidate* (London: Allen Lane, 1979), pp. 75–76. The virus was also used as a short-term immobilizer by the CIA. Several reports on vaccines against VEEV, and viral strains of differing pathogenicity, are contained in "Commission on Epidemiological Survey; Armed Forces Epidemiological Board, Annual Report 1959–60," which appears to be the first such publicly available AFEB report to discuss frankly its role in biological warfare, both defensive and offensive. The report also reveals that Koprowski's collaborator on the VEEV work, Edwin Lennette, was by then considered a potentially key player in a planned "testing program with regard to civilian and military interests" of "diseases of importance to the military."

5.   Norton was apparently given the vaccine on January 16, 1951, and Cox on March 2, 1951 — roughly a year after the feeding of the six-year-old boy. See H. Koprowski, G. A. Jervis, and T. W. Norton, "Immune Responses in Human Volunteers upon Oral Administration of a Rodent-Adapted Strain of Poliomyelitis Virus," *Am. J. Hyg.*, 1952, 55, 108–126.

6.   H. Koprowski, G. A. Jervis, and T. W. Norton, "Oral Administration of a Rodent-Adapted Strain of Poliomyelitis Virus to Chimpanzees," *Arch. Ges. Virusforsch.*, 1954, 5, 413–424; H. Koprowski, G. A. Jervis, and T. W. Norton, "Oral Administration of Poliomyelitis Virus to Man and Ape — A Comparative Study," *Proc. Natl. Acad. Sci.*, 1954, 40, 36–39.

7.   Later in the interview, Koprowski claimed that the first chimp testing they had done in the United States had been in 1954 or 1955.

8. The presence of Koprowski and Norton at the first OPV feeding featured at the beginning of Norton and Koprowski's draft manuscript tentatively titled "Polio — An Adventure."

9. The first ever pool of SM, fed to three individuals in 1953, was the only exception, for this was made in rodent brain. See H. Koprowski, G. A. Jervis, and T. W. Norton, "Administration of an Attenuated Type 1 Poliomyelitis Virus to Human Subjects," 1954, *Proc. Soc. Exp. Biol. Med.*, 86; 244–247.

10. See T. Curtis, "The Origin of AIDS," *Rolling Stone*, March 19, 1992, pp. 54–61, 106–108, in which Koprowski claims that kidneys from either rhesus or African green monkeys were used (p. 59), and also that the kidneys were already removed from their hosts (p. 61). However, in "AIDS and the Poliovaccine" (letter), *Science*, 1992, 257, 1024–1027, Koprowski claims (p.1024) that all his polio vaccines after the early TN "were produced in kidney tissue obtained from rhesus monkeys (*Macaca mulatta*) captured either in India or the Philippines." In fact, macaques from the Philippines are cynomolgus, not rhesus macaques.

11. Koprowski et al., "Oral Administration of Poliomyelitis Virus to Man and Ape."

12. *NYAS* 57.

13. A. A. Smorodintsev et al., "Material for the Study of the Harmlessness of the Live Poliomyelitis Vaccine Prepared from Sabin Strains," *PAHO1*, 324–332. This account describes the first eight human passages.

14. B. F. Elswood and R. B. Stricker, "Polio Vaccines and the Origin of AIDS" (letter), *Res. Virol.*, 1993, 144, 175–177; B. F. Elswood and R. B. Stricker, "Polio Vaccines and the Origin of AIDS," *Med. Hypotheses*, 1994, 42, 347–354.

15. R. B. Stricker, D. I. Abrams, L. Corash, and M. A. Shuman, "Target Platelet Antigen in Homosexual Men with Immune Thrombocytopenia," *N. Engl. J. Med.*, 1985, 313, 1375–1380.

16. M. A. Shuman, L. Corash, and D. I. Abrams, Retraction, *N. Engl. J. Med.*, 1991, 325(21), 1487.

17. "NIH Guide for Grants and Contracts," 1993, 22(23), Final Findings of Scientific Misconduct; entry for Raphael B. Stricker on p. 3.

18. In 1996 I discussed this episode with Blaine Elswood, who said that he had not known about it at the time they had cowritten the letters and articles, and that he too had been shocked when he found out. He added that the papers that came out under both their names between 1992 and 1994 had been predominantly his own work.

CHAPTER 30: *The West Coast Trials*

1. *NYAS* 57, see pp. 128–133.

2. Anon., "Live Virus in the Jungle," *Time*, August 11, 1958, p. 30.

3. A contemporary book by Greer Williams provided a slightly different version, claiming that Koprowski had "recaptured the virus from the feces of one person, C80, whose name he abbreviated as 'Chat.'" (G. Williams, *Virus Hunters* [London: Hutchinson, 1960], p. 283.)

4. L. Pascal, "What Happens When Science Goes Bad. The Corruption of Science and the Origin of AIDS: A Study in Spontaneous Generation," University of Wollongong Working Paper No. 9, December 1991.

5. See M. Vogt, R. Dulbecco, and H. A. Wenner, "Mutants of Poliomyelitis Viruses with Reduced Efficiency of Plating in Acid Medium and Reduced Neuropathogenicity,"

*Virol.,* 1957, 4, 141–155. This describes an *in vitro* marker of poliovirus virulence, which the authors were proposing as an alternative to the monkey safety test. This paper, as it happens, is also interesting for another reason. Of the ten attenuated vaccine viruses tested by Renato Dulbecco, only one showed the "D+" character that was thought to be typical of a wild poliovirus. This was the other Type 1 vaccine submitted by Koprowski — SM N-90, pool 21.

6. Discussion by Dulbecco in *NYAS* 57, see pp. 138–139.

7. *NYAS* 57, see pp. 128–133.

8. J. L. Melnick et al., "Environmental Studies of Endemic Enteric Virus Infections. I. Community Seroimmune Patterns and Poliovirus Infection Rates," *Am. J. Hyg.,* 1957, 65, 1–28.

9. P. De Somer et al., "Determination de la valeur antigenique du vaccin antipoliomyeletique," *Bull. WHO,* 1960, 22, 295–305.

10. P. De Somer et al., "Resultants du programme de vaccination contre la poliomyelite en Belgique," *Rev. Med. Louvain,* 1957, 21; 341–355. This shows that "an experimental [IPV] vaccine containing the Charleston strain" of Dr. Melnick had been tested on "a limited number of subjects" in Belgium by June 1957.

11. Jack London, "Told in the Drooling Ward," found in A. Calder-Marshall (editor), *The Bodley Head Jack London* (London: Bodley Head, 1963).

12. In 1952, Smadel was chief of the department of viral and rickettsial diseases and director of the division of communicable diseases, at the graduate school of Walter Reed Army Medical Center. See J. Cattell (editor), *American Men of Science* (Lancaster, PA: The Science Press, 1955).

13. Anon., "New Antipolio Product Reported," *Flint Journal,* May 22, 1955. Other information from Dr. David Chadwick.

14. H. Koprowski, T. W. Norton, T. L. Nelson, K. F. Meyer et al., "Clinical Investigations on Attenuated Strains of Poliomyelitis Virus. Use as a Method of Immunization of Children with Living Virus," *JAMA,* 1956, 160, 954–966. Also see M. Roca-Garcia, H. Koprowski, T. W. Norton, T. L. Nelson et al., "Immunization of Humans with a Chick Embryo Adapted Strain of MEF1 Poliomyelitis Virus," *J. Immunol.,* 1956, 77 (2), 123–131.

15. During a lengthy phone call with Dr. Chadwick, I learned various other important details about the trial. During that period, there were apparently epidemics of rubella and chicken pox at Sonoma, and although Chadwick observed several of the vaccinees getting fevers and rashes, he believed that rubella was responsible in most cases. Intriguingly, Dr. Chadwick stated more than once that his recollection was that his own personal checks were paid by the Wistar Institute (this, of course, was in the summer of 1955, two years before Koprowski moved to the Wistar and, if correct, raises the question of whether Koprowski had links with the Wistar long before he took over that institution).

16. Anon., "Sonoma Polio Test Cleared in 4 New Cases," *San Francisco Call-Bulletin,* undated (but clearly early 1953), p. 6.

17. H. Koprowski, G. A. Jervis, T. W. Norton et al., "Further Studies on Oral Administration of Living Poliomyelitis Virus to Human Subjects," *Proc. Soc. Exp. Biol. Med.,* 1953, 82, 277–280. The article was *submitted* on December 1, 1952, but there can be little doubt that its authors would have learned of the polio outbreak (which occurred in October or November) from Nelson or Meyer before that date. The vaccinations in Cromwell were with Type 2 OPV (a relatively rare virus, compared to the other two polio types), so it certainly would have been useful had Koprowski detailed in his paper which poliovirus type had caused the outbreak.

18. T. L. Nelson and H. Koprowski, "Serial Passage of Attenuated Poliomyelitis Virus (SM Type 1) in Man," read at the Western Society for Pediatric Research meeting, San Francisco, October 29, 1957.

19. *NYAS* 57, see Table 3 on p. 130.

20. The fecal virus from C81 was even more virulent, both paralyzing and causing lesions in six out of twelve monkeys injected intraspinally, and causing lesions in two of twelve injected in the brain. Only the fecal virus of child C82 was entirely innocuous intraspinally.

21. Full name withheld at the request of Dr. Charlton.

22. This is because details of the third serial passage (i.e., involving C79) are included in a discussion contribution by Koprowski at a conference held in May 1956. J. Stokes, H. Koprowski, T. W. Norton et al., "Passive-Active Immunization of Infants with Attenuated Poliomyelitis Viruses Administered Orally," *Am. Ped. Soc. Trans.*, 66th annual meeting (Buck Hill Falls, PA, May 9–11, 1956), published in [*Am. Med. Assoc.*] *J. Dis. Child.*, 1956 (December), pp. 452–454.

23. This comes from Professor Bill Hamilton who, after learning from Greer Williams (see footnote 3) that the source of the CHAT virus was patient C80, interpreted it as meaning that C80 had been rendered phonetically, as "C-A-T," and that — perhaps during the visit by Koprowski and Norton to the Francophone Belgian Congo — the feline had been lightheartedly translated into French.

24. These three, incidentally, provide another possible (albeit far-fetched) explanation for the naming of CHAT — Courtois, Hilary And Tom.

25. During my first interview with Hilary Koprowski, he had told me that his former assistant, Stanley Plotkin, thought that "CHAT" was the name of a child, "abbreviated of course." He himself could not recall the details, however.

## CHAPTER 31:
### *The East Coast Trials — And the Question of Informed Consent*

1. H. Koprowski, G. A. Jervis, and T. W. Norton, "Immune Responses in Human Volunteers upon Oral Administrations of a Rodent-Adapted Strain of Poliomyelitis Virus," *Am. J. Hyg.*, 1952, 55, 108–126.

2. Later in the article, in a footnote, we are informed that "For obvious reasons, the age, sex and physical status of each volunteer are not mentioned."

3. Anon., "Poliomyelitis: A New Approach," *Lancet*, 1952, 1(i), 552.

4. A. Chase, *Magic Shots* (New York: William Morrow, 1982), p. 295.

5. H. Koprowski, T. L. Nelson et al., "Clinical Investigations on Attenuated Strains of Poliomyelitis Virus. Use as a Method of Immunization of Children with Living Virus," *JAMA*, 1956, 160, 954–966.

6. See previous reference, and M. Roca-Garcia, H. Koprowski, G. A. Jervis, T. W. Norton, T. L. Nelson, and H. R. Cox, "Immunization of Humans with a Chick Embryo Adapted Strain of MEF1 Poliomyelitis Virus," *J. Immunol.*, 1956, 77, 123–131. Apparently both parents and public health authorities approved the Woodbine trials in 1954–1956.

7. Elizabeth McGee worked for Joe Stokes only between 1954 and 1956, so her memories of these events all stemmed from the time when Koprowski was still at Lederle, a year or more before he moved to the Wistar.

8. The birth records show that between August 1955 and April 1958, more than a third of all Clinton infants were born to under-eighteen mothers, and that juvenile mothers consented to vaccination for their babies much more frequently than adults, by a ratio of 3:2.

9. Between August 1955 and April 1958, 175 babies were born at Clinton, 60 percent of whom were black.

10. "Formula" is a mixture of canned milk, maltose, and water.

11. "Clinton Farms Physician on Polio Virus Mission," *Democrat* (Flemington, NJ), February 27, 1958. The scenario described was obviously the original plan, and represents a substantial difference from the eventual vaccination of 215,000 in Ruzizi and southwestern Burundi.

12. H. Koprowski et al., "Immunization of Infants with Living Attenuated Poliomyelitis Virus: Laboratory Investigations of Alimentary Infection and Antibody Response in Infants under Six Months of Age with Congenitally Acquired Antibodies," *JAMA*, 1956, 162(14), 1281–1288; S. A. Plotkin, H. Koprowski, and J. Stokes, "Clinical Trials in Infants of Orally Administered Attenuated Poliomyelitis Viruses," *Pediatrics*, June 1959, pp. 1041–1062; H. Koprowski, "Vaccination with Modified Active Viruses," *Papers and Discussions Presented at the Fourth International Poliomyelitis Conference* (Geneva, July 8–12, 1957) (Philadelphia: J. B. Lippincott, 1958), pp. 112–123; J. Stokes, "The Prospect for Control of Poliomyelitis: The Combined Approach of Oral Attenuated Virus Vaccine and Parenteral Inactivated Virus Vaccine," *Ann. Paediatr. Fenn*, 1957, 3(4), 658–665; S. A. Plotkin, H. Koprowski et al., "Persistence of Antibodies after Vaccination with Living Attenuated Poliovirus," *JAMA*, 1959, 170(1), 72–76.

13. "Immunization of a Population of an Institution with an Attenuated Type 1 Poliomyelitis Vaccine," submitted by H. Koprowski to the WHO Expert Committee on Poliomyelitis, WHO/Polio/30, June 28, 1957.

14. The cardiac check was made on March 14, 1956, five months after the boy's birth, and he was transferred to the Crippled Children's Hospital on April 5, 1956. However, it was later revealed that there was another possible explanation for his health problems (see chapter 51).

15. Important CHAT vaccinations in Clinton and Stanleyville were staged on February 27 in 1957 and 1958, and Koprowski named his opening address to the 1960 Washington conference on OPVs "The Tin Anniversary of the Development of Live Poliovirus Vaccine," in its honor [*PAHO2*, 5–11].

16. S. A. Plotkin et al., "Clinical Trials in Infants of Orally Administered Attenuated Poliomyelitis Viruses."

17. Another paper indicated that the calf in question had first been fed CHAT, but we now know that cows cannot develop antibodies to poliovirus, so the actual source of this vaccine virus remains a mystery. H. Koprowski, "Counterparts of Human Viral Disease in Animals," *Ann. N.Y. Acad. Sci.*, 1958, 70, 369–382; see pp. 372–373. Stanley Plotkin later confirmed that Wistar was not a genuine calf-adapted strain.

18. Anon., "Progress on a Better Polio Vaccine," *Life*, October 29, 1956, pp. 61–66.

19. Anon., "New Technique in Polio Protection Developed by Moorestown Families Test," *Moorestown News Chronicle*, February 19, 1959, p. 1.

20. Anon., "Wistar Institute Is Both Monument and Prototype of Modern Research," *Scope Weekly*, May 21, 1958, pp. 6–7.

21. A note in one of the reports states that "type 2 vaccination was discontinued in the 18th week, due to a shortage of supply." This was in mid-May, 1959, which was just eight

weeks after the publication of an article by Sabin in the *British Medical Journal,* in which he roundly criticized CHAT (A. B. Sabin, "Present Position of Immunization against Poliomyelitis with Live Virus Vaccines," *BMJ,* 1959, 1(ii), 663–682). Koprowski's reply was published in the *Journal* later in May (H. Koprowski, "Live Poliomyelitis Vaccine," *BMJ,* 1959, 1(ii), 1349–1350). However, he and Sabin might have had words before then, and the sudden nonavailability of P-712 might not be unrelated.

22. J. S. Pagano, S. A. Plotkin, H. Koprowski et al., "Routine Immunization with Orally Administered Attenuated Poliovirus," *JAMA,* 1960, 173(17), 1883–1889.

23. The study found that such babies could be successfully immunized during the first five days of life, but after that it became more difficult to establish immunity until the infant was two months old and began to lose maternal antibodies.

24. Apart from 4B-5, the only other CHAT pools that had been developed when the Philadelphia trials started, in January 1959, would seem to have been 10A-11 and 13, both of which had been tested on a large scale in Africa, and among small trial groups in Europe, but apparently not in the United States (except perhaps on a limited scale at Clinton). For additional reasoning on 4B-5, see chapter 28, note 37.

25. This was confirmed by a paper by Ikic, which revealed that although vaccine prepared in HDCS and MKTC was given in early 1963 to a total of eleven thousand children, the Croatian team did not administer a placebo, which would have constituted a good control for this first mass trial of OPV made in HDCS. See D. Ikic, "Poliovaccines Prepared in Human Diploid Cell Strains," *First International Conference on Vaccines Against Viral and Rickettsial Diseases of Man* (November 1966), PAHO Scientific Publications No. 147, 1967, 185–189.

26. As clinician Wilson Carswell commented in 1997: "It is for the reasons enunciated [in this paragraph] that Good Clinical Practice has been introduced for clinical trials. These require both internal and external monitoring . . . usually carried out by clinical trial organizations rather than academics or clinicians."

27. D. E. Jeremiah, "Development of Live Polio Vaccine" (letter), *BMJ,* 1960, 2(i), 468.

28. I. Koprowska, *A Woman Wanders through Life and Science* (Albany: State University of New York Press, 1997), p. 298.

29. Duncan Jeremiah, personal communication, March 1995.

CHAPTER 32: *At the CDC*

1. Shortly after our last interview, in 1995, Dr. Curran left the CDC to join Emory University.

2. For two less than complimentary accounts of Curran's time in charge of AIDS, see R. Blow, "Critical Condition," *Rolling Stone,* March 26, 1987, pp. 67–70 and 150; J. Kwitny, "At CDC's AIDS Lab: Egos, Power, Politics and Lost Experiments," *Wall St. Journal,* December 12, 1986.

3. Letter dated November 20, 1992, from Walter R. Dowdle, deputy director of the CDC, to Giovanni Rovera, director of the Wistar Institute.

4. Ronald Desrosiers later denied this. "I was never charged with organizing the testing," he told me in 1998. "I maybe raised the issue of whether it [the CHAT sample] should be tested, and made a few phone calls about that testing."

5. The CDC indices actually read "Wistar, Pool No. 13," not CHAT pool 13. However, "Wistar-CHAT pool 13" had been tested by the National Institutes of Health a month or

so earlier; see S. Baron, R. M. Friedman, R. Murray et al., "Laboratory Investigation of the Attenuated Poliovirus Vaccine Strains. II. Tissue Culture Characteristics Before and After Gastrointestinal Passage," *PAHO2*, 124–131. It therefore seems likely that Kew's sample is also of CHAT, rather than of Wistar, Koprowski's other experimental Type 1 vaccine. If correct, this means that it was from the same pool of poliovirus used in Leopoldville and Wyszkow.

6. Fox pool 12 was first produced in late 1956, at the same time as the original version of CHAT, plaque 20, so it is intriguing that no early sample of CHAT is part of the collection. See M. Vogt, R. Dulbecco, and H. Wenner, "Mutants of Poliomyelitis Viruses with Reduced Efficiency of Plating in Acid Medium and Reduced Neuropathogenicity," *Virol.*, 1957, 4, 141–155.

7. A. B. Sabin and L. R. Boulger, "History of Sabin Attenuated Poliovirus Oral Live Vaccine Strains," *J. Biol. Stand.*, 1973, 1, 115–118.

8. E. C. Dick, "Chimpanzee Kidney Tissue Cultures for Growth and Isolation of Viruses," *J. Bacteriol.*, 1963, 86, 573–576. The data in the article reveal that with chimpanzee kidney tissue cultures, previous inoculation caused cytopathic effect within two days, which is as fast — if not even faster — than with rhesus MKTC.

9. S. E. Luria, "Cell Susceptibility to Viruses," *Ann. N.Y. Acad. Sci.*, 1955, 61, 852–855.

10. Later, I interviewed the author of the paper on chimpanzee kidney tissue culture, Elliott Dick (no relation to George), in Madison, Wisconsin. He told me that in the early sixties he had been searching for a suitable tissue culture system for the rhinoviruses — "common cold viruses" — and while he had six fresh chimp kidneys at his disposal, he decided to investigate the response of several other viruses to this culture system. He found that CKTC grew most viruses as well as rhesus MKTC or human diploid cell strains and told me that "apart from the cost . . . chimp kidney tissue culture may very well be the perfect substrate [for human viruses] . . . simply because it's the closest to us genetically."

11. L. R. Smith and C. L. Heaton, "Actinomycosis Presenting as Wegener's Granulomatosis," *JAMA*, 1978, 240(3), 247–248.

12. J. Oleske et al., "Immune Deficiency Syndrome in Children," *JAMA*, 1983, 249(17), 2345–2349.

13. An alternative explanation would be that the patient was someone who had had sex, or shared a needle, with a former Clinton baby.

14. I would be glad to share the data that I have gathered about the Clinton infant vaccinees with an official investigative team of this type.

CHAPTER 33: *Tom Norton*

1. Anon., "7 David's Island Children First Test New Polio Cure," *Boothbay Register* (Bar Harbor, Maine), July 31, 1958. This claimed that an oral polio vaccine had been "first tested" on Norton's three daughters in 1953. The early rodent-adapted version of SM was indeed fed to three individuals for the first time in 1953, but they were reported to have had terminal cancer. (H. Koprowski, G. A. Jervis, and T. W. Norton, "Administration of an Attenuated Type 1 Poliomyelitis Virus to Human Subjects," *Proc. Soc. Exp. Biol. Med.*, 1954, 86, 244–247.) We must therefore presume that the vaccine that Tom Norton fed to his children in 1953 was the one named after himself: TN. This was three years after the first TN feedings.

2. Koprowski himself commented, in 1959: "Indeed, the loose affiliation between the Institute and the University of Pennsylvannia is ideal for both organizations." R. E. Billingham and H. Koprowski, "The Wistar Institute of Anatomy and Biology, Philadelphia," *Nature*, 1959, 184, 6–10.

3. The camp, together with an inn, a zoo, and a hospital, had been run by a spirited American artist named Anne Putnam, who had later written a book, *Madami*, about her experiences there, which Tom had apparently read and enjoyed before his departure. A. E. Putnam and A. Keller, *Madami — My Eight Years of Adventure with the Congo Pygmies* (New York: Prentice-Hall, 1954). One passage describes a pygmy child who is mauled by a pet chimpanzee, and who later develops polio (pp. 106–111). This highlights the possibility that chimps can be naturally infected with polio, or even that they could represent a reservoir for the virus.

4. The captions on the back of the photos referred to 1956, but I later discovered that they had been written in the eighties, when the prints had been made from slides.

5. The *Times* leader opened as follows: "The report of the reckless and illegal release of a genetically engineered virus in Argentina raises the spectre of a biological version of Chernobyl." (Anon., "Dangers in Gene Research" (editorial), *Times* (U.K.), April 11, 1988, p. 11.) Also see J. Palca, "Inquiry into Argentine Trials," *Nature*, 1986, 324, 609.

6. A. Tyler, "Monkey Business," *Independent* (U.K.), September 19, 1992, magazine section, pp. 22–29. Tyler reported: "Last year, Wistar fired him [Koprowski] as its director, making serious allegations against him. Koprowski maintains that he was removed by the institute's board of managers because of age discrimination and animosity between himself and the board's president."

7. The out-of-court settlement was agreed in April 1993, on terms that were "confidential but . . . acceptable to both parties." This was just over two years after Koprowski's removal as director (in March 1991). Although he and the Wistar were in dispute throughout 1992, when the *Rolling Stone* controversy was most intense, he still apparently retained an office at the institute, and spent a day or two there each week. "Settlement Reached on Wistar/Koprowski Lawsuit," Wistar Institute press release, April 7, 1993.

8. J. E. Conant, "Polio Answer Seen in Use of Live Virus," *San Francisco Call-Bulletin*, March 13, 1956.

9. G. B. Lal, "Live Virus Vaccine for Polio Now in Use," *San Francisco Examiner*, March 1, 1956, sect. 2, p. 3.

10. B. W. Hotchkiss, "Babies Being Fed Live Polio Virus," *Newark Evening News*, October 24, 1956. The article emphasized that the mothers of all the infants involved in the study had provided written consent, including those who were still juveniles — who were treated, in this instance, as if they had attained the age of legal responsibility.

11. No details were given about the location of these alleged June 1956 feedings of Fox, and since other references to Fox refer to the Clinton feedings of October 1956 as the first, it is possible that the reporter was misinformed. If not, we have to presume that feedings of an early pool of Fox may have occurred at Letchworth Village or Clinton.

12. This information is interesting, because these nine can only have been the Clinton infants coded C26 to C34, about whom relatively little is known. C33 and C34 were the ones fed Fox in October 1956, and infants C26 and C32 were later reported as having been fed SM, but the remaining five are not documented in the literature. Presumably they were fed with early versions of CHAT, SM-45, or Fox between June and October 1956.

13. This apparent reticence by Koprowski about his employers is hinted at by the Nairobi newspaper article below, but became more pronounced when he and Norton arrived in Stanleyville a few days later — as will be detailed in chapter 39.

14. Anon., "City Polio Proposal," *East African Standard,* February 1, 1957, p. 1.

15. We know this because some of the vaccine virus that they were carrying with them to test in the spines of the five Lindi chimps was material from "Plaque 20," which would be identified by Dulbecco as pertaining to the Charlton strain. See M. Vogt, R. Dulbecco, and H. Wenner, "Mutants of Poliomyelitis Viruses with Reduced Efficiency of Plating in Acid Medium and Reduced Neuropathogenicity," *Virol.,* 1957, 4, 141–155.

16. These two vaccinees would later be referred to as BO and GA in Koprowski's paper "Vaccination with Modified Active Viruses," published in *Fourth International Polio-myelitis Conference* (Geneva, July 1957) (Philadelphia: J. P. Lippincott, 1958), pp. 112–123. I later discovered that BO was fed in November 1956 and GA in January 1957. They were probably the first two trial vaccinees with material from CHAT Plaque 20.

17. Anon., "Polio Vaccine" (editorial), *East African Standard,* February 1, 1957, p. 8.

18. Anon., "Scientist Back from Africa Talks at Radrock," unknown New Jersey paper, April 11, 1957.

19. Anon., "7 David's Island Children First Test New Polio Cure."


CHAPTER 34: *Hilary Koprowski — End Game*

1. Anon., "'Origin of AIDS' Update" (clarification), *Rolling Stone,* December 9, 1993, p.39. This postdated issue hit the streets in late November 1993, enabling my second interview with Dr. Koprowski to take place at the start of December.

2. This was highlighted by the subtitle. T. Curtis, "The Origin of AIDS: A Startling New Theory Attempts to Answer the Question 'Was It an Act of God or an Act of Man?'" *Rolling Stone,* March 19, 1992, 626, 54–108.

3. *Philadelphia* (Tri-Star Productions), the first big Hollywood movie to tackle the subject of AIDS, won Oscars for Best Actor (Tom Hanks) and Best Original Song (Bruce Springsteen, "Streets of Philadelphia").

4. Sources close to *Rolling Stone* dispute that this was the case.

5. Koprowski said the article would be easy to find, and mentioned one or two newspapers in which it might have appeared, but I have not managed to locate any such article.

6. George Dick and David Dane *did* passage SM in MKTC, but only as part of the monkey safety tests (so SM and excreted SM could be compared at the same titer). They *did not* passage in MKTC the vaccine that was fed to humans. (G. W. A. Dick, D. S. Dane et al., "Vaccination against Poliomyelitis with Live Virus Vaccines. 2. A Trial of SM Type I Attenuated Poliomyelitis Virus Vaccine," *BMJ,* 1957, 1(i), 65–70.) The TN vaccine virus, by contrast, would not grow in MKTC (even if the highly pathogenic excreted virus did), showing that the version sent to Belfast was not monkey-adapted. (D. S. Dane, G. W. A. Dick et al., "Vaccination against Poliomyelitis with Live Virus Vaccines. 1. A Trial of TN Type II Vaccine," *BMJ,* 1957, 1(i), 59–65.)

7. J. R. Wilson, *Margin of Safety* (London: Collins, 1963), pp. 166–167.

8. In fact, Koprowski denied that it was at the New York Academy of Sciences (NYAS) con-ference in January 1957 that Dr. Dick made his "hullabaloo." He did recall, however, that the conference in question had been staged at a big New York hotel — probably the Waldorf-Astoria. This detail (and the evidence of George Dick's passport, which reveals

that the only times he entered the United States between March 1956 and March 1961 were on January 6, 1957 — for *NYAS 57* — and on June 19, 1959 — for *PAHO1*) confirms that Koprowski was wrong and that Dick's speech *was* made at the NYAS conference. See G. Williams, *Virus Hunters* (London: Hutchinson, 1960), p. 278.

9. In 1993, Bill Boland, executive editor of New York Academy of Science Publications, told me that authors are allowed to revise their speeches for the published proceedings, and added that this would have been especially likely, given that Koprowski was then director of the section on biology (and, as it later transpired, president-elect). It was not clear, however, whether speakers were normally allowed to redraft the major part of their speeches retrospectively.

10. Apart from David Dane's recollection of Koprowski's conceding that excreted TN vaccine virus *was* noncytopathogenic, nobody with whom I have spoken recalls anything of the content of Koprowski's speech at the January 1957 conference in New York. (There is no mention of TN in the published version of Koprowski's speech.)

11. For example: H. Koprowski, "Immunization against Poliomyelitis with Living Attenuated Virus," *Am. J. Trop. Med. Hyg.*, 1956, 5, 440–452; and G. W. A. Dick, D. S. Dane et al., "Vaccination against Poliomyelitis with Live Virus Vaccines. 2. A Trial of SM Type I Attenuated Poliomyelitis Virus Vaccine," *BMJ*, 1957, 1(i), 65–70, see especially Table 1 on p. 66. Both state clearly that SM vaccine was made in chick embryo tissue culture.

12. *BMJ 58*, which states that Koprowski "had the opportunity, through the kindness of Dr T. J. Wiktor . . . to contact [Courtois] and to propose a programme of experiments for the evaluation of attenuated strains of poliovirus in chimpanzees."

13. H. Koprowski, G. A. Jervis, and T. W. Norton, "Oral Administration of Poliomyelitis Virus to Man and Ape — A Comparative Study," *Proc. Natl. Acad. Sci.*, 1954, 40, 36–39. See also, on the same research, H. Koprowski, G. A. Jervis, and T. W. Norton, "Oral Administration of a Rodent-Adapted Strain of Poliomyelitis Virus to Chimpanzees," *Arch. Virus*, 1954, 5, 413–424.

14. Anon. "7 David's Island Children First Test New Polio Cure," *Boothbay Register* (Bar Harbor, Maine), July 31, 1958.

15. I have since checked the tape again, and Koprowski says clearly that the records were lost during the move *to* the Wistar. Furthermore, he blames the Wistar staff for the loss, and given the circumstances of his departure from Lederle, it seems logical that it would have been Wistar (rather than the Lederle) staff who would have collected any records left behind at Lederle after his departure (on or about April 30, 1957).

16. Both the papers about Lindi (like *BMJ 58*) and those who worked there (like Ninane) describe vaccination and challenge experiments, rather than merely vaccinating and checking for antibodies.

17. The first such article was probably A. B. Sabin, "Behavior of Chimpanzee-Avirulent Poliomyelitis Viruses in Experimentally Infected Human Volunteers," *Am. J. Med. Sci.*, 1955, 230, 64–72.

18. A. B. Sabin, "Properties of Attenuated Polioviruses and Their Behavior in Human Beings," *NYAS 57*, 5, 113–127. Also important is another article from January 1957: A. B. Sabin, "Present Status of Attenuated Live Virus Poliomyelitis Vaccine," *Bull. N.Y. Acad. Med.*, 1957, 33(1), 17–39, which reported on Sabin's experiments on a total of 150 chimpanzees over two years. It featured the observation that even chimps infected with large doses of poliovirus, which demonstrated viral multiplication in the throat, did not present any demonstrable virus in the stools, and added: "This is the main reason why ultimate definitive studies on attenuated strains [have] to be carried out in human beings."

The importance of this article is underlined by the fact that it came out shortly before Koprowski and Norton's departure for the Congo — and that Tom Norton had a copy among his papers, almost the only article he had by an author who was not part of Koprowski's group.

19. Gabu-Nioka is just under two hundred miles east of Epulu, but in those days the roads were good, especially during the dry season, which was when Koprowksi and Norton visited. The trip would probably have taken only about four hours by car.

20. Odette Osterrieth recalled Koprowski's visit to Stanleyville with Tom Norton (early 1957) and his attendance at the opening of the virus lab (September 1957). Paul Osterrieth thought that Koprowski might have made one further visit.

21. All other observers agreed that Norton had visited Africa just the once.

22. Letter from P. Van De Perre to H. Koprowski, dated May 25, 1992.

23. H. Koprowski, "AIDS and the Polio Vaccine" (letter), *Science,* 1992, 257, 1024–1027.

24. It is important to examine Philippe Van De Perre's claims in some detail, especially since Koprowski used them so extensively in his response in *Science* to Curtis. Van De Perre correctly points out that Biggar's article about Kivu (R. J. Biggar et al., "Seroepidemiology of HTLV-III Antibodies in a Remote Population of Eastern Zaire," *BMJ,* 1985, 290, 808–810) was discredited, in that it had included a lot of false positives. He writes that some of the early AIDS cases in the Sonnet article, which Curtis quoted (J. Sonnet et al., "Early AIDS Cases Originating from Zaire and Burundi [1962–1976]," *Scand. J. Infect. Dis.,* 1987, 19, 511–517), were only clinically defined, and claims that in any case most of the patients came from districts that were "many thousands [of] kilometers from the Kivu region," such as Kinshasa and Shaba. (In fact, both places are less than fifteen hundred kilometers from Kivu. But far more important, all of Sonnet's cases came from areas very close to where CHAT trials *had* been staged, though Van De Perre would not have know this.) Van De Perre adds, with regard to Ruzizi, that "With no doubts, in the case several thousands of children had been accidentally infected by HIV in the fifties, one should probably observe a major local epidemic in adults of this rural area." This contention is highly debatable, in that it is far more likely that AIDS cases would first become visible in the local towns. In any case, it is rather more likely that, if the vaccine had been contaminated with a low titer of SIV, then only a few infant or immunocompromised vaccinees would have become infected — and AIDS witnessed only sporadically thereafter. Van De Perre cites seroprevalence figures of between 0.7 percent and 3.7 percent for rural Burundi, Rwanda, and Kivu province — figures that are correct, albeit rather selective. However, had he been aware of the true location of the Ruzizi trial, one would presume that he would have been rather less sanguine — for those HIV-prevalence figures that exist for the vaccinated areas like Bujumbura and Rumonge (especially the early figures, from 1980/1) are very high indeed. (See J. Morvan et al., "Enquête séro-épidémiologique sur les infections à HIV au Burundi entre 1980 et 1981," *Bull. Soc. Path. Exot.,* 1989, 82, 130–140.)

25. 215,504 people, to be precise.

26. S. A. Plotkin, A. Lebrun, and H. Koprowski, "Vaccination with the CHAT Strain of Type 1 Attenuated Poliomyelitis Virus in Leopoldville, Belgian Congo. 2. Studies of the Safety and Efficacy of Vaccination," *Bull. WHO,* 1960, 22, 215–234.

27. As I discovered later, this too was incorrect. CHAT was also fed to most of the population in Stanleyville and Bukavu, and to an unspecified number in Kikwit and Coquilhatville (now Mbandaka). It was also used in several of the smaller towns in the Congo.

28. In fact his NIH grant E-1799, for "Study of attenuated strain of poliomyelitis virus" did not become operative until 1958, seven months after his arrival at the Wistar. He was, however, in receipt of two NIH grants at the Wistar in 1957, both for "Biological prospects of normal and malignant cells."

29. F. Przesmycki et al., "Report on Field Trials with Live Attenuated Poliomyelitis Vaccine of Koprowski in Poland," *Am. J. Hyg.*, 1960, 71(3), 275–284. 2,888 children from Wyszkow and surrounding villages, 32 children from a Wyszkow boarding school, and 22 kids from Warsaw were vaccinated with pool 13, making a grand total of 2,942 Polish vaccinees with that pool. (See *PAHO1*, pp. 497–507.)

30. Undoubtedly the incidence of polio dropped dramatically, but this would seem to be an exaggerated claim. In S. A. Plotkin, "Recent Results of Mass Immunization against Poliomyelitis with Koprowski Strains of Attenuated Live Poliovirus," *Am. J. Public Health*, 1962, 52(6), 946–960, the annual figures for polio cases in Poland were 1,112 in 1959, and 275 in 1960.

31. S. A. Plotkin, B. J. Cohen, and H. Koprowski, "Intratypic Serodifferentiation of Polioviruses," *Virol.*, 1961, 15, 473–485. See pp. 477 and 478.

32. When he next referred to this ampoule, Koprowski said that "they" had found it — by which he presumably meant officials from the Wistar Institute.

33. "Advisory Committee Studying Origin of AIDS Theory Issues Final Report," Wistar Institute press release, October 22, 1992. "The Wistar Institute of Anatomy and Biology Responds to Advisory Committee's Report on the Origin of AIDS," Wistar Institute press release, October 22, 1992.

34. A. B. Sabin, "Present Position of Immunization against Poliomyelitis with Live Virus Vaccines," *BMJ*, 1959, 1(i), 663–682; see especially pp. 677–678.

35. H. Koprowski, "Vaccination with Modified Active Viruses," *Papers and Discussions Presented at the Fourth International Poliomyelitis Conference* (Philadelphia: Lippincott, 1958), pp. 112–123.

36. Koprowski said the following in a statement to *Science*: "Immunization of children in Africa against polio could be used as a model for the approach to the mass-immunization against AIDS once a vaccine becomes available." (J. Cohen, "Debate on AIDS Origin: Rolling Stone Weighs In," *Science*, March 20, 1992, 255, 1505.)

37. Later, I was to discover even more dramatic correlations between CHAT feeding and AIDS — see chapter 54.

38. See chapter 45.

39. See chapter 20.

40. See David Ho's account of Koprowski's comment to Frank Lilly in chapter 36.

41. PCR could, in other words, be used to test the mitochondrial DNA (mtDNA) of the host.

CHAPTER 35: *Other Views, Other Voices — From Lederle to the Wistar*

1. He was implying that plaque purification, which technically isolated a single virion of poliovirus, would presumably involve the selection of one or other of the parent strains.

2. *NYAS* 57.

3. This was later confirmed by David Dane, who said that Max Theiler told him he believed that TN and his own Type 2 strain were identical. George Dick also spoke of this episode on several occasions.

4. Cabasso gave three examples. First was the time at the start of the fifties, when Koprowski claimed that he had obtained his Type 2 polio strain by passaging a Type 1 poliovirus, a transmutation that is clearly impossible. (H. Koprowski, G. A. Jervis, and T. W. Norton, "Immune Responses in Human Volunteers upon Oral Administration of a Rodent-Adapted Strain of Poliomyelitis Virus," *Am. J. Hyg.,* 1952, 55, 108–126; see especially p. 109.) Second was an occasion when Koprowski apparently reported that West Nile virus (an arbovirus spread by insects) was present in several different cancer tissues, "as a sort of universal cancer-producing virus." (I have not managed to find a source for this.) And third was a time when Koprowski claimed that rabies virus was not pathogenic unless there was a coinfection with another virus called LCM. (H. Koprowski, T. J. Wiktor, and M. M. Kaplan, "Enhancement of Rabies Virus Infection by Lymphocytic Chorio-meningitis Virus," *Virol.,* 1966, 28(4), 754–756.)

5. The third instance, involving LCM.

6. Because he was born in Indiana.

7. These were Robert Phillips's photos of the Ruzizi trial, as featured in the *Rolling Stone* article.

8. In those days, what is now known as hepatitis A was called infectious hepatitis, while hepatitis B was known as serum hepatitis.

9. The Henles, I later discovered, had given "hot shots" of hepatitis virus to over 150 female volunteers from Clinton Farms, in the course of eight experiments conducted between 1949 and 1953. Joe Stokes once again helped set up the study (M. Q. Hawkes, *Excellent Effect: The Edna Mahan Story* [Laurel, MD: The American Correctional Association, 1994], pp. 135–136).

10. F. Deinhardt et al., "Studies of Liver Function Tests in Chimpanzees after Inoculation with Human Infectious Hepatitis Virus," *Am. J. Hyg.,* 1962, 75, 311–321. (I later discovered that the kidneys came from chimps that had already been used in the polio vaccine studies, and that were scheduled for sacrifice. The kidneys were removed, minced, and then mixed with "isologous sera" and Hanks' solution. Each kidney shipment — the number of kidneys was not vouchsafed — was then dispatched to Philadelphia in an insulated box, without refrigeration. See W. Henle, G. Henle, and F. Deinhardt, "Studies on Viral Hepatitis," March 1958–February 1959, in *Annual Report to the Commission on Viral Infections of the Armed Forces Epidemiological Board.*)

11. Second and third passages were made from the chimp kidney cultures, and attempts were then made to infect the different passage levels with hepatitis virus, as an *in vitro* follow-up of the *in vivo* experiments at Lindi. Among these experiments were challenges of the (presumably hepatitis-infected) cultures with other cytopathogenic viruses (including Type 1 polio), but the tests showed no evidence of viral interference. W. Henle et al., "Studies on Viral Hepatitis," see p. 5.

12. The first suspicions of adventitious viruses in chimp kidney cultures were voiced in E. C. Dick, "Chimpanzee Kidney Tissue Cultures for Growth and Isolation of Viruses," *J. Bacteriol.,* 1963, 86, 573–576; For confirmation, see N. G. Roberts, C. J. Gibbs Jr. et al., "Latent Viruses in Chimpanzees with Experimental Kuru," *Nature,* 1967, 216, 446–449; S. Kalter and R. Heberling, "Comparative Virology of Primates," *Bacteriol. Rev.,* 1971, 35(3), 310–364, especially Table 6, or p. 321–323; J. Hooks and C. Gibbs, "The Foamy Viruses," *Bacteriol. Rev.,* 1975, 39(3), 169–185.

13. Later evidence suggested that at least two of the six shipments had been sent later, but the important detail is that Deinhardt dispatched at least some of the cultures himself.

14. The only alternative view that any of the parties involved has offered was Paul Osterrieth's feeling that the kidneys of baboons had probably been used to produce a small amount of tissue culture at the Stanleyville lab. None of the other scientists working there has confirmed this claim.

15. Hayflick had first investigated the possibility of making cell cultures from normal human tissue by using the umbilical cord of his own daughter Susan, born in November 1958. However, after thirty-five days the cells began to immortalize — into a cell line, rather than a cell strain. None the less, WISH (Wistar Institute Susan Hayflick) was used as a cell line for many years until it was shown to be contaminated by HeLa. (L. Hayflick, "The Establishment of a Line [WISH] of Human Amnion Cells in Continuous Cultivation," *Exp. Cell Res.*, 1961, 23, 14–20; W. A. Nelson-Rees and R. R. Flandermeyer, "HeLa Cultures Defined," *Science*, 1976, 191, 96–98.)

16. L. Hayflick, S. A. Plotkin, T. W. Norton, and H. Koprowski, "Preparation of Poliovirus Vaccines in a Human Fetal Diploid Cell Strain," *Am. J. Hyg.*, 1962, 75, 240–258. Whereas a *cell line* (like HeLa) is derived from abnormal tissue (like a tumor), and consists of cells with abnormal karyology, which are immortal, grow in suspension culture, and almost always produce tumors when injected into an animal, a *cell strain* consists of karyologically normal cells, is mortal, cannot grow in suspension (only when attached to a surface), and cannot grow when injected experimentally into animals. Hayflick agreed that it was perhaps unfortunate, in retrospect, that the name he chose, cell strain, was so similar to cell line, thus encouraging confusion between these two very different types of cultures.

17. Hayflick explained that earlier reports of successful passages of poliovirus in rodent and chick embryo cells were probably mistaken, and were merely recording the progressive dilution of the virus with each passage.

18. L. Hayflick, "Human Diploid Cell Strains as Hosts for Viruses," chapter 13 in M. Pollard (editor), *Perspectives in Virology III* (New York: Hoeber, 1963), pp. 213–237; see p. 234. Later, Hayflick summarized the political, economic, and scientific reasons that, he said, had determined why WI-38 had failed to become the substrate for all human vaccine requirements. One of the key reasons was the fear that it might contain a latent human cancer virus lurking unseen, one that would be revealed only decades later. In actual fact, he claimed, there are far more legitimate grounds for concern over simian viruses, which tend to produce tumors or disease in species other than the normal host — as evidenced, he said, by HIV, and by monkey B and Marburg viruses (both of which had killed several lab technicians and monkey handlers).

19. The Wistar Institute was granted a patent for the hybridoma process in the United States and Japan, but refused one in the United Kingdom on grounds of "obviousness." See P. W. Grubb, *Patents in Chemistry and Biotechnology* (Oxford: Clarendon Press, 1986), pp. 165–166.

## CHAPTER 36: *David Ho*

1. David Ho, interviewed at the 9th International Conference on AIDS (in Berlin, July 1993), as featured in Part 4 of a TV documentary series on AIDS, called *The Plague* (Barraclough Carey Productions), shown on Channel Four (U.K.), December 16, 1993 — and on similar dates in the United States and other countries.

2. The extrapolation that Ho's findings disproved the OPV theory of origin was made in Part 4 of *The Plague*, although the statement was made by the narrator, rather than by Ho himself.

3.  M. Eigen and K. Nieselt-Struwe, "How Old Is the Immunodeficiency Virus?" *AIDS*, 1990, 4 (suppl. 1), S85–S93. Although this brilliant article postulates that the divergence between HIV-1, HIV-2, and SIV probably occurred a long time ago (600 to 1,200 years), because rates of mutation have been nonlinear, it does not make it sufficiently clear that much of the evolution thereafter must have occurred in nonhuman primates. Almost hidden in the article (in Table 1) is the detail that the divergence of the earliest African isolates of HIV-1 (from the Congo) probably occurred between 1945 and 1960.

4.  G. Bell, "Revealed: David Carr, the West's First Aids Victim," *Sunday Express* (U.K.), July 29, 1990. C. Mihill, "Manchester Man Had HIV 31 Years Ago," *Guardian* (U.K.), July 6, 1990. Anon., "Aids Traced to Death in 1959," *Daily Telegraph* (U.K.), July 6, 1990. All these claimed that David Carr had visited Africa.

5.  George Williams, personal communication, 1993.

6.  E. Hooper and W. D. Hamilton, "1959 Manchester Case of Syndrome Resembling AIDS," *Lancet,* 1996, 348, 1363–1365. Where the Manchester contamination occurred has never been established.

7.  The concept of viral quasispecies — the cloud of closely related viral sequences that develops in the body of a person infected with a highly mutable virus (like HIV) — had first been published by Nobel Prize–winner Manfred Eigen just a few months earlier. See M. Eigen, "Viral Quasispecies," *Scientific American,* July 1993, pp. 32–39.

8.  In an interview conducted at his house in March 1994, George Williams confirmed that he had been storing the tissues at his home since "just after the case was confirmed" (in about July 1990), but that this was no longer the case. (The tissues were apparently still at his home when Ho contacted him in 1993.)

9.  See further details in chapter 38.

10. "HIV/AIDS Surveillance Database," U.S. Department of Government, Bureau of the Census, June 1994.

11. J. A. Pineda et al., "Prevalencia de anti-LAV/HTLV-III en prostitutas de Sevilla," *Med. Clin.* (Barcelona), 1986, 86, 498–500.

12. J. A. Pineda et al., "HIV-1 Infection among Non-intravenous Drug User Female Prostitutes in Spain. No Evidence of Evolution to Pattern II," *AIDS,* 1992, 6, 1365–1369.

13. R. F. Garry et al., "Documentation of an AIDS Virus Infection in the United States in 1968," *JAMA,* 1988, 260(14), 2085–2087.

14. Dr. Preston Marx, as I was later to learn. Z. Chen, P. A. Marx et al., "Museum Specimens from 1918 Contain HIV-2 Related DNA in a New Species of Mangabey," 1st National Conference on Human Retroviruses and Related Infections (Washington, D.C., 1993), abstract 151, p. 81.

15. Preston Marx, personal communication, 1995.

16. In a letter to Frank Lilly written by Koprowski on December 3, 1992, after the Wistar committee had delivered its report, Koprowski congratulated Lilly on the report, adding that he would like to clarify "only one important point" concerning which monkeys had been used for preparing the polio vaccine used in Africa. These were, he wrote, rhesus monkeys "originating from India or the Philippines." However, Ho's comment to me, and the text of the Wistar report, make it clear that in a previous conversation with Lilly Koprowski had revealed that he could not be sure which monkey kidneys had been used.

17. S. Connor, "World's First Aids Case Was False," *Independent* (U.K.), March 24, 1995, pp. 1–3.

CHAPTER 37: *Bill Hamilton*

1. In 1993, there were just seventeen British scientists receiving Royal Society grants, which effectively allowed them to concentrate purely on research, without having to devote time to teaching duties.

2. In December 1991.

3. R. Preston, *The Hot Zone* (New York: Doubleday, 1994).

4. "Ebola Haemorrhagic Fever in Sudan, 1976: Report of a WHO/International Study Team," *Bull. WHO*, 1978, 56(2), 247–270; "Ebola Haemorrhagic Fever in Zaire, 1976: Report of an International Commission," *Bull. WHO*, 1978, 56(2), 271–293.

5. Hamilton had heard about films shown at primate conferences, featuring pygmy chimps (or bonobos) doing "all the things which humans do in bed" — including heterosexual and homosexual oral sex, masturbation, and incest. Not only did *Pan paniscus*, like *Homo sapiens*, enjoy sex in lots of different positions, but sexual contact seemed to be an integral component of almost every pygmy chimp activity, with genital, oral, and manual stimulation seemingly taking place between pairs or groups every few minutes. A good example of a film that graphically depicts bonobo sexuality was "Monkey in the Mirror," shown as part of the *Natural World* series on BBC1 (U.K.) on February 18, 1995.

6. For evidence of this, see H. Vervaecke and L. van Elsacker, "Hybrids between Common Chimpanzee (*Pan troglodytes*) and Pygmy Chimpanzee (*Pan paniscus*) in Captivity," *Mammalia*, 1992, 56(4), 667–669.

7. Martha Lubell, personal communication, August 1993.

8. In fact, the diagnostics, epidemiology, and vaccine research branches of the SBL had been renamed the Swedish Institute of Infectious Disease Control (SIIDC) in July 1993.

9. This letter was formally submitted to *Science* on January 27, 1994.

10. B. Martin, "Stifling the Media" (letter), *Nature*, 1993, 363, 202.

11. H. Koprowski, "AIDS and the Polio Vaccine" (letter), *Science*, 1992, 257, 1024–1027.

12. The material in this covering letter, Hamilton emphasized, was definitely not for publication.

13. For a discussion of the treatment of the OPV/AIDS theory by *Science*, see J. Cribb, *The White Death* (Sydney: Angus and Robertson, 1996), pp. 189–190.

14. Letter from W. D. Hamilton to D. Koshland, February 23, 1994, after *Science* rejected Hamilton's letter on February 16. Hamilton wrote: "Even the prospect of nuclear war cannot match the destructive potential of such an event [a hypothetical future zoonosis, which might combine the destructiveness of AIDS with the infectiousness of influenza]. Thus I think you as editor of *Science* have a grave responsibility to humanity to see that these issues are as fully discussed as is possible."

15. W. D. Hamilton, "AIDS Theory vs. Lawsuit," draft letter submitted to *Nature* on March 11, 1994. A slightly earlier version of this letter is published in full in J. Cribb, *The White Death*, pp. 254–257; see also pp. 182–184, for Cribb's excellent analysis of the episode. To avoid confusion, I have used quotations from the final version of the *Nature* letter, rather than any of the earlier drafts sent to *Science*.

16. Letter from Maxine Clarke, executive editor of *Nature*, to Bill Hamilton, May 25, 1994.

17. Galileo Galilei (1564–1642), Italian astronomer and philosopher, and one of the founders of modern science, was compelled by the Inquisition to repudiate the Copernican theory, whereas Giordano Bruno (1548–c.1599), another Italian philosopher, who regarded God

as the unity reconciling spirit and matter, was condemned to death by burning. This heretical metaphor originally featured in Hamilton's unpublished letter to *Nature*.

18. For the text of Curtis's reply to Koprowski's letter to *Science*, itself submitted to *Science* on September 30, 1992, but rejected by that journal, see J. Cribb, *The White Death*, pp. 258–262.

## CHAPTER 38: *The Two Sailors*

1. *The Pawel Koprowski Memorial Vacation Awards* (Manchester: University of Manchester Press, 1991).

2. The date of death is recorded as March 1, 1957, in the memorial book, though it was actually February 28, as confirmed by the death certificate. The Manchester *Guardian* of March 1, 1957 (death notices, p. 16) shows that it was the funeral that took place on March 1. The death certificate also reveals that Koprowski's father's surgery, a prostatectomy, occurred in December 1956.

3. An earlier report that Dave had been inducted at H.M.S. *Victory,* in Portsmouth, was now revealed to be a misreading of Victoria Barracks in Devonport.

4. This is further confirmed by members of the *Whitby*'s crew.

5. I began to suspect that Kevin's and Clive's memories of forty years earlier had become entwined with the 1990 newspaper reports proposing that Dave Carr had visited Africa.

6. Intriguingly, Dave's initial medical check before entry to the navy, conducted in September 1955, had revealed no such problems, and had assigned him to "Grade 1." Similarly, no skin ailments were reported in his discharge medical in November 1957.

7. M. M. Eibl et al., "Abnormal T-Lymphocyte Subpopulations in Healthy Subjects after Tetanus Booster Immunization" (letter), *N. Engl. J. Med.,* 1984, 310(3), 672–673. Also relevant: H. G. Kingston et al., "Cellular and Human Responses to Poliovirus and Tetanus following Primary Immunization of SIV-infected Macaques," in P. Racz (editor), *Animal Models of HIV and Other Retroviral Infections* (Basel: Karger, 1993), pp. 75–85.

8. Some examples: G. Finger, "Le problème des vaccinations dans les Unites Militaires," *Rev. Int. Serv. Santé Armées Terre,* 1960, 33(4), 247–260. "Update: Vaccine Side Effects, Adverse Reactions, Contraindications, and Precautions," by the Advisory Committee on Immunization Practices; *MMWR,* 1996, 45, RR-12; 1–35.

9. R. Norton-Taylor, "MoD Ignored Warning on Gulf Drugs," *Guardian* (U.K.), October 29, 1997.

10. Michael Grosse (quoting a magazine article from 1969 or 1970, entitled "Verdens Lengste Trailerute"), personal communication, 1994.

11. Arvid apparently left the international haulage company in 1973 or 1974, because his wife's deteriorating health meant that he needed to be based nearer home. He then started work with another haulage firm serving towns in southern Norway, but had to resign in 1975, when he himself fell sick again.

12. H. Heimpel, personal communication, 1995.

13. W. Sterry et al., "Kaposi's Sarcoma, Aplastic Pancytopenia, and Multiple Opportunistic Infections in a Homosexual (Cologne, 1976)," *Lancet,* 1983, 1(i), 924–925.

14. Arvid delivered to many towns around Gelsenkirchen, and used to pick up consignments of metal granules from Oberhausen, which lies less than a dozen miles away. The German chef may also, of course, have been bisexual.

15. Formal letters to doctors Frøland, Wefring, and Rasokat dated June 1993, were sent from the MRC Centre, Cambridge, where Dr. Tristem was then working. Tristem sent further letters to Frøland and Rasokat from Imperial College (where he had moved) in 1994.

16. Interview with the brother of "Arvid," February 1994.

17. Karl Wefring, personal communication, May 1993. (None of the other ports visited during those journeys — in the Middle and Far East, Australia, Europe, North America, and the Caribbean — were convincing venues for HIV infection in the sixties.)

18. The earliest recorded AIDS case in Kenya was a Ugandan journalist who fell sick in 1984.

19. N. R. E. Fendall, "Poliomyelitis in Kenya — the 1960 Epidemic and Oral Vaccine Campaign," *J. Trop. Med. Hyg.*, 1962, 62, 245–255.

20. G. Lecatsas and J. J. Alexander, "Origins of HIV" (letter), *Lancet*, 1992, 339, 1427. See also G. Lecatsas and I. Kaiser, "Cercopithecus Monkeys Seropositive for HIV," abstract presented at 8th International Congress of Virology (Berlin, August 1990).

21. The Mauritius and Kenya campaigns are described in J. Gear, "Live Virus Vaccine Studies in Southern Africa," *PAHO2*, 474–479. A series of articles in the *South African Medical Journal*, 1963, 37(19), 497–518 gives the details of the South African vaccination campaign, and why Sabin's vaccine was preferred to Koprowski's. Page 497 also refers to a small-scale vaccination in the face of an epidemic in Uganda in 1959, using the South African vaccine. This appears to have involved people in Kampala (see annual report of the South African Institute for Medical Research, 1960, pp. 177 and 183).

22. Fergal Hill, personal communications, 1995 and 1996. Indeed, by 1995 the Lecatsas team seemed less confident of its findings. See T. K. Smit, G. Lecatsas et al., "Simian Immunodeficiency Virus (SIVagm) in Vervet Monkeys in South Africa: A Case History," poster presented at the 5th International Congress on the Impact of Viral Diseases in the Developing World (Johannesburg, July 1995), p. P3–35.

23. See T. Curtis, "The Origin of AIDS," *Rolling Stone*, March 19, 1992, pp. 54–61, 106–108.


CHAPTER 39: *From the Archives*


1. Anon., "A propos de poliomyélite," *Le Stanleyvillois*, November 14, 1956, p. 9.

2. Anon., "La Mission Courtois-Koprowski et la lutte contre la Poliomyélite," *Le Stanleyvillois*, February 12, 1957.

3. Anon., "City Polio Proposal," *East African Standard*, February 1, 1957, pp. 1, 8, and 17.

4. By which the writer clearly means the University of Pennsylvania, situated in Philadelphia.

5. It is unclear who was responsible for these errors — the reporter, Ghislain Courtois, who introduced the American to the audience, or Koprowski himself.

6. Hilary Koprowski, personal communication, December 1993.

7. Anon., "Guerre à la polio dans la brousse stanleyvilloise," *Le Stanleyvillois*, February 11, 1957, pp. 1 and 4; E.-L. Bouffa, "Les savants américain et belges lutte victorieusement contre la polio," *L'Echo de Stan*, February 11, 1957, pp. 1 and 3. The former was the article previously sent me by Gaston Ninane.

8. Anon., "Inauguration du nouveau Laboratoire," *Le Stanleyvillois*, September 30, 1957, p. 1. Most of the speeches delivered at the symposium are published in "Symposium sur les maladies à virus en Afrique centrale, organisé à l'occasion de l'inauguration du nouveau laboratoire médical de Stanleyville," *Ann. Soc. Belg. Méd. Trop.*, 1958, 38, 241–386.

9. Norton's photos from February and March 1957 showed that the main buildings, including the windows, were already complete by then, although the surrounding bush had still to be cleared.

10. Laboratoire Médical Provincial, Stanleyville, Rapport Annuel, 1957, p. 82.

11. This response was later reinforced when I saw contemporary film of the old and new Stanleyville laboratories, highlighting how much money had been spent on the latter.

12. L.-J. André and E. André-Gadras, "16 cas de poliomyélite observés dans un district de brousse du Gabon," *Méd Trop.*, 1958, 18, 638–641. Dr. L.-J. André is described as a *"Médecin Capitaine"* (a doctor-captain) from the overseas branches of the Pasteur Institute.

13. Discussion by P. Lépine, *NYAS* 57, pp. 148–149; and Anon., "Le vaccin du professeur Lépine sera vendu par une firme pharmaceutique americaine," *L'Echo de Stan,* June 24, 1957, citing an Agence France Presse report.

14. Anon., "On Vaccine," *Le Stanleyvillois,* March 7, 1958. The same pool of CHAT 10A-11 had been given to about four hundred Swiss infants and children at about this time — but this hardly means that it had been "adopted in Switzerland."

15. Anon., "Vaccination massive contre la poliomyélite," *Centre Afrique* (Bukavu), April 8, 1958, p. 1, and Anon., "Campaign de vaccination massive contre la poliomyélite," *Temps Nouveau d'Afrique* (Usumbura), April 13, 1958. These reports reveal that apart from Bugarama (in present-day Rwanda), the so-called Ruzizi Valley vaccination was staged entirely in the Congo and Burundi.

16. Anon., "Vaccination massive contre la poliomyélite."

17. The "polio in Lindi chimps" article (which never appeared) was also cited in the two published reports of the vaccinations: *BMJ* 58; and G. Courtois, "Vaccination antipoliomyélitique par virus vivant au Congo Belge," *Ann. Soc. Belg. Méd. Trop.*, 1958, 38, 805–816.

18. By contrast, the *BMJ* 58 article claimed that intraspinal safety tests on Fox Type 3 vaccine had already been conducted at Lindi.

19. G. Courtois, "Previsions experimentation — Station Lindi," October 1, 1957, continues as G. Courtois, "Projet de travail scientifique à executer en collaboration entre le Laboratoire de Stanleyville et le Wistar Institute de Philadelphie (U.S.A.)," file H4475/984, Ministry of Foreign Affairs archives (Belgium).

20. A. B. Sabin, "Properties of Attenuated Polioviruses and Their Behavior in Human Beings," *NYAS* 57, 113–127; A. B. Sabin, "Attenuated Live Virus Poliomyelitis Vaccine," *Bull. N.Y. Acad. Med.*, 1957, 33(1), 17–39.

21. The first article (see n.20, above) constituted the speech that Sabin delivered at the New York Academy of Sciences conference that Koprowski helped organize in early January 1957; the second article (published in the same month) was almost the only polio article by someone outside the Koprowski group to be found among Norton's papers.

22. Letter from M. Van den Abeele to the governor-general of the Belgian Congo, dated August 6, 1958, available in "Poliomyélite: correspondance," file H4484/1058, Ministry of Foreign Affairs archives (Belgium).

23. "Proces — Verbal de Réunion," July 9, 1956, file H4484/1058, Ministry of Foreign Affairs archives (Belgium).

24. M. Agerholm, "Arresting an Outbreak of Poliomyelitis" (letter), *BMJ,* 1958, 2(i), 638–639. See also M. Agerholm, "Live Polio Vaccine" (letter), *BMJ,* 1960, 1(i), 966–967; and W. C. Fothergill, "Live Polio Vaccine" (letter), *BMJ,* 1960, 1(ii), 1278. Working under Professor Trueta at the Wingfield Morris Hospital in Oxford during the fifties, Agerholm took over the treatment of many of Ritchie Russell's polio patients after they became noninfectious.

Although it is not known whether she was one of those whom Russell vaccinated with TN in Oxford in 1956, she would undoubtedly have been familiar with the debacle that followed that vaccination, and Dick's discovery that TN reverted to virulence after human passage. John Spalding, personal communication, October 1996.

25. It was a reasonable proposal, and Agerholm would probably have been even more alarmed had she had all the relevant facts. CHAT vaccinations in Stanleyville began in February 1957 and continued throughout the year; the Aketi schoolchildren were fed CHAT in May 1957. Banalia, where eight children were paralyzed between November 1957 and January 1958, is 80 miles north of Stanleyville. Also in early January, there were seven polio cases at Bambesa, which is 220 miles north of Banalia (and 140 from Aketi, with a railway connection for most of the way). Later in January 1958, polio also struck in the military camps at Gombari (twelve cases) and Watsa (two cases). Although these are situated between 400 and 500 miles from Stanleyville, it is quite possible that vaccinees would have traveled there from Stanleyville, the regional capital.

26. Letter from Bervoets to De Brauwere, September 17, 1958, file H4484/1058, Ministry of Foreign Affairs archives, Brussels. The figures for each vaccination varied slightly from those published in *BMJ* 58, although the grand total matched quite well. The only instance in which the *BMJ* 58 figures were apparently more accurate was Aketi, for which Bervoets quoted "around 2000" — instead of the *BMJ* 58 figure of 1978.

27. Bervoets's letter reveals that the vaccine ran out before all the Bambesa villagers had been vaccinated, something directly contradicted in *BMJ* 58, which states that every inhabitant of the village received the vaccine.

28. Partial vaccinations such as those in Bambesa and among the Kilo miners, which allowed for the spread of excreted viruses from vaccinees to nonvaccinees, may have provided the ideal conditions for polio reversions to occur.

29. Bervoets appears to have been sidetracked by the discovery that all five CHAT vaccinees who went on to contract polio did so within nine days of vaccination, which probably meant that they had been infected with wild virus shortly before vaccination, rather than by vaccine virus that had reverted. However, he completely ignores the possibility that nonvaccinees could have been infected by reverted vaccine virus.

30. Letter from De Brauwere to Médicin en chef; September 1, 1959, file H4484/1058, Ministry of Foreign Affairs archives (Belgium).

31. A. Lebrun et al., "Vaccination with the CHAT Strain of Type 1 Attenuated Poliomyelitis Virus in Leopoldville, Belgian Congo. 1. Description of the City, Its History of Polio-myelitis, and the Plan of the Vaccination Campaign," *Bull. WHO,* 1960, 22, 203–213; S. A. Plotkin, A. Lebrun, and H. Koprowski, "Vaccination with the CHAT Strain of Type 1 Attenuated Poliomyelitis Virus in Leopoldville, Belgian Congo. 2. Studies of the Safety and Efficacy of Vaccination," *Bull. WHO,* 1960, 22, 215–234; S. A. Plotkin, A. Lebrun, G. Courtois, and H. Koprowski, "Vaccination with the CHAT Strain of Type 1 Attenu-ated Poliomyelitis Virus in Leopoldville, Congo. 3. Safety and Efficacy during the First 21 Months of Study," *Bull. WHO,* 1961, 24, 785–792.

32. S. Gard, "Immunological Strain Specificity within Type 1 Poliovirus," *Bull. WHO,* 1960, 22, 235–242.

33. S. A. Plotkin et al., "Vaccination with the CHAT Strain of Type 1 Attenuated Poliomyelitis Virus in Leopoldville, Congo. 3," see page 788. See also Anon., "Vaccination par voie buc-cale contre la poliomyélite," *L'Essor du Congo* (Elisabethville), August 13, 1959, p. 5.

34. H. Koprowski, "Historical Aspects of the Development of Live Virus Vaccines in Polio-myelitis," *Am. J. Dis. Child.,* 1960, 100, 428–439; see p. 436. Koprowski's comment, made

at the Alvarenga Prize Lecture in October 1959, was clearly based on information from the Belgian Congo, where the intention by August 1959 was to proceed with a mass vaccination of the entire indigenous child population.

35. Letter from Dr. André Lebrun to Dr. Kivits, February 10, 1960, file H4484/1060, Ministry of Foreign Affairs archives (Belgium).

36. This figure, however, was inappropriate for Ruanda-Urundi, in that more than seventy-three thousand of the total had consisted of vaccinees from the Congolese side of the border. See G. Courtois, "Vaccination antipoliomyélitique par virus vivant au Congo Belge."

37. This turned out to be Professor Daniel Vangroenweghe, from the Department of African Studies at the University of Ghent, the only other researcher whom I know to have interviewed Gaston Ninane about the incidents at Lindi. Vangroenweghe eventually published a book that contains a chapter on the OPV hypothesis, and concludes that it is the most plausible hypothesis for the origin of AIDS. See D. Vangroenweghe, *Aids in Afrika* (Breda: De Geus, 1997).

## CHAPTER 40: *Ghislain Courtois*

1. Save for 1946–1949, when he was director of the small medical laboratory at Blukwa, near Gabu Nioka and Lake Albert.

2. The official account is that the colonial government financed all aspects of the chimp camp. Nonetheless, André Courtois's close friendship with Koprowski suggests that his account of the funding may have some merit.

3. André Courtois also said that at the old medical laboratory in Stanleyville there had been some fifteen cages to house chimps, together with a few baboons and rhesus macaques. This was before the building of the new lab and animal house.

4. G. Courtois, J. C. Levaditi et al., "Mycose cutanée à corps levuriformes observées chez des singes Africains en captivité," *Ann. Institut Pasteur,* 1955, 89, 124–127.

5. I later discovered that in May 1958, Courtois paid a visit to Clinton, and that in August, in Brussels, he personally handed over the CHAT vaccine to be used in the Leopoldville campaign to Henry Gelfand from Tulane, who was en route from the United States to the Congo. (Clinton archives, minutes of board meeting of May 14, 1958, and Henry Gelfand, personal communication, 1996.)

6. G. Courtois, "Vaccinations antipoliomyélitique par virus vivant au Congo Belge," *Ann. Soc. Belg. Méd. Trop.,* 1958, 38, 805–816. Interestingly, this account of the vaccinations by Courtois was never cited by Koprowski in any of his subsequent articles.

7. International Association of Microbiological Societies, *Minutes of the Fourth Meeting of the Committee of Cell Cultures* (London, September 1967), (Geneva: IABS; 1968).

8. Also present on the committee was Leonard Hayflick from the Wistar, and Koprowski's collaborator, Drago Ikic, from Zagreb. The three men again proposed the use of characterized human cell strains like WI-38.

9. D. I. H. Simpson, G. Courtois et al., "Congo Virus: A Hitherto Undescribed Virus Occurring in Africa," *E. Af. Med. J.;* 1967, 44(2), 87–98.

10. G. Courtois and A. de Wewer, "Campagne de vaccination de masse par le poliovirus vivant atténué et problèmes posés par sa réalisation," *Brux.-Méd.,* 1964, 44, 415–426.

11. G. Courtois, "Present Day Progress in Our Knowledge of the Enterovirus," *Bulletin des Grands Endemies en Afrique,* 1960, 2, 271–281.

12. D. Bodian, "Poliovirus in Chimpanzee Tissues after Virus Feeding," *Am. J. Hyg.,* 1956, 58, 81–100. Bodian's work was mentioned (and praised) by Courtois, but later in his speech (note 11), and in a different context.

13. G. Courtois, "Sur la réalisation d'une singerie de chimpanzés au Congo," *Symposium internationale sur l'avenir des animaux de laboratoires* (Lyon: Institut Pasteur, 1967), pp. 235–244.

14. G. Courtois and J. Mortelmans, "Apes," *Primates in Med.,*1969, 2, 75–86.

15. A. Kortlandt, "Chimpanzee Ecology and Laboratory Management," *Laboratory Primate Newsletter,* 1966, 5(3), 1–11; see p. 8.

16. As an aside, Courtois added that they had never had any case of tuberculosis among the Lindi chimps, although they had seen several cases among the Asian macaques, imported via Holland, which were held at the Stanleyville laboratory.

17. Anon., "La lutte contre la polio au Congo: une nouvelle étape," *Courrier d'Afrique* (Leopoldville), May 4, 1959, pp. 4 and 6. Also see Anon., "La vaccination massive contre la polyo," *L'Avenir* (Leopoldville), May 2/3, 1959.

18. Anon., "Congo May Lead World in Fight against Polio," *Uganda Argus* (Kampala), undated, but clearly 1958.

19. P. Osterrieth, "Propriétés biochimiques des Klebsiella," *Ann. Soc. Belg. Méd. Trop.,* 1958, 38, 721–730.

20. R. V. Henrickson et al., "Epidemic of Acquired Immunodeficiency in Rhesus Monkeys," *Lancet,* 1983, 1(i), 388–390. This article specifically mentions both *Klebsiella pneumoniae* and *Candida* infections as being two of the principal infections of both simian and human AIDS.

### CHAPTER 41: *Stanley Plotkin*

1. Anon., "Congo May Lead World in Fight against Polio," *Uganda Argus* (Kampala), unknown date in 1958.

2. By this stage, I had found one document that provided partial support to Plotkin's claim. In a paper entitled "Factors Influencing a Successful Vaccination with Live Poliovirus" (WHO/BS/IR/84), which he submitted to the Study Group on Requirements on Poliomyelitis Vaccine in October 1960, Plotkin wrote that the discovery of SV40 "in almost all Rhesus monkey kidney tissue cultures" was likely to have a considerable impact on vaccine production. He added that at the Wistar they were just now beginning to look for the presence of SV40 antibodies in the sera of their vaccinees, but that they had already investigated the incidence of serious illness in approximately two hundred children, now aged between one and three-and-a-half, who had been fed as infants with "live virus vaccines which presumably contained the vacuolating agent [SV40]." (These were presumably the infants fed at Clinton, about two hundred of whom would have been fed different OPVs made in monkey kidney — CHAT, Wistar, P-712, Jackson, and Fox — between May 1957 and late 1959.) Plotkin's comment was intriguing, for although it did not clearly state the fact, it implied that rhesus monkey kidney tissue culture had been used at some stage during vaccine manufacture. When this submission was made, three years (1957–1960) had passed since CHAT was first described, and during that time the substrate had never been identified. It is therefore remarkable that despite his hints about rhesus, Plotkin failed to provide a definitive

statement. If ever there was a time to state unequivocally the species in which the principal Koprowski vaccines, CHAT and Fox, were normally made, then this moment — just after the discovery of SV40 — was surely it. Why the reticence? Of course, Plotkin became involved with the Wistar's polio vaccine program only in late 1957 or early 1958, and may not have been certain about the species (singular or plural) used to make CHAT and Fox prior to that date. Furthermore, it is worth noting that this paper does not report the finding of SV40 in the Wistar's vaccines — only the *expectation* of finding SV40 — and recalling that Meinrad Schar, in interview, said he thought that Koprowski's vaccines were *not* contaminated with SV40. (If correct, this suggests that they were not made in rhesus or cynomolgus kidneys.)

3.  Anon., "La vaccination massive contre la polyo," *L'Avenir* (Leopoldville), May 2–3, 1959.

4.  Letter from Stanley Plotkin to Fritz Deinhardt, May 28, 1959, made available by Dr. Jean Deinhardt; this letter had been typed on Public Health Service headed notepaper. However, at the press conference he had described himself as being present "only as a scientific observer for the University of Philadelphia [sic] and its Wistar Institute."

5.  Sven Gard was less confident that there had been no reversion. See S. Gard, "Immunological Strain Specificity within Type 1 Poliovirus," *Bull. WHO,* 1960, 22, 235–242.

6.  S. A. Plotkin, H. Koprowski et al., "Intratypic Serodifferentiation of Polioviruses," *Virol.,* 1961, 15, 473–485.

7.  After this interview, I became quite excited about the possibility that the CHAT pool numbers might simply reflect the plaques from which pools were prepared. Further reflection, however, did not provide support for this interpretation. For a start, why was Plaque 20 (which clearly represented material derived from that plaque) always referred to as a plaque, whereas the other vaccine feeding lots were referred to as "pools"? Second, if Plotkin was right, then pool 10A-11 would have been made from plaques 10 and 11 on the plaque chart and therefore only single plaque purified, while pool 13 would have been double plaque purified. By contrast, the claim had always been that all pools of CHAT were triple plaque purified, to meet WHO requirements.

8.  R. McKie, "Ethical Dilemma May Thwart Drive for Aids Vaccine," *Observer* (U.K.), September 12, 1993, p. 10; N. Hawkes, "First Test of Aids Vaccine Offers Hope for Treatment," *Times* (U.K.), September 11, 1993, p. 3.

9.  H. J. Hearn Jr., "A Variant of Venezuelan Equine Encephalomyelitis Virus Attenuated for Mice and Monkeys," *J. Immunol.,* 1960, 84, 626–634.

10. P. S. Brachman, S. A. Plotkin et al., "An Epidemic of Inhalation Anthrax: The First in the Twentieth Century. II. Epidemiology," *Am. J. Hyg.,* 1960, 72, 6–23.

11. The Johns Hopkins University (similarly supported by a Chemical Corps contract) was also involved in the research. See P. S. Norman, J. G. Rey Jr., P. S. Brachman, S. A. Plotkin, and J. S. Pagano, "Serologic Testing for Anthrax Antibodies in Workers in a Goat Hair Processing Mill," *Am. J. Hyg.,* 1960, 72, 32–37.

12. S. A. Plotkin, P. S. Brachman, et al., "An Epidemic of Inhalation Anthrax: The First in the Twentieth Century. I. Clinical Features," *Am. J. Med.,* 1960, 29, 992–1001.

13. P. S. Brachman, S. A. Plotkin et al., "Field Evaluation of a Human Anthrax Vaccine," *Am. J. Public Health,* 1962, 52(4), 632–645.

14. The vaccine had been prepared at Fort Detrick, where the injection of six hundred scientific personnel had apparently demonstrated its suitability for human use. G. G. Wright et al., "Studies on Immunity in Anthrax. V. Immunizing Activity of Alum-Precipitated Protective Antigen," *J. Immunol.,* 1954, 73, 387–391.

15. J. M. Barnes, "The Development of Anthrax Following the Administration of Spores by Inhalation," *Br. J. Exp. Pathol.*, 1947, 28, 385–394.

16. This prompts Brachman and Plotkin to observe that "only by extraordinary means, of which there was no record," could this man's infection (and later death) have been linked to the introduction of the new detergent. It is possible, of course, that the victim simply visited another part of the mill — and died before this fact could be checked.

17. Commission on Epidemiological Survey, (U.S.) Armed Forces Epidemiological Board, Annual Report 1959–60, Minutes of March 23, 1960, pp. 1–11.

18. Anon., "Wistar Institute Names Chief," *New York Times*, March 27, 1957, p. 6.

19. For further details, see R. E. Billingham and H. Koprowski, "The Wistar Institute of Anatomy and Biology, Philadelphia," *Nature*, 1959, 184 (4688), B. A. 6–10.

20. W. S. Albrink et al., "Experimental Inhalation Anthrax in the Chimpanzee," *Am. J. Pathol.*, 1959, 35(5), 1055–1065. This article refers to three of the four experimental chimpanzees as being *Pan troglodytes (Schwarz)*, and the fourth as *Pan troglodytes troglodytes*. In fact, Albrink almost certainly means that the three were *Pan paniscus*, for Schwarz is the primatologist who first reported *Pan paniscus* as a separate species. See R. L. Susman, *The Pygmy Chimpanzee — Evolutionary Biology and Behavior* (New York: Plenum Press, 1984), p. xii.

21. J. Goldstein, "Vietnam Research on Campus: The Summit/Spicerack Controversy at the University of Pennsylvania, 1965–67," *Peace and Change*, 1986, 11(2), 27–49, especially pp. 31–32. My thanks also to Julian Perry Robinson, Science Policy Research Unit, University of Sussex, U.K.

22. J. Aber, J. Benjamin, and R. Martin, *Germ Warfare Research for Vietnam* (Philadelphia Area Committee to End the War in Vietnam, 1966), pp. 1–31, see especially p. 7. See also S. Stern, "War Catalog of the University of Pennsylvania," *Ramparts*, August 1966, pp. 32–40, especially p. 38, and Anon., "Research Supported by Pentagon Stirs Germ Warfare Accusations," *New York Times*, March 19, 1989, p. 30.

CHAPTER 42: *Le Laboratoire Médical de Stanleyville*

1. *BMJ* 58. See also G. Courtois, "Vaccination antipoliomyélitique par virus vivant au Congo Belge," *Ann. Soc. Belg. Med. Trop.*, 1958, 38, 805–816.

2. Hubert Caubergh, personal communication, 1997.

3. Paul Osterrieth, personal communication, 1994.

4. Rollais discovered a few of their special foods, like very young shoots of bamboo, which persuaded them to offer the chimps sugarcane, which was popular, even if it was not part of their natural diet.

5. P. Doupagne, "The identification of 113 strains of 'Candida.' 'Levine E.M.B.A.,' the ideal medium for the identification of Candida albicans in hot countries," *Bull. des Grands Endemies en Afrique*, 1960, 2, 262–264.

6. A. André, G. Courtois, G. Ninane, P. Osterrieth et al., "Mise en évidence d'antigènes de groupes sanguins A, B, O et Rh chez les singes chimpanzés," *Ann. Institut Pasteur*, 1961, 101, 82–95.

7. My guess was that the samples might well have been sent in August 1957, when Robert Daenens said that there had been 175 chimps at Lindi, the most there had ever been at one time.

8.  J. P. Delville and S. R. Pattyn, "Epidémiologie de la poliomyélite au Congo Belge et au Ruanda-Urundi. Etat actuel de nos connaissances," *Ann. Soc. Belg. Méd. Trop.*, 1958, 38, 283–292.

9.  Anon., "La lutte contre la polio au Congo: une nouvelle étape," *Courrier d'Afrique* (Leopoldville), May 4, 1959, pp. 4 and 6.

10. S. R. Pattyn, "A Review of Enteroviruses in the Congo," *Trop. Geogr. Med.*, 1962, 14, 71–79. This article reports the work that Pattyn and Delville conducted in E'ville in 1957–1959, and the fact that polio isolations were very few in those years.

11. A newspaper article places this event in August 1959. Anon., "Vaccination par voie buccale contre la poliomyélite," *L'Essor du Congo* (Elisabethville), August 13, 1959, p. 5.

12. F. Deinhardt, G. Courtois et al., "Studies of Liver Function Tests in the Chimpanzee after Inoculation with Human Infectious Hepatitis Virus," *Am. J. Hyg.*, 1962, 75, 311–321. G. Courtois, discussion in R. Sohier and O. G. Gaudin, "Monkey Cell Cultures in Virology," *Primates in Med.*, 1969, 3, 80–92; especially p. 91.

13. I later learned that Ninane was right — and that the doctors' reunion had taken place in Leuven, rather than Liège. P. Doupagne, personal communication, 1997.

## CHAPTER 43: *The Chimpanzees*

1.  Discussion by G. Courtois after R. Sohier and O. G. Gaudin, "Monkey Cell Cultures in Virology," *Primates in Med.*, 1969, 3, 80–92; see p. 91.

2.  As evidenced by the precise times for the journey recorded in Agnes Flack's diary entries for February 1958.

3.  See F. Deinhardt, G. Courtois et al., "Studies of Liver Function Tests in the Chimpanzee after Inoculation with Human Infectious Hepatitis Virus," *Am. J. Hyg.*, 1962, 75, 311–321.

4.  Robert Gallo apparently once said that five hundred chimps would be enough to "guarantee a vaccine against AIDS." See D. Blum, *The Monkey Wars* (New York: Oxford University Press, 1994), p. 209.

5.  In the early fifties, Bugyaki had taken over the Elisabethville vet lab from Jezierski, whom he found "a very scientific man," but also very nervous, someone who lost his temper easily.

6.  I went back to see Louis Bugyaki thirty months later, in November 1996, in order to check this key point about the excision of chimp kidneys so that cultures could be made therefrom. On this occasion, however, he told me that his memory was failing, and that he could not be certain.

7.  This closely reflected what Courtois had written in his 1966 speech at Lyon. See G. Courtois, "Sur la réalization d'une singerie de chimpanzés au Congo," *Symposium internationale sur l'avenir des animaux de laboratoires* (Lyon: Institut Pasteur, 1967), pp. 235–244.

8.  Fluency in English would help the American doctors working on polio at Lindi.

9.  My own information suggested that most of the remaining chimps were transferred to the animal house at the laboratory early in 1960, and that in February 1961 Ghislain Courtois, then back in Belgium, recommended that some be released into the bush, and some couples onto Liculi, an island in the Congo River (presumably in the hope that they would breed, and could perhaps be utilized at a later date). Adriaan Kortlandt, personal communication, 1995, and letter from G. Courtois to J. Stijns, February 1961. However, Gilbert Rollais thought that the final Lindi chimps were transferred to Leopoldville Zoo.

10. I later wrote to Gilbert Rollais, asking him exactly where he had caught his chimps during this period. He sent back a map, which marked an area in western Congo Brazzaville, not far from where one of Martine Peeters' SIV-positive chimps was caught. This raises the intriguing possibility that the first chimp in space might have had SIV.

11. One article claims that in West Africa between two and three adults had to be killed to capture one young chimpanzee. A. Kortlandt, "Chimpanzee Ecology and Laboratory Management," *Laboratory Primate Newsletter,* 1966, 5(3), 1–11.

12. This alternative method of chimp capture is described in Gilbert Rollais's only published article: "Notes sur la capture des chimpanzés," *Service des Eaux et Forêts, Chasse et Pêche, Bull.* (Belgian Congo), 1959, 6(24), 595–602.

13. Most of the modern charts drawn up by primatologists fail to show any *Pan paniscus* in the area due south of Kisangani and east of the Lomami River. But until recently, at least, there were many to be found there, as confirmed not only by Gilbert Rollais but also by zoologist Sinclair Dunnett, a member of the Zaire River Expedition of 1974/5.

14. For the sake of the chimpanzees, it seems prudent to withhold such details from the present text. There are plans afoot to mount an expedition to these areas, so that specimens for SIV studies can be procured.

15. Discussion by G. Courtois at the end of his article "Apes," in *Primates in Medicine;* see p. 85.

16. Rollais said the locals from this part of Africa called a chimpanzee *nyama,* which is the Kiswahili and Lingala word for both "animal" and "meat." However, there are certainly many African peoples who will not eat chimpanzee (or even monkey) meat, considering it "too human."

CHAPTER 44: *The Belgian Vaccine*

1. *BMJ* 58.

2. S. A. Plotkin, H. Koprowski et al., "Intratypic Serodifferentiation of Polioviruses," *Virol.,* 1961, 15, 473–485. The full name of the pool ("De Somer") is given in another paper by Plotkin, namely: "Factors Influencing a Successful Vaccination with Live Polio Virus," *6th International Congress on Biological Standardization* (Wiesbaden, 1960), (Berlin: HoffmannVerlag, 1961), pp. 48–73, see Table 5.

3. H. Koprowski, "Live Poliomyelitis Vaccine" (letter), *BMJ,* 1959, 1(ii), 1349–1350.

4. Abel Prinzie says that Huygelen proposed to De Somer that he could run the department more efficiently and cheaply than Lamy, and was given the chance to do so; he succeeded. Lamy left soon afterward, disillusioned.

5. This process is described in P. De Somer, A. Prinzie, M. Lamy, and N. Dufrane, "Résultats du programme de vaccination contre la poliomyélite en Belgique," *Rev. Méd. Louvain,* 1957, 21, 341–355.

6. In this brief statement, Peetermans was effectively contradicting both of the points that his then-boss, Monique Lamy, had made to me. RIT had both manufactured Koprowski's vaccines — and tested them and found them safe (otherwise they would undoubtedly not have released them).

7. However, De Somer might have felt that making vaccine free of charge would stand RIT in good stead, should the Koprowski strains ever be licensed. Koprowski had told me in interview that Wyeth had manufactured the Polish vaccine for no fee.

8. F. Przesmycki et al., "Vaccination against Poliomyelitis in Poland with Types 1 and 3 Attenuated Viruses of Koprowski," *Bull. WHO,* 1962, 26, 733–743. When speaking to

Peetermans, I forgot that Koprowski had already told me that Wyeth of Pennsylvania had produced the vaccines used in Poland.

CHAPTER 45: *The Threats Begin*

1.  I closed the letter by stating that I had also made copies of the tapes of the first interview, but that since Sprague had not included these in his request, I would wait to hear from him about these.

2.  S. A. Plotkin, B. J. Cohen, and H. Koprowski, "Intratypic Serodifferentiation of Polioviruses," *Virol.*, 1961, 15, 473–485.

3.  Osterrieth went on to write that if he had said that he had used chimp kidneys for tissue culture during our first meeting, then "it was an error, perhaps due to a misunderstanding of the question." He was wrong — for he had never said this, and I had not claimed that he had.

4.  Certainly only one previous letter from Sprague had arrived at my house, not two separate letters on behalf of Koprowski and Plotkin, as he claimed. Surprisingly, it had been sent in the open mail, rather than by special delivery requiring a signature on receipt.

5.  J. Cribb, *The White Death* (Sydney: Angus and Robertson, 1996), p. 187.

6.  This claim, which had featured in my second interview with Koprowski, had also featured an unpublished manuscript by Blaine Elswood entitled "Origins: The Beginning of the AIDS Pandemic," dated April 30, 1995. On page 4, Elswood writes: "All records of Koprowski's Congo vaccine field tests, including records of the preparation of the vaccine at the Wistar Institute, have been 'lost in a move' according to sworn declarations submitted to attorneys in a concluded legal matter (Koprowski vs. Straight Arrow Publications, et al.)."

7.  See, for instance, G. Lecatsas and J. J. Alexander, "Safe Testing of Poliovirus Vaccine and the Origin of HIV Infection in Man" (letter), *S. Af. Med. J.*, 1989, 76, 451, which states: "Most virologists would agree that 'clean cells' are for practical purposes non-existent."

8.  As it later transpired, the only CHAT protocols that the Wistar Institute was able to supply (for pools 23 and 24) applied to versions of CHAT made in the sixties. Koprowski himself, in a subsequent deposition, acknowledged that these protocols applied to the period 1961–1963. See Hilary Koprowski v. The Associated Press, deposition of Hilary Koprowski, M.D., March 27, 1996, pp. 91–92.

9.  Indeed, in the very first report of HIV (though not then called by that name) in the medical literature, the virus was grown without T-cell growth factor. See F. Barré-Sinoussi, L. Montagnier et al., "Isolation of a T-Lymphotropic Retrovirus from a Patient at Risk for Acquired Immune Deficiency Syndrome (AIDS)," *Science*, 1983, 220, 876–871.

10. Affidavit of Joseph Melnick, Ph.D., October 25, 1993, Koprowski vs. Straight Arrow Publishers Inc., Civil Action No. 92-CV-743, U.S. District Court, Eastern District of Pennsylvania, p. 3.

11. M. K. Curtis, "Monkey Trials: Science, Defamation, and the Suppression of Dissent," *William and Mary Bill of Rights J.*, 1995, 4(2), 507–593.

12. Letter from Cecil H. Fox to Michael K. Curtis, January 1996.

13. Cecil Fox, personal communication, 1998.

14. R. Gallo, *Virus Hunting — AIDS, Cancer and the Human Retrovirus: A Story of Scientific Discovery* (New York: Basic Books, 1991), pp. 315 and 274–275. When comparing the

three men, Gallo described Koprowski as "the most responsive to doing laboratory experiments and . . . full of ideas and energy (he is the youngest)."

15. H. Koprowski, C. W. Saxinger, R. C. Gallo et al., "Multiple Sclerosis and Human T-Cell Lymphotropic Viruses," *Nature*, 1985, 318, 154–160.

16. "Viruses, Immunoresponse and Cancer. A Special Symposium in Honor of Hilary Koprowski," *AIDS Res. Human Retro.*, 1987, 3(suppl. 1); see the whole volume, but especially pp. v-x of the preface.

17. For further references in the literature to the Koprowski/Gallo relationship, see N. Hodgkinson, *AIDS — The Future of Contemporary Science* (London: Fourth Estate, 1996), p. 49, in which Koprowski is described as a "Gallo friend and collaborator." See also "Introduction to Annual Laboratory Meeting — 1995," *AIDS Res. Human Retro.*, 1995, 11(suppl. 1). In his introduction to this, the last of the annual lab meetings on AIDS held by the Laboratory of Human Tumor Cell Biology of the NIH, Gallo acknowledged that the highlight of these select invitation-only meetings had always been the banquet lectures, featuring "Hilary Koprowski at the piano." See also J. Seligmann, "Tracing the Origin of AIDS," *Newsweek*, May 7, 1984, pp. 62–63, which reports that "Gallo and other AIDS researchers met last week at Philadelphia's Wistar Institute for a 'brainstorming' session on AIDS therapy."

18. An accompanying sheet from Professor Albert gave very precise details of the PCR techniques used to test for HIV-1, HIV-2, and SIV. These had also included positive control samples, made by "spiking" aliquots of the vaccines with a minute amount (about 100 virions) of HIV RNA. All the original samples had tested negative for immunodeficiency virus, and all the control samples had tested positive.

19. G. Courtois, "Vaccination antipoliomyélitique par virus vivant au Congo Belge," *Ann. Soc. Belg. Méd. Trop.*, 1958, 38, 805–816.

20. M. Böttiger et al., "Vaccination with Attenuated Type 1 Poliovirus, the Chat Strain. III. Antibody Response and Spread of Virus in Schoolchildren," *Acta Paed. Scand.*, 1966, 55, 1–10.

21. Brian Mahy, personal communication, December 1994.

22. David Heymann and Julie Milstein, personal communications, July 1993.

23. Giovanni Rovera, personal communication, November 1995.

24. Meinrad Schar, personal communication, August 1993.

25. Constant Huygelen and Julian Peetermans, personal communications, May 1994.

26. S. Connor, "World's First AIDS Case Was False," *Independent* (U.K.), March 24, 1995, p. 1.

27. David Ho, personal communication, March 1994.

28. In this article, Conner stated Ho had concluded "that the authenticity of the research is not only in doubt, but that there has been either a monumental mixup or a deliberate switch of experimental material." However, Ho was apparently less positive about how the contamination had occurred than he had seemed two years earlier, for he also told Conner: "We even discussed wild ideas that someone intentionally provided us with a sample that just came from a contemporary Aids [sic] patient." There are also certain other possible explanations, as examined in E. Hooper and W. D. Hamilton, "1959 Manchester Case of Syndrome Resembling AIDS," *Lancet*, 1996, 348, 1363–1365. But as of the date of publication of this book, the question of how the contamination occurred has never been resolved.

29. S. Connor, "Admission of False Aids Case Suppressed by NHS," *Independent* (U.K.), April 6, 1995, p. 1.

30. S. A. Moore, "Academic Freedom for Aids Doctor" (letter), *Independent* (U.K.), April 26, 1995.

31. L. K. Altman, "Earliest Documented AIDS Case Is Called into Doubt," *New York Times*, April 4, 1995, pp. C1 and C3.

32. S. Connor, "New Tests to Help Solve Dispute Over 'First Aids Case,'" *Independent* (U.K.), April 10, 1995.

33. T. Zhu and D. D. Ho, "Was HIV Present in 1959?" (letter), *Nature*, 1995, 374, 503–504. For further analysis, see S. Connor, "Researchers in U.S. Dispute First Case of AIDS," *BMJ*, 1995, 310, 957.

34. The two Manchester virologists, Bailey and Corbitt, responded to Ho's letter in January 1996 (A. S. Bailey and G. Corbitt, "Was HIV Present in 1959?" [letter], *Lancet*, 1996, 347, 189). Their letter stated that the Forensic Science Service had not found evidence to support Ho's claim that tissues from more than one individual had been involved, but they seconded Ho's finding that the HIV-1 they had isolated had to be modern. They stated that the most likely source of contamination was from within their own laboratory, but rejected suggestions that the results had been "in some way synthesised," adding that the work had been done in good faith. This, of course, begged further questions, such as why only the patient samples and not those from the control had tested positive in a double-blind study. These were examined in E. Hooper and W. D. Hamilton, "1959 Manchester Case of Syndrome Resembling AIDS."

35. David Ho, personal communication, June 1995.

36. Steve Connor, personal communication, 1996.

CHAPTER 46: *Alexandre Jezierski*

1. A. Jezierski and J. P. Delville, "Sensibilité de divers animaux à un virus neurotrope isolé des selles d'un enfant presumé atteint de poliomyélite," *Ann. Soc. Belge Méd. Trop.*, 1950, 30, 479–482.

2. G. Barski and P. Lépine, "Recherche des anticorps neutralisants de la poliomyélite chez les Africains (noirs et pygmés) du Congo Belge," *Bull. WHO*, 1956, 14, 119–128.

3. A. Jezierski, "Action cytopathogène des trois prototypes de virus de la poliomyélite *in vitro* sur les tissus de differentes espèces de singes d'Afrique centrale. Non receptivité des tissus de certains animaux," *Ann. Inst. Past.*, 1955, 89, 78–82.

4. A. Jezierski, "Preparation du serum contre la poliomyélite sur l'âne. Séparation de l'immuno-gamma-globuline et sa valeur," *Ann. Inst. Past.*, 1955, 89, 206–215.

5. A. Jezierski, "Immunisation active des singes contre la poliomyélite au moyen d'un vaccin formolé et d'un vaccin vivant," *Bull. Soc. Pathol. Exot.*, 1955, 48, 79–89. The paper featured the following observation: "It must be pointed out that the tissue culture technique is an extremely important method presenting unlimited possibilities, particularly in the field of research, because it can be applied to a number of different problems such as the isolation, identification and multiplication of viruses."

6. Later, the Sabin strains were apparently passaged in both cynomolgus and rhesus MKTC. See J. L. Melnick, "Live Attenuated Poliovirus Vaccines," in S. A. Plotkin and E. A. Mortimer (editors), *Vaccines* (Philadelphia: W. B. Saunders, 1994), pp. 155–204.

7. Interestingly, Salk himself does not seem to have identified in his articles the species of monkey he used for culturing poliovirus — but it was widely known to be rhesus, and was so described in the articles of several contemporaries, including Jezierski.

8. H. Koprowski, G. A. Jervis, T. W. Norton, and K. Pfeister, "Adaptation of Type 1 Strain of Poliomyelitis Virus to Mice and Cotton Rats," *Proc. Soc. Exp. Biol. Med.,* 1954, 86, 244–247.

9. A. Jezierski, "Attenuation des trois types de virus de la poliomyélite sur les tissus de singes de l'espèce Colobus. Virus vivants modifiés et leur application par différentes voies sur les singes," *Ann. Soc. Belg. Méd. Trop.,* 1959, 39, 69–96.

10. H. Koprowski, G. A. Jervis, and T. W. Norton, "Oral Administration of Poliomyelitis Virus to Man and Ape: A Comparative Study," *Proc. Natl. Acad. Sci.,* 1954, 40(1), 36–39; H. Koprowski, G. A. Jervis, and T. W. Norton, "Oral Administration of a Rodent-Adapted Strain of Poliomyelitis Virus to Chimpanzees," *Arch. Ges. Virusforsch.,* 1954, 5(5), 413–424.

11. A. Jezierski, "Destruction of Poliovirus in the Digestive Tract of Chimpanzees by Means of Specific High-Titre Gamma-Globulin," *Ann. Soc. Belge Méd. Trop.,* 1960, 40, 169–172; see also discussion by J. Mortelmans, P. Brutsaert, and A. Jezierski, pp. 172–181. The paper makes it clear that Jezierski had experimented on at least twenty chimps. At least four were fed virulent virus, and the rest were fed attenuated strains.

12. Brutsaert visited an INEAC establishment during that visit, which may well have been Jezierski's lab at Gabu.

13. Another ten primates were donated by Jezierski to the Virus Research Institute at Entebbe, Uganda. East African Virus Research Institute, Entebbe, Annual Report No. 8, 1957–1958, p. 44.

14. Bror Morein, personal communication, 1993.

15. V. Turco, A. Jezierski, G. R. Scott, T. J. Wiktor et al., "La vaccination anti-pestique dans la lutte contre la peste bovine," *Bull. Agricole de Congo Belge,* 1957, 48(4), 935–980. See also G. R. Scott, "Impressions of the 1954 Rinderpest Outbreak in the Belgian Congo," *Bull. of Epizootic Diseases of Africa,* 1954, 2, 399–400.

16. East African Veterinary Research Organization, annual report 1954–1955, East African High Commission (Nairobi, Kenya), 1955, pp. 14–15.

17. Koprowski's speech of January 30, 1957, was described as having been about "the present position on the use of living attenuated virus for immunisation against poliomyelitis" in the honorary secretary's report (1957) to the AGM of the British Medical Association (Kenya branch), March 22, 1958.

18. Gordon Scott, personal communications, 1996. (In the end, of course, Koprowski conducted his vaccine field trial just over a year later, in Congo and Burundi, when he fed CHAT to 215,000 Africans.)

19. Sabena timetable, 1957, p. 15, available from the archives section at Sabena headquarters, Brussels airport.

20. Anon., "City Polio Proposal — Talks Held on Trial of New Vaccine in Kenya," *East African Standard* (Nairobi), February 1, 1957, p. 1.

21. Nothing about trying to make tissue culture from crocodile kidney is recorded in Jezierski's published papers. However, it is a credible scenario, given that he tried making cultures from the tissues of various other reptiles.

22. L. J. Lowenstine, P. Marx, M. Gardner et al., "Seroepidemiologic Survey of Captive Old-World Primates for Antibodies to Human and Simian Retroviruses, and Isolation of a Lentivirus from Sooty Mangabeys (*Cercocebus atys*)," *Intl. J. Cancer,* 1986, 38, 563–574. Lowenstine et al. identified this species as *Colobus guereza,* though the more normal scientific name is *Colobus abyssinicus abyssinicus.*

23. By coincidence, the first two epidemiological studies from the area, both conducted in 1986, one in Aru (a town one hundred miles by road to the north) and the other from

the neighboring Ugandan province of West Nile, both testify to there having been a relatively low HIV prevalence of 1.4 percent among the indigenous inhabitants. L. Aktar et
al., "Distribution of Antibodies to HIV-1 in an Urban Community (Aru, Zaire)," *3rd
International Conference on AIDS in Africa* (Naples, 1987), Abstract TH-34; J. W.
Carswell, "HIV Infection in Healthy Persons in Uganda," *AIDS*, 1987, 1, 223–227.

24. This was F. K. Sanders's trip to Gambia, when he sent back kidneys from four different
African monkeys, and they were found to provide tissue culture suitable for poliovirus
growth by, among others, Bill Wood of Glaxo.

25. "Committee on Laboratory Investigations of Poliomyelitis," Minutes of the First Meeting,
July 14, 1955, Medical Research Council document MRC.55.658 LIP.min.1.

26. The Kampala campaign is mentioned in passing in "The Poliomyelitis Research
Foundation," *Annual Report of the South African Institute for Medical Research,* 1960,
pp. 171–183. Dr. Ronald Huckstep, an orthopedic surgeon who arrived in Uganda in
February 1960 to help with polio cases, has confirmed that "a very limited vaccination
scheme" (presumably with the South African OPV) was in operation at the time of his
arrival (letter of September 1995).

27. E. D. Cooper et al., "Problems Resulting from the Use of Live Attenuated Poliomyelitis
Virus Type 1 in a Mass Campaign in a Large Urban Area," *S. Af. Med. J.,* 1960, 1961, 35,
232–235.

28. Geoffrey Timms, personal communication, July 1995. This version of events is largely
confirmed by a subsequent review of the polio situation in Kenya, so it seems that
CHAT was never used in any open trial in that country. N. R. E. Fendall, "Poliomyelitis
in Kenya," *E. Af. Med. J.,* 1960, 37(2), 89–103. See also N. R. E. Fendall, "Poliomyelitis in
Kenya — The 1960 Epidemic and Oral Vaccine Campaign," *J. Trop. Méd. Hyg.,* 1962, 62,
245–255.

29. L. J. André and E. André-Gadras, "16 cas de poliomyélite observés dans un district de
brousse du Gabon," *Méd. Trop.,* 1958, 18, 638–641.

30. L. J. André, personal communication, July 1997.

31. "Poliomyelitis Vaccination — A Review of the Present Position at a Meeting of Experts
Convened by WHO" (Stockholm, November 21–25, 1955), Medical Research Council
document MRC.55/1013, LIP.55/11, pp. 6 and 7. Also published as WHO document
WHO/Polio/17, dated November 29, 1955.

32. Interestingly, two Belgian researchers who feature prominently in this story, Monique
Lamy and Ghislain Courtois, were also on secondment at the Pasteur at the time of
Jezierski's secondment there. Monique Lamy worked with Georges Barski on a tissue culture study involving his pygmy blood samples (G. Barski and M. Lamy, "Etude en cultures
cellulaires du virus encephalomyélitique 'Mengo,'" *Ann. Inst. Past.,* 1955, 89, 318–326),
and also cowrote another article with Barski and Lépine. Ghislain Courtois wrote an
article about the presence of yeast-like bodies in the tissues of a Guinea baboon from the
Pasteur colony in Paris (where baboons were already being used to prepare tissue culture). G. Courtois, J.-C. Levaditi et al., "Mycose cutanée à corps levuriformes observée
chez des singes Africains en captivité," *Ann. Inst. Past.,* 1955, 89, 124–127.

33. W. Janssens et al., "Phylogenetic Analysis of a New Chimpanzee Lentivirus SIVcpz-gab2
from a Wild-Captured Chimpanzee from Gabon," *AIDS Res. & Human Retro.,* 1994,
10(9), 1191–1192.

34. P. Lépine et al., "Presence apparemment insolite et conservation de microfilaires du
singe dans des cultures de tissus," *Bull. Soc. Pathol. Exot.,* 1955, 48, 838–843. See also
P. Lépine, "Sur l'antigenicité des vaccins contre la poliomyélite. Vaccins inactivés et

vaccinations par virus vivants attenués," *Bull. Acad. Natl. Méd.*, 1960, 144, 480–498; especially p. 489.

35. H. Tsujimoto et al., "Isolation and Characterization of Simian Immunodeficiency Virus from Mandrills in Africa and Its Relationship to Other Human and Simian Immuno-deficiency Viruses," *J. Virol.*, 1988, 62, 4044–4050.

36. See G. Barski, A. Jezierski, and P. Lépine, "Sensibilité au virus de la poliomyélite *in vitro* des tissus de differentes espèces de singes d'Afrique centrale. Non receptivité des tissus de certains mammifères," *Ann. Inst. Past.*, 1954, 86, 243–247 (poliovirus grown in nine species). A. Jezierski, "Action cytopathogène des trois prototypes de virus de la polio-myélite *in vitro* sur les tissus de differentes espèces de singes d'Afrique centrale. Non receptivité des tissus de certains animaux," *Ann. Inst. Past.*, 1955, 89, 78–82 (six species). G. D. Hsiung and J. L. Melnick, "Comparative Susceptibility of Kidney Cells from Different Monkey Species to Enteric Viruses (Poliomyelitis, Coxsackie, and ECHO Groups)," *J. Immunol.*, 1957, 78, 136–146 (thirteen species — plus three cited by Jezierski). Several reports claim that capuchin monkeys from South America are not susceptible to poliovirus, but one disagrees: A. S. Kaplan, "Comparison of Susceptible and Resistant Cells to Infection with Poliomyelitis Virus," *Ann. N.Y. Acad. Sci.*, 1955, 61(4), 830–839. See also P. Lépine et al., "Presence apparemment insolite et conservation de microfilaires du singe dans des cultures de tissus," *Bull. Soc. Pathol. Exot.*, 1955, 48, 838–843 (one species).

CHAPTER 47: *The HIV-2 Enigma*

1. As mentioned previously, Pascal's explanation for HIV-2 involved an immunization trial with a yellow fever vaccine (17E) in Brazil in 1936, which had included monkey hyperimmune serum from rhesus monkeys (F. L. Soper, H. H. Smith, "Yellow Fever Vaccination with Cultivated Virus and Immune and Hyperimmune Serum," *Am. J. Trop. Med.*, 1938, 18(2), 111–134). The theory was intriguing, not least because early versions of a similar yellow fever vaccine had been contaminated with hepatitis virus, a disas-trous event that had been investigated by, among others, Edwin Lennette of the Yellow Fever Research Service of Rio and Karl Meyer of the G. W. Hooper Foundation. (See, for instance, W. A. Sawyer, K. F. Meyer et al., "Jaundice in Army Personnel in the Western Region of the United States and Its Relation to Vaccination against Yellow Fever [Parts 2, 3, and 4]," *Am. J. Hyg.*, 1944, 40, 35–107; see also related articles referenced in end-notes.) Nonetheless, for the hypothesis to make sense for HIV-2, the rhesus monkeys involved in making 17E would first have had to have been contaminated with an SIV from sooty mangabeys — and there is no evidence that the latter species was even pres-ent in the United States, where the vaccine was made, in the thirties. Furthermore, one would then have to explain how the presence of HIV-2 was confirmed in Brazil only in 1991, whereas it clearly emerged decades earlier in another Lusophone country on the other side of the Atlantic — Guinea-Bissau. To me, Pascal's HIV-2/yellow fever vaccine theory seemed implausible.

2. E. Hooper, "The Proof of the Pudding," December 1994 (unpublished manuscript sent to Bill Hamilton, Brian Martin and Louis Pascal for comment).

3. F. Barin, F. Denis, and J. S. Allan, "Serological Evidence for Virus Related to Simian T-Lymphotropic Retrovirus III in Residents of West Africa," *Lancet*, 1985, 2(ii), 1387–1389.

4.  F. Clavel et al., "Isolation of a New Human Retrovirus from West African Patients with AIDS," *Science*, 1986, 233, 343–346.

5.  P. J. Kanki and K. M. De Cock, "Epidemiology and Natural History of HIV-2," *AIDS*, 1994, 8 (suppl.1), S85-S93.

6.  K. M. De Cock, F. Brun-Vezinet et al., "HIV-1 and HIV-2 Infections and AIDS in West Africa," *AIDS*, 1991, 5 (suppl.1), S21–S28.

7.  HIV/AIDS Surveillance Database, U.S. Bureau of the Census, June 1996 issue.

8.  R. T. Espejo et al., untitled letter to the editor, *N. Engl. J. Med.*, 1989, 321(12), 830–831, plus letters following by T. R. O'Brien and D. D. Ho, on pp. 831–832. On the basis of this research, I have taken "dual reactivity" to equate with HIV-1 infection in this analysis.

9.  Data obtained from Table 2 in K. M. De Cock et al., "HIV-1 and HIV-2 Infections and AIDS in West Africa," and from HIV/AIDS Surveillance Database, U.S. Department of Commerce, Bureau of the Census, 1991 issue. Using this method, the percentage of AIDS attributable to HIV-2 in the West African region in 1990 varied from Ghana, at 12 percent, to Guinea-Bissau, at 100 percent.

10. B. Le Guenno et al., "HIV-1 and HIV-2: Two Ancient Viruses for a New Disease?" (letter), *Trans. R. Soc. Trop. Med. Hyg.*, 1989, 83, 847. See also Y. Robin et al., "Les arbovirus en Côte d'Ivoire. Enquête sérologique dans la population humaine," *Bull. Soc. Pathol. Exot.*, 1968, 61, 833–845. Sassandra region is a credible venue for a first sighting of HIV-2 in that there is a very mobile population of hired workers in rural areas, and HIV prevalence among women born in Sassandra subprefecture has been recorded as a worrying 16.1 percent (compared to 6.1 percent among those born in Sassandra town). B. Soro, J.-L. Rey et al., "L'infection par le VIH chez les femmes en âge de procréer à Sassandra (Côte d'Ivoire)," *Cahiers Santé*, 1993, 3, 31–36.

11. Le Guenno identified bands typical for *gag, pol*, and *env* on Western blot, and confirmed the findings through peptide analysis. In December 1994, he wrote me: "I have diagnosed many HIV-2 patients (confirmed by clinical and immunological evolution) during the years spent in Dakar, and the Western blot pattern of the 2 Ivorian sera was identical to those sera."

12. See A. H. Booth, "The Zoogeography of West African Primates: A Review," *Bull. IFAN*, 1958, 20A(2), 587–622, especially pp. 604–605. C. Tahiti-Zagret, "Les *Cercopithecidae* de Côte d'Ivoire," *Bull. IFAN*, 1976, 38A(1), 206–230, pp. especially 223–225.

13. B. Le Guenno et al., "HIV-2 Prevalence in Three Rural Regions of Senegal: Low Levels and Heterogeneous Distribution" (letter), *Trans. R. Soc. Trop. Med. Hyg.;* 1992, 86, 301–302. Further details from Bernard Le Guenno, personal communication, February 1995.

14. The official figures for Guinea-Bissan refugees in Casamance in 1971 were 55,000, but the true total was believed to run into six figures.

15. In 1973, the French zoologist A. R. Dupuy declared that the sooty mangabey "probably" lived in the tiny Basse-Casamance national park — because it was suitable terrain. The park is situated ten miles to the east of Kabrousse. (See A. R. Dupuy, "Premier inventaire des mammifères du Parc National de Basse Casamance (Senegal)," *Bull. IFAN*, 1973, 35A(1), 186–197.) However, the only positive sightings of live sooty mangabeys in Senegal occurred in December 1969 in the Bissine Forest, some sixty miles east of Kabrousse by road. (See T. T. Struhsaker, "Notes on *Cercocebus a. atys* in Senegal, West Africa," *Mammalia*, 1971, 35, 343–344.)

16. M. Kawamura, M. Hayami et al.; "HIV-2 in West Africa in 1966" (letter), *Lancet*, 1989, 1(i), 385.

17. Altogether 84 sera were positive by ELISA, but 74 of these were not confirmed by Western blot. Forty-eight of these presented only core but not envelope proteins of HIV, and the writers suggested that the serum donors "probably lost their antibody response to *env* proteins about the stage of AIDS development or had been infected with another virus related to HIV." However, these nonspecific reactions are fairly common in Africa, and are normally viewed simply as false positives.

18. The *Lancet* letter merely stated: "Specific antibody to *env* products of HIV-2 was detected in 10 sera," which might mean that a single *env* protein typical of HIV-2 was considered sufficient. By 1991, however, it was widely accepted that at least two *env* bands were needed for HIV-2 confirmation. (See K. M. De Cock et al., "HIV-1 and HIV-2 Infections and AIDS in West Africa," p. S22.) In May 1995, Dr. Masanori Hayami, a coauthor of the paper, wrote to me to say that he had been unable to locate either the original sera or the Western blot data. He added: "I believe that most of them [the ten sera], but not all of them, are truly HIV-2 positive." However, because we cannot be sure which are, and which are not, it is not safe to accept any of these purported HIV-2-positive sera as "confirmed sightings."

19. One doctor suggested to me that the frequent electricity cuts experienced in Guinea-Bissau meant that few archival sera had survived in freezers. However, more than nine thousand sera from different ethnic groups in Portuguese Guinea were collected in 1957/8 by scientists from the Institute of Tropical Medicine in Lisbon. (See C. Trincao et al., "A Survey of Abnormal Hemoglobins in Portuguese Guinea," *Nature*, 1960, 185, 326–327.) If these samples still exist, they could provide a fascinating insight into the prehistory of HIV-2 in the country (though I was unable to locate them during a visit to Lisbon in 1997).

20. In addition to other references cited in this section, see J. Botas et al., "HIV-2 Infection: Some Clinical and Epidemiological Aspects in Portugal," *5th International Conference on AIDS* (Montreal, 1989), abstract M.A.P.77.

21. The exception is a bisexual French sailor who frequently visited West Africa during the first five years of the seventies. D. Boudart et al., "Serological Evidence of Successive HIV-2 and HIV-1 Infection in a Bisexual Man," *AIDS*, 1992, 6, 593.

22. "Immunodeficiency and Cryptosporidiosis" (Clinicopathological Conference), *BMJ*, 1980, 281, 1123–1127; see Dr. Bryceson's contribution on p. 1126.

23. A. Bryceson et al., "HIV-2-Associated AIDS in the 1970s" (letter), *Lancet*, 1988, 2(i), 221.

24. A. G. Saimot et al., "HIV-2/LAV-2 in Portuguese Man with AIDS (Paris, 1978) Who Had Served in Angola in 1968–74," *Lancet*, 1987, 1(i), 688. The patient was admitted to hospital in Paris in 1978, and was often included in lists of early (HIV-1-related) AIDS cases before it was realized that he had been infected with HIV-2.

25. N. Burin des Roziers, L. Montagnier et al., "Infection par le virus HIV-2 avec longue période d'incubation," *Presse Méd.*, 1987, 16(39), 1981.

26. R. Ancelle et al., "Long Incubation Period for HIV-2 Infection" (letter), *Lancet*, 1987, 1(i), 688–689.

27. G. Dufoort et al., "No Clinical Signs 14 Years after HIV-2 Transmission after Blood Transfusion" (letter), *Lancet*, 1988, 2(i), 510.

28. There could have been more, however, since one paper described fifteen men from northern Portugal who had become infected with HIV-2 after serving in West Africa (which was defined as "Guinea Bissau and Angola"). A. Mota-Miranda et al., "HIV-2 Infection in the North of Portugal," 9th International Conference on AIDS (Berlin, 1993), Abstract PO-C09–2798.

29. It is not recorded that any of the infectees were gay, but if they were then clearly the number of transmission steps can be reduced accordingly.

30. M. O. Santos-Ferreira, L. Montagnier et al., "A Study of Seroprevalence of HIV-1 and HIV-2 in Six Provinces of People's Republic of Angola: Clues to the Spread of HIV Infection," *J. AIDS*, 1990, 3, 780–786.

31. Interestingly, the only Mozambican province in which HIV-2 prevalence was less than 1 percent, Pemba, is one of only two provinces that were taken by the liberation movement, FRELIMO, in 1966, and held until independence in 1975. (Notes taken by Wilson Carswell from a poster shown at the 3rd International Conference on AIDS and Associated Cancers in Africa [Arusha, 1988].) The poster was not included in the abstracts volume, but may have involved the same study as that reported in 1989: F. De la Cruz, "HIV in Mozambique, a General Overview," 5th International Conference on AIDS (Montreal, 1989), Th.G.P.22.

32. A paper describing this as the first HIV-2 epidemic outside Africa emphasizes the fact that Portugal used to move African troops from one territory to another (including Goa) during the sixties. H. Rubsamen-Waigmann et al., "High Proportion of HIV-2 and HIV1/2 Double-Reactive Sera in Two Indian States, Maharashta and Goa: First Appearance of an HIV-2 Epidemic Along with an HIV-1 Epidemic Outside of Africa," *Zbl. Bakt.*, 1994, 280, 398–402.

33. B. Davidson, "Portuguese-Speaking Africa," chapter 15 in M. Crowder (editor), *The Cambridge History of Africa, Volume 8 (from about 1940 to about 1975)* (Cambridge: Cambridge University Press, 1984), pp. 755–806. See also G. Chaliand, *Armed Struggle in Africa — With the Guerillas in "Portuguese" Guinea* (New York: MR, 1967), pp. ix–xvi, and 3–27.

34. A. Naucler, "HIV-2 Infection and AIDS" (thesis) (Lund, Sweden, 1991), pp. 20–30. The rural area is believed to have been in Biombo district, immediately to the west of Bissau.

35. P. A. Andreasson et al., "HIV-2 Infection in Pre-natal Women and Vertical Transmission of HIV-2 in Guinea-Bissau," 4th International Conference on AIDS and Associated Cancers in Africa (Marseilles, 1989), poster 052.

36. A. Shoumatoff, *African Madness* (New York: Knopf, 1988), p. 142.

37. P. A. Andreasson et al., "HIV-2 Infection in Pre-natal Women and Vertical Transmission of HIV-2 in Guinea-Bissau." In addition, studies conducted on pregnant women in the late eighties reported HIV-2-prevalence of between 3.5 percent and 12.3 percent in various of Bissau's suburbs. See M. Smallman-Raynor, A. Cliff, and P. Haggett, *Atlas of AIDS* (Oxford: Blackwell, 1992), pp. 312–313.

38. A. Wilkins et al., "The Epidemiology of HIV Infection in a Rural Area of Guinea-Bissau," *AIDS*, 1993, 7(8), 1119–1122.

39. See W. F. Canas Ferreira et al., "Epidemiology of HIV 1 and HIV 2 in West Africa," 3rd International Conference on AIDS and Associated Cancers in Africa (Arusha, 1988), TP6. J. Piedade, W. F. Canas Ferreira et al., "Seroprevalence and Risk Factors Associated with HIV Infection in Guinea-Bissau," 7th International Conference on AIDS in Africa (Yaoundé, 1992), TP072. The latter reference reveals that overall prevalence was HIV-2 only (8.2 percent), HIV-1 only (0.2 percent), and dually reactive (0.8 percent), making a total HIV prevalence of 9.2 percent. Another survey found HIV-2 prevalence of over 10 percent in two other villages in late 1985, see F. Antunes et al., "HIV Infection in Rural Areas of West Africa (Guinea Bissau)," 3rd International Conference on AIDS (Washington, D.C., 1987), Abstract THP.88.

40. See HIV/AIDS Surveillance Database, U.S. Dept. of Commerce, Bureau of the Census, June 1996, which cites results from the individual areas. All twelve sampling points mentioned had at least three HIV-2-positive persons, and one, Galomaro, in the Bafata area, had nineteen, with a HIV-2-prevalence of over 26 percent.

41. As with the Kawamura paper earlier, we cannot be certain whether one protein band or two was considered sufficient confirmation on Western blot. (Nowadays, two are required.) In 1997, the lead author on most of these papers, Wanda Canas Ferreira, told me that she herself could no longer remember.

42. J. M. Amat-Roze et al., "La géographie de l'infection par les virus de l'immunodéficiencé humaine (VIH) en Afrique noire: mise en evidence de facteurs d'épidémisation et de régionalisation," *Bull. Soc. Pathol. Exot.,* 1990, 83, 137–148.

43. See HIV/AIDS Surveillance Database for Senegal. Further detailed analysis featured in P. Kanki et al., "Prevalence and Risk Determinants of Human Immunodeficiency Virus Type 2 (HIV-2) and Human Immunodeficiency Virus Type 1 (HIV-1) in West African Female Prostitutes," *Am. J. Epidem.,* 1992, 136(7), 895–907.

44. For further helpful discussion and a map, see M. Smallman-Raynor et al., *Atlas of AIDS,* pp. 310–312.

45. Immigration policy in Nigeria (which contains almost a quarter of the total population of sub-Saharan Africa) changed again in the late eighties, and prevalences of both HIV-1 and HIV-2 in blood donors and hospital patients all increased two- to fourfold between 1989 and 1990. See O. D. Olaleye et al., "Prevalence of Human Immunodeficiency Virus Types 1 and 2 Infections in Nigeria," *J. Infect. Dis.,* 1993, 167, 710–714.

46. Taking the West African region as a whole, less Nigeria (which, because of its huge population and low AIDS incidence, would otherwise skew the results), Liberia has fourteen times fewer HIV-2-related AIDS cases than the regional average, Sierra Leone five times, and Guinea-Conakry three times. Sources K. M. De Cock et al., "HIV-1 and HIV-2 Infections and AIDS in West Africa," and HIV/AIDS Surveillance Database, U.S. Dept. of Commerce, Bureau of the Census, 1991 issue.

47. F. Gao, P. M. Sharp, B. H. Hahn et al., "Human Infection by Genetically Diverse SIVsm-Related HIV-2 in West Africa," *Nature,* 1992, 358, 495–499.

48. D. D. Ho et al.; "HIV-2 in Los Angeles" (letter), *AIDS,* 1990, 4, 1301–1302.

49. F. Gao, P. M. Sharp, B. H. Hahn et al., "Genetic Diversity of Human Immunodeficiency Virus Type 2: Evidence for Distinct Sequence Subtypes with Differences in Virus Biology," *J. Virol.,* 1994, 68(11), 7433–7447. Plus Paul Sharp, personal communications, July and September 1995.

50. See, for instance, Y. Li, R. C. Desrosiers et al., "Genetic Diversity of Simian Immunodeficiency Virus," *J. Med. Primatol.,* 1989, 18, 261–269; and M. Smallman-Raynor et al., *Atlas of AIDS,* p. 134. An incorrect map, which places sooties in Guinea-Bissau, features in F. Kirchoff, G. Hunsmann et al., "Genomic Diversity of an HIV-2 from a German AIDS Patient Probably Infected in Mali," *AIDS,* 1990, 4(9), 847–857.

51. Two reports claim that the two *Cercocebus torquatus* subspecies have been identified in the relatively small area lying between the Nzo and Sassandra rivers, and there is some evidence that limited interbreeding may have occurred in this zone. A. H. Booth, "The Zoogeography of West African Primates," especially pp. 604–605. C. Tahiti-Zagret, "Les *Cercopithecidae* de Côte d'Ivoire," especially pp. 223–225.

52. K. Tonomaga, M. Hayami et al., "Isolation and Characterization of Simian Immunodeficiency Virus from African White-Crowned Mangabey Monkeys (*Cercocebus torquatus lunulatus*)," *Arch. Virol.,* 1993, 129, 77–92.

53. P. M. Sharp, D. L. Robertson, B. H. Hahn et al., "Cross-Species Transmission and Re-combination of 'AIDS' Viruses," *Philos. Trans. R. Soc. London (Biol.)*, 1995, 349, 41–47.

54. T. T. Struhsaker, "Notes on *Cercocebus a. atys* in Senegal, West Africa." In 1997, I spoke with Gerard Wartraux, a zoologist and zookeeper who had spent twenty years living in Casamance; he told me that in that time he had seen a sooty mangabey only once (between 1980 and 1982), just to the south of the Bissine Forest.

55. A. R. Dupuy, "Premier inventaire des mammifères du Parc National de Basse Casamance (Senegal)." See also A. R. Dupuy, "State actuel des primates au Senegal."

56. F. Frade et al., "Trabalho de missão zoologica da Guiné. Relatorio e contribuicão para o conhecimento da fauna da Guiné-Portuguesa," *Anais da Junta de Investigacoes Colonais,* 1946, I, 261–415.

57. B. Limoges (editor), *Résultats de l'inventaire faunique au niveau naturel et propositions de modifications à la loi sur la chasse* [CECI (Canada)/IUCN (Switzerland), 1989], pp. 15–22 and 98. A further investigation by an IUCN team in southern Guinea-Bissau in late 1997 found no traces of the sooty mangabey. E. Féron, personal communication, 1998.

58. M.-J. Robillard (editor), *Utilisation et perception de la faune et du milieu naturel en Guinea-Bissau* (CECI/IUCN, 1989), pp. 46–58.

59. A. Gessain, R. C. Gallo et al., "Low Degree of Human T-Cell Leukemia/Lymphoma Virus Type 1 Genetic Drift In Vivo as a Means of Monitoring Viral Transmission and Move-ment of Ancient Populations," *J. Virol.,* 1992, 66(4), 2288–2295. This article illustrates that an HTLV-1 isolate from Guinea-Bissau was "virtually identical" to others from the French West Indies, Haiti, and South America, indicating that the virus probably crossed the Atlantic with the slave trade.

60. Most of these Brazilian slaves originated from present-day Guinea-Bissau and Angola.

61. E. Cortes, D. Ho et al., "HIV-1, HIV-2, and HTLV-1 Infection in High-Risk Groups in Brazil," *N. Engl. J. Med.,* 1989, 320(15), 953–958.

62. D. Caussy, W. A. Blattner et al., "Changes in HIV-2 Seroprevalence in Cape Verde, West Africa," *J. AIDS,* 1993, 6(4), 432–433. In the year of the first survey, 1963, a massive Portuguese military base was established on the islands, a stopover point for those trav-eling to and from the African wars. Knowing what we do about the early epidemiology of HIV-2, it could be that HIV-2 arrived on Cape Verde soon after.

63. Neither was there any evidence of HIV infection in Liberia until the latter half of the eighties; 593 sera collected from workers on plantations and mines in 1973, and 2,000 collected from plantation workers in 1986, all subsequently proved to be negative for HIV on ELISA and Western blot assays (though it is possible that these early assays might have failed to pick up HIV-2 infections). A prostitute who died of TB in 1986, and one person tested in 1987 (out of 241 persons thought to be at high risk) were the first two confirmed seropositives in Liberia. See E. Mintz et al., "A Serological Study of HIV Infection in Liberia," *J. AIDS,* 1988, 1, 67–68.

64. J. Hudgens and R. Trillo, *West Africa — the Rough Guide* (London: Rough Guides, 1993), pp. 538 and 552.

65. These include a transfer of SIVagm to the yellow baboon (*Papio hamadryas cyno-cephalus*) in the wild in Tanzania (M. J. Jin, R. C. Desrosiers, P. M. Sharp, B. H. Hahn et al., "Infection of a Yellow Baboon with Simian Immunodeficiency Virus from African Green Monkeys: Evidence for Cross-Species Transmission in the Wild," *J. Virol.,* 1994, 68(12), 8454–8460), and of SIVagm to *Cercocebus torquatus lunulatus* in the primate colony in Kenya (either through fighting, or artificially — through the reuse of a con-taminated needle).

66. C. and H. Boesch, "Hunting Behavior of Wild Chimpanzees in the Tai National Park," *Am. J. Phys. Anthropol.*, 1989, 78, 547–573.

67. P. N. Fultz et al., "Transient Increases in Numbers of Infectious Cells in an HIV-Infected Chimpanzee Following Immune Stimulation," *AIDS Res. Hum. Retro.*, 1992, 8(2), 313–317.

68. For example: S. W. Barnett, J. A. Levy et al., "An AIDS-Like Condition Induced in Baboons by HIV-2," *Science*, 1994, 266, 642–646; B. A. Castro, J. A. Levy et al., "Persistent Infection of Baboons and Rhesus Monkeys with Different Strains of HIV-2," *Virol.*, 1991, 184, 219–226.

69. It is also relevant to mention that many local Moslems have up to four wives, meaning there is less sexual networking outside marriage, and less opportunity for the unbridled spread of HIV.

70. A.-G. Poulsen, P. Aaby, F. Dias et al., "HIV-2 in People over 50 Years in Bissau: Prevalence and Risk Factors," 8th International Conference on AIDS (Amsterdam, 1992), poster PoC 4032, full text kindly provided by Dr. Poulsen.

71. The Portuguese and PAIGC sides gave very different versions of who controlled which areas. But for a good idea of their relative holdings in 1967 and 1973, see M. J. Glantz, "The War of the Maps: Portugal vs PAIGC," *Pan-Af. J.*, 1973, 6(3), 285–296 (especially the maps on pp. 290 and 294). This article compares the two sides' claims with commendable balance, and finds those of the PAIGC more tenable. Glantz's findings are largely supported by the map in B. Davidson, *The Liberation of Guinea* (London: Penguin, 1969).

72. These seventeen are Bissau city and its suburbs, Caio, São Domingos, Djugul, and Ingoré (in Cacheu district to the northwest), Cupedo (in Biombo district, west of Bissau), Bubaque (in Bolama district — the offshore islands), Bafata, Bambadinca, Bricama, Xitole, and Galomaro (in Bafata district in the center of the country), Gabú, Paunca, Sonaco, and Pirada (in Gabú district in the east), and Catio (in Tombali district in the south). I have been unable to confirm that Djugul, Bricama, and Xitole were Portuguese garrisons, but they seem likely to have been. The other fourteen were definitely under Portuguese control.

73. See B. Davidson, *The Liberation of Guinea*, pp. 104–105, for more details of Arnando Schultz and his "strategic hamlets" policy.

74. Schultz and Spinola apparently received military advice, materiel, and bombers from the United States, and borrowed many of the disastrous counterinsurgency tactics that had been employed in Vietnam and Cambodia. See, for instance, A. J. Venter, *Portugal's Guerilla War — The Campaign for Africa* (Cape Town: John Malherbe Pty, 1973), pp. 176–178.

75. Basil Davidson, personal communication, April 1997.

76. B. Davidson, *No Fist Is Big Enough to Hide the Sky* (London: Zed Press, 1981), pp. 13–14.

77. A. J. Venter, *Portugal's Guerilla War — The Campaign for Africa*, pp. 124–143 and 63.

78. A.-G. Poulsen et al., "Prevalence of and Mortality from Human Immunodeficiency Virus Type 2 in Bissau, West Africa," *Lancet*, 1989, 1(ii), 827–830.

79. In women of childbearing age in Abidjan, HIV-2 peaks among thirty- to thirty-nine-year-olds (K. M. De Cock et al., "Epidemiology and Transmission of HIV-2," *JAMA*, 1993, 270(17), 2083–2086). In hospitalized patients it peaks among forty to forty-nine-year-olds (K. M. De Cock et al., "A Comparison of HIV-1 and HIV-2 Infections in Hospitalized Patients in Abidjan, Côte d'Ivoire," *AIDS*, 1990, 4, 443–448).

80. One factor that has to be taken into account, however, is "survivor bias": doctors can only investigate those patients who are still alive.

81. Guinea, Angola, and Mozambique were officially reclassified from colony to overseas territory in 1951. Indeed, part of the reason for Portugal's decision to reclassify her African colonies was to reduce international and U.N. monitoring of what was going on there. See B. Davidson in M. Crowder, *The Cambridge History of Africa, Volume 8 (from about 1940 to about 1975)*, p. 763.

82. With smallpox, for instance, the official Final Report on Smallpox Eradication does not include figures for Guinea-Bissau. However, the local report for the West African region does record that 200,000 smallpox jabs were administered between 1967 and 1971 — which indicates very poor coverage, with less than a quarter of the population being inoculated.

83. A. Garrett, "A immunizacão contra a poliomielite," *Portugal Medico*, 1955, 39(6), 327–349. Lépine's virology unit at the Pasteur and the Institute of Tropical Medicine in Lisbon later collaborated on a polio serosurvey in Cape Verde; it is not known if this was ever followed up by a vaccination campaign. See J. C. De Sousa, "Contribution à l'étude de la poliomyélite dans les îles du Cap-Vert," *Ann. Inst. Past.*, 1960, 99, 202–209.

84. A. Sampaio, "Progressos recentes no estudo da poliomielite e sua profilaxia," *Bol. Serv. Saúde Publica*, 1962, 8(4), 465–485.

85. F. A. Goncalves Ferreira, "Vacinas vivas contra a poliomielite," *Portugal Medico*, 1960, 44(2), 75–96.

86. A. B. de Castro Soares, "Vaccination against poliomyelitis in Portugal," 9th Conference of the European Association Against Poliomyelitis (Stockholm, 1963), 58–62.

87. M. de L. da Silva Ferreira, "L'évolution de la poliomyélite en Angola," *Arch. Franc. Pediatr.;* 1959, 16, 780–789.

88. G. D. Hsiung, "Comparative Susceptibility of Kidney Cultures Derived from Different Animal Species to Enteric Viruses," 6th International Congresses on Tropical Medicine and Malaria (Lisbon, September 1958), pp. 346–347.

89. G. D. Hsiung and J. L. Melnick, "Comparative Susceptibility of Kidney Cultures from Different Monkey Species to Enteric Viruses (Poliomyelitis, Coxsackie and Echo Groups)," *J. Immunol.*, 1957, 78, 137–146.

90. A paper about IPV in the main Portuguese medical journal in 1957 revealed that the writer was aware that the *Cercocebus* family was sensitive to poliovirus — and this was even before the Melnick/Hsiung paper had appeared. See J. G. Lacorte, "A poliomielite e a vacina Salk," *Portugal Medico*, 1957, 41(5), 273–288.

91. J. H. Wolfheim, *Primates of the World* (Seattle: University of Washington Press, 1983), pp. 356–360. By contrast the Diana monkey was already, by 1956, defined as rare in Sierra Leone, Liberia, and Ivory Coast (pp. 381–384).

CHAPTER 48: *Infection by Mouth*

1. According to the philosopher of science Karl Popper, a theory — to be scientific — must be falsifiable. By this criterion at least, the natural transfer theory is unscientific.

2. W.-H. Li and P. Sharp, "Rates and Dates of Divergence between AIDS Virus Nucleotide Sequences," *Mol. Biol. Evol.*, 1988, 5(4), 313–330.

3. J. K. Kelly, "An Application of Population Genetic Theory to Synonymous Gene Sequence Evolution in the Human Immunodeficiency Virus (HIV)," *Genet. Res.*, 1994, 64, 1–9. This paper comes up with evolutionary rates which are within 7 percent of Li and Sharp's calculations, which would translate into a starburst date not quite two years

later — circa 1962. Also: G. Myers, "HIV: Between Past and Future," *AIDS Res. Human Retro.,* 1994, 10(11), 1317–1324.

4. P. M. Sharp, W.-H. Li, "Understanding the Origins of AIDS Viruses" (letter), *Nature,* 1988, 336, 315.

5. M. J. Jin, P. M. Sharp, B. H. Hahn et al., "Mosaic Genome Structure of Simian Immuno-deficiency Virus from West African Green Monkeys," *EMBO J.,* 1994, 13(12), 2935–2947.

6. P. Emau, P. N. Fultz et al., "Isolation from African Sykes' Monkeys (*Cercopithecus mitis*) of a Lentivirus Related to Human and Simian Immunodeficiency Viruses," *J. Virol.,* 1991, 65(4), 2135–2140.

7. F. Gao, P. M. Sharp, B. H. Hahn et al., "Genetic Diversity of Human Immunodeficiency Virus Type 2: Distinct Sequence Subtypes with Differences in Virus Biology," *J. Virol.,* 1994, 68(11), 7433–7447.

8. P. M. Sharp, F. Gao, B. H. Hahn et al., "Origins and Diversity of Human Immuno-deficiency Viruses," *AIDS,* 1994, 8(suppl. 1), S27–S42.

9. G. Lecatsas, J. J. Alexander, "Origins of HIV" (letter), *Lancet,* 1992, 339, 1427. In fact, there has never been any confirmation of the HIV-1-like nature of the South African AGM virus by PCR. Furthermore in 1995, Teresa Smit, from Lecatsas's laboratory, reported that the antibody response was now more typical of HIV-2 than HIV-1, which suggested problems with the new Western blot assay being used. T. K. Smit et al., "Simian Immunodeficiency Virus (SIVagm) in Vervet Monkeys in South Africa: A Case History," poster presented at the 5th International Congress on the Impact of Viral Diseases in the Developing World (Johannesburg, 1995). Later, Smit analyzed one of these samples by PCR and sent the products to Fergal Hill for sequencing and characterization; they turned out to be a labo-ratory contamination. (Fergal Hill, personal communication, 1996.)

10. M. J. Jin, P. M. Sharp, B. H. Hahn et al., "Infection of a Yellow Baboon with Simian Immunodeficiency Virus from African Green Monkeys: Evidence for Cross-Species Transmission in the Wild," *J. Virol.,* 1994, 68(12), 8454–8460.

11. F. Gao, B. H. Hahn et al., "Human Infection by Genetically Diverse SIVsm-Related HIV-2 in West Africa," *Nature,* 1992, 358, 495–499.

12. Albert T. White, who helped collect the samples, told me that the two new isolates, rep-resenting HIV-2 subtypes C and D, had come from workers at the giant Firestone plan-tation at Harbel, north of Monrovia, and that one of the two — he could not recall which — originated from Voinjama, in the extreme northwest of Liberia. Voinjama, he told me, was also the source of the other three HIV-2-positive sera discovered in the study, but because of the distance of this area from Monrovia, they did not have time to go back and take further samples from which virus might be isolated.

13. S. C. Knight, "Infection of Dendritic Cells with HIV Type 1," *AIDS Res. Human Retro.,* 1994, 10(12), 1591–1592. L. R. Braathen et al., "Langerhans' Cells as Primary Target Cells for HIV Infection" (letter), *Lancet,* 1987, 2(ii), 1094. The importance of both Langerhans' cells and dendritic cells was spectacularly confirmed by a paper that appeared shortly after my conversation with Hahn, which demonstrated that these were not only impor-tant targets of HIV-1 infection, but that they may play the key role in passing HIV-1 on to lymphocytes. See S. Ayehounie, R. M. Ruprecht et al., "Acutely Infected Langerhans' Cells Are More Efficient than T Cells in Disseminating HIV Type 1 to Activated T Cells Following a Short Cell-Cell Contact," *AIDS Res. Human Retro.,* 1995, 11(8), 877–884.

14. By this time, the subtypes of HIV-1 Group M had got as far as H.

15. F. Barré-Sinoussi, J. C. Chermann et al., "Resistance of AIDS Virus at Room Tempera-ture," *Lancet,* 1987, 2(i), 721–722.

16. Brian Martin of Wollongong University provided further perspective in 1997, when he explained that although it is quite usual for the burden of proof to lie with the challenger of an established theory, it is unjustifiable in this instance, because the natural transfer theory has so little supporting evidence that it cannot be considered more established or successful than the OPV theory. Therefore, there is presumably a social reason why natural transfer is assumed to be the established theory, which may be that it is less threatening to key interest groups, especially those in the medical research community.

17. P. N. Fultz et al., "Identification and Biologic Characterization of an Acutely Lethal Variant of Simian Immunodeficiency Virus from Sooty Mangabeys (SIV/SMM)," *AIDS Res. Human Retro.*, 1989, 5(4), 397–409.

18. W. A. Sawyer, K. F. Meyer et al., "Jaundice in Army Personnel in the Western Region of the United States and Its Relation to Vaccination against Yellow Fever (Parts 2, 3, and 4)," *Am. J. Hyg.*, 1944, 40, 35–107.

19. See P. N. Fultz, "Superinfection of HIV-1 Infected Chimpanzees with a Second Unrelated HIV-1," [9th] *Colloque des Cent Gardes*, 1994, 257–262.

20. Q. Wei and P. N. Fultz, "Extensive Diversification of Human Immunodeficiency Virus Type 1 Subtype B Strains during Dual Infection of a Chimpanzee That Progressed to AIDS," *J. Virol.*, 1998, 72(4), 3005–3017.

21. "The Apocalypse Bug," shown on CNN, May 20, 1995.

22. M. D. Daniel, R. C. Desrosiers et al., "Protective Effects of a Live Attenuated SIV Vaccine with a Deletion in the *nef* Gene," *Science*, 1992, 258, 1938–1941.

23. T. W. Baba, R. M. Ruprecht et al., "Pathogenicity of Live, Attenuated SIV after Mucosal Infection of Neonatal Macaques," *Science*, 1995, 267, 1820–1825.

24. M. D. Daniel, R. C. Desrosiers et al., "Protective Effects of a Live Attenuated SIV Vaccine with a Deletion in the *nef* Gene."

25. T. Curtis, "AIDS Theories" (letter), *Science*, 1993, 259, 14.

26. W. J. Whelan, "Asilomar: 20 Years On" (editorial), *FASEB J.*, 1995, 9, 295.

27. R. C. Desrosiers, "Non-Human Primate Models for AIDS Vaccines," *AIDS*, 1995, 9(suppl. A), S137–S141.

28. H. Koprowski, "Vaccination with Modified Active Viruses," *Papers and Discussions Presented at the Fourth International Poliomyelitis Conference (Geneva, 1957)* (Philadelphia: J. B. Lippincott, 1958), pp. 112–123.

29. To be fair, there are also logical reasons for mounting vaccine trials in Third World countries. In countries where HIV prevalence is higher, fewer test participants are needed to show positive results, which may therefore be obtained more quickly. See M. Essex, "Confronting the AIDS Vaccine Challenge," *Technology Rev.*, October 1994, pp. 23–29.

30. T. W. Baba, R. M. Ruprecht et al., "Infection and AIDS in Adult Macaques after Nontraumatic Oral Exposure to Cell-Free SIV," *Science*, 1996, 272, 1486–1489.

31. R. M. Ruprecht et al., "Murine and Simian Retrovirus Models: The Threshold Hypothesis," *AIDS*, 1996, 10(suppl. A), S33–S40.

32. Data further supporting the hypothesis that some humans are effectively immunized by their exposure to HIV was published in 1995. See S. Rowland-Jones, K. Ariyoshi et al., "HIV-Specific Cytotoxic T-cells in HIV-Exposed but Uninfected Gambian Women," *Nature Med.*, 1995, 1(1), 59–64.

33. R. M. Ruprecht et al., "Live Attenuated HIV as a Vaccine for AIDS: Pros and Cons," *Seminars in Virol.*, 1996, 7, 147–155.

34. L. Resnick et al., "Stability and Inactivation of HTLVIII/LAV under Clinical and Laboratory Environments," *JAMA*, 1986, 255(14), 1887–1891.

35. Personal communications, David Dane and Philip Minor, September 1997. Dr. Dane, an expert in vaccines since the fifties, wrote me: "We used to spin very slowly to avoid damage to cells. This would be most unlikely to have done any damage to SIV/HIV inside or outside cells."

36. J. L. Melnick, "Tissue Culture Methods for the Cultivation of Poliomyelitis and Other Viruses," in *Diagnostic Procedures for Virus and Rickettsial Diseases* (New York: American Public Health Association, 1956), pp. 97–151. This article is the best summary of the different ways of making tissue culture in 1956 — suspended-cell, roller-tube, or stationary-tube techniques, and trypsinization.

37. T. H. Weller, J. F. Enders et al., "Studies on the Cultivation of Poliomyelitis Viruses in Tissue Culture. 1. The Propagation of Poliomyelitis Viruses in Suspended Cell Cultures of Various Human Tissues," *J. Immunol.,* 1952, 69, 645–671.

38. "Expert Committee on Poliomyelitis, Third Report," *WHO Tech. Rep. Ser.,* 1960, 203, 1–53, especially p. 36. See also "Expert Committee on Poliomyelitis, Second Report," *WHO Tech. Rep. Ser.,* 1958, 145, 1–83, especially pp. 39–40.

39. R. Dulbecco and M. Vogt, "Plaque Formation and Isolation of Pure Lines with Poliomyelitis Viruses," *J. Exp. Med.,* 1954, 99, 167–182. See also J. S. Youngner, "Monolayer Tissue Cultures 1: Preparation and Standardization of Suspensions of Trypsin-Dispersed Monkey Kidney Cells," *Proc. Soc. Exp. Biol. Med.,* 1954, 85, 202–205.

40. D. Bodian, "Simplified Version of Dispersion of Monkey Kidney Cells with Trypsin," *Virol.,* 1956, 4, 575–576; C. Rappaport, "Trypsinization of Monkey-Kidney Tissue: An Automatic Method for the Preparation of Cell Suspensions," *Bull. WHO,* 1956, 14, 147–166; J. Gear, "The South African Poliomyelitis Vaccine," *S. Af. Med. J.,* 1956, 30, 587–594.

41. V. J. Cabasso, G. A. Jervis, H. R. Cox et al., "Cumulative Testing Experience with Consecutive Lots of Oral Poliomyelitis Vaccine," *BMJ,* 1960, 1(i), 373–387.

42. We do not know when CHAT was first developed, though it was unlikely to have been before August 1956; the first trial feeding of the vaccine, at Clinton, appears to have taken place in November 1956.

43. Indeed, the only poliomyelitis articles by Koprowski in which trypsinization is mentioned are two research papers, published in 1960 and 1962, which primarily deal not with polio vaccines, but with genetic markers of virulence. It may not be coincidental that these are the only two papers in which the source of the kidneys is also identified, for they were bought from Microbiological Associates Ltd of Bethesda. In the first instance, trypsinization was performed after arrival in the laboratory (H. Koprowski, S. Gard et al., "Genetic Markers and Serological Identity of Wild and Attenuated Strains of Type 1 Poliovirus, with Special Emphasis on Strains Isolated from Patients During an Epidemic in the Belgian Congo," *Bull. WHO,* 1960, 22, 243–253). In the second, the monkey kidney cells were already trypsinized (R. I. Carp and H. Koprowski, "Investigations of the Reproductive Capacity Temperature Marker of Polioviruses," *Virol.,* 1962, 16, 371–383). Microbiological Associates are not, however, cited in the papers that deal directly with polio vaccines and the trials of same.

44. *NYAS* 57, p. 129.

45. S. A. Plotkin, H. Koprowski et al., "Clinical Trials in Infants of Orally Administered Attenuated Poliomyelitis Viruses," *Pediatrics I,* 1959, 23, 1041–1060.

46. A. J. Garrett et al., "Retroviruses and Poliovaccines," *Lancet,* 1993, 342, 932–933.

47. 0.25 percent is the standard strength of trypsin for tissue culture work.

48. A. J. Garrett, "HIV Contamination of Poliovaccines" (author's reply), *Lancet,* 1994, 343, 52–53.

49. Such findings have also been repeated by other scientists, e.g., S. Tang and J. A. Levy, "Inactivation of HIV-1 by Trypsin and Its Use in Demonstrating Specific Virus Infection of Cells," *J. Virol. Meth.*, 1991, 33, 39–46.

50. Garrett left the cells in culture for ten days — much longer than the four days that would normally have applied when making polio vaccine in the fifties, for it takes from two to four days for poliovirus to lyse, or kill, the monkey kidney cells.

51. John Garrett, personal communication, June 1997.

52. CHAT was not one of the fifteen vaccines tested, and the CHAT/AIDS theory does not propose that HIV-1 would survive in tissue cultures of cynomolgus kidney.

53. K. Shah and N. Nathanson, "Human Exposure to SV40: Review and Comment," *Am. J. Epidem.*, 1976, 103, 1–12, see especially p. 4.

54. Philip Minor, personal communication, June 1997.

55. Furthermore, there are real grounds for doubting whether in 1957, the term "mono-layer" automatically involved breaking down the cells with trypsin. A Medical Research Council memo from 1955 reveals that versene, as well as trypsin, was then being used for breaking down primary tissues (see A. D. Macrae, "VERSENE," note prepared for the Committee on Laboratory Investigations of Poliomyelitis, Medical Research Council (U.K.), 1955, MRC document MRC.55/666; LIP.55/8). Versene (now called EDTA) is a gentler agent (which, according to David Dane, would almost certainly not have inacti-vated SIV or HIV), but in the memo the technique is still referred to as "trypsinization." American histologist Cecil Fox, who has worked with tissue cultures since the fifties, insists that monolayers can be made with or without trypsin, and that in the fifties mak-ing tissue culture was not a precise science.

56. Garrett told me that the limits of the detection system in this experiment were ten virions per milliliter.

57. J. Gear, "The South African Poliomyelitis Vaccine," *S. Af. Med. J.*, 1956, 30, 587–594, see p. 589. The method also involved three centrifugings, but since these were relatively gentle, they would be unlikely to harm any SIVs or HIVs that might be present.

58. K. Konopka et al., "Long-Term Noncytopathic Productive Infection of the Human Monocytic Leukemia Cell Line THP-1 by Human Immunodeficiency Virus Type 1 (HIV-1-IIIB)," *Virol.*, 1993, 193, 877–887. J. Blom et al., "An Ultrastructural Study of HIV-Infected Human Dendritic Cells and Monocytes/Macrophages," *APMIS* (Denmark), 1993, 101, 672–680.

59. Cecil Fox, communication to Michael Kent Curtis, January 1996.

60. This comment was made by one of the anonymous referees of Bill Hamilton's letter on OPV/AIDS (rejected by *Science* in February 1994), who had also been watching time-lapse films of primary monkey kidney monolayers.

61. John Garrett, personal communication, 1997, quoting a 1985 letter from Robin Weiss, of the Chester Beatty Cancer Research Institute in London. The dangers of using such *primary* cultures for human vaccines are highlighted in Victor Grachev's chapter in A. Mizrahi (ed.), *Viral Vaccines* (New York: Wiley-Liss, 1990), pp. 38–67; see especially pp. 39–40.

62. These are important virological questions that would benefit from further experimen-tal work. The key experiment would involve trypsinizing SIV-infected macrophages, washing away any trypsin, and then finding out if any infectious SIV was released/pro-duced in the days following. Indeed Tang and Levy, who show that HIV-1 in the super-natant is sensitive to trypsin, also demonstrate that infected T-cells, like lymphocytes and macrophages, produce infectious HIV-1 after trypsinization. See Tang and Levy,

"Inactivation of HIV-1 by Trypsin and Its Use in Demonstrating Specific Virus Infection of Cells."

63. O. Bagasra et al., "Detection of Human Immunodeficiency Virus Type 1 Provirus in Mononuclear Cells by in Situ Polymerase Chain Reaction," *N. Eng. J. Med.,* 1992, 326(21), 1385–1391. This important paper shows that in asymptomatic HIV-positive persons, as few as 0.1 percent of lymphocytes contained HIV-1 provirus, whereas when HIV-positive persons with lymphadenopathy or AIDS were tested, up to 13.5 percent and 11.8 percent of lymphocytes, respectively, were infected with the virus.

64. R. B. Stricker, B. Elswood et al., "HIV Contamination of Poliovaccines" (letter), *Lancet,* 1994, 343, 52–53, including reply by A. J. Garrett.

65. R. B. Stricker and B. Goldberg, "Polio Vaccines and Retroviral Contamination" (letter), *J. Inf. Dis.,* 1997, 176, 545.

66. Although it has been discovered that pig-tailed macaques can also be infected with HIV-1, and therefore can be used as an infection model, this seems to be an atypical, transient infection, leaving chimpanzees, despite their rarity, the preferred animal for HIV-1 research *in vivo.* See D. Blum, *The Monkey Wars* (Oxford: Oxford University Press, 1994), p. 213, and M. B. Agy et al., "Serial in Vivo Passage of HIV-1 Infection on Macaca nemestrina," *Virol.,* 1997, 238(2), 336–343.

67. S. K. Ghosh, P. N. Fultz, P. M. Sharp, B. H. Hahn et al., "A Molecular Clone of HIV-1 Tropic and Cytopathic for Human and Chimpanzee Lymphocytes," *Virol.,* 1993, 194, 858–864.

68. B. A. Castro et al., "Persistent Infection of Baboons and Rhesus Monkeys with Different Strains of HIV-2," *Virol.,* 1991, 184, 219–226.

CHAPTER 49: *Preston Marx and an Alternative Hypothesis*

1. Gordon told me that the Kansas City and Fort Knox sooties arrived in 1966/7. A report on the formation of the mangabey group at Yerkes refers to the introduction of three separate groups of mangabeys in 1968 and 1969, but makes no reference to source, other than stating that one group was "made available on loan" by another worker at Yerkes. See I. S. Bernstein, "The Influence of Introductory Techniques on the Formation of Captive Mangabey Groups," *Primates,* 1971, 12(1), 33–44.

2. This is the closely related mangabey species that comes from the Ivory Coast and Ghana, *Cercocebus torquatus lunulatus,* which is not known to be *naturally* infected with SIV.

3. N. L. Letvin, R.D Hunt et al., "Acquired Immunodeficiency Syndrome in a Colony of Macaque Monkeys," *Proc. Soc. Acad. Sci.,* 1983, 80, 2718–2722. The Type D retrovirus causation was first reported in M. Daniel et al., "A New Type D Retrovirus Isolated from Macaques with an Immunodeficiency Syndrome," *Science,* 1984, 223, 602–605. See also P. A. Marx, M. B. Gardner et al., "Simian AIDS: Isolation of a Type D Retrovirus and Transmission of the Disease," *Science,* 1984, 223, 1083–1086.

4. M. D. Daniel, R. C. Desrosiers et al., "Isolation of T-Cell Tropic HTLV-III-Like Retrovirus from Macaques," *Science,* 1985, 228, 1201–1204.

5. Y. Ohta, M. Hayami et al., "Isolation of Simian Immunodeficiency Virus from African Green Monkeys and Seroepidemiological Survey of the Virus in Various Non-Human Primates," *Intl. J. Cancer,* 1988, 41, 115–122.

6. However, Pat Fultz thought that the original transfer of SIV to stump-tails could well have taken place either at one of the primate holding centers like those in Florida and California, or during onward shipment to the primate research facilities, for on at least

one occasion the two species were shipped together. Back in the fifties and sixties, when the dangers of cross-species transmission of viruses were only dimly realized, procedures at the holding centers were apparently not strictly controlled or monitored, and it might be that needles were passed from the arm of one monkey to another during inoculations or blood extractions — for instance during the tuberculin testing that is carried out on all new arrivals. L. J. Lowenstine, P. N. Fultz, M. B. Gardner et al., "Evidence for a Lentiviral Etiology in an Epizootic of Immune Deficiency and Lymphoma in Stump-Tailed Macaques (*Macaca arctoides*)," *J. Med. Primatol.*, 1992, 21, 1–14.

7. D. Blum, *The Monkey Wars* (New York: Oxford University Press, 1994), p. 204. Patricia Fultz, personal communication, May 1995.

8. M. Murphey-Corb, B. J. Gormus et al., "Isolation of an HTLV-III-Related Retrovirus from Macaques with Simian AIDS, and Its Possible Origin in Asymptomatic Mangabeys," *Nature*, 1986, 321, 435–437.

9. M. D. Daniel et al., "Isolation of T-Cell Tropic HTLV-III-Like Retrovirus from Macaques."

10. H. W. Kestler et al., "Comparison of Simian Immunodeficiency Virus Isolates" (letter), *Nature*, 1988, 331, 619–622.

11. R. E. Bienveniste, L. O. Arthur et al., "Isolation of a Lentivirus from a Macaque with Lymphoma: Comparison with HTLV-III/LAV and Other Lentiviruses," *J. Virol.*, 1986, 60(2), 483–490.

12. F. J. Novembre, P. N. Fultz, P. R. Johnson et al., "SIV from Stump-Tailed Macaques: Molecular Characterization of a Highly Transmissible Lentivirus," *Virol.*, 1992, 186, 783–787.

13. At the time of my visit, LEMSIP was home to 220 chimpanzees, many held on behalf of AIDS vaccine researchers such as Pat Fultz, and — Marx told me with some pride — was an open facility, with facilities for genuinely interested parties, like journalists and animal activists, to stay overnight in the compound.

14. Kuru was encountered only in the Fore tribe of New Guinea, whose tradition it was for the women and children to eat the uncooked flesh (including the brains) of the recently deceased.

15. See R. Rhodes, *Deadly Feasts: Tracking the Secrets of a Terrifying New Plague* (New York: Simon and Schuster, 1997).

16. However, I have not managed to find anything in the literature to support Marx's claim. Gadjusek's own summary of the experiments reports that kuru was transmissible to sooties, and to rhesus, pig-tailed, and stump-tailed macaques, and refers to other cross-species transfers of "slow virus"-infected brain, but does not refer to the specific transfers that Marx mentioned to me. D. C. Gadjusek, "Unconventional Viruses and the Origin and Disappearance of Kuru," *Science*, 1977, 197, 943–960.

17. K. G. Mansfield, N. W. Lerche, M. B. Gardner et al., "Origins of Simian Immunodeficiency Virus Infection in Macaques at the New England Regional Primate Research Center," *J. Med. Primatol.*, 1995, 24(3), 116–122.

18. G. Greene, *Journey Without Maps* (London: William Heinemann, 1936), pp. 116–117, and 233.

19. P. A. Marx, R. C. Desrosiers et al., "Isolation of a Simian Immunodeficiency Virus Related to Human Immunodeficiency Virus Type 2 from a West African Pet Sooty Mangabey," *J. Virol.*, 1991, 65(8), 4480–4485.

20. Z. Chen, P. A. Marx et al., "Human Immunodeficiency Virus Type 2 (HIV-2) Seroprevalence and Characterization of a Distinct HIV-2 Genetic Subtype from the Natural

Range of Simian Immunodeficiency Virus-Infected Sooty Mangabeys," *J. Virol.*, 1997, 71(5), 3953–3960. In this article, Marx reveals that the donor of "Lua" (or 93SL2, as it is now designated) was a fifty-two-year-old woman who had had multiple sexual partners and eaten sooty mangabey meat. He suggested that 93SL2 represented cross-species transfer of SIVsm to humans.

21. D. D. Ho et al., "HIV-2 in Los Angeles" (letter), *AIDS*, 1990, 4, 1301–1302.

22. Z. Chen, D. D. Ho, P. A. Marx et al., "Genetic Characterization of New West African Simian Immunodeficiency Virus SIVsm: Geographic Clustering of Household-Derived SIV Strains with Human Immunodeficiency Virus Type 2 Subtypes and Genetically Diverse Viruses from a Single Feral Sooty Mangabey Troop," *J. Virol.*, 1996, 70(6), 3617–3627.

23. L. J. Lowenstine, P. Marx et al., "Seroepidemiologic Survey of Captive Old-World Primates for Antibodies to Human and Simian Retroviruses, and Isolation of a Lentivirus from Sooty Mangabeys (*Cercocebus atys*)," *Intl. J. Cancer*, 1986, 38, 563–574, see p. 572. For more details see "Status Report on Simian Retroviruses," WHO Biologicals Report; 1987, BLG/Polio/87.2

24. Z. Chen, D. D. Ho, P. A. Marx et al., "Genetic Characterization of New West African Simian Immunodeficiency Virus SIVsm: Geographic Clustering of Household-Derived SIV Strains with Human Immunodeficiency Virus Type 2 Subtypes and Genetically Diverse Viruses from a Single Feral Sooty Mangabey Troop."

25. Another example, of course, would be Marx's HIV-2 subtype F.

26. Z. Chen, P. A. Marx et al., "Museum Specimens from 1918 Contain HIV-2 Related DNA in a New Species of Mangabey," *Proceedings of the First National Conference on Human Retroviruses and Related Infections* (Washington, D.C.), 1993, Abstract 151, p. 81.

27. The proof of the contamination, Marx said, was that although the museum specimens were positive for SIV, they were negative for mitochondrial DNA (which is present in every cell in the body). He now realized that this meant that all the DNA had been degraded.

28. R. F. Khabbaz, T. M. Folks et al., "Simian Immunodeficiency Virus Needlestick Accident in a Laboratory Worker," *Lancet*, 1992, 340, 271–273. Retrovirus Diseases branch, CDC, "Seroconversion to Simian Immunodeficiency Virus in Two Laboratory Workers," *MMWR*, 1992, 41(36), 678–681. R. F. Khabbaz, T. M. Folks et al., "Brief Report: Infection of Laboratory Worker with Simian Immunodeficiency Virus," *N. Engl. J. Med.*, 1994, 330(3), 172–177.

29. "Report of the WHO International Commission for Certification of Smallpox Eradication from West Africa," WHO document AFR/SMALLPOX/80, 1980, p. 16. Table 1 shows that Sierra Leone, Guinea-Conakry, and Ivory Coast received more than one smallpox vaccination per head of population, Liberia had 67 percent of the population vaccinated, while Guinea-Bissau (presumably because of the war) had just 29 percent. See also *Annual Epidemiological and Vital Statistics* (Geneva: WHO, published annually).

CHAPTER 50: *Natural or Iatrogenic Transfer?*

1. C. Fyfe, "The Dynamics of African Dispersal: The Transatlantic Slave Trade," in M. L. Kilson and R. I. Rotberg (editors), *The African Diaspora — Interpretive Essays* (Cambridge: Harvard University Press, 1976), pp. 57–74. This figure of ten million is based on Philip Curtin's careful reassessment of available data; previous assessments of the numbers shipped ranged from fifteen million to upward of fifty million. See B. Davidson,

*The African Slave Trade — Precolonial History 1450–1850* (Boston: Little, Brown, 1961), pp. 79–113.

2.  C. Plimmer and D. Plimmer, *Slavery — The Anglo-American Involvement* (New York: Barnes and Noble, 1973), p. 7.

3.  D. P. Mannix, *Black Cargoes* (London: Longmans, 1962), p. 264.

4.  P. D. Curtin, "Epidemiology and the Slave Trade," *Polit. Sci. Q.,* 1968, 83(2), 190–216; J. Walvin, *Black Ivory — A History of British Slavery* (London: HarperCollins, 1992), pp. 134–154.

5.  One must bear in mind Marx's hypothesis that transient SIV infections could have infected the first generation of slaves, but thereafter would not be passed on.

6.  The slave trade was officially abolished by Britain and the United States in 1807. Slavery itself was abolished in British colonies in 1838, in the United States in 1865, in Cuba in 1886, and in Brazil in 1888. In reality, most transatlantic slaving came to an end in the early 1860s, although some Portuguese vessels continued taking slaves from Angola to Brazil for some years afterward.

7.  R. Harms, "Sustaining the System: Trading Towns along the Middle Zaire," in C. C. Robertson and M. A. Klein (editors), *Women and Slavery in Africa* (Madison: University of Wisconsin Press, 1983), pp. 95–110.

8.  "Geography and Some Explorers" in J. Conrad, *Tales of Hearsay and Last Essays* (London: J. M. Dent, 1928), p. 17. Reshid may have been another name for Tippu Tib.

9.  F. McLynn, *Hearts of Darkness — The European Exploration of Africa* (London: Pimlico, 1992), pp. 189–212.

10. R. Harms, *River of Wealth, River of Sorrow* (New Haven: Yale University Press, 1981), p. 232.

11. J. C. Miller, "The Slave Trade in Congo and Angola," in M. L. Kilson and R. I. Rotberg, *The African Diaspora — Interpretive Essays,* pp. 75–113.

12. *The New Encyclopaedia Britannica, Macropedia* (Chicago: Encyclopaedia Britannica, 1997), vol. 29, p. 894. Fernando Po is now the island of Bioko, in Equatorial Guinea.

13. J. Walvin, *Black Ivory — A History of British Slavery,* pp. 214–229.

14. M. Strobel, "Slavery and Reproductive Labor in Mombasa," in C. C. Robertson and M. A. Klein (editors), *Women and Slavery in Africa,* pp. 111–129.

15. Basil Davidson reckons that at least five million slaves were taken from the Congo and Angola between 1680 and 1836. See B. Davidson, *The African Slave Trade,* p. 160.

16. M. W. DeLancey, "Health and Disease on the Plantations of Cameroon, 1884–1939," in G. W. Hartwig and K. D. Patterson, *Disease in African History* (Durham: Duke University Press, 1978), pp. 152–179.

17. C. Perrings, *Black Mineworkers in Central Africa* (London: Heinemann, 1979), pp. 73–105 and 165–182.

18. A. D. Roberts (editor), *The Cambridge History of Africa, Volume 7, from 1905 to 1940* (Cambridge: Cambridge University Press, 1986), p. 478.

19. A. D. Roberts, *The Cambridge History of Africa, Volume 7,* pp. 422–423, 664–667, 352, 357.

20. M. Crowder (editor), *The Cambridge History of Africa, Volume 8, from about 1940 to about 1975* (Cambridge: Cambridge University Press, 1984), pp. 8–40.

21. N. Nzilambi, K. M. De Cock, J. B. McCormick et al., "The Prevalence of Infection with Human Immunodeficiency Virus over a 10-Year Period in Rural Zaire," *N. Engl. J. Med.,* 1988, 318, 276–279.

22. L. Vail, "HIV Infection in Zaire" (letter), *N. Engl. J. Med.,* 1988, 319(5), 309.

23. A. D. Roberts, *The Cambridge History of Africa, Volume 7*, pp. 370–371.

24. C. J. Hackett, "Private Medical Practice and Anti-Yaws Campaigns in South Eastern Nigeria 1925–1950," *Trop. Doctor*, 1980, 10, 129–132.

25. Manpower was at a premium; for instance in 1920 French West Africa only had half of the 130 doctors required. A. D. Roberts, *The Cambridge History of Africa, Volume 7*, p. 369.

26. The British virologist and polio expert John O'Hare Tobin tells me that before 1945, nobody would have been concerned about changing syringes and needles between jabs. He describes vaccination procedures that he and his colleagues used in the British army during the Second World War, including vaccinating an entire battalion of nine hundred men against typhoid using just three syringes, and changing to a newly boiled needle roughly once every ten jabs (personal communication, January 1995). Others say needles were usually waved briefly over a small methylated spirits burner. (Wilson Carswell, personal communication, November 1997.)

27. By contrast, Mount Nimba's unique virgin forest contains some two hundred species found nowhere else in the world, and it is a protected nature reserve in Guinea Conakry and the Ivory Coast. K. Curry-Lindahl, "Report to the Government of Liberia on Conservation, Management and Utilization of Wildlife Resources," *IUCN Publications New Series* (suppl. paper No. 24), 1969, 23–24.

28. P. T. Robinson, "Wildlife Trends in Liberia and Sierra Leone," *Oryx*, 1971, 11(2/3), 117–122; M. Coe, "Mammalian Ecological Studies on Mount Nimba, Liberia," *Mammalia*, 1975, 39(4), 527–575. During Coe's seven months in the area, he saw one single monkey (bought from a hunter), and heard the cries of a few chimpanzees.

29. Malcolm Coe, personal communication, January 1995.

30. A. D. Roberts, *The Cambridge History of Africa, Volume 7*, p. 136.

31. H. H. Gunson and H. Dodsworth, "Fifty Years of Blood Transfusion," *Transfusion Med.*, 1996, 6 (Supp. 1), 1–88.

32. Jack Davies, Hector Meyus, personal communications, September 1996 and February 1998.

33. N. Burin des Roziers et al., "Infection par le virus HIV-2 avec longue periode d'incubation" (letter), *Presse Méd.*, 1987, 16(39), 1981. J. Botas, F. Antunes et al., "HIV2 Infection. Some Clinical and Epidemiological Aspects in Portugal," 5th International Conference on AIDS (Montreal, 1989), abstract M.A.P.77.

34. The earliest known HIV-1-related AIDS case with a transfusion link is that of the Canadian flight engineer who was apparently infected in Kisangani in 1976 and died in 1980.

35. "A New King for the Congo: Mobutu and the Nihilism of Africa," in V. S. Naipaul, *The Return of Eva Peron, with The Killings in Trinidad* (London: Andre Deutsch, 1980), pp. 171–204, especially pp. 182–186. See also V. S. Naipaul, *A Bend in the River* (London: Penguin, 1979), pp. 11–15.

36. I have come across a few reports that might help, involving large-scale blood surveys from potential target areas. These include 900 samples from Harbel, Liberia, in 1956 (A. R. Robinson et al., "Two 'Fast' Hemoglobin Components in Liberian Blood Samples," *Blood*, 1956, 11, 902–906); 9,200 from all regions of Guinea-Bissau in (1957/8) (C. Trincao et al., "A Survey of Abnormal Haemoglobins in Portuguese Guinea," *Nature*, 1960, 185, 326–327); 11,000 blood samples from Coquilhatville, Belgian Congo, in 1958 and 500 from Elisabethville, Congo, in 1952 (J. Vandepitte and J. Stijns, "Les hémoglobinoses au Congo (Leopoldville) et au Rwanda-Burundi," *Ann. Soc. Belge Méd. Trop.*, 1963, 43,

271–282). My own attempts to follow up on some of these cohorts have not been successful, but there are other series to be found in the literature, and there is little doubt that early
African blood samples are still to be found in medical freezers, if one searches hard
enough.

37.  W.-H. Li, P. M. Sharp et al., "Rates and Dates of Divergence between AIDS Virus Nucleotide Sequences," *Mol. Biol. Evol.,* 1988, 5 (4), 313–330.

38.  R. F. Doolittle, "The Simian-Human Connection," *Nature,* 1989, 339, 338–339.

39.  G. Querat et al., "Nucleotide Sequence Analysis of SA-OMVV, a Visna-Related Ovine
Lentivirus: Phylogenetic History of Lentiviruses," *Virol.,* 1990, 175, 434–447.

40.  M. Eigen et al., "How Old Is the Immunodeficiency Virus?" *AIDS,* 1990, 4(suppl.1),
S85–S93. This article is often cited as favoring an older origin of AIDS, but in fact it
merely proposes an age of 600 to 1,200 years for the position of the oldest PIV node, the
ancestor of all the known HIVs and SIVs.

41.  G. Myers, "HIV: Between Past and Future," *AIDS Res. Human Retro.,* 1994, 10(11),
1317–1324.

42.  C. L. Kuiken and B. T. M. Korber, "Epidemiological Significance of Intra- and Inter-
Person Variation of HIV-1," *AIDS,* 1994, 8(suppl.1), S73-S83.

43.  P. Kasper, E. C. Holmes et al., "The Genetic Diversification of the HIV Type 1 gag p17
Gene in Patients Infected from a Common Source," *AIDS Res. Human Retro.,* 1995,
11(10), 1197–1201.

44.  F. Barré-Sinoussi, "HIV as the Cause of AIDS," *Lancet,* 1996, 348, 31–35.

45.  J. Goudsmit, *Viral Sex — The Nature of AIDS* (New York: Oxford University Press,
1997).

46.  B. Auvert et al., "Dynamics of HIV Infection and AIDS in Central African Cities," *Intl.
J. Epidem.,* 1990, 19(2), 417–428.

47.  A. Flahault and A.-J. Valleron, "A Method for Assessing the Global Spread of HIV-1
Infection Based on Air Travel," *Math. Pop. Stud.,* 1992, 3(3), 161–171. This model correctly predicted the exponential rise of HIV-1 in Asia in the mid-nineties.


CHAPTER 51: *What Happened at Letchworth and Clinton*

1.  Ann's husband had by this stage shown me the documents that Koprowski had returned,
and they consisted of six or seven files that made up a pile less than two inches deep,
which included more than one copy of certain papers. I was also shown a letter from
Koprowski's wife, Irena Koprowska, dated July 12, 1994, which explained that she had
had to abandon her "excessively ambitious plan ... to write the history of Poliomyelitis." A previous letter, dated June 2, 1994, from Koprowski himself, had explained
that "a woman is coming from Poland to write my biography," and that he was keeping
the papers in case *she* wanted to peruse them. It is not known if the biography was ever
published.

2.  Simian kidneys would often be dispatched separately, so that if one set of kidneys was
virally or bacterially contaminated, it would not ruin the others.

3.  I needed to determine if Priscilla Norton could have been mistaken on this point — and
if, for instance, Jim could have been a driver for Lederle rather than the Wistar. I therefore asked Stewart Aston to tell me the names of the Lederle drivers in the fifties. He
recalled various Christian names, but assured me that there had never been a driver
there called Jim.

4. H. Koprowski, "Historical Aspects of the Development of Live Virus Vaccines in Polio-myelitis," *Am. J. Dis. Child.*, 1960, 100, 428–439.

5. Anon., *Forty-Second Annual Report of the Board of Visitors of Letchworth Village for the Fiscal Year Ended March 31, 1950* (Utica, NY: State Hospitals Press, 1951), p. 41.

6. To begin with, Mrs. Jervis said she guessed that the chimps had been kept in the small animal house in the Letchworth grounds, but when I asked for more details she became uncertain, and eventually said she doubted that there had ever been any monkeys or chimps at the Village.

7. Neither was this fact mentioned in the Letchworth annual reports for 1950 and 1951.

8. M. Roca Garcia and G. A. Jervis, "Experimentally Produced Poliomyelitis Variant in Chick Embryo," *Ann. N.Y. Acad. Sci.*, 1955, 61, 911–922. This paper reports that fifteen further children (including three with "incurable diseases" who died a year or two later) had been fed with two new pools of TN, twenty with new versions of SM, and two with a different version of MEF1. These were almost certainly from Letchworth.

9. G. A. Jervis, "Comparative Susceptibility of Tissue Culture Cells in Experimental Animals and Man," *Ann. N.Y. Acad. Sci.*, 1955, 61, 848–851.

10. At the same conference, Jervis reported giving MEF1 Type 2 virus to four young chim-panzees and several cynomolgus monkeys — indicating that these primates were almost certainly then resident at the Letchworth animal house.

11. H. R. Cox, "Trial Vaccines and Human Welfare," *Lancet*, 1953, 2(i), 1–5.

12. S. A. Plotkin, H. Koprowski et al., "Vaccination of Families against Poliomyelitis by Feeding and by Contact Spread of Living Attenuated Virus," *Pediatrics*, 1960, 49, 551–571, especially Table 18 on p. 564, and acknowledgments, p. 570.

13. New Jersey State Archives, 185 West State Street, Trenton, NJ 08625-0307, U.S.A. In fact, my visit to the Trenton archives was not made until this book was almost completed, late in 1998, but the information is included here for reasons of narrative fluency.

14. M. Q. Hawkes, *Excellent Effect — The Edna Mahan Story* (Arlington, VA: American Correctional Association, 1994), pp. 109–110 and 135–136. Typhus experiments (in-volving infection with lice) were carried out by researchers from the University of Pennsylvania in 1946/7, and Werner and Gertrude Henle, from the same university, con-ducted eight experiments on infectious hepatitis between 1949 and 1953 on behalf of the army. In the latter research, inmates "became seriously ill and felt miserable for a long time, some well after the study ended. They did not complain. There were deep feelings of pride at the significant contribution they made to the military, medical research and society." On both occasions it was Joe Stokes who helped to make the ini-tial arrangements, just as he was to do for Koprowski in 1955.

15. In the minutes of the meeting of the Clinton board of governors, dated July 6, 1955 (p. 9), it was stated that during this initial phone call to Edna Mahan, Dr. Stokes informed her that similar vaccination programs were already in effect at Woodbine and New Lisbon. If correct, this was the first time I had heard of polio vaccinations being carried out at New Lisbon (which is another New Jersey state school for disabled chil-dren, situated some forty miles due east of Philadelphia).

16. Anon., "Progress on a Better Polio Vaccine," *Life*, October 29, 1956, pp. 61–66.

17. B. W. Hotchkiss, "Babies Being Fed Live Polio Virus," *Newark Evening News*, October 24, 1956.

18. Minutes of the meeting of the Clinton board of governors, dated February 8, 1956, p. 5.

19. H. Koprowski, T. W. Norton, J. Stokes Jr. et al., "Immunization of Infants with Living Attenuated Poliomyelitis Virus: Laboratory Investigations of Alimentary Infection and

Antibody Response in Infants under Six Months of Age with Congenitally Acquired Antibodies," *JAMA*, 1956, 162(14), 1281–1288.

20. See p. 9 of the minutes of the Clinton board of governors meeting of April 10, 1957, p. 7 of that of May 15, p. 5 of that of June 12, and p. 4 of that of July 10, 1957.

21. Minutes of the meeting of the Clinton board of governors, dated November 13, 1957, p. 7; and March 12, 1958, p. 7.

22. M. Q. Hawkes, *Excellent Effect — The Edna Mahan Story,* p. 137.

23. H. Koprowski, "Vaccinations with Modified Active Viruses," in *Papers and Discussions Presented at the Fourth International Poliomyelitis Conference (Geneva, July 1957)* (Philadelphia: J. B. Lippincott, 1958), pp. 112–123.

24. S. A. Plotkin, H. Koprowski, and J. Stokes Jr., "Clinical Trials of Orally Administered Attenuated Poliomyelitis Viruses," *Pediatrics,* 1959, 23, 1041–1062. None of the Fox vaccinations took at the first feeding, which meant that the Type 3 vaccine had to be refed in November and December 1956.

25. WHO document WHO/Polio/30 (see above) indicates that two Clinton children were fed "SM Pool 45" at ages of 14 days and 39 days. I deduce that the latter must have been fed on February 27, 1957, and the former in October or November 1956, when the first trial feedings of CHAT and Fox also took place.

26. My own research shows that six infants must have been fed CHAT (and one SM-45) on February 27, 1957. It is not clear why the official report of the feedings (see n.19, above) and the "History of the Use of CHAT Strain 'Type 1' Attenuated Polio Virus in Humans" paper (see n.42, below) mentions only five Clinton infants having been fed this "first pool." What is possible, however, is that the feedings of BO, GA, and perhaps the sixth CHAT vaccinee of February 27 (who must have been infant No. 43) may have involved an even earlier version of CHAT than the one based on Plaque 20. Perhaps it was based on another CHAT plaque, or even made in a different substrate. What this highlights, once again, is that not all of the more experimental feedings at Clinton were recorded in the scientific literature.

27. H. Koprowski, "Vaccination with Modified Active Viruses," *Papers and Discussions Presented at the Fourth International Poliomyelitis Conference (Geneva, July 1957),* pp. 112–123, see especially Table 33 on p. 115.

28. It may well be that the experiments on excreted CHAT virus were only staged in response to Dick's adverse report about the virulence of excreted TN at the New York conference on January 7–9, 1957, and in the *BMJ* report of January 12. Whether or not this is so, a maximum of just two CHAT vaccinees (BO and GA) can have been assessed for the virulence of excreted virus before Koprowski and Norton set off for Africa in late January 1957 and began feeding CHAT. (In fact, the records suggest that only a single infant, BO, had been assessed by that stage.)

29. "TA" (who equates to Infant No. 46) was fed CHAT on February 27, 1957.

30. GA was in fact the second CHAT vaccinee, being fed on January 3, 1957, but the Geneva paper makes it clear that GA was the "third infant" to be assessed for the virulence of the excreted virus. If, as seems likely, this occurred after TA's adverse results became apparent, the GA results cannot have been known before April 1957. Nowhere in the Geneva paper, or in Plotkin's subsequent paper on Clinton, is it suggested that the excreted viruses of the other five infants fed CHAT on February 27, 1957, were safety tested prior to the Aketi trial in May. This suggests that only three infants (BO, TA, and GA) were assessed for fecal virus before some 2,000 Congolese children were fed CHAT.

31. S. A. Plotkin, H. Koprowski et al., "Vaccination of Full-Term Infants with Attenuated Polioviruses," *PAHO2*, 294–301.

32. T. Norton, R. Carp and S. A. Plotkin, "Summary of feeding results with attenuated polioviruses grown in human diploid cell strains," WHO internal document "Virus Diseases/WP/6," 1962.

33. R. I. Carp and H. Koprowski, "A New Test of the Reproductive Capacity Temperature Marker of Poliovirus: the Limited Thermal Exposure Test," *Virol.*, 1962, 16, 71–79.

34. R. I. Carp and H. Koprowski, "Mutation of Type 3 Poliovirus with Nitrous Acid," *Virol.*, 1962, 16, 99–109.

35. J. Oleske et al., "Immune Deficiency Syndrome in Children," *JAMA*, 1983, 249(17), 2345–2349.

36. David Ho confirmed in July 1997 that the papers sent me represented *all* the papers that had been made available to the expert committee from the Wistar Institute. He also told me: "I think what they [the Wistar Institute] sent out [to the expert committee] was just a . . . sample of what they had."

37. The paper actually stated the figures the other way around. However, *BMJ* 58 shows that the figure of 1,978 applied to the Aketi schoolchildren. The figure of 80 presumably applied to the Lindi staff and their families and the few people vaccinated at Stanleyville lab in February 1957.

38. However, Ghislain Courtois did report this in the literature: G. Courtois, "Vaccination antipoliomyélitique par virus vivant au Congo Belge," *Ann. Soc. Belg. Méd. Trop.*, 1958, 38, 805–816.

39. Letter from Bervoets to De Brauwere, dated September 17, 1958, found in file H4484/1058 at the Ministry of Foreign Affairs archives, Brussels.

40. Jean Deinhardt, personal communication, 1994. In a letter written in April 1997, she confirmed that she had no idea whether Fritz had also delivered polio vaccine to Stanleyville in January 1957.

41. The Moorestown paper says the index feedings occurred in "mid-January 1958," but details supplied by Dr. Edmund Preston, and by the mother of one of the Moorestown vaccinees indicates that the first feedings of CHAT actually took place on the same date as Gombari: January 27, 1958.

42. The reasoning here is rather convoluted, but is basically: (a) since the Moorestown trials began at latest on January 27, 1958, they must surely have employed either pool 4B-5 or 10A-11 of CHAT, since — as far as I know — no others were then in production; (b) this is supported by *PAHO1*, 135–139, especially Table 5 on p. 138, which strongly suggests that the vaccine used at Moorestown was "4B," (c) in *Pediatrics*, 1960, 49, 551–571, Jervis's contribution (Table 18 on p. 564) records that the titer of the CHAT fed at Moorestown was log 7.5, which is exactly the same as that in "the first pool" of CHAT mentioned in the "History of the Use of CHAT Strain 'Type 1' Attenuated Polio Virus in Humans" paper supplied to the Wistar expert committee by the Wistar Institute.

43. A scribbled note in the CHAT pool 23 protocol claimed that pages 4 and 5 were the same as the equivalent pages in the Type 3 protocol (presumably WM-3 pool 17), but the relevant pages were not included in the Type 3 protocol either.

44. Instructions for poliovirus production from this period indicate that the streptomycin concentration is wrong: it should read 100 micrograms (not grams) per milliliter. See J. L. Melnick, "Tissue Culture Methods for the Cultivation of Poliomyelitis and Other

Viruses," in *Diagnostic Procedures for Virus and Rickettsial Diseases* (New York: American Public Health Association, 1956), pp. 97–151, especially p. 102.

45. C. Basilico, C. Buck, R. Desrosiers, D. Ho, F. Lilly, and E. Wimmer, "Report from the AIDS/Poliovirus Advisory Committee," September 18, 1992, released at a press conference in New York on October 22, 1992; available from Brian Martin, Department of Science and Technology Studies, University of Wollongong, NSW 2522, Australia; fax: +61-2-4221 3452; e-mail: brianmartin@uow.edu.au.

46. Luc Montagnier, personal communication, 1993.

47. Also included in the packet were a very general four-page "Resumé of live virus vaccination in polio," apparently written in early 1959, and a one-page protocol for a clinical trial of CHAT and Fox among infants at the Hospital of the University of Pennsylvania, from around the same period. These, however, were of little relevance to the issue of substrate.

48. Anon., "Zahtjevi za proizvodnju atenuirane vakcine protiv poliomijelitisa (sojevi Koprowski), *Immunolski. Zavod. Radovi* (Yugoslavia), 1964, 2, 124–125.

49. *BMJ* 58.

50. H. Koprowski, "AIDS and the Polio Vaccine" (letter), *Science*, 1992, 257, 1024–1027.

51. This information (that all infants born at Clinton during this period were vaccinated) is not confirmed by any articles in the mainstream medical literature, but it is apparently confirmed by Hilary Koprowski's submission to the WHO Expert Committee on Poliomyelitis. See H. Koprowski, "Immunization of a Population of an Institution with an Attenuated Type 1 Poliomyelitis Vaccine," WHO document WHO/POLIO/30, dated June 28, 1957.

52. The Clinton archives reveal two examples. In the minutes of the board meeting of July 6, 1955 (page 9), there is a reference to two females, both wards of the State Board of Child Welfare (and therefore presumably "Clinton babies"), who had been moved, respectively, to eight and seventeen different foster homes, before themselves being sent to Clinton.

53. This was confirmed by Mrs. Lorenzo, who recalled that, in the early days of the study, the staff had had to change their shoes and outside clothes when entering the nursery, to wash with disinfectant, and to autoclave the babies clothes and bed linen.

54. As it happened, yet more details about this child emerged from the minutes of the monthly meetings of the Clinton board of governors. He was one of the original six Clinton vaccinees who, according to Agnes Flack, had received the vaccine on November 16, 1955 (though, according to my calculations, he must have been fed on November 10). Of the first six, five were fed with SM and one with TN; and this boy, alone among the SM vaccinees, did not receive TN two months later. This was probably because he was still excreting Type 1 virus, which he did for more than 100 days. In March 1956, the boy spent ten days at the Hunterdon Medical Center having a heart evaluation, and then on April 5, he was transferred to Newark Babies' Hospital for plastic surgery on his webbed fingers. Presumably he was transferred from there to the Crippled Children's Hospital. Given Ruth Lorenzo's testimony, it seems likely that his primary health problems related to developmental abnormalities precipitated by his mother's bout of measles. However, that there is no mention of his health problems in the detailed scientific report of the vaccinations, which there perhaps should have been — albeit within the context of the mother's illness.

55. This photo was later published in *Life* magazine: "Progress on a Better Polio Vaccine," October 29, 1956, p. 64 (middle photograph).

CHAPTER 52: *What Happened at Lindi*

1.  It is mentioned in the footnotes of two articles by G. Courtois, "Vaccination anti-poliomyélitique par virus vivant au Congo Belge," *Ann. Soc. Belge Méd. Trop.*, 1958, 38, 805–816; and *BMJ* 58. It is also alluded to in the 1958 annual report of the Laboratoire Médical de Stanleyville.

2.  The much-promised article was mentioned once again in 1960, in a letter dated November 12 from Osterrieth to Courtois, which says: "Ninane tells me that you will be putting together an article about the experiments carried out on the chimps. I would like to have a copy." There was no evidence among Courtois's papers of any such article, even in draft form.

3.  *BMJ* 58.

4.  *PAHO1*, pp. 201 and 227.

5.  The D+ marker was thought to characterize a wild, rather than a vaccine virus. See M. Vogt, R. Dulbecco, and H. A. Wenner, "Mutants of Poliomyelitis Viruses with Reduced Efficiency of Plating in Acid Medium and Reduced Neuropathogenicity," *Virol.*, 1957, 4, 141–155.

6.  *BMJ* 58 and *NYAS* 57.

7.  *PAHO1*, p. 201. (One chimp was paralyzed, and one developed lesions.) In addition, see A. Lebrun, G. Courtois, H. Koprowski et al., "Vaccination with the CHAT Strain of Type 1 Attenuated Poliomyelitis Virus in Leopoldville, Belgian Congo. 1. Description of the City, Its History of Poliomyelitis, and the Plan of the Vaccination Campaign," *Bull. WHO*, 1960, 22, 203–213, which refers to the intraspinal testing of five chimps with CHAT, but fails to make clear whether this refers to the original Plaque 20 test or an additional test on pool 13, as used in the Leopoldville trial.

8.  Deduced by subtracting the details in *BMJ* 58 from Koprowski's *PAHO1* total.

9.  Courtois fed the chimps 10cc of tissue culture fluid containing 10 million viral particles, for both the YSK and Mexican wild viruses.

10. Ninane's annual report for the Laboratoire Médical for 1959 says that five more chimps (which may or may not have been included in Koprowski's thirty-nine) were tested intraspinally in that year, and that another five were due to be similarly used for the testing of a Type 2 vaccine in 1960. We do not know whether the latter testing ever took place.

11. F. Deinhardt, G. Courtois, P. Dherte, P. Osterrieth, G. Ninane, G. Henle, and W. Henle, "Studies of Liver Function Tests in Chimpanzees after Inoculation with Human Infectious Hepatitis Virus," *Am. J. Hyg.*, 1962, 75, 311–321.

12. W. Henle, G. Henle, and F. Deinhardt, "Studies on Viral Hepatitis," *Annual Report to the Commission on Viral Infections of the Armed Forces Epidemiological Board*, March 1958–February 1959.

13. This was reinforced by a later paper about arteriosclerosis in the chimpanzee, which confirmed that 47 of the 63 Lindi chimps used had previously been involved in research into polio, scarlet fever, and hepatitis. The other 16, being recent captures, had — to quote the authors — "escaped these experiments." See R. Delcourt, G. Ninane, P. Osterrieth, and M. Vastesaeger, "Le métabolisme lipidique du chimpanzé," *Acta Cardiol.*, 1964, 19, 531–545.

14. That most of the databook was the work of one or both of these people is strongly suggested by a letter from Stanley Plotkin to Deinhardt dated May 28, 1959, and another from Paulette Dherte to Deinhardt dated June 20, 1959.

15. Chimps number 1, 2, and 5 (the pets) were apparently not used in any of the experiments.

16. R. Lefebvre, "Note concernant le soixantième anniversaire des experiences de domestication de l'éléphant au Congo Belge et les activités durant la dernière décennie de la Station de la Chasse (Gangala na Bodio et Epulu)," *Bulletin, Service des Eaux et Forets, Chasse et Peche* (Leopoldville, Belgian Congo), 1960, 7, 655–661. The information about research into arteriosclerosis and cancer comes from the 1959 annual report of the Laboratoire Médical de Stanleyville.

17. This tremendous rate of intake into the camp is supported by an article that may well refer to this very period. P. Osterrieth and P. Deleplanque-Liegois, "Presence d'anticorps vis-à-vis des virus transmis par arthropodes chez le chimpanzé (*Pan troglodites*). Comparaison de leur état immunitaire à celui de l'homme," *Ann. Soc. Belg. Méd. Trop.,* 1961, 41, 63–72, refers to ninety-four chimps having been brought to the camp in less than two months.

18. The Daenens family, personal communications, May 1994. It may be no coincidence that exactly the same number of sera (175) were sent from Stanleyville to Liège in Belgium for a blood group study that was eventually published in 1961. A. André, G. Courtois, G. Lennes, G. Ninane, and P. M. Osterrieth, "Mise en évidence d'antigènes de groupes sanguins A, B, O et Rh chez les singes chimpanzés," *Ann. Inst. Past.,* 1961, 101, 82–95.

19. At this stage, even pet animals that were often afforded the freedom of the camp — such as Djamba (2) and Marie Paulin (5), together with Lindi's very first resident, Simbangai — were submitted to biopsies, and considered for inclusion in the trial. (They were, however, rejected, and allowed to resume their favored-chimp status.)

20. These twenty-seven would not have been eligible for the third trial, but it is not known if they were still alive at the time of that trial.

21. It would seem that during his six weeks in Stanleyville, Tom Norton injected CHAT, Fox, and maybe SM N-90 into the spines of ten or fifteen chimps, and monitored their health status, as well as monitoring those chimps that had been fed YSK on his arrival.

22. The 30 animals thus would have comprised 25 fed YSK, of which 5 were paralyzed, and 5 replacements fed only with "Mexican." Presumably some chimps would have died in the course of the following year, and would therefore not feature in the Deinhardt databook.

23. For probably the first mention of Koprowski's theory, see H. Koprowski, G. A. Jervis, and T. W. Norton, "Oral Administration of a Rodent-Adapted Strain of Poliomyelitis Virus to Chimpanzees," *Arch. Ges. Virusforsch.,* 1954, 5(5), 413–424. Koprowski mentioned the idea again at his speech at the nurses' school on February 7, 1957, when he told the audience that "experiments are being done to see if attenuated Type 1 virus can immunize human beings against the other [polio] viruses." See Anon., "La Mission Courtois-Koprowski et la lutte contre la Poliomyélite," *Le Stanleyvillois,* February 12, 1957.

24. Indeed, in his 1959 lab report, Ninane announced that the Stanleyville doctors intended to safety test a Type 2 polio vaccine on five chimps in 1960 (which may well have been one of Koprowski's new "temperature-adapted" Type 2 strains, TN-19 or TN-21). See R. I. Carp and H. Koprowski, "A New Test of the Reproductive Capacity Temperature Marker of Poliovirus: the Limited Thermal Exposure Test," *Virol.,* 1962, 16, 71–79.

25. One suspects that if intracerebral safety testing had been conducted, it would have been mentioned in the *BMJ* 58 report.

26. Furthermore, even when fed large doses, chimps do not demonstrate excreted virus in the stools. See A. B. Sabin, "Present Status of Attenuated Live Virus Poliomyelitis Vaccine," *Bull. N.Y. Acad. Med.,* 1957, 33(1), 17–39, in which Sabin concludes: "This [the lack of excreted poliovirus in the stools of chimps fed OPV] is the main reason why ultimate

definitive studies on attenuated strains had to be carried out in human beings." Norton had a copy of this article in his stored papers. Also see Stanley Plotkin's retrospective comments about the lack of relevance of the chimp work at Lindi, in chapter 41.

27. "Service de virologie — Compte rendu analytique du travail effectué dans le service," in *1958 Annual Report of Laboratoire Médical de Stanleyville.*

28. These experiments being: feeding Types 1 and 2 wild virus; vaccination with Type 1 and challenge with Type 2; and the intraspinal safety tests.

29. The figure of 94 breaks down into 30 fed virulent viruses, 25 vaccinated with Type 1 and challenged with Type 2, and 39 injected intraspinally.

30. Anon., "Mort ou Vif. Un bock avec Ghislain Courtois, Directeur du Laboratoire de Stanleyville," *Pourqoui Pas* (Belgian Congo), exact date unknown, but apparently April–May 1958.

31. Anon., "Dans la plaine de la Ruzizi: Vaccination massive contre la poliomyélite," *Centre Afrique,* April 8, 1958, p. 1.

32. Lefebvre, "Note concernant le soixantième anniversaire des experiences de domestication de l'éléphant au Congo Belge et les activités durant la dernière décennie de la Station de la Chasse (Gangala na Bodio et Epulu)."

33. One or two of the numbers are chronologically slightly out of order, and it seems possible that some of the early chimps were given replacement numbers (presumably of chimps that had died); one chimp, for instance, is numbered "4 bis" (4 twice). This suggests that the grand total may have been even higher.

34. G. Courtois, "Sur la réalisation d'une singerie de chimpanzés au Congo," *Symposium International sur l'avenir des animaux de laboratoire,* Lyon, September 18–20, 1966 (Lyon: Institut Mérieux, 1967), pp. 235–244.

35. This suggestion correlates quite well with the experience of the chimp and baboon colony at Pastoria, in French West Africa, which admitted an average of forty-two chimps a year between 1950 and 1956, of which one-third died of natural causes. See G. Lefrou and V. Michard, "Etude sur les causes de mortalité des chimpanzés en captivité à l'Institut Pasteur de Kindia (1950–1956)," *Ann. Inst. Past.,* 1957, 93(4), 502–516.

36. G. Courtois, "Sur la réalisation d'une singerie de chimpanzés au Congo," see p. 243. Interestingly, it was the isolation of the *Klebsiella* organism from the chimps in 1956/7 that led to the discovery that it was also locally widespread in humans. P. Osterrieth, "Propriétés biochimiques des Klebsiella," *Ann. Soc. Belg. Méd. Trop.,* 1958, 38, 721–730.

37. P. Doupagne, "The Identification of 113 Strains of 'Candida'. 'Levine E.M.B.A.', the Ideal Medium for the Identification of Candida Albicans in Hot Countries," *Bulletin des Grands Endemies en Afrique,* 1960, 1, 262–264.

38. When questioned on this point thirty-four years later, Doupagne was unable to say for certain whether any of the *Candida* isolates might have come from the Lindi chimps.

39. Anon., "1993 Revised Classification System for HIV Infection and Expanded Surveillance Case Definition for AIDS Among Adolescents and Adults," *MMWR,* 1992, 41 (RR-17), 1–19; see p. 17.

40. R. V. Henrickson, M. B. Gardner et al., "Epidemic of Acquired Immunodeficiency in Rhesus Macaques," *Lancet,* 1983, 1(i), 388–390.

41. In his *Klebsiella* article (see note 36), Osterrieth writes that the organism was isolated from sick persons with urinary infections and fatal pneumonias at Stanleyville hospital. He provided no figures for the deaths.

42. Martine Peeters and colleagues tested 95 chimpanzees, of which 2 were found to be positive. M. Peeters et al., "Isolation and Partial Characterization of an HIV-Related Virus

Occurring Naturally in Chimpanzees in Gabon," *AIDS,* 1989, 3, 625–630. Later, they
tested a chimp brought illegally into Brussels airport, and found that to be SIV-positive
too, making a total of 3 positives out of 96 chimps tested. M. Peeters et al., "Isolation and
Characterization of a New Chimpanzee Lentivirus (Simian Immunodeficiency Virus
Isolate cpz-ant) from a Wild-Captured Chimpanzee," *AIDS,* 1992, 6, 447–451.

43. Gilbert Rollais, personal communications, 1994, 1995, 1996. For the present, I feel it
    is better not to divulge publicly the specific areas where Rollais mounted his chimp
    capture operations, though there may come a time when such information can be
    responsibly and usefully followed up.

44. Z. Chen, D. D. Ho, P. A. Marx et al., "Genetic Characterization of New West African
    Simian Immunodeficiency Virus SIVsm: Geographic Clustering of Household-Derived
    SIV Strains with Human Immunodeficiency Virus Type 2 Subtypes and Genetically
    Diverse Viruses from a Single Feral Sooty Mangabey Troop," *J. Virol.,* 1996, 70(6),
    3617–3627.

45. The chimp that provided the SIVcpz-gab-1 isolate was four years old, the host of
    SIVcpz-gab-2 was two years old, while that of SIVcpz-ant was about five; all were there-
    fore juveniles.

46. For interspecies SIV transmission in an African primate colony, through male/male
    aggression, see E. Nevrienet et al., "Phylogenetic Analysis of SIV and STLV Type 1 in
    Mandrills (*Mandrillus sphinx*): Indications That Intracolony Transmissions Are Pre-
    dominantly the Result of Male-to-Male Aggressive Contacts," *AIDS Res. Hum. Retro.,*
    1998, 14(9), 785–796. M. J. Jin, P. M. Sharp, B. H. Hahn et al., "Infection of a Yellow
    Baboon with Simian Immunodeficiency Virus from African Green Monkeys: Evidence
    for Cross-Species Transmission in the Wild," *J. Virol.,* 1994, 68(12), 8454–8460. It should
    be added that, of the hundred-plus chimpanzees infected experimentally with a
    lentivirus from a closely related species (HIV-1), just one (infected with three different
    strains of HIV-1) has gone on to get AIDS — though another chimp transfused with its
    blood sustained a rapid decline in CD4+ cells. (F. J. Novembre et al., "Development of
    AIDS in a Chimpanzee Infected with Human Immunodeficiency Virus Type 1," *J. Virol.;*
    1997; 71[5]; 4086–4091.) Similarly, multiple infections with lentivirus strains from a
    related species (*Pan paniscus?*) and onward passage could have served to trigger simian
    AIDS in the Lindi *Pan troglodytes* chimps.

47. C. Djerassi, *The Pill, Pygmy Chimps and Degas' Horse: The Autobiography of Carl Djerassi*
    (New York: Basic Books, 1992), see p. 240. See also F. B. M. De Waal, "Bonobo Sex and
    Society," *Scientific American,* March 1995, 58–64; and F. J. White, "Pygmy Chimpanzee
    Social Organization: Variation with Party Size and between Study Sites," *Am. J. Primatol.,*
    1992, 26, 203–214.

48. Anon., "Belgian Scientists Have High Hopes of New Vaccine" (this version from *Iraq
    Times,* March 15, 1959).

49. G. Courtois, "Sur la réalization d'une singerie de chimpanzés au Congo."

50. A year later, when the *BMJ* 58 article came out, Hillaby wrote an article about the Congo
    trials: "Live Polio Virus in Vaccine Tested," *New York Times,* July 26, 1958, p. 17.

51. See A. Kortlandt, "Statements on Pygmy Chimpanzees" (letter), *Laboratory Primate
    Newsletter,* 1976, 15(1), 15. However, in another unpublished manuscript (A. Kortlandt,
    "A Survey of Islands Where a Primate Laboratory Might Be Founded," Paper No. 3 on an
    I.L.P.B. [International Laboratory of Primate Biology], May 1960) he writes: "There are
    rumors according to which all 86 paniscus chimpanzees captured for the Laboratoire
    Medical died within a few weeks. (These rumors may exaggerate, and I was unable to

check them exactly, but I presume the core of them is true.)" Dr. Kortlandt tells me that his sources for this information about the pygmy chimp deaths were Madame Liegois (who by 1960 was helping to take care of the chimps at the lab) and Paul Osterrieth.

52. Open letter by Adriaan Kortlandt to various primatologists, dated March 18, 1960, and made available by the author. In fact, by 1960, most of the chimps would have been intended for cancer and arteriosclerosis research, rather than polio.

53. W. Henle et al., "Studies on Viral Hepatitis."

54. This was pointed out to me by Elliot Dick, who, in the early sixties, tested chimp kidneys for their ability to grow many different viruses. His experiments included the three polioviruses and, like Jezierski before him, he found chimp kidneys to be as productive as macaque kidneys. E. C. Dick, "Chimpanzee Kidney Tissue Cultures for Growth and Isolation of Viruses," *J. Bact.*, 1963, 86, 573–576; plus E. C. Dick, personal communication, 1994.

55. G. Courtois and J. Mortelmans, "Apes," *Primates in Medicine*, 1969, 2, 75–86.

56. W. Henle et al., "Studies on Viral Hepatitis," see p. 3.

57. G. Courtois and J. Mortelmans, "Apes," see p. 82.

58. H. Vagtborg (editor), *The Baboon in Medical Research* (Austin: University of Texas Press, 1965). See Deinhardt's comment in discussion session, p. 418.

59. G. Courtois, "Previsions experimentation: Station Lindi," *Laboratoire Médical Provinçal de Stanleyville*, 73/001033, October 1 1957, in file H4475/984 of the Belgian Foreign Ministry archives. The total annual budget was calculated at 2,195,400 Bf — or approximately $40,000 U.S. or £15,000 sterling. This included all the African wages, provisions and medicaments for the chimps, and the purchase of a truck.

60. The great microbiologist S. E. Luria had advised that the last host cell in which a virus was grown determined its host range thereafter. S. E. Luria, "Cell Susceptibility to Viruses," *Ann. N.Y. Acad. Sci.*, 1955, 61, 852–855.

61. Anon., "India Cuts Export of Some Monkeys," *New York Times*, March 11, 1955, p. 27. See also Anon., "India Will Permit the Export of Monkeys to be Used in Genuine Medical Research," *New York Times*, April 14, 1955, p. 21.

62. D. Bodian, "Poliovirus in Chimpanzee Tissues after Virus Feeding," *Am. J. Hyg.*, 1956, 64, 181–197. That Courtois was familiar with this research was proven in 1960, when he made a lengthy (albeit unreferenced) allusion to it in a speech about enteroviruses in Leopoldville, published in English as G. Courtois, "Present Day Progress in our Knowledge of the Enterovirus," *Bull. des Grands Endemies en Afrique*, 1960, 2, 271–285.

63. W. Henle et al., "Studies on Viral Hepatitis."

64. Kidneys are one of the easiest organs to remove from a body. As surgeon Wilson Carswell explains: "You push the colon to one side, and make one cut . . . each side, and you're down in the kidney. It's snip, snip, snip, snip, and it's in your hand."

65. A. B. Sabin, "Properties and Behavior of Orally Administered Attenuated Poliovirus Vaccine," *J. Am. Med. Assoc.*, 1957, 164(11), 1216–1223.

66. This was the less virulent Type 1 strain, Brunhilde, modified by John Enders, and passed through a chimpanzee by Albert Sabin. See J. Gear, "The South African Poliomyelitis Vaccine," *S. Af. Med. J.*, 1956, 30, 587–594, and W. Wood, "The Production of Poliomyelitis Vaccine in 1956," *Proc. Roy. Soc. Med.*, 1957, 50, 1068–1070.

67. The proportion of kidney weight to total body weight is even higher in the chimpanzee than in man. See G. H. Bourne (editor), *Physiology, Behavior, Serology, and Diseases of Chimpanzees — Volume 2* (Basel: S. Karger, 1970), especially the chapter entitled "Renal Function in the Chimpanzee," by J. A. Gagnon, pp. 69–99.

68. For instance, the definition of monkey in *The Shorter Oxford English Dictionary* (Guild Publishing, 1983, 3rd edition), p. 1348, is "An animal of any species of the group of mammals closely allied to and resembling man, and ranging from the anthropoid apes to the marmosets; any animal of the order *Primates* except man and the lemurs. In a more restricted sense, the term is taken to exclude the anthropoid apes and the baboons." The usage of monkeys as including all nonhuman primates (including chimps) is even more common in French, in which the term *"singes"* embraces *"chimpanzés"* also.

69. L. Quersin-Thiry, "Action of Anticellular Sera on Virus Infections. 1. Influence on Homologous Tissue Cultures Infected with Various Viruses," *J. Immunol.*, 1958, 81, 253–260. L. Quersin-Thiry, "Action of Anticellular Sera on Virus Infections. 2. Influence on Heterologous Tissue Cultures," *J. Immunol.*, 1959, 82, 542–552.

70. They were listed as 49 *Pan paniscus* and 30 *Pan troglodytes.* However, the localities listed for each skull suggest that some of the chimps may have been mislabeled at source, and that the real totals should have been 47 *paniscus* and 32 *troglodytes.*

71. We know that two hundred tubes and ten bottles of baboon kidney tissue culture were prepared at the Stanleyville lab, but that was in 1958. (See p. 95 of the 1958 annual report of the Service Médicale de Province Orientale.) Given the fact that hundreds of chimps were used in 1957, during the early days of Lindi camp, it seems more likely that the kidneys sent by Courtois in that year would have been chimp kidneys.

72. Henry Gelfand, personal communication, 1996.

73. Letter from G. Courtois to J. Stijns dated February 17, 1961, made available by Dr. André Courtois.

74. It is hard to know which version of events is correct as regards the fate of the last group of Lindi chimps — this one, Gaston Ninane's belief that they were either shot or eaten, or Gilbert Rollais's recollection that some were released to the bush, while others were transported to Leopoldville Zoo. It may be that some chimpanzees met with each of these fates.

75. A. Kortlandt, "A Survey of Islands Where a Primate Laboratory Might be Founded," pp. 4 and 5. This unpublished 1960 memorandum was posted to fifty-three scientists, mainly primatologists.

76. Madame Brakel, personal communication, January 1997. No other Stanleyville resident has suggested that Jamba (or Djamba) was *born* at Lindi, but it is certainly possible.


CHAPTER 53: *Where CHAT Was Fed*

1. Anon., "Live Virus in the Jungle," *Time,* August 11, 1958, p. 30.

2. G. Courtois, "Vaccination antipoliomyélitique par virus vivant au Congo Belge," *Ann. Soc. Belg. Méd. Trop.,* 1958, 38, 805–816. This account of the Stanleyville vaccinations of 1957/8, which includes "the children of the military camps," matches what I was told by the Belgian doctors far more closely than does the account provided (by Koprowski?) in *BMJ* 58. The latter states that "infants, children and adults of European and native origin living in Stanleyville," and "a large group of schoolchildren, mostly of European origin," were vaccinated.

3. W. Bervoets, personal communication, 1996.

4. Sister Amelia, personal communication, 1994.

5. Alex Forro, personal communication, 1994. According to one source, Vicicongo's responsibility for medical services in Aketi may also have terminated shortly before the end of 1957. See Service de l'Hygiene Publique de Stanleyville, 1957 annual report, p. 169.

6. There had previously been mass feedings of OPV in Morocco in the early fifties, but this involved a French-made vaccine prepared in rabbit tissues. See M. Blanc and L.-A. Martin, "Premiers essais de prophylaxie de la poliomyélite par virus vivant fixé au lapin. Innocuité de la méthode," *Bull. Acad. Med.*, 1953, 137, 230–234. I have been unable to determine exactly when in 1957 Sabin's OPV trials began in the Soviet Union, but it was probably in the second half of the year.

7. S. R. Pattyn, "Anti-Poliomyelitic Vaccination in Tropical Countries," *Trop. Geogr. Med.*, 1964, 14, 4–9. Dr. Pattyn emphasized that the "Koprowski system" allowed the vaccine to be transported in concentrated form and diluted at the last minute, one day at a time, because "vaccine which remains at the end of the day is generally contaminated and had better not be used the following day."

8. Letter dated September 17, 1958, from Bervoets to De Brauwere, in file H4484/1058, Ministry of Foreign Affairs archives (Belgium).

9. G. Courtois, "Vaccination antipoliomyélitique par virus vivant au Congo Belge." See also Anon., "Dans la plaine de la Ruzizi: Vaccination massive contre la poliomyélite," *Centre Afrique*, April 8, 1958. This article contains one important error, for it claims that both Koprowski and Sabin vaccines were being tried in Ruzizi — a claim not corroborated by other sources.

10. Just three towns are shown in the map in *BMJ* 58: Bukavu, Kabunambo, and Usumbura. Kabunambo was indeed fed in the Ruzizi Valley campaign, and Usumbura was fed during the Meyus/Ninane vaccination that immediately followed. But Bukavu was not vaccinated until later in 1958, after the article had been published. The map is poorly drawn, and suggests that Kabunambo lies on Lake Tanganyika; it is actually fifty miles north of there, in the Ruzizi Valley.

11. The largest Vicicongo depot outside Aketi, the main center for distribution of goods coming from the east coast ports to eastern Congo, was at Kamanyola, just a few miles north of Kabunambo on the west side of the Ruzizi Valley. There was also a military camp at Kamanyola, and Ninane recalled vaccinating there.

12. In a letter to a friend written on February 26, 1958, Dr. Flack describes the first day of vaccination. "Monday we were greeted at a village by a horde of humans — babies, old men, women, etc etc — and immunized 2,579. They are like . . . chickens [and] run in all directions — all anxious to get the miracle medicine. I measured and delivered into a tablespoon each dose, which was poured into each mouth by four workers (2 doctors, 2 natives). The spoons were resterilized and used over and over. What a system, a real production." Later in the day, organization must have improved, for she writes: "The natives wait patiently and eagerly in the sun. They stand in long rows or sit while waiting their turn." (Copy of a letter from Agnes Flack to "Bee," a friend at Clinton Farms.)

13. G. Courtois, "Vaccination antipoliomyélitique par virus vivant au Congo Belge," p. 811.

14. Letter from Dr. Flack to "Lois," dated March 19, 1958.

15. Quite possibly Dr. Flack's version of Kuryange, north of Bujumbura in present-day Burundi.

16. The Phillipses (she a journalist, he a well-known freelance photographer) apparently went to the Belgian colonies "at the behest of the Belgian government, against which there was a condemnation resolution before the U.N.," and part of their travel expenses was paid by the Belgians. Most of their time was spent at big projects like the Inga dam and the mines in Katanga, and they apparently "fell into the polio story quite by accident." They spent a day in the Ruzizi Valley, having dinner with Agnes Flack on the

shores of Lake Tanganyika, and they also met Fritz Deinhardt in Stanleyville. (Joan Phillips, personal communication, August 1995.)

17. This detail is provided by an early draft of Koprowski's response to Curtis in *Science* (H. Koprowski, "AIDS and the Polio Vaccine" [letter], *Science*, 1992, 257, 1024–1027), which was given to me by Stanley Plotkin.

18. Anon., "On Vaccine," *Le Stanleyvillois*, March 7, 1958.

19. See G. Courtois, "Vaccination antipoliomyélitique par virus vivant au Congo Belge," p. 811. The deference to Jervis suggests that it was he who was seen as Koprowski's representative at Ruzizi.

20. Anon., "Ruzizi. Campagne de vaccination massive contre la poliomyélite," *Temps Nouveau d'Afrique*, April 13, 1958.

21. In fact, 15,000 (not 10,000) further people were fed CHAT in Stanleyville.

22. This may refer to the region of Kabare, near Bukavu in Kivu province, and that of Lubudi, in Katanga province (now Shaba). However, these towns are hundreds of miles apart, and it would seem possible that "Kabare" was either misheard or misprinted, for Lake Kabwe and the town of Kalule are both near Lubudi. If correct, then Lubudi would appear to be the only major feeding of CHAT in Katanga. The provincial director of medicine from the end of the fifties, Dr. Jean Delville, tells me that his doctors first used the Salk vaccine and then that of Sabin, rather than Koprowski. He believes, however, that individual areas like Lubudi might well have made other arrangements, either through the initiative of a local mining or agricultural company (which tended to carry out their own vaccinations), or of an enterprising missionary.

23. Anon., "La lutte contre le polio au Congo: une nouvelle étape," *Courrier d'Afrique* (Leopoldville), May 4, 1959, pp. 4 and 6.

24. Laboratoire Médical Provincial, Stanleyville, *Rapport Annuel*, 1959, penultimate page.

25. Mary Fagg and Dr. Jim Bishop, personal communications, December 1996. Ms. Fagg worked for the BMS at Yakusu as a senior registered nurse between 1951 and 1972. She recalls that the vaccine was provided by Dr. Courtois (which dates the event as occurring before September 1959), and fed in drop form to children at all the clinics that the BMS ran between Yakusu (ten miles west of Lindi camp) and Yaselia, near Yangambi, the INEAC headquarters.

26. The Coquilhatville campaign was mentioned in Ghislain Courtois's letters.

27. These were the inspector general of *hygiène* for the Belgian Congo (Wilfried Bervoets), the director of the Marcel Wanson Institute of Hygiene in Leopoldville (André Lebrun), and the chief of the Service d'Hygiène in Leo (Jacques Cerf), all of whom were interviewed in person.

28. I have also come across one reference (in a letter of October 10, 1959, from Dr. Dricot to De Brauwere in Brussels, in file H4484/1058 at the Belgian Ministry of Foreign Affairs) to a planned vaccination in Luluabourg (now Kananga), the largest town in Kasai province. However, this was at the time that there were frequent references to a nationwide CHAT vaccination of Congolese children, and since I have come across no confirmation of this campaign, I have treated it as anecdotal and omitted it from the final list.

29. The paper was dated February 1961, and Caubergh confirmed that it provided a retrospective overview of *all* the CHAT vaccinations that had taken place in Urundi.

30. Ghislain Courtois, in his French-language account of the Ruzizi vaccinations, had detailed the Ruanda-Urundi side of the campaign as involving 59,772 children and 81,913 adults. See G. Courtois, "Vaccination antipoliomyélitique par virus vivant au Congo Belge."

31. This involved a total of some 272,000 infant and child vaccinations in the six *territoires* of Ngozi, Muhinga, Ruyigi, Kitega, Muramvya, and Rutana.

32. In 1960, some 50,000 children were fed in 36 centers in the *territoires* of Bubanza and Usumbura, including 18 centers where CHAT had already been fed in 1958.

33. The 1960 report of the medical services of Ruanda-Urundi features a figure of 382,638 for "anti-polio vaccinations." This is close enough to the total of 379,077 in Caubergh's paper (which included the Urundi CHAT campaigns of both 1958 and 1959/60) to suggest that Caubergh's grand total for 1958–1960 was carelessly used as the basis for the annual total for 1960. The alternative explanation is that some 60,000 adult vaccinations were included in the 1960 figure.

34. Populations are as given in *Chambers's World Gazetteer and Geographical Dictionary* (London: Chambers, 1957).

35. Caubergh is not certain, but believes that by the time of the 1959 Ruanda vaccination, they may still have been vaccinating all those who turned up (including accompanying adults), rather than just the children. He recalls, however, that by 1959/60 the vaccine supplies from Stanleyville were beginning to run low, and so the Burundi teams would only feed parents and siblings when spare vaccine was left over at the end of a day.

36. This total applies if the 64,000 mooted vaccinations in "Kabare-Lubudi" are included, and if one assumes an average of 5,000 vaccinees for each of the campaigns for which there are no numerical details.

37. This is a minimum total for adults. The total may be many more than 60,000 if adults were also fed in 1959/60.

38. This speech was also published in English as G. Courtois, "Present Day Progress in Our Knowledge of the Enterovirus," *Bull. des Grands Endemies en Afrique*, 1960, 2, 271–285.

39. Anon., "History of the Use of CHAT Strain 'Type 1' Attenuated Polio Virus in Humans," undated, though it appears to have been written in January 1958. This single page of text was submitted by the Wistar Institute to the Wistar expert committee. It is the only salient information about the history of the African pools of CHAT to be submitted to that committee, and it was released to me in 1995 by David Ho.

40. This was how Koprowski described the form of CHAT vaccine that was injected into five of the Lindi chimps. See his discussion in *NYAS* 57, especially p. 129.

41. This hypothesis is supported by two undated articles ("Call to Duty" and "Dr. Flack Is Assigned to Belgian Congo") from late 1957 in local Pennsylvania newspapers (one the *Wilkes-Barre Record*), which report that Agnes Flack was originally scheduled to leave for Stanleyville to participate in the mass trial on December 7, 1957. The articles reported that Dr. Flack would oversee immunizations to be conducted on about 75,000 persons in four areas of the Congo, including Stanleyville, Bukavu, and Elisabethville (Lubumbashi). This suggests that a large batch of 10A-11 had already been prepared by that date, even though the first trials at Clinton of this pool began only in mid-November 1957. It may be that although the Ruzizi trial was delayed until February 1958, some of the vaccine was air-freighted out to Stanleyville in December or early January, and was used in Banalia from January 8 to January 12, 1958. The same vaccine may have been used for the three epidemic feedings in Gombari, Watsa, and Bambesa (fed between January 27 and February 1), or this latter batch of CHAT may have arrived courtesy of Deinhardt.

42. G. Courtois, "Vaccination antipoliomyélitique par virus vivant au Congo Belge," *Ann. Soc. Belg. Méd. Trop.*, 1958, 38, 805–816.

43.   The *BMJ* 58 article about the Ruzizi campaign clearly states: "The large pools representing
      each strain [CHAT and Fox] were prepared in the Laboratories of the Wistar Institute,
      Philadelphia." This is confirmed by a contemporary newspaper article from Philadelphia,
      which states that the vaccine used in Ruzizi (and in Province Oriental) had been grown in
      flasks containing tissue culture at the Wistar's laboratories and flown out to Africa in con-
      centrated form, to be diluted there. See P. C. Fraley, "Polio Vaccine Made Here Given to
      244,596 in Africa," *Sunday Bulletin* (Philadelphia), July 27, 1958, p. 19. In his own report
      of the campaign, Ghislain Courtois identifies the pool used as 10A-11; see G. Courtois,
      "Vaccination antipoliomyélitique par virus vivant au Congo Belge." However, other clues
      suggest that whereas the CHAT 10A-11 virus strain was developed at the Wistar, not all of
      the vaccine pool 10A-11 was made there. An article from Stanleyville published soon after
      the start of the campaign forecasts that the campaign will involve 150,000; see Anon., "On
      Vaccine," *Le Stanleyvillois,* March 7, 1958. Furthermore, we know from Agnes Flack's diary
      that 150,000 was the approximate running total of vaccinees when she ended her partici-
      pation in the campaign on March 30. The remaining vaccinees therefore seem likely to
      have been fed with another batch during the final eleven days of the campaign. This is
      confirmed by a later article: Anon., "Ruzizi. Campagne de vaccination massive contre
      la poliomyélite," *Temps Nouveau d'Afrique,* April 13, 1958. This account, published in
      Usumbura just as the campaign was ending, makes it clear that the vaccinations were cov-
      ering the entire population between Bugarama, in the Ruzizi Valley, as far south as Nyanza
      Lac on Lake Tanganyika, and that a total of some 220,000 were being vaccinated. In other
      words, the intended total of vaccinees had risen by roughly 70,000 from that mentioned
      in *Le Stanleyvillois* a month earlier.

44.   Henry Gelfand, personal communications; 1995, 1996. It seems likely that this same
      pool of CHAT, 13, was also used for the immunization campaign in the economically
      important town of Bukavu, which Gelfand visited later in his Congo journey, and where
      he thinks he may also have delivered vaccine.

45.   A press conference held in Leopoldville in 1959 by Courtois, Lebrun, and Plotkin about
      the vaccination campaign in the city (Anon., "La vaccination massive contre la polyo,"
      *L'Avenir,* May 2–3, 1959) states clearly that the Wistar Institute makes the Koprowski
      vaccine. There is no mention of Belgian involvement.

46.   S. A. Plotkin, B. J. Cohen, and H. Koprowski, "Intratypic Serodifferentiation of Polio-
      viruses," *Virol.,* 1961, 15, 473–485.

47.   This was presumably the CHAT pool made at RIT in 1959, which was mentioned by
      Huygelen and Peetermans, though both claimed it had been used in Poland, not the
      Congo.

48.   H. Koprowski, "AIDS and the Polio Vaccine" (letter), *Science,* 1992, 257, 1024–1027.

49.   F. Przesmycki, J. Georgiades et al., "Report on Field Trials with Live Attenuated
      Poliomyelitis Vaccine of Koprowski in Poland," *Am. J. Hyg.,* 1960, 71, 275–284. See also
      J. Georgiades, "Research on the Penetration of the Attenuated Polio Virus Strain Type 1
      (CHAT) into an Unvaccinated Population in Wyszkow and the Surrounding District,"
      *Bull. Inst. Med. Morsk.,* 1959, 10(5/6), 75–82. There is no evidence that AIDS emerged
      early in Poland. However, the Polish pool 13 trial was actually very minor, with just
      2,888 children being fed in Wyszkow and neighboring villages — a fact sometimes over-
      looked by detractors of the OPV theory, who recall only that some seven million chil-
      dren received CHAT in Poland. (In fact, the seven million were fed with CHAT pool 18.)

50.   The Swedes accurately reported that they had made a further passage of CHAT 10A-11
      in cynomolgus tissue — but they were not, it would seem, aware of which species of

primate Koprowski had been using to make the tissue culture for his version of the vaccine. The corollary is that different vaccine production lots, prepared in different substrates, can be prepared from the same numbered pool of attenuated poliovirus.

51. D. Ikic, "Polio Vaccines Prepared in Human Diploid Cells," in 1st International Conference on Vaccines against Viral and Rickettsial Diseases of Man (Washington, D.C., November 7–11, 1967), published as PAHO Scientific Publication 147, May 1967, 185–189.

52. Many might find it remarkable that production lots of a vaccine pool are not given separate designations — such as 13 (P-Cy) and 13 (L-Ch) — to identify the place of manufacture, and the substrate used.

53. Marie Antoinette Bossut, personal communication, 1994.

54. Gaston Ninane, personal communication, 1992.

55. From Agnes Flack's diary. Similarly, in a letter to "Bee," a friend at Clinton Farms, dated February 26, 1958, she writes: "Each village chief brings his people, and those that object get 'what for' in no uncertain terms with much shouting." In a postcard to Ruth Lorenzo from the same period, Dr. Flack wrote: "Whole villages turn out with their chief. He doesn't ask for their request [i.e. compliance]."

56. A. Lebrun, J. Cerf, H. M. Gelfand, G. Courtois, S. A. Plotkin, and H. Koprowski, "Vaccination with the CHAT Strains of Type 1 Attenuated Poliomyelitis Virus in Leopoldville, Belgian Congo. 1. Description of the City, Its History of Poliomyelitis, and the Plan of the Vaccination Campaign," *Bull. WHO*, 1960, 22, 203–213; see p. 210.

57. *BMJ* 58.

58. H. Koprowski, "Etat actuel de l'immunisation contre la poliomyélite avec des virus vivants atténués," *Rev. Lyon. Méd.*, January 1959, pp. 39–40, which is the transcript of a short speech he gave at the Symposium Internationale de Virologie, held in Lyon between June 7 and 9, 1958.

59. S. A. Plotkin, A. Lebrun, and H. Koprowski, "Vaccination with the CHAT Strain of Type 1 Attenuated Poliomyelitis Virus in Leopoldville, Belgian Congo. 2. Studies of the Safety and Efficacy of Vaccination," *Bull. WHO*, 1960, 22, 215–234; see p. 218.

60. Stanley Plotkin, personal communication, 1994.

61. B. K. Nottay et al., "Molecular Variation of Type 1 Vaccine-Related and Wild Polioviruses during Replication in Humans," *Virol.*, 1981, 108, 415–423; M. Nakano et al., "Genetical Analysis on the Stability of Poliovirus Type 3 Leon 12a1b," *J. Biol. Stand.*, 1979, 7, 157–168; WHO Consultative Group, "Evidence on the Safety and Efficacy of Live Poliomyelitis Vaccines Currently in Use, with Special Reference to Type 3 Poliovirus," *Bull. WHO*, 1969, 40, 925–945.

62. J. R. Wilson, *Margin of Safety — The Story of Poliomyelitis Vaccine* (London: Collins, 1963), pp. 213–219.

63. D. S. Dane, G. W. A. Dick et al., "Vaccination against Poliomyelitis with Live Virus Vaccines. 1. A Trial of TN Type II Vaccine," *BMJ*, 1957, 1(i), 59–65; G. W. A. Dick and D. S. Dane, "3. The Evaluation of TN and SM Virus Vaccines," *BMJ*, 1957, 1(i), 70–74.

64. Anon., "Sonoma Polio Test Cleared In 4 New Cases," *San Francisco Call-Bulletin*, 1953 (date unknown), p. 6.

65. Letter from Dr. W. P. Bervoets to the Belgian inspector general of hygiene, dated September 17, 1958, found in file H4484/1058 at the Belgian Ministry of Foreign Affairs.

66. Also in 1960, the stools from two contacts of a person fed CHAT pool 10A-11 in Switzerland were tested by Roderick Murray and colleagues from the NIH's Division of Biologics Standards. They found that these stool viruses had an altered character in

MKTC, and caused a higher level of paralysis when inoculated into monkeys. In the same report, they found that two further tissue culture passages of another Koprowski Type 1 vaccine, Wistar, at the raised temperature of 40°C, resulted in a marked increase in neurovirulence. S. Baron et al., "Laboratory Investigations of the Attenuated Poliovirus Vaccine Strains. II. Tissue Culture Characteristics before and after Gastrointestinal Passage," *PAHO2*, 124–131. What would be interesting, of course, would be if the viruses from these polio cases could be sequenced and compared to the vaccine viruses by modern phylogenetic analysis.

67. S. A. Plotkin, A. Lebrun, G. Courtois, and H. Koprowski, "Vaccination with the CHAT Strain of Type 1 Attenuated Poliomyelitis Virus in Leopoldville, Congo. 3. Safety and Efficacy during the First 21 Months of Study," *Bull. WHO*, 1961, 24, 785–792.

68. H. Plotkin et al., "Vaccination with the CHAT Strain of Type 1 Attenuated Poliomyelitis Virus in Leopoldville, Belgian Congo. 2."

69. S. Gard, "Immunological Strain Specificity within Type 1 Poliovirus," *Bull. WHO*, 1960, 22, 235–242. See also H. Koprowski, T. W. Norton, E. Wecker, and S. Gard, "Genetic Markers and Serological Identity of Wild and Attenuated Strains of Type 1 Poliovirus, with Special Emphasis on Strains Isolated from Patients During an Epidemic in the Belgian Congo," *Bull. WHO*, 1960, 22, 243–253, which is especially interesting. The authors write that present analysis of viruses from the paralytic cases suggests that they are distinct from the vaccine virus, and that no reversion has occurred, but then concede: "It is possible to argue that the attenuated virus lost its original characteristics after, let us say, ten human passages and became indistinguishable from wild virus." When I interviewed Sven Gard in 1993, he was extremely skeptical about the safety of CHAT and other OPVs, from the perspective both of reversion and freedom from contamination.

70. Anon., "Prolonged Poliovirus Excretion in an Immunodeficient Person with Vaccine-Associated Paralytic Poliomyelitis," *MMWR*, 1997, 46(28), 641–643.

71. This comment is taken from a previous draft of De Moor's article, given me by André Courtois. The published version of the article (J. De Moor, "Evolution de la poliomyélite à Leopoldville de 1951 à 1963," *Ann. Soc. Belg. Méd. Trop.*, 1965, 45[6], 651–664) is slightly less forthright.

72. J. De Moor, "Evolution de la poliomyélite à Leopoldville de 1951 à 1963," p. 659. See also Anon., "Polio Vaccine Donated to the Congo (Leopoldville)," *WHO Chronicle*, 1961, 15(10), 388, which reports that the Wellcome Foundation had donated doses of the trivalent (Sabin) vaccine.

73. De Moor reports that the population of Leo rose from 550,000 in 1960 to 850,000 in 1962 and an estimated 1.3 million in 1964.

74. Lebrun et al., "Vaccination with the CHAT Strain of Type 1 Attenuated Poliomyelitis Virus in Leopoldville, Belgian Congo. 1."; see especially p. 209.

75. *BMJ 58*. See also G. Courtois, "Vaccination antipoliomyélitique par virus vivant au Congo Belge."

76. See file H4484/1058 ("Poliomyélite: Correspondance") at the Belgian Ministry of Foreign Affairs archives, which covers the period 1956–1960, but has no entries for this key period.

77. Anon., "Expert Committee on Poliomyelitis: Second Report," *WHO Tech. Rep. Ser.*, 1958, 145, 1–83; see p. 25.

78. Anon., "U.N. Group Urges Wide Trials of a Live-Virus Polio Vaccine," *New York Times*, July 20, 1957, pp. 1 and 4.

79. *BMJ 58*.

80. A.M.-M. Payne, "Poliomyelitis Vaccine" (letter), *BMJ,* 1958, 2(ii), 1472–1473.

81. Anon., "Expert Committee on Poliomyelitis: Second Report"; see pp. 25–27.

82. Plotkin et al., "Vaccination with the CHAT Strain of Type 1 Attenuated Poliomyelitis Virus in Leopoldville, Belgian Congo. 2." Plotkin's name is followed by a similar disclaimer in the Moorestown paper.

83. Anon., "La lutte contre le polio au Congo: une nouvelle étape." See also Anon., "La vaccination massive contre le polyo," *L'Avenir* (Leopoldville), May 2–3, 1959.

84. One of the articles about Agnes Flack's assistance with the Ruzizi vaccinations states baldly: "The polio immunization program in the Belgian Congo was a joint undertaking of the Belgian and United States Public Health Services." (See Anon., "Wilson to Honor Physician Agnes Flack," *Wilson College Bull.,* April 1959, 4, 1.) And when Ghislain Courtois sought further funding from the Congo authorities for Lindi camp, he wrote of the collaboration between the Stanleyville laboratory and the Wistar Institute: "We can count on this collaboration over the years to come because the work . . . is supported by the U.S. Public Health Service." (See G. Courtois, "Projet de travail scientifique à executer en collaboration entre le laboratoire de Stanleyville et le Wistar Institute de Philadelphie (U.S.A.)," memorandum dated October 7, 1957, file H4475/984, available in Ministry of Foreign Affairs archives [Belgium].)

85. "Public Health Service Grants and Fellowships, Awarded by the National Institutes of Health: Fiscal Year 1958 Funds," published by PHS NIH Division of Research Grants, 1958, p. 271. By the standards of the times, this was a generous grant. In the first year, for instance, it was set at $66,000, making it the fourth largest research grant out of 191 awarded to institutions in Philadelphia. By 1963, the grant was worth over $180,000. Barbara Kempner of the NIH grant management branch informs me that the grant applications forms for E-1799 were forwarded to Federal Records in 1974, and would have been destroyed seven years later. I have therefore been unable to obtain details about the specific research that the grant supported.

86. This was highlighted by a ten-minute film of the Lindi operation, which I received in 1997 from one of the former members of the Stanleyville lab. It captures many aspects of life at the chimp camp, but it also shows the old medical laboratory, a rather lovely mission-style building of brick and tile entwined by creeper, and the new lab — a huge concrete structure, seemingly far larger than required for a town the size of Stanleyville. Almost half of the building was devoted to an *animalier,* or animal house, and it seems probable that it was viewed (by whoever provided the funds) as a significant (and probably long-term) research investment.

87. G. Courtois, "Sur la réalisation d'une singerie de chimpanzés au Congo," *Symposium Internationale sur l'Avenir des Animaux de Laboratoires* (Lyon, September 18–20, 1966). Karl Meyer was director of the George Williams Hooper Foundation, a charitable organization based at the University of California, which often channeled funds to worthy research efforts — such as Koprowski's Sonoma studies. It is also possible that it helped provide informal American funds for the chimp research at Lindi.

88. Anon., "Ferme d'elevage chimpanzés," file H4487/1087, Ministry of Foreign Affairs archives (Belgium). In the end, Koprowski and Andrus did not go to Leopoldville. However, Fred Stare, a nutrition expert at Harvard (and one or two others) took their places. Fred Stare and Arthur Riopelle, personal communications, 1995.

89. Letter from Dr. G. Courtois to Dr. J. Stijns (February 17, 1961). However, in a later letter to Dr. Demarchi (April 19, 1961), Courtois explains that he has not, after all, found anybody to examine the samples.

90. Anon., "Wistar Institute Is Both Monument and Prototype of Modern Research," *Scope Weekly,* May 21, 1958, pp. 6–7. The photocopy I have of this article is indistinct toward the margins, so the words "top" and "post" of this quotation are likely, but not certain.

91. Later on, both Plotkin and Pagano left government service and formally joined the Wistar staff.

92. Joseph Pagano told me that Plotkin's effective boss at the CDC, Alex Langmuir, was left weeping with rage after one altercation with Koprowski. Apparently Langmuir suspected that Koprowski was using the presence of Plotkin and Pagano in order to obtain a de facto CDC seal of approval for the Wistar's work. Joseph Pagano, personal communication, 1993.

93. Stanley Plotkin, personal communication, April 1994.

## CHAPTER 54: *Correlation with Early HIV and AIDS*

1. G. Myers, "HIV: Between Past and Future," *AIDS Res. Human Retro.,* 1994, 10(11), 1317–1324.

2. Sharp initially used the term "starburst" to describe the sudden explosion of subtype B viruses in the United States. (P. M. Sharp et al., "Origins and Diversity of Human Immunodeficiency Viruses," *AIDS,* 1994, 8(suppl. 1), S27–S42). But I believe that it is equally applicable to the phylogenetic picture of the explosions of subtypes in Group M and Group O.

3. These cases were Montreal (1945) and New York (1959).

4. T. Zhu, B. T. Korber, A. J. Nahmias, E. Hooper, P. M. Sharp, and D. Ho, "An African HIV-1 Sequence from 1959 and Implications for the Origin of the Epidemic," *Nature,* 1998, 391, 594–597.

5. This case has never been convincingly confirmed by PCR, despite repeated attempts, although in 1997 Robert Garry claimed that he had finally obtained a PCR sequence. See T. O. Jonassen, S. S. Frøland, B. Grinde et al., "Sequence Analysis of HIV-1 Group O from Norwegian Patients Infected in the 1960s," *Virol.,* 1997, 231, 43–47; and also chapter 55.

6. Originally, Ninane was unsure whether the feeding had taken place at Lisala or the nearby town of Bumba — but eventually he decided that Lisala was almost certainly the correct venue.

7. There are in fact many more likely AIDS cases from Kinshasa from the year 1978 onward, as suggested by the 44 cases of fatal cryptococcal meningitis that occurred between 1978 and 1984, and 15 cases of the same disseminated condition that were reported in 1982, some of which occurred in 1980 or earlier. These have not, however, been included in the table in this chapter because the specific year of getting disease is unknown. See J. Vandepitte, H. Taelman et al., "Cryptococcal Meningitis and AIDS in Kinshasa, Zaire," 1st International Conference on AIDS and Associated Cancers in Africa (Brussels, 1985), abstract 04/II; and B. Lamey and N. Melameka, "Aspects cliniques et epidemiologiques de la cryptococcose à Kinshasa," *Méd. Trop.,* 1982, 42(5), 507–511.

8. Of the remainder, four involve Zambia, and one each Rwanda, Burundi, Uganda, Tanzania, and either Kenya or Cameroon. In most cases, this indicates where the patient fell ill, but in three cases involving non-Africans, it indicates the country where HIV exposure probably occurred.

9. The fact that the preponderance of cases came from Kinshasa was undoubtedly partly because it was the capital and by far the largest city, but it also reflected the fact that Kinshasa had the most doctors actively monitoring the syndrome.

10. These being the thirteen cases from Kinshasa, the two from Kisangani, and single cases from Bujumbura, Bukavu, and Lisala.

11. Uvira is ten miles from the nearest vaccination point in the Ruzizi Valley; Kigali is some fifty miles from Butare (Astrida), and less from Nyanza. Yambuku and Abumonbazi are some 90 and 140 miles, respectively, from Lisala. Likasi and Lumumbashi are 125 and 175 miles, respectively, from Lubudi, where a mass feeding of CHAT was planned. (I was unable to find out if it actually happened.)

12. A. J. Nahmias et al., "Evidence for Human Infection with an HTLV III/LAV-Like Virus in Central Africa, 1959" (letter), *Lancet,* 1986, 1(ii), 1279–1280.

13. J. Desmyter, L. Montagnier et al., "Anti-LAV/HTLV-III in Kinshasa Mothers in 1970 and 1980" (abstract), 2nd International Conference on AIDS in Africa (Paris, 1986), communication 110: S17g.

14. N. Nzilambi et al., "The Prevalence of Infection with Human Immunodeficiency Virus over a 10-Year Period in Rural Zaire," *N. Engl. J. Med.,* 1988, 318(5), 276–279. Two of the sera were positive for HIV-1 antigen, rather than antibodies.

15. J. Morvan et al., "Enquête séro-épidémiologique sur les infection à HIV au Burundi entre 1980 et 1981," *Bull. Soc. Pathol. Exot.,* 1989, 82, 130–140.

16. The two other HIV-positive samples originated from either Muramvya or Ijenda, both in the central mountains, but within thirty miles of the capital, Bujumbura.

17. P. Piot, F. A. Plummer et al., "Retrospective Seroepidemiology of AIDS Virus Infection in Nairobi Populations," *J. Infect. Dis.,* 1987, 155(6), 1108–1112. All nine HIV-positives came from high-risk groups (female prostitutes, or persons with STDs).

18. I. Wendler, A. F. Fleming, H. Schmitz et al., "Seroepidemiology of Human Immunodeficiency Virus in Africa," *BMJ,* 1986, 293, 782–785. Herbert Schmitz says that the Senegalese serum probably came from Dakar.

19. Joe McCormick claims that 0.9 percent of sera taken from around Nzara in southern Sudan in either 1976 or 1979 (he names both years) were HIV-positive. See J. B. McCormick and S. Fisher-Hoch, *The Virus Hunters — Dispatches from the Frontline* (London: Bloomsbury, 1996), pp. 185 and 190. However, since this claim appears to be based on one of the very earliest ELISA serosurveys, and since the details are confused with regard to year and seem never to have been reported in the literature, I have felt it best to omit them from the list.

20. Other papers show that it was only the Bujumbura blood samples from the Morvan survey (see n.15) that were taken in 1980; the other Burundian samples were taken in 1981.

21. Kihanga was fed again in 1959/60, but this time only 935 children were fed, as compared to 2,891 in 1958.

22. Although Kihanga lies in the Ruzizi Valley, it is only some fifteen miles northwest of Bujumbura, so HIV could alternatively have spread there from the capital in the course of twenty years.

23. J. Sonnet, J.-L. Michaux et al., "Early AIDS Cases Originating from Zaire and Burundi (1962–1976)," *Scand. J. Infect. Dis.,* 1987, 19, 511–517.

24. Anon., "La lutte contre la polio au Congo: une nouvelle étape," *Courrier d'Afrique* (Leopoldville), May 4, 1959, p. 4.

25. This suggests that several thousand people were vaccinated, not "a couple of hundred," as Plotkin claimed to me in interview.

26. Michel Vandeputte, personal communication, September 1997; André Lebrun, personal communication, May 1995.

27. S. A. Plotkin, A. Lebrun, G. Courtois, and H. Koprowski, "Vaccination with the CHAT Strain of Attenuated Poliomyelitis Virus in Leopoldville, Congo. 3. Safety and Efficacy during the First 21 Months of Study," *Bull. WHO*, 1961, 24, 785–792; see pp. 789–790. André Lebrun confirmed that this report of 364 Europeans of all ages and 253 African children being fed CHAT in November 1959 in a group of "villages" actually referred to a vaccination in and around Kikwit.

28. See also A. Lebrun, J. Cerf, H. M. Gelfand, G. Courtois, S. A. Plotkin, and H. Koprowski, "Vaccination with the CHAT Strain of Type 1 Attenuated Poliomyelitis Virus in Leopold-ville, Belgian Congo. 1. Description of the City, Its History of Poliomyelitis, and the Plan of the Vaccination Campaign," *Bull. WHO*, 1960, 22, 203–213, see p. 210, footnote 1. This note makes it clear that every Congolese inhabitant in the capital had by law to have a certificate showing that he or she was free of sleeping sickness, leprosy, tuberculosis, and VD, which was obtained from the Marcel Wanson Institute of Hygiene. One wonders, however, whether such strict measures were enforced outside the capital, even before 1958.

29. A. Lebrun, H. Koprowski et al., "Vaccination with the CHAT Strain of Type 1 Attenuated Poliomyelitis Virus in Leopoldville, Belgian Congo. 1."

30. J. De Moor, "Evolution de la poliomyélite à Léopoldville de 1951 à 1963," *Ann. Soc. Belge Méd. Trop.*, 1965, 45(6), 651–664.

31. J. Mann, J. McCormick, J. W. Curran et al., "Surveillance for AIDS in a Central African City," *JAMA*, 1986, 255(23), 3255–3259. Unofficial estimates put the 1984 population of Kinshasa even higher than 2.5 million.

32. Anon., "Vaccination par voie buccale contre la poliomyélite," *L'Essor du Congo* (Elisabeth-ville), August 13, 1959, p. 5, suggests August 1959 for the start of European feeding of the Koprowski strains, but S. Plotkin et al., "Vaccination with the CHAT Strain of Attenuated Poliomyelitis Virus in Leopoldville, Congo. 3," claims September.

33. D. K. Dube et al., "Serological and Nucleic Acid Analyses for HIV and HTLV Infection on Archival Human Plasma Samples from Zaire," *Virol.*, 1994, 202, 379–389.

34. See chapter 55.

35. Anon., "The Medieval Pattern," *Time*, November 7, 1960, p. 73.

36. Burundi also suffered a civil war, though it began in 1972.

37. Ruprecht found that nine out of ten infant macaques fed orally with an attenuated, multiply-deleted form of SIV (SIVΔ3) developed simian AIDS, and later in 1997 that two adult macaques also developed signs of simian AIDS after the same treatment. T. W. Baba, R. M. Ruprecht et al., "Pathogenicity of Live, Attenuated SIV after Mucosal Infection of Neonatal Macaques," *Science*, 1995, 267, 1820–1825. R. M. Ruprecht et al., "Longterm Follow-up of Rhesus Macaques Infected with Live Attenuated SIVmac239Δ3" (abstract 163), Institute of Human Virol., 2nd Annual Meeting (Baltimore, September 15–21, 1997).

38. R. Taylor, "Histocompatibility Antigens, Protective Immunity, and HIV-1," *J. NIH Res.*, 1994, 6, 68–71; J. A. Levy, "HIV Pathogenesis and Long-Term Survival," *AIDS*, 1993, 7, 1401–1410; R. Colebunders, "Long-time Survivors: What Can We Learn from Them?" chapter 11 in J. M. Mann and D. J. M. Tarantola, *AIDS in the World II: Global Dimensions, Social Roots, and Responses: The Global AIDS Policy Coalition* (New York: Oxford University Press, 1996), pp. 165–170.

39. R. M. Ruprecht, T. W. Baba et al., "Murine and Simian Retrovirus Models: The Threshold Hypothesis," *AIDS*, 1996, 10(suppl. A), S33–S40; R. M. Ruprecht, T. W. Baba et al., "Attenuated Vaccines for AIDS?" (letter), *Lancet*, 1995, 346, 177–178.

40. D. D. Ho et al., "Long-Term Survivors of Human Immunodeficiency Virus Type 1 Infection," *N. Engl. J. Med.*, 1995, 332, 1647–1648.

41. L. Garrett, *The Coming Plague — Newly Emerging Diseases in a World out of Balance* (New York: Farrar, Straus and Giroux, 1995), pp. 378–379.

42. A. Lebrun et al., "Vaccination with the CHAT Strain of Type 1 Attenuated Poliomyelitis Virus in Leopoldville, Belgian Congo. 1.," see p. 204.

43. Note the model of the wild sooty mangabey troop studied by Preston Marx, three of which proved to be infected with highly divergent strains of SIVsm, each differing by 20 percent from the other. Z. Chen, D. D. Ho, P. A. Marx et al., "Genetic Characterization of New West African Simian Immunodeficiency Virus SIVsm: Geographic Clustering of Household-Derived SIV Strains with Human Immunodeficiency Virus Type 2 Subtypes and Genetically Diverse Viruses from a Single Feral Sooty Mangabey Troop," *J. Virol.*, 1996, 70(6), 3617–3627.

44. It is difficult, so many years afterward, to gauge how many pairs of chimp kidneys would have been needed to produce, say, a million vaccine doses. Using modern techniques, it might require up to four pairs — but using older, less efficient methods (e.g., Maitland cultures), it could require ten or twenty times as many. Clearly there is the potential for several different SIV variants to be introduced into a single vaccine batch — and, as has been shown, several different batches (and lots) of vaccine were used in central Africa between 1957 and 1960.

45. F. Gao, B. H. Hahn, P. M. Sharp et al., "The Heterosexual Human Immunodeficiency Virus Type 1 Epidemic in Thailand Is Caused by an Intersubtype (A/E) Recombinant of African Origin," *J. Virol.*, 1996, 70(10), 7013–7029. An example of an individual recombinant virus is Z321, for so many years the oldest HIV-1 isolate (from Yambuku in 1976), which turned out to be a G/A recombinant.

46. Perhaps the second scenario is better able to explain the sudden emergence of HIV-1 subtypes differing by 20 percent or so from each other.

47. R. Colebunders, J. W. Curran, P. Piot et al., "Slow Progression of Illness Occasionally Occurs in HIV Infected Africans" (letter), *AIDS*, 1987, 1(1), 65. In interview, the lead author, Robert Colebunders, confirmed the patient details, including dates of birth. Patient 1 had had symptoms suggestive of AIDS since 1978, was HIV-positive, had lost a baby in 1982 and had suffered four miscarriages, but was still alive (albeit suffering from polyadenopathy and weight loss) in 1985. Patient 3, born in 1957, had had symptoms typical of AIDS since 1976, was HIV-positive, had suffered two spontaneous abortions, and had lost both her husband and child — apparently to AIDS — in 1979. She was still alive in 1986 (but also suffering polyadenopathy and weight loss). Patient 2 in the letter, apparently born in 1952, gave birth to an HIV-positive child in 1980, and died of AIDS in 1986. She could have been aged five when the CHAT vaccinations in Leo began in August 1958, and could therefore have been among the child vaccinees.

48. Other slow progressors might include the Belgian cartographer and his Congolese wife from Kikwit (Sonnet's patients 6 and 7), as well as "Maria," his patient 3, who could have been vaccinated near Astrida in 1959. (J. Sonnet et al., "Early AIDS Cases Originating from Zaire and Burundi [1962–1976]"). Another example could be the Rwandese mother who first demonstrated symptoms of AIDS in 1977, but was still alive more than

six years later. T. Jonckheer et al., "Cluster of HTLV-III/LAV Infection in an African Family" (letter), *Lancet*, 1985, 1(i), 400–401.

49. Many different hypotheses have been advanced to explain why some persons get AIDS much more slowly than others — including the HLA-haplotype (immunological makeup) of the host, the amount of the initial virus load, and infection with a less cytopathic or genetically defective strain of virus. See R. Colebunders, "Long-time Survivors: What Can We Learn from Them?" This article claims that the term "nonprogressors" is probably a misnomer, in that "over time, all HIV-infected individuals may eventually develop AIDS."

50. In Kinshasa, the earliest reliable evidence of AIDS is from 1973, thirteen years after the last CHAT vaccination; in Rwanda, the first evidence of AIDS is in 1977, some eighteen years after the Rwanda CHAT feedings.

51. A few more details are available for a subset of 47 of the 78 males; ten of these (21 percent) were hospital patients, and the age range was 17 to 60, with a mean of 31.1 years. A. G. Motulsky, J. Vandepitte et al., "Population Genetic Studies in the Congo. 1. Glucose-6-Phosphate Dehydrogenase Deficiency, Hemoglobin S, and Malaria," *Am. J. Hum. Gen.*, 1966, 18(6), 514–537. See also E. R. Giblett, A. G. Motulsky et al., "Population Genetic Studies in the Congo. 4. Haptoglobin and Transferrin Serum Groups in the Congo and in Other African Populations," *Am. J. Hum. Gen.*, 1966, 18(6), 553–558.

52. This is not unreasonable, for one of the other series reported in the paper, "Leo V," consisted of finger-prick specimens taken by Vandepitte from hospital staff and patients — again presumably at Lovanium, the hospital where he worked. The "Leo V" series would have been reported separately from the "Leo" group (which were collected by venepuncture and sent to Seattle by air), because they were only analyzed in Africa.

53. Jean Vandepitte has never contacted me again, as he promised to do if he ever came across further details.

54. Motulsky reports bleeding only two groups from the Stanleyville area: one involving 98 hospital patients from Stanleyville itself, and the other including some 70 pygmies working on a nearby plantation, so it would appear that Ninane vaccinated at least one of these groups at the same time. Ninane also thought that Motulsky had been prompted to visit the Congo in 1959 after speaking with Hilary Koprowski, and hearing from him about his collaboration with the Belgian doctors there. In December 1996, Motulsky told me he thought that he had met Koprowski for the first time only *after* his Congo visit.

55. These were bloods taken from schoolboys in Usumbura, and village boys from around Popokabaka (a small Yaka town some 250 miles southeast of Leopoldville). Delaisse provided Motulsky with blood specimens from Tutsi children in four Usumbura schools — all of whom would presumably have been vaccinated in April 1958. Similarly, Motulsky and Vandepitte collected blood samples in early 1959 from boys in villages near Popokabaka. It appears that CHAT had been fed to the same population, for Dr. Jacques Cerf, the director of hygiene for Leopoldville between 1958 and 1960, recalls participating in a pre-vaccination blood collection in the district of Kwango, between Kenge and Popokabaka, at around the time of Gelfand's visit in August 1958. Although all of Motulsky's Popokabaka and Usumbura samples were finger-prick specimens, which were tested on the spot and not sent back to Seattle by air, the fact that they were taken from the same populations that had been fed CHAT establishes the principle that post-vaccination blood samples might have been taken by Belgian doctors at the same time as samples for genetic studies.

56. Michel Vandeputte, personal communication, September 1997.

57. Anon., "Nationalism's Rapid Growth in Congo — Arrests Continue," *Times* (U.K.), February 2, 1959, p. 6.

58. A. Lebrun, J. Cerf, H. M. Gelfand, G. Courtois, and H. Koprowski, "Preliminary Report on Mass Vaccination with Live Attenuated Poliomyelitis Virus in Leopoldville, Belgian Congo," *PAHO1*, pp. 410–418; see p. 416.

59. Compare table 1 in A. G. Motulsky, J. Vandepitte et al., "Population Genetic Studies in the Congo. 1. Glucose-6-Phosphate Dehydrogenase Deficiency, Hemoglobin S, and Malaria," *Am. J. Human Gen.*, 1966, 18(6), 514–537, with table 2 in J. Vandepitte and J. Stijns, "Haemoglobulinopathies in the Congo (Leopoldville) and Ruanda-Urundi, a Progress Report," in J. H. P. Jonxis (editor), *Abnormal Haemoglobins in Africa* (Oxford: Blackwell, 1965). Eight of the twelve series featured in Motulsky's paper involved Motulsky himself, often in concert with others like Vandepitte or Ninane; while three were provided by Belgian collaborators (Delaisse and, in two instances, doctors Sonnet and Michaux, the same men who later wrote the seminal paper on early AIDS cases in the Belgian colonies). There is no specific information about the twelfth series (Leo), though that group appears similar to one featured in table 2 of the Vandepitte/Stijns paper, this being 106 males assessed by Stijns for G6PD deficiency. Stijns also bled 2,160 men and women in the same year to test for the sickling trait. Both Stijns and Courtois are thanked at the end of Motulsky's paper, and we know that all the others so thanked (Sonnet, Ninane, Dherte, and Delaisse) had helped with the collection of blood samples.

60. Arno Motulsky, personal communication, December 1996.

61. One piece of evidence that would strongly support such a hypothesis would be if an SIV isolate from a chimpanzee from the Kisangani region, one thousand miles from Leopoldville, was ever sequenced and found to resemble the L70 isolate.

CHAPTER 55: *Starburst and Dispersal*

1. Peter Aaby, personal communication, August 1997.

2. P. Mauclere, F. Brun-Venizet et al., "Serological and Virological Characterization of HIV-1 Group O Infection in Cameroon," *AIDS*, 1997, 11, 445–453 and its footnotes 27–34 for geographically dispersed cases. The lack of Group O infections in western Cameroon may merely be due to a lack of testing in that region, but it is noticeable that most of the other countries where Group O has appeared are former French colonies.

3. The epidemic among South African blacks is mainly of clade C, whereas the gay epidemic among white South African males involved clade B.

4. M. S. Broder, "HIV Subtypes Migrate to the U.S.," *Harvard AIDS Rev.*, Fall 1998, pp. 14–15.

5. L. Garrett, *The Coming Plague — Newly Emerging Diseases in a World out of Balance* (New York: Farrar, Straus & Giroux, 1994), p. 387 and footnote 111 on p. 658.

6. M. Essex, "Heterosexual Transmission Efficiency: Another Determinant of HIV Phenotype?" *IAS Newsletter*, July 1995, 2, 10–11. S. Connor, "AIDS Expert Warns of New Threat," *Independent* (U.K.), October 23, 1995.

7. F. Gao, P. M. Sharp et al., "The Heterosexual Human Immunodeficiency Virus Type 1 Epidemic in Thailand Is Caused by an Intersubtype (A/E) Recombinant of African Origin," *J. Virol.*, 1996, 70 (10), 7013–7029.

8.  J. Louwagie et al., "Phylogenetic Analysis of *gag* Genes from 70 International HIV-1 Isolates Provides Evidence for Multiple Genotypes," *AIDS,* 1993, 7, 769–780.

9.  B. S. Hersh, D. L. Heymann et al., "Acquired Immunodeficiency Syndrome in Romania," *Lancet,* 1991, 338, 645–649; O. Dumitrescu, J. A. Levy et al., "Characterization of Human Immunodeficiency Virus Type 1 Isolates from Children in Romania: Identification of a New Envelope Subtype," *J. Infect. Dis.,* 1994, 169, 281–288.

10. Wilson Carswell, personal communication, November 1997.

11. M. Smallman-Raynor, A. Cliff, and P. Haggett, *Atlas of AIDS* (Oxford: Blackwell, 1992), p. 333.

12. W. Janssens et al., "Genetic and Phylogenetic Analysis of *env* Subtypes G and H in Central Africa," *AIDS Res. Hum. Retro.,* 1994, 10(7), 877–879.

13. L. G. Kostrikis, D. Ho et al., "Genetic Analysis of Human Immunodeficiency Virus Type 1 Strains from Patients in Cyprus: Identification of a New Subtype Designated Subtype I," *J. Virol.,* 1995, 69(10), 6122–6130.

14. T. Leitner et al., "Yet Another Subtype of HIV Type 1?" *AIDS Res. Hum. Retro.,* 1995, 11(8), 995–997.

15. To serve the Greek community, Sabena flights between Kisangani/Stanleyville and Brussels had, for many years, a stopover in Athens, but probably more important, a private company, Sobelair, operated a schedule from Johannesburg to Brussels, which called at Stanleyville, and which featured a one- or two-day stopover for flight crews in Cyprus. Paul Osterrieth, personal communication, 1994. Supporting the hypothesis of a Kisangari/Cyprus link was a paper published in late 1998, which reported that subtype I was actually a multiple recombinant strain of HIV-1, one that "must have existed in Central Africa prior to [1976]." See F. Gao, P. M. Sharpe, B. H. Hahn et al., "An Isolate of Human Immunodeficiency Virus Type 1 Originally Clarified as Subtype I Represents a Complex Mosaic Comprising Three Different Group M Subtypes (A, G, and I)," *J. Virol.,* 1998, 72(12), 10,234–10,241.

16. Subtype information from HIV Sequence Database, December 1995 and December 1994 editions, and from P. M. Sharp, B. H. Hahn et al., "Origins and Diversity of Human Immunodeficiency Viruses," *AIDS,* 1994, 8(suppl. 1), S27-S42. By 1999, the diversity of subtypes found in the Congo was even more pronounced, for eight of the ten Group M subtypes had been found there, including seven detected in Kimpese, a small town near Kinshasa. For subtype J, see J. L. K. Mokill et al., "Genetic Heterogeneity of HIV Type 1 Subtypes in Kimpese, Rural Democratic Republic of Congo," *Aids Res. Hum. Retro.,* 1999, 15(7), 655–664, and for E, see F. Simon et al., "HIV Type 1 Diversity in Northern Paris, France," *AIDS Res. Hum. Retro.,* 1996, 12(15), 1427–1433. A ninth subtype (I), found in Cyprus, was clearly related to (and predated) the Z321 (recombinant A/G) isolate from rural Yambuku, taken in 1976 (see n. 15); and the only "missing subtype" was still clade B.

17. By contrast, Cameroon and Gabon, which have recently been proposed as representing the hearth of the HIV-1 Group M epidemic (as well as the Group O outbreak) by the Dutch researcher Jaap Goudsmit, have between them produced isolates from only seven of the ten subtypes. J. Goudsmit, *Viral Sex — The Nature of AIDS* (New York: Oxford University Press, 1997), p. 81.

18. Anon., "8,000 Watusis Reported Slain in Tribal Strife," *New York Times,* January 22, 1964, p. 2.

19. H. L. Vis et al., "Aspects cliniques et biochimiques de la malnutrition proteique au Kivu Central," *Ann. Soc. Belg. Méd. Trop.,* 1965, 45, 607–628.

20. A. C. Templeton, "Generalized Herpes Simplex in Malnourished Children," *J. Clin. Pathol.*, 1970, 23, 24–30. Many Bahutu from Rwanda and Burundi used to come to Uganda to work, often on a seasonal basis. See F. J. Bennett, "Preliminary Observations on the Relationship between the Ecology of Rwandans Living in Buganda and Their Disease Pattern," *E. Af. Med. J.*, 1966, 43(11), 508–514.

21. This was apparently *Klebsiella pneumoniae;* could this have been recalled by Jack Davies as *Pneumocystis carinii* pneumonia (PCP)?

22. Bill Hamilton, personal communications, 1995.

23. P. Van de Perre et al., "Female Prostitutes: A Risk Group for Infection with Human T-Cell Lymphotropic Virus Type III," *Lancet*, 1985, 2(i), 524–526.

24. There may even have been another link, in that during the fighting in the early sixties the bodies of many Tutsis were hurled into the Kagera, and would have been carried down to the mouth of that river, to be washed up around Lukunyu and Kasensero. (See A. L. Latham-Koenig, "Attempted Genocide in Ruanda," *World Today* [London], March 1964, pp. 97–100.) The same thing happened on an even larger scale in 1994, when the hundreds of corpses washed up along the shores of Lake Victoria were acknowledged to pose a considerable health risk to those collecting them for burial. See R. Dowden, "'The Graves of the Tutsi Are Only Half Full — We Must Complete the Task,'" *Independent* (U.K.), May 24, 1994, p. 1 (with photo and map). We know that "wet" HIV can survive at room temperature for up to fifteen days; if a member of the burial team had cuts on the hands, could he or she have gotten infected? (L. Resnick et al., "Stability and Inactivation of HTLVIII/LAV under Clinical and Laboratory Environments," *JAMA*, 1986, 255(14), 1887–1891.)

25. Hubert Caubergh, personal communication, November 1996.

26. In one village, a woman of seventy-two years recalled having to walk in to Astrida, and of being given a "drop in the mouth"; she spoke of this having happened "when the white man came." In another nearby village, some four miles from Butare, a seventy-one-year-old man spoke of having walked in to the *Centre de Santé* in 1957, or so he thought, to be vaccinated against a disease that left you with paralyzed legs. Both informants apparently recognized photos of oral vaccination by Ninane's syringe method.

27. R. Yeld, *Rwanda — Unprecedented Problems Call for Unprecedented Solutions* (Oxford: Refugee Studies Programme, 1996), pp. 34 and 50.

28. R. Lemarchand, *Rwanda and Burundi* (London: Pall Mall Press, 1970), pp. 171–173 and 206–216. H. Christensen, "The Progress of Refugee Settlements in Africa," Copenhagen University thesis (available from UNHCR library, Geneva), 1977, see pp. 37–44. R. Yeld, *Implications of Experience with Refugee Settlements* (East African Institute of Social Research Conference Papers, 1965). The best source of all is the excellent 128-page dissertation by Rachel Yeld: "Refugee Resettlement in Tanganyika," 1964, now revised and published as R. Yeld, "Rwanda: Unprecedented Problems Call for Unprecedented Solutions." See especially Map 3, showing the site of Rwandan settlements in Bukoba district, and chapter 6 (pp. 49–52). I am indebted to Ms. Van Der Meeren (née Yeld) for her sustained assistance with this area of the research.

29. In December 1966, a team of scientists from Entebbe, Uganda, went to Bukoba district to investigate the unusually high incidence of KS (twelve reports in the space of four years). They only managed, however, to follow up the Ngando case on the ground. See A. W. R. McCrae, M. C. Pike et al., "Studies Concerning Cancer: Kaposi's Sarcoma — Simulium and Kaposi's Sarcoma in Bukoba District, Tanzania," *Annual Report of the Ugandan Virus Research Institute*, 1966, pp. 19–21. See also A. W. R. McCrae et al., "*Simulium* and Kaposi's

Sarcoma," in P. Clifford, C. A. Linsell, and G. A. Timms, *Cancer in Africa* (Nairobi: East African Publishing House, 1968), pp. 436–444, especially map on page 437, which shows that four of the twelve cases of KS came from the Kagera Salient or from Kiamtwara chiefdom (where Tutsi refugees were scatter settled in 1962), two more cases came from near Kamuchumu, where self-settled Tutsis were living in 1966.

30. R. Colebunders, J. M. Mann, P. Piot et al., "Slow Progression of Illness Occasionally Occurs in HIV-Infected Africans" (letter), *AIDS,* 1987, 1, 65.

31. C. Watson, "Aids-Hit Uganda Learns to Love Carefully," *Independent* (U.K.), December 4, 1986.

32. D. Low-Beer, R. L. Stoneburner, and A. Mukulu, "Empirical Evidence for the Severe but Localized Impact of AIDS on Population Structure," *Nature Med.,* 1997, 3(5), 553–557. Katera was the base camp of the Amin forces, which the 207th Brigade captured first and where a battalion of soldiers was left behind to guard the rear of the brigade; Kyebe is the trading center three miles down the road, where most of the TPDF were in fact based during 1979 and 1980, and Kibale is the village where the Kasensero road rejoins the main road from Bukoba north to Masaka, and where the 207th was reunited with the rest of the TPDF.

33. T. Avirgan and M. Honey, *War in Uganda — The Legacy of Idi Amin* (Dar es Salaam: Tanzanian Publishing House, 1982), see pp. 79–81, 86, 89–90, 154, 174–196.

34. E. Hooper, *Slim* (London: The Bodley Head, 1990), pp. 18–23.

35. J. Goudsmit, *Viral Sex — The Nature of AIDS* (New York: Oxford University Press, 1997), pp. 53 and 74.

36. The rest of the Arvid Noe/subtype B hypothesis ran as follows: After being infected for six to nine years, Arvid perhaps infected a female prostitute in the Ruhr, during one of his truck journeys to Germany in the early seventies. Perhaps she in turn infected Herbert H., the bisexual violin player from Cologne who recruited bosomy female prostitutes for his orgies, and who presented his first symptoms of AIDS in 1976. Indeed, this might have been the moment at which HIV-1 entered the gay community for the first time — and with a variant that by now was more like subtype B than subtype D. Perhaps other gay Germans (like the chef from Gelsenkirchen in the Ruhr) also became infected, and later helped transport subtype B to Haiti and the United States. As revealed later, however, this hypothesis was proved comprehensively wrong.

37. Rachel Van Der Meeren personally knows several Astrida/Nyanza Tutsi who went to Kampala to settle (she even gave lifts to some of them), and believes it "more than likely" that others went to Kenya, where at that time the Mwami of the Tutsi was living with many of his followers. All this suggests that the proportion of the refugees from Astrida/Nyanza who "disappeared from the system" and either dispersed in Bukoba district, or to other countries in East Africa, may actually have been quite high. This is in contrast to what Ms. Van Der Meeren initially reported in "Implication of Experience with Refugee Settlements."

38. E. Hooper, *Slim,* p. 298; see also pp. 312, 243, and 246.

39. E. Huxley, *The Sorcerer's Apprentice — A Journey through East Africa* (London: Chatto and Windus, 1948), pp. 190–194. Forty-five years later, another great female travel writer, Dervla Murphy, visited Bukoba by means of the same lake ferry, and found that the same tradition continued. "In my clean and comfortable cabin," she wrote, "the other five berths were occupied by a group of friends, luscious teenage girls going to seek their fortunes in, they hoped, Mombasa — 'where is many tourists, Bukoba have none'. . . . The Bahaya women, I was told all over East and Central Africa, are famous for

their beauty and amatory skills." (D. Murphy, *The Ukimwi Road — From Kenya to Zimbabwe* [London: Flamingo, 1994], pp. 160–161.)

40. T. O. Jonassen, S. S. Frøland, B. Grinde et al., "Sequence Analysis of HIV-1 Group O from Norwegian Patients Infected in the 1960s," *Virol.,* 1997, 231, 43–47.

41. There has only been one Group O infection detected from Kenya, and that was a dually reactive O/M isolate from 1995/6. See E. M. Songok et al., "Surveillance for HIV-1 Subtypes O and M in Kenya," *Lancet,* 1996, 347, 1700.

42. E. Hooper, "Sailors and Star-Bursts, and the Arrival of HIV," *BMJ,* 1997, 315, 1689–1691.

43. In Douala and Yaounde, the two main Cameroonian cities, Group O viruses comprise over 5 percent of all HIV infections. P. Mauclere, F. Brun-Venizet et al., "Serological and Virological Characterization of HIV-1 Group O Infection in Cameroon."

44. Jo Griffin, personal communication, April 1998.

45. T. Zhu, B. T. Korber, A. J. Nahmias, E. Hooper, P. M. Sharp, and D. D. Ho, "An African HIV-1 Sequence from 1959 and Implications for the Origin of the Epidemic," *Nature,* 1998, 391, 594–597.

46. J. Goudsmit, *Viral Sex — The Nature of AIDS,* p. 110. As Goudsmit puts it: "When a virus enters an unaccustomed host and starts to produce disease, the viral DNA suddenly changes to make new proteins." Bill Hamilton, as demonstrated in chapter 37, shares this opinion.

47. In fact, Paul Sharp now believes that the *forties* is the most likely date for the introduction of the ancestral virus to humans, because of the nonlinear evolution of HIV. Paul Sharp, personal communication, May 1998.

48. Paul Sharp, personal communication, May 1998.

49. Goudsmit, *Viral Sex — The Nature of AIDS.*

50. In fact, as my friend Kamil Kucera has documented, the first convincing evidence of epidemic PCP in an institution actually comes from Rostock in northern Germany; the report of these cases contains convincing photographs of the *Pneumocystis* cysts in the alveoli of the lungs. E. Benecke, "Eigenartige Bronchiolenerkrankung im ersten Lebensjahr," *Virchows Arch. Path. Ges.,* 1939, 31, 402–406. In this paper, Benecke retrospectively diagnoses ten children with PCP during the years 1935–1938. In order to connect these children to West Africa, one would have to postulate that the return of German settlers from Kamerun to Europe in 1916 was the crucial factor.

51. If Dr. Goudsmit would like to test any one of the other four slides for HIV, he is welcome to try.

52. T. O. Jonassen, B. Grinde, S. S. Frøland et al., "Sequence Analysis of HIV-1 Group O from Norwegian Patients Infected in the 1960s."

53. One of the inventors of PCR, John Sninsky, who tried to isolate a virus from the Robert R. sample over the course of several years, was always wary about the possibility of contamination; he has not contributed to this latest study. It is also worth noting that neither Goudsmit nor Garry knew about the L70 sequence when they advanced their theories about HIV-1 being an "ancient virus."

54. R. Shilts, *And the Band Played On* (New York: St. Martin's Press, 1987), pp. 392–393.

55. Anon., "History of the Use of CHAT Strain 'Type 1' Attenuated Polio Virus in Humans," date unknown, but clearly late January 1958; Wistar Institute document provided to the Wistar expert committee.

56. J. Oleske et al., "Immune Deficiency Syndrome in Children," *JAMA,* 1983, 249(17), 2345–2349 (see case 6, p. 2346).

57. R. M. Ruprecht et al., "Murine and Simian Retrovirus Models: The Threshold Hypothesis," *AIDS*, 1996, 10(suppl. A), S33–S40.


CHAPTER 56: *Dead Ends and Hidden Bends*

1. L. Quersin-Thiry, "Action of Anticellular Sera on Virus Infections. I. Influence on Homologous Tissue Cultures Infected with Various Viruses," *J. Immunol.*, 1958, 81, 252–260. L. Quersin-Thiry, "Action of Anticellular Sera on Virus Infections. II. Influence on Heterologous Tissue Cultures," *J. Immunol.*, 1958, 82, 542–552.

2. I write "presumably" because at this time Dr. Thiry had two posts in Brussels. Ninane says that he studied under Thiry at the Université Libre de Bruxelles, but Thiry's work on CHAT was reported from the Pasteur Institute of Brabant.

3. HeLa is the lab substrate par excellence, but being a cell line derived from a human cancer, would not be suitable for the production of vaccines.

4. Dr. Flack's handwriting was rather ornate, and spelling foreign names was not her forte. By the time of her return to Brussels in mid-April, she was referring to her friend as "Dr. Liesa Thiery."

5. Ruth Jervis, personal communication, 1995; Mary Hawkes, personal communication, 1998.

6. Pieter De Somer's brother's widow had no recollection of any polio vaccination happening in Lusambo, which fitted with my finding that CHAT had not been fed in Kasai district, and that the only places where CHAT had been fed in central Congo were at Kikwit and Lisala.

7. D. Bodian, "Poliovirus in Chimpanzee Tissues after Virus Feeding," *Am. J. Hyg.*, 1956, 58, 81–100.

8. Study group on requirements for poliomyelitis vaccine (oral), "Requirements for Biological Substances. 7. Requirements for Poliomyelitis Vaccine (Oral)," *WHO Tech. Rep. Ser.*, 1962, 237, 1–27; see p. 13. Compare this with the previous requirements report on OPV (Expert Committee on Poliomyelitis, Third Report, *WHO Tech. Rep. Ser.*, 1960, 203, 1–53). In 1962, for the first time, a new phrase entered the OPV requirements published by the WHO. For the production of seed virus and vaccine, it declared, "monkeys of a suitable species, in good health, and which have not previously been used for experimental purposes of significance to the safety of the vaccine shall be used." This suggested that previously the kidneys of experimental monkeys could have been reused to make tissue culture.

9. G. Courtois, "Present Day Progress in Our Knowledge of the Enterovirus," *Bulletin des Grands Endemies en Afrique*, 1960, 2, 271–281. This speech mentions David Bodian by name, and the latter's work is clearly the source of several of the ideas that Courtois presents.

10. Because of the problems during our previous interview, on this occasion a French-speaking friend interviewed Dr. Lamy on my behalf.

11. Both Jezierski and Lamy appear to have been at the Pasteur working with Lépine and Barski between late 1954 and early 1955.

12. Edward De Maeyer says that at least one of the Lépine strains was given to De Somer by Barski at the time that he and Lépine acrimoniously parted company in 1955. Lépine was apparently furious, accusing Barski of stealing his vaccine.

13. It was noticeable, however, that later in the interview, when Monique Lamy reviewed the dates of her career, she now said that production of the Sabin vaccines had started at RIT in 1959. According to Prinzie and several others, it was in 1959 that RIT started making *Koprowski's* vaccines.

14. The phrase used in *BMJ* 58.

15. This was hinted at by the journalist Joan Phillips, who told me that Fritz Deinhardt had been "present at the trials." As far as is known, Deinhardt was not present at Ruzizi, but Ms. Phillips also specifically mentioned "field trials that took place around Stanleyville." This presumably means the vaccination at the nearby military camp on February 27, 1958. Paul Osterreith told me that he and Paulette Dherte had carried out certain vaccinations in Stanleyville, and it is known that Dherte helped Deinhardt with much of his work.

16. Osterrieth told me: "He [Vandepitte] came for six months and he wanted to change everything. Everything which was done by Courtois was badly done, according to him. And he tried to change things. I can tell you that he had a lot of problems with that. Because I simply refused. I didn't refuse, I said 'yes,' but I didn't do it ... looking him straight in the eyes, [I'd] say 'I forgot.'" Paul Osterrieth, personal communication, April 1993.

17. From records provided by the Central Africa Museum at Tervuren.

18. This information is from Paul Osterrieth, and is supported by Agnes Flack's diary, which has Professor Welsch visiting Ruzizi on February 25, and by a photo of the staff of the Stanleyville lab, which features both Welsch and Vandepitte, and which therefore can only have been taken on or after March 25. It appears that Welsch must have spent at least a month out in Africa — and probably longer.

19. Anon., "Nationalism's Rapid Growth in the Congo: Arrests Continue," *Times* (U.K.), February 2, 1959, p. 6.

CHAPTER 57: *The Rechanneling of History*

1. H. Koprowski, "Living Attenuated Poliomyelitis Virus as an Immunizing Agent of Man," *S. Af. Med. J.*, 1955, 29, 1134–1142.

2. P. J. Kanki, J. Alroy and M. Essex, "Isolation of T-Lymphotropic Retrovirus Related to HTLV-III/LAV from Wild-Caught African Green Monkeys," *Science*, 1985, 230, 951–954.

3. John Seale, "The Origins of Human Lentiviruses and the AIDS Epidemic," unpublished manuscript, dated January 12, 1990. Seale and Pascal had corresponded since 1987, but much of this paper contained Seale's original ideas. He did not, however, credit Pascal as the author of the hypothesis that the early CHAT vaccinations might have started AIDS, an omission that prompted an angry letter from Pascal in March 1990. (John Seale, personal communications and copies of his archives, 1995 and 1996.)

4. G. Lecatsas and J. J. Alexander, "Safe Testing of Oral Poliovirus Vaccine and the Origin of HIV Infection in Man" (letter), *S. Af. Med. J.*, 1989, 76, 451. Response: B. D. Schoub, C. J. Dommann, S. F. Lyons, "Safety of Live, Oral Poliovirus Vaccine and the Origin of HIV Infection in Man" (letter), *S. Af. Med. J.*, 1990, 77, 51–52.

5. J. Cribb, *The White Death* (Sydney: Angus and Robertson, 1996). This, the only other book to seriously examine the OPV hypothesis, is beautifully written and provides an excellent summary of the investigations by Pascal, Curtis, Hamilton, and others — even if it features

little in the way of new research. Of particular value are the chapters on plagues in history (chapter 2), and on the evolution of the CHAT hypothesis (chapter 8 and chapter 9).

6. There is, admittedly, no published evidence that SIV can survive the process of vaccine manufacture (or that it could have done so in the fifties). However, a spokesman for Lederle Laboratories admitted to Tom Curtis that "since 1985, when sensitive new testing procedures were instituted, Lederle has sometimes found SIV in the early stages of its vaccine production process." (T. Curtis, "Did a Polio Vaccine Experiment Unleash AIDS in Africa?" *Washington Post,* April 5, 1992.) Some might feel, of course, that before 1985 some SIV might have got through — and that it is hard, in the nineties, to simulate experimentally the vaccine production methods of the fifties.

7. B. Martin, "The Political Refutation of a Scientific Theory," *Health Care Analysis,* 1998, 6, 175–179.

8. In December 1994, more than two years after the Wistar committee issued its report, Dr. Brian Mahy of the CDC wrote me to confirm that "we have not received any polio vaccine sample from the Wistar Institute for testing."

9. Giovanni Rovera, personal communication, November 1995.

10. Memorandum from Steven Holloway, April 20, 1992, included in material submitted by the Wistar Institute to the Wistar expert committee, July 30, 1992.

11. H. Koprowski, "AIDS and the Polio Vaccine" (letter), *Science,* 1992, 257, 1024–1027.

12. As revealed earlier, Olen Kew at the CDC appears to have a sample of CHAT (or "Wistar") pool 13, but this is seed virus rather than vaccine.

13. Meinrad Schar, personal communication, August 1993.

14. Hans Wigzell and Jan Albert, personal communications, January 1995.

15. Letters from Bill Hamilton to Hans Wigzell dated March 3, 1995 and July 5, 1995.

16. In our January 1994 meeting, Wigzell had said that he might send some of the CHAT vaccine samples to be tested at the (U.K.) National Institute of Biological Standards and Control laboratories near Potter's Bar, on the outskirts of London.

17. Letter from author to Hans Wigzell, dated July 10, 1996.

18. Wigzell was also by then the chairman of the Steering Committee on Vaccine Development convened by the WHO Global Program on AIDS — a group that would help decide whether or not to proceed with human trials of a live attenuated AIDS vaccine. WHO Working Group, "Feasibility of Developing Live Attenuated HIV Vaccines: Conclusions and Recommendations," *AIDS,* 1994, 10(2), 221–222.

19. Fax from Hans Wigzell, dated July 27, 1996.

20. This was strange, for on two of the five occasions, Hamilton had left specific messages with Wigzell's secretary, asking him to phone back.

21. Letter from author to Hans Wigzell, dated July 28, 1996.

22. David Ho, personal communication, July 1997.

23. Hilary Koprowski, in collaboration with Stanley Plotkin, "History of Koprowski Vaccine against Poliomyelitis," in S. Plotkin and B. Fantini (editors), *Vaccinia, Vaccination and Vaccinology: Jenner, Pasteur and Their Successors* (Paris: Elsevier, 1996), 229–240.

24. Irena Koprowska, *A Woman Wanders through Life and Science* (Albany, NY: State University of New York Press, 1997), pp. 297–303. This very human account of Irena's own scientific work and of her life with Hilary frankly documents many intriguing details about the Koprowski personality, including glimpses of his relationships with other women — most notably his mother, whose domineering presence looms throughout. But apart from the appendix (penned by Koprowski himself), the book is disappointingly lacking in information about Hilary's polio work. Those details that are included

are frequently inaccurate, such as a reference to his visit to Africa to work with chimps that places it in 1951, six years before it actually happened. This lack of familiarity with the subject is remarkable, given that the alleged reason for Hilary's suddenly needing to obtain Tom Norton's papers from his widow in 1992 was that Irena was "now ready to start with the history of oral polio vaccine, bringing it up to date, inclusive of all the nonsense about the relationship of AIDS to the polio vaccine." Quotation from letter from Hilary Koprowski to Ann, Tom Norton's daughter, July 1992.

25. CHAT is not the set of initials of the child from whose stool the virus was taken, as they claim, but rather an abbreviation of the child's surname. We still do not know why they decided to change the name of the vaccine from the original version, which was "Charlton," especially when another of their vaccines was named "Jackson," after the first human vaccinee.

26. WHO Expert Committee on Poliomyelitis, Second Report, *WHO Tech. Rep. Ser.,* 1958, 145, 1–83; see p. 24. David Dane, George Dick's former collaborator, told me that the increase in virulence was one hundred times greater than he had come across in any other polio vaccine. Furthermore, it would seem that TN was not the only problem strain. See S. Baron, R. Murray et al., "Laboratory Investigations of the Attenuated Vaccine Strains. II. Tissue Culture Characteristics Before and After Gastrointestinal Passage," *PAHO1,* 124–131, for further evaluation of the Wistar and CHAT strains.

27. The 1980 lecture implies that the entire Ruzizi campaign was staged in order to combat a polio epidemic, and Koprowski concludes: "To tell you that it stopped an epidemic would be very difficult, because trial conditions allowed cases to escape." By contrast, the chapter in the Plotkin book claims that, during the Ruzizi campaign, Flack and Jervis heard of a polio epidemic in a nearby village of four thousand people, rushed there, and stopped the epidemic with vaccine. Both these versions seem to confuse Ninane's epidemic vaccinations of January 1958 with Flack and Jervis's huge Ruzizi trial in February and March.

28. See chapters 34 and 41.

29. The Sabin-Koprowski papers were kindly made available by the Sabin archives at the University of Cincinnati. My thanks to Billi Broadus, archivist, for locating and faxing the relevant pages to me.

30. In his letter to Koprowski, Sabin also pointed out that the Congo vaccine had been used in Poland — although, as explained in an earlier chapter, the CHAT vaccine that he himself tested was probably pool 10A-11, which was never used in Poland.

31. It will be recalled that the principal source for this information was Chuck Cyberski, the San Francisco TV producer, who wrote to Louis Pascal on May 17, 1992, telling him that Hayflick had told him that he had been in Paris two weeks earlier, meeting with Montagnier, Koprowski, and Plotkin — and that in the same interview, Hayflick had told him that the French had been experimenting with a polio vaccine made in baboon kidney in French Equatorial Africa at the end of the fifties.

32. It was not until February 1999 that I came across a reference (by Pascal) to Curtis also having interviewed Hayflick in 1992, and being told about the Paris meeting. I promptly phoned Curtis to check, and although at short notice he was unable to locate his original interview notes, he phoned me back the following day to relate his "best recollections" of his conversation with Hayflick. This quote is taken from the phone call. This would appear to be the correct version of this much-rumored event, because when I interviewed Luc Montagnier for the second time, in September 1997, he told me that he had no recollection of meeting with Hayflick during 1992 (I did not ask about

Koprowski), but added that he might have had a private talk with Plotkin on the subject of the OPV/AIDS theory, though it was not an official meeting. He said that he thought Plotkin was wrong, and that he personally didn't pay too much attention to the theory. He went on to say that since *Research in Virology* is an open journal, they went on to print Elswood and Stricker's argument (albeit as a letter, not a paper).

33.  B. F. Elswood and R. B. Stricker, "Polio Vaccines and the Origin of AIDS," *Res. Virol.,* 1993, 144, 175–177.

34.  H. Koprowski, "AIDS and the Polio Vaccine" (letter), *Science,* 1992, 257, 1024–1027. Throughout the last seven years (1992–1999), I have searched for some documentary evidence of the monkey species used to make the CHAT and Fox vaccines fed in Africa in the fifties, and I have not managed to find anything. It is worth recording, however, what I have located. There are two photos from the fifties featuring Koprowski holding monkeys, both of which appear to be macaques. However, the caption of one photo makes it clear that the monkey had been used "to test vaccine's safety" (H. Earle, "On the Way: A Pill for Polio," *Today's Health,* May 1959, pp. 40–41 and 60), while the fact that the other was taken by a *Life* photographer in 1956, while Koprowski was still working at Lederle — where Cox opposed the use of monkey kidney tissue culture for vaccine manufacture — leads to the inevitable conclusion that this monkey, too, was employed in vaccine safety testing (photo reprinted in A. Tyler, "Monkey Business?" *Independent* (U.K.), magazine section, September 19, 1992, pp. 24–29). I also recalled that in 1992, in rejection of the OPV/AIDS theory, Koprowski had told a reporter that seed stocks for his polio vaccine strains were available for study at the American Type Culture Collection (ATCC) in Rockville, Maryland, and could be "tested for the presence of any virus." (Anon., "In the Beginning," *Economist* [U.K.], March 14, 1992, pp. 123–124.) I therefore checked the official entries for Koprowski's CHAT and Fox vaccines in the ATCC catalogue, which features many samples of viruses and vaccines from this era (C. Buck, G. Paulino [editors], *Catalogue of Animal Viruses and Antisera, Chalmydiae and Rickettsiae, Sixth Edition* [Rockville, Maryland: American Type Culture Collection, 1990], pp. 110–111). This compendium records one attenuated poliovirus sample identified as Chat [WCH Wy 4B-5], which has a "host of choice" and a "host range" of monkey kidney and diploid, and another attenuated poliovirus sample named Fox (Wy 3), which has monkey kidney as its host of choice, and a host range of monkey kidney and HDCS. The suffixes attached to the two vaccine strains seemed to indicate that both had been produced at Wyeth. (This is the vaccine house that had previously been mentioned by Koprowski, but only in the context of producing CHAT pool 18, or 18 G-I, which was first used in Poland in June 1959.) Later, I applied to the ATCC for further details of the passage histories of CHAT, Fox, and other poliovirus strains, and was sent several typed sheets, which were described as file copies of product sheets. To my surprise, they related not to poliovirus pools (as in the catalogue), but to individual frozen lots of vaccine. One sheet was for "Chat (WCH Wy 4B-5) lot 11W," and recorded the passage history as follows: the SM strain had been passed 28 times through monkeys, 14 times through chick embryo tissue culture, 5 times alternately through monkey kidney and chick embryo tissue culture, 4 times through man, 4 times (plaqued) through monkey kidney, twice more in monkey kidney, once in rhesus monkey kidney cells, and finally in a rhesus monkey kidney continuous cell line (CCL); the latter passage had been performed at the ATCC itself. Another undated product sheet for Fox (Wy 3) lot 3 recorded a passage history of 5 passes in monkey kidney (including four plaqued passages), followed by 2 passes in rhesus monkey kidney cells. Although I had been told in my interview with Richard Roblin, the ATCC vice-president of research and

development, that the passage histories they held would certainly include the passages carried out at the ATCC itself (presumably to replenish stocks, and boost titer), there were no indications on the product sheets about when the samples had been deposited with the ATCC, or which passages had been carried out by Koprowski, which by Wyeth, and which by the ATCC itself. Two further attempts to find out more information from the ATCC drew a blank, but in February 1999 I contacted the associate collection manager, Charles Buck, who went back through the archives to locate the original records of the two vaccines. He told me that both the CHAT and Fox strains had been deposited by Dr. Koprowski in 1960. For CHAT, the start of the 1960 passage history was the same as that on the product sheet I had received, up to and including the 2 passages in monkey kidney; however, the last 2 passages (in rhesus monkey kidney cells, and in rhesus monkey kidney CCL) had clearly been carried out after that, almost certainly at the ATCC itself. It was the same for the Fox strain — both the final passages in rhesus monkey kidney cells had been carried out after the vaccine had been deposited by Dr. Koprowski in 1960. In other words, Koprowski's two vaccines, CHAT and Fox, had been made in a tissue culture from an unspecified monkey species, whereas the ATCC had specified that for their passages, rhesus TC had been employed. (They used the same species to passage all their polioviruses, whether Koprowski's, or the other attenuated or virulent reference strains.) Even if the mystery of substrate was not solved, the ATCC records did effectively confirm certain other relevant details about Koprowski's poliovirus pools, and the manufacturers of the vaccines used in specific campaigns. I had already come across a record of Fox WFX, pool Wy 3-3, being fed to 79 persons in Bern, Switzerland, between November 1958 and April 1959 (F. Buser and M. Schar, "Poliomyelitis Vaccination with Live Poliovirus," *Am J. Dis. Child.*, 1961, 10, 568–574); this appeared to be the same vaccine as Fox (Wy 3), lot 3. The sole reference to CHAT "vaccine lot 4B" (which may well be a reference to a vaccine lot made from pool 4B-5) comes in a 1959 article on genetic markers (H. Koprowski, "The Role of Markers of Poliovirus in Attempts to Identify Strains Isolated from Man During a Mass Vaccination Program," *PAHO1*, pp. 135–139, see p. 138), which suggests that this material may have been fed in the small trials in Moorestown (89 persons, starting in January 1958) and Philadelphia (850 persons, starting in January 1959). (For reasoning, see chapter 28, n.37.) Material from the same pool (4B-5) may have been fed to the first 2,000 vaccinees in Africa — those in Stanleyville and Aketi, between February and May, 1957. (For reasoning, see chapter 51, especially n.42.) What all this seems to indicate is that Wyeth, a commercial vaccine house, produced the vaccines that were used in the very first African trials, plus the only open trials in the United States, and the Type 3 trials in Switzerland. By contrast, different pools (10A-11 and 13), each made partly at the Wistar (see S. A. Plotkin et al., "Intratypic Serodifferentiation of Polioviruses," *Virol.* 1961, 15, 473–485; see especially 477–478), and partly in De Somer's labs, were used in the mass trials at Ruzizi and Leopoldville, which took place at exactly the same time as the American and Swiss trials. The reasons for the use of different pools in different continents are not known.

35. A. Giri, R. C. Gallo et al., "Isolation of a Novel Simian T-Cell Lymphotropic Virus from *Pan paniscus* That Is Distantly Related to the Human T-Cell Leukemia/Lymphotropic Virus Types I and II," *J. Virol.*, 1994, 68, 8392–8395.

36. A. M. Vandamme, J. Desmyter, P. Goubau et al., "The Presence of a Divergent T-Lymphotropic Virus in a Wild-Caught Chimpanzee (*Pan paniscus*) Supports an African Origin for the Human T-Lymphotropic/Simian T-Lymphotropic Group of Viruses," *J. Gen. Virol.*, 1996, 77, 1089–1099.

37. Stewart Aston, personal communication, June 1995.

38. As soon as I was round the corner, I jotted down these final words. Since then, I have considered how best to deal with the interview. Much of it was on the record, whatever the speaker said at the end. On the other hand, some of the more remarkable comments had been made off the record, and I could not include those if I named the interviewee. I have finally decided not to identify him. However, what he said is recorded in my notebooks, and all but one brief section is on tape.

39. P. Manson, "Theories Tying AIDS to Contaminated Vaccines Date Back to 1988," *Houston Post,* August 19, 1992, A14. This fine summary of the OPV/AIDS controversy also records that Nobel Prize–winner Frederick Robbins and AIDS researcher Anthony Fauci of the NIH also believe that old vaccine stocks should be tested for HIV and other retroviruses.

40. Affidavit of Joseph Melnick, Ph.D., October 25, 1993, Koprowski vs. Straight Arrow Publishers Inc. (Civil Action No. 92-CV-743, U.S. District Court, Eastern District of Pennsylvania). Most of the quote (plus further discussion) features in M. K. Curtis, "Monkey Trials: Science, Defamation and the Suppression of Dissent," *William and Mary Bill of Rights J.,* 1995, 4(2), 507–593; see p. 593. This excellent summary of the ethical and legal issues arising from the Koprowski lawsuit is written by Tom Curtis's brother. Other mandatory reading on the issue of free speech in science, with special reference to the OPV/AIDS case, includes the following two articles by Brian Martin: "Sticking a Needle into Science: The Case of Polio Vaccines and the Origin of AIDS," *Soc. Stud. Sci.,* 1996, 26, 245–276; and "Peer Review and the Origin of AIDS — A Case Study in Rejected Ideas," *BioScience,* 1993, 43(9), 624–627.

41. According to sources such as Blaine Elswood and Julian Cribb, Curtis's livelihood as a freelance journalist was almost destroyed, because he had to devote so much time to his defense case. (See J. Cribb, *The White Death,* p. 186.) However, he is now (1999) the editor of an impressive journal, *Biomedical Inquiry,* which is published by the University of Texas Medical Branch.

CHAPTER 58: *When the Levee Breaks*

1. Anon., "Update: Trends in AIDS Incidence — United States, 1996," *MMWR,* 1997, 46(37), 861–867. Anon., "A New Lease of Life," *Guardian* (U.K.), May 12, 1997, section 2, p. 2; S. M. Hammer et al., "A Trial Comparing Nucleotide Monotherapy with Combination Therapy in HIV-Infected Adults with CD4 Cell Counts from 200 to 500 per Cubic Millimeter," *N. Engl. J. Med.,* 1996, 335(15), 1081–1090. However, by late 1998, many scientists were proposing that the way that HIV disrupts the immune system is not explicable merely by a massive daily level of HIV virion production and CD4 cell death, as proposed — for instance — by David Ho's group. If correct, this would have important long-term implications for combination therapies, and would suggest — for instance — that immune-restoring treatments should be taken alongside antiviral drugs. See M. Day, "Guerilla Warfare," *New Sci.,* November 28, 1998, 42–46.

2. M. Waldholz, "Scientists Find 'Sleeping' HIV, Deferring Cure," *Wall Street J.,* November 14, 1997, pp. B1 and B13; M. Day, "AIDS Drug Cocktails Fail in the Real World," *New Sci.,* October 11, 1997, p. 11. R. McKie, "The Killer That Will Strike Again," *Observer* (U.K.), February 28, 1999, p. 15. Commenting on these new drug-resistant HIV strains, a doctor from the U.K. Public Health Laboratory Service said: "[T]he problem . . . has not gone away. Deaths are just being postponed."

3. D. Usborne, "Aids in US Is Spreading Faster among Women Than Men," *Independent* (U.K.); September 18, 1997, p. 5.

4. P. Burton, "Of Vice and Men," *Independent on Sunday* (U.K.); October 12, 1997, review, pp. 4–9.

5. The Status and Trends of the Global HIV/AIDS Pandemic Symposium Final Report, Vancouver, July 5-6, 1996, AIDSCAP/Family Health International, Harvard School of Public Health and UNAIDS (1996), pp. 15–20.

6. P. Thomas, "The Quest for an AIDS Vaccine," *Harvard AIDS Rev.,* Winter 1998, pp. 11–14.

7. The figures in December 1998 were 33.4 million living with HIV/AIDS globally, 22.5 million of whom were from sub-Saharan Africa. Anon., "AIDS Epidemic Update — December 1998," report issued by UNAIDS, December 1, 1998, p. 5.

8. T. E. Mertens and A. Burton, "Estimates and Trends of the HIV/AIDS Epidemic," *AIDS,* 1996, 10(suppl. A), S221–S228.

9. Anon., "AIDS Epidemic Update — December 1998," p. 15.

10. J. Cribb, *The White Death* (Sydney: Angus and Robertson, 1996), pp. 38–42. In the two preceding paragraphs, I have borrowed heavily from Cribb's excellent analysis of the impact of AIDS.

11. Anon., "Paralytic Poliomyelitis — United States, 1980–1994," *MMWR,* 1997, 46(4), 79–83. This paper also reveals that all the 133 confirmed polio cases in the United States since 1979 have been vaccine associated (i.e., caused by reversion and spread of the live vaccine virus). To combat this, the Advisory Committee on Immunization Practices now recommends two doses of IPV followed by two of OPV for routine vaccination of U.S. children, until such time as poliovirus be eradicated globally.

12. Anon., "Polio-free Europe," *New Scientist,* September 27, 1997, p. 5.

13. Anon., "Progress toward Poliomyelitis Eradication — Africa, 1996," *MMWR,* 1997, 46(15), 321–325.

14. David Dane once discussed the problem of viral contamination of polio vaccines with Albert Sabin, who pointed out that "one can only try to eliminate the dangers one knows about." David Dane, personal communication, 1998.

15. WHO Expert Committee on Poliomyelitis, Third Report, *WHO Tech. Rep. Ser.,* 1960, 203, 1–53; see especially pp. 35–36.

16. Study Group on Requirements for Poliomyelitis Vaccine (Oral), "Requirements for Biologic Substances. 7. Requirements for Poliomyelitis Vaccine (Oral)," *WHO Tech. Rep. Ser.,* 1962, 237, 3–29, especially p. 13.

17. R. Murray, "Recommendations Relating to the Manufacture of Poliovirus Vaccine, Live Oral," in *Proceedings of 6th International Congress of Microbiological Standardization* (Berlin: Hoffmann Verlag, 1961), pp. 37–43.

18. C. L. Greening, "The Controlled Collection, Holding, Transport and Stock Housing of Monkeys Intended for Tissue Culture Production," in *Proceedings of 6th International Congress of Microbiological Standardization* (Berlin: Hoffmann Verlag, 1961), pp. 111–117.

19. Lord Cohen of Birkenhead, "Address by the President of the Congress," in A. F. B. Standfast et al. (editors), *Proceedings of 7th International Congress for Microbiological Standardization* (Edinburgh: E. & S. Livingstone, 1962), pp. 1–4.

20. K. Shah and N. Nathanson, "Human Exposure to SV40: Review and Comment," *Am. J. Epidem.,* 1976, 103(1), 1–12.

21. M. Carbone et al., "Simian Virus 40-like DNA Sequences in Human Pleural Mesothelioma," *Oncogene,* 1994, 9, 1781–1790.

22. See P. Brown, "Mystery Virus Linked to Asbestos Cancer," *New Scientist*, May 21, 1994, p. 4; and P. Brown, "Polio Vaccine Linked to Cancer," *New Scientist*, August 24, 1996, p. 16.

23. J. Tratschin et al., "Canine Parvovirus: Relationship to Wild-Type and Vaccine Strains of Feline Panleukopenia Virus and Mink Enteritis Virus," *J. Gen. Virol.*, 1982, 61, 33–41.

24. J. Seale, "Crossing the Species Barrier — Viruses and the Origins of AIDS in Perspective," *J. R. Soc. Med.*, 1989, 82, 519–523. With this excellent article, John Seale redeemed himself for much of the confusion caused by his earlier assertions that AIDS was the result of a germ warfare experiment.

25. M. Watts, "The Birth of BSE," *Independent on Sunday* (U.K.), March 31, 1996, p. 17.

26. J. Walsh, "A Fatal Beef Crisis," *Time*, April 1, 1996, pp. 20–24. C. Mihill, "Mad Cow Disease Linked to New CJD," *Guardian* (U.K.), September 30, 1997.

27. N. Schoon, "CJD Could Be Spread through Blood Transfusions," *Independent* (U.K.), October 8, 1997, p. 1.

28. A. F. Hill, J. Collinge et al., "Diagnosis of New Variant Creutzfeldt-Jakob Disease by Tonsil Biopsy" (letter), *Lancet*, 1997, 349, 99–100.

29. J. Nichol, "Stranger than Fiction," *Guardian* (U.K.), November 5, 1997, G2 magazine section, p. 9. Mr. Nichol, an ex-soldier, recalls how he was called up for Gulf War service in 1990, at the age of 45, and that within three days of arriving in the Gulf, had been given "18 inoculations, most of which went unrecorded, a few of which were secret." Since returning from the Gulf, he apparently "has violent mood swings, sleeps little, and his memory has all but gone." Other veterans have apparently found that their medical records for the period of Gulf service, and their military vaccination records, have been "wiped clean." See also R. Norton-Taylor, "MoD Ignored Warning on Gulf Drugs," *Guardian* (U.K.), October 29, 1997.

30. Anon., "U.S. Presidential Gulf War Investigation Extended," *Lancet*, January 18, 1997, 349, 188; M. Braid, "MoD Accused of Turning Blind Eye to Stricken Troops," *Independent* (U.K.), November 8, 1995.

31. Anon., "Open the Files on Gulf War Syndrome" (editorial), *Independent* (U.K.), November 21, 1994.

32. R. J. Manchee et al., "*Bacillus anthracis* on Gruinard Island," *Nature*, 1981, 294, 254–255.

33. G. Lardner Jr., "Army Report Details Germ War Exercise In N.Y. Subway in '66," *Washington Post*, April 22, 1980.

34. R. Watson et al., "Nuclear Secrets," *Newsweek*, January 3, 1994, pp. 22–25.

35. S. Miller, "Testing on Human Guinea Pigs," *Newsweek*, January 3, 1994, p. 25; V. Kiernan, "Radiation Doctors Abused Trust in the Name of Science," *New Scientist*, October 14, 1995, p. 8.

36. J. H. Cushman Jr., "204 Secret Nuclear Tests by U.S. Are Made Public," *New York Times*, December 8, 1993, p. A20.

37. S. Tisdall, "U.S. Admits Years of Atomic Radiation Tests on People," *Guardian* (U.K.), December 30, 1993. This article mentions 250 deliberate overground radiation releases staged in Nevada, New Mexico, Utah, and Washington state between 1944 and 1961, presumably partly in order to research a usable radiation weapon. One wonders again whether the tale of a neutron bomb experiment along the Snake River in Washington in 1958 might have any substance.

38. With a nod to C. Bukowski, *Tales of Ordinary Madness* (San Francisco: City Lights, 1967).

39. A meeting about the chimp breeding station went ahead in Leopoldville in February 1960, preceeded by a field trip to the IRSAC field station at Lwiro (near Bukavu). The U.S. delegation was led by Karl Meyer, and included Willard Eyestone (NIH), Fred Stare (Harvard), Art Riopelle (Yerkes Primate Center), and George Burch (Tulane); the Belgian side was led by Ghislain Courtois, and included primatologist Urs Rahm from IRSAC and Charles Cordier, the chimp catcher. The delegates apparently rejected Lindi as a site for the chimp farm, instead settling on an island below Idjwi in Lake Kivu. Apparently the plan never materialized, though others (unnamed) later apparently arranged for a supply of chimps from the Congo to a Department of Defense unit based in Texas. "Ferme d'elevage chimpanzés," file H4487/1087, Ministry of Foreign Affairs archives (Belgium). Fred Stare and Arthur Riopelle, personal communications, 1995.

40. C. H. Kratochvil, "Introduction [to 1st Holloman Symposium on Primate Immunology and Molecular Genetics]," *Primates in Med.*, 1968, 1, VII–XV.

41. K. Reemstma et al., "Renal Heterotransplantation in Man," *Ann. Surg.*, 1964, 160, 384–410; T. E. Starzl et al., "Renal Heterotransplantation from Baboon to Man: Experience with 6 Cases," *Transplantation*, 1964, 2, 752.

42. B. Hahn, personal communication, 1995.

43. R. G. Gosden, "AIDS and Malaria Experiments," *Nature*, 1992, 355, 305.

44. C. Gilks, "AIDS, Monkeys and Malaria," *Nature*, 1991, 354, 262.

45. L. L. Bailey et al., "Baboon-to-Human Cardiac Xenotransplantation in a Neonate," *JAMA*, 1985, 254(23), 3321–3329.

46. T. E. Starzl et al.; "Clinical Xenotransplantation," *Xenotransplantation*, 1994, 1, 3–7.

47. R. P. Lanza et al., "Xenotransplantation," *Scientific American*, July 1997, pp. 40–45.

48. D. Blum, *The Monkey Wars* (New York: Oxford University Press, 1994), pp. 221–241.

49. B. Holmes, "Baboon Man Leaves Hospital," *New Scientist*, January 13, 1996, p. 6.

50. F. Koechlin, "The Animal Heart of the Matter — Xenotransplantation and the Threat of New Diseases," *Ecologist*, 1996, 26(3), 93–97.

51. L. E. Chapman, T. M. Folks et al., "Xenotransplantation and Xenogenic Infections," *N. Engl. J. Med.*, 1995, 333, 1498–1501.

52. T. Wilkie, "Could a Pig Save Your Life?" *Independent* (U.K.), May 1, 1996, p. 15.

53. M. Day, "Tainted Transplants," *New Scientist*, October 18, 1997, p. 4.

54. For a detailed discussion of these issues, see Nuffield Council on Bioethics, *Animal-to-Human Transplants — The Ethics of Xenotransplantation* (London: Nuffield Council on Bioethics, 1996), available from Nuffield Council on Bioethics, 28 Bedford Square, London WC1B 3EG, U.K.

55. Anon., "An Uncalculated Risk" (editorial), *New Scientist*, October 18, 1997, p. 3.

56. M. Kettle, "Doctors to Be Guinea Pigs in Tests of HIV Vaccine," *Guardian* (U.K.), September 23, 1997, p. 1.

57. This information was later confirmed in K. Kleiner, "Live and Dangerous; Fresh Safety Doubts Emerge over Plans for HIV Vaccine Trial," *New Scientist*, October 4, 1997, p. 5, and in "Don't Die of Recklessness," the editorial on p. 3 of the same issue. See also M. Day, "Vaccine Setback," *New Scientist*, October 18, 1997, p. 7.

58. W. J. Whelan, "Asilomar; Twenty Years On" (editorial), *FASEB J.*, 1995, 9, 295.

59. Perhaps the nadir came in an interview broadcast on British television in October 1997. Dr. Desrosiers was asked whether he was willing to take his vaccine himself; to which he replied: "It's not been decided yet." The reporter, Susan Watts, asked the question once more on camera (and apparently about a dozen times off camera) and never elicited a

clear response. Interview broadcast on *Newsnight*, BBC2 (U.K.), October 21, 1997. When I reminded him of this episode, Ron Desrosiers complained that it was not a fair question: whether or not he was prepared to take the vaccine was not the real issue.

60. R. Desrosiers, "Prospects for Live Attenuated HIV" (letter), *Nature Med.*, 1998, 4(9), 982.

61. R. C. Desrosiers, L. O. Arthur, R. C. Johnson et al., "Identification of Highly Attenuated Mutants of Simian Immunodeficiency Virus," *J. Virol.*, 1998, 72(2), 1431–1437.

62. Desrosiers said that he considered Ruprecht's attitude toward himself unduly *ad hominem* (something that had never struck me when I had interviewed her on the phone), and added, *inter alia*, that she had obtained the attenuated strains that she was now criticizing direct from him.

63. P. Thomas, "The Quest for an AIDS Vaccine." For a good review of AIDS vaccine trials, see J. Esparza et al., "HIV Vaccine Development: from Basic Research to Human Trials," *AIDS*, 1996, 10(suppl. A), S123–S132.

64. J. Crewdson, "New Doubts on AIDS Vaccine," *Chicago Tribune*, May 29, 1994, p. 1. J. Cohen, "Will Media Reports KO Upcoming Real-Life Trials?" *Science*, 1994, 264, 1660.

65. P. Brown, "Will Third World Gamble on HIV Vaccines?" *New Scientist*, October 8, 1994, p. 4.

66. S. Berkley, "The International AIDS Vaccine Initiative," *J. Intl. Assoc. Phys. AIDS Care*, November 1997, pp. 30–34.

67. R. McKie, "Vaccine for Aids Set Back a Decade," *Observer* (U.K.), April 10, 1994, p. 1.

68. R. Marlink, "Achieving an HIV Vaccine: The Need for an Accelerated National Campaign," *J. Intl. Assoc. Phys. AIDS Care*, November 1997, 35–37. Other information: Richard Marlink, personal communication, October 1998.

69. John Rowan Wilson, *Margin of Safety* (London: Collins, 1963), p. 26.

70. For further background on the possibility that new, modified variants of HIV could be introduced into *Homo sapiens*, some of which could combine with existing strains to produce even more devastating HIV variants, see P. Brown, "How the Parasite Learnt to Kill," *New Scientist*, November 16, 1996, pp. 32–36. For good discussion on recombination, see P. M. Sharp, D. L. Robertson, and B. H. Hahn, "Cross-species Transmission and Recombination of 'AIDS' Viruses," *Phil. Trans. Roy. Soc. Lond. B.*, 1995, 349, 41–47.

71. Example: S. Bosely, "Doctor to Be HIV Guinea Pig in Hunt for Vaccine," *Guardian* (U.K.), December 20, 1997, p. 20.

72. J. Zuniga, "Setting the Record Straight: IAPAC's HIV Vaccine Initiative," *J. Intl. Assoc. Phys. AIDS Care*, November 1997, pp. 38–39.

73. M. Kettle, "Doctors to Be Guinea Pigs in Tests of HIV Vaccine."

74. For IAPAC's view, see J. Zuniga, "Setting the Record Straight: IAPAC's HIV Vaccine Initiative."

75. Fortunately, Dr. Mann was not alone in his concerns. For an example of the useful collaborative discussions that have taken place on this issue, see P. Lurie et al., "Ethical, Behavioral and Social Aspects of HIV Vaccine Trials in Developing Countries," *JAMA*, 1994, 271(4), 295–301.

76. David Dane, personal communication, November 1994. This conversation occurred shortly after articles had appeared discussing whether developing countries would proceed with trials of the vaccines that had been rejected by the United States, and warning of the dangers of testing live attenuated vaccines in Africa. See P. Brown, "Will Third World Gamble on HIV Vaccines?"; R. McKie, "AIDS Vaccine Hits Ethical Hurdle," *Observer* (U.K.), October 3, 1994, p. 28.

## POSTSCRIPT

1. F. Simon, F. Barré-Sinoussi, F. Brun-Vezinet et al., "Identification of a New Human Immunodeficiency Virus Type I Distinct from Group M and Group O," *Nature Med.,* 1998, 4(9), 1032–1037.
2. "N" was chosen for "New," and because it falls between "M" and "O" (the other two groups of HIV-1) in the alphabet.
3. See, for example H. J. A. Fleury et al., "Virus Related To but Not Identical with LAV/ HTLV-III in Cameroon" (letter), *Lancet,* 1986, 1(ii), 854; E. Delaporte et al., "HIV-Related Virus in Gabon," 3rd Conference on AIDS in Africa (Naples, 1987), TH-28.
4. S. Wain-Hobson, "More Ado about HIV's Origins," *Nature Med.,* 1998, 4(9), 1001–1002.
5. Preceding quotations from Hahn, Gao, and Sharp taken from BBC television and radio news reports broadcast on February 1, 1999.
6. By that stage, it had been established for well over ten years that all nonhuman African primates that host SIVs are apparently "immune" to these viruses (an indicator of how long host and virus have evolved together), whereas when SIVs are transferred to other species — like macaques and humans — they cause disease.
7. S. Connor and L. Gregoriadis, "Aids Virus Is Thousands of Years Old," *Independent* (U.K.), February 1, 1999, p. 1; P. Brown, "Chimp Close to Being Wiped Out Was Source of HIV Virus," *Guardian* (U.K.), February 1, 1999, p. 9; L. K. Altman, "H.I.V. Is Linked To a Subspecies of Chimpanzee," *New York Times,* February 1, 1999, pp. A1 and A18; C. Clover and R. Highfield, "Aids Started by Humans Eating Chimps," *Daily Telegraph* (U.K.), February 1, 1999, p. 9; N. Nuttall, "Chimpanzee Meat Blamed for Aids Epidemic," *Times* (U.K.), February 1, 1999, p. 1 and 2.
8. F. Gao, D. L. Robertson, L. B. Cummins, L. O. Arthur, M. Peeters, G. M. Shaw, P. M. Sharp, B. H. Hahn et al., "Origin of HIV-1 in the Chimpanzee *Pan troglodytes troglodytes,"* *Nature,* 1999, 397, 436–441. See also R. A. Weiss and R. W. Wrangham, "From *Pan* to Pandemic" (News and Views), *Nature,* 1999, 397, 385–386.
9. The taxonomy was something that most people had long suspected, and that had been confirmed to me in writing in 1994 by one of the Belgian researchers, Luc Kestens. I had told Hahn and Gao about this during my 1995 visit, and they had now gone one stage further by confirming the species by DNA analysis.
10. Charles Arthur had himself inherited the tissues from Holloman some time after Marilyn's death, and had tried — apparently unsuccessfully — to grow the "HIV-1-like" virus. L. K. Altman, "H.I.V. Is Linked to a Subspecies of Chimpanzee."
11. I also had several other reservations about the paper. The first was the author's failure to mention the fact that Marilyn had been injected with human blood at Holloman between 1966 and 1969, as part of hepatitis experiments. Even if (as is demonstrated in this book) HIV-1 was most unlikely to have been present in North America at that time, this is a detail that should surely have been reported in the paper. Another important and relevant point was that — as I told both Hahn and Gao in 1995 — since Marilyn was brought to the United States in 1963, she is very likely to have originated from Cameroon, as indicated by a detailed report about the Holloman chimps that reveals that in the early sixties nearly all of them were being brought in from that country. (W. D. Hillis, "An Outbreak of Infectious Hepatitis among Chimpanzee Handlers at a United States Air Force Base," *Am. J. Hyg.,* 1961, 73, 316–328.) Third is the fact that,

according to primatologist Bill Hillis, who was personally involved with importing many of the Holloman chimps, one local vet in Cameroon "on several occasions" injected chimps in his care with whole human blood taken from "native Africans," in order to "protect the animals against human diseases to which they will likely be exposed during captivity." (See Hillis article, above, p. 317, but also J. Held, "Hepatitis in Humans Associated with Chimpanzees," *Lab. Primate News,* 1962, 1(4), 8–14, especially p. 10, which reports that "as far as can be determined, only this one individual practiced this procedure [injecting the chimps with human blood].") This historical detail is clearly of potential relevance — and, once again, I told Hahn about this in 1995.

12. The earliest anecdotal indication of an HIV-1 Group M infection in these countries would appear to pertain to a blood transfusion given in Congo Brazzaville in 1981 (see n.25, below).

13. T. Huet, S. Wain-Hobson et al., "Genetic Organization of a Chimpanzee Lentivirus Related to HIV-1," *Nature,* 1990, 345, 356–359.

14. M. Peeters et al., "Isolation and Partial Characterization of an HIV-Related Virus Occurring Naturally in Chimpanzees in Gabon," *AIDS,* 1989, 3, 625–630.

15. S. Connor and L. Gregoriadis, "Aids Virus Is Thousands of Years Old."

16. The fact that both the first two SIV-infected chimps came from Gabon (or Cameroon) has long excited researchers, and prompted some of them to propose that this could be the area where AIDS began. In 1994 and 1996, two articles written mainly by Belgian researchers observed that the HIV infections found in Cameroon and Gabon, respectively, were characterized by relatively low prevalence in the general population, but a high diversity of subtypes (five Group M subtypes and Group O, in each instance). (J. N. Nkengasong, P. Piot et al., "Genotypic Subtypes of HIV-1 in Cameroon," *AIDS,* 1994, 8, 1405–1412; E. Delaporte, W. Janssens, M. Peeters et al., "Epidemiological and Molecular Characteristics of HIV Infection in Gabon, 1986–1994," *AIDS,* 1996, 10, 903–910.) This might indicate, Delaporte suggested, that the viruses had been present in the country longer than elsewhere, and indeed that "the HIV viruses [might] somehow originate from this part of Africa." A similar hypothesis was proposed the following year by Jaap Goudsmit, in his book *Viral Sex* (Oxford: Oxford University Press, 1997). Goudsmit even drew a map showing where he thought the sources of the Group M and Group O epidemics might be. (For Group M, he rather hedged his bets, including southwestern Congo, southern Congo Brazzaville, all of Gabon and Equatorial Guinea, and southern Cameroon in his oval of origin; his Group O oval paralleled and overlapped that of Group M, but was sited about 250 miles to the northeast.) Origin theories like these seem to me to be based heavily on hypothesis, but to be light on data. I would propose that the number of HIV-1 subtypes detected in Cameroon and Gabon is partly related to observer bias, in that both countries are popular work venues for Francophone researchers. The Congo, by contrast, is generally viewed as a much riskier place to work, especially since the closure of Projet SIDA in 1991, and the start of the civil war in 1996. Despite this, six subtypes of HIV-1 have been identified in the Congo, one in Congolese living in Sweden, one in Bangui (which faces the Congo border), and one in Cyprus, with which the Congo has strong traditional links. In terms of Group M subtype diversity, therefore, the Congo would seem to be a more plausible site for the origin of Group M than either Cameroon or Gabon. (See chapter 55.)

17. L. K. Altman, "H.I.V. Is Linked To a Subspecies Of Chimpanzee." For good source material on this subject nearly five years earlier, see S. Connor, "Great Apes Face Extinction as Food Trade Grows," *Independent* (U.K.), October 26, 1994, p. 7, and the various press

releases issued in (and since) 1994 by the World Society for the Preservation of Animals, 2 Langley Lane, London SW 8 ITJ, U.K.

18. The range of *Pan troglodytes troglodytes* embraces the southern half of Cameroon, virtually all of Gabon and Equatorial Guinea, and the west and north of Congo Brazzaville (see map). The demands of zoos and laboratories in the fifties and sixties, just like the escalating bush-meat trade of the eighties and nineties, have severely affected the numbers, but chimps apparently still exist in most of these areas today. Until recently, at least, *troglodytes* were also found in small corners of southeastern Nigeria and southwestern Central African Republic — and in Cabinda, the oil terminal enclave (officially part of Angola) that lies north of the mouth of the Congo River. J. H. Wolfheim, *Primates of the World* (Seattle: University of Washington Press, 1983), pp. 701–719; J. Dorst and P. Dandelot, *A Field Guide to the Larger Mammals of Africa* (London: Collins, 1983), pp. 80, 88–90, 100. In addition, in the 1950s *troglodytes* were still being found around Tshela — the extreme west of the Congo, near the border with Cabinda.

19. M. Crowder (editor), *The Cambridge History of Africa, Volume 8, from about 1940 to about 1975* (Cambridge: Cambridge University Press, 1984), pp. 31–40.

20. The official records for these countries have the first reported AIDS case in Congo Brazzaville in 1983, Cameroon in 1985, and Gabon in 1987; Equatorial Guinea had still not had a case by 1988. (Panos Institute, *AIDS and the Third World,* third edition [London: Panos Institute, 1988], pp. 156–167, and J. P. Durand et al., "AIDS in Cameroon," 2nd International Conference on AIDS [Paris, 1986], poster 377.) However, records from France reveal some earlier traces, for of eighteen African AIDS patients seen by 1983 (three of which pertained to "before 1980"), four were from Congo Brazzaville, one from Cameroon, and one from Gabon. For comparison, nine were from the Congo — which, alone of the countries cited, was not a former French colony; moreover, in those days most Congolese AIDS patients who attended European hospitals went to Brussels, not Paris. (See J. B. Brunet, "Acquired Immune Deficiency Syndrome in France," *Eur. J. Clin. Microbiol.,* 1984, 3(1), 66; J. Leibowitch, *A Strange Virus of Unknown Origin* [New York: Ballantine, 1985], p. 21–26; and J. B. Brunet, D. Klatzmann et al., "AIDS in France: The African Hypothesis," in A. E. Friedman-Kien (editor), *The Epidemiology of Kaposi's Sarcoma and Opportunistic Infections* [New York: Year Book Medical Publishers, 1984], pp. 317–321.) On the other hand, a more recent report (encountered as I was revising this postscript) claimed that "the first three patients with AIDS, described in France in 1978 (i.e., before the AIDS epidemic), came from Gabon and Congo [Brazzaville]." (E. Delaporte, W. Janssens, M. Peeters et al., "Epidemiological and Molecular Characteristics of HIV Infection in Gabon, 1986–1994," see p. 909.) I have since learned from the lead author, Eric Delaporte, that the apparently positive sera (originating from AIDS-like cases seen in France, and only tested retrospectively for HIV in around 1994) have not been analyzed genetically, and that the viruses may, therefore, have been from any of the HIV-1 groups, including O and N. Neither do I know which assays were used for the testing. But even if one or more of these three cases should turn out to have been caused by a Group M virus, this would not be unexpected based on normal spread from a Group M epicenter in the Congo.

21. C. Rouzioux, L. Montagnier et al., "Absence of Antibody to LAV/HTLV-III and STLV-III(mac) in Pygmies," 2nd International Conference on AIDS (Paris, 1996), poster 378.

22. F. Louis et al., "HIV Seroprevalence Levels Among Bantous and Pygmies in South Cameroon: A Comparison Study at Four Years Interval (1990–1993)," 9th International Conference on AIDS (Berlin, 1993), poster PO-C07-2754.

23. B. Lamey et al., "Aspects Cliniques et Epidemiologiques de la Cryptococcose a Kinshasa," *Med . Trop.,* 1982, 42(5), 507–511. P. Piot et al., "Acquired Immunodeficiency Syndrome in a Heterosexual Population in Zaire," *Lancet,* 1984, 2(i), 65–69.

24. See map and chart of HIV-1-related AIDS in Africa in Chapter 54.

25. A Soviet man was apparently infected through a blood transfusion given in Congo Brazzaville in 1981. See M. Smallman-Raynor, A. Cliff, and P. Haggett, *Atlas of AIDS* (Oxford: Blackwell, 1992), pp. 332–334. The infected man's wife later gave birth to a perinatally infected baby, who — in one of the saddest and most extraordinary stories of the AIDS pandemic — was the source of a nosocomial outbreak of Group M–related AIDS at Elista Hospital in the south of the U.S.S.R. This epidemic resulted in the infection of 57 infants (probably due to the use of inadequately sterilized needles) and eight mothers — who may have contracted the virus from their infants, as a result of breast-feeding with cracked nipples.

26. Although there is no record of *Pantroglodytes troglodytes* being present at Lindi, it is not impossible. Jos Mortelmans recalls that Courtois was already working with chimps in Stanleyville before Lindi opened in June 1956, and these animals might have come from Leopoldville or Coquilhatville (where both *troglodytes* and *schweinfurthi* were available). And the Lindi databook reveals that during 1957 and 1958, two chimps arrived at Lindi from the Stanleyville zoo, and one from Coquilhatville. The species and subspecies were not identified.

27. F. Gao et al., "Origin of HIV-1 in the Chimpanzee *Pan troglodytes troglodytes,*" see p. 440.

28. See annual editions of the HIV/AIDS Surveillance Database, available from International Programs Center, U.S. Bureau of the Census, Washington, D.C. 20233. Journalists who attended Hahn's press conference acquired a slightly different impression, and several wrote reports such as the following: "the natural habitat of this chimpanzee sub-species [*P. t. troglodytes*] overlaps precisely with the region of west-central Africa where HIV-1 was first recognised." (C. Clover and R. Highfield, "Aids Started by Humans Eating Chimps.") This claim of geographical symmetry is correct for the minor two variants of HIV-1 (the earliest likely sighting of HIV-1 Group O relates to Douala, Cameroon, in 1961 or 1962 — as evidenced by the tale of Arvid Noe, while the first evidence of HIV-1 Group N also emanates from Cameroon, in 1992). However, it is incorrect for Group M.

29. N. Nuttall, "Chimpanzee Meat Blamed for Aids Epidemic."

30. E. Delaporte, personal communication, March 1999.

31. Frequent visitors to Kinshasa zoo in the eighties and nineties speak of chimps being kept in appalling conditions, sometimes two or three to a small iron cage, and of extremely high death rates. "It's the absolute worst zoo I have ever seen," said one European animal specialist, who had spent many months trying to arrange for some of the chimps to be relocated.

32. "B," personal communication, February 1999.

33. The other omnivorous nonhuman African primates are of course the baboons (which include the mandrills of west central Africa).

34. A. André, G. Courtois, G. Lennes, G. Ninane, and P. M. Osterreith, "Mise en évidence d'antigènes de groupes sanguins A, B, O et Rh chez les singes chimpanzés," *Ann. Inst. Past.,* 1961, 101, 82–95.

35. The English summary of the André paper (cited above) reports: "These findings suggest that different varieties might exist in the group *Pan troglodytes* . . . they might be related to the *Pan verus and Pan schweinfurti* [sic] varieties." (Here, it is apparent that the taxonomy has become confused, and that the researchers have mistakenly referred to

*P. t. troglodytes* when they mean *P. t. schweinfurthi,* and vice versa. Nonetheless, their central hypothesis — that certain chimpanzee groups living a thousand miles apart might be closely related — is clear.) In fact, this hypothesis is not as incredible as it might at first sound, for a paper published by Vanessa Hirsch (with Paul Sharp as last author) in February 1999 provided a remarkably precise model for just this kind of transcontinental connection. Hirsch and Sharp reported the sequencing of a new form of SIV (effectively a sixth PIV lineage) from a zoo specimen of the l'Hoest monkey (*Cercopithecus l'hoesti l'hoesti*), the natural range of which, they reported, was "a localized area of central Africa" that, according to their map, was positioned somewhere in central Congo. (V. M. Hirsch, P. M. Sharp et al., "Characterization of a Novel Simian Immunodeficiency Virus (SIV) from l'Hoest Monkeys (*Cercopithecus l'hoesti*): Implications for the Origins of SIVmnd and Other Primate Lentiviruses," *J. Virol.,* 1999, 73[2], 1036–1045. For the initial report of SIV-positivity in l'Hoest monkeys, see I. Nicol, D. Messinger et al., "Use of Old World Monkeys for Acquired Immunodeficiency Syndrome Research," *J. Med. Primatol.,* 1989, 18, 227–236.) Hirsch and Sharp found, surprisingly, that the l'Hoest SIV sequence clustered — not closely, but distinctively — with the SIV of the mandrill, which is found only in a small part of the Cameroon/ Gabon/Equatorial Guinea rain forest, nearly a thousand miles to the west. They suggested a possible solution to the mystery, by revealing that a close relative to the l'Hoest monkey, which they referred to as the preussis monkey (*Cercopithecus preussi preussi*), is found in the west central African rain forest, and suggesting that the mandrill (which is from the baboon family) could have acquired its virus through attacking and/or eating a preussis in the past. J. Dorst and P. Dandelot, in *A Field Guide to the Larger Mammals of Africa,* pp. 68 and 87, actually define the preussis monkey as a subspecies of the l'Hoest (*Cercopithecus l'hoesti preussi*), which renders the cross-species transmission hypothesis even more plausible. Dorst and Dandelot describe the habitat of the l'Hoest monkey as "montane forest," and their map on page 87 suggests that the range comprises Mount Cameroon and Bioko Island in west central Africa, and — in the east — a square with two hundred mile sides, with its eastern edge running along the mountain spine that separates eastern Congo from western Uganda, Rwanda, and Burundi. The relevance of all this for SIV research is that the eastern and western branches of the l'Hoest monkey (*l'hoest* and *preussi*) afford a remarkably precise model for the eastern and western branches of the chimpanzee (the Mambasa group, presently defined as *schweinfurthi,* and the *troglodytes* from west central Africa). If the l'Hoest monkeys once occupied a range that extended from the Congo-Uganda border to Cameroon, then perhaps one group of chimpanzees did so also, which — indeed — is exactly what the Belgian chimp researchers were postulating back in 1961. Furthermore, this hypothesis is ecologically viable, for until recent times the rain forest in the south of the present-day Central African Republic was a continuous strip, one that linked Cameroon to the northeast of the Congo, but which was separated from the main habitat of *schweinfurthi* in northern Congo by the wide expanse of the Oubangui River. The rub of course is that if the two groups (Cameroonian *troglodytes,* and Mambasa *schweinfurthi*) are in reality more closely related than present-day chimp taxonomy would suggest, then the two groups may also be hosting more closely related strains of SIV.

36. This information was confirmed by Paul Osterrieth in 1993. For the dating, refer to chapter 52, especially n.18.
37. Since the closure of Lindi camp in around 1960, the Mambasa chimps would be more likely to be sent to the animal center at Epulu, which is just fifty miles from Mambasa.

It may even be, therefore, that Noah is a Mambasa chimp, and that it is the Mambasa group (rather than "normal" *schweinfurthi*) that is host to divergent SIVs such as SIVcpz-ant.

38. As detailed above, I have heard anecdotally that Noah's cage mate, Nico, was tested and found to be SIV-negative. It addition, it has been suggested to me by an anonymous Belgian primatologist that after the Noah sample tested positive, other *schweinfurthi* blood samples available in Belgium may well have been assayed for SIV. Whether or not that is the case, nothing has been published. By contrast, most of the chimpanzees in research labs in America and Europe (apart from Belgium) are either *P. t. troglodytes* or *P. t. verus* (from West Africa). Simon Wain-Hobson tells me that Fred Prince tested 200 *verus* chimps from Liberia for SIV, and failed to find any positives. (It is, however, conceivable that some could have been infected with a highly divergent form of SIVcpz — one that would not have been picked up by the standard HIV-1 assays.)

39. I also have more specific details of where Rollais conducted his capture operations.

40. The four pygmy chimps (three of which had come direct from the Congo, and the fourth of which had spent some time in Frankfurt Zoo) were tested for HIV-1, HIV-2, and SIV by a new generation ELISA-type assay called MPEA; all tests were negative. Albert Osterhaus, personal communication, February 1999. Professor Osterhaus also mentioned, in passing, that his team had found a new SIV in the talapoin — another primate from west central Africa — and that sequencing was under way.

41. In addition to *P. t. verus* (from Pastoria) and *P. t. troglodytes* (from Brazzaville), Lépine's lab also had access to the third subspecies of common chimp — *P. t. schweinfurthi* from Jezierski at Gabu-Nioka.

42. P. Lépine et al., "Presence apparemment insolite et conservation de microfilaires du singe dans des cultures de tissus," *Bull. Soc. Pathol. Exot.,* 1955, 48, 838–843.

43. Examples of new research and ideas in the field emerge on a regular basis. For instance, on May 6, 1999, as I was completing the proofreading of this book, I received a fax from Brian Martin, which contained an e-mail from Julian Cribb, advising him (Brian) to get hold of a new book (Omar Bagasra, *HIV and Molecular Immunology: Prospects for an AIDS Vaccine* [Lincoln University, PA: BioTechniques Books/Eaton Publishing, 1999]). According to Cribb, the book has an introduction by Luc Montagnier, and Bagasra is "a distinguished Indian-born U.S. scientist, whose main claim to fame — prior to this — was the invention of the *in situ* PCR technique. . . . In the book, [Bagasra] argues the case for a new form of immunity, molecular immunity, which he says has protected humans against retroviruses and lentiviruses for eons." Cribb continues: "[Bagasra] accepts that AIDS probably began in the CHAT-1 polio vaccine (because it would take a mass experiment like this to break down the long-established molecular immunity which kept humans comparatively safe from retroviral invasion). He argues that monkey kidney cultures probably contained numerous strains of SIV, and that during the vaccine process these were able to combine with one another — and maybe with native human retroviruses — to give rise to new forms of deadly virus, the HIVs. . . . He believes that HIV-1 and HIV-2 were introduced to humans at the same time, probably stemming from different recombinants. . . . But the OPV theory is less important than the conclusion he draws from it. The vaccine recipients would have been infected with recombinants of varying pathogenicity. The bad ones would have killed their hosts — and died with them. The more weakly pathogenic strains would have outlived their hosts and been passed on as HIV/AIDS. And the nonpathogenic ones would have immunized their recipients. [Bagasra's] punchline: 'I believe that the live attenuated

vaccine against HIV-1 already exists in the bloodstreams of those individuals who received CHAT-1 live polio vaccine in the Ruzizi Valley, near Lake Tanganyika. These individuals carry the sort of viral particles that we can utilize for future AIDS vaccines. If these individuals have survived for over 50 years with a kind of attenuated lentivirus related to HIV-1, we should explore the possibility of using these lentiviruses for mass vaccination.' Bagasra also sounds a very strong warning against current AIDS vaccine projects, arguing that using bits of the really pathogenic virus will, owing to its powerful ability to recombine (as seen in the enormous array of HIV strains which have already emerged worldwide), give rise to fresh and maybe even deadlier strains of HIV." Neither Cribb nor I feel qualified to comment on the author's "molecular immunity" hypothesis, and I have not yet had a chance to view the book. Nonetheless, the passages on OPV/AIDS and AIDS vaccines sound intriguing, and would seem to tie in rather well with some of the arguments advanced in this book. Cribb comments at the end of his e-mail that Bagasra's book "demonstrates that there is a darn good reason to hope that the OPV theory is correct — because it may also lead to a way to curb the epidemic."

*Glossary*

**Acquired** — Obtained during the life of an organism, not inherited; for example: immunity.

**Adenovirus** — A group of DNA viruses that mainly causes respiratory disease and conjunctivitis.

**Adventitious agent** — A contaminant (e.g., in tissue culture).

**AGM** — African green monkey

**AIDS (acquired immune deficiency syndrome)** — The disease caused by HIV, which typically occurs when a patient's T-cell count drops to 200 or below. Common presentations ("opportunistic infections") of AIDS include the following: PCP; toxoplasmosis; tuberculosis; disseminated herpes infections, atypical candidiasis; cryptococcal meningitis; aggressive KS, etc. Other, less specific symptoms may include lymphadenopathy, uncontrolled bacterial infections, and weight loss.

**Antibody** — Protein secreted by the immune system, which interacts with a specific invading antigen in an immune response. The presence of antibodies is used as a test for infection by a virus.

**Antigen** — Any foreign substance that, if present in the body, stimulates the immune system to produce antibodies. Each antigen stimulates specific antibodies.

**Apathogenic** — Not causing disease.

**ARC (AIDS-related complex)** — A prodromal (early) AIDS condition involving mild symptoms, such as lymphadenopathy, skin and respiratory infections, and sometimes *Herpes zoster*.

**Assay** — Test to determine the content or concentration of a substance.

**Asymptomatic** — Infected, but without symptoms of infection.

**Attenuate** (virus) — To reduce the virulence of a virus, achieved by passaging the virus through tissue culture or live animals. The attenuated virus can be used as a vaccine if it infects and immunizes without causing disease.

**Autoimmune disease** — Disease caused when an organism's immune system responds to molecules normally regarded as "self" but which instead act as antigens.

**Batch** — In this book, a small quantity of vaccine made in a single process, as part of a production lot.

**BSE** — Bovine spongiform encephalopathy ("mad cow disease").

**Cancer** — Disease caused by a benign or malignant growth resulting from abnormal and uncontrolled division of body cells.

**Candidiasis** — "Thrush"; yeast-like infection, often of the mouth or vagina, caused by *Candida* fungus.

**Carcinogen** — Any substance that causes transformation of a normal cell to a cancer cell.

**Cell** — The smallest living membrane-bound unit capable of independent reproduction.

**CD4 Cell** — A type of T-cell, or lymphocyte, that is a receptor for HIV.

**CDC (Centers for Disease Control)** — located in Atlanta, Georgia.

**Cell culture** — See tissue culture.

**Cell line** — A group of dividing cells derived from abnormal tissue (e.g., a tumor). The cells are immortal; they have abnormal nuclei and almost always produce tumors when injected into an animal. Example: HeLa cells.

**Cell strain** — A group of dividing cells derived from normal tissue. The cells are mortal (they die after a certain number of cell divisions), and they cannot grow when injected into animals. Example: WI-38 cells.

**CETC (chick embryo tissue culture)** — An *in vitro* system used to study and grow viruses.

**Challenge** — To administer virulent virus to a test animal that has previously been vaccinated, to check whether the vaccine was effective, and immunity has been established.

**CHAT** — An oral polio vaccine against Type 1 poliovirus, developed in the 1950s by Dr. Hilary Koprowski.

**Chronic** — Persisting for a long time.

**CJD (Creutzfeldt-Jakob disease)** — a fatal degenerative brain disease of humans, believed to be caused by a prion.

**Clade** — A group of organisms that share a common ancestor and form a phylogenetic lineage. In terms of HIV, the term "clade" is interchangeable with "subtype."

**CMV (cytomegalovirus)** — A common, normally harmless virus, which can cause disease in immunosuppressed patients.

**Cohort** — A trial group.

**Congenital** — Present at birth.

**Congo** — Until 1960 called Belgian Congo; then called Republic of the Congo, or Congo Kinshasa, until 1972, when its name was changed to Zaire. In 1997 the name reverted to the Republic of the Congo. Not to be confused with Congo Brazzaville.

**CPE (cytopathic effect)** — The visible abnormality of, or destruction caused to, cells in tissue culture by viruses (e.g., polioviruses).

**Cryptococcal meningitis** — Inflammatory disease of the membranes of the brain and spinal cord (meninges) caused by fungi of the *Cryptococcus* genus.

**DNA (deoxyribonucleic acid)** — Double-stranded molecule that is the genetic material of all organisms (except RNA viruses).

**Dysfunction** — An abnormality or impairment of function.

**ELISA (enzyme-linked immunosorbent assay)** — A technique used for testing sera for viral antibodies.

**Endemic** — An endemic infection is one that is present on a stable basis in a community, without causing epidemics.

**Endogenous Virus** — Virus incorporated into the host cell DNA; generally noninfectious, but capable of replication; only transmitted vertically (from parent to child).

**Enteropathic** — Pertaining to disease of the alimentary tract.

**Enzyme** — Protein that catalyzes biological reactions, e.g., reverse transcriptase.

**Epicenter** — Geographical area of highest incidence, e.g., of a disease.

**Epidemic** — Outbreak of a disease in a region, affecting many people at the same time.

**Epidemiology** — The study of epidemics: their origin, distribution, control, etc.

**Epidemiology Intelligence Service (EIS)** — The department of the CDC that investigates outbreaks of new diseases; formerly, in the fifties, concerned with biowarfare research.

**Etiology** — The cause of a disease.

**Exogenous virus** — Infectious particle, capable of horizontal transmission (contagious spread from one individual to another).

**Explant** — Fragment of animal or plant tissue from which tissue culture is made.

**Factor VIII** — One of the proteins involved in blood clotting, deficiency in which causes hemophilia.

**Fibroblast** — Characteristic cell type of the connective tissue.

**Formalin** — Chemical used to inactivate poliovirus to produce IPV.

**Founder effect** — Evolution of a closely related population in a geographical region following the initial introduction of a "founder" pathogen (such as a virus that has been carried there by a human host).

**Gene** — Unit of hereditary information. One gene usually contains the information required to make one protein.

**Genetic engineering** — Manipulation of genetic material.

**Genetics** — The study of heredity and its variations in biological systems.

**Genome** — Total genetic material of a cell or virus.

**Genotype** — Genetic constitution, or makeup, of a cell or individual.

**Germ Line** — The cells in an organism that have the potential to form gametes (sperm and eggs).

**Group M** — HIV-1 main group.

**Group N** — HIV-1 new group.

**Group O** — HIV-1 outlier group.

**HDCS (human diploid cell strain)** — A tissue culture system based on a cell strain of semi-stable, mortal human cells that, because they are diploid (containing pairs of identical chromosomes), can reproduce by division. Such cells will die after about fifty doublings, by which time they can theoretically have produced several tons of cells for tissue culture. Example: WI-38 cells.

**Hearth** — The place where a disease seems to have originated.

**HeLa** — A vigorous human cell line originating from the cervical tumor of American Henrietta Lacks, who died in 1951.

**Hemophilia** — Hereditary disease in which blood fails to clot at normal speed, due to absence of Factor VIII.

**HIV (human immunodeficiency virus)** — A type of lentivirus, or lentiretrovirus, that is the cause of AIDS. The virus attacks the body's T-cells, so impairing the immune system. The major variants of HIV are: HIV-1 Group M, the most common cause of AIDS, with an apparent epicenter in central Africa; HIV-1 Group O, with an apparent epicenter in Cameroon; and HIV-2, with an apparent epicenter in western Africa.

**Homologous** — Genetically related and therefore similar.

**Host** — Organism or cell that supports a parasite or other organism (such as a virus).

**HTLV (human T-cell lymphotropic virus)** — An oncogenic retrovirus. One type, HTLV-I, causes adult T-cell leukemia. HTLV-III was one of the original names for HIV-1, as proposed by Robert Gallo.

**Hypothesis** — A set of proposed ideas to be used as the basis for further reasoning, without assumption of its truth; a postulated solution used as the basis for investigation or experiment.

**Iatrogenic disease** — Disease caused by medical intervention.

**ICL (idiopathic CD4+ lymphocytopenia)** — General immunosuppression similar to AIDS but caused by unknown factors other than HIV.

**IFA (immunofluorescence assay)** — An assay that employs fluorescently labeled antibodies to detect presence of antigens in a sample.

**Immune system** — Animal system that resists infection by pathogens. It involves the production of antibodies by lymphocytes, which bind to antigens, marking them for destruction by other cells.

**Immunization** — Administration of antigens to create immunity.

**Immunocompromised** — Having a defective immune system.

**Immunodeficiency** — Condition resulting from a defective immune system.

**Immunosuppression** — Reduction in the immune system's response to antigens.

**Incidence** — Rate of occurrence, e.g., annually.

**Index case** — First case in a group to come to medical/scientific attention; case being studied.

**Infection** — Invasion and growth of a microorganism in a host.

**Infectious particle (of virus)** — An individual virion capable of both infecting a cell and reproducing.

**Inoculate** — To introduce a pathogen (living or dead) into a human or animal, usually by injection (e.g., when immunizing with a vaccine).

**Intracerebral** — (Injection) into the brain.

**Intraspinal** — (Injection) into the spinal cord.

**Intravenous** — (Injection) into the bloodstream.

*In vitro* — In the test tube — literally, "in glass."

*In vivo* — In the living creature.

**IPV (inactivated polio vaccine)** — Vaccine containing killed poliovirus.

**Isolate** — Microorganism found in an infectee and cultivated on tissue culture.

**IVDU (intravenous drug user)** — Generally applies to nonmedicinal use.

**Karyology** — The study of cell nuclei.

**KS (Kaposi's sarcoma)** — Type of cancer that can be a symptom of AIDS, particularly in homosexual patients. Discovered in 1995 to be caused by a herpes virus.


**Labile** — Unstable.

**Lentivirus** (also **lentiretrovirus**) — Type of "slow virus" in the retrovirus family; includes the immunodeficiency viruses (HIV, SIV).

**Leo** — Leopoldville; present-day Kinshasa, Congo.

**Leukemia** — Malignant disease in which bone marrow and other blood-forming organs produce white blood cells in excess.

**Lot** — (or **production lot**) — A quantity of virus (often vaccine virus) that has been grown from a viral seed pool, usually by one or two further passages in tissue culture. In this book, as in the literature of the fifties and sixties, the word "pool" is sometimes used loosely, instead of "lot," to describe a quantity of vaccine — thus "Pool 1A of vaccine" would actually mean a vaccine lot produced from the 1A viral seed pool.

**Lymphadenopathy** — Disease causing enlargement of the lymph nodes, often characteristic of **AIDS**.

**Lymphocyte** — Type of white blood cell, including T-cells.

**Lymphoma** — Cancer of the lymph tissue.


**Macrophage** — Large white blood cells produced by the immune system to engulf and destroy foreign bodies.

**Malignant** — (Of a disease) virulent; exceptionally contagious or infectious. (Of a tumor) tending to spread and recur after removal.

**Mitochondrion** — A highly specialized part of the cell containing enzymes for respiration and energy production.

**MKTC (monkey kidney tissue culture)** — An *in vitro* system used to study and grow viruses. Still today the substrate of choice for most polio vaccines.

**Molecular clock** — A theoretical tool used by geneticists in an attempt to determine the rate at which mutations occur.

**Monocyte** — Type of white blood cell; differentiates into macrophages.

**Monolayer** — Tissue culture consisting of a single layer of cells.

**Mutable** — Liable to mutate.

**Mutation** — An inheritable alteration in the DNA of an organism (or RNA if that is the genetic material); the presentation thereof.

**Mycoplasma** — Any of a group of microscopic organisms; includes certain parasites and saprophytes. Considered to be the smallest free-living organisms.


**Natural transfer hypothesis** — Theory that the four HIVs were introduced to *Homo sapiens* during the "natural" process of hunting and butchering certain African primates for food. By itself, this theory fails to explain the apparently recent emergence of the AIDS epidemics.

**NFIP (National Foundation for Infantile Paralysis)** — A private charity that bankrolled polio research in the United States in the forties and fifties, largely through fund-raising campaigns like the March of Dimes.

**Neoplasm** — New growth; a tumor.

**Neurotropic** — (Virus) affecting the brain.

**Neurovirulent** — Causing damage to the central nervous system (often leading to paralysis or brain dysfunction).

**NIH (National Institutes of Health)** — Bethesda, Maryland.

**Nosocomial** — (Infection) acquired in a hospital.

**Nucleotide** — The "building blocks" that make up DNA; the four types are called adenine, thymine, cytosine, and guanine, and are abbreviated to A, T, C, and G. The order in which they appear in an organism is the DNA sequence. In RNA, the thymine is replaced by uracil.

**Nucleotide substitution** (also **base substitution**) — Mutation that becomes fixed in the genome and passed on to the next generation.


**Oncogene** — Genes that render cells malignant.

**Oncogenic** — Any substance capable of inducing malignant transformation cells.

**Oncovirus** — Type of retrovirus responsible for causing cancer.

**Opportunistic infection (OI)** — Infection with agent that is normally apathogenic, but that causes disease in cases of immunodeficiency.

**OPV (oral polio vaccine)** — Vaccine containing live, attenuated poliovirus.

**OPV/AIDS hypothesis** — Theory that a contaminated oral polio vaccine was responsible for introducing HIV to *Homo sapiens*. Louis Pascal's version is also sometimes known as "the CHAT hypothesis."

**Outlier** — In phylogeny, an isolate that is only distantly related, or that lies outside the main cluster of isolates.


**Pandemic** — Epidemic of a disease that spreads to more than one continent. Most commonly, however, used to describe a global epidemic.

**Parenteral** — Pertaining to the blood stream.

**Parenteral administration** — By injection, not via the alimentary canal.

**Passage** — A passage of virus through a living creature, or through tissue culture, involves inoculating the virus into the chosen medium, allowing it to multiply, and then harvesting it again. The process often causes genetic changes to the virus.

**Pathogen** — Disease-causing agent.

**PCP (*Pneumocystis carinii* pneumonia)** — Infection of the lungs caused by a fungal microorganism, *Pneumocystis carinii*; the major presentation of AIDS in the Western world.

**PCR (polymerase chain reaction)** — Process involving isolation and amplification of a specific DNA sequence, which can then be studied.

**Perinatal** — Pertaining to the moment of birth, or the few weeks before or after birth.

**Phylogenetic tree** — A family tree constructed by comparing the genetic differences between species, to determine the possible evolutionary history.

**Phylogeny** — Evolutionary history.

**Picornavirus** — A member of a family of small RNA viruses, e.g., poliovirus.

**PIV (primate immunodeficiency virus)** — SIV or HIV.

**Plaque purification** — Technique for purification of viruses. A single virion is selected from a culture, then grown up on a fresh tissue culture. This process is usually repeated three times.

**Plasma** — Liquid component of blood; what remains when cells (but not clotting factors) are removed.

**Poliomyelitis (polio)** — Viral disease caused when poliovirus invades the central nervous system; can cause paralysis if the spinal cord becomes infected. Formerly also called infantile paralysis.

**Poliovirus** — Virus that normally lives in the gastrointestinal tract, but that can cause disease if it migrates to the central nervous system.

**Pool (or seed pool)** — A term used to identify the passage level of a virus (e.g., poliovirus) that has been manipulated (or attenuated) in the laboratory. Sometimes also used, loosely, to describe the production lots (of vaccine) made from a numbered viral pool (e.g., Pool 2A of vaccine would mean vaccine produced from the 2A viral seed pool).

**Prevalence** — Frequency of disease or infection found in a group, expressed as a proportion or percentage.

**Primer** — Short fragment of DNA that is introduced into a PCR reaction in order to define the sequence that one wishes to multiply.

**Prion** — A tiny infectious protein particle, smaller than a virus, that entirely lacks genetic material such as DNA. Prions are thought to be the cause of BSE in cows, scrapie in sheep, and the human diseases CJD and kuru.

**Prodrome** — Early symptom indicating onset of disease.

**Production lot** — see lot.

**Provenance** — Chain of ownership from origin (or birth) to present (or death).

**Quasispecies** — The cloud of slightly different viral mutations that have evolved in a living host, as distinct from a laboratory clone of a single variant of virus.

**Recombination** — Process by which genetic material of a cell is exchanged and thus reorganized, for example between two viruses that both infect the same cell.

**Retrovirus** — Virus with RNA as its genetic material, which uses an enzyme, reverse transcriptase, to convert the RNA to DNA so that it can become incorporated into the host genome.

**Reverse transcriptase** — Retroviral enzyme that converts viral RNA into DNA.

**RIPA (radioimmunoprecipitation assay)** — A technique used to confirm antibody presence.

**RNA (ribonucleic acid)** — Type of genetic material present in all living cells, where its role is in the synthesis of proteins from the DNA template. RNA is also the genetic material of RNA viruses (including retroviruses).

**Ruanda-Urundi** — U.N. trusteeship in central Africa administered by Belgium until July 1962, when it split into independent Rwanda and Burundi.

**Saprophyte** — An organism that lives off dead or decaying matter.

**Sarcoma** — Cancer of the connective tissue.

**Sequence** — The order of the nucleotides in a strand of DNA or RNA.

**Sequencing** — Technique used to determine the sequence of nucleotides in fragments of DNA.

**Seroconversion** — Point at which the first antibodies against a pathogen are produced (and detected).

**Seroconversion illness** — Mild, often flu-like illness sometimes occurring at the time of HIV seroconversion.

**Seroepidemiology** — Epidemiology based on serological data.

**Serology** — The study of sera to determine presence of antibodies — or antigens.

**Seronegative** — Lacking antibodies against (and therefore, usually, immunity to) a specific pathogen.

**Seropositive** — Possessing antibodies against (and, therefore, usually immunity to) a specific pathogen.

**Seroprevalence** — Frequency of occurrence of antibodies in a sample, expressed as a proportion or percentage.

**Serosurvey** — Survey conducted to detect antibodies (e.g., against HIV) in a group of sera.

**Serum** (plural **sera**) — Liquid component of blood that remains when blood cells and clotting factors are removed.

**SIV (simian immunodeficiency virus)** — Group of lentiviruses found naturally in many monkeys and apes in Africa in which they appear not to cause disease. When acquired by other primates (e.g., Asian monkeys), SIVs often cause disease. The SIVs are the closest known relatives of the HIVs.

**Slim** — Common name given to AIDS in parts of eastern Africa where the main symptoms are wasting and diarrhea.

**Speciation** — The generation of two different species from a common ancestor.

**Spirochete** — Large, spirally twisted, unicellular bacterium, e.g., *Treponema pallidum,* which causes syphilis.

**Stan** — Stanleyville; present-day Kisangani, Congo.

**Starburst** — The divergence of a species into different subgroups at around the same time, as represented on a phylogenetic tree. This formation may indicate a time of rapid passage (and mutation), for instance, as a virus spreads in a new host, or an unusual occurrence around the time of divergence.

**STD** — Sexually transmitted disease.

**Strain** (viral) — Group of closely related viruses.

**Substrate** — The medium in which a reaction takes place; in the context of this book, the tissue culture used in vaccine production.

**Subtype** (viral) — Group of viral isolates that are genetically closely related.

**Supernatant** — The liquid above a tissue culture preparation.

**SV40 (Simian Virus 40)** — Tumorigenic monkey virus. It contaminated batches of IPV and OPV in the fifties and early sixties.

**Symbiosis** — Relationship between two organisms that benefits each one.

**Syndrome** — Disease characterized by a range of symptoms rather than a single presentation.

**T-cell** — Type of lymphocyte; target cell of HIV.

**Tissue Culture** — Material made by culturing certain animal or plant cells under appropriate conditions to maintain them. Used for cultivating other organisms, such as viruses, *in vitro.* Also called cell culture.

**Titer** — Measure of the amount of virus, or antibody, present in a given amount of fluid (such as blood).

**Titrate** — To assess the concentration of a substance in solution.

**Toxoplasmosis** — Fungal infection, typically of the brain, caused by *Toxoplasma gondii.*

**Transmissible** — Capable of being transmitted; infectious.

**Tuberculosis** — Infectious disease caused by *Mycobacterium tuberculosis*: the classic opportunistic infection of AIDS in Africa.

**Tumorigenic** — Tumor-causing.

**Vaccine** — Preparation that produces immune reaction and acquired immunity to a pathogen, often a virus such as polio. Inactivated vaccine consists of killed pathogen and live vaccine consists of an attenuated pathogen.

**Viral load** — Amount of virus in the blood.

**Viremia** — Presence of virus in the bloodstream.

**Virion** — Single, complete virus particle, consisting of a core of nucleic acid, within a protein envelope.

**Virulence** — The destructive or malignant properties of a disease.

**Virus** — Minute infectious agent, only able to multiply inside a living host cell.

**Western Blot** — Technique used to confirm presence of a disease; it identifies the presence in the blood of antibodies to proteins of specific size.

**WI-38** — A human diploid cell strain developed in 1961 by Leonard Hayflick.

**Zoonosis** — A human disease acquired from animals (e.g., AIDS, new variant CJD).